# American Trypanosomiasis Chagas Disease

# American Trypanosomiasis Chagas Disease

## One Hundred Years of Research

### Second Edition

*Edited by*

## Jenny Telleria

Unité Mixte de Recherche: Institut de Recherche pour le Développement (IRD)/CIRAD (La recherche agronomique pour le développement), Montpellier Cedex, France

## Michel Tibayrenc

Maladies Infectieuses et Vecteurs Ecologie, Génétique, Evolution et Contrôle MIVEGEC (Institut de Recherche pour le Développement 224- Centre National de la Recherche Scientifique 5290-Universités de Montpellier 1 and 2), Centre IRD, Montpellier, France

ELSEVIER        elsevier.com

Elsevier
Radarweg 29, PO Box 211, 1000 AE Amsterdam, Netherlands
The Boulevard, Langford Lane, Kidlington, Oxford OX5 1GB, United Kingdom
50 Hampshire Street, 5th Floor, Cambridge, MA 02139, United States

**Notices**
Knowledge and best practice in this field are constantly changing. As new research and experience broaden
our understanding, changes in research methods, professional practices, or medical treatment may become
necessary.

Practitioners and researchers must always rely on their own experience and knowledge in evaluating
and using any information, methods, compounds, or experiments described herein. In using such
information or methods they should be mindful of their own safety and the safety of others, including
parties for whom they have a professional responsibility.

To the fullest extent of the law, neither the Publisher nor the authors, contributors, or editors, assume
any liability for any injury and/or damage to persons or property as a matter of products liability,
negligence or otherwise, or from any use or operation of any methods, products, instructions, or ideas
contained in the material herein.

**British Library Cataloguing-in-Publication Data**
A catalogue record for this book is available from the British Library

**Library of Congress Cataloging-in-Publication Data**
A catalog record for this book is available from the Library of Congress

ISBN: 978-0-12-801029-7

For Information on all Elsevier publications
visit our website at https://www.elsevier.com

  **Working together
to grow libraries in
developing countries**

www.elsevier.com • www.bookaid.org

*Publisher*: Sara Tenney
*Acquisition Editor*: Linda Versteeg-Buschman
*Editorial Project Manager*: Halima Williams
*Production Project Managers*: Karen East and Kirsty Halterman
*Cover Designer (Elsevier)*: Greg Harris

Typeset by MPS Limited, Chennai, India

# Contents

# List of Contributors

**W. Apt** University of Chile, Santiago, Chile

**T. Araujo-Jorge** Fundação Oswaldo Cruz, Rio de Janeiro, Brazil

**F.J. Ayala** University of California, Irvine, CA, United States

**C. Aznar** Université des Antilles et de la Guyane, Cayenne, French Guyana

**M.D. Bargues** Universidad de Valencia, Burjassot Valencia, Spain

**E.S. Barrias** Instituto nacional de Metrologia, Normalização e Qualidade - Inmetro, Rio de Janeiro, Brazil; Avenida Nossa Senhora das Graças, Rio de Janeiro, Brazil

**D.C. Bartholomeu** University of Minas Gerais, Belo Horizonte, MG, Brazil

**M.A. Basombrío** Universidad Nacional de Salta, Salta, Argentina

**C.P. Brandan** Universidad Nacional de Salta, Salta, Argentina

**S.F. Brenière** Institut de Recherche pour le Développement (IRD), Montpellier, France

**Y. Carlier** Université Libre de Bruxelles (ULB), Brussels, Belgium; Tulane University, New Orleans, LA, United States

**S.S. Catalá** CRILAR-CONICET, Centro Regional de Investigación Científica de La Rioja, Anillaco (La Rioja), Argentina

**M. Corti** Infectious Diseases Hospital "F. J. Muñiz," Buenos Aires, Argentina

**J.A. Costales** Pontificia Universidad Católica del Ecuador, Quito, Ecuador

**J.R. Dalenz** Universidad Mayor de San Andrés, La Paz, Bolivia

**T.U. de Carvalho** Instituto de Biofísica Carlos Chagas Filho, Universidade Federal do Rio de Janeiro, Rio de Janeiro, Brazil

**M. de Lana** Federal University of Ouro Preto, Minas Gerais, Brazil

**E.M. de Menezes Machado** Federal University of Ouro Preto, Minas Gerais, Brazil

**J.M. de Rezende**[†] Federal University of Goias, Goias, Brazil

**W. de Souza** Universidade Federal do Rio de Janeiro, Rio de Janeiro, Brazil; Instituto Nacional de Ciência e Tecnologia em Biologia Estrutural e Bioimagens, Rio de Janeiro, Brazil

**M. Desquesnes** CIRAD-Bios, UMR177-Trypanosomes, Montpellier, France; Kasetsart University, Bangkok, Thailand

**J.C.P. Dias** Emerit Research of the Oswaldo Cruz Foundation, Centro de Pesquisa René Rachou, Belo Horizonte, MG, Brazil

**R. Docampo** University of Georgia, Athens, GA, United States

**P.L. Dorn** Loyola University New Orleans, New Orleans, LA, United States

**J.-P. Dujardin** Institut de Recherche pour le Développement (IRD), UMR 177 Intertryp, Montpellier, France

**N.M.A. El-Sayed** University of Maryland, College Park, MD, United States

**D. Gorla** Universidad Nacional de Córdoba, Consejo Nacional de Investigaciones Científicas y Técnicas, Argentina; Consejo Nacional de Investigaciones Científicas y Técnicas, Universidad Nacional de Córdoba, Argentina

**F. Guhl** Universidad de los Andes, Centro de Investigaciones en Microbiología y Parasitología Tropical, Bogotá, Colombia

**P.B. Hamilton** University of Exeter, Exeter, United Kingdom

**K. Hashimoto** Freelance Global Health Consultant, Japan

**A.M. Jansen** Oswaldo Cruz Institute, Rio de Janeiro, Brazil

**M.D. Lewis** London School of Hygiene and Tropical Medicine, London, United Kingdom

[†] Deceased

**M.S. Llewellyn** University of Glasgow, Glasgow, United Kingdom

**A.O. Luquetti** Federal University of Goias, Goias, Brazil

**L.A. Messenger** London School of Hygiene and Tropical Medicine, London, United Kingdom

**M.A. Miles** London School of Hygiene and Tropical Medicine, London, United Kingdom

**Á. Moncayo** Academia Nacional de Medicina, Bogotá, Colombia

**S.N.J. Moreno** University of Georgia, Athens, GA, United States

**F. Noireau** Institute de Recherche pour le Ddéveloppement (IRD), UMR 177 Intertryp, Montpellier, France

**A.M. Padilla** University of Georgia, Athens, GA, United States

**A. Rassi** Federal University of Goias, Goias, Brazil

**A. Rassi Jr** Anis Rassi Hospital, Goias, Brazil

**A.L.R. Roque** Oswaldo Cruz Institute, Rio de Janeiro, Brazil

**G.A. Schmuñis** Regional Office of the World Health Organization for the Americas

**C.J. Schofield** London School of Tropical Medicine and Hygiene and ECLAT Net Work, United Kingdom

**M.-A. Shaw** University of Leeds, St James's University Hospital, Leeds, United Kingdom

**A.C. Silveira**[†]

**J.R. Stevens** University of Exeter, Exeter, United Kingdom

**L. Stevens** University of Vermont, Burlington, VT, United States

**M. Svoboda** Université Libre de Bruxelles, Brussels, Belgium

**S.M.R. Teixeira** Federal University of Minas Gerais, Belo Horizonte, MG, Brazil

[†] Deceased

**J. Telleria** Institute for Research for Development (IRD), Montpellier, France

**M. Tibayrenc** Maladies Infectieuses et Vecteurs Ecologie, Génétique, Evolution et Contrôle MIVEGEC (Institut de Recherche pour le Développement 224- Centre National de la Recherche Scientifique 5290-Universités de Montpellier 1 and 2), Centre IRD, Montpellier, France

**C. Truyens** Université Libre de Bruxelles (ULB), Brussels, Belgium

**A. Villacis** Center for Infectious and Chronic Disease Research, School of Biological Sciences, Pontifical Catholic University of Ecuador, Quito, Ecuador

**M.F. Villafañe** Infectious Diseases Hospital "F. J. Muñiz," Buenos Aires, Argentina

**E. Waleckx** Universidad Autónoma de Yucatán, Mérida, Mexico

**S.C.C. Xavier** Oswaldo Cruz Institute, Rio de Janeiro, Brazil

**M. Yeo** London School of Hygiene and Tropical Medicine, London, United Kingdom

# Preface

In 1909, Carlos Chagas identified *Trypanosoma cruzi* as the agent of Chagas disease. In 1910, Chagas discovered that *Triatoma* bugs are vectors of the parasite and that various animals (first, the armadillo) are wild reservoirs for the parasite. The parasite was named in honor of Oswaldo Cruz, the great Brazilian epidemiologist of yellow fever, smallpox, and bubonic plague. In 1986, Michel Tibayrenc and collaborators discovered that the reproduction of the parasite is clonal, rather than sexual. The disease is, of course, much older than Chagas' discovery. It may have been associated with humans shortly after they arrived in the Americas some 15,000 years ago. *T. cruzi* has been found in mummies from northern Chile and southern Peru that are nearly 9000 years old.

Chagas disease is endemic in Mexico and Central and South America, with significant prevalence of human infection in 22 Latin American countries, where it affects 10−12 million people and kills more than 10,000 humans each year. There are several hundred thousand people infected with *T. cruzi* in other parts of the world. Mostly, in the United States, Canada, Australia, Japan, Spain, and Portugal, where the carriers are typically Latin American immigrants, who are often unaware of their infection, but cause the infection of others through blood transfusions and otherwise. In the United States, the annual cost of treatment is about $900 million. The global cost is estimated to be more than $7 billion.

In spite of counting among mankind's worst scourges, Chagas disease has received relatively little attention from investigators and institutions. Pharmaceutical corporations typically have little or no interest in diseases that affect the world's poorest. In the United States, Europe, and other industrialized countries, Chagas is largely perceived as a foreign disease, which does not motivate government agencies, foundations, and other institutions to invest substantial resources to discover curative drugs and medical treatments.

This neglect has been changing. In 1943, the Oswaldo Cruz Institute's Prophylaxis and Study Center for Chagas Disease was created in Bambuí, Brazil. In 1974, the World Health Organization set a special program for the study of Chagas disease. In 1991, Argentina, Bolivia, Brazil, Chile, Paraguay, and Uruguay started the Southern Cone initiative for vector control. The Drugs for Neglected Diseases Initiative (DNDi) was established the same year to promote research against Chagas and other tropical diseases. In 2013, the DNDi received the Carlos Slim Health Award, as well as a Next Century Innovator's Award from the Rockefeller Foundation. The first complete genome sequence of *T. cruzi* was published in 2005, culminating an effort pioneered since 1998 by Björn Andersson and others. There are now very few treatment drugs in use, notably benznidazole and posaconazole, but research and testing of several other drugs are in the pipeline.

*American Trypanosomiasis Chagas Disease: One Hundred Years of Research* is a wonderful addition to current efforts. The coverage is broad, almost all-inclusive: from history and geography—through vectors and nonhuman hosts, the biology and modes of transmission of the parasite, and the host—parasite immune interactions— to the pathology, diagnosis, and treatment of the disease. I anticipate that this Second Edition will be hailed as a landmark in the history and control of Chagas disease, as the First Edition was also recognized.

**Francisco J. Ayala**
University of California, Irvine, United States

# History of the discovery of the American Trypanosomiasis (Chagas disease)

T. Araujo-Jorge[1], J. Telleria[2,3] and J.R. Dalenz[4]

[1]Fundação Oswaldo Cruz, Rio de Janeiro, Brazil, [2]Institute for Research for Development (IRD), Montpellier, France, [3]Pontifical Catholic University of Ecuador, Quito, Ecuador, [4]Universidad Mayor de San Andrés, La Paz, Bolivia

## Chapter Outline

## A beautiful history of life and work

American Trypanosomiasis was named Chagas Disease in honor of its discoverer Carlos Ribeiro Justiniano Chagas,[1] who was born in a coffee farm at Oliveira (Fig. 1.1), state of Minas Gerais, on July 9, 1878.[1−4] His father was a tradesman named José Justiniano Chagas and his mother was Maria Ribeiro de Castro, born into a traditional family of coffee producers (Fig. 1.2).

Carlos Chagas suffered three important family losses: his father and his two brothers. Soon, he assumed the responsibility as the head of the family, helping his mother and sister. He spent his childhood (Fig. 1.3) in the farm and his youth in a catholic school in São João del Rey, where the priest João Sacramento exerted an enormous influence on his education.[2,3]

His mother wanted him to be an engineer but he did not pass the entrance exams, and in consequence, he experienced a severe depression. Carlos Chagas then decided to break with his mother's expectations and settled in Rio de Janeiro to study medicine, 3 years before the end of the 19th century. Two uncles from his mother' family profoundly influenced him in finding his medical vocation.

American Trypanosomiasis Chagas Disease. DOI: http://dx.doi.org/10.1016/B978-0-12-801029-7.00001-0

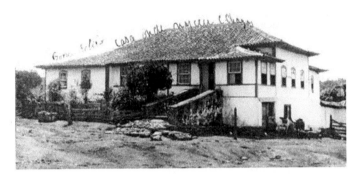

**Figure 1.1** The house in Oliveira, state of Minas Gerais, Brazil, where Carlos Ribeiro Justiniano Chagas was born (July 9, 1878) (Archives of the Instituto Oswaldo Cruz).

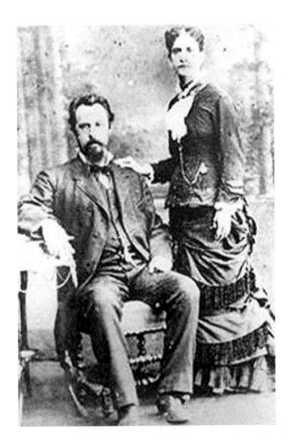

**Figure 1.2** The parents of Carlos Ribeiro Justiniano Chagas: José Justiniano Chagas and Maria Ribeiro de Castro (Archives of the Instituto Oswaldo Cruz).

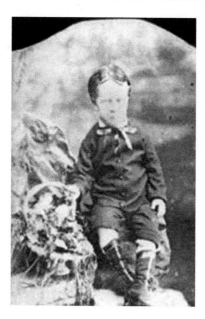

**Figure 1.3** Carlos at the age of about 5, in the farm where he was born (Archives of the Instituto Oswaldo Cruz).

During his childhood and youth, his curiosity was awakened; moreover, Sacramento introduced him to the delights of the discovery of the natural world and the art world.

Carlos Chagas exercised all the important mental tools for educating his imagination, as summarized in 1999 by Robert and Michelle Root-Bernstein[5]: to observe, to evoke images, to abstract, to recognize and to form patterns, to think with the body, to empathize, to think in a dimensional way, to establish analogies, to create models, to play, to transform, and to synthesize. These are some of the tools that explain how creative thinking emerges and we can recognize them in his scientific work.

Carlos Chagas graduated in Medicine in 1903, concluding his clinical training under the influence of Professor Miguel Couto and with a well-grounded laboratory experience in the Manguinhos Institute, where he studied malaria. He accepted the invitation of Oswaldo Cruz and got a contract to work as a doctor at the Hygiene and Public Health Office/Ministry, because of his expertise in malaria and also because he needed to take a job with a fixed salary to marry the woman he had fallen in love with, Miss Iris Lobo (Fig. 1.4) from a rich family in Rio de Janeiro. With her he had his two sons, Evandro and Carlos (Figs. 1.4 and 1.5).

He was then commissioned by Oswaldo Cruz to lead a campaign against malaria in Itatinga, state of São Paulo. In this and other situations, he advocated a strategy of prevention based on the intrahousehold combat of the mosquito and succeeded in his goal of controlling malaria. Thereafter, a series of events characterize a successful scientific career. Carlos Chagas became member of the Brazilian National

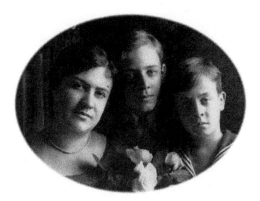

**Figure 1.4** The family founded by Carlos Ribeiro Justiniano Chagas [his wife, Iris Lobo (married in July 1904), and his two sons: Evandro and Carlos] (Archives of the Instituto Oswaldo Cruz).

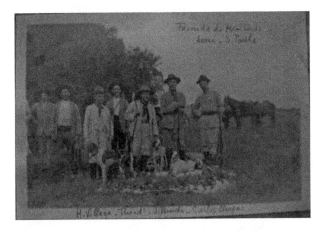

**Figure 1.5** Carlos Ribeiro Justiniano Chagas (in center) with a group of friends after a hunting expedition, on a property at Rio Pardo, Avaré, Sao Paolo (Archives of the Instituto Oswaldo Cruz).

Academy of Medicine in a place especially created for him, received numerous awards and titles of Doctor Honoris Causa (including Harvard, Paris, Lima, and Belgium Universities), was nominated twice for the Nobel Prize (in 1913 and 1921), directed the Oswaldo Cruz Institute for 17 years, and coordinated the campaign against the epidemic of Spanish influenza in Brazil. Several biographers registered these stories, but we especially like two books written by his son, Carlos Chagas Filho,[3] where the human and emotional aspects of the scientist do appear very clearly. Two picturesque aspects have been reported by his son: Chagas loved to hunt (Fig. 1.6) and enjoyed football, supporting the football club Botafogo in Rio de Janeiro.

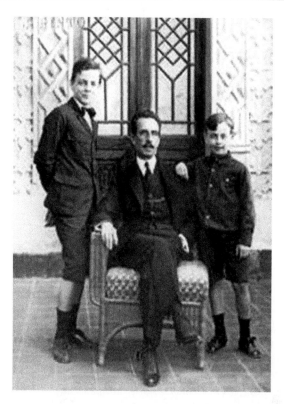

**Figure 1.6** Carlos Ribeiro Justiniano Chagas' sons: Evandro and Carlos (Archives of the Instituto Oswaldo Cruz).

The political, scientific, and cultural context in which Carlos Chagas was immersed and made his discovery was a very rich one. Politically, it was the end of the era of the Brazilian empire, with the abolition of slavery and the proclamation of the Republic of Brazil. Successive presidential elections and popular rebellions occurred.

The American Trypanosomiasis discovery also was determined by a peculiar health context in Brazil. In the Institute of Manguinhos, Oswaldo Cruz implanted a virtuous triad articulating assistance, research, and education. This public health model remains until now at the current Fiocruz, which continues today as an institution of science, technology, and innovation in health linked to the Ministry of Health. After the campaign against the Spanish flu in 1918, Chagas created the National Department of Public Health, giving rise to the future Ministry of Health, and implicating the presence of the State all over the Nation due to the creation of the Sanitary Code, thus expanding the assistance to other diseases such as tuberculosis, venereal diseases, and workers' health, creating the School of Nursing and creating a program for prophylaxis in endemic areas with "endemic guards." A strong cooperation with the Rockefeller Foundation was initiated. Formal science education started in 1911 with the first "Course of Application" at the Institute, and in 1925 Carlos Chagas began the first Special Course in Hygiene and Public Health. He became Professor of Tropical Medicine at the Faculty of Medicine in 1928.[3]

## The history of a significant discovery

In 1987 the great science sociologist Bruno Latour[6] said, "The more controversy we articulate, the broader becomes the world." Carlos Chagas and his colleagues precisely articulated controversies and discovered a new world of research and of political action in public health.

The disease had already existed in the Americas for over 9000 years.[7] Mummies were found in Peru with physical evidence of clinical signs of Chagas disease from which samples of *Trypanosoma cruzi* DNA were recovered. In Brazil, paleoparasitology studies conducted by Adauto Araujo, Luiz Fernando Ferreira, and his group have confirmed *T. cruzi* DNA in mummies dating back to 7000 years. These findings changed the assumptions about the emergence of Chagas disease in the Americas, dating it back to the contact of hunters and gatherers with mammalian reservoirs and insect vectors, much earlier than the period when Andean men started home breeding small animals, as it was thought previously. This means that the disease had already been in Latin America for 9000 years and that no one had seen or detected it before Carlos Chagas in 1909. Even Charles Darwin registered the presence of triatomines during his stay in South America in 1835 (Darwin 1899, cited in Neiva & Lent, 1943),[8] but this was not associated to any specific disease: "The night I experienced an attack (for it deserves no less a name) of the Vinchuca (a species of Reduvius) the great black bug of the Pampas. It is most disgusting to feel soft wingless insects, about an inch long, crawling over one's body. Before sucking, they are quite thin, but afterwards became round and bloated with blood, and in this state they are easily crushed. One which I caught at Iquique was very empty. When placed on a table, and though surrounded by people, if a finger was presented, the bold insect would immediately draw its sucker, make a charge, and if allowed, draw blood. No pain was caused by the wound. It was curious to watch its body during the act of sucking, as it changed in less than 10 minutes, from being as flat as a wafer to a globular form." Darwin's biographers suspect that he also had contacted Chagas disease in the Beagle voyage.[9]

Was Carlos Chagas different? Why and how could he make the triple discovery: the parasite, the vector, and the disease? All other parasitic diseases took years or decades to get their cycle completely elucidated, from the etiological agent, to the vector(s), the reservoir(s), and the clinical manifestations. How did Carlos Chagas do all that in less than 5 months?

First, Carlos Chagas was educated as a scientist, with a mind trained in the tools that educate the imagination, as we said before, in association with a lot of solid experience in scientific method and reasoning. Second, he had an excellent clinical training as a physician, associated with excellent training in the laboratory, being a skillful examiner of blood smears for the diagnosis of malaria that was the subject

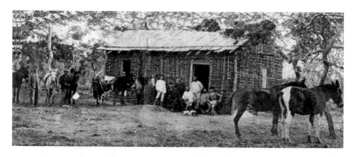

**Figure 1.7** Carlos Chagas with his work team at the railway station in Lassance—Minas Gerais, Brazil (1908) (Archives of the Instituto Oswaldo Cruz).

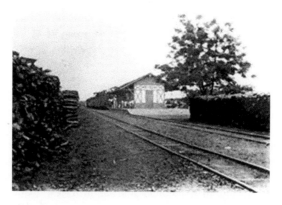

**Figure 1.8** View of the railway station in Lassance—Minas Gerais (1908) (Archives of the Instituto Oswaldo Cruz).

of his MD thesis. Third, the scientific environment of the Manguinhos Institute allowed him to follow the development of medical entomology and the development of literature on tropical medicine and microbiology. And finally, at the Institute, he had laboratories to do experimental animal testing under controlled conditions. That is why, while on a mission for malaria control in the region of Itatinga, São Paulo, then in Xerém, Rio de Janeiro, and later in Lassance, Minas Gerais (Figs. 1.7 and 1.8), he articulated the daily work of the prophylaxis of malaria with the work of an investigator.

Chagas worked in two ways, first as a health professional and second as a health researcher. He was trained embracing the idea of Patrick Manson's School of Hygiene and Tropical Medicine in London[10] that a tropical disease is "a more convenient than accurate concept" because bacteriology is cosmopolitan, with variations in climate and geography, and protozoa and helminths are prominent in tropical climates where many vectors and hosts live. According to him, the concept of tropical medicine in Brazil reconciles the microbiology laboratory with the entomological collection, based on the classification of naturalists. All this gave him a more holistic environmental approach.

With these ideas in mind, when Chagas studied the real health situation in the interior of Brazil, he transformed science and public health into a tool for building a Nation.[4] He rethought the Nation among its "hinterlands" and its people. Carlos Chagas took advantage of the period of modernization of Rio de Janeiro, then the capital of the New Republic, to call for the integration of the entire country.

The discovery took place in the context of expanding Brazilian economic frontiers, following the need for installation of railways for transportation of agricultural production, along with the intense collection of biological material that Carlos Chagas promoted during his missions.[4,11] In Lassance the engineer of the train company showed him an insect. Carlos Chagas had already discovered a *Trypanosoma* when he examined the blood of monkeys in the region (it was not *T. cruzi*, but *T. minasense*[12]). He had sent the infected insects to Manguinhos, asking Oswaldo Cruz to perform experimental infections that confirmed that the parasite could cause disease in monkeys. After a train journey lasting more than 70 hours, Chagas went to the laboratory in the middle of the night. He had realized that the protozoon was not *T. minasense* but a new species, which he called *T. cruzi* in honor of the master Oswaldo Cruz.

His work described, with beautiful plates, all the stages of the evolution of *T. cruzi* in the insect, in cultures, and in organs of infected animals.[1] Chagas had a certainty in his mind: a new parasite, a vector, wild reservoirs, and only the human cases were missing. He then returned to Lassance and began to look careful at every febrile child, always examining blood smears. In his work,[1] he described the finding of a trypanosome in the blood of a cat, defining a domestic reservoir, and in the sequence he found *T. cruzi* in the blood of Berenice, case number 1 (Fig. 1.9).

In the article published in a medical journal in 1909,[13] Chagas wrote: "In a febrile patient, deeply anaemic and with oedema, engorged with multiple ganglia,

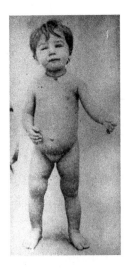

**Figure 1.9** Berenice, Carlos Chagas' first patient (Archives of the Instituto Oswaldo Cruz).

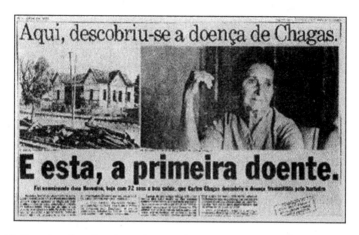

**Figure 1.10** Berenice, found again at the age of 78 for further clinical studies (Archives of the Instituto Oswaldo Cruz).

we found trypanosomes, whose morphology is identical to that of *Trypanosoma cruzi*. In the absence of any other aetiology for the morbid symptoms observed and in accordance with previous experiments in animals, we believe this is a human trypanosomiasis, the disease caused by *Trypanosoma cruzi*, transmitted by *Conorrhinus sanguissuga*."

Carlos Chagas examined many other children because he did not find circulating trypanosomes in adults. Berenice, his first patient, was found (Fig. 1.10) and restudied at the age of 78 by Lana et al.[14] and still had circulating trypanosomes, remaining asymptomatic, in the indeterminate chronic form of Chagas disease, just as 75% of patients with Chagas disease. Berenice did not die from *T. cruzi* infection but from other causes.

This was therefore the natural path traced by Carlos Chagas, in which the scientific fact was the result of a social construction caused by a public health problem. It begins with the identification of a vector, then the causative agent and the epidemiological characteristics, in the search for an associated disease without previous clinical evidence.

The disease was described in the initial period, without definitive evidence of etiological and epidemiological studies. Ten years after the description, only 40 cases had been confirmed by laboratory procedures. Carlos Chagas claimed that the disease was a major public health problem and a major obstacle to the country's progress, but the final acceptance of the existence of a new disease led to a social and cognitive process which spanned over three decades. In publications such as in 1911,[15] in photos and films, Carlos Chagas showed the whole country that this "new trypanosomiasis reached vast areas of Minas Gerais and other Brazilian states, giving rise to a degenerate population seriously jeopardizing the vitality and productivity of rural persons in the country." And he made an error, associating the trypanosomiasis to the goiter, which was endemic in this area of iodine deficiency. That was later revised and corrected by several researchers.

From 1916 to 1920, Carlos Chagas led a large national campaign for rural sanitation, entering then into a phase of both glory and ordeal. In 1917, after the death of Oswaldo Cruz, Carlos Chagas at the age of 39 became director of the Oswaldo Cruz Institute.

Glory from 1909 to 1913, when Brazilian science was recognized internationally for its excellence, when the Oswaldo Cruz Institute was consolidated, when the flag of the "Movement of Rural Hygiene" was created, public health in Brazil was founded, and a Nation began to be built and prepared to face the health challenges for economic and social development. He was thus twice nominated for the Nobel Prize.

The ordeal began when part of the medical and political community doubted on clinical aspects, on epidemiological data, and on the scale of the disease, claiming that it was a "rare disease entity" and not a "national evil." There was a political dimension concerning a possible negative image of Brazil abroad, questioning the project of tropical medicine.

During this period Carlos Chagas and his assistants worked hard to achieve a double translation of the parasitic thyroiditis,[4] with multinodule goiter and cretinism, for the chronic heart and nervous disease.[16] The acute and chronic diseases were also determined as two different entities. The silent indeterminate clinical form, "the potential cardiac patients," was also described. So it then changed from a "Brazilian disease" into "American Trypanosomiasis." To overcome these ordeals it was essential to develop clinical simplified diagnostic features such as the Romanha's sign, which describes the swelling around the eyes and face,[17] the reports of cases found by Mazza in Argentina,[18] and the electrocardiogram.[19] In the 1940s, after the identification of cases in Argentina, after several scientific expeditions to the interior of Brazil, after the creation of the Centre for the Study and Prevention of Chagas disease in 1943 in Bambuí, the prevalence and relevance of Chagas disease was finally proved and the strategic method to control transmission using insecticides and house improvement was implemented.[20,21]

Carlos Chagas made many important discoveries such as the theory on the intradomicile transmission of malaria,[22] which was fundamental for its prophylaxis, and the description of *Pneumocysti carinii*, which was confused with a cystic form of *T. cruzi*.[1,3] But, history will acknowledge him for this unique achievement in biomedical science: his 1909 description of a new etiological agent, the hemoflagellate *T. cruzi*, its life cycle, vectors, domestic and sylvatic reservoirs, and corresponding human disease.[1] This brilliant scientist was more than a member of the "microbe hunter" generation, but decades were required for international recognition of the dramatic epidemiological picture of Chagas disease. He died at the age of 56, after 32 years of a hard and fruitful scientific career and 17 years of active direction of the Oswaldo Cruz Institute.

## Salvador Mazza: marked the history of the knowledge of his disease

In 1915 and 1916, Maggio and Rosenbusch with Kraus noticed the absence of a link between infected bloodsucking insects and the goiter and cretinism, which constituted the basis of a set of doubts relating to the pathogenic conceptions proposed by Carlos Chagas.

This decade saw the beginning of the work by Salvador Mazza (1886–1946) on Chagas disease, which profoundly marked the history of knowledge of the disease.

Mazza, born in Rauch, Buenos Aires, Argentina, graduated from the School of Medicine in 1910 and was a specialist in chemical and bacteriological pathology. During his career, he was a member of the National Department of Hygiene, Minister of Health, then, appointed professor of Bacteriology at UBA, and Director of the Central Laboratory of the Clinics Hospital in Buenos Aires. Thus, in 1926, he founded the Jujuy Scientific Society. Between 1926 and 1927, subsidiaries of the society were created in Salta, Tucumán, Catamarca, Santiago del Estero, La Rioja, and in Corrientes. The year 1928 saw the creation, with the support of Dr José Arce, of an official extension of the universities dependent on the Institute of Clinical Surgery of the Faculty of Medicine of the University of Buenos Aires, called MEPRA (Mission de Estudios de Patologia Régional Argentina). During this time, Mazza had met Carlos Chagas in Germany, and had been impressed by the clarity and strength of his arguments concerning the disease. Consequently, he initiated many studies which confirmed the existence and the importance of this pathology. In 1926, Mazza found a dog infected with *T. cruzi* and in 1927, he diagnosed clinically the first acute case in Argentina.[18]

During the 1930s, at the head of MEPRA, Mazza guided studies of this affection confirming its multiple aspects, the insect vectors, the mammal hosts, the epidemiology, and the pathogenesis. This work, carried out with tenacity, enabled the diagnosis of several hundred cases, both clinical and parasitological. Furthermore, the verification of Chagas disease in the zones where the goiter is endemic, enabled him to overcome the obstacles that Carlos Chagas had confronted. Following this work, Trypanosomiasis Americana was the main theme of the Sixth National Congress of Medicine in 1939. In 1940, Mazza and Jörg defined the three anatomo-clinical periods of the disease which remain valid to this day. In 1946 Mazza died from a heart attack. MEPRA, which had become a multidisciplinary team carrying out treatment, teaching, and research, was temporarily directed by Jörg. However, he was unable to overcome the institutional and political vicissitudes which finally led to its closure in 1958.

## Cecilio Romanha: his contribution to the identification of the disease

Research carried out at MEPRA during the 17 years that Mazza worked for the mission, enabled him to observe men and animals in the zone infected by *T. cruzi*, also the infestation of the bloodsucking bugs in the homes, and, among the descriptions of the clinical manifestations of the disease, a crucial point in its identification, the observation of an ocular edema (known as the Romanha's sign, in honor of the doctor—a disciple of Mazza—who suggested it) was crucial in the diagnoses of infected patients.

The Romanha's sign[17] is a pathognomonic early sign of Chagas disease: unilateral severe conjunctivitis and swelling of the eyelid for more than 30 days, inflammation of the tear gland, and swelling of regional lymph glands, caused by the entry of *T. cruzi*. The sign has proved of great value in the identification of the infection in its acute phase. It constituted a fundamental element to establish a rapid diagnosis and a clinical characterization of the disease and it enabled the confirmation of many cases, finally putting an end to doubts concerning its spread.

In 1946, the year of the transfer of MEPRA to Buenos Aires, Mazza and his collaborators had registered 1400 cases of Chagas disease of which the parasite in the blood could be proved for 1100.[23] During the same period, the Regional Medicine Institute had been founded at the National University of Tucuman, directed by Cecilio Romanha. The institute dealt with the more precise characterization of the clinical symptoms of the disease, as well as trials on the efficiency of hexachlorocyclohexane, an insecticide capable of killing the bloodsucking bug.

During the first Panamerican meeting of Chagas disease, organized by Romanha in Tucuman in 1949, a decision was taken to create, in 1950, a management committee for research and Prophylaxis on Chagas disease at the Ministry of Health and the coordination was entrusted to Cecilio Romanha. This was an important step because it constituted the first institutional organization concerning Chagas disease, outside the university research institutes already mentioned.[24]

# First evidence of Trypanosomiasis Americana (Chagas disease) in various countries of Latin America

Thus, slowly the discovery of Chagas disease spread across various countries of Latin America.

In Central America, the first report of human Trypanosomiasis Americana was made by Segovia in El Salvador in 1913.[25] Subsequently other Salvadorian researchers reported on new cases: Reina Guerra (1939),[26] Castro, Fasquelle, Garcia Montenegro. In 1956, renowned researchers[27] described in detail the epidemiological and clinical symptoms of this disease.

In Costa Rica, the disease was originally described in 1922 by Picado (doctoral thesis) and later studied by Von Bullon, Cespedes, Chen, and Zeledon. In Guatemala,[28] the disease was first encountered by Reichnow in 1933. Subsequently, the work of De Leon in 1935 highlighted the importance of this disease in this country.[29] However, it is important to emphasize the considerable contributions to the understanding of this disease realized by Montenegro, Esteres, Blanco, and Peñalver.

In Panama in 1931, the presence of the disease was proven with the report of 19 human cases in the area of the Panama Canal. Later on, other research was carried out by Calero, Johnson, and Rivas.

In Honduras, the disease was not officially reported until the first case came to light in 1960, on which the doctors A. Leon Gomez, A. Flores Fiallo, E. Poujeol, and M. Barilla reported in the Seventh Day of Honduran Medicine which took place in San Pedro Sula.[29] In 1961, the same authors communicated seven cases of Chagas' chronic myocarditis[30] and in 1965, Duron, in a postmortem study, encountered numerous pseudocysts of Leishmania in the myocardium of a girl suffering from acute Chagasic myocarditis who died suddenly. Nevertheless, already in 1950, Zepada had observed the existence of a vector in various zones of the country and in 1939 an opossum infected with *T. cruzi* was discovered.[31] In 1968, Fernandez and Lainez reported for the first time the first two cases of the acute form of the disease, with the discovery of *T. cruzi* in peripheral blood, whose clinical characteristics presented a unilateral conjunctive reaction, temperature above 39°C, palpebral edema, hemifacial edema, and cervical adenitis.

It was in 1949 that the first native case of the disease was described in Nicaragua and as recently as 1969 that Fray Bernadini de Schagen reported on the infestation of homes by vectors described as bloodsucking insects like cockroaches with wings and very poisonous (the Chagas Space Group).

In Mexico, Hoffman published in 1928 a document describing the great abundance and domiciliation of *Triatoma dimidiata* in Choapas, Veracruz and in 1938, the same author spoke of a case native of the same region that was described by Luis Mazzotti, who, in 1936 identified the first two officially recognized cases originating from Oaxaca as being abundantly infected with triatomine bugs.[32] In 1938, Bernal Flandes published on transmitter insects and trypanosomatides in Veracruz, and in 1940 Palomo Eroso described two other new cases in Yutacan. But, it was only in 1972 that the first formal identification of the disease was carried out with reports by Eugenio Palomo and Luis Mazzotti.[33]

In South America, the first case of Chagas disease reported in Venezuela was by Enrique Tejera, in the state of Zulia,[34] 10 years after Carlos Chagas discovery. Pioneer studies were carried out in Venezuela, directed by José Francisco Torrealba, who, from 1932, initiated studies in the state of Guàrico[35] and introduced the xenodiagnosis, invented by Emile Brumpt, while in 1941 Pifano[36] studied the epidemiology of the disease in the state of Yaracuy. Both authors highlighted its importance as a public health problem and a social one with the maintenance of this zooanthroponosis. In the Institute of Tropical Medicine of the Central University of Venezuela, Maekelt in 1960 had developed a protocol for the preparation of antigen which is still used in the country and Pifano in 1960 published the first figures of national prevalence. As recently as in 1961, the Ministry of Health and Social Welfare allocated budgets, effort, and expertise to fight Chagas Disease, and initiated the Campaign which in 1966 was officially proclaimed as the program to control Chagas disease.[37]

In Colombia,[38] Ignacio Moreno Perez observed in Cali in 1939 for the first time, the pathogenic parasite provoking the disease, according to a report by Hernando Ucros in 1971. In 1947, J. Caicedo and C. Hernandez wrote a report describing the first proven chronic case of the disease in Colombia originating from Fusagasuga in Cundinamarca and in 1961, Marcos Duque began studies on Chagas' cardiopathy. Ten years later, Hernando Rocha communicated his discoveries on the megaesophagus which is a consequence of the disease.[38]

The first research on the epidemiology of Chagas disease in Chile[39] is attributed to Prof. Juan Noe, who, in 1921, observed for the first time, the presence of *T. cruzi* in the evidence of many samples of *Triatoma infestans*, coming from the outskirts of the town of Santiago. Later, in 1931, Dr Miguel Massa, under the authority and direction of Prof. Noe, demonstrated the specificity of the parasite in cardiac fibers in animals used for experimentation. With the creation of the Department of Parasitology of the State Health Office in 1937, began the systematic investigations leading to the demonstration of the first human cases of this disease.[39]

In Peru, in 1919, E. Escomel described the first human case demonstrating the presence of *Trypanosoma* in human blood, in a border zone between Brazil and Bolivia where species of the flora and fauna are very abundant. Escomel said that predecessors had described *T. infestans* in the Vitor and Majes valleys which was suspected of being the cause of certain patients' clinical symptoms which were, in fact, those of trypanosomiasis; however, the confirmation of the parasite had not been able to be made.[40] Roughly 25 years after Escomel's cited publication, the second human case of Chagas disease was verified in Peru, and at the same time the first epidemiological research was realized.

In Paraguay, in 1924 the first discoveries were made with studies by Lutz, Sousa, Araujo, de Fonseca, and Migone, which showed the first infected bloodsucking insects (the Chagas Space Group). In this way, Gamiro in Uruguay, carried out studies on the infection of these insects in his country.

In Bolivia, in the 16th century, when Bolivia was part of the Spanish Viceroyalty of Peru, a priest, Fray Reginaldo de Lizarraga traveling to inspect the convents of this region, noticed that in the valleys of Cochabamba bloodsucking insects like cockroaches, called "vinchucas" by natives, fell, during the night, from the ceiling of houses of the poor and bit the people while sleeping, particularly in the face and other exposed parts of the body. This was a description of the Triatominae, as was discovered later.[41]

In 1916, in Sococha, a small town of the Department of Potosi and near the border with Argentina, the Brazilian Artur Neiva, from the group of the Manguinhos Institute of Rio de Janeiro later named as the Oswaldo Cruz Institute, found these Triatominae, similar to the ones called "barbeiros" in Brazil, infected with the parasite *T. cruzi*.[42] Later, in 1929, the Bolivian Felix Veintimillas, claimed that he found Triatominae with *T. cruzi* in the area of Yungas of La Paz as he reported in 1930.[43]

The Argentinean Salvador Mazza who studied Chagas disease in the northern region of Argentina, did expeditions to several regions of Bolivia from 1937 to 1943 and found infected triatomine bugs, of the species *T. infestans*, in 22% of the cases studied in Vitichi, Potosi, 50% in the small village of Mollegrande, Potosi, and found a very thin 2-year-old girl, who died a few days later, with *T. cruzi* in smears of her blood.[44,45]

Rafael Torrico (Fig. 1.11) returned to Bolivia in 1943, after postgraduate studies at the Oswaldo Cruz Institute of Brazil, became Professor of Parasitology at the Medical School in Cochabamba and director of the Central Laboratory of Interamerican Cooperative Public Health Service of the Ministry of Health, where

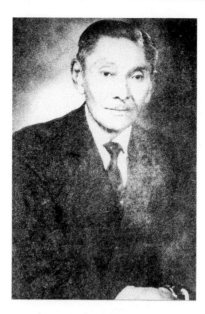

**Figure 1.11** Rafael Torrico, 1943, the father of Chagas disease in Bolivia.

he did several studies on Chagas disease. With M. Dias he published work, in 1943, relating to infected triatomine bugs of the species *T. infestans* in several towns of the Department of Cochabamba.[42]

In 1946 he described a 14-year-old girl from Capinota (Fig. 1.12), a rural area of the Department of Cochabamba, as the first case in Bolivia of an acute form of Chagas disease with edema on the eyelid, the site of the bite by a triatomine bugs, identified as *T. infestans*, and a preauricular lymphadenopathy as described by Romanha in Argentina.[46,47]

In this area, where the patient lived, Torrico found in 427 insects, of the species *T. infestans*, 84.9% infected with *T. cruzi*. However, a Bolivian student in Chile, C.L. Ponce Caballero,[48] published in 1946 a study of seven cases of Chagas disease from the town of Colcapirhua, Cochabamba, confirmed, as he claimed by xeno-diagnosis, that did not have any clinical manifestations of the disease according to one of the participants of this study.[48] Romanha, in 1947, with students of the University of Chile, including Ponce Caballero, reported 122 cases, confirmed by xenodiagnosis, in several areas of Bolivia.[49]

At the first Panamerican Meeting of Chagas disease, held in Argentina in 1949, Torrico presented a paper about the knowledge of Chagas disease in Bolivia up to that year. He stated that *T. infestans* was the principal and the most important vector because of its high infection index, its prevalence, and wide distribution, predominantly in the valleys, where it was an obliged host in most houses. He stated also that guinea pigs (*Cavia cobaya*), dogs, and cats were the only parasite reservoirs known of *T. cruzi* in Bolivia, particularly the guinea pigs that are seen in houses inhabited by peasants where they live together. Regarding human morbidity, he

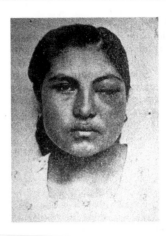

**Figure 1.12** First case of Chagas disease in Bolivia, reported in a girl aged 14 in Capinota, Department of Cochabamba, Bolivia.

presented 211 cases collected, most of which were acute ones, either studied by him or published by others, diagnosed by blood examination and mostly by xenodiagnosis, from many areas of the country.[50]

Finally, Torrico presented an up-to-date study of the situation of Chagas disease in Bolivia, at the International Congress of Chagas disease in 1959, held in Rio de Janeiro, confirming his observations of the vectors, the reservoirs, and human cases, acute or chronic, which had increased to 342 patients, including cases of Chagasic myocardiopathy, with its classic electrocardiography, studied by J. Rodriguez Rivas.[51,52]

## Chagas disease 100 years after the discovery

What is Chagas disease now, 100 years after its discovery? It remains a neglected and silent disease of poverty.[53] Millions of people are infected in Latin America and thousands of others in Europe, Asia, and North America.

The centenary of the discovery of Chagas disease[54] led us to reflect on the evolution of ideas and concepts about it.[55−57] The first phase from 1909 to 1934, mainly through the work of Chagas and the team of scientists from Manguinhos, which ended immersed in controversies; the second phase, from 1935 to 1960, after the death of Chagas, when Mazza and Romanha confirmed acute Chagas disease in Argentina and when Evandro Chagas (Chagas' elder son) and his student Emmanuel Dias deepened studies and confirmed the concept of endemic chronic disease; and finally a third phase, in which political awareness about Chagas disease, associated to the need for control and to the implementation of national and international policies of vector control and corresponding challenges, paved the way for more work to be done in the 21st century.

The control program brought many advances, because there were about 200,000 new cases per year in 2000 while in 1983 this picture was 700,000 per year.[58] Today there are less than 100,000 per year. These numbers are possibly underestimated due to lack of attention to Chagas disease in health information systems that mainly report injuries.

In recent years, the effectiveness of the two main drugs—benznidazole and nifurtmox—for the treatment of Chagas disease in the chronic phase, has produced a regain in interest due to (1) the new observational data, showing that nontreated chronic cases had worse clinical outcomes, higher serological levels, and a higher number of parasites recovered by hemoculture and detected by PCR[59]; (2) the large studies conducted by Médicins sans Frontières showing much less incidence of side effects and higher evidence of effectiveness[60]; and (3) the reviews indicating the emergence of a paradigm shift in the treatment of chronic Chagas disease.[61] In 2015, a benefit trial (Benznidazole Evaluation for Interrupting Trypanosomiasis), a double-blind, placebo-controlled trial on cardiac patients, was conducted. This study (1) confirmed that the etiological treatment led to negative *T. cruzi* DNA blood detection and (2) confirmed the tolerability of the drug, but did not show an increase in the benefit of treatment in cardiac complications, probably due to the advanced heart disease stages of the cases included in the studied cohort.[62] This will probably be the bottom line of many other studies needed to answer dozens of open questions raised in the first decade of precise clinical trials involving chronic Chagas disease patients. A new profile of oral transmission predominates in the scenario and, therefore, this disease still needs a lot of attention. With the Worldmapper tool[63] it is possible to display the country areas proportions comparing the relative burden of various diseases and the existing epidemiological data. The reality of cases of Chagas disease in the Americas can be seen at the site www.worldmapper.org/display_extra.php?selected=392.

A very important and new issue in the scenario of Chagas disease is the organization of many associations of patients and affected people, claiming to fight against negligence and for their rights to have access to diagnosis and treatment. In 2009, during the meeting celebrating 100 years of Chagas disease discovery in Uberaba, Brazil, a work group formed by almost a dozen associations worldwide decided to create the International Federation of Patients Associations, named FINDECHAGAS (http://www.findechagas.com), and supported by associations from every city where affected people found a way to meet and talk about their problems and the consequences of the different dimensions of Chagas disease as a neglected illness.[64,65] These new protagonists on the Chagas disease scene will certainly influence research choices, priorities, and outcomes.

All Latin America has to honor the Carlos Chagas legacy and face such challenges. His old institution and many others on the continent are actively engaged in research on several topics concerning Chagas disease.

In 2009 the clinical trials website (www.clinicaltrials.gov) showed very few studies are devoted to infectious diseases clinical trials: 390 on malaria, 336 on tuberculosis, but only 10 on Chagas disease: 5 on diagnosis and 5 on treatment. This expresses the real definition of a neglected disease. Neglected by the pharmaceutical industry, which does not invest in research and technological development of drugs for the treatment of Chagas disease because it does not provide a rich market for buying future products. In 2016 those numbers changed respectively to 976 for malaria, 887 for tuberculosis, but only 98 for Chagas disease, thus confirming negligence.

Chagas disease is still the most neglected among the kinetoplastid infectious diseases (Leishmaniasis and African trypanosomiasis). From the total amount of resources invested in 2007 (over US$125 million) only 8% were for Chagas disease. This leads, of course, to a lack of research on interventions and therapeutic innovations in Chagas disease and emphasizes the need for public policies to help the affected countries to face their problems.

Chagas disease has poverty as its major social determinant and has the vector and the susceptibility of human host as its major biological determinants. The affected countries need policies not only for studies and development of drugs and vaccines, but also for the reduction of poverty and social disparities which expose the poor to risks of contamination. So here we highlight the words of Peter Hotez[66]: "We have the technology available to develop new drugs, vaccines and diagnostics to combat poverty. However, what is needed is more innovation to enable financial institutions to be able to lead the intensification of the process of developing manufacturing and clinical testing, in order to ensure global access to these new products." It is worth remembering the legacy of Carlos Chagas: his son Evandro Chagas[67] wrote in 1935 that "for Chagas, science was valid only if it was directed toward the welfare of humanity."

Carlos Chagas began in 1909: the joy of broad social commitment. And the words of Chagas fill us with hope and renew our commitment to the struggle for control of the disease and care for people: "It won't take long for us to pass on a beautiful and strong science which creates art in the support of life."

## Acknowledgments

We wish to extend our thanks to Paulo Ernani Vieira, the president of Fiocruz, for all his help in the writing of this chapter and acknowledge him as a coauthor. Equally to Tania Araujo-Jorge, Director of the Oswaldo Cruz Institute, Oswaldo Cruz Foundation—Fiocruz, Brazil and also attached to the Conselho Nacional de Pesquisas (CNPq) for productivity in science. Our thanks also to the following people: Joseli Lannes-Vieira, Maria de Nazaré Soeiro, Nara Azevedo, Simone Kropf, Lisabel Klein, Luiz Fernando Ferreira, Joao Carlos P. Dias, José R. Coura, and Rodrigo Correa-Oliveira.

## References

1. Chagas CRJ. Nova tripanosomiase humana. Estudos sobre a morfolojia e o ciclo evolutivo do *Schizotrypanum cruzi* n.g., n.sp., ajente etiolojico de nova entidade morbida do
   homem. *Mem Inst Oswaldo Cruz* 1909;**1**:159—218.

2. Chagas Filho C. Cenas da vida de Carlos Chagas. *Ciên Cult* 1979;**31**(Suppl):5−14.
3. Chagas Filho C. *Meu pai*—Casa de Oswaldo Cruz/Fiocruz, Rio de Janeiro; 1993.
4. Kropft SP, Sá MR. The discovery of *Trypanosoma cruzi* and Chagas disease (1908−1909): tropical medicine in Brazil. *Hist Cien Saúde-Manguinhos* 2009;**16** (Suppl. I):13−34.
5. Root-Bernstein R, Root-Bernstein M. *Sparks of Genius: the Thirteen Thinking tools of the World's Most Creative People.* New York: Mariner Books Ed; 1999.
6. Latour B. *Science in Action: How to Follow Scientists and Engineers Through Society.* Cambridge: Harvard Univ. Press; 1987.
7. Araújo A, Jansen AM, Reinhard K, Ferreira LF. Paleoparasitology of Chagas' disease: a review. *Mem Inst Oswaldo Cruz* 2009;**104**(Suppl. I):9−16.
8. Neiva A, Lent H. Triatomídeos do Chile. *Mem Inst Oswaldo Cruz* 1943;**39**:43−75.
9. Bernstein RE. Darwin's illness: Chagas' disease resurgens. *J R Soc Med* 1984;**77**: 608−9.
10. Riley EM. The London School of Hygiene and Tropical Medicine: a new century of malaria research. *Mem Inst Oswaldo Cruz* 2000;**95**(Suppl. 1):25−32.
11. Sá MR. The history of Tropical Medicine in Brazil: the discovery of *Trypanosoma cruzi* by Carlos Chagas and the German School of Protozoology. *Parasitologia* 2005;**47**:309−17.
12. Chagas C. *Trypanosoma minasense*: Nota preliminar. *Brasil Méd* 1908;**22**(48):471.
13. Chagas C. Nova espécie mórbida do homem, produzida por um *Trypanozoma (Trypanozoma cruzi)*: Nota prévia. *Brasil Med* 1909;**23**(16):161.
14. Lana M, Chiari CA, Chiari E, Morel CM, Gonçalves AM, Romanha AJ. Characterization of two isolates of *Trypanosoma cruzi* obtained from the patient Berenice, the first human case of Chagas' disease described by Carlos Chagas in 1909. *Parasitol Res* 1996;**82**:257−60.
15. Chagas C. Nova entidade morbida do homem: rezumo geral de estudos etiolojicos e clinicos. *Mem Inst Oswaldo Cruz* 1911;**3**:219−75.
16. Chagas CRJ, Villela E. Cardiac form of American Trypanosomiasis. *Mem Inst Oswaldo Cruz* 1922;**14**:3−54.
17. Romanha C. Acerca de um sintoma inicial de valor para El diagnóstico de forma aguda de La enfermedad de Chagas. La conjuntivitis esquizotripanosica unilateral (hipotesis sobre puerta de entrada conjuntival de La enfermedad). *Misión Estud Pat Reg Argent* 1935;**22**:16−28.
18. Mazza S. La enfermedad de Chagas em La Republica Argentina. *Mem Inst Oswaldo Cruz* 1949;**47**:273−88.
19. Laranja FS, Dias E, Nobrega GC, Miranda A. Chagas' disease. A clinical, epidemiologic, and pathologic study. *Circulation* 1956;**14**:1035−60.
20. Dias E, Peregrino J. Alguns ensaios sobre o "gamexanne" no combate aos transmissores da doença de Chagas. *Brasil Med* 1948;**18−20**:1−20.
21. Dias JC. Elimination of transmission in Chagas' disease: Perspectives. *Mem Inst Oswaldo Cruz* 2009;**104**(Suppl. I):41−5.
22. Chagas C. Prophylaxia do impaludismo. *Brazil Med* 1906. 20 (31, 33, 41): 315−17, 337−40, 419−22.
23. Sierra Iglesias JP. *Salvador Mazza, redescubridor de la enfermedad de Chagas: su vida, su obra.* San Salvador de Jujuy: Universidad Nacional de Jujuy; 1990.
24. Kreimer P, Zabala JP. Quelle connaissance et pour qui? Problèmes sociaux, production et usage social de connaissances scientifiques sur la maladie de Chagas en Argentine. *Rev Anthropol Connais* 2008;**2**:413−39.

25. Segovia JC. Un caso de trypanosomiasis. *Arch Hosp Rosales San Salvador* 1913;**10**:249–54.
26. Reina Guerra A. Contribución al estudio de la Trypanosomiasis en El Salvador. *Folleto* 1939;29.
27. Peñalver LM. Estado actual de la E. de Chagas en Guatemala. *Rev Col Méd Guatemala* 1953. Vol. IV, No. A. Guatemala.
28. De León JR. Nota preliminar acerca de la enfermedad de Chagas en Guatemala. *Rev. Cruz Roja Guatemalteca* 1942;**5**(9).
29. León Gómez A, Flores Fiállos A, Reyes Quesada L, Bonilla M, Poujol ER, Gómez C. La enfermedad de Chagas en Honduras. *Comunicación preliminar*. Tegucigalpa, DC: Publicación del Hospital General; 1960.
30. León Gómez A, Flores Fialols A, Poujol ER, Bonilla M. La cardiopatía chagásica crónica en Honduras. *Bol Soc Hond Méd Int* 1961;**1**:1.
31. Robertson A. Nota sobre un trypanosoma morfológicamente semejante al *Trypanosoma cruzi* encontrado en una zarigüeya capturada en Tela, Honduras. *Rev Méd Hond* 1931;**2**:3–13.
32. Mazzotti L. Dos casos de enfermedad de Chagas en el estado de Oaxaca. México. *Gac Med Mex* 1940;**70**:417–20.
33. Academia Nacional de Medicina. Simposium sobre la lucha palúdica en el mundoy en México. *Gac Med Mex* 1975;**6**:389–408.
34. Tejera E. La trypanosomose americaine ou maladie de Chagas au Venezuela. *Bull Soc Pathol Exot* 1919;**12**:509–13.
35. Torrealba J.F. *La maladie de Chagas au Venezuela*. Otras Notas Científicas. Recopilación Vargas. Caracas, Venezuela. Fascículo VII: 203–43; 1935.
36. Pifano F. La epidemiología de la Enfermedad de Chagas en el estado Yaracuy. *Rev San Asist Soc* 1941;**6**:303–10.
37. Feliciangeli MD. Controle da doença de Chagas na Venezuela: sucessos passados e actuais desafios. *INCI* 2009;**34**:393–9.
38. Serpa Florez. Historia de la trypanosomiasis americana en Colombia. *Medicina* 2000;**22**:53–78.
39. Gasic G, Bertin V. Epidemiologia de la enfermedad de chagas en Chile. *Rev Chil Ped* 1940;**11**:561–84.
40. Ayulo VM, Herrer A. Estudios sobre trypanosomiasis americana en el Perú: I. Observaciones en el departamento de Arequipa. *Rev Perú Med Exp Salud Pub* 1944;**3**:96–117.
41. De Lizarraga R. *Descripcion Colonia*, Libro Primero, 2 ed. Buenos Aires, Lib. La Facultad, p. 220–1; 1928.
42. Dias E, Torrico RA. Estudios preliminares sobre doença de Chagas na Bolivia. *Mem Inst Oswaldo Cruz* 1939;**38**:165–73.
43. Veintenillas F. La tripanosomiasis en Bolivia. *Bol Direc Sanidad* 1931;**3**(6).
44. Mazza S. Consideraciones sobre la enfermedad de Chagas en Bolivia. *Prensa Med Arg* 1942;**29**:51.
45. Mazza S, Chacon R. Primeros animales domesticos y seres humanos con *S. cruzi* comprobados en Bolivia. *Prensa Med Arg* 1943;**30**:9.
46. Torrico EA. Primer caso agudo de forma oftalmoganglionar de la enfermedad de Chagas comprobado en Bolivia. *Anales Lab Central SCISP, Cochabamba* 1946;**1**:3–10.
47. Romanha C. Epidemiologia y distribucion geografica de la enfermedad de Chagas. *Bol Ofic Sanit Panamer* 1961;**5**:390–403.
48. Ponce Caballero L. Enfermedad de Chagas en Bolivia. *Rev Med Chile* 1946;**74**:349.

49. Roman JP. Consideraciones al estudio de la enfermedad de Chagas en Bolivia. *Rev Chil Hig Med Prev* 1947;**9**:61−79.
50. Torrico RA. *Conocimientos anuales sobre la epidemiologia de la enfermedad de Chagas en Bolivia.* Tucuman: Anales Primera Reunion Panamericana de la Enfermedad de Chagas; 1949.
51. Torrico R.A. *Enfermedad de Chagas en Bolivia.* Anais do Congresso International sobre Doença de Chagas. Rio de Janeiro, Ofic. Grafica de Universidade do Brasil 1−13; 1959.
52. Rodriguez Rivas J. Primeros casos de miocarditis chagasica en Bolivia. *Prensa Med (La Paz)* 1957;**11**−41.
53. Hotez PJ, Bottazzi ME, Franco-Paredes C, Ault SK, Periago MR. The neglected tropical diseases of Latin America and the Caribbean: a review of disease burden and distribution and a roadmap for control and elimination. *PLoS Negl Trop Dis* 2008;**2**(9):e300.
54. Lannes-Vieira J, de Araújo-Jorge TC, Soeiro MN, Gadelha P, Corrêa-Oliveira R. The centennial of the discovery of Chagas disease: facing the current challenges. *PLoS Negl Trop Dis.* 2010;**4**(6):e645.
55. Morel CM. Chagas disease: from discovery to control—and beyond: history, myths and lessons to take home. *Mem Inst Oswaldo Cruz* 1999;**94**(Suppl):3−16.
56. Coura JR. Present situation and new strategies for Chagas' disease chemotherapy—a proposal. *Mem Inst Oswaldo Cruz* 2009;**104**:549−54.
57. Coura JR, Dias JCP. Epidemiology, control and surveillance of Chagas' disease—100 years after its discovery. *Mem Inst Oswaldo Cruz* 2009;**104**(Suppl. I):31−40.
58. Moncayo A, Silveira AC. Current epidemiological trends for Chagas' disease in Latin America and future challenges in epidemiology, surveillance and health policy. *Mem Inst Oswaldo Cruz* 2009;**104**(Suppl. I):17−30.
59. Machado-de-Assis GF, Diniz GA, Montoya RA, Dias JC, Coura JR, Machado-Coelho GL, et al. A serological, parasitological and clinical evaluation of untreated Chagas' disease patients and those treated with benznidazole before and thirteen years after intervention. *Mem Inst Oswaldo Cruz* 2013;**108**(7):873−80. Available from: http://dx.doi.org/10.1590/0074-0276130122.
60. Yun OI, Lima MA, Ellman T, Chambi W, Castillo S, Flevaud L, et al. Feasibility, drug safety, and effectiveness of etiological treatment programs for Chagas' disease in Honduras, Guatemala, and Bolivia: 10-year experience of Médecins Sans Frontières. *PLoS Negl Trop Dis* 2009;**3**(7):e488. Available from: http://dx.doi.org/10.1371/journal. pntd.0000488.
61. Viotti R, Alarcón de Noya B, Araujo-Jorge T, Grijalva MJ, Guhl F, López MC, et al. Towards a paradigm shift in the treatment of chronic Chagas' disease. *Antimicrob Agents Chemother* 2014;**58**:635−9. Available from: http://dx.doi.org/10.1128/ AAC.01662-13.
62. Morillo CA, Marin-Neto JA, Avezum A, Sosa-Estani S, Rassi Jr A, Rosas F, et al. Randomized trial of benznidazole for chronic Chagas' cardiomyopathy. *N Engl J Med* 2015;**2015**(373):1295−306.
63. Dorling D. Worldmapper: the human anatomy of a small planet. *PLoS Med* 2007;**4**(1).
64. Camargo AMA, Guariento ME. Associações civis e garantia de direitos em saúde: experiência de um grupo de portadores da doença de Chagas. *Universitas* 2011;**4**(7):21−35.
65. Sanmartino M, Avaria Saavedra A, Gómez i Prat J, Parada Barba MC, Albajar-Viñas P. Do not be afraid of us: Chagas' disease as explained by people affected by it. *Interface (Botucatu)* 2015;**19**. Available from:http://dx.doi.org/10.1590/1807-57622014.1170/.

66. Morel C, Broun D, Dangi A, Elias C, Gardner C, Gupta RK, et al. Health innovation in developing countries to address diseases of the poor. *Innov Strategy Today* 2005;**1**:1−15.
67. Chagas E. Summula dos conhecimentos actuaes sobre a *Trypanosomiasis americana*. *Mem Inst Oswaldo Cruz* 1935;**30**:387−416.

# Chagas disease in pre-Colombian civilizations*

F. Guhl

Universidad de los Andes, Centro de Investigaciones en Microbiología y Parasitología Tropical, Bogotá, Colombia

## Chapter Outline

## Introduction

Chagas disease caused by the parasite *Trypanosoma cruzi* is a complex zoonosis that is widely distributed throughout the American continent. More than 150 species of triatomine bugs and more than 100 species of mammals, mostly wild species, maintain *T. cruzi* infection in nature. The infection can be acquired by infected triatomine feces, blood transfusion, oral and vertical transmission. Chagas disease represents an important public health problem, with estimates by the World Health Organization in 2015 of at least 6 million people having *T. cruzi* infection in 21 Latin American countries and 25% of Latin America's population being at risk due to the geographical distribution of insect vectors.

---

*In memoriam to Arthur Aufderheide who opened a new research field in ancient medicine and parasitology.

American Trypanosomiasis Chagas Disease. DOI: http://dx.doi.org/10.1016/B978-0-12-801029-7.00002-2

Also, immigration of infected people from endemic countries is now making Chagas disease a relevant health issue in other regions, including Europe and the United States.[1]

Chagas disease comprises two stages where the acute phase occurs about 1 week after initial infection, and about 30—40% of the infected patients develop the chronic phase of the disease when the cardiomyopathy is the most frequent and severe clinical manifestation.

Reconstruction of the behavior of a modern disease during antiquity is a formidable challenge. However, success in such an endeavor would allow for the creation of a new database, and this new information could then spawn new hypotheses. Their results could then be blended with our present knowledge to produce an unbroken history of infectious diseases from deep antiquity to the present. Paleoecological integration of such data could help explain chronological changes, whose causes could be exploited for novel modern therapeutic or preventive control of the condition.

However, there are currently only three methodological tools that can be used in such searches: genetic variation, archeology, and biochemistry.

## Genetic variation

A nomenclature for *T. cruzi* has been adopted since 2009 and includes six discrete taxonomic units (DTUs), namely, *T. cruzi* I (TcI), *T. cruzi* II (TcII), *T. cruzi* III (TcIII), *T. cruzi* IV (TcIV), *T. cruzi* V (TcV), and *T. cruzi* VI (TcVI), based on different molecular markers and biological features.[2] Recently, *T. cruzi* bat has been described as an independent DTU, based on phylogenetic and phylogeographical analyses, multiple molecular markers, and degrees of sequence divergence between *T. cruzi* bat and the six already reported DTUs.[3]

Many eukaryotic pathogenic microorganisms that were previously assumed to propagate clonally have retained cryptic sexual cycles. The *T. cruzi* parasite comprises a heterogeneous population that displays clonal propagation due to the different cycles of transmission, and also the possibility of recombination exchange that can be found in nature. Several reports indicate that natural hybridization in *T. cruzi* may be frequent, potentially involving independent exchange of kinetoplast and nuclear genetic material as well as canonical meiotic mechanisms.[4]

Different molecular markers including a 48 set of microsatellite loci have shown the great diversity in TcI.[5−7] Primers designed based on the sequences of TcI confirmed the existence of three genotypes (Ia, Ib, and Id) and a new genotype found in the Southern Cone countries named as TcIe.[8] Genetic variability has also been clearly demonstrated, reporting homogeneous (TcII) and heterogeneous groups considered hybrids due to recombination events (TcIII−TcVI).[9,10] Hybrids are considered within *T. cruzi* showing TcIII and TcIV probably as a product of recombination of TcI and TcII and TcIV−TcVI as a product of recombination of *T. cruzi* II and *T. cruzi* III/*T. cruzi* IV,[11] although this last statement is still controversial.

The molecular epidemiology and distribution of *T. cruzi* genotypes may have important implications on the disease features. However, a few correlations have been relating *T. cruzi* genetic variability and the disease outcome, showing *T. cruzi* I more related to patients with cardiomyopathy in Colombia and Venezuela and *T. cruzi* II−*T. cruzi* VI more related to patients with digestive syndrome.[12]

For triatomines, susceptibility or resistance to trypanosome infections seems to be modulated by the intestinal symbionts, which are vital for development. *T. cruzi* is considered to be subpathogenic to triatomines, whereas *Trypanosoma rangeli* is another species that commonly infects *Rhodnius* species and causes pathogenicity based on a reduction of the number of symbionts Some studies using different species of triatomines, such as *R. pallescens*, *T. dimidiata*, *R. colombiensis*, and *P. geniculatus*, have shown the affinity of TcI to infect these species in comparison with TcII transmitted by *Triatoma infestans* in the southern countries of South America.[13]

# Archeology

The modern domestic cycle is the common environment in which humans are exposed to reduviid bugs, usually *T. infestans* and *Rhodnius prolixus*. These insects hide in the cracks and defects of a house's roof and wall during the day, emerging at night to obtain a blood meal from their prey. That prey includes not only humans, but also domestic animals. Thatched roofs are especially attractive for these insects.[14] Even today, many families supplement their meals by raising guinea pigs and chickens in cages in the home as well as wild animals such as armadillos and small mammals, a high fraction of which can become infected by *T. cruzi*.

One of the best-studied populations with regard to Chagas disease is from the coastal area of northern Chile at the foot of the western Andean slopes between about 19 and 23 degrees of south latitude. The extremely arid climate here generates rapid, spontaneous desiccation of buried bodies, arresting the decay process. The absence of rainfall then preserves these dried bodies (mummies) for millennia, these conditions allow to elucidate the transmission dynamics and determinants of ancient genotypes, and to try to unravel the natural history of the *T. cruzi* taxon and Chagas disease. Interestingly, *T. cruzi* bat, the recently described Discrete Taxonomic Unit, emerges as the plausible ancestor of *T. cruzi*. The findings allow us to present a plausible model of *T. cruzi* transmission in pre-Columbian civilizations.

# Biochemistry (Bioarcheology)

Our attempt to reconstruct the behavior of Chagas disease in antiquity was based on the assumption that the soft tissues of naturally desiccated human remains (mummies) would also preserve trypanosomes that were present at the time of death. We had already demonstrated the survival of the tubercle bacillus in one of these mummies. We had dry soft tissue samples from several hundred mummies in our files; these spanned an interval of 9000 years until the 19th century. We felt that we could make a major contribution to our understanding of Chagas disease if we could identify the presence of *T. cruzi* in those individuals who were infected at the time of their death.

While the biochemical methods of dealing with ancient DNA (aDNA) were still evolving at the time of this study (and are evolving even still), we approached it by targeting a segment of mitochondrial DNA that was unique to *T. cruzi*; i.e., found in no other plant, animal, or human.[15,16] We pulverized 400 mg of each sample of dried mummy. We then extracted the sample's aDNA content and amplified this minute amount by subjecting it to nested PCR (polymerase chain reaction). The sequence of the amplified aDNA was then determined.[17]

The results indicated that an average of 40% of these mostly prehistoric people were infected with *T. cruzi* at the time of their death. That frequency was common to all cultural groups studied, and did not differ between time periods.

We wondered whether it was really possible that nearly half of ancient South Americans were suffering from Chagas disease. To answer this question, we examined the available literature to compare modern frequencies with our results.[18,19]

Recently, we developed a Whole-Genome Amplification (WGA) strategy in order to detect *T. cruzi* DNA in mummified bodies.[20]

Anatomic dissection was performed in human spontaneously mummified remains from the coastal regions of Atacama desert in Northern Chile corresponding to The Chinchorro culture. The Chinchorro culture colonized this area from about 7500 BC until 1500 BC. These sample specimens were obtained by cautiously dissection of the remains in communities near the site and maintained at water proof and airtight containers at $-80°C$ temperature until analysis. The mummified remains were obtained from Chiribaya Alta sites near the city of Ilo, the Alto Ramírez site near Pisagua, and sites near Arica (Azapa, Camarones, and Morro). We selected 43 mummified tissues (heart, stomach, esophagus, colon, intestine, rib, and sternum) corresponding to 19 mummified bodies from the same geographical area (Fig. 2.1).

We also included as a positive control, one Peruvian (c. AD 1400) mummified tissue from an adult female where *T. cruzi* amastigotes were previously described by electron microscopy and immunostaining.[21] Additionally, specimens from a spontaneously mummified ancient Egypt mummy (about 200 BC) from the Dakhleh Oasis was included as negative control since American Trypanosomiasis is restricted to the New World (detailed information about these mummies can be retrieved from Refs. [16,18,19]).

In the 43 tissues corresponding to 19 mummies we were able to amplify *T. cruzi* DNA in 31 remains (72%) by the two molecular targets (kDNA and nDNA). To ensure that the absence of amplification was not attributed to PCR inhibitors we performed β-actine assays which were positive for all the samples analyzed. Appropriate positive and negative controls were included in the diagnostic PCR assays validating the results. Regarding the nuclear (SL-IR, GPI, 18S, and HSP60) and mitochondrial (Cytb, COII, ND1, and ND4) sequences, we were able to discriminate *T. cruzi* DTUs. *T. cruzi* gene fragments were only amplified from 26 (60%) mummified tissues despite having used the WGA strategy.

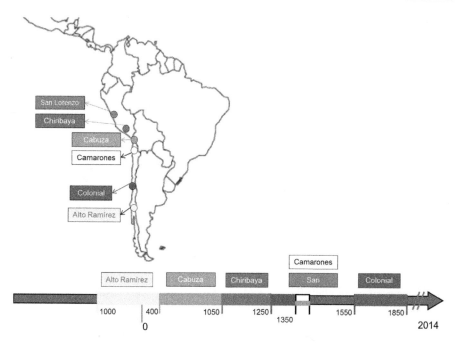

**Figure 2.1** Geographical and chronological information on the cultures used for the paleoepidemiological study of *Trypanosoma cruzi* discrete typing units (DTUs). The succession of cultures is shown on the timescale with the numbers indicating years AD and BC from zero. *Source*: After Guhl F, Aufderheide A, Ramirez J.D. From ancient to contemporary molecular eco-epidemiology of Chagas disease in the Americas. Int J Parasit 2014;44:605–12.

The occurrence of *T. cruzi* I was observed in four (15%) tissues corresponding to three mummified bodies from Chinchorro, San Lorenzo, and Colonial cultures. *T. cruzi* II in nine (35%) tissues from six distinct mummified bodies belonging to Chiribaya, San Lorenzo, Alto Ramírez, and Colonial cultures. The presence of *T. cruzi* IV in four (15%) tissues from the Chinchorro culture and from three different mummified bodies. Likewise, *T. cruzi* V was described in four (15%) tissues from four different mummies that corresponded to San Lorenzo, Cabuza, and Colonial cultures. One (4%) tissue was identified as *T. cruzi* VI from Camarones culture. Interestingly, the novel genotype *T. cruzi* bat was detected in three (11%) tissues from three different bodies dissected from the Cabuza and Camarones cultures.

## The parasite transmission cycle

The epidemiological pattern of *T. cruzi* reveals that primitive transmission was restricted to established cycles in tropical environments. The parasite was spread via anal gland secretions and urine from opossums and later via triatomine insects that fed on small mammals in broad areas of the South American continent, with no human intervention in this natural cycle.[22]

Because of long periods of adaptation, the parasite has a wide range of wild mammal reservoirs, including *Didelphis marsupialis*, *Philander opossum*, *Dasypus novemcinctus*, *Tamandua tetradactyla*, *Saimiri sciurius*, *Chiropotes satanas*, and bats of the genus *Phyllostomus* and others. The same situation persists today in the wild, where the disease maintains an enzootic character. The presence of *T. cruzi* does not seem to significantly affect triatomines nor does it impact mammals that have been naturally infected. Humans might then have become infected as a single addition to the already extensive host range of *T. cruzi*, which also includes other primates.[23]

Estimates have been made about the age of the order Xenarthra (which contains armadillos, anteaters, and sloths), one of the four major clades of placental mammals reported to be hosts for *T. cruzi*. All four of these clades were isolated in South America following its separation from the other continental land masses. Xenarthrans diverged over a period of about 65 million years, leaving more than 200 extinct genera and only 31 living species.

The next placental mammal *T. cruzi* reservoirs to emerge in South America were the caviomorph rodents and platyrrhine primates during the Eocene.[24] These clades appear following colonizations by rafting or island hopping across the Atlantic Ocean from Africa by their respective most recent ancestors. The continental isolation ended when the Isthmus of Panama land connection between South and North America emerged approximately 3.5 Mya in the Pliocene, marking the beginning of the Great American Biotic Interchange.[25]

The northern invaders of South America included carnivores, insectivores, noncaviomorph rodents, lagomorphs, artiodactyls, and perisodactyls. Bats contribute to 20% of the mammalian species diversity. Based on molecular dating, interordinal diversification occurred in Laurasia during the Cretaceous, including the appearance of bats estimated at 85 Mya.[26]

*T. cruzi* was originally transmitted directly between marsupials, but was subsequently vectored to other mammals through the advent of the blood-sucking Hemiptera (Triatominae) that are now considered the major vectors. This transfer from marsupials to other mammals may have been the main factor promoting adaptation of the parasite from the original widespread form (*T. cruzi* I) to a range of other lineages.

Current estimates suggest that the first divergence from *T. cruzi* I to *T. cruzi* II (mainly human), occurred about 10 Mya.[2] The epidemiological pattern of *T. cruzi* reveals that primitive transmission was restricted to established cycles in tropical forest environments. Triatomine insects fed on small mammals in broad areas of the South American continent, with no human involvement in the natural cycle. The same situation persists today in the wild, where the disease maintains enzootic epidemiological character. The presence of *T. cruzi* does not seem to affect triatomines significantly, nor does it impact the mammals that have been naturally infected, suggesting that a balance exists between species as a result of long periods of adaptation and coevolution.[23]

Although in general the Hemiptera represent an ancient order, with fossilized remains dating from the Permian, nearly 232−280 Mya, it is possible that the triatomines evolved later starting at different times and from diverse ancestral forms.

The Hemiptera comprise a large order with over 80,000 species widely distributed in all tropical and temperate areas. Ancestral predatory habits among the triatomines can be inferred from the fact that some species occupy a relatively wide spectrum of ecotopes and are able to exploit different species of hosts, while others occupy restricted habitats and hosts.[27] The vectorial transmission of *T. cruzi* is restricted to the New World.

## Insect vectors associated with the human habitats

*T. infestans* is the *T. cruzi* vector with the widest distribution in South America, occupying the geographic regions that today belong to Argentina, Bolivia, Brazil, Chile, Paraguay, Uruguay, and southern Peru, usually found in rural dwellings inside the cracks of walls and roofs.

In the 1970s and 1980s, surveys of poorly constructed houses were carried out in endemic areas. In northern Chile, houses were inspected to determine whether they contained living vectors of Chagas disease. About one-third housed the vector, and a fifth of these insects were infected with *T. cruzi*. All of the houses inspected in some endemic areas of Argentina contained the vector. Between one-fourth and one-half of domestic animals (such as Guinea pigs, cats, and dogs) were found to be infected.[27] Not unexpectedly, humans living in these areas were also commonly infected. About 40−80% of rural Bolivians were shown to be infected; infection was also detected in northern Chile (20%), southern Peru (12−20%), and endemic areas of Venezuela (54%).[28,29]

As a result, this domiciliated insect has been targeted for vector control activities in the past decade and has been eliminated from Chile, Uruguay, and Brazil, as well as large areas of Argentina and Paraguay.

*T. infestans* reaches high population densities in human dwellings, maintaining similarly sized populations from year to year. Its generation time is about 6 months, so it is possible to have two generations per year. Unlike other medically important insects such as mosquitoes, triatomines tend to adapt to efficiently exploit a stable environment like the nest of a mammal or a human habitation.

These insects were undoubtedly present in the human environment in pre-Colombian times and effectively transmitted *T. cruzi* as we will see. The dispersion of the vectors is a high risk factor for human settlements. Historical reconstructions suggest that the dispersal of *T. infestans* from its supposed origin in central Bolivia was associated with documented human migration.[30]

This also is true for *R. prolixus*, the primary domiciliated-vector in regions of Colombia, Venezuela, and the vast majority of Central American countries. The development of *R. prolixus* from egg to adult takes 3−4 months whereas for species such as *Triatoma dimidiata*, a peridomiciliary/domiciliary species, this may take 1−2 years.

Triatomines show a high degree of dispersion, which involves two different mechanisms: (1) passive, by the vertebrate host and (2) active by walking or in the

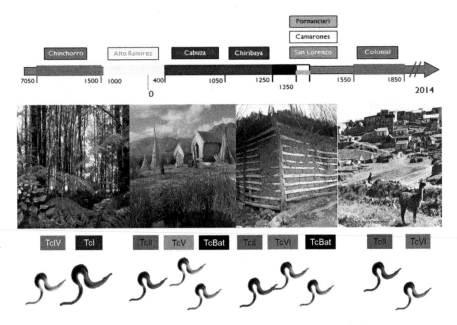

**Figure 2.2** Distribution of different triatomine species restricted to particular geo-ecoepidemiological factors.

case of adult insects flying. Several authors have reported the passive transport of triatomines in clothing, baggage, and transport and even the transport of eggs and nymphs in the feathers of birds.[31]

The geographic distribution of triatomine species extends from the Neotropics to Neoarctic regions and is closely related to environmental and ecological factors (Fig. 2.2).

Historical data indicate that the disease was transmitted in South America and seriously affected the inhabitants of endemic regions, who referred to the insects with vernacular names. The many indigenous names for the insect vectors such as vinchuca, hita, and chirimacha demonstrate the frequency with which pre-Colombian civilizations encountered these insects.

The Quechua word vinchuca, for example, means "bug that lets itself fall" which describes the behavior of domiciliated insect after feeding on blood. Hita is also a Quechua word that means "bedbug" and the chirimacha meaning is "which fears the cold." These Quechua words clearly evoke the domiciliated behavior of triatomines.

Quechua ("qheshwa") is an indigenous language of the Andean region, spoken today by approximately 13 million people in Bolivia, Peru, Ecuador, Northern Chile, Argentina, and Southern Colombia. It was the official language of Tawantinsuyu, the Inca Empire, which was the largest empire in pre-Colombian America. The administrative, political, and military center of the empire was located in Cusco in modern day Peru. The Inca civilization arose in the highlands of Peru sometime in the early 13th century (Table 2.1).

**Table 2.1 List of the vernacular names for triatomine insects in South American geographical areas and cultures**

| Region | Names | Meaning |
|---|---|---|
| Argentina, Chile, Uruguay | vinchuca[a] | bug that lets itself fall |
| Belize | bush chinche[h] | (implies absence of domestic Triatominae in Belize) |
| Bolivia | vinchuca[a] | bug that lets itself fall |
| | uluchi[a] | bug without wings; refers to nymphal stages |
| | timbucú | |
| Brazil | Barbeiro[b] | barber shaver |
| | furão[b] | big piercing bug |
| | chupão[b] | big sucking bug |
| | bicudo | beaked bug |
| | fincão[b] | big piercing bug |
| | cascudo[b] | thick-skinned bug, used mainly for nymphs |
| | chupança[b] | sucking bug |
| | procotó[b] | bug that hides in cracks |
| | Gigolô[b] | exploiter of women |
| | percevejo[b] | wall bedbug |
| | gaudério[b] | indigent thief |
| | rondão[b] | big bug that observes from hiding |
| | percevejão[b] | big bedbug |
| | percevejo do sertão[b] | bedbug from the sertão, Sertão = interior of Brazil |
| | percevejo das pedras[b] | bedbug amongst the stones |
| | piolho de piassava[b] | louse from the piassaba palm, refers to *R. brethesi* in Amazon region |
| | vunvum[b] | probably onomatopoeic for the sound of bug flight |
| | josipak | Matacos indians, Roraima |
| | îipi | Macuxi Indians, Roraima and Venezuela, refers specifically to *T. maculata* |
| Colombia | Pito[c] | whistle or horn |
| | chupasangre[c] | Blood sucker |
| | kajta in kággaba[d] | Kogi Indians, refers to the spirit of the insect |
| | kajta chiguibu[d] | the eggs of the triatomines |
| | kajta bulo[d] | first nymph star |
| | kajta yagua[d] | second nimph star |
| | kajta tema[d] | other star and adults |
| | kajta ungaga[d] | the place for payment, where the spiritual Leader (Mamo) after consultation with the spirit of the triatomines, pays with offerings that vary greatly depending on the query in order to restore the natural balance |

*(Continued)*

**Table 2.1 (Continued)**

| Region | Names | Meaning |
|--------|-------|---------|
| Cuba | sangrejuela[c] | Bloodstealer |
| Ecuador | Chinchorro[c] | large bug |
| Central | chinche besucona[c] | kissing bug |
|   America | talaje[c] | cutting bug |
| | chuluyu | needle |
| | polvoso[c] | dusty |
| | chinche bebe sangre[c] | blood-drinking bug |
| | chinche picuda[c] | biting bug |
| Mexico | chinche besucona[c] | kissing bug |
| | chinche hosicona[c] | trunked bug |
| | chinche picuda[c] | biting bug |
| | chinchona[c] | big bug |
| | pech[e] | onomatopoeic for the sound of bug flight |
| | Texcan[f] | |
| Paraguay | chichá guazú[g] | big ug |
| | Itchajuponja[g] | bug sucker |
| | sham bui tá[g] | insect that does harm by its dejections |
| | timbucú[g] | long beak |
| Peru | chirimacha[a] | bug that dislikes the cold |
| | Yta[a] | |
| USA | kissing bug[h] | cone-nose bug, big bedbug |
| | China bug[h] | refers to *T. protracta* on Pacific coast, once assumed to come from the orient |
| | red-banded | cone-nose refers to *T. rubrofasciata* and/or *T. sanguisuga* |
| Venezuela | chipo[c] | little bug |
| | îipi | Macuxi Indians; refers specifically to *T. maculate* |

[a]Quechua, a native American language family spoken primarily in the Andes of South America, derived from an original common ancestor language, Proto-Quechua. It is the most widely spoken language family of the indigenous peoples of the Americas.
[b]Portuguese.
[c]Spanish.
[d]Kogui language, Colombia.
[e]Maya language.
[f]Azteca (Nahuatl) language.
[g]Guaraní.
[h]English.
*Source*: Adapted, modified, and expanded from Schofield CJ, Galvao C. Classification evolution and species groups within the Triatominae. *Acta Trop* 2009;**110**:88–100.[32]

# Historical overview

Historical data allow us to infer that when the Europeans arrived in the New World, there was already a local knowledge of triatomine insects, including their habits and some biological characteristics directly related to man; however, these insects were not known to be associated with the disease first described by Carlos Chagas in 1909.

Geronimo de Bibar, Chilean author of a chronicle from early 1500, writes "for six years now there is a type of bugs that sting very badly and give little itching, they are as big as cockroaches and their time is in summer."[33] Various chroniclers, such as Antonio de Ciudad Real, also make references to bugs with wings. There are other references to bugs with wings that correspond to Triatominae (i.e., kissing bugs, pitos hyphae, hocicones) (texcan in Nahuatl, pec in Maya, and yta in Quechua). Lizárraga also refers to this group of insects saying the following about Bolivia and Argentina:

> Here called hyphae, cockroaches (black), as large as the insects found in the ships of the North Sea, and that color, with wings: but with the difference that they are almost invisible, they sting and bite so delicately at night that it is not felt after the fire is finished, however after two days a welt rises as a bean, so itchy it is insufferable (...) The insects are afraid of fire, and when the fire goes out they fall down the walls or from the ceiling and bite the sleeper in the legs, in the head and face (...) They have clumsy feet, and when they have filled their bellies with the blood they have sucked, cannot walk.

Felix de Azara also describes these bugs "like flat beetles," adding the important observation that "when defecating on the wound, they leave an indelible stain."

When describing the existence of "vinchucas" in Venezuela, the Jesuit José Gumilla, reports that the bite is painless, however, once the arthropod detaches, unbearable itching pain occurs. In Peru, especially in the area of Charcas, Bernabé Cobo comments that they are harmful, locate their victims by scent, and are known by the natives as hyphae.[34]

Archeological excavations have been carried out along the Aleutian Islands and the west coasts of Canada and the United States, as well as on the west coasts of Central and South America. The origin and spread of humans coincided with the latter part of the Pleistocene ice ages, and the geographical distribution of early humans was influenced by these ice ages in a number of ways. All of the excavations have yielded evidence of the presence of human activity since nearly 15,000 years ago. However, the precise date of the first human presence on the continent may be even earlier, as far back as 20,000–25,000 years, although this is still a matter of debate among archeologists. For the purpose of this chapter, it is safe to conclude that humans were spreading south and east of North America and that these small bands of hunter gatherers had reached the northern tip of South America around 10,000–12,000 years ago.[23]

This amount of time was enough for the adaptation of various parasitic diseases to their new hosts. Cultural developments, such as agriculture and permanent or semipermanent settlement patterns, created an ideal environment for the spread of infectious diseases, including tuberculosis and syphilis. Human cultural adaptation to warm and humid environments allowed Chagas disease to spread widely.

The epidemiological pattern of *T. cruzi* reveals that primitive transmission was restricted to established cycles in tropical forest environments. The parasite was spread via anal gland secretions and urine from opossums and later via triatomine insects that fed on small mammals in broad areas of the South American continent, with no human intervention in this natural cycle. This would suggest a balance between species.

Because of long periods of adaptation, the parasite has a wide range of wild mammal reservoirs, including *D. marsupialis*, *P. opossum*, *D. novemcinctus*, *T. tetradactyla*, *S. sciurius*, *C. satanas*, and bats of the genus *Phyllostomus*. The same situation persists today in the wild, where the disease maintains an enzootic epidemiological character. The presence of *T. cruzi* does not seem to significantly affect triatomines nor does it impact mammals that have been naturally infected. Humans might then have become infected as a single addition to the already extensive host range of *T. cruzi*, which also includes other primates.

Human Chagas disease is a purely coincidental occurrence. As humans came into contact with the natural foci of infection and caused different degrees of ecological transformations, infected triatomine insects were forced to occupy their dwellings.[23,35]

Thus began a process of adaptation and domiciliation to human habitations through which the vectors had direct access to abundant food as well as protection from climatic changes and predators. A good example of this adaptation is *T. infestans*, the main vector of *T. cruzi* in the Southern Cone countries of South America. *T. infestans* is considered to be an almost exclusively domiciliary species, and the same is true for *R. prolixus* in the northern region of South America and Central America.[23]

Estimates have been made about the age of the order Xenarthra (which contains armadillos, anteaters, and sloths), one of the four major clades of placental mammals reported to be hosts for *T. cruzi*. All four of these clades were isolated in South America following its separation from the other continental land masses. Xenarthrans diverged over a period of about 65 million years, leaving more than 200 extinct genera and only 31 living species.

The next placental mammal *T. cruzi* reservoirs to emerge in South America were the caviomorph rodents and platyrrhine primates during the Eocene. These clades appear following colonizations by rafting or island hopping across the Atlantic Ocean from Africa by their respective most recent ancestors. The continental isolation ended when the Isthmus of Panamá land connection between South and North America emerged approximately 3.5 Mya in the Pliocene, marking the beginning of the Great American Biotic Interchange.[25] In regard to mammals, the northern invaders of South America included carnivores, insectivores, noncaviomorph rodents, lagomorphs, artiodactyls, and perissodactyls. However, bats are conspicuously absent in this scenario despite their contribution to 20% of the mammalian species diversity.

Based on molecular dating, interordinal diversification occurred in Laurasia during the Cretaceous, including the appearance of bats estimated at 85 Mya[26] (Fig. 2.3).

# Pre-Hispanic settlements in areas of transmission of *T. cruzi*

The process of triatomine domiciliation occurred simultaneously with the process of human settlement near zoonotic transmission cycles of *T. cruzi*. The process was

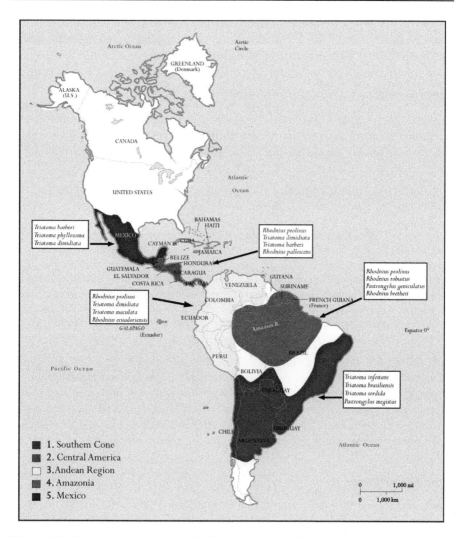

**Figure 2.3** Migration routes and spread of modern humans. Hypothesized evolutionary sylvatic cycle of *Trypanosoma cruzi* in America. Human contact with *T. cruzi* occurred as a simple addition to the already extensive host range around 8−10,000 years ago.

gradual, as has been demonstrated with other species of Triatominae today. The insects found enough food sources, feeding on men and domestic animals such as dogs, chickens, and guinea pigs. There is evidence that, as in modern times, people living with pets in their homes in endemic areas enhanced the transmission of the parasite. By comparing the migration patterns of pre-Colombian cultures in different areas of Latin America with the distribution of triatomine species, it is possible to infer the degree of passive dispersion between the parasite/insect vector and pre-Hispanic settlements.

One of the most extensive and detailed studies of this type was performed by Viana and Carpintero,[35−37] from which one can draw the following information relating to the major pre-Hispanic cultures in the Americas:

## Argentine-Bolivian Altiplano, Northwest Argentina

This area received direct and indirect influences from the high Andean cultures and had a society based on an intensive agricultural economy, with a variety of vegetables, livestock, and advanced bronze metallurgy. These cultures survived for a period of just over 1700 years, which was grouped into three stages:

- *Early period*: From the appearance of the earliest civilizations to the year 650 AD Cultures: Tafi, Cienaga, Candelaria, and Condorhuasi.
- *Middle period*: From 650 to 850 AD. La Aguada Culture.
- *Late period*: From the 850 AD until about 1480 AD, beginning in the Inca period, ranging from the arrival of the Incas to the first entry of the Spanish conquerors. In the course of human settlements, natural pathways were formed, by which they conducted a lively exchange that enabled the economic complementarity of the different cultures. The most important archeological sites (Quebrada de Humahuaca) show that the houses were important community nuclei and were built of stone walls and roofs of branches and mud, very good niches for triatomines. The economy was based on agricultural farming supplemented by the raising of Llamas (*Lama glama*).

Remains of *T. infestans* (which can easily be recognized by an expert eye) were found in the detritus deposited in urns of Tafi, Santamaría, and Aguada cultures.

The sealing and subsequent burial of the urns would have prevented any triatomine penetration a posteriori. Clearly, the insects were buried at the same time, probably hidden in the clothes of the corpses, which obviously suggests a close contact between the vector and pre-Columbian aboriginal communities.

## Sierras Centrales

This region, comprising the central region of Argentina-Sierras de Córdoba, San Luis, and Santiago del Estero, has been inhabited since the year 6000 BC. Interestingly the region of Santiago del Estero continues to have one of the highest prevalences of Chagas disease in Argentina and is one of most triatomine-infested areas.

## Sur del Perú

For the purposes of this chapter, we will highlight the Chilca culture (3800 BC) and Nasca culture (2500 BC). In Huanuco, Peru's Eastern Sierra, buildings were found that confirm the domestication of "cui" (*Cavia* sp.), dating to 1200 BC.

In the Formative Period (1200 BC−100 AD), and continuing through the Regional Development Period (100−800 AD), the Wari Old Empire (800−1200 AD), and the Empire Tawantisuyo (1430−1532 AD), the human migration of these populations increased in northwest Argentina. The construction of large cities that still surprise us, agriculture, and the breeding of llamas and other mammals were all good environments for domiciliated populations of *T. infestans*.

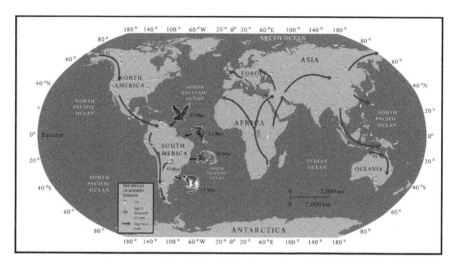

**Figure 2.4** The origin and dispersal of *T. infestans* in South America.

New settlements and the displacement of entire villages, as a result of wars of conquest, facilitated the dispersion of triatomines into new areas. The mechanism of *T. infestans* adaptation to human habitats was probably facilitated by the custom of pet storage near or even inside houses. This custom still persists in many parts of Bolivia, Peru, and Ecuador, where guinea pigs are bred in homes for human consumption.

These mechanisms of domiciliation helped *T. infestans* became one of the first insects to adapt to human habitats in South America, and it remains probably the most widespread and numerous. Although its settlement of Uruguay and Brazil occurred more recently (probably through Argentina), its dispersion increased, spreading northeast into Bahia (Brazil). *T. infestans* was one of the main vectors in the country (with *Panstrongylus megistus*), until a decade ago when efficient vector controls were established. Paraguay could be settled from the Provinces of Northwest Argentina and across the Gran Chaco (Fig. 2.4).

## Meso-America, Mayan culture

The great Mayan culture in the Peten region (northern Guatemala) lasted from 300 to 900 AD. However, the different communities that made up the amazing Mayan Empire seem to have originated from what is now northern Honduras (Santa Rosa de Copan). In the Early Formative Period (1200 BC−300 AD) the society was agricultural and built ceremonial buildings in stone. Constructions of this type also housed chiefs, priests, and dignitaries, although in most of the towns people occupied dwellings made of boughs and straw-reinforced adobe and poles, an environment conducive to the establishment of triatomines.

After an intermediate period (900−1000 AD) the New Empire or Mexican Period began, which took place primarily in Yucatan, Quintana Roo, Campeche, Tabasco, and Chiapas (1000−1200 AD). The disintegration of the Empire began

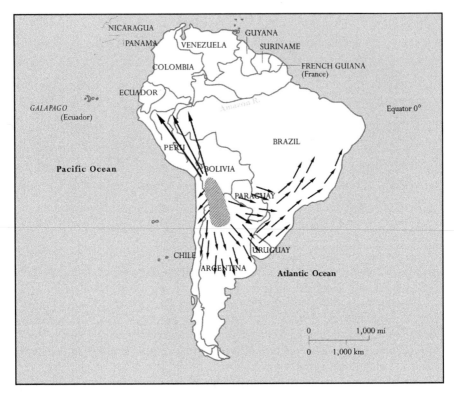

**Figure 2.5** The origin and dispersal of *T. dimidiata* in Mesoamerica and northern South America region.

due to internal wars and was completed by the arrival of the Spanish (1450–1550 AD). The economy, mainly agricultural, reached a high level, and trade with the cultures of Central Mexico was frequent and important. There is also sufficient evidence of an active relationship, mostly commercial, with the northern cultures of South America.

The keeping of poultry among the Toltecas, a Mayan village dominated by the Aztecs in the 14th century, certainly led to the adaptation of *T. dimidiata* and subspecies to human habitats by a mechanism similar to that for *T. infestans*.

Although its geographical distribution is wide, *T. dimidiata* is less efficient in transmitting the *T. cruzi*. It range extends north into Mexico, and south to Colombia and Ecuador.[38]

Interestingly, a culture akin to the Maya flourished in the area occupied by the current state of Oaxaca: the Zapotec culture. This area is inhabited by *Triatoma barberi*, the Protracta complex species that is best adapted to human habitats.

The adaptation of species and subspecies of the Phyllosoma complex, which is found around dwellings and in domiciliary environments in southern and central Mexico, seems to have been more recent occurring by a mechanism similar to that of the species mentioned so far (Fig. 2.5).

## Andean region, Northern South America

The Chibcha tribes, stretched from Colombia to Ecuador and Nicaragua. Their houses were built of posts or poles, with or without added adobe, and the roofs were built with palm leaves. The domiciliation process of *R. prolixus* from its wild habitat occurred as it does today. Genetic studies of these insects have shown the identity of genotypes among domiciled insects and insects found in the wild, especially those nesting in palm trees of the genus *Attalea*.[39]

One of the most prominent Chibcha groups inhabiting the highlands of Bogota and its nearby valleys, were the Muiscas (men), who built several large communities (100 AD). They grew corn, potatoes, sweet potatoes, cotton, and cassava in the lower valleys, and their extensive housing groups formed stable communities for the creation of a solid economy based on trade with neighboring villages, primarily those to the north and west. Domiciliated *R. prolixus* penetrated into Colombia and Venezuela and then expanded northward reaching Guatemala (Fig. 2.6).

# Oral infection by *T. cruzi*

In addition to insect transmission, Chagas disease may be acquired by ingestion. *T. cruzi* oral transmission is possible through food contamination by the feces of the vector or by the ingestion of raw meat from infected sylvatic reservoirs.

From its initial diagnosis in 1967, tens of oral outbrakes have been reported mostly in the Brazilian Amazon and subsequently in other countries of South America. Environmental imbalance caused by man through the invasion and deforestation of woodlands, results in reduction of biodiversity of mammals as food source for triatomines, affecting the dilution effect of *T. cruzi* in nature, thus increasing the risk of human infection. Many aboriginal cultures and rural populations in South America today still have the habit of eating raw or semiraw meat from wild animals, which are reservoirs of the parasite.

In the last 10 years, for example, many outbreaks of orally acquired acute Chagas disease have been reported in different geographical areas in South America. 152 cases, including 5 deaths and 121 acute cases in Brazilian Amazonia, 34 case including 4 deaths in Colombia, and a large urban outbreak of orally acquired acute Chagas disease at a school in Caracas, Venezuela that affected 103 schoolchildren.[40–42]

In general, these outbreaks lead to the death of a percentage of infected individuals, which indicates a high pathogenicity of the parasites and demonstrates its capacity to penetrate through the gastric mucosa, despite the presence of gastric acid. Additionally the presence of metacyclic forms of *T. cruzi* in anal gland secretions of the opossum (*D. marsupialis*), an animal with wild and peri-urban habits, cannot be overlooked as a source of oral transmission in the outbreaks.[43] The traditional mechanism of transmission of Chagas disease, which involves contact with metacyclic forms in the feces of wild triatomines, may not be the most common type of transmission in wild ecotopes like the Amazon where several other types of transmission appear to be occurring.

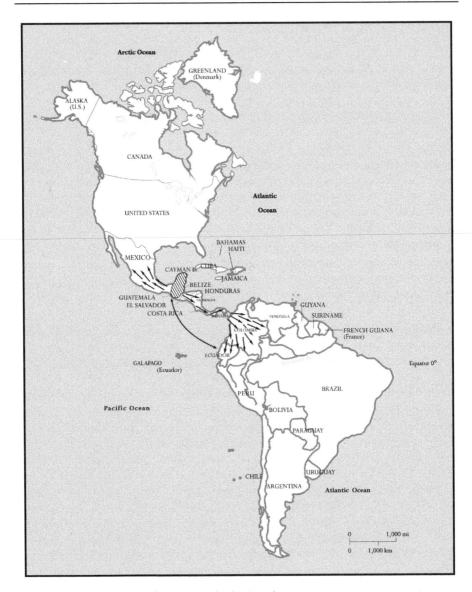

**Figure 2.6** The dispersion of *R. prolixus* in the Americas.

# Evidence of human *T. cruzi* infection in pre-Colombian civilizations

For more than a century, examination of skeletal tissue from ancient human remains has demonstrated information useful for the understanding of some diseases in antiquity.[18] Unfortunately, only a minority of human diseases leave a detectable impact on bone. Hence, during the past few decades, efforts have been made to evaluate whether other diseases could be detected by examination of the soft (i.e., nonskeletal) tissues in mummified human remains.

One of the first reports related to Chagas disease in human remains from South America was from Rothhammer et al.,[44,45] which describes cardiac lesions compatible with the chronic clinical picture of the disease. The evidence was obtained from 35 bodies dating from 470 BC to 600 AD that were mummified in the desert of Atacama in Chile.

A Peruvian Inca mummy was studied by Fornaciari et al. in 1992,[21] who showed evidence of Chagas disease in the lesions described; additionally they demonstrated the presence of amastigote nests in the heart muscle of the mummy.

In 1997 and 1999, molecular studies of mummies from the Atacama desert was performed. For the first time, they isolated *T. cruzi* DNA from 4000-year-old mummified tissue.[16]

Ferreira et al.[46] published an article on mummies from San Pedro de Atacama, which confirmed chagasic infection in specimens up to 2000 years old. All of these reports confirm the hypothesis discussed in this chapter on human migration and Chagas disease.

Most of these studies have taken the form of individual case reports. These are valuable and will remain so for a long time; however, the study reported herein represents an effort to determine whether examination of such mummified human soft tissues can reconstruct the behavior of a disease in entire ancient populations.[19]

We selected American trypanosomiasis, more popularly known as Chagas disease, as an appropriate candidate because of its high prevalence in the area of our study.

Initially, we attempted to detect the presence of *T. cruzi* using molecular biology methods that targeted a segment of the parasite's DNA in excess of 300 base pairs. Although we succeeded in that effort, the target segment proved to be too long for the sensitivity needed for a study involving a large number of specimens. A shorter segment involving a probe had the necessary sensitivity, but required considerable manipulation of the amplified product.[17]

Our final effort, described in detail in this report, used a short segment of kinetoplast DNA with less handling of our amplicon. This technique proved to have the sensitivity we needed with minimal manipulation to bring about the hybridization reaction. This was then applied to extracts of tissue specimens from 283 mummified human remains from a South Andean coastal zone. The results enabled us to construct the paleoepidemiology of Chagas disease in that area over a period of 9 millennia, from the appearance of the first humans in that region to the near present.[19]

Members of the Chinchorro cultural group were the first to settle this coastal segment. The oldest body from this group was radiocarbon-dated to about 9000 years ago. Stable isotope reconstruction of their diet indicates that approximately 90% of their diet was of marine origin, consistent with some of their grave artifacts. We have only a few samples of their housing because of lack of rain, which meant they did not need a waterproof shelter. Reconstruction of several of these shelters indicates that a series of slender wood poles were arranged in a circular pattern, and the top ends were gathered together in the form of a wooden tepee. The cover of the pole skeleton did not survive, but was most probably composed of intertwined reeds harvested from the brackish water at the river mouth. Such a dwelling would be ideal for nesting by the Chagas insect vector.

After more than 5000 years of residence with this type of a marine-based strategy, the Chinchorros were replaced by highland migrants, who we call Alto Ramirez. Arriving at the coast in about 1000 BC, they introduced agriculture. Their shelters were slightly larger than those of the Chinchorros, with walls of cane and reeds; however, because they still employed plant products in parts of their structures, these remained attractive for insect nesting.

By 4000 BC, the rapidly expanding highland population called Tihuanaco extended their territory to the sea, where it remained the dominant force until their empire crumbled in about 1000 AD. Emerging from the resulting politicocultural chaos of small, fragmented groups, were the people now known as Maitas Chiribaya. By this time, they had drifted from a mixture of marine and agricultural strategies more toward the latter, and this remained the case until the Incas arrived, preceding the Spanish.

Beginning at the end of the Chinchorro period the trend in these societies was one of progressive technology development, particularly in textile production. Their shelters also slowly increased in sturdiness. However, local resources were limited, so opportunities remained available for insect vectors to move in permanently. The arrival of the Spanish initiated the historic period. The following cultural and societal chaos rarely offered the native populations improvements with respect to living quarters.

Thus, the picture painted by archeological findings of events in the past nine millennia begins with primitive dwelling structures that were altered by the succession of cultural groups until historic times, but not to a degree that would prevent infestation by the Chagas disease's insect vector.

Our results corroborate the high genetic diversity of the *T. cruzi* taxon and demonstrates the ancient pattern displayed by this pathogen, suggesting that bats are the key reservoir in understanding the diversification of this microorganism. The rise of whole-genome sequencing for ancient genomes allows a better understanding of the evolution of the pathogens and to determine whether or not there is a coevolution process within *T. cruzi* and its human host (Fig. 2.7).

The intervention of the pre-Hispanic cultures in their environment over time resulted in different types of housing and land management, which led to the emergence of new *T. cruzi* genotypes in the transmission cycles of the parasite.[20]

Another interesting study of *T. cruzi* was in human remains dating back 4500−7000 years obtained from a Brazilian archeological site. From these remains the analyses of an aDNA sequence corresponding to the *T. cruzi* I was recovered. The mummy was a woman of ∼35 years of age from a hunter-gatherer population. She was found in the Abrigo Malhador archeological site, Peruaçu Valley, Minas Gerais State. In this region, the semiarid ecosystem is predominant, thus it has a dry climate, and soil with a basic pH. These conditions have contributed to the preservation of specimens.

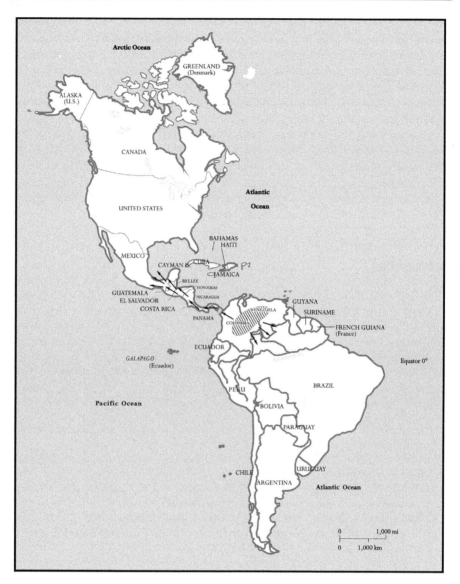

**Figure 2.7** *T. cruzi* DTUs association with human natural history in the past 9 millennia. *Source*: After Guhl F, Aufderheide A, Ramirez J.D. From ancient to contemporary molecular eco-epidemiology of Chagas disease in the Americas. Int J Parasit 2014;44:605−12.

This report[47] showed that *T. cruzi* human infection in Brazil is ancient, dating back at least 4500 years and therefore occurring in hunter-gatherer populations largely preceding *T. infestans* domiciliation. The presence of the *T. cruzi* I in humans 4500−7000 years ago in Minas Gerais State, where this genotype is currently absent, suggests that the distribution pattern of *T. cruzi* genotypes in humans has changed over time. Moreover, the recovery of an aDNA sequence and the possibility of genotyping parasites from human remains make it possible to reconstruct the early dispersion patterns of *T. cruzi* subpopulations. On the basis of these results, one may speculate that the current outbreaks of human *T. cruzi* infection, independent of triatomine domiciliation, are reemergences of the ancient epidemiologic scenario of Chagas disease in Brazil.

Paleoparasitological studies of Chagas disease may clarify the antiquity of this disease in the Americas through extraction and amplification of *T. cruzi* aDNA from human remains, other animal hosts, and vectors fragments found in archeological findings.

Phylogenetic analysis of this material would also shed light on different aspects of host–parasite coevolution and parasite transmission cycles.

# References

1. World Health Organization. Chagas disease in Latin America: an epidemiological update based on 2010 estimates. *Week. Epidemiol. Record* 2015;**90**:33–44.
2. Zingales B, Andrade S, Briones RS, Campbell DA, Chiari E, Fernandes O, et al. A new consensus for *Trypanosoma cruzi* intraspecific nomenclature: second revision meeting recommends TcI to TcVI. *Mem Inst Oswaldo Cruz* 2009;**104**(7):1051–4.
3. Lima L, Espinosa-Alvarez O, Ortiz PA, Trejo-Varón JA, Carranza JC, Pinto CM, et al. Genetic diversity of *Trypanosoma cruzi* in bats, and multilocus phylogenetic and phylogeographical analyses supporting Tcbat as an independent DTU (discrete typing unit). *Acta Trop* 2015;**151**:166–77.
4. Messenger LA, Miles MA. Evidence and importance of genetic exchange among filed populations of *Trypanosoma cruzi*. *Acta Trop* 2015;**151**:150–5.
5. Guhl F, Ramirez JD. *Trypanosoma cruzi* I diversity: towards the need of genetic subdivision? *Acta Trop* 2011;**119**:1–4.
6. Lewellyn MS, Miles MA, Carrazco HJ, Lewis MD, Yeo M, Vargas J, et al. Genome-scale multilocus microsatellite typing of *Trypanosoma cruzi* discrete typing unit I reveals phylogeographic structure and specific genotypes linked to human infection. *Plos Path* 2009;**5**(5):e1000410. Available from: http://dx.doi.org/10.1371/journalppat.100410/
7. Ramirez JD, Duque MC, Guhl F. Phylogenetic reconstruction based on Cytochrome b (Cytb) gene sequences reveals distinct genotypes within Colombian *Trypanosoma cruzi* I populations. *Acta Trop* 2011;**119**:61–5.
8. Falla A, Herrera C, Fajardo A, Montilla M, Vallejo GA, Guhl F. Haplotype identification within *Trypanosoma cruzi* I in Colombian isolates from several reservoirs, vectors and humans. *Acta Trop* 2009;**110**(1):15–21.
9. Gaunt MW, Yeo M, Frame IA, Tothard JR, Carrazco HJ, Taylor MC, et al. Mechanism of genetic exchange in American trypanosomes. *Nature* 2003;**421**:936–9.
10. Westenberger SJ, Sturm NR, Campbell DA. *Trypanosoma cruzi* 5S rRNA arrays define five groups and indicate the geographic origin of an ancestor of the heterozygous hybrids. *Int. J. Parasit* 2006;**36**:337–46.

11. Brisse S, Henriksson J, Barnabé C, Douzery EJP, Berkvens D, Serrano M, et al. Evidence for genetic exchange and hybridization in *Trypansoma cruzi* based on nucleotide sequences and molecular karyotype. *Infect Genet Evol* 2003;**2**(3):173−83.
12. Rassi Jr. A, Marin-Neto JA. Chagas disease. *Lancet* 2010;**375**(9723):1388−402.
13. Vallejo GA, Guhl F, Schaub GA. Triatominae−*Trypanosoma cruzi*/*T. rangeli*: vector−parasite interactions. *Acta Trop* 2009;**110**:137−47.
14. Edgcomb J, Johnson C. American Trypanosomiasis (Chagas disease). In: Chapman Binford and Daniel Connor, editor. *Pathology of tropical and extraordinary diseases*, Vol. I. Washington, DC: Armed Forces Institute of Pathology; 1976. . p. 244−51.
15. Guhl F, Jaramillo C, Yockteng R, Vallejo GA, Cárdenas-Arroyo F. *Trypanosoma cruzi* DNA in human mummies. *Lancet* 1997;**349**(9062):1370.
16. Guhl F, Jaramillo C, Vallejo GA, Yockteng R, Cárdenas-Arroyo F, Fornaciari G, et al. Isolation of *Trypanosoma cruzi* DNA in 4000 year-old mummified human tissue from Northen Chile. *Am J Phys Anthrop* 1999;**108**:401−7.
17. Madden M, Salo LW, Streitz J, Auderheide AC, Fornacieri G, Guhl F, et al. Hybridization screening of very short PCR products for paleoepidemiological studies of Chagas disease. *Bio-Tech* 2000;**1**(1):102-4, 106, 108-9.
18. Aufderheide A. *The scientific study of mummies*. Cambridge: University Press; 2003. p. 608.
19. Aufderheide AC, Salo LW, Madden M, Streitz J, Buikstr J, Guhl F, et al. A 9000 year record of Chagas disease. *Proc Natl Acad Sci* 2004;**101**(7):2034−9.
20. Guhl F, Aufderheide A, Ramirez JD. From ancient to contemporary molecular eco-epidemiology of Chagas disease in the Americas. *Int J Parasit* 2014;**44**:605−12.
21. Fornaciari G, Castagna M, Viacava P, Tognetti A, Bevilacqua G, Segura E. Chagas disease in a Peruvian Inca mummy. *Lancet* 1992;**257**:1933−6.
22. Deane MP, Lenzi HL, Jansen AM. *Trypanosoma cruzi*: vertebrate and invertebrate cycles in the same mammal host, the opossum *Didelphis marsupialis*. *Mem Inst Oswaldo Cruz* 1984;**79**:513−15.
23. Guhl F, Jaramillo C, Vallejo GA, Cardenas F, Aufderheide A. Human migration and Chagas disease. *Mem Inst Oswaldo Cruz* 2000;**95**(4):553−5.
24. Poux C, Chevret P, Huchon D, de Jong WW, Douzery EJP. Arrival and diversification of caviomorph rodents and platyrrhine primates in South America. *Syst Biol* 2006;**55**: 228−44.
25. Stehli FG, Webb SD, editors. *The Great American biotic interchange*. New York: Plenum Press; 1985.
26. Springer MS, Murphy WJ, Eizirik E, O'Brien SJ. Placental mammal diversification and the Cretaceous-Tertiary boundary. *Proc Natl Acad Sci USA* 2003;**100**:1056−61.
27. Schofield CJ, Matthews JNS. Theoretical approach to active dispersal and colonization of houses by *Triatoma infestans*. *J Trop Med Hyg* 1985;**88**:211−22.
28. Bastein JW. *The kiss of death: Chagas disease in the Americas*. Salt Lake City: University of Utah Press; 1998.
29. Briceño-Leon R. Rural housing for control of Chagas disease in Venezuela. *Parasit Today* 1987;**3**:384−7.
30. Schofield CJ. *Triatominae Biología y control*. UK: Eurocommunica Publications; 1994 ISBN 1 898763 01 1.
31. Foratini OP, Ferreira OA, Rocha e Silva EO, Rabello EX, Ferreira do santos JL. Aspectos ecologicos da tripanosomose americana II: Distribucao e dispersao local de triatominos, em ecotopos naturais e artificiais. *Rev Saud Publ* 1971;**5**:193−205.

32. Schofield CJ, Galvao C. Classification evolution and species groups within the Triatominae. *Acta Trop* 2009;**110**:88−100.
33. Bibar G de. *Crónica y relación copiosa y verdadera de los Reinos de Chile (1558). Edición de Leopoldo Sáez-Godoy, Biblioteca Ibero- Americana.* Berlín: Colloquium Verlag; 1966. p. 181−2.
34. Gumilla J. *El Orinoco ilustrado y defendido.* Caracas, Venezuela: Academia Nacional de Historia; 1963. p. 519.
35. Araújo A, Ferreira LF. Paleoparasitology and the antiquity of human host−parasite relationships. *Mem Inst Oswaldo Cruz* 2000;**95**(Suppl. 1):89−93.
36. Viana MJ, Carpintero DJ. *Aporte al conocimiento de los Triatominos en la Argentina. I Com. Rev. Museo Arg. Cienc. Nat.* Argentina: Buenos Aires; 1977. p. 161−74 V (8).
37. Carpintero DJ, Viana EJ. *Hipótesis sobre el desarrollo de la Trypanosomiasis Americana. Resúmenes (No. 376) II Simposio Internacional de Chagas.* Argentina: Buenos Aires; 1979 Noviembre−Diciembre.
38. Bargues MD, Klisiowicz DR, Gonzalez-Candelas F, Ramse J, Monro C, Ponce C, et al. Phylogeography genetic variation of *Triatoma dimidiata*, the main Chagas disease vector in Central America, and its position within the genus Triatoma. *PLoS Negl Trop Dis* 2008;**2**(5):e233 101371.
39. Pinto N, Marín D, Herrera C, Vallejo GA, Naranjo JM, Guhl F. Comprobación del ciclo silvestre de *Rhodnius prolixus* Stall en reductos de Attalea butyracea, en el departamento de Casanare. Memorias XII Congreso Colombiano de Parasitología y Medicina Tropical. *Biomédica* 2005;**25**(Suppl. 1):159.
40. Alarcón de Noya B, Noya Gonzalez O. An ecological overview on the factors that drives to *Trypanosoma cruzi* oral transmission. *Acta Trop* 2015;**151**:94−102.
41. Alarcón de Noya B, Díaz-Bello Z, Colmenares C, Ruiz-Guevara R, Mauriello L, Zavala-Jaspe R, et al. Large urban outbreak of orally acquire acute Chagas disease at a school in Caracas, Venezuela. *J Infect Dis* 2010;**201**(19):1308−15.
42. Coura JR. Chagas disease as endemic to the Brasilian Amazon: risk or hypothesis? *Rev Soc Bras Med Trop* 1990;**23**:67−70.
43. Lainson R, Shaw JJ, Fraiha H, Miles MA, Draper CC. Chagas disease in the Amazon Basin. I. *Trypanosoma cruzi* infections in silvatic mammals, triatomine bugs and man in the State of Pará, North Brazil. *Trans Roy Soc Trop Med Hyg* 1979;**73**:193−204.
44. Rothhammer F, Allison MJ, Núñez L, Staden V, Arriza B. Chagas disease in pre-Colombian South America. *Am J Phys Anthropol* 1985;**68**:495−8.
45. Rothhammer F, Standen V, Nuñez L, Allison MJ, Arriza B. Origen y desarrollo de la Tripanosomiasis en el área Centro-Sur Andina. *Rev Chungara* 1984;**12**:155−60.
46. Ferreira LF, Britto C, Cardoso MA, Fernandes O, Reinhard F, Araújo A. Paleoparasitology of Chagas disease revaled by infected tissues from Chielan mummies. *Acta Trop* 2000;**75**:79−84.
47. Lima VS, Iniguez AM, Otsuki K, Ferreira LF, Araújo A, Vicente ACP, et al. Chagas disease in ancient hunter-gatherer population. *Emerg Infect Dis* 2008;**14**(6):101−2.

# Social and medical aspects on Chagas disease management and control

*J.C.P. Dias[1] and C.J. Schofield[2]*

[1]Emerit Research of the Oswaldo Cruz Foundation, Centro de Pesquisa René Rachou, Belo Horizonte, MG, Brazil, [2]London School of Tropical Medicine and Hygiene and ECLAT Net Work, United Kingdom

## Chapter Outline

## Introduction

In their recent publication about Human Chagas Disease (HCD), the Médecins Sans Frontières (MSF) declared that "when we say that Chagas disease is a silent disease, we are simply stating a fact: in most cases it is a disease that presents no suspicious signs or symptoms for several years. Patients who suffer from it are not often aware that they are infected until heart or digestive dysfunction develops in its chronic stage. However, when we say that Chagas is a silenced disease we want to stress that there are those who wish to silence it."[1-3]

In reality, both aspects remain associated with the social context of HCD. Poverty, huts, economic instability, lacking of favorable production relations, and the usual absence of political and social priorities by the Latin American governments are some of the general factors involved in the history and the expansion of HCD and its control.[4-7] In spite of several evidences of its existence among very ancient indigenous settlements in South America, e.g., by the detection of *Trypanosoma cruzi* DNA in Chilean and Peruvian mommies aging up to eight centuries before Christ, HCD dispersion occurred mainly after the Columbus discovery. Its epidemiological apex occurred during the 20th century, as a result of extremely deep social and economic changes through the whole region.[8-10]

American Trypanosomiasis Chagas Disease. DOI: http://dx.doi.org/10.1016/B978-0-12-801029-7.00003-4

The appearance of the disease as endemic depended basically on the economic and social scenery of Latin American colonization, involving complex and different anthropic factors such as migration, inequity in the productive/extractive process, and a very unstable and precarious way of living. In addition, other social and political factors have been associated with the tragedy of HCD in Latin America, following the independence of the countries, in the 19th century. Among others, political factors made the difference, resulting, for instance, in the complete absence of official planning for human settlement, mainly in terms of public health, public education, and environmental policy.[4,6,11]

The classical pattern of HCD has been expanded throughout the poorest Latin American rural areas during many decades, particularly in the period between the end of the 19th century and the years 1970−90 when the insecticide campaigns were launched in several endemic countries and the classical rural to urban migration process began to be reversed in all the regions.[12] Since then, from its original frame, HCD began to modify its general epidemiology. Important demographic changes such as globalization and rural to urban migration were involved in this process, in which "chagasic" individuals have been detected in almost all Latin American urban centers, as well as in Europe and other nonendemic regions. Another new epidemiological fact concerns the growing detection of acute cases due to oral *T. cruzi* transmission in Brazilian Amazon region.[2,9,13,14] Looking at the future, the main challenges regarding HCD as a public health problem may be considered as (1) to consolidate vector and blood banks control in Latin American countries still without regular control programs; (2) to implement a regular and sustainable epidemiological surveillance in those countries with advanced control programs; and (3) to detect and to take medical and social attention to around 12−14 million of infected people both in endemic and nonendemic countries.[2,14−16]

A very crucial point in the history of HCD control has been the political priority of the official control programs and their sustainability. In most situations, the population under transmission risk remains very poor, so dependent of continuous governmental public actions for disease prevention and medical attention. By another angle, disease transmission has been controlled in many areas of the endemic region, by means of intensive control of triatomines and blood banks.[12,16] As a consequence, the present and future scenarios involve a progressive reduction of disease visibility and the need of a permanent surveillance regarding savage triatomines and new possible epidemiological situations. Such risks cannot be ignored and will require adequate approaches in a foreseeable context of reduced political interest and consequent lower operational budgets.[3,14,16]

In this context, the political activity of many scientists involved in the fight against HCD has been decisive in order to create and to maintain the priorities for HCD control. The basic strategy in this task was basically the research and the publication of epidemiological data, pointing out the medical and social frame of the disease, in terms of its geographical distribution, incidence, prevalence, morbidity, mortality, and social costs.[8,12,14]

In the last three decades, it has been recognized that the social and economic aspects of HCD were extremely important in the production and in the dispersion of the disease. Moreover, such a "contextual" frame showed to be clearly linked with the clinical aspects, also being determinant of the possibilities of disease controlling and management.[2,6,10,17] It is consensual that the definitive fight against HCD cannot be focused simply on the traditional biologic angle, but must involve all those aspects and determinants of its occurrence, "understanding the 'chagasic' patient in his bio-psycho-social and cultural reality, in a political and economic context in which the common denominator is poverty"[10] (p. 527). In the present chapter, we intend to reinforce some yet traditional ideas of such a context, focusing the main discussion on the related medical dimension, including some disease prevention aspects.

## General frame and costs of HCD

Three major parameters define the social context of HCD in endemic areas.

1. From the viewpoint of disease spreading, the general picture of poverty can be represented by the typical Latin American rural huts (extremely easy to be invaded and colonized by triatomine bugs), by the weakness of local and regional Public Health Systems (with serious problems of access, expertise, and sustainable actions, including the control of blood banks), and by the general inequity involving the production relationship throughout the whole region.[9,13,16]
2. By the cultural and sociologic standpoint, HCD is characterized by illiterate individuals, generally without a positive political expression, by the very low self-appraisal of the infected or those individuals under disease risk.[2,6,10]
3. At the political and economic side, the disease does not have the necessary governmental priority, and in the endemic countries there is a chronic lacking of human and financial resources to disease control, frequently generating program discontinuity.[3,10]

Another important aspect concerns the very poor involvement of regular national education systems in the campaign against HCD, throughout the endemic area. At the same time, the disease does not represent a good market, with regard to either the political or the common capitalistic interests.[1,13,18]

The costs of the disease have been estimated in several studies. In general, the authors agree that the costs of the chronic disease are higher than the acute one, mainly in terms of mortality and morbidity. Most studies have shown that the principal element of cost remains in severe chronic Chagas heart disease, leading the affected people to premature death, to high medical and hospital expenditures, and to working absenteeism. They also agree that the costs of prevention (triatomine and blood banks control) are relatively low in comparison with the financial loss due to HCD in endemic areas.[8,19,20]

## The medical burden of HCD in endemic and nonendemic areas

According to recent PAHO data, 21 countries must be considered endemic for HCD in the Americas, with a general prevalence rate of 1.448 by 100,000 inhabitants, meaning at least 7,694,500 infected individuals. Between 60 and 80 million suscep-tible individuals remain under the risk of *T. cruzi* transmission, in endemic countries.[21]

The annual incidence rate was calculated as 0.008 cases by 100,000 inhabitants, meaning a number of 41,200 cases of vectorial transmission and 14,385 cases of congenital transmission yearly.[21] Since the morbidity of HCD is different according to different geographical regions and age groups, general data have been restricted to estimate the impact of HCD in terms of cardiac involvement and premature deaths, both in the acute and in the chronic phase of the infection. For the acute disease, it is accepted that the mortality of nontreated individuals will depend on the intensity and the virulence of the infection, producing an acute myo-cardiopathy associated or not with a meningo-encephalic compromise. Deaths in acute HCD occur basically in children up to 3 years of age, a fact that means a very high pressure of transmission, chiefly of "domiciliated" infected triatomines.[4,8,22]

The general rate in nontreated individuals comprises between 2% and 12% of mortality in the acute phase, being higher in low age groups. A correlated conse-quence of severe acute HCD has been demonstrated in longitudinal studies, in which the worst evolution of HCD at long term (50 years of follow-up) corresponds exactly to those cases with severe acute onset detected in ages below 3 years.[18] On the other hand, acute HCD has shown to be curable with the current available drugs (nifurtimox and benznidazole).[14,15]

The adequate treatment reaches the betterment of the clinical picture and the parasitological cure in about 80—90% of the cases. Nevertheless, three major con-straints involve acute treatment: (1) the great shortage of medical expertise in endemic areas, making the correct diagnosis difficult and rare; (2) the problem of correct and early diagnosis, because of the laboratory difficulties and of the clinical picture, which is often not apparent or too similar to other several febrile diseases; and (3) the difficulties of medical access for the poor and rural populations of endemic countries.[18] An additional problem remains in the progressive loss of interest and visibility of this disease, which is occurring in endemic areas following the control implementation.[16]

The chronic phase constitutes nowadays the major problem of HCD in all endemic and nonendemic countries. Among the millions of infected individuals, at least 20% will develop a chronic heart disease and/or a digestive form. All of them are potential transmitters of the parasite by means of blood and organ transplanta-tion. And those patients suffering from Chagas heart disease will certainly have severe working limitations, high costs concerning medical attention, and reduction of life expectation according to several studies.[10,13,14,22]

Another aspect concern the superposition of coinfections and/or chronic degener-ative diseases in individuals primo-infected with *T. cruzi*. Both these situations are related to social and demographic factors involving the migration to urban centers and the survival of "chagasic" people.[2,13] At the present, the possibilities for chronic infected individuals have been considered much more optimistic, in com-parison with the medical and social situation 30 years ago. Not only the specific treatment, but also the supportive management for chronic cardiopathy and digestive "megas" have been considerably improved in recent decades.[13,14] Following the evolution of disease management, according to the recent consensus of several scientific working groups, it is possible to improve the quality and quantity of life of the infected individuals, regarding chiefly the prevention of severe arrhythmias, the progression of cardiac failure, and the occurrence of sudden death. The same is valid for the "mega" syndromes, since a precocious intervention at the beginning of the symptoms can be used to delay or even to prevent late severe complications. At this point, the social and political aspects can be crucial for the prognosis and the follow-up of thousands of patients: We must consider, above all, that the "chagasic" people are generally very poor, illiterate, and politically weak, a context extremely traditional among the "neglected diseases."[2,8,22]

The correct management of HCD presupposes continuity for several years, with regular medical supervision, including for indeterminate chronic patients. In this context, three main elements must be considered for an effective sector management policy: access, expertise, and drug availability. On the other hand, the social security is deeply involved with the evolution of the chronic HCD, mainly for those patients who demonstrate initial and severe degrees of cardiac failure and complex arrhythmias. When adequately managed and detected early, these classical heart disturbances of HCD can be effectively controlled by means of modern drugs and other medical interventions such as pace-makers, defibrillators, and (of course) rest and physical adequacy.[1,13,14,22] Obviously, social security is strictly involved with social, administrative, and economic aspects.

For instance, in Brazil, with about 2.5 chronic infected individuals, it can be calculated that 20% of them will develop a cardiac disease (500,000 individuals) and, among these, 5–10% (25,000−50,000) of individuals will develop severe degrees of "chagasic" cardiopathy.[9,23] All of them will require not only permanent medical but also social attention, involving the traditional problems of medical access and expertise, as well as the budgetary constraints of social security in poor countries. In such a context, probably the half of Brazilian individuals who deserve the benefit will never receive it, a fact clearly linked with the reduction of their survival. In our framework, the social consequences of HCD are mainly due to chronic cardiopathy, involving work limitation and quality and quantity of life, thus generating severe social consequences at the individual and group level. Besides the *T. cruzi* infection and some biological characteristics, some social factors are recognized as determinants of Chagas heart disease, such as physical effort, undernourishment, alcoholism, and the lacking of medical attention.[3,23]

The more severe "chagasic" cardiopathy used to kill very early the affected patients, generally of the male gender, of age 35−50 years. The immediate social and group consequences involve a significant population of orphans, widows, and children who must prematurely leave school to help the family survive.[3,9,10] On the other hand, the majority of infected individuals remain several years in the chronic indeterminate clinical form. Most of them never will be diagnosed since neither symptoms nor physical signs are present. Some of them will be diagnosed by means of blood banks serological screening, others by population serology, presurgical procedures, or special public health programs (e.g., pregnant women screening).[15,17,22]

The conspicuous consequence will be the lost opportunity to treat precociously such individuals and to interview clinically at the beginning of a cardiac or digestive disturbance. Nowadays, especially in low age groups, specific treatment is being considered as a very promising procedure, able to achieve the delay of severe chronic forms or even the parasitological cure of the infection.[1,22] In the case of nonendemic areas, the social and macropolitical aspects involving globalization, underemployment, and immigration of people from endemic countries have been the main causes for the detection of thousands of infected individuals in several countries of Europe, Oceania, Asia, and North America (mainly the United States). This relatively new situation involves serial problems concerning medical attention, labor affairs, and concrete possibilities of disease transmission, chiefly by blood transfusion, congenital, and organ transplantation mechanisms. Two correlated and crucial problems involved are medical expertise to diagnose and treat the disease, and the clandestine situation of thousands of individuals who are socially unprotected.[2,3,17,23]

## The particular question of specific treatment of Chagas disease

Since some years ago, the scientific community who deals with HCD has been more and more involved with the theme of specific treatment: the classical drugs (nifurtimox and benznidazole) were employed over many years and several experimental, clinical, and epidemiological evidences of concrete benefits for acute cases were well established. Moreover, recent data have shown that parasitological cure is possible in young chronic patients and in a minor proportion (20%) of chronic older individuals.[14,15,22]

The social aspects related to specific treatment correspond mainly to drug availability, medical expertise, and the political and administrative problem concerning case detection and the organization of a public system for treatment provision. Drug production also has been a social problem, since the market is very weak, considering the miserable chagasic population and the lack of political priority in endemic regions.[1,14]

The possibility of new and more effective drugs has been also a considerable constraint since the research for new molecules is very expensive and HCD does not interest the pharmaceutical industry. The particular strategy to take advantage of already existing products which would be effective against *T. cruzi* has been attempted and shows good possibilities. For example, third-generation antimycotic drugs are able to inhibit the sterol metabolism of the parasite. The problem once more has been social and economic since these drugs are very expensive and the pharmaceutical industry absolutely has no interest in the making of "social" (philanthropic) products.[1,23]

## Some social remarks concerning the control of HCD

Many years ago, a PAHO scientific group, which took place in Caracas and was organized by Jorge Rabinovich and Robert Tonn, put into an ancient computer thousands of pieces of data concerning the available strategies for HCD control in a typical Latin American rural situation. Considering a projection for 20 years, the results showed that the adequate and sustainable triatomine chemical control would provide the best short-term impact, reaching the interruption of vector transmission in the first 4 or 5 years and sustaining this situation for the rest of the prospective period. House betterment came in second place, reaching considerable reduction of transmission in the medium term. An ideal vaccine and patient-specific treatment did not work.[12]

The only alternative would be social development, which provided similar results to insecticide, over the long term. Regarding this theoretical approach, 28 years later, we can confirm absolutely the projection made in 1979. In several areas of endemic countries, in which regular chemical programs were undertaken, not only was the incidence of HCD stopped, but the degrees of prevalence, morbidity, and mortality are also falling down.[12,14,22,23] Naturally, in the scope of such results, there is a clear association between the chemical strategy and the social and economic development.

Regular insecticide spraying and the sustained entomological surveillance produced naturally the first and more bruising impact, cutting down dramatically the indoors population of *Triatoma infestans* and *Rhodnius prolixus*. This impact can be particularly certified in very poor and underdeveloped communities of Argentina, Bolivia, Brazil, Honduras, Paraguay, and even Venezuela, where social development did not arrive in the last decades.[16,24] On the other side, it is unquestionable that the social improvement of several Latin American communities, a consequence of the regional economical development, is also contributing with house improvement, better local health services, reduction of rural density, etc. Some examples can be easily observed in the State of São Paulo, Brazil, where industry and extensive crops of sugarcane and soybean rapidly improved the social status of the whole population. Thus, the challenge for the future will necessarily involve the social and the political affairs, side by side with insecticides, and medical attention. In both areas of the question (transmission control and medical attention), the problems concerning sustainability, access, expertise, and public health systems will be crucial to consolidate the overcoming of HCD in Latin America. All of these goals are absolutely attainable, according to current observations, but all of them are dependent on political will.[14,16,24]

Since 1990, a new social and political figure appeared in the scenery of HCD control, the so-called "Intergovernmental Initiatives," sharing resources, expertise, policies, and political reinforcement among the countries of different regions (Southern Cone, Andean, Central America and Mexico, and Amazon, the latter being added as the "nonendemic" countries).[12,25] With the involvement of the WHO and PAHO, a schedule of continuous supervision, operational and epidemiological criteria homogenization, rationality of costs and prices, general research, and intensive communication was implemented and regularly reviewed, generating significant impacts, mainly in terms of vector and blood banks control. Additionally, new aspects of disease management have been incorporated, such as congenital transmission, diagnosis, clinical management, and specific treatment.[14,23] In spite of natural problems, chiefly in terms of financial constraints, human resources turnover, and the evolution of the programs to decentralized models, the Initiatives remain active and can be considered as an exceptional advance in terms of the macropolicies required to face neglected diseases.[14]

## Final remarks

It was not our purpose to make a deep discussion of the social aspects involving HCD, but to summarize, in few words, how much they are present in the production, in the impact, and in the management and control of this so important and so neglected disease. It can be expected for the endemic countries that over the next 20 years, if the control actions and strategies are sustained, transmission will be controlled in most parts of the region.

Other consequences concerning the reduction of morbidity and mortality will also depend on the improvement of the public health system. Undoubtedly, we need more research to face new epidemiological and clinical situations, as well as to improve specific treatment and cure assessment. On the control side, the key words will be sustainable epidemiological surveillance, effectiveness of actions in peridomestic ecotopes, and, particularly, a better approach to congenital disease prevention.[16,23,26] All these questions involve naturally the regional capacity of research, since HCD does not have an exciting market and does not affect the so-called First World.[1,23] Finally, considering the next future of HCD in the Americas, some risks and challenges must be pointed out in this small discussion:

a. The disease will be definitely controlled in endemic areas according to political sustainability, which means[2]:
   * Economic development
   * Social development
   * Environmental protection
   * Cultural diversity.
b. As a price of the reached success and of the decreasing of disease visibility, as well as of the political and administrative inconsistency in endemic regions, some risks must be appointed[18,23,27]:
   * The loss of regular structure of the programs and of the surveillance
   * The progressive loosing of human resource
   * The loss of epidemiological information
   * The absence or weakness of the educative component
   * Several difficulties for the counter reference of cases
   * The absence of a "basic basket" for "chagasic" people
   * The difficulty to maintain regular programs in the present decentralized health systems
   * The loss of research priority
   * The loss of consistency in the university curricula.
c. Some very concrete constraints can be detected both at control and clinical programs at the present moment, such as[16]:
   * The punishment of success
   * *External enemies*: They do not provide more support; they withdraw resources

- *Internal enemies*: The programs are not changed to the new phase and they do not adapt to the risks of success; the same continues to be done
- Risks are based on believing that success is permanent and that it's unnecessary to adapt.

Finally, we have evidence that all these constraints and risks can be overcome by means of the technical and political association of the more authentic protagonists. On the side of the war against HCD, the primary round did not emerge from the politicians, the health authorities, or the "chagasic" people. Since Carlos Chagas, the main efforts for HCD recognition and control resulted from the Latin American scientific community, also incorporating valorous partners from Europe and the United States. In the last two decades, such efforts have been directed by other very important partners and strategies, with a special distinction for the so-called Intergovernmental Initiatives for Chagas Disease Control. Such a framework represents a new logic for a sustainable and more effective control approach.[16] The association among endemic countries can be considered the most visible political advance since Carlos Chagas stated, in 1911, that HCD might be considered a problem for the State.[28] In particular, the role of WHO, PAHO, and some NGO associations like MSF has been more and more fundamental for the sustainability of the fight against HCD.[1,22,27] It will be a real human and social tragedy if these organizations withdraw Chagas disease from their agenda over the next 20 years. In conclusion, we must admit that the overcoming of Chagas disease clearly involves not only a technical logistic and a political affaire, but also several aspects of social ethics.[1−3,23]

# Abbreviations

**HCD**    Human Chagas Disease
**MSF**    Médecins Sans Frontières
**OPS**    Organización Panamericana de Salud
**PAHO**   Pan American Health Organization
*T. cruzi*  *Trypanosoma cruzi*
**TDR**    Tropical Diseases Research (WHO/UNDP/WB)
**WHO**    World Health Organization

# References

1. MSF (Medécins Sans Frontieres). *Chagas, a silent tragedy*. Buenos Aires: Editorial Losada; 2005. p. 2005.
2. Briceño-León R. La enfermedad de Chagas y las transformaciones sociales de América Latina. In: OPS-Fundación Mundo Sano, editor. *La enfermedad de Chagas a la puerta de los 100 años del conocimiento de una endemia americana ancestral*. Washington: OPS/CD/426-06; 2007. p. 219−30.
3. Ault SK. Chagas disease and neglected diseases: challenging poverty and exclusion. In: OPS-Fundación Mundo Sano, editor. *La enfermedad de Chagas a la puerta de los 100 años del conocimiento de una endemia americana ancestral*. Washington: OPS/CD/426-06; 2007. p. 13−15.

4. Bucher EH, Schofield CJ. Economic assault on Chagas disease. *New Sci* 1981;**92**: 321−4.
5. Briceño-León R. *La casa enferma. Sociología de la enfermedad de Chagas*. Caracas: Carriles Ed; 1990.
6. Dias JCP, Borges Dias R. Aspectos sociais, econômicos e culturais da doença de Chagas. *Ciên Cult* 1979;**31**(Suppl):105−17.
7. Dias JCP. Rural resource development and its potential to introduce domestic vectors into new epidemiological situation. *Rev Argent Microbiol* 1988;**20**(Suppl.):81−5.
8. Antunes CMA. The epidemiology of Chagas disease. In: Gilles HM, editor. *Protozoal Diseases*. London: Arnold; 1999. p. 351−69.
9. Carlier Y, Dias JCP, Luquetti AO, Honteberye M, Torrico F, Truyens C. *Trypanosomiase Américaine ou Maladie de Chagas*. Paris: Elsevier; 2002.
10. Dias JCP, Briceño-León R, Storino R. Aspectos sociales, económicos, políticos, culturales y psicológicos. In: Storino R, Milei J, editors. *Enfermedad de Chagas*. Buenos Aires: Mosby; 1994. p. 527−48.
11. Candioti CA. *Santa Fé del Norte, Santa Fe del Sur. La desigualdad social*. Santa Fe (Argentina): Universidad Nacional del Litoral; 1989.
12. Dias JCP, Schofield CJ. The evolution of Chagas disease (American Trypanosomiasis) control after 90 years since Carlos Chagas discovery. *Mem Inst Oswaldo Cruz* 1999;**94** (Suppl. I):103−22.
13. Dias JCP. Enfermedad de Chagas: epidemiología y control. *Enf Emerg* 2005;**8** (Suppl. 1):10−17.
14. Coura JR, Albajar-Vinas P, Junqueira AV. Ecoepidemiology, short history and control of Chagas disease in the endemic countries and the new challenge for non-endemic countries. *Mem Inst Oswaldo Cruz* 2014;**109**:856−62.
15. CDC 2013. http://www.cdc.gov/parasites/chagas/ [accessed February 2016].
16. Schofield CJ, Jannin J, Salvatella R. The future of Chagas disease control. *Trends Parasitol* 2006;**22**:583−8.
17. WHO (World Health Organization). *Control of Chagas Disease*. Geneva: WHO Technical Report Series 905; 2002.
18. Dias JCP. Chagas disease: successes and challenges. *Cad S Públ* 2004;**22**:2020−1.
19. Akhavan D. *Análise do custo-efetividade do programa de controle da doença de Chagas no Brasil*. Brasília: OPS/OMS; 2000.
20. Schofield CJ, Dias JCP. A cost−benefit analysis of Chagas disease control. *Mem Inst Oswaldo Cruz* 1991;**86**:285−95.
21. OPS (Organización Panamericana de la Salud). *Estimación cuantitativa de la enfermedad de Chagas en las Américas*. Montevideo: OPS/HDM/CD/425-06; 2006.
22. Brasil. Consenso Brasileiro em Doença de Chagas. *Rev Soc Bras Med Trop* 2005;**38** (Suppl. III):4−29.
23. Dias JCP. Enfermedad de Chagas. Las etapas recorridas y las perspectivas futuras. In: OPS-Fundación Mundo Sano, editor. *La enfermedad de Chagas a la puerta de los 100 años del conocimiento de una endemia americana ancestral*. Washington: OPS/CD/ 426-06; 2007. p. 37−50.
24. Dias JCP, Silveira AC, Schofield CJ. The impact of Chagas disease control in Latin America: a review. *Mem Inst Oswaldo Cruz* 2002;**97**:603−12.
25. Figueroa R. Cooperación técnica regional y sub-regional. In: OPS-Fundación Mundo Sano, editor. *La enfermedad de Chagas a la puerta de los 100 años del*

*conocimiento de una endemia americana ancestral*, 2007. Washington: OPS/CD/ 426-06; 2007. p. 187–95.

26. WHO. Chagas disease in Latin America: an epidemiological update based on 2010 estimates. *WER* 2015;**2015**(6):33–44.

27. WHO. Chagas disease (American trypanosomiasis). http://www.who.int/mediacentre/ factsheets/en/; 2016 [updated March 2016].

28. Chagas 1911. Moléstia de Carlos Chagas. Segunda Conferência realizada na Academia Nacional de Medicina. In: Prata AR (organ.). *Carlos Chagas, coletânea de trabalhos científicos*. Brasília; UNB Edit; 1981. p. 167–92.

# Current epidemiological trends of Chagas disease in Latin America and future challenges: epidemiology, surveillance, and health policies*

*Á. Moncayo and A.C. Silveira†*
Academia Nacional de Medicina, Bogotá, Colombia

## Chapter Outline

* This paper did not receive any financial support.
† Dr. Antonio Carlos Silveira was deceased in 2012.

American Trypanosomiasis Chagas Disease. DOI: http://dx.doi.org/10.1016/B978-0-12-801029-7.00004-6

# Introduction

Chagas disease, named after Carlos Chagas who first described it in 1909, exists only on the American Continent.[1] It is caused by a flagellate parasite, *Trypanosoma cruzi,* transmitted to humans by blood-sucking triatomine bugs and by blood transfusion, the two main ways of transmission.

Chagas disease has two successive phases, acute and chronic. The acute phase lasts 6−8 weeks. Once the acute phase subsides, most of the infected patients recover an apparent healthy status, where no organ damage can be demonstrated by the current standard methods of clinical diagnosis. The infection can only be verified by serological or parasitological tests. This form of the chronic phase of Chagas disease is called indeterminate form. Most patients remain in this form of the disease.

However, after several years of starting the chronic phase, 20−35% of the infected individuals, depending on the geographical area will develop irreversible lesions of the autonomous nervous system in the heart, esophagus, colon, and the peripheral nervous system. The chronic phase lasts the rest of the life of the infected individual.

Chagas disease represents the first cause of cardiac lesions in young, economically productive adults in the endemic countries in Latin America.

Thanks to a coordinated multicountry program in the Southern Cone countries the transmission of Chagas disease by vectors and by blood transfusion has been interrupted in Uruguay in 1997, Chile in 1999, and in Brazil in 2006.

# Modes of transmission

## Transmission through vectors

Chagas disease is a zoonosis transmitted in natural foci or ecological units within a well-defined geographical environment. The ecological unit is composed of sylvan or domestic mammals and of sylvan Triatoma bugs, both infected with *T. cruzi.* Continuous transmission is assured with or without the involvement of human beings.

These conditions of transmission are present from latitude 42°N to latitude 40°S and so *T. cruzi* infection occurs from the south of the United States to the south of Argentina.

There are two stages of the human disease: the acute stage, which appears shortly after the infection; and the chronic stage, which may last several years and after several years of a silent asymptomatic period, 25% of those infected develop cardiac symptoms that may lead to chronic heart failure and sudden death, 6% develop digestive damage, mainly mega-colon and mega-esophagus, and 3% will suffer peripheral nervous involvement.[2−4]

## Transmission via blood transfusion

The rural-to-urban migration movements that occurred in Latin America in the decades of the 1970s and 1980s changed the traditional epidemiological pattern of Chagas disease as a rural condition and transformed it into an urban infection that can be transmitted by blood transfusion.

In most countries in Latin America it is now compulsory to screen for infected blood in blood banks and systems have been established to do so.

## Methods and measurement of epidemiological trends in the continent from 1980 to 2006

It should be noted that the prevalence and incidence of the disease as well as the mortality are constantly changing as a consequence of the impact of control programs, people migration, and changes in socioeconomic conditions of the population.

Data on the decrease of the frequency of new cases of infection by *T. cruzi* in the last decade as a result of vector control are presented below in the sections on the Sub-regional Initiatives for the Interruption of Transmission of Chagas disease.

The estimation of the decrease in the incidence rates of infection by *T. cruzi* in the period under study was made by comparing the age-specific prevalence rates of infection in a given age group in the period 1980−85 (at the time when the cross-sectional studies were carried out in the different countries) and the age-specific prevalence rates in the **same** age group in the period 1997−2006, i.e., 20 years later (see Fig. 4.1 and Table 4.1).

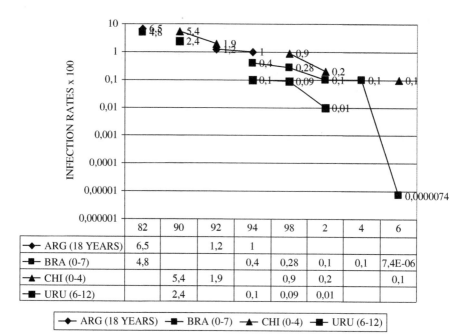

| | 82 | 90 | 92 | 94 | 98 | 2 | 4 | 6 |
|---|---|---|---|---|---|---|---|---|
| ◆ ARG (18 YEARS) | 6,5 | | 1,2 | 1 | | | | |
| ■ BRA (0-7) | 4,8 | | | 0,4 | 0,28 | 0,1 | 0,1 | 7,4E-06 |
| ▲ CHI (0-4) | | 5,4 | 1,9 | | 0,9 | 0,2 | | 0,1 |
| ■ URU (6-12) | | 2,4 | | 0,1 | 0,09 | 0,01 | | |

◆ ARG (18 YEARS)   ■ BRA (0-7)   ▲ CHI (0-4)   ■ URU (6-12)

**Figure 4.1** Interruption of transmission of Chagas disease, infection rates × 100 Southern Cone countries, 1982−2006.
*Source*: World Health Organization. Report of the Expert Committee on the control of Chagas disease. *Technical Report Series 905*, Geneva; 2002. p. 85; INCOSUR, 1993−2006.

Table 4.1 **Prevalence of human *T. cruzi* infection in Latin America, 1975—85**

| Country | Population at risk (thousands) | Percentage of total population | Number of infected persons (thousands) |
|---|---|---|---|
| Argentina | 6900 | 23 | 2640 |
| Brazil | 41,054 | 32 | 6180 |
| Bolivia | 1800 | 32 | 1300 |
| Chile | 11,600 | 63 | 1460 |
| Paraguay | 1475 | 31 | 397 |
| Uruguay | 975 | 33 | 37 |
| Colombia | 3000 | 11 | 900 |
| Ecuador | 3822 | 41 | 30 |
| Perú | 6766 | 39 | 621 |
| Venezuela | 12,500 | 72 | 1200 |
| Costa Rica | 1112 | 45 | 130 |
| El Salvador | 2146 | 45 | 900 |
| Guatemala | 4022 | 54 | 1100 |
| Nicaragua | ND | ND | |
| Honduras | 1824 | 47 | 300 |
| Panamá | 898 | 47 | 200 |
| México | ND | ND | |
| Total | 99,895 | 25 | 17,395 |

ND, no data.

## Transmission through vectors

Data on the prevalence and distribution of Chagas disease improved in quality during the 1980s as a result of the demographically representative cross-sectional studies carried out in countries where accurate information was not available. A group of experts met in Brasilia in 1979 and devised standard protocols to carry out countrywide prevalence studies on human *T. cruzi* infection and triatomine house infestation.

These studies were carried out during the 1980s in collaboration with the Ministries of Health of Argentina, Bolivia, Brazil, Chile, Colombia, Costa Rica, Ecuador, El Salvador, Guatemala, Honduras, Panama, Paraguay, Peru, Uruguay, and Venezuela. The accurate information obtained has made it easier for individual countries to plan and to evaluate the effectiveness of national control programs[5-20] (Table 4.1).

On the basis of these individual countrywide cross-sectional surveys, it was estimated that the overall prevalence of human *T. cruzi* infection in the 18 endemic countries reaches 17 million cases. Some 100 million people (25% of all the inhabitants of Latin America) were at risk of contracting *T. cruzi* infection (Table 4.1).

The incidence was estimated at 700–800,000 new cases per year and the annual deaths due to the cardiac form of Chagas disease at 45,000.[21]

The originally endemic area with vectorial transmission in the human domicile comprised 18 countries with higher *Trypanosoma cruzi* infection rates in the regions infested by *Triatoma infestans* (Southern Cone countries) and *Rhodnius prolixus* (Andean countries and Central America) which were the triatomine species best adapted to the human domicile.

The epidemiological quantification was one of the reasons to prioritize the control of the disease but the final political decision came from the demonstration of the high cost–benefit ratio of the control programs versus the costs of the medical care and the social security of the infected patients (Akhavan, 1998).

## Transmission through blood transfusion

The figures in Table 4.2 show the extent of the problem of transmission via blood transfusion in some selected cities of the continent between 1980 and 1989.[31] While it varies between 1.3% and 51.0%, the prevalence of *T. cruzi* infection in blood was much higher than that of Hepatitis or HIV infection.

The transmission of Chagas disease via blood transfusion is a real threat even for countries where the disease is not transmitted by vector, such as the United States and Canada, where cases of acute Chagas disease have been documented[32,33] (Kichkoff, 1989).

The prevalence of infected blood samples in the Southern Cone countries has decreased as shown by the consistently decreasing trend in all six countries of this subregion since 1994 (Table 4.3).

# Feasibility of interruption of transmission

The tools for interrupting the domestic cycle of *T. cruzi* transmission, such as chemical control, housing improvement, and health education, are available. In fact, the prevalence of the infection has decreased in countries that have consistently applied control measures. For example, after 20 years of control programs in Argentina, positive serology in 18-year-old males has significantly decreased since 1980, and the number of reported new acute cases decreased since the 1970s.[34] In Brazil, transmission by vector has been interrupted in the whole state of Sao Paulo since the mid-1970s. Decreasing rates of seropositive school children has paralleled the above control efficacy: in 1976, the incidence rate was 60% and in 1983 it dropped to 0%.[35]

Transmission through transfusion could be prevented if blood is screened by serology and positive units are discarded. In most countries of the region, serology for *T. cruzi* is mandatory for blood donors.

Table **4.2** **Prevalence of *T. cruzi* infected blood in blood banks of selected countries, 1980−89**

| Country | Number of samples tested | Percentage positive | Reference |
|---|---|---|---|
| **Argentina** | | | |
| Buenos Aires (1987) | 58,284 | 4.9 | [22] |
| Santiago Estero (1987) | 2003 | 17.6 | [22] |
| Córdoba (1982) | 2441 | 8.4 | [22] |
| **Bolivia** | | | |
| Santa Cruz (1990) | 205 | 51.0 | [23] |
| **Brazil** | | | |
| Brasilia (1984) | 2413 | 14.6 | Pereira 1984 |
| Paraná (1987) | 3000 | 4.8 | [24] |
| Sao Paulo (1982) | 56,902 | 2.9 | [25] |
| **Chile** | | | |
| Santiago (1983) | 214 | 3.7 | [26] |
| Vicuña (1983) | 62 | 14.5 | [26] |
| **Colombia** | | | |
| Bogotá (1990) | 1128 | 2.5 | [27] |
| Cúcuta (1987) | 491 | 7.5 | [27] |
| **Costa Rica** | | | |
| San José (1985) | 602 | 1.6 | [28] |
| **Ecuador** | | | |
| Guayaquil (1971) | 1054 | 3.2 | Reports Ministry of Health |
| **Honduras** | | | |
| Tegucigalpa (1987) | 1225 | 11.6 | [29] |
| **México** | | | |
| Puebla (1986) | 200 | 17.5 | [30] |
| **Peru** | | | |
| Tacna (1972) | 329 | 12.9 | Reports Ministry of Health |
| **Paraguay** | | | |
| Asunción (1972) | 562 | 11.3 | Reports Ministry of Health |

(*Continued*)

Table 4.2 **(Continued)**

| Country | Number of samples tested | Percentage positive | Reference |
|---------|--------------------------|---------------------|-----------|
| **Uruguay** | | | |
| Paysandú (1983–84) | 445 | 4.7 | [6] |
| Salto (1983–84) | 71 | 4.2 | [6] |
| Tacuarembó (1983–84) | 699 | 7.7 | [6] |
| **Venezuela** | | | |
| Various cities | 195,476 | 1.3 | [31] |

*Source*: Schmunis GA. Trypanosoma cruzi, the etiologic agent of Chagas' disease: status in the blood supply in endemic and non endemic countries. *Transfusion* 1991;**31**:547–57.

Table 4.3 **Estimated number of infections by *T. cruzi* and annual incidence in Latin America, 1975–2005**

| Country or region | Total number of infections | | | New cases | | |
|-------------------|---------|---------|---------|---------|---------|---------|
| | 1975/85 | 1995 | 2005 | 1990 | 1995 | 2005 |
| Central America and Mexico | 1,935,000[a] | ... | 1,906,600 | 209,187 | 72,677 | 16,200 |
| Argentina | 2,333,000[b] | 2,100,000 | 1,600,000 | ... | ... | 1300 |
| Brazil | 4,500,000 | 1,900,000 | 1,900,000 | ... | ... | 0 |
| Bolivia | 1,134,000 | ... | 620,000 | 86,676 | ... | 10,300 |
| Chile | 1,239,000 | 157,000 | 160,200 | ... | ... | 0 |
| Colombia | 900,000 | ... | 436,000 | 39,162 | 31,330 | 5250 |
| Ecuador | 300,000 | 450,000 | 230,000 | 7488 | 13,365 | 2350 |
| Paraguay | 397,000 | ... | 150,000 | 14,680 | ... | 900 |
| Peru | 643,000 | ... | 192,000 | 24,320 | 19,072 | 3100 |
| Uruguay | 37,000 | ... | 21,700 | ... | ... | 0 |
| Venezuela | 1,200,000 | ... | 310,000 | 179,703 | 22,960 | 1400 |

(...) No data.
[a]Except Mexico 1995.
[b]1990.
[c]Vectorial transmission.

Available knowledge therefore indicates that the most common ways of transmission of human *T. cruzi* infection could be interrupted by:

- Implementation of vector control activities in houses in order to first reduce and then eliminate the vector-borne transmission of *T. cruzi*
- Strengthening the ability of blood banks to prevent transmission of Chagas disease by blood transfusion through development and implementation of a policy for screening blood for human use.

# Current control programs

The traditional vertical control programs in the Latin American countries have focused on the spraying of insecticides on houses and household annexes and buildings. National control programs aimed at the interruption of the domestic and peridomestic cycles of transmission involving vectors, animal reservoirs, and man are feasible and have proven to be very effective. Reaching the goal of eliminating vector borne transmission is more feasible in areas where the vector is domiciliated like *T. infestans* and *R. prolixus*.

Twelve countries of the Americas have active control programs that combine insecticide spraying with health education. The common pattern of the vertical, centralized control programs follows several operational steps or phases, namely:

- Preparatory phase for mapping and general programing of activities and estimation of resources
- Attack phase during which a first massive insecticide spraying of houses takes place and is followed by a second spraying 6−12 months later, with further evaluations for selective respraying of reinfested houses
- Surveillance phase for the detection of residual foci of Triatomines after the objective of the attack phase has been reached. In this last phase, the involvement of the community and the decentralization of residual control activities are essential elements.

A prime example is the program which has been operating in Brazil since 1975 when 711 Brazilian municipalities had Triatomine-infested dwellings that were the objective of the control program. Ten years later, in 1986, only 186 municipalities remained infested. This represents a successful accomplishment of the program objectives in 74% of the originally infested municipalities. In 1993 there were only 83 municipalities infested which represents a reduction of 86%. In 1983, 84,334 *T. infestans* bugs were captured by field workers but in 1998 only 485 insects were found in the whole country.

In large parts of the Southern Cone countries, programs have entered the surveillance phase characterized by monitoring of house infestation, and where necessary, focal spraying.

# Economic impact

## Program costs and cost-effectiveness of control interventions

The countries of the Southern Cone Initiative have spent in the period 1991−2000 more than US$345 million from their national budgets to finance the vector control activities in their territories since the launching of the Initiative.

The Ministry of Health of Brazil carried out a study aimed at the analysis of the cost-effectiveness and cost−benefit of the Chagas Disease Control Program in Brazil. Due to the chronic nature of the disease and the protracted period of evolution, a period of 21 years was chosen for the analysis. The time interval from 1975 to 1995 includes data from different sources of information that were used to carry out this evaluation.[36]

Effectiveness was defined using various parameters, but the main one was the measurement of the burden of disease prevented in DALYs (Disability-Adjusted Life Years). From 1975 to 1995, the Program (excluding blood banks) prevented an estimated 89% of potential disease transmission, avoiding some 2,339,000 new infections and 337,000 deaths. This translated into the prevented loss of 11,486,000 DALYs, 31% from averted deaths, and 69% from averted disability, showing the large role of disability in the overall burden of disease caused by Chagas disease.

The estimated benefits (expenditures prevented) of the Program (excluding blood banks) were US$7,500,000,000, 63% of the savings being health-care expenditures and 37% social security expenditures (disability insurance and retirements).

The cost-effectiveness analysis demonstrated that for each US$39 spent on the Program, 1 DALY was gained. This places the Program and its activities in the category of interventions with a very high cost-effectiveness. The results of the cost–benefit analysis indicated savings of US$17 for each dollar spent on prevention, also indicating that the Program is a health investment with good return. The analysis of other diseases with socioeconomic causes demonstrated that the decline in Chagas disease infection rates is due to the preventive activities, and not due to general improvement in life conditions.

The economic impact of the disease during the chronic stage is very high as shown by data from Brazil. If we consider that about 30% of the infected persons will develop severe cardiac and digestive lesions such as cardiac arrhythmia (75,000 cases), mega-esophagus (45,000 cases), and mega-colon (30,000 cases) per year, the estimated costs for pacemaker implants and corrective surgery (average US$5000) would amount to approximately US$750 million per year, which would be enough for the improvement or construction of more than 700,000 rural dwellings at a minimum estimated cost of US$1000 each in Brazil in 2000.

Between 1979 and 1981, 14,022 deaths were due to Chagas disease in Brazil which represented approximately 259,152 years of potential life lost (YPLL) before the age of retirement. Assuming that all the patients were unqualified rural workers only and that the minimum daily wage was at the time US$2.5, the total economic loss due to premature deaths would amount to US$237 million.

# Epidemiological impact in the region

The average reduction of incidence in the Southern Cone countries is 94% as shown in Table 4.4. By cutting the transmission of the disease in the countries of the sub-region in this proportion, the incidence of Chagas disease in the whole of Latin America has been reduced by 70%: the number of incident cases was reduced from an estimated 700,000 new cases per year in the whole region in 1983 to less than 200,000 new cases per year in 2000 and to 41,200 in 2006. Also the annual number of deaths dropped

Table 4.4 **Changes in epidemiological parameters due to interruption of transmission and decrease of incidence, 1990−2006**

| Epidemiological parameters | 1990 | 2000 | 2006 |
|---|---|---|---|
| Annual deaths | >45,000 | 21,000 | 12,500 |
| Annual new cases | 700,000 | 200,000 | 41,200 |
| Prevalence (million) | 30 | 18 | 15 |
| Population at risk (million) | 100 | 40 | 28 |
| Distribution | 18 countries | 16 countries | 15 countries (transmission interrupted in Uruguay in 1997, Chile in 1999 and Brazil in 2006) |

*Source*: World Health Organization/TDR. Report of the Scientific Working Group on Chagas disease, Buenos Aires, Geneva; 2006. p. 7.

from more that 45,000 to 12,500. The number of endemic countries was 18 in 1983 and in 2006 it was reduced to 15, as shown in Table 4.4.[37]

The intradomiciliary infestation by *T. infestans* has been eliminated in Brazil in 2006, in Chile in 1999, and in Uruguay in 1997.

At present, the major challenge is to ensure the sustainability of this program in an epidemiological context with very low *T. cruzi* infection rates and a political−institutional context of health sector reforms, where the decentralization of operations may result in the risk of the activities losing priority. The new institutional order requires that Chagas disease control be integrated into other services, and programs, and become part of a broader scheme for meeting the health needs of the population. In these circumstances the integrated activities must sustain the significant progress so far achieved in the way of elimination of Chagas disease.

## *Initiative of the Southern Cone countries: epidemiological trends*

Accepting that the epidemiological and entomological spaces did not overlap with political divisions, in Brasilia in June 1991, the Ministers of Health of Argentina, Brazil, Bolivia, Chile, Paraguay, and Uruguay launched the "Initiative for the Elimination of transmission of Chagas Disease."[38] Since the vector of *T. cruzi*, in these countries, *T. infestans*, is intradomiciliary, sustained implementation of control measures have successfully interrupted transmission of Chagas disease as indicated below.

At the time, in these countries there were 11 million infected persons and 50 million were at risk. This represented 62% of the prevalence of infected individuals of the whole continent.

Technical representatives of each Ministry were designated to constitute an Intergovernmental Commission in charge of implementation and evaluation of the control programs. The Pan American Health Organization (PAHO) was appointed as the Secretariat of this Commission and has played a leading role of promotion and coordination.

A program guide was designed by the Commission incorporating revisions submitted by the professional staff of the control programs and was used for the development of the country programs. The proposed plans for Argentina, Brazil, Bolivia, Chile, Paraguay, and Uruguay are approved on a yearly basis by their respective governments.

The objectives of the "Southern Cone Initiative" were clearly established on their inception and comprised the interruption of vectorial and transfusional transmission. The cooperation among countries was ensured by the formal commitments of the countries which introduced the agreed activities in their national control programs. Later, other objectives of this Initiative were introduced, such as etiological treatment and medical care of the infected patients as an ethical imperative.

Current data[37,39−46,47] on disinfestations of houses, blood bank screening, and incidence of infection in the under-5 years age group, indicate that the vector borne and transfusional transmission of Chagas disease were interrupted in Uruguay in 1997, in Chile in 1999, and in Brazil in 2006. Chagas disease has been targeted for elimination by the World Health Assembly in Resolution WHA51.14 approved in May 1998[48] and recently reviewed by the WHO Executive Board in January 2009.[49]

The model implemented in the Southern Cone was adapted to the Initiatives of the Andean Countries in 1996 (IPA) and Central America in 1997 (IPCA).[50] and more recently the Amazon Initiative in 2004 (AMCHA).

The advances in control of Chagas disease accomplished in the period 1991−2006 changed the epidemiological model of the disease.

From a general point of view the most important changes obtained by the Southern Cone Initiative are:

- Interruption of transmission of *T. cruzi* by *T. infestans* certified in Brazil, Chile, and Uruguay, in the eastern region of Paraguay, and in 10 of the 13 endemic provinces of Argentina. (Misiones, Santa Fe, San Luis, Santiago del Estero, Jujuy, Entre Rios, La Pampa, Neuquén, and Rio Negro.)[51]
- Important reduction of vectorial transmission in Bolivia due to the coverage of house spraying with insecticides in the endemic area and regular activities of vector control in southern Peru where the house infestation is also caused by *T. infestans.*
- Reduction of the transmission by secondary species in Brazil.
- Coverage of blood screening close to 100% in all the countries as shown in Table 4.2.
- Systematic screening in blood banks is carried out routinely in 20 out of 21 countries.
- The prevalence of infection in young children has been substantially reduced throughout the continent and the number of people at risk of infection by the parasite has decreased in 40%, from 108 million in 2006 to 65 million in 2010.

Progress in control in each country is reported as follows:

## Argentina

The area of transmission covered 60% of the country north of parallel 44 degrees. The main vector is *T. infestans*. In 1980 the average house infestation rate for the country as a whole was 30%; in 1998 it was 1.2%; and in 2002 it dropped to 1.0% which is equivalent to 98% reduction in house infestation by the main vector.

The seroprevalence rates for the whole country for the age group 0−4 years is 0.9% which confirms the very low number of acute cases among children in this age group. In the age group 0−14 years the rate is 1.9%. In the age group of 18-year-old males the seroprevalence rates have dropped from 5.8% in 1981 to 1.0% in 1993 and 0.5% in 2002. The interruption of vectorial transmission has been achieved in 10 of the 13 endemic provinces of the country.[52]

Finally, there is 100% coverage of the blood donations screened against Chagas disease in the blood banks of the public sector and 80% coverage in the private ones.[41]

## *Bolivia*

The endemic area covers 80% of the extension of the country which corresponds to seven of the nine Departments. *T. infestans* is the main vector. In 1982 it was estimated there were a total of 1,300,000 infected persons and in 26% of them electrocardiograph alterations were observed. The house infestation rate for the whole country was 41.2% in that year and the infection rate in the vectors was 30.0%. Infection rates of more than 50.0% have been reported in blood donors in Santa Cruz.[23]

Data on serological prevalence shows a rate of 28.8% in the general population while in the age group of 0−4 years it is 22.0% in Cochabamba but 0.0% in Potosi where there is an active vector control program. In Tupiza, another department where there is an active control program, the house infestation rate is 0.8%.[53]

## *Brazil*

The main vector was *T. infestans*. Other two common species, *Triatoma brasiliensis* and *Panstrongilus megistus* are less important in disease transmission.

In 1975 the endemic area comprised 3,600,000 km$^2$ or 36% of the total extension of the country and the most extensive endemic area on the continent. This area included 2493 municipalities in the States of Alagoas, Bahía, Ceará, Espirito Santo, Goiás, Piauí, Mato Grosso, Mato Grosso do Sul, Maranhao, Paraiba, Paraná, Pernambuco, Río de Janeiro, Río Grande do Norte, Río Grande do Sul, Sergipe, Tocantins, and the Federal District of Brasilia. At present only the States of Bahía and Rio Grande do Sul are still considered infested by the main vector in residual foci with low density.

House infestation due to *T. infestans* has been reduced from 166,000 insects captured in the endemic areas by the control program in 1975 to 611 insects captured in 1999 in the same areas which corresponds to a reduction of 99.7% of the infestation by this vector. This represents an average of 1 insect per 10,000 houses surveyed, i.e., an infestation rate far below the minimum required for effective transmission of the parasite into new patients.

The prevalence of human *T. cruzi* infection in the 7−14 year group in 1999 was 0.04% as compared with 18.5% in 1980. This represents a 99.8% reduction of incidence of infection in this age group.

Results of 94,000 serological tests carried out in a population sample in the population of the 0−5 year group in 2007 indicate that the seroprevalence in this age group is 0.0% which can be interpreted as a proof of the interruption of vectorial transmission of Chagas disease in Brazil (Luquetti, 2007).

The above data confirms the interruption of transmission of Chagas disease by *T. infestans* vectors in Brazil. Based on the above epidemiological and entomological data an international commission in charge of evaluating the interruption of vectorial transmission in this country issued a certification to declare the country as free of transmission in 2006.[42,46,47,53,54]

## Chile

The vector responsible for disease transmission was *T. infestans* which has been eliminated from human dwellings and hence the transmission has been interrupted.

The overall infestation rate for the country has been reduced from 3.2% in 1994 to 0.14% in 1999, a reduction of 99.8%. In 1999 there were just 26 *T. infestans* insects were captured in the interior of dwellings of the endemic areas in the whole country which represents 2.5 insects in every 1000 houses, an infestation rate far below the threshold required for effective transmission of the parasite to new persons.

The infection rate in the age group 0−4 years in 1999 was 0.016% which represents a reduction of 98.5% as compared to 1.12% that was found in the same age group in 1995.

The screening in blood banks in the endemic areas has been mandatory since 1996 and the prevalence of infected samples has been reduced to 0.5%.

An independent commission visited the endemic areas of the country in November 1999 and based on the above data certified the interruption of vectorial transmission.[44,45]

## Paraguay

The main vector is *T. infestans*. Chagas disease is endemic in all rural areas of the country and the house infestation rate in 1982 varied from 10% in the Department of Misiones to 20% in Cordillera.

In a serological survey carried out in 1997 in a representative sample (940 individuals) of children less than 13 years old in marginal areas of the capital city of Asuncion a significant decrease of prevalence rates was observed in all age groups when compared with data of 1972.

Rural/urban migration to these marginal areas of Asuncion comes mainly from Paraguari, Cordillera, and Central which have the highest domiciliary infestation rates by triatomines. However, the fact of the 0 prevalence rate in the age group of less than 4-years-old indicate interruption of transmission by triatomines in the urban areas of the capital.[53,54]

## Uruguay

*T. infestans* was the only intradomicile vector. Since 1997 this species has been eliminated from the intradomiciles in the whole country. In 1975 the endemic area comprised the Departments of Artigas, Cerro Largo, Colonia, Durazno, Flores, Florida, Paysandú, Rio Negro, Rivera, Salto, San José, Soriano, and Tacuarembó.

The house infestation rate dropped from 5.65% in 1983 to 0.30% in 1997.

The interruption of vectorial and transfusional transmission was certified in 1997 and the whole country is under surveillance. There is 100% coverage of blood screening in blood banks.

The incidence of infection in the age group of 0–12 years was 0%, which confirms the interruption of vectorial and transfusional transmission of Chagas disease in Uruguay since 1997.[43]

## Initiative of the Andean countries: epidemiological trends

In these countries there are 5 million infected individuals and 25 million are at risk of contracting the infection. This represents 27% of the prevalence of infected individuals of the whole continent.

As the vectors of Chagas disease in these countries are not strictly domiciliated, it is necessary to adapt and test the vector control strategies to the local entomological conditions.

In the Andean countries of Colombia, Ecuador, Peru, and Venezuela, the elimination of the vectorial transmission was launched at an Intergovernmental meeting held in Bogotá in February 1997, where detailed country by country plans of action including annual goals, budgetary needs, evaluation mechanisms, and research needs were prepared.[55]

The advances made in these countries, both in the development of new methods for evaluation and in control activities, include:

- Development of methodologies for risk stratification
- Stratification of vectorial transmission risks and limited control programs in Colombia
- Establishment of a national control program in Ecuador and implementation of activities following risk stratification criteria
- Implementation of regular control activities in the MACROSUR region of Peru
- Reestablishment of activities of vector control and entomological surveillance in Venezuela
- Screening of blood for transfusion close to 100% as shown in Table 4.1.

Progress in control in each country is reported as follows:

## Colombia

The main vector is *Rhodnius prolixus* but *Triatoma dimidiata* has also been described as an effective *Trypanosoma cruzi* vector.

It has been estimated that a 5% of the population living in the endemic areas is infected or approximately 700,000 persons. The Departments with higher infection rates are Arauca (21.1%), Casanare (10.0%), Santander (6.3%), Norte de Santander (5.2%), Boyacá (3.7%), Cundinamarca (1.9%), and Meta (1.7%).

The screening in blood banks has been mandatory since 1995 and there is 100% coverage in the whole country. In 2001 the prevalence in blood donors was 0.65% as compared with 2.1% in 1998.

The preparatory phase of the national Chagas disease control program has been advanced and a map of the country featuring the risk municipalities has been prepared. The vector control activities with insecticide sprayings have been decentralized to the Departments but there are no data available to monitor the impact of the control programs.

## Ecuador

The main vector is *T. dimidiata*. The transmission occurs in the Provinces of the Pacific coast including El Oro, Manabí, and Guayas. It is estimated that between 30,000 and 50,000 persons are infected. However there are no data on prevalence of infection by age groups or on house infestation rates by Province.

The preparatory phase of the national Chagas disease control program has been advanced. The law reorganizing the control program was issued in December 1998 and places the program under the Secretary of Tropical Medicine with specific functions and budget. The law for compulsory blood screening against *T. cruzi* was issued in August 1998. The seroprevalence of infected blood in blood banks for the whole country is 0.2%.

## Peru

The highest prevalence of human infection is found in the Departments of Arequipa, Moquegua, Ica, and Tacna, which together comprise 8% of the total population of the country. The main vector is *T. infestans* and it is estimated that there are some 394,000 houses infested with 24,000 persons infected with the parasite. Acute cases are regularly reported from this endemic area which indicates active transmission. There are no screening programs in blood banks in spite of a prevalence of infected donations estimated in 2.4% in 1993.

## Venezuela

The main vector is *R. prolixus*. The endemic area comprised in 1987 591 municipalities in an area of 700,000 km$^2$ with a population of 12 million.

The control program was officially established in 1966. The objective of the Program was to interrupt intradomestic transmission through vector control by insecticide spraying. The Program for improvement of rural housing, originally initiated in the 1960s, assists the rural inhabitants to substitute palm roofs, to plaster adobe walls, and to cement earthen floors. In addition, routine screening for *T. cruzi* in blood banks has been mandatory since 1988.

In children under 10 years, the figures of seroprevalence rates for *T. cruzi* infection have decreased steadily in the last four decades from 20.5% (1958−68) to 3.9% (1969−79) and further on to 1.1% (1980−89) and to 0.8% (1990−99).

The incidence of infection in the age group 0–4 year old was reduced by 90% to less than 1.0% from 1990 to 1999. The geographical distribution of *T. cruzi* transmission is restricted to the States of Portuguesa, Barinas, and Lara.[56]

The prevalence of infected blood in blood banks was reduced from 1.16% in 1993 to 0.78% in 1998 (Aquatella, 1987).[57]

## Initiative of the Central American countries: epidemiological trends

In these countries there are 2 million infected individuals and 26 million are at risk of contracting the infection. This represents 11% of the prevalence of infected individuals of the whole continent.

As the vectors of Chagas disease in these countries are not strictly domiciliated, it is necessary to adapt and test the vector control strategies to the local entomological conditions.

In the Central American countries, Belize, Costa Rica, El Salvador, Guatemala, Honduras, Mexico, Nicaragua, and Panama, progress in blood banks control is also proceeding well and all of them except one have issued legislation for compulsory blood screening against blood infected by *T. cruzi*.

Similarly, the elimination of the vectorial transmission was launched at an Intergovernmental meeting held in Tegucigalpa in October 1997 where detailed country by country plans of action including annual goals, budgetary needs, evaluation mechanisms, and research needs were prepared.[55]

The advances made in vector control and in control of blood transfusions in these countries include[58]:

- The interruption of transmission of the parasite by *R. prolixus* in all endemic countries of Central America has been accomplished.
- Interruption of transmission of *T. cruzi* by *R. prolixus* certified in Guatemala.
- Interruption of transmission of *T. cruzi* by *R. prolixus* in Honduras and Nicaragua in the process of certification.
- Reduction of transmission by *T. dimidiata* in several countries.
- Testing of alternative methodologies for control of *Rhodnius pallescens*.

Progress in control in each country is reported as follows:

### Belize

The only vector species of epidemiological importance is *T. dimidiata*, but it is restricted to the wild environment. There are sporadic reports of insect adults attracted by light that are frequently found in the periphery of the cities and villages. The seroprevalence in the general population is very low and the seropositives found are migrants from neighboring countries. The screening of blood banks has 100% coverage and the prevalence among blood donors in 2000 was 0.5%.

## Costa Rica

The main vector is *T. dimidiata*. The vectors are found in the central plain, extending primarily to the northwest and southwest regions of the country. Seroprevalence of 1.94% was found in some blood banks of the country that participated in one study in 2000. A survey carried out in the Heredia Province in 2001 in school children aged 7–12 years showed an infection rate of 0.2%. Chagas disease is not considered a public health problem.[59]

## El Salvador

*T. dimidiata* is the main vector. *R. prolixus* was detected in the country in the 1980s, but this species has since disappeared from El Salvador. *T. dimidiata* is the only vector currently detected in all Departments with a house infestation rate of 21% in the dwellings in rural areas and in the small or medium townships. In 2000 the prevalence of the infection in school children aged 7–14 years was 0.3% and 2.1% in the population older than 14 years.

The blood screening coverage was 100% in 2000 when the prevalence of infected blood was 2.48%. The vector control program treated in that year 67.3% of infested dwellings in areas where there is coexistence of infestation by anophelins and triatominos.

## Guatemala

*T. dimidiata* is found in 18 of the 22 departments and *R. prolixus* in 5 departments. The infestation rate varies from 12% to 35%. The infection rate in school children in the five most endemic departments, namely, Zacapa, Chiquimula, Jalapa, Jutiapa, and Santa Rosa was 4.9% in a survey carried out in 2000. There is a poor blood bank control system and prevalence of seropositive blood donations in 2000 was 0.84%.

Vector control activities are carried out by the control program of the Ministry of Health in the mentioned Departments with highest house infestation rates.[59] Interruption of transmission of *T. cruzi* by *R. prolixus* was certified in 2005.

## Honduras

The main vector *R. prolixus* is present in 11 departments of the country and the second vector *T. dimidiata* is present in 16 departments. Vectors are present in the departments of Choluteca, Comayagua, Copan, Francisco Morazan, Intibuca, Lempira, Ocotepeque, Olancho, El Paraiso, La Paz, Santa Barbara, and Yoro. In 1983, the highest infection rates were found in the western and eastern departments and in the southern region. About half of the population is estimated to be at risk. Infection rates of 32% or more in the vectors have been reported. The most frequent clinical manifestation is cardiopathy.

Vector control activities are carried out in six of the nine Health Regions of the country.

A recent seroepidemiological survey carried out in areas under chemical control in children aged less than 5 years was 0.36% and in school children aged 7−14 years was 3.3%. The coverage of the control of transfusional transmission is 100% and the national seroprevalence in blood donors in 2000 was 1.53% as compared to 11% in 1985.[59] Interruption of transmission of *T. cruzi* by *R. prolixus* is in the process of certification.

## Mexico

Vectors and infected mammals are found in the states of Chiapas, Guanajuato, Guerrero, Hidalgo, Jalisco, Mexico, Michoacan, Morelos, Nayarit, Oaxaca, Puebla, Sonora, Yucatan, and Zacatecas. The prevalence of the disease is highest in the pacific coast states from Chiapas to Nayarit, in the Yucatan peninsula, and in some areas of the central part of the country. Although most of the human infections and clinical forms in Mexico are considered to be mild, there have been recent reports of some cases of mega-viscera. Mexico has not introduced routine screening for *T. cruzi* in blood banks where 850,000 donations are made every year and where around 12,760 units of blood could be infected.

There is no vector control program although there is a renewed interest of the health authorities to organize national and state vector control activities.

## Nicaragua

*T. dimidiata* is present in 14 of 17 departments of the country and *R. prolixus* in five departments. The control of transfusional transmission is made in 70% of the blood banks with a prevalence of infected blood of 0.33%. A seroepidemiological survey carried out in 2000 in school children showed a prevalence rate of 3.3% in this age group.[59] Interruption of transmission of *T. cruzi* by *R. prolixus* is the process of certification.

## Panama

The main vector is *R. pallescens* found inside the dwellings of the Chorrera district. This vector is present also in palms in the wild environment. *T. dimidiata* is also an important vector. There is no compulsory screening in blood banks or vector control programs.

## Amazon initiative

The "Initiative for Surveillance of Chagas disease in the Amazon Region" (AMCHA) was launched in 2004.

The epidemiological data are scanty to assess the magnitude of the problem. In the report of the first meeting held in Bogota there is no mention of the burden of disease except for a mention of the presence of 279 autochthon cases (252 acute cases and 27 chronic cases) in the whole of the 5,000,000 km$^2$ extensive territory of the Brazilian Amazon region. In addition it is mentioned that in the national serological survey (1975—81) the rate of positivity by State oscillated between 0.0% in Amapá and 1.9% in Amazonas. There are no data for tendencies or data of annual incidence (Guhl, 2004, pp. 17, 103).

In the same report it is only mentioned that in the Colombian Amazon region, there are positive serology in nine communities of the Department of Guainía but there are no indications as to the methodology of selection of the population samples (Guhl, 2004, pp. 27, 102). On the other hand, for Guyana, Surinam, and French Guyana it is concluded that Chagas disease "is not a public health problem for these three countries" (Guhl, 2004, p. 36). Ecuador, Peru, and Bolivia do not have information on the morbidity by Chagas disease in the Departments or Provinces of their respective Amazon regions.

In the report of the second meeting held in Manaus in September 2004, the risk of the establishment of endemic Chagas disease is discussed and it is mentioned that up to 1998, 17 episodes with 85 cases have occurred of possible oral transmission of *Trypanosoma cruzi* due to the ingestion of açai juice (*Euterpa catinga*) in the States of Pará, Acre, Amapá, and Amazonas. Apart from the above information there are no further epidemiological data on the trends in Brazil or in any of the countries (http://cdiaecuniandes.edu.co/AMCHA.htm).

The advances made in vector control and in control of blood transfusions in these countries include:

* Development and standardization of a surveillance model based on the detection of antibodies against *T. cruzi* through serological analysis of samples collected for the diagnosis of malaria.
* This surveillance model has been evaluated in Brazil and partially in Ecuador.

# Epidemiological impact

The most significant results in the interruption of transmission have been achieved in the Southern Cone and the Central American countries. The national programs of Argentina, Brazil, Chile, and Uruguay had shown important results even before the launching of the Initiative. Fig. 4.1 shows the current trends of the incidence of infections in the Southern Cone countries as a consequence of elimination of vectorial transmission in Uruguay, Chile, and Brazil.[60,61]

In Central America, after the creation of the IPCA, the response of the governments was very effective and complemented by the participation of international cooperation agencies in the financing and execution of control activities. In the Andean countries the difficulties encountered by the IPA were twofold: on the one hand the variety of epidemiological and entomological situations and on the other side the different degrees of political commitment of the governments. The concept of risk stratification was developed in the context of this Initiative and was an important contribution to the other ones.[62–64] In addition it was felt the need to define better the objectives such as the elimination of *T. dimidiata* in Ecuador, of *R. ecuadoriensis* in Peru, and of *R. prolixus* in Colombia.

With respect of the Amazon Initiative (AMCHA) it is recognized that it is still in an initial phase of generation of knowledge on the magnitude of the problem and development of control methodologies, in particular in Brazil and to a lesser extent in Ecuador.

The impact of vector control programs and the possible influence of other variables, such as the general socioeconomic development of the populations at risk, can be better evaluated by the trends of the number of infected cases in different moments. Table 4.1 shows those data in three different moments: 1975−85, 1995, and 2005 to estimate the prevalence and 1990, 1995, and 2005 to estimate the incidence.

As the information compiled in this table has different sources (WHO/OPS, 2006[65]), the interpretation should be cautious and should be considered as the best estimation of the real epidemiological situation.

The impact on the decrease of the burden of disease measured in DALYs lost due to Chagas disease has been the most important in the period 1990−2001 for Latin America and the Caribbean. The number of DALYS dropped from 2.8 million in 1990 to 0.8 in 2001, a reduction of 78%, the highest among the top eight communicable diseases in the region.[65,66]

The impact on mortality due to Chagas disease is evidenced by the reduction in mortality from 45,000 annual deaths in 1980 (Moncayo, 1993) to 14,000 in 2001 (World Bank, 2006) a net decrease of 70%. Table 4.3 summarizes the reduction in incidence, prevalence, mortality, and distribution of Chagas disease on the continent.[37]

In Table 4.5 the data on coverage of blood Banks screening and the percentage of positive samples for 2005 are shown. The sources of this information are the official reports of the governments to the meetings of the Intergovernmental Commissions of the Subregional Initiatives. The high coverage and low percentage of seroreactivity in the different countries can be observed.

# Future challenges

In spite of the progress achieved there are a number of future challenges to pursue on the way ahead. They can be divided into three categories: epidemiological, technical, and political.

## Epidemiological

### Oral transmission

This route of transmission is well established and documented[67,68] (Ministerio da Saúde/Brasil 2005[69,70]). The most salient characteristic of the oral transmission is the fact that several persons are affected simultaneously pointing to the occurrence of a common source outbreak through contaminated food.

Table 4.5 **Coverage of screening of blood for transfusion for T. cruzi (%) and proportion of positive samples in endemic countries, 2005**

| Country | Coverage of screening for *T. cruzi* (%) | Positive samples (%) |
|---|---|---|
| **Southern cone** | | |
| Argentina | 100 | 2.47 |
| Bolivia | 80 | 8.0 |
| Brazil | 100 | 0.21 |
| Chile | 87 | 0.6 |
| Paraguay | 99 | 3.2 |
| Uruguay | 100 | 0.47 |
| **Andean countries** | | |
| Colombia | 100 | 0.44 |
| Ecuador | 100 | 0.15 |
| Peru | 99 | 0.57 |
| Venezuela | 100 | 0.6 |
| **Central America and Mexico** | | |
| Belice | ND | 0.4 |
| Costa Rica | 100 | 0.09 |
| El Salvador | 100 | 2.4 |
| Guatemala | 100 | 0.79 |
| Honduras | 100 | 1.4 |
| Nicaragua | 100 | 0.9 |
| Panama | 97.6 | 1.4 |
| Mexico | 100 | 0.51 |

ND, no data.
*Source*: Document OPS/HDM/CD/425-06, Reunión Iniciativa de los Países de Centroamérica 2006, Reunión Iniciativa de los Países Andinos 2006.

The challenge here is the prevention of the oral transmission via the ingestion of beverages such as the açai juice (*Euterpe oleracea, Euterpa catinga*) in the Brazilian Amazon region.

In other documented cases of outbreaks of oral transmission the contaminated food was served in family celebrations and in circumstances that were unpredictable. This was the case in the outbreaks of Teotonia, Catolé do Rocha and Santa Catarina in Brazil (Nery-Guimarães et al., 1968,[67] Ministerio da Saúde/Brasil 2005) and in Caracas, Venezuela.[70]

The approach for prevention of these outbreaks is based on surveillance, prevention, and management similar to the control of diseases transmitted by food as recommended by a group of experts convened by the Pan American Health Organization (PAHO) in Brasilia in 2006.[71]

## Transmission in the Amazon region

The patterns of vectorial transmission in this region are unusual and different from those that were recognized as necessary to maintain the endemic levels such as the presence and colonization of the household by the vectors. So, the few known cases of infection by *T. cruzi* are being transmitted (1) by the oral route; (2) by vectors that enter the dwelling but do not develop intra domicile colonies; and (3) by infection of persons that enter the jungle and have contact with sylvan triatomines such as *Rhodnius brethesi* in the extraction of "piaçaba," a vegetal fiber (*Leopoldinia piassaba*).[72,73]

Most of the documented cases are due to the ingestion of "açai" juice and are concentrated in the States of Pará and Amapá where the production of this fruit is intensive.

Fig. 4.2 depicts the number of cases by year since the first ones were reported in 1969.[74] These cases were the result of outbreaks and hence produced by oral transmission.

The especial characteristics of the transmission of the disease in this region, required a new model of epidemiological surveillance adapted from the traditional used in the endemic areas that is based on the detection of the intradomicile vector, the screening of blood for transfusion, and the identification and treatment of the congenital form. In addition, it was necessary to take into account the enormous extension of the territory of this region which implied very serious operational difficulties.

However, there were other favorable factors to be considered such as the financial resources allocated by the Brazilian government for malaria surveillance and the feasibility of the parasitological diagnosis of *T. cruzi* to be carried out simultaneously in the same slide as for *Plasmodium falciparum*. However, it is recognized that the sensitivity of this examination for the detection of *T. cruzi* is low.

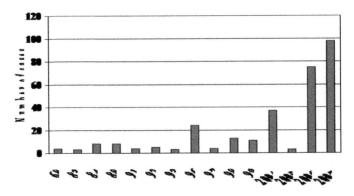

**Figure 4.2** Cases of acute Chagas disease reported from the Brazilian Amazon region, 1968/2007.
*Source*: Gerencia Técnica de Doença de Chagas/Secretaria de Vigilância em Saúde/Ministério da Saúde-Brasil, 2007.

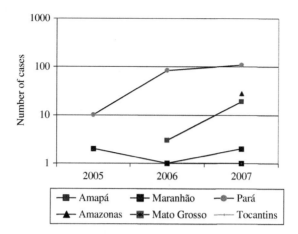

**Figure 4.3** Cases of acute Chagas disease reported by the States of the Brazilian Amazon region, 2005−7.
*Source*: Gerência Técnica de Doença de Chagas/SVS/M. da Saúde/Brasil, 2009.

The following surveillance activities were proposed at the meeting held in Cayenne in 2005 that were accepted by the Pan American Health Organization[75]:

- Detection of cases using the infrastructure of malaria surveillance
- Identification and mapping of environmental markers for the identification of current or potential vector species
- Research and monitoring of entomological situations when vector colonization is suspected by some species such as *Triatoma maculata*, *Panstrongylus geniculatus*, *Panstrongylus herreri*, *Rhodnius neglectus*, and *Rhodnius stali*.

The increase in the number of cases in the Amazon States in recent years can be observed in Fig. 4.3. This increase coincides with the fact that the surveillance program has been fully operational in the same period.

## Globalization of transmission

The increasing mobility of populations and the migration toward nonendemic countries have extended the infection to these countries through blood transfusion, organ transplantation, and the congenital form among migrants. The risk is related with the country of origin of the migrants and the rate of prevalence in that given country.

However, the advances observed in control of the transmission indicate that this potential extension to Europe, the United States, and Canada might be transitory or decreasing.

The World Health Organization recently launched the Global Network for Chagas disease elimination (WHO Global Network for Chagas Elimination— GNChE) to meet this situation.

## Local epidemiological situations

There are a number of situations that depend of localized circumstances that have implications for vector control operations in the following areas:

### The Chaco region

In spite of the sustained regular activities of vector control in this territory that is shared by Argentina, Bolivia, and Paraguay, the rates of infestation by *T. infestans* remain high. The reasons are associated to the complex peridomiciles of the rural houses, the emergence of resistance of the vector to the pyrethroid insecticides in the Provinces of La Rioja and Salta in Argentina and the Departments of Tarija and Cochabamba in Bolivia, and the presence of sylvan foci of *T. infestans* in Bolivia.

An integrated approach is being proposed that includes the improvement of peridomiciles and the use of higher doses of insecticide in these peridomiciles.[76]

### Areas with vectorial transmission without intradomicile colonization

In these areas the transmission occurs because of the "visit" of the vector to the houses from the natural ecotopes to feed on the inhabitants after which the insect comes out. This form of transmission has been documented for *R. pallescens* in Panama and Colombia where the natural ecotopes of this species are several types of palm trees which are planted around the rural dwellings. The infection rates of this insect with the parasite are very high.

The surveillance and control in these particular situations are based on the analysis of variables that influence transmission such as the ratio houses/ecotopes, the insect infection rates by *T. cruzi*, the vulnerability of the dwelling to the insect "visit" and the frequency of these "visits."[77]

Several alternatives of control have been proposed including physical or chemical barriers and the use of light sources that are not attractive to the insects.

## Technical

### Chemical vector control in the peridomicile

The peridomicile comprises the annexes, fences, corrals, and poultry yards that are built around the rural dwellings. The efficacy of the insecticides sprayed in this part of the house is low due to the degradation of the active principle by the rains and the continued exposure to sunlight. Other reasons of this low efficacy include the operational difficulties for spraying and the lack of order and cleanness in these spaces. So, residual infestations are invariably situated in the peridomicile.

It seems that the only alternative is the physical management of these spaces including reordering of the structures and the objects found there.

### Resistance of vector populations to insecticides

"Control failures" that evidence the cross-resistance of vectors to pyrethroids have been documented in areas of Tarija and Cochabamba in Bolivia and in Salta and La Rioja in Argentina. Some field tests have been carried out with other insecticides such as carbamates and phosforates with poor results. It is necessary to develop and test new molecules to overcome the emerging resistance.

## Low sensitivity of entomological methods

The available methods for direct detection of domiciled triatomines have a low sensitivity especially in circumstances where the insect densities are low as it is the case in advanced control phases. The direct reporting by the inhabitants of the presence of domiciled vectors is more effective and there are studies to evaluate the efficacy of traps with and without attractants such as pheromones.

## Political and structural factors

These factors refer to the ranking of disease control priorities within the national health policies.

## Maintaining the political priority

At present, the major challenge is to ensure the sustainability of the national control programs in an epidemiological context with very low *T. cruzi* infection rates in the younger age groups of the populations of several countries and negligible house infestation rates.

The national programs should be adapted to the new epidemiological circumstances but should be maintained with emphasis in entomological surveillance to avoid that the government efforts, financial and otherwise, to attain the interruption of transmission, be lost. The successes accomplished in this respect should not be "punished" but maintained.

It is proposed the stratification of the risk be the central criterion to shape the required surveillance and control activities.[63,64]

## Decentralization of control programs

Since the 1980s the traditional vertical programs for disease prevention and control are being dismantled in accordance to the current political and institutional context of health sector reforms, where the decentralization of operations may result in the risk of the activities losing priority.

The vertical programs were characterized by high specificity of activities, strict planning, and clear definition of measurable goals and investment of important financial resources.

The decentralization of programs has resulted in the lack of recognition by the local authorities of the priority given to Chagas disease control in view of more pressing needs for immediate attention.

The new institutional order requires that Chagas disease control be integrated into other services and programs and become part of a broader scheme to meet the health needs of the population. In these circumstances the integrated activities must sustain and expand the significant progress so far achieved in the interruption of transmission of Chagas disease in several countries of Latin America.

**Dr. Alvaro Moncayo** was secretary of the TDR Steering Committee on Chagas disease from 1979 to 1997; chief, Control of Trypanosomiasis and Leishmaniasis 1990—98; and manager of the TDR Task Force on Intervention Research on Chagas disease from 1998 to 2001 at the World Health Organization, Geneva, Switzerland. Currently he is the vice president of the Academia Nacional de Medicina, Bogotá, Colombia.

**Dr. Antonio Carlos Silveira** was director of the Chagas Disease Division (1977—84); director of the National Epidemiology Division (1986—88); director of the Health National Foundation Operational Department (1992); coordinator of the Vector-Borne Diseases Control Coordination (1994—98) of the Ministry of Health/ Brazil and national consultant of the Pan American Health Organization/WHO. PWR-Brazil (1998—99). Doctor Silveira was deceased in 2012.

# References

1. Chagas C. Nova tripanozomiase humana. Estudos sobre a morfolojía e o ciclo evolutivo de *Schizotrypanum cruzi* n. gen., n.sp., ajente etiolójico de nova entidade morbida do homen. *Mem Inst Oswald Cruz* 1909;**1**:159—218.
2. Pereira JB, Willcox HP, Coura JR. Morbidade da doenca de Chagas. III. Estudo longitudinal de seis anos, em Virgen da Lapa, MG, Brasil. *Mem Inst Oswald Cruz* 1985;**80**(1):63—71.
3. Coura JR, Anunziato N, Willcox HPF. Morbidade da doenca de Chagas I. Estado de casos procedentes de varios estados de Brasil, observados no Rio de Janeiro. *Mem Inst Oswald Cruz* 1983;**78**:363—72.
4. Coura JR, et al. Morbidade da doenca de Chagas'. IV. Estudo Longitudinal de dez anos em Pains e Iguatama, Minas Gerais, Brasil. *Mem Inst Oswald Cruz* 1985;**80**:73—80.
5. Cordova E, et al. Enfermedad de Chagas en el Sur del Perú. *Bol Peru Parasitol* 1980;**2**(1—2):46—50.
6. Franca ME. Chagas disease in Uruguay in the last twenty years. *Rev Méd Uruguay* 1986;**2**:125—31.
7. Acquatella H, et al. Encuesta epidemiológica en sujetos con serología positiva para Enfermedad de Chagas. *Cien Tecnol Venezuela* 1987;**4**:185—200.
8. López L. *Encuesta serológica de prevalencia de la Enfermedad de Chagas en Paraguay.* Asunción, Paraguay: Ministerio de Salud, SENEPA, Informe de Proyecto; 1985.
9. Marinkelle C. *Aspects of Chagas disease in Colombia. American Trypanosomiasis Research.* Washington, DC: PAHO Scientific Publication No. 318; 1976. p. 340—6.
10. Matta V, et al. *Seroepidemiología de la Enfermedad de Chagas en Guatemala. Memorias VII Congreso Centroamericano de Microbiología.* San José: Costa Rica; 1985. p. 17.
11. Pan American Health Organization. Aspectos Clínicos de la Enfermedad de Chagas. *Bol Ofic Sanitaria Panamericana* 1974;**76**:141—55.
12. Camargo M, et al. Inquérito Sorológico da Prevalencia de Infeccao Chagásica no Brasil 1975/80. *Rev Inst Med Trop Sao Paulo* 1984;**26**(4):192—204.
13. Ponce C. *Prevalencia de la Enfermedad de Chagas en Honduras.* Tegucigalpa, Honduras: Ministerio de Salud; 1984.

14. Reyes Lituma V. *Estudio de Prevalencia de Enfermedad de Chagas en Ecuador.* Guayaquil, Ecuador: Ministerio de Salud, Programa de Control de Vectores; 1984.
15. Salvatella R, Calegari L, Casserone S, et al. Seroprevalencia de anticuerpos contra *Trypanosoma cruzi* en 13 departamentos del Uruguay. *Bol Of Sanitaria Panamericana* 1989;**107**:108−17.
16. Schenone H, et al. Enfermedad de Chagas en Chile. Sectores rurales y periurbanos del área de endemo-enzootia. Relaciones entre condiciones de la vivienda, infestación triatomídea domiciliaria e infección por *Trypanosoma cruzi* del vector, del humano y de mamíferos domésticos. 1982−1985. *Bol Chil Parasitol* 1985;**40**:58−67.
17. Sousa O. *Encuesta serológica de prevalencia de la Enfermedad de Chagas en Panamá Laboratorio de Biología.* Ciudad de Panamá: Universidad de Panamá, Informe de Proyecto; 1985.
18. Cedillos RA. Chagas disease in El Salvador. *Bull Pan Amer Health Org* 1975;**9**:135−41.
19. Valencia A. *Investigación Epidemiológica Nacional de la Enfermedad de Chagas.* La Paz, Bolivia: Ministerio de Previsión Social y Salud Pública, PL-480 Title III; 1990.
20. Zeledón R, et al. Epidemiological pattern of Chagas disease in an Endemic Area of Costa Rica. *Am J Trop Med Hyg* 1976;**24**(2):214−25.
21. UNDP/WORLD BANK/WHO. Special Programme for Research and Training in Tropical Diseases. In *Eleventh programme report*, Geneva; 1991. p. 67.
22. Pérez A, Segura EL. Blood transfusion and transmission of Chagas infection in Argentina. *Rev Arg Trans* 1989;**15**:127−32.
23. Carrasco R. Prevalence of *Trypanosoma cruzi* infection in blood banks of seven departments of Bolivia. *Mem Inst Oswald Cruz* 1990;**85**:69−73.
24. Marzochi MCA. Chagas disease as an urban problem. *Cad Saúd Públ* 1981;**2**:7−12.
25. Dias JCP, Brener Z. Chagas disease and blood transfusion. *Mem Inst Oswald Cruz* 1984;**79**(Supl):139−47.
26. Liendo F, et al. Enfermedad de Chagas en Chile. Sectores urbanos. XIII. Prevalencia de infección por *Tripanosoma cruzi* en donantes de sangre del sector sur del área metropolitana de Santiago, 1985. *Bol Chil Parasitol* 1985;**40**:82−4.
27. Guhl F, et al. Rastreo seroepidemiológico de donantes de sangre chagásicos enuna zona endémica (Norte de Santander, Colombia). *Rev Latinoam Microbiol* 1987;**29**:63−6.
28. Urbina A, et al. Serologic prevalence of infection with *T. cruzi* in blood donors in Costa Rica. In *Abstracts VII Congreso Centroamericano de Microbiología y Parasitología No. 18*; 1991. p. 204.
29. Ponce C, Ponce E. Infección por Tripanosoma cruzi en donantes de sangre de diferentes hospitales de Honduras. In *8th Latin American congress of parasitology*, Guatemala, November 1987; 1987. p. 260.
30. Velasco Castrejón O, Guzmán Bracho C. Importance of Chagas disease in México. *Rev Latin Am Microbiol* 1986;**28**:275−83.
31. Schmunis GA. *Trypanosoma cruzi*, the etiologic agent of Chagas' disease: status in the blood supply in endemic and non endemic countries. *Transfusion* 1991;**31**:547−57.
32. Grant IH, Gold JW, Wittner M. Transfusion-associated acute Chagas disease acquired in the United States. *Ann Int Med* 1989;**111**:849−51.
33. Nickerson P, Orr P, Schroeder ML, et al. Transfusion-associated *Trypanosoma cruzi* infection in a non-endemic area. *Ann Int Med* 1989;**111**:851−3.
34. Segura EL, Pérez A, Yanovsky JF, et al. Decrease in the prevalence of infection by *Trypanosoma cruzi* (Chagas disease) in young men of Argentina. *Bull Pan Amer Health Org* 1985;**19**:252−64.
35. Souza AG, Wanderley DMV, Buralli, et al. Consolidation of the control of Chagas disease vectors in the State of Sao Paulo. *Mem Inst Oswald Cruz* 1984;**79**(Suppl):125−31.

36. Akhavan D. *Analysis of cost-effectiveness of the Chagas disease control programme.* Brasilia: Ministry of Health, National Health Foundation; 1997.
37. World Health Organization/TDR. *Report of the Scientific Working Group on Chagas disease.* Geneva: Buenos Aires; 2006. p. 72005.
38. MERCOSUR. Reunión de Ministros de Salud del MERCOSUR, Brasilia, Junio 1991, Resolución 04-3-CS; 1991.
39. World Health Organization. Chagas disease, elimination of transmission in Uruguay. *Weekly Epidemiological Record* 1994;**6**:38−40.
40. World Health Organization. Chagas disease, interruption of transmission in Chile. *Weekly Epidemiological Record* 1995;**3**:13−16.
41. World Health Organization. Chagas disease, progress towards elimination of transmission in Argentina. *Weekly Epidemiological Record* 1996;**2**:12−15.
42. World Health Organization. Chagas disease, interruption of transmission in Brazil. *Weekly Epidemiological Record* 1997;**72**:1−5.
43. World Health Organization. Chagas disease, interruption of transmission in Uruguay. *Weekly Epidemiological Record* 1998;**73**:1−4.
44. World Health Organization. Chagas disease, interruption of transmission in Chile. *Weekly Epidemiological Record* 1999;**2**:9−11.
45. World Health Organization. Chagas disease, certification of interruption of transmission in Chile. *Weekly Epidemiological Record* 2000;**2**:10−12.
46. World Health Organization. Chagas disease, interruption of transmission in Brazil. *Weekly Epidemiological Record* 2000;**19**:153−5.
47. Pan American Health Organization. XVI Reunión de la Comisión Intergubernamental de la Iniciativa del Cono Sur, Brasilia, Junio de 2007; 2007. www.paho.org.
48. World Health Organization. 51st World Health Assembly, Resolution WHA51.14; 1998b.
49. World Health Organization. Document EB 124/17, January 2009. Available from: www. who.int.
50. World Health Organization. Report of the Expert Committee on the control of Chagas disease. *Technical Report Series 905*, Geneva; 2002. p. 85.
51. Spillmann CA. Situación actual del programa nacional de Chagas. Avances y logros alcanzados en el marco del "Plan Nacional de Chagas 2011-2016." *Rev Arg Salud Públ, Agosto* 2012;14−15 2012.
52. Ministerio de Salud Argentina. Informe del Ministerio de Salud, Buenos Aires; 2002.
53. Pan American Health Organization. *Report of the VII Meeting of the Intergovernmental Commission of the Southern Cone Initiative.* Argentina: Buenos Aires; March 1998, OPS/HPC/HCT/98.114, Washington, DC.
54. Pan American Health Organization. *Report of the VI Meeting of the Intergovernmental Commission of the Southern Cone Initiative.* Chile: Santiago; March 1997, OPS/HPC/ HCT/98.102, Washington, DC, 33−36.
55. OPS/OMS. Informes de las Iniciativas de los Países Andinos, Bogotá, Febrero 1997 y Tegucigalpa, Octubre 1997.
56. World Health Organization. Chagas disease, progress towards interruption of transmission in Venezuela. *Weekly Epidemiological Record* 1999;**35**:289−92.
57. Aché A, Matos A. Interrupting Chagas disease transmission in Venezuela. *Rev Inst Med Tropical Sao Paulo* 2001;**43**(1):37−43.
58. Salvatella R. Control de la enfermedad de Chagas en las sub-regiones de América. *Rev Arg Salud Públ Agosto* 2012;13−14.

59. OPS/OMS. Informe de la IV Reunión de la Comisión Intergubernamental de la Iniciativa de Centro América, Ciudad de Panamá, 2001.
60. Moncayo A. Progress towards elimination of transmission of Chagas disease in Latin America. *WHO World Health Stat Quarter* 1997;**50**:195−8.
61. Moncayo A. Chagas disease: current epidemiological trends after the interruption of vectorial and transfusional transmission in the southern cone countries. *Mem Inst Oswald Cruz Rio de Janeiro* 2003;**98**(5):577−91.
62. Guhl F. Programas en la eliminación de la transmisión de la enfermedad de Chagas en Colombia. *Medicina* 2000;**22**(53):95−103.
63. Organización Panamericana de la Salud (OPS/OMS). Definición de variables y Criterios de Riesgos para la Caracterización Epidemiológica e Identificación de Áreas Prioritarias en el Control y Vigilancia de la Transmisión Vectorial de la Enfermedad de Chagas. Ed. OPS/DPC/CD/302/04; 2004.
64. Silveira AC. Enfoque de riesgo en actividades de control de triatominos. *Rev Patol Trop* 2004;**33**(2):193−206.
65. Schmunis GA. Enfermedad de Chagas en un mundo global. In: Silveira AC, editor. *La enfermedad de Chagas a la puerta de los 100 años del conocimiento de una endemia americana ancestral.* Buenos Aires: OPS (OPS/CD/426-06)/Fundación Mundo Sano; 2007. p. 251−66.
66. Schmunis GA. Epidemiology of Chagas disease in non-endemic countries: the role of international migration. *Mem Inst Oswald Cruz* 2007;**102**(Suppl. I):75−85.
67. Shikanai-Yasuda MA, Marcondes CB, Guedes AS, Siqueira GS, Barone AA, Dias JCP, et al. Possible oral transmission of acute Chagas' disease in Brazil. *Rev Inst Med Trop São Paulo* 1991;**33**:351−7.
68. Valente SAS, Valente VC, Fraiha Neto H. Transmissão da doença de Chagas: como estamos? Considerações sobre a epidemiologia e a transmissão da doença de Chagas na Amazônia Brasileira. *Rev Soc Bras Med Tropical* 1999;**32** (Suppl. 2):51−5.
69. Camandaroba ELP, Pinheiro Lima CM, Andrade SG. Oral transmission of Chagas' disease: importance of *Trypanosoma cruzi* biodeme in the intragastric experimental infection. *Rev Inst Med Trop São Paulo* 2002;**44**:97−103.
70. Rodríguez-Morales AJ. Chagas disease: an emerging food-borne entity?. *J Infect Developing Countries* 2008;**2**(2):149−50.
71. Organización Panamericana de la Salud/ Unidad Regional de Prevención y Control de Enfermedades Transmisibles (DPC/CD/CHA). *Grupo Técnico Especializado en Inocuidad de Alimentos (DPC/VP/FOS 2006). Informe de la Consulta Técnica en Epidemiología. Prevención y Manejo de la Transmisión de la Enfermedad de Chagas como Enfermedad Transmitida por Alimentos (ETA).* Rio de Janeiro: Organización Panamericana de la Salud; 2006. p. 46.
72. Coura JR, Barrett TV, Arboleda-Naranjo M. Ataque de populações humanas por triatomíneos silvestres no Amazonas: Uma nova forma de transmissão da infecção chagásica? *Rev Soc Bras Med Trop* 1994;**27**(4):251−3.
73. Silveira AC, Passos ADC. Altos índices de prevalência sorológica da infecção chagásica em área da Amazônia. In *Programa e Resumos do XXII Congresso da Sociedade Brasileira de Medicina Tropical*; 1986.
74. Shaw J, Lainson R, Frahia H. Considerações sobre a epidemiologia dos primeiros casos autóctones de doença de Chagas registrados em Belém, Pará, Brasil. *Rev Saúd Públ São Paulo* 1969;**3**:153−7.

75. Organización Panamericana de la Salud (OPS/OMS). Conclusiones y recomendaciones generales 2a. Reunión de la Iniciativa Intergubernamental de Vigilancia y Prevención de la Enfermedad de Chagas en la Amazonía (AMCHA) (Cayenne, Guayana Francesa). Available from http://www.paho.org/spanish/ad/dpc/cd/dch-amcha-2-recom.pdf; 2005.

76. Gürtler RE, Uriel Kitron U, Cecere MC, Elsa L, Segura EL, Cohen JE. Sustainable vector control and management of Chagas disease in the Gran Chaco, Argentina. *PNAS* 2007;**104**(41):6194−16199.

77. Zeledón R. A new entomological indicator useful in epidemiological studies and in control campaigns against Chagas disease. *Entomol Vect* 2003;**10**:269−76.

# Geographical distribution of Chagas disease

*F. Guhl*

Universidad de los Andes, Centro de Investigaciones en Microbiología y Parasitología Tropical, Bogotá, Colombia

## Chapter Outline

## Introduction

Just over a century ago, the Brazilian physician Carlos Chagas was the first to describe the disease that was to subsequently take his name. He went much further than recognizing the clinical aspects of the disease; he also isolated and described the etiological agent (*Trypanosoma cruzi*) and identified the insect vector, triatomine bugs (blood-feeding true bugs of the family Reduviidae).

A full understanding of the etiology and epidemiology of Chagas disease across its distribution was to prove elusive and complex, and remains under intense investigation to the present day. The difficulty in completely defining the epidemiology of Chagas disease is attributable to several factors. Firstly, Chagas disease is a zoonosis, and a variety of widely distributed mammals serve as reservoirs for *T. cruzi*.

Moreover, all mammals are susceptible to infection. A further factor that contributes to the complexity of Chagas disease as a zoonosis is the variety of vectors involved, being not simply represented by a range of related species or genera, as is the case for all other insect vectors, associated with any given disease.

American Trypanosomiasis Chagas Disease. DOI: http://dx.doi.org/10.1016/B978-0-12-801029-7.00005-8

Triatomine bugs are a subfamily of insects and across this relatively broad taxonomic range there are members from all groups that can harbor *T. cruzi*. Most transmission, however, is attributable to three main genera: *Rhodnius*, *Panstrongylus*, and *Triatoma*, but this diversity still represents two different tribes of the subfamily (Rhodniini and Triatomini). Furthermore, the insects vary in more than ancestry, having a diverse range of vertebrate host and ecological associations. The third factor that complicates Chagas disease epidemiology and accounts for variation in the clinical manifestation of the disease is the subspecific diversity of *T. cruzi* itself. Much work has been conducted over the past years to elucidate the variation of *T. cruzi* across its geographical distribution and associations with hosts and vector species.

Even the basic epidemiology was elusive at first, as it was not until the mid-1920s was it resolved that transmission occurs via contamination with feces of infected triatomine bugs rather than by the bite, as is the usual route of transmission of protozoa transmitted by insects. This key epidemiological factor limits those at risk to vectorial transmission to people living in infested houses with prolonged exposure, essentially poor rural communities. However, this factor, which in most scenarios limits transmission to rural communities, historically caused the disease to have a limited political impact and low profile and priority as a public health issue. This hurdle was difficult to overcome, and appropriate recognition was not forthcoming until scientists began to demonstrate the economic impact of the disease.

In addition to vector transmission, a small percentage of cases are attributable to unscreened blood transfusions, congenital transmission, and incidences of oral transmission by contamination of food. In the 1990s, it was estimated that greater than 80% of transmission was due to vectors and approximately 16% were due to blood transfusion.[1] Most endemic countries have since implemented approaching 100% screening of donated blood.

# Vector phylogeography and ecology

The endemic transmission of Chagas disease in humans and wild hosts is restricted to the Americas and corresponds largely with the distribution of triatomine bugs approximately from latitudes 42°N to 46°S (i.e., from the mid-United States to Patagonia).

The triatomines constitute a subfamily of an otherwise predatory group of bugs, and is relatively small compared to the thousands of predatory reduviids. The Triatominae comprises some 150 species. This diversity is classified into 6 tribes and 19 genera.

Importantly, the main factor that constrains Chagas disease to the Americas is the same reason that African trypanosomiasis is restricted to Africa—the vectors are solely endemic to their respective continents. This is certainly true for tsetse flies, but strictly speaking not entirely the case for triatomine bugs. Seven endemic species of Triatoma are reported from Southeast Asia,[2] and one genus (*Linshcosteus*) is endemic to India.

A further species, *Triatoma rubrofasciata*, has a global tropicopolitan distribution and is recorded from port areas throughout the tropics and subtropics in Africa and the Americas and from various islands in the Caribbean, Pacific, and Indian oceans. *T. rubrofasciata* is frequently found in coastal cities of Brazil, especially the city of Sao Luis, Maranhao, where it causes public concern.

Natural infection of *T. rubrofasciata* with *T. cruzi* has been reported in Brazil, although the feeding and defecation habits of this species make it a relatively inefficient vector.[3] Most reports of *T. rubrofasciata* in the Old World are old. Indeed, the oldest description of any triatomine refers to a specimen of *T. rubrofasciata* collected in the then Dutch East Indies (now Indonesia).[4]

A review about Triatominae in Asia presents comparisons using morphometry, cytogenetics, and new DNA sequences data, to clarify their relationship with each other and with the better-known American species, and the authors deduce that all Asian Triatominae have probably derived from forms originally spread during the 15th to 18th centuries on sailing ships, from the area that now forms the southern United States.[5]

There are no records of any triatomine infected with *T. cruzi* beyond the Americas. Furthermore, the recent migratory trends of human populations pose little or no threat to the establishment of transmission cycles beyond the American continent.

However, there has been a trend in recent years for immigrant-descended Latin American populations to return to their countries of ancestry. If this should ever become the case for the large ethnically Indian populations of the Guyanas to migrate back to southern India, it is possible that they could take infected *T. rubrofasciata* (or another species) back with them, and endemic Asian triatomine species could theoretically be involved in initiating sylvatic and domestic *T. cruzi* transmission cycles outside of the Americas. There are some general trends in the geographical distribution of triatomine bugs.

Fundamentally, it has been established that there is a relationship between latitude and species richness, with increasing diversity toward the equator and easterly in latitude, thus corresponding to the Amazon.

There are also some patterns in geographical distribution that can be related to the taxonomic groups. For example, *Rhodnius* species are mostly associated with the Amazon and Orinoco regions. Abad-Franch et al.[6] published a comprehensive overview of palm infestation by triatomines in the Americas using site-occupancy modeling (SOM) to examine 3590 palms sampled with nondestructive methods and standard statistics to describe and compare infestation in 2940 palms sampled by felling-and-dissection. Thirty-eight palm species (18 genera) have been reported to be infested by 39 triatomine species (10 genera) from the United States to Argentina. Palms offer suitable habitat for triatomines and for *T. cruzi* mammalian hosts. Wild triatomines often invade houses by flying from nearby palms potentially leading to new cases of human Chagas disease.

Rendón et al.[7] evaluate the population densities and relative abundance of triatomines and mammals involved in the sylvatic cycle of Chagas disease to clarify the epidemiological scenario in an endemic area in the Orinoco region in Colombia.

Insect vectors on *Attalea butyracea* palms were captured and report an infestation index of 88.5% in 148 palms and an index of *Trypanosoma cruzi* natural infection of 60.2% in 269 dissected insects and 11.9% in 160 captured mammals. No evidence of insect domiciliation was found, suggesting that eco-epidemiological factors shape the transmission dynamics of *T. cruzi*, creating diverse scenarios of disease transmission.

In general, any given species of triatomine bugs has a relatively limited distribution. This is evident in some of the taxonomic nomenclature, where a number of species are named after countries or regions. One notable exception is *Panstrongylus geniculatus*, which has the most extensive continuous distribution of any triatomine species, from the Atlantic to Pacific coasts and from mid-Central America to northern Argentina. Its region of origin is thought to be the Amazon. *P. geniculatus* has a strong association with subterranean burrowing mammals, such as armadillos. Subsequently, it has been speculated that after initial adaptation to environments of high humidity in the Amazon, association with the humid microclimate of armadillo burrows has facilitated its observed broad geographical distribution well beyond the limits of the Amazon.[8]

A few other species also have broader distributions, possibly due to their potential to exploit a broader range of habitats, or because their ecological niche is widespread. The potential to exploit and adapt to a variety of environments is one of the factors that might facilitate some species to invade domestic environments and initiate disease transmission. Certainly, three of the most important vector species, *Triatoma infestans*, *Rhodnius prolixus*, and *Triatoma dimidiata*, have distributions across several countries (Fig. 5.1).

Most of the 150 Triatominae species occupy sylvatic ecotopes in association with their respective vertebrate hosts. Examples include palm crowns, bird nests, possum lodges, rock piles, hollow trees, rodent nests, and bat caves. In most cases triatomine species are exquisitely adapted to their ecotopes with little propensity to invade human habitations. Therefore, there are only some 10−15 species of triatomines that show anthropophilic tendencies and are regularly implicated in disease transmission. Several factors can initiate the development of domestic tendencies in wild populations of triatomines, such as a successful control of one species in houses can offer an open niche for other species to invade. Another factor is habitat destruction, in particular deforestation, which can potentially drive species toward invading domestic environment. Cordovez and Guhl[9] discuss the process of domestication and highlight that when domesticated populations undergo a process of simplification through adaptation to the stable domestic environment, the resulting optimum genotypes would offer reduced fitness in sylvatic ecotopes. This has proven to be the case for *T. infestans*, which until recently had a huge distribution across Brazil and occurred in all Southern Cone countries. However, through most of its range it was solely domestic, having originally adapted to domestic environments from a relatively small sylvatic distribution in Bolivia. As a result of the Southern Cone program, it has largely been eliminated from much of its previous range (Fig. 5.3).

There have been numerous studies to assess the relationships between domestic and sylvatic populations of triatomines in attempts to address the question of

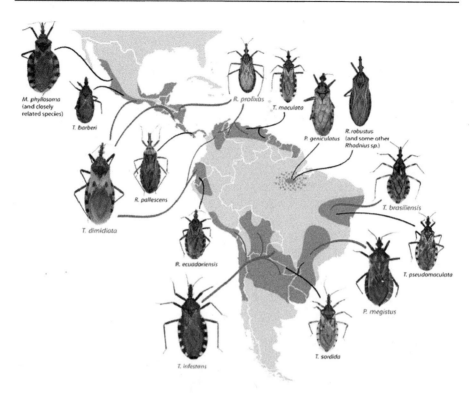

**Figure 5.1** Map of Chagas-endemic regions of Central and South America showing respective associations with the 14 most important vector species. The five most important vector species and their associated regions are indicated in red. Genera are *Triatoma*, *Rhodnius*, *Panstrongylus*, and *Meccus* (*Meccus* is synonymous with *Triatoma* in some literature).

whether there is population differentiation due to domestication. Also, other studies have been concerned with establishing the extent of gene flow across geographical areas to help plan a strategy for control.

With the eminent success of controlling predominantly domestic species, such as *T. infestans* in the Southern cone countries and *Rhodnius prolixus* in the Central American countries, there is an increasing emphasis on defining the role that invasive species play in Chagas disease transmission.[10] Careful surveillance of potential vectors ecology and distribution[11,12] are important for the identification of trends leading to the domestication or potential proximity to human habitations and activity.

A prominent example is that proximity of human settlements to sylvatic foci, palm trees in particular, poses a risk of invasion and colonization in the Andean and Amazon regions.

For example, in the case of *R. prolixus* in Venezuela and Colombia[7,9,13] and other palm-dwelling triatomines related to incidences of transmission by contamination in food production in the Amazon. Such factors need to be considered long term in the context of surveillance and control.[10]

Risk mapping using distribution records, bioclimatic data, and geographical information systems has recently been developed to aid the design of intervention.

Examples of risk mapping triatomine species' distributions include *T. dimidiata* in Mexico,[14] *R. prolixus* in Colombia[15] and Central America,[16] and *T. infestans* in the Southern Cone countries.[17] Also, detailed ecological analysis and niche characterization can be used to estimate areas at risk, according to sylvatic ecology such as for *Rhodnius ecuadoriensis*[18] and other *Rhodnius* species[19] and domestic ecology.[20,21] Finally, predictive ecological niche modeling algorithms have been applied to the Brazilian species *Rhodnius neglectus*[22] and *Triatoma brasiliensis*, and to the Triatominae of North America[23] and Mexico.[11,24] Dispersal of triatomines can be either passive or active, and there are clear examples of both in the literature. The most striking example of passive dispersal is the earlier discussed global dispersal of *T. rubrofasciata*. Another long-distance dispersal associated with human movements is the introduction of *T. dimidiata* to Ecuador from Central America (this will be addressed in more detail in a later section). Passive dispersal can also be facilitated by sylvatic vertebrate hosts; small nymphs can be carried in fur or feathers, some species have been observed to attach their eggs to feathers.[1,25] Active dispersal by flight is observed to be seasonal for some species, brought on by hot dry weather.

Other related factors that may trigger dispersal are high densities,[1] and for several triatomine species it has been observed that starvation is the main factor that initiates dispersal by flight.[26,27]

## Parasite phylogeography and ecology

*T. cruzi* is genetically diverse and is classified into a series of strains or subtypes. This genetic diversity was initially discovered using a panel of isoenzyme markers to investigate differences between parasites involved in the domestic and sylvatic cycles in Bahia state of Brazil.[28,29] This study was a breakthrough, revealing that in Bahia there were substantial genetic differences between the parasites in sympatric sylvatic and domestic transmission cycles. These described variants were designated zymodemes I and II (ZI and ZII). It was soon after revealed that the widespread strain associated with the sylvatic cycle in Brazil (ZI) was the predominant cause of human disease in Venezuela.[29] These groundbreaking findings opened the door to investigating the etiology of Chagas disease, allowing host—vector—parasite associations and comparative geographical distributions to be explored, as reviewed by Miles et al.[30] In the following two decades, various authors proceeded to characterize strains, applying other molecular methods as they became available. As a result, further diversity within the original zymodemes was discovered. However, designations of subtypes in the literature started to become confusing. To standardize the nomenclature, it was decided by the scientific community to formally recognize two main groups that corresponded with the original zymodemes; these were called TcI and TcII.[31] Most recently, the scientific community has redesignated the six genotypes as TcI to VI discrete typing units (DTUs).[32]

The ordering of the current nomenclature better indicates the perceived phylogenetic relationships between the strains: TcI and TcII are the most anciently divergent.[33] TcIII and TcIV show similarities. Some argue that they represent the result of ancient hybridization events between TcI and TcII,[34] alternatively they could represent a separate lineage.[35] Finally, TcV and TcIV are generally accepted to be hybrids derived from parental stocks of TcII and TcIII.[33] TcI has remained a constant grouping in the nomenclature since first described.

However, in recent years at least four subgroupings within TcI have been identified,[36–38] with further characterization with microsatellite markers.[39] Both sequence variation[37] and microsatellite markers demonstrate that genotypes/haplotypes involved in human infections in Venezuela and Colombia are distinct from sympatric sylvatic variants. This is intriguing as it was recently demonstrated that the main vector in the region, *R. prolixus*, demonstrates panmixia between domestic and sylvatic environments across the western endemic region in Venezuela.[40]

# Epidemiological implications of parasite distributions

*T. cruzi* presents great genetic diversity and is classified by consensus into six DTUs named TcI to TcVI.[32] The relevance of *T. cruzi* genetic diversity in Chagas disease should be examined further but existing evidence supports the importance of this diversity in terms of epidemiology and its association with clinical presentation and outcomes.

Different DTUs are associated with different biological cycles of transmission and seem to have varying geographical distributions.[41] TcI, the most frequent and widely distributed DTU, has been found from the South of the United States to the North of Chile and Argentina, and can be transmitted both in sylvatic and domestic cycles. TcIII and TcIV have been more frequently associated with sylvatic cycles, and have been implicated as a cause of acute outbreaks in the Amazon basin.[42,43] TcIII has also been found in armadillos,[44] although it has been identified from domestic dogs as well,[45] and associated to the terrestrial niche even in the Chaco region.[46,47] While TcIV seemed to have an arboreal ecotope[45] and is the second most frequent DTU detected in Venezuela.[48] TcII, TcV, and TcVI have been more often associated with domestic cycles in the Southern Cone countries. Some authors have identified a differential tissue tropism among these DTUs and linked some of them to specific clinical presentations. For instance, TcI has been associated with cardiac disease in Colombia, Argentina, Venezuela, and Brazil[49,50]; TcII, TcV, and TcVI can cause both cardiac and digestive disease, even causing megasyndromes. In addition, *T. cruzi*'s genetic diversity seems to confer different drug susceptibility both in vitro,[51,52] although this does not seem to influence the clinical outcome,[53] and in vivo[54] (Fig. 5.2).

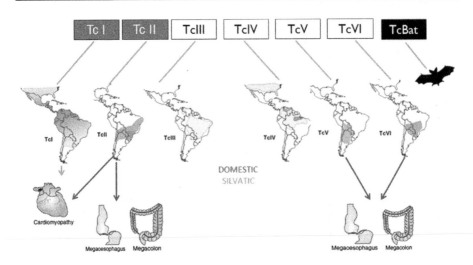

**Figure 5.2** Geographical distributions of *Trypanosoma cruzi* discrete typing units (DTUs) and its association with the domestic and silvatic cycles and human pathogenesis.

# Vector—parasite—host interactions and implications for Chagas disease distribution

There have been relatively few in-depth investigations to test coevolutionary relationships between triatomines, *T. cruzi*, and vertebrate hosts. There is a close association among TcI, *Rhodnius* species (and other arboreal triatomines), and arboreal marsupials, in particular *Didelphis marsupialis*. There is also a close association between TcII—TcVI Triatoma (and other terrestrial triatomines) and armadillo species, particularly *Dasypus*.[55]

However, the associations are not absolute, and in the case of TcI, there was no apparent clustering of particular TcI genotypes with *Didelphis* in comparison to isolates from other arboreal mammals.[39] Also for phylogeographical analyses of TcIII, the results indicate that isolates cluster according to geography rather than host association. Two interesting studies of host response to different strains have confirmed, by comparative artificial infection, that in the southern United States two species of opossum (*Monodelphis domestica* and *Didelphis virginiana*) seem to be resistant to TcIV.[56,57] This highlights a mechanism for the association of a vertebrate host with one strain over others. The strong association between TcI and *Rhodnius* species can also be explained by a similar mechanism: comparative artificial infection studies of *R. prolixus* with various strains revealed a tendency for it to be resistant to infection by TcII.[58] For triatomines, susceptibility or resistance to trypanosome infections seems to be modulated by the intestinal symbionts, which are vital for development. *T. cruzi* is considered to be subpathogenic to triatomines, whereas *Trypanosoma rangeli* is another species that commonly infects *Rhodnius* species and causes pathogenicity based on a reduction of the number of symbionts.[59]

A study of four *Rhodnius* species artificially infected with different strains of *T. rangeli* showed a measurable difference in response and indicated adaptation of trypanosome strains to the local vector species.[33] At least half of all species of triatomine bugs have been found naturally infected with *T. cruzi*.[60] Unfortunately the vast majority of these records do not include specific genotype associations. Clearly this is an area of potential research.

In the context of dispersal triggered by starvation, there is evidence that starvation decreases *T. cruzi* infection in triatomines[61] and in some species starvation may clear infection altogether.[62,63] This factor could go toward explaining paradigms such as in Venezuela where sylvatic and domestic bugs seem to be in panmixia but TcI shows discrete general clustering of sylvatic and domestic cycles.

Triatomine bugs directly determine the etiology of the strains of *T. cruzi* involved in human transmission cycles. This is clear because despite TcI and *Didelphis* being widespread, it is the northern distribution of *Rhodnius* that corresponds with occurrence in human cycles. Overall, the aspects of epidemiological relevance are the associations between terrestrial ecology, *T. infestans*, terrestrial mammals, and *T. cruzi* genotypes.

TcII–TcIV have lead to the prominence of TcII, TcV, and TcIV in human infections in the southern region of South America. In the northern regions human infections stem from TcI associated with arboreal *Rhodnius* and arboreal mammals.

Jansen et al.[64] report the results generated from over 20 years of studies of the *T. cruzi* sylvatic transmission cycle. Using serological and parasitological tests they examined *T. cruzi* infection in 7285 mammalian specimens from nine mammalian orders dispersed all over the Brazilian biomes. The obtained *T. cruzi* isolates were characterized by mini-exon gene sequence polymorphism and PCR RFLP to identify DTUs. *Didelphis* spp. are able to maintain high and long-lasting parasitemias (positive hemocultures) caused by TcI but maintain and rapidly control parasitemias caused by TcII to almost undetectable levels. In contrast, the tamarin species *Leontopithecus rosalia* and *L. chrysomelas* maintain long-lasting and high parasitemias caused by TcII similarly to *Philander sp.* The coati *Nasua nasua* maintains high parasitemias by both parental *T. cruzi* DTUs TcI or TcII and by TcII/TcIV at detectable levels. TcI predominates throughout (58% of the *T. cruzi* isolates); however, in spite of being significantly less frequent (17%) TcII is also widely distributed. Concomitant DTU infection occurred in 16% of infected mammals of all biomes and included arboreal and terrestrial species as well as bats. Taking together the published results, the authors demonstrate the complexity of the *T. cruzi* reservoir system and its transmission strategies, indicating that there is considerably more to be learned regarding ecology of *T. cruzi*.

# Assessment of regions affected by Chagas disease

In the last 10 years, due to the successful interruption of the vectorial and transfusional transmission of infection by *T. cruzi*, its incidence has been dramatically reduced in the entire American continent and the raising of awareness of Chagas disease has globalized due to migration to nonendemic countries. Fig. 5.3 shows the approximate distribution of the main active triatomine domiciliated foci that still requires control actions.

According to WHO,[65] the estimates based on 2010 data, 5,742,167 people were infected with *T. cruzi* in 21 Latin American countries, of which 62.4% (3,581,423 people) were from countries of the Southern Cone Initiative. Argentina, Brazil, and Mexico were the three countries with the highest estimated number of infected people (1,505,235, 1,156,821, and 876,458, respectively), followed by Bolivia (607,186). In the Andean Region, which accounts for 958,453 infected people, 45.7% of these (437,960) were from Colombia. Countries with 100,000−200,000 infected people included 2 in the Southern Cone subregion (Chile and Paraguay), 3 in the Andean subregion (Bolivarian Republic of Venezuela, Ecuador, and Peru), and 1 in Central America (Guatemala).

Of new cases due to vectorial transmission, Bolivia had the highest estimated number (8087), followed by Mexico (6135) and Colombia (5274). Between 850 and 2055 new cases were found in 7 countries: Peru (2055), Ecuador (2042), Guatemala (1275), Argentina (1078), El Salvador (972), Honduras (933), and Venezuela (873).

Bolivia accounted for 92.6% of all new cases in the Southern Cone Subregion, and Argentina and Bolivia together accounted for 30.62% of the new cases in Latin America. The Andean subregion, comprising Colombia, Ecuador, Peru, and Venezuela, accounted for 34.23% of the new cases in that Region. Guatemala, El Salvador, and Honduras accounted for 84.62% of the new cases in the seven Central American countries.

In the United States, Chagas disease exists almost exclusively as a zoonosis; only six autochthonous cases have been reported in humans, and the two most recent[66] were both attributable to *Triatoma sanguisuga. T. sanguisuga* has a broad distribution across the south from Texas to Maryland. *T. gerstaekeri* also shows anthropophilic tendencies and is found in Texas and New Mexico.[67]

The southern states of the United States have an active sylvatic transmission cycle involving numerous wild animal reservoirs. Recent serological surveys suggest that raccoons and possums are the main hosts[68] with prevalences as high as 68%. Different *T. cruzi* strains have been associated with these two main hosts[57]: TcI and TcIV with raccoons and TcI with possums. A recent report[69] shows 61% of *Triatoma rubida* collected in Texas infected with TcI. In another study conducted in Arizona,[70] 41.5% of the 164 triatomine insects were infected with *T. cruzi* (no DTU was reported). In the United States, based on population figures from countries where Chagas disease is endemic, it is estimated that in 2011 there were about 300,000 people infected with *T. cruzi*.[71]

In nonendemic countries, migration flows have been the key for the emergence of Chagas disease in areas where it was not previously reported. The importance of Chagas disease in this new scenario is directly related to the volume of migration flows received by each host country and also related to the specific origin of migrants received, since the distribution of Chagas disease is not homogeneous within endemic countries.[72] It is estimated that in Europe there are between 68,000 and 123,000 infected people with *T. cruzi*, most of them living in Spain.

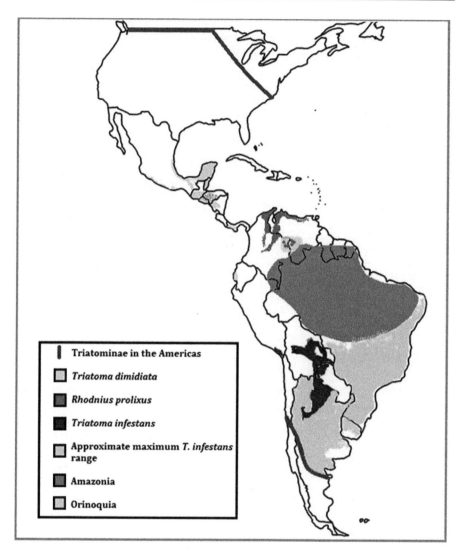

**Figure 5.3** Approximate distribution of the main insect vectors associated with the human habitat that still require control activities in the Americas.

Spain has by far the most Latin American immigrants in Europe, with annual numbers increasing dramatically almost fivefold over the past decade from 446,000 in 2001 to more than 2 million in 2008.[73] Another estimate for 2008 is slightly lower, stating that Spain has approximately 1.7 million Latin American immigrants. Of these, an estimated 5.2% were potentially infected with *T. cruzi*, approximately 17,000 of whom may be expected to eventually present with Chagas disease.[74] The same study suggested that there may have been as many as 92 congenital infections of newborns in Spain in 2007. A survey of recent literature[72] reveals that numerous cases have been reported from the immigrant population, mostly by congenital (vertical) transmission and by contaminated blood transfusion.

A case study[75] assessed the prevalence of Chagas disease in Bolivian pregnant women in a Spanish hospital for 2 years and found a 17.7% rate (71/401), with a 1.4% vertical transmission rate (1/71). Screening for *T. cruzi* has been implemented in Spain since 2005.

The survey of literature by Castro et al.[76] reveals that Chagas disease has been reported from immigrants in Denmark, Germany, Italy, Netherlands, and Switzerland, and congenital cases have been documented in Romania and France.

Estimates as of 2008 state that Italy has 230,000 Latin American immigrants from Chagas disease endemic countries, while Portugal has 121,001 and Switzerland has 57,000 such immigrants.[73] The estimated number of Latin Americans living in France has risen from 27,400 in 1999 to 105,000 in 2005.[77] The varying estimates and recent increases in immigration trends to Europe in general highlight the need for European Union-centered assessment of Chagas disease for the region, including comprehensive efforts to halt transfusional and congenital transmission. The number of people infected by *T. cruzi* ranges from 140 (Austria) to over 12,000 (England).

## Oceania and Asia

Australia has an estimated 80,579 Latin American immigrants with an estimated 1392 cases of *T. cruzi* infection. Japan accommodates some 371,700 people from Chagas-endemic regions, 84% of whom are from Brazil with an estimated 3592 *T. cruzi*-infected residents.[77] These immigrants represent the descendants of people that migrated to Brazil in the early 20th century to work on coffee plantations. The 1980s saw a reversal of this migration back to Japan. In Brazil, these immigrant Japanese were called dekasseguis, and now more than 300,000 dekasseguis Brazilians live in Japan.[76] Several cases of Chagas cardiomyopathy have been reported in Brazilian immigrants in Japan[78,79] (Fig. 5.4).

From a recent update of the epidemiological information on Chagas disease from the 21 Latin American countries,[65] based on the available 2010 demographic and epidemiologic information, with the direct participation of their governmental, academic, and scientific institutions, for each country, the following demographic and epidemiologic data were compiled:

(1) Population by country; (2) Annual number of births by country; (3) Estimated number of people infected with *T. cruzi*; (4) Estimated annual number of new cases of *T. cruzi* infection due to vectorial transmission; (5) Estimated number of women aged 15−44 years with *T. cruzi* infection; (6) Estimated annual number of cases of *T. cruzi* infection due to congenital transmission; (7) Estimated prevalence of *T. cruzi* infection per 100 habitants; (8) Estimated incidence due to vectorial transmission per 100 habitants; (9) Estimated incidence of *T. cruzi* infection due to congenital transmission per 100 live births; (10) Estimated population at

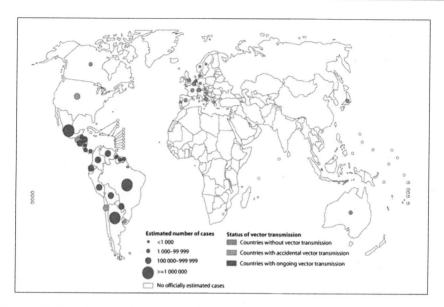

**Figure 5.4** Global distribution of cases of Chagas disease based on official estimates and status of vector transmission.
*Source*: WHO/DCO/WHD/2014.1.

risk of *T. cruzi* infection due to the existence of domicile infestation or active transmission of infection in the country; (11) Estimated number of people with Chagasic cardiopathy; (12) Estimated prevalence of *T. cruzi* infection among blood donors (Table 5.1).

# Chagas disease in Mexico and Central America

*R. prolixus* appears to be exclusively associated with domestic environments in Central America and is thought to have been introduced from domestic South American populations, as has been demonstrated through morphometric and genetic comparisons of samples from Honduras and Colombia.[80] The other two main species implicated in transmission in Central American countries are *T. dimidiata* and *R. pallescens*. *T. dimidiata* is endemic to the region and the most widespread vector species; it regularly invades domestic and peridomestic ecotypes from a variety of natural habitats including rock piles, palms, and caves.

It has been linked to rural and recently to urban transmission in Merida City, Yucatan, Mexico.[81] *R. pallescens* occurs in Panama, where it is associated with Attelea palm trees and domestic infestations; recent reports demonstrate that TcI circulates in both domestic and sylvatic *R. pallescens*.[82,83] Mexico has some 30 vector species (including *T. dimidiata*), with 8 that pose a risk to transmission.[11] They are members of the *Triatoma* (*Meccus*) phyllosoma complex and *Triatoma barberi* (Fig. 5.2).

# Table 5.1 Estimated demographic and epidemiological parameters of Chagas disease in Latin America by country

| Latin American countries | Population | Estimated no. of people infected by *T. cruzi* | Estimated annual no. of new cases due to vectorial transmission | Estimated no. of women aged 15–44 years with *T. cruzi* infection | Estimated annual no. of cases of *T. cruzi* infection due to congenital transmission | Estimated prevalence of *T. cruzi* infection per 100 habitants | Estimated incidence due to vectorial transmission per 100 habitants | Estimated incidence of *T. cruzi* infection due to congenital transmission per 100 live births | Estimated population at risk of *T. cruzi* infection | Estimated no. of people with Chagasic cardiopathy | Estimated prevalence of *T. cruzi* infection among blood donors |
|---|---|---|---|---|---|---|---|---|---|---|---|
| Argentina | 41,343,000 | 1,505,235 | 1078 | 211,102 | 1457 | 3.640 | 0.0020 | 0.210 | 2,242,528 | 376,309 | 3.130 |
| Belize | 315,000 | 1040 | 10 | 272 | 25 | 0.330 | 0.0030 | 0.333 | 70,252 | 200 | N/A |
| Bolivia | 9,947,000 | 607,186 | 8087 | 199,351 | 616 | 6.104 | 0.0810 | 0.235 | 586,434 | 121,437 | 2.320 |
| Brazil | 190,755,799 | 1,156,821 | 46 | 119,298 | 571 | 0.03 | 0.084 per 1000–0.084 | 0.020 | 25,474,365 | 231,364 | 0.180 |
| Chile | 17,095,000 | 119,660 | 0 | 11,771 | 115 | 0.699 | 0 | 0.046 | 0 | 35,898 | 0.160 |
| Colombia | 45,805,000 | 437,960 | 5274 | 116,221 | 1046 | 0.956 | 0.0110 | 0.114 | 4,813,543 | 131,388 | 0.410 |
| Costa Rica | 4,516,000 | 7667 | 10 | 1728 | 61 | 0.169 | 0.0002 | 0.080 | 233,333 | 2300 | 0.045 |
| Ecuador | 14,483,499 | 199,872 | 2042 | 62,898 | 696 | 1.379 | 0.0140 | 0.317 | 4,199,793 | 40,384 | 0.190 |
| El Salvador | 6,952,000 | 90,222 | 972 | 18,211 | 234 | 1.297 | 0.0130 | 0.187 | 1,019,000 | 18,044 | 1.610 |
| Guatemala | 13,550,000 | 166,667 | 1275 | 32,759 | 164 | 1.230 | 0.0090 | 0.035 | 1,400,000 | 20,833 | 1.340 |
| French Guyana & Surinam | 1,501,962 | 12,600 | 280 | 3818 | 18 | 0.838 | 0.0180 | 0.075 | 377,258 | 882 | N/A |
| Honduras | 7,989,000 | 73,333 | 933 | 16,149 | 257 | 0.917 | 0.0110 | 0.126 | 1,171,133 | 14,667 | 1.650 |
| Mexico | 112,468,855 | 876,458 | 6135 | 185,600 | 1788 | 0.779 | 0.0050 | 0.089 | 23,474,780 | 70,117 | 0.390 |
| Nicaragua | 5,604,000 | 29,300 | 383 | 5822 | 138 | 0.522 | 0.0060 | 0.124 | 642,750 | 5990 | 0.220 |
| Panama | 3,557,687 | 18,337 | 175 | 6332 | 40 | 0.515 | 0.0040 | 0.056 | 466,667 | 3667 | 0.500 |
| Paraguay | 8,668,000 | 184,669 | 297 | 63,385 | 525 | 2.130 | 0.0030 | 0.340 | 1,703,659 | 32,974 | 2.550 |
| Peru | 28,948,000 | 127,282 | 2055 | 28,132 | 232 | 0.439 | 0.0070 | 0.038 | 1,290,415 | 25,456 | 0.620 |
| Uruguay | 3,301,000 | 7852 | 0 | 1858 | 20 | 0.237 | 0 | 0.040 | 0 | 615 | 0.230 |
| Venezuela (Bolivarian Republic of) | 27,223,000 | 193,339 | 873 | 40,223 | 665 | 0.710 | 0.0030 | 0.110 | 1,033,450 | 38,668 | 0.320 |
| Total | 543,877,115 | 5,742,167 | 29,925 | 1,124,930 | 8668 | 1.055 | 0.0050 | 0.089 | 70,199,360 | 1,171,193 | 0.930 |

As in northern South America, TcI predominates in Central America and Mexico in both sylvatic and domestic cycles. However, recent reports from Guatemala found domestic *T. dimidiata* harboring TcI and TcII concurrently.[84] This surprising finding highlights a need for further molecular epidemiological studies in the region.

The Central American countries initiative (Belize, Costa Rica, El Salvador, Guatemala, Honduras, Panamá) was inaugurated in 1996. This program, like the Central American countries, has more complications than the Southern Cone initiative because there are more vector species other than *Rhodnius prolixus* involved that maintain peridomestic habitats and pose the threat of reinvasion post control, such as *Triatoma dimidiata*.

## Chagas disease in the Amazon region

The Amazon region is vast, extending across much of northwestern Brazil, the Guyanas, northern Bolivia, eastern Peru and Ecuador, and southern Colombia and Venezuela. The region has a high number of sylvatic triatomine species.[8,85] However, only the following seven (mostly *Rhodnius* species) have been implicated in disease transmission: *R. prolixus*, *R. pictipes*, *R. robustus*, *R. stali*, *P. geniculatus*, *P. herreri*, and *T. maculata*. There are also a plethora of reservoir hosts (e.g., marsupials, bats, rodents, edentates, carnivores, and primates). In the Amazon, the observed tendency is that infestation by triatomine species is occasional and sporadic. Most Amazon species seem to be constrained from readily exploiting domestic environments by preadaptation to humid environments.

Human activities that negatively impact the natural ecology of triatomines species, such as deforestation, are likely to drive adaptation to the domestic environment.[85]

There is a diverse range of *T. cruzi* strains reported from the Amazon from TcI to TcV. Predominantly TcI and TcIII circulate,[55] and both have been associated with human infections along with TcIV.[42,47] There are many reports of acute cases of disease in humans,[86] but chronic forms of the disease are considered to be relatively rare in the region.[87] As described by Miles et al.,[30,87] currently the main type of transmission cycle in the Amazon region is enzootic (i.e., no/few domestic colonies of triatomines exist), but infrequent, sporadic cases of Chagas disease may occur due to bugs sporadically flying into houses and infecting people or contaminating food. There are numerous reports of small epidemics in the Brazilian Amazon, mainly attributed to oral transmission.[29,87−91]

Often oral contamination involves palm-dwelling species (most likely *Rhodnius* species) that are accidentally collected along with palm fruits, such as acai, and subsequently pressed to make juice. The most recent outbreaks was reported by de Noya and Gonzalez.[91] Another paradigm is communities are frequently attacked by *R. brethesi* when venturing into the forest along the Rio Negro (Brazil, Colombia, and Venezuela) to harvest piassaba palm fibers.[86] There are also reports of foci of transmission associated with vector infestation, such as *P. geniculatus* in the Amazon basin, *R. stali* in Bolivia, and *P. herreri* in Peru. An initiative for Chagas disease surveillance and prevention in the Amazon (AMCHA) was officially launched with the backing of Pan American Health Organization (PAHO) in 2004.[92]

## Chagas disease in the Andean region

The main vector in the Andean region is *R. prolixus*, principally in Venezuela and Colombia where it is mainly associated with the foothills of the Andes and adjacent plains (Llanos). *R. prolixus* is a close relative of the Amazon species *R. robustus*,[93,94] and it seems probable that *R. prolixus* represents a lineage that adapted to exploit drier environments north of the Amazon, thereby predisposing it to be an efficient invader of domestic environments. However, unlike *T. infestans*, *R. prolixus* has widespread sylvatic foci that pose the threat of reinvasion of houses postintervention; this was demonstrated by a population genetics study comparing domestic and sylvatic samples in Venezuela[40] and by the identification of palm trees as a risk factor to domestic infestations.[13] However, previous studies have suggested that the risk of invasion by sylvatic *R. prolixus* is unlikely.[7,95] *T. dimidiata* is implicated in transmission in Colombia and Ecuador. However, there is strong evidence to suggest that *T. dimidiata* in Ecuador was introduced from mid-Central America in association with human migration patterns.[96,97] Therefore, it may represent a more domiciliated population with fewer sylvatic refuges and better prospects for control.

*R. ecuadoriensis* is an important vector implicated in transmission in Ecuador and northern Peru.[18,98] Like *R. prolixus*, it maintains sylvatic populations in palm trees that pose the risk of reinvasion after the control of domestic populations.[19] The Andean initiative (Colombia, Ecuador, Peru, and Venezuela) was inaugurated in 1997. This program, like the Central American countries, has more complications than the Southern Cone initiative because there are more vector species involved which maintain sylvatic habitats and pose the threat of reinvasion post control.[94]

## Chagas disease in the Southern Cone countries

Historically the main vector for the region was *T. infestans*. However, with the eminent success of the Southern Cone program, having effectively eliminated *T. infestans* from Brazil, Chile, and Uruguay, and many parts of Argentina, it has been demonstrated that the center of radiation for the species is in Bolivia,[99] where it most likely continues to cause a problem due to ready reinvasion from sylvatic foci. Domestic infestations continue to persist in the Chaco region where sylvatic foci of *T. infestans* are present. Several other species are implicated as secondary vectors, particularly since the control of *T. infestans*, and the presentation of the niche to other species. In northeastern Brazil, *T. brasiliensis* and *T. psuedomaculata* show strong tendencies to colonize domestic habitats along with *Panstrongylus megistus* in southern Brazil. Other species that have shown some potential to domiciliation are *R. neglectus*, *T. vitticeps*, and *T. rubrovaria* in Brazil. *Triatoma sordida* is an important secondary vector in Paraguay, Bolivia, northern Argentina, and southern Brazil. *T. sordida* and a related species, *T. guasayana*, demonstrate mass dispersal during the dry season, which can result in the invasion of domestic environments.[100]

*T. cruzi* subtypes TcII and TcVI predominate in both sylvatic and domestic cycles in this region. Interestingly TcI is also present in many arboreal hosts, such as *Didelphis* species. The absence of *Rhodnius* species in the southern part of this region and the lack of data for other triatomines carrying TcI present the possibility that transmission of TcI, in *Didelphis* at least, commonly occurs without vectors by direct contamination from the anal scent glands.[101] However, *P. megistus* has been implicated with TcI transmission in southern central Brazil,[102] as has as a species of *Rhodnius*, *R. neglectus*,[103] which has a distribution extending from the Amazon to southern Brazil. Also, *Triatoma (Mepraia) spinolai* in Chile has been reported to be infected with TcI.[104] Other vector species may yet to be implicated in TcI transmission because it is often difficult to sample from sylvatic habitats directly. Table 5.2 summarizes the actions and strategies to be taken for controlling triatomine species in the different initiatives in the Americas.

**Table 5.2 Action to be taken for controlling autoctonous or introduced triatomine species in different control initiatives in the Americas[a]**

| Region | Perspectives |
| --- | --- |
| Southern countries and Southern Perú | Introduced triatomine species present a high degree of domiciliation (i.e., *Triatoma infestans*) and are vulnerable to latest generation insecticide action and can thus be eliminated, as has been demonstrated in Brazil, Chile and Uruguay. It is totally feasible that the other countries involved in the Southern Cone and Southern initiative can achieve this goal in the short- and medium-term. Autochthonous species (such as *Triatoma brasiliensis*, *Panstrongylus megistus*, and *Triatoma sordida*) require an ongoing entomological surveillance given that they can adapt to human habitat |
| Andean and Central-American countries' initiatives | Introduced triatomine species presenting a high degree of domiciliation (such as *Rhodnius prolixus*) in extensive areas of Colombia, Venezuela, and in most Central America countries (except for El Salvador and Panamá), the same as *Rhodnius ecuadoriensis* in Ecuador and Northern Peru, are vulnerable to insecticide action and can thus be eliminated as has been demonstrate with *R. prolixus* in some regions of Guatemala and Venezuela. Peridomiciliated species |

*(Continued)*

**Table 5.2 (Continued)**

| Region | Perspectives |
| --- | --- |
|  | (such as *Triatoma dimidiata*) require the physical management of human habitations and the peridomiciliary environment, as well as sustained entomological surveillance programmes. Some species from sylvatic habitats represent a challenge for future control action, as in the case of silvatic *R. prolixus* populations in Venezuela and Colombia |
| Amazonian countries' initiatives | The Amazonian initiative for vectorial control of Chagas' disease is formed by nine South American countries, representing an important challenge in terms of entomological surveillance and merits special attention in the immediate future. Different *Rhodnius* and *Panstrongylus* species present in the Amazon Region must be considered to be epidemiologically important potential vectors |
| All continental initiatives | It must be born in mind that, in spite of the achievements made in different regional initiatives, Chagas disease persist in Latin America given that it represents a silvatic enzooty and anthropozoonosis and therefore requires long-term surveillance and control action |

# References

1. Schofield CJ. *Triatominae—biology & control*. Bognor Regis, West Sussex: Eurocommunica Publications; 1994.
2. Ryckman RE, Archbold EF. The Triatominae and Triatominae borne trypanosomes of Asia, Africa, Australia and the East Indies. *Bull Soc Vector Ecol* 1981;**6**:43−166.
3. Braga MV, Lima MM. Feeding and defecation patterns of nymphs of *Triatoma rubrofasciata* (De Geer, 1773) (Hemiptera: Reduviidae), and its potential role as vector for *Trypanosoma cruzi*. *Mem Inst Oswaldo Cruz* 1999;**94**:127−9.
4. DeGeer C. *Mémoires pour servir a l'histoire des Insectes*, vol. 3. Stockholm: Pierrer Hesselberg; 1773. p. 696.
5. Dujardin JP, PhamThi K, Truong Xuan L, Panzera F, Pita S, Schofield CJ. Epidemiological status of kissing-bugs in South East Asia: a preliminary assesment. *Acta Trop* 2015;**151**:142−9.
6. Abad-Franch F, Lima MM, Sarquis O, Gurgel-Goncalves R, Sánchez-Martin M, et al. *Acta Trop* 2015;**151**; 126−14.
7. Rendón L, Guhl F, Cordovez JM, Erazo D. New scenarios of *Trypanosoma cruzi* transmission in the Orinoco región of Colombia. *Mem Inst Oswaldo Cruz* 2015;**110**(3):283−8.
8. Abad-Franch F, Monteiro FA. Biogeography and evolution of Amazonian triatomines (Heteroptera: Reduviidae): implications for Chagas disease surveillance in humid forest ecoregions. *Mem Inst Oswaldo Cruz* 2007;**102**:57−69.

9. Cordovez JM, Guhl F. The impact of landscape transformation on the reinfestation rates of *Rhodnius prolixus* in the Orinoco Region, Colombia. *Acta Trop* 2015;**151**:73−9.

10. Guhl F, Pinto N, Aguilera G. Sylvatic triatominae: a new challenge in vector control transmission. *Mem Inst Oswaldo Cruz* 2009;**104**(Suppl.1):71−5.

11. Cruz-Reyes A, Pickering-Lopez JM. Chagas disease in Mexico: an analysis of geographical distribution during the past 76 years—a review. *Mem Inst Oswaldo Cruz* 2006;**101**:345−54.

12. Guhl F, Aguilera G, Pinto N, Vergara D. Updated geographical distribution and ecoepidemiology of the triatomine fauna (Reduviidae: Triatominae) in Colombia. *Biomedica* 2007;**27**(Suppl. 1):143−62.

13. Sanchez-Martin MJ, Feliciangeli MD, Campbell-Lendrum D, Davies CR. Could the Chagas disease elimination programme in Venezuela be compromised by reinvasion of houses by sylvatic *Rhodnius prolixus* bug populations?. *Trop Med Int Health* 2006;**11**:1585−93.

14. Dumonteil E, Gourbiere S. Predicting *Triatoma dimidiata* abundance and infection rate: a risk map for natural transmission of Chagas disease in the Yucatan Peninsula of Mexico. *Am J Trop Med Hyg* 2004;**70**:514−19.

15. Guhl F, Restrepo M, Angulo VM, Antunes CMF, Campbell-Lendrum D, Davies C. Lessons from a national survey of Chagas disease transmission in Colombia. *Trends Parasitol* 2005. Available from: http://dx.doi.org/10.1016/j.pt.2005.04.11.

16. Arboleda S, Gorla DE, Porcasi X, Saldana A, Calzada J, Jaramillo ON. Development of a geographical distribution model of *Rhodnius pallescens* Barber, 1932 using environmental data recorded by remote sensing. *Infect Genet Evol* 2009;**9**:441−8.

17. Gorla D. Variables ambientales registradas por sensores remotos como indicadores de la distribución geográfica de *Triatoma infestans* (Heteroptera: Reduviidae). *Ecol Aust* 2002;**12**:117−27.

18. Abad-Franch F, Aguilar HM, Paucar A, Lorosa ES, Noireau F. Observations on the domestic ecology of *Rhodnius ecuadoriensis* (Triatominae). *Mem Inst Oswaldo Cruz* 2002;**97**:199−202.

19. Abad-Franch F, Palomeque FS, Aguilar HMT, Miles MA. Field ecology of sylvatic Rhodnius populations (Heteroptera, Triatominae): risk factors for palm tree infestation in western Ecuador. *Trop Med Int Health* 2005;**10**:1258−66.

20. Cohen JE, Gurtler RE. Modeling household transmission of American trypanosomiasis. *Science* 2001;**293**:694−8.

21. Campbell-Lendrum DH, Angulo VM, Esteban L, Tarazona Z, Parra GJ, Restrepo M, et al. House-level risk factors for triatomine infestation in Colombia. *Int J Epidemiol* 2007;**36**:866−72.

22. Gurgel-Goncalves R, Cuba CA. Predicting the potential geographical distribution of *Rhodnius neglectus* (Hemiptera, Reduviidae) based on ecological niche modeling. *J Med Entomol* 2009;**46**:952−60.

23. Ibarra-Cerdena CN, Sanchez-Cordero V, Townsend Peterson A, Ramsey JM. Ecology of North American Triatominae. *Acta Trop* 2009;**110**:178−86.

24. Sandoval-Ruiz CA, Zumaquero-Rios JL, Rojas-Soto OR. Predicting geographic and ecological distributions of triatomine species in the southern Mexican state of Puebla using ecological niche modeling. *J Med Entomol* 2008;**45**:540−6.

25. Forattini OP, Ferreira OA, Da Rocha e Silva EO, Rabello EX, dos Santos JL. Ecological aspects of American trypanosomiasis. II. Distribution and local dispersion of triatominae in natural and artificial ecotopes. *Rev Saude Publ* 1971;**5**:163−92.

26. Ekkens DB. Nocturnal flights of Triatoma (Hemiptera: Reduviidae) in Sabino Canyon, Arizona. *J Med Entomol* 1981;**18**:211−27.

27. Lehane MJ, Schofield CJ. Field experiments of dispersive flight by *Triatoma infestans*. *Trans R Soc Trop Med Hyg* 1981;**75**:399−400.

28. Miles MA, Toye PJ, Oswald SC, Godfrey DG. The identification by isoenzyme patterns of two distinct strain-groups of *Trypanosoma cruzi*, circulating independently in a rural area of Brazil. *Trans R Soc Trop Med Hyg* 1977;**71**:217−25.

29. Miles MA, Souza A, Povoa M, Shaw JJ, Lainson R, Toye PJ. Isozymic heterogeneity of *Trypanosoma cruzi* in the first autochthonous patients with Chagas' disease in Amazonian Brazil. *Nature* 1978;**272**:819−21.

30. Miles MA, Llewellyn MS, Lewis MD, Yeo M, Baleela R, Fitzpatrick S, et al. The molecular epidemiology and phylogeography of *Trypanosoma cruzi* and parallel research on Leishmania: looking back and to the future. *Parasitology* 2009;**136**:1509−28.

31. Anon. Recommendations from a satellite meeting. *Mem Inst Oswaldo Cruz* 1999;**94**:429−32.

32. Zingales B, Andrade SG, Briones MR, Campbell DA, Chiari E, Fernandes O, et al. A new consensus for *Trypanosoma cruzi* intraspecific nomenclature: second revision meeting recommends TcI to TcVI. *Mem Inst Oswaldo Cruz* 2009;**104**:1051−4.

33. Machado CA, Ayala FJ. Nucleotide sequences provide evidence of genetic exchange among distantly related lineages of *Trypanosoma cruzi*. *Proc Natl Acad Sci USA* 2001;**98**:7396−401.

34. Westenberger SJ, Barnabe C, Campbell DA, Sturm NR. Two hybridization events define the population structure of *Trypanosoma cruzi*. *Genetics* 2005;**171**:527−43.

35. De Freitas JM, Augusto-Pinto L, Pimenta JR, Bastos-Rodrigues L, Goncalves VF, Teixeira SM, et al. Ancestral genomes, sex, and the population structure of *Trypanosoma cruzi*. *PLoS Pathog* 2006;**2**:e24.

36. Herrera C, Bargues MD, Fajardo A, Montilla M, Triana O, Vallejo GA, et al. Identifying four *Trypanosoma cruzi* I isolate haplotypes from different geographic regions in Colombia. *Infect Genet Evol* 2007;**7**:535−9.

37. Herrera C, Guhl F, Falla A, Fajardo A, Montilla M, Vallejo GA, et al. Genetic variability and phylogenetic relationships within *Trypanosoma cruzi* I isolated in Colombia based on miniexon gene sequences. *J Parasitol Res* 2009. 2009, Article ID 897364, doi:897310.891155/892009/897364.

38. Falla A, Herrera C, Fajardo A, Montilla M, Vallejo GA, Guhl F. Haplotype identification within *Trypanosoma cruzi* I in Colombian isolates from several reservoirs, vectors and humans. *Acta Trop* 2009;**110**:15−21.

39. Llewellyn MS, Miles MA, Carrasco HJ, Lewis MD, Yeo M, Vargas J, et al. Genome-scale multilocus microsatellite typing of *Trypanosoma cruzi* discrete typing unit I reveals phylogeographic structure and specific genotypes linked to human infection. *PLoS Pathol* 2009;**5**:e1000410.

40. Fitzpatrick S, Feliciangeli MD, Sanchez-Martin MJ, Monteiro FA, Miles MA. Molecular genetics reveal that sylvatic *Rhodnius prolixus* do colonise rural houses. *PLoS Negl Trop Dis* 2008;**2**:e210.

41. Zingales B, Miles MA, Campbell DA, Tibayrenc M, Macedo AM, Teixeira MMG, et al. The revised *Trypanosoma cruzi* subspecific nomenclature: rationale, epidemiological relevance and research application. *Infect Genet Evol* 2012;**12**(2):240−53.

42. Marcili A, Valente VC, Valente SA, Junqueira AC, da Silva FM, Pinto AY, et al. *Trypanosoma cruzi* in Brazilian Amazonia: lineages TCI and TCIIa in wild primates,

Rhodnius spp. and in humans with Chagas disease associated with oral transmission. *Int J Parasitol* 2009;**39**:615−23.

43. Monteiro WM, Magalhaes LK, de Sa AR, Gomes ML, Toledo MJ, Borges L, et al. *Trypanosoma cruzi* IVcausing outbreaks of acute Chagas disease and infections by differenthaplotypes in the Western Brazilian Amazonia. *PLoS One* 2012;**7**(7):e41284.

44. Yeo M, Acosta N, Llewellyn M, Sanchez H, Adamson S, Miles GA, et al. Origins of Chagas disease: didelphis species are natural hosts of *Trypanosoma cruzi* I and armadillos hosts of *Trypanosoma cruzi* II, including hybrids. *Int J Parasitol* 2005;**35**(2):225−33.

45. Cardinal MV, Lauricella MA, Ceballos LA, Lanati L, Marcet PL, Levin MJ, et al. Molecular epidemiology ofdomestic and sylvatic *Trypanosoma cruzi* infection in rural northwestern Argentina. *Int J Parasitol* 2008;**38**(13):1533−43.

46. Llewellyn MS, Lewis MD, Acosta N, Yeo M, Carrasco HJ, Segovia M, et al. *Trypanosoma cruzi* IIc: phylogenetic and phylogeographic insights from sequence and microsatellite analysis and potential impact on emergent Chagas disease. *PLoS Negl Trop Dis* 2009;**3**:e510.

47. Marcili A, Lima L, Valente VC, Valente SA, Batista JS, Junqueira AC, et al. Comparative phylogeography of *Trypanosoma cruzi* TCIIc: new hosts, association with terrestrial ecotopes, and spatial clustering. *Infect Genet Evol* 2009;**9**(6):1265−74.

48. Carrasco HJ, Segovia M, Llewellyn MS, Morocoima A, Urdaneta-Morales S, Martínez C, et al. Geographical distribution of *Trypanosoma cruzi* genotypes in Venezuela. *PLoS Negl Trop Dis* 2012;**6**(6):e1707.

49. Burgos JM, Diez M, Vigliano C, Bisio M, Risso M, Duffy T, et al. Molecular identification of *Trypanosoma cruzi* discrete typing units in end-stage chronic Chagas heart disease and reactivation after heart transplantation. *Clin Infect Dis* 2010;**51**(5):485−95.

50. Ramírez JD, Guhl F, Rendón LM, Rosas F, Marin-Neto JA, Morillo CA. Chagas cardiomyopathy manifestations and *Trypanosoma cruzi* genotypes circulating in chronic chagasic patients. *PLoS Negl Trop Dis* 2010;**4**(11):e899.

51. Moraes CB, Giardini MA, Kim H, Franco CH, Araujo-Junior AM, Schenkman S, et al. Nitroheterocyclic compounds are more efficacious than CYP51 inhibitors against *Trypanosoma cruzi*: implications for Chagas disease drug discovery and development. *Sci Rep* 2014;**4**:4703.

52. Zingales B, Miles MA, Moraes CB, Luquetti A, Guhl F, Schijman AG, et al. Drug discovery for Chagas disease should consider *Trypanosoma cruzi* strain diversity. *Mem Inst Oswaldo Cruz* 2014;**109**(6):828−33.

53. Moreno M, D'Avila DA, Silva MN, Galvao LM, Macedo AM, Chiari E, et al. *Trypanosoma cruzi* benznidazole susceptibility in vitrodoes not predict the therapeutic outcome of human Chagas disease. *Mem Inst Oswaldo Cruz* 2010;**105**(7):918−24.

54. Teston AP, Monteiro WM, Reis D, Bossolani GD, Gomes ML, de Araujo SM, et al. In vivo susceptibility tobenznidazole of *Trypanosoma cruzi* strains from the western Brazilian Amazon. *Trop Med Int Health* 2013;**18**(1):85−95.

55. Gaunt M, Miles M. The ecotopes and evolution of triatomine bugs (triatominae) and their associated trypanosomes. *Mem Inst Oswaldo Cruz* 2000;**95**:557−65.

56. Roellig DM, Ellis AE, Yabsley MJ. Genetically different isolates of *Trypanosoma cruzi* elicit different infection dynamics in raccoons (*Procyon lotor*) and Virginia opossums (*Didelphis virginiana*). *Int J Parasitol* 2009;**39**:1603−10.

57. Roellig DM, McMillan K, Ellis AE, Vandeberg JL, Champagne DE, Yabsley MJ. Experimental infection of two South American reservoirs with four distinct strains of *Trypanosoma cruzi*. *Parasitology* 2009;1−8.

58. Mello CB, Azambuja P, Garcia ES, Ratcliffe NA. Differential in vitro and in vivo behavior of three strains of *Trypanosoma cruzi* in the gut and hemolymph of *Rhodnius prolixus*. *Exp Parasitol* 1996;**82**:112−21.

59. Vallejo GA, Guhl F, Schaub GA. Triatominae—*Trypanosoma cruzi/T. rangeli*: vector−parasite interactions. *Acta Trop* 2009;**110**:137−47.

60. Lent H, Wygodzinsky P. Revision of the Triatominae (Hemiptera, Reduviidae) and their significance as vectors of Chagas' disease. *Bull Am Mus Nat Hist* 1979;**163**:123−520.

61. Kollien AH, Schaub GA. Development of *Trypanosoma cruzi* after starvation and feeding of the vector—a review. *Tokai J Exp Clin Med* 1998;**23**:335−40.

62. Phillips NR, Bertram DS. Laboratory studies of *Trypanosoma cruzi* infections in *Rhodnius prolixus*—larvae and adults in *Triatoma infestans, T. protracta* and *T. maculata* adults. *J Med Entomol* 1967;**4**:168−74.

63. Vargas LG, Zeledon R. Effect of fasting on *Trypanosoma cruzi* infection in *Triatoma dimidiata* (Hemiptera: Reduviidae). *J Med Entomol* 1985;**22**:683.

64. Jansen AM, Xavier SCC, Roque ALR. The multiple and complex and changeable scenarios of the *Trypanosoma cruzi* transmission cycle in the sylvatic environment. *Acta Trop* 2015;**51**:1−15.

65. WHO. Weekly Epidemiological Record. No. 6, 90, 33−44; 2015.

66. Herwaldt BL, Grijalva MJ, Newsome AL, McGhee CR, Powell MR, Nemec DG, et al. Use of polymerase chain reaction to diagnose the fifth reported US case of autochthonous transmission of *Trypanosoma cruzi*, in Tennessee, 1998. *J Infect Dis* 2000;**181**:395−9.

67. Dorn PL, Perniciaro L, Yabsley MJ, Roellig DM, Balsamo G, Diaz J, et al. Autochthonous transmission of *Trypanosoma cruzi*, Louisiana. *Emerg Infect Dis* 2007;**13**:605−7.

68. Brown EL, Roellig DM, Gompper ME, Monello RJ, Wenning KM, Gabriel MW, et al. Seroprevalence of *Trypanosoma cruzi* among eleven potential reservoir species from six states across the Southern United States. *Vector Borne Zoonotic Dis* 2009. Available from: http://dx.doi.org/10.1089/vbz.2009.0009

69. Buhaya MH, Galvan S, Maldonado RA. Incidence of *Trypanosoma cruzi* infection in triatomines collected at Indio Mountains Research Station. *Acta Trop* 2015;**150**:97−9.

70. Reisenman CE, Lawrence G, Guerenstein PG, Gregory T, Dotson E, et al. Infection of kissing bugs with *Trypanosoma cruzi*, Tucson, Arizona, USA. *Emerg Infect Dis* 2010;**16** (3):400−5.

71. Bern C, Montgomery SP. An estimate of the burden of Chagas disease in the United States. *Clin Infect Dis* 2009;**49**:e52−4.

72. Pinazo MJ, Gascon J. The importance of multidisciplinary approach to deal with the new epidemiological scenario of Chagas disease (global health). *Acta Trop* 2015;**151**:16−20.

73. Gascon J, Bern C, Pinazo MJ. Chagas disease in Spain, the United States and other non-endemic countries. *Acta Trop* 2010;**115**:22−7.

74. Schmunis GA, Yadon ZE. Chagas disease: a Latin American health problem becoming a world health problem. *Acta Trop* 2010;**115**:14−21.

75. Gonzalez-Granado LI, Rojo-Conejo P, Ruiz-Contreras J, Gonzalez-Tome MI. Chagas disease travels to Europe. *Lancet* 2009;**373**:2025.

76. Castro AM, Vinaud M, Teixeira A. Chagas disease: a global health problem. In: Teixeira A, Vinaud M, Castro AM, editors. *Emerging Chagas disease*. BenthamBooks; 2009.

77. Lescure FX, Canestri A, Melliez H, Jaureguiberry S, Develoux M, Dorent R, et al. Chagas disease, France. *Emerg Infect Dis* 2008;**14**:644−6.
78. Ueno Y, Nakamura Y, Takahashi M, Inoue T, Endo S, Kinoshita M, et al. A highly suspected case of chronic Chagas' heart disease diagnosed in Japan. *Jpn Circ J* 1995;**59**:219−23.
79. Nishimura A, Ueno Y, Fujiwara S, Nushida H, Tatsuno Y. An autopsy case of sudden death due to Chagas' disease. *Nihon Hoigaku Zasshi* 1997;**51**:39−43.
80. Falta referencia.
81. Guzman-Tapia Y, Ramirez-Sierra MJ, Dumonteil E. Urban infestation by *Triatoma dimidiata* in the city of Merida, Yucatan, Mexico. *Vector Borne Zoonotic Dis* 2007;**7**:597−606.
82. Sousa OE, Samudio F, de Junca C, Calzada JE. Molecular characterization of human *Trypanosoma cruzi* isolates from endemic areas in Panama. *Mem Inst Oswaldo Cruz* 2006;**101**:455−7.
83. Samudio F, Ortega-Barria E, Saldana A, Calzada J. Predominance of *Trypanosoma cruzi* I among Panamanian sylvatic isolates. *Acta Trop* 2007;**101**:178−81.
84. Pennington PM, Messenger LA, Reina JG, Juarez GG, Lawrence EM, et al. The Chagas disease domestic transmission cycle in Guatemala: parasite-vector switches and lack of mitochondrial co-diversification between *Triatoma dimidiata* and *Trypanosoma cruzi* subpopulations suggest non-vectorial parasite dispersal across the Motagua valley. *Acta Trop* 2015;**151**:80−7.
85. Abad-Franch F, Ferraz G, Campos C, Palomeque FS, Grijalva MJ, Aguilar HM, et al. Modeling disease vector occurrence when detection is imperfect: infestation of Amazonian palm trees by triatomine bugs at three spatial scales. *PLoS Negl Trop Dis* 2010;**4**:e620. Available from: http://dx.doi.org/10.1371/journal.pntd.0000620.
86. Coura JR, Junqueira ACV. Ecological diversity of *Trypanosoma cruzi* transmission in the Amazon basin. The main scenarios in the Brazilian Amazon. *Acta Trop* 2015;**151**:32−50.
87. Aguilar HM, Abad-Franch F, Dias JC, Junqueira AC, Coura JR. Chagas disease in the Amazon region. *Mem Inst Oswaldo Cruz* 2007;**102**(Suppl.1):47−56 106 American Trypanosomiasis.
88. Beltrao H de, B, Cerroni Mde P, Freitas DR, Pinto AY, Valente Vda C, Valente SA, et al. Investigation of two outbreaks of suspected oral transmission of acute Chagas disease in the Amazon region, Para State, Brazil, in 2007. *Trop Doct* 2009;**39**:231−2.
89. Valente VC, Valente SA, Noireau F, Carrasco HJ, Miles MA. Chagas disease in the Amazon basin: association of *Panstrongylus geniculatus* (Hemiptera: Reduviidae) with domestic pigs. *J Med Entomol* 1998;**35**:99−103.
90. Valente SA, da Costa Valente V, das Neves Pinto AY, de Jesus Barbosa Cesar M, dos Santos MP, Miranda MP, et al. Analysis of an acute Chagas disease outbreak in the Brazilian Amazon: human cases, triatomines, reservoir mammals and parasites. *Trans R Soc Trop Med Hyg* 2009;**103**:291−7.
91. De Noya B, Gonzalez ON. An ecological overview on the factors that drives to *Trypanosoma cruzi* oral transmission. *Acta Trop* 2015;**151**:94−102.
92. Guhl F, Schofield CJ. International workshop on Chagas Disease surveillance in the Amazon Region. In: Guhl F, Schofield CJ, editors. *Proceedings ECLAT-AMCHA*. Bogota, Colombia: Universidad de los Andes; 2004. p. 174.
93. Monteiro FA, Barrett TV, Fitzpatrick S, Cordon-Rosales C, Feliciangeli D, Beard CB. Molecular phylogeography of the Amazonian Chagas disease vectors *Rhodnius prolixus* and *R. robustus*. *Mol Ecol* 2003;**12**:997−1006.

94. Guhl F. Chagas disease in Andean countries. *Mem Inst Oswaldo Cruz* 2007;**102** (Suppl.1):29−38.

95. Feliciangeli M.D., Campbell-Lendrum D, Martinez C, Gonzalez D, Coleman P, Davies C. Chagas disease control in Venezuela: lessons for the Andean region and beyond. *Trends Parasitol* 2003;**19**:44−9.

96. Bargues MD, Klisiowicz DR, Gonzalez-Candelas F, Ramsey JM, Monroy C, Ponce C, et al. Phylogeography and genetic variation of *Triatoma dimidiata*, the main Chagas disease vector in Central America, and its position within the genus *Triatoma*. *PLoS Negl Trop Dis* 2008;**2**:e233.

97. Bargues MD, Marcilla A, Ramsey JM, Dujardin JP, Schofield CJ, Mas-Coma S. Nuclear rDNA-based molecular clock of the evolution of triatominae (Hemiptera: reduviidae), vectors of Chagas disease. *Mem Inst Oswaldo Cruz* 2000;**95**:567−73.

98. Cuba CAC, Abad-Franch F, Rodriguez JR, Vasquez FV, Velasquez LP, Miles MA. The triatomines of northern Peru, with emphasis on the ecology and infection by trypanosomes of *Rhodnius ecuadoriensis* (Triatominae). *Mem Inst Oswaldo Cruz* 2002;**97**:175−83.

99. Bargues MD, Klisiowicz DR, Panzera F, Noireau F, Marcilla A, Perez R, et al. Origin and phylogeography of the Chagas disease main vector *Triatoma infestans* based on nuclear rDNA sequences and genome size. *Infect Genet Evol* 2006;**6**:46−62.

100. Noireau F, Dujardin JP. Flight and nutritional status of sylvatic *Triatoma sordida* and *Triatoma guasayana*. *Mem Inst Oswaldo Cruz* 2001;**96**:385−9.

101. Carreira JC, Jansen AM, de Nazareth Meirelles M, Costa e Silva F, Lenzi HL. *Trypanosoma cruzi* in the scent glands of *Didelphis marsupialis*: the kinetics of colonization. *Exp Parasitol* 2001;**97**:129−40.

102. Diotaiuti L, Pereira AS, Loiola CF, Fernandes AJ, Schofield JC, Dujardin JP, et al. Interrelation of sylvatic and domestic transmission of *Trypanosoma cruzi* in areas with and without domestic vectorial transmission in Minas-Gerais, Brazil. *Mem Inst Oswaldo Cruz* 1995;**90**:443−8.

103. Fernandes AJ, Chiari E, Rodrigues RR, Dias JCP, Romanha AJ. The importance of the opossum (*Didelphis albiventris*) as a reservoir for *Trypanosoma cruzi* in Bambui, Minas-Gerais state. *Mem Inst Oswaldo Cruz* 1991;**86**:81−5.

104. Miles MA, Apt BW, Widmer G, Povoa MM, Schofield CJ. Isozyme heterogeneity and numerical taxonomy of *Trypanosoma cruzi* stocks from Chile. *Trans R Soc Trop Med Hyg* 1984;**78**:526−35.

# Classification and systematics of the Triatominae

*M.D. Bargues[1], C. Schofield[2] and J.-P. Dujardin[3]*
[1]Universidad de Valencia, Burjassot Valencia, Spain, [2]London School of Tropical Medicine and Hygiene and ECLAT Net Work, United Kingdom, [3]Institut de Recherche pour le Développement (IRD), UMR 177 Intertryp, Montpellier, France

## Chapter Outline

American Trypanosomiasis Chagas Disease. DOI: http://dx.doi.org/10.1016/B978-0-12-801029-7.00006-X

# Introduction

In understanding biodiversity, taxonomy (classification) and systematics (including phylogenetics) work together, although the two terms are often confused. The objective of systematics is to understand the natural mechanisms responsible for the biodiversity, while the task of taxonomy is to set up a useful classification of the organisms concerned. In a sense, systematics provides guidelines for taxonomy to classify organisms according to accepted rules of nomenclature.[1] But nevertheless, the two concepts face an inevitable conflict because classification and nomenclature are designed to be stable (ICZN) and of use to those considering other aspects of the organisms, whereas systematics is essentially a dynamic approach suggesting changes and adjustments as new data become available, and also inherently considering a dynamic system in which the units of study species or populations are liable to change with time and circumstance.

Divergence between the modern concepts of systematics starts at the definition given to the taxa they want to analyze, either single individuals,[2] reproductively isolated populations,[3,4] populations,[5] or agglomerations of populations.[6] In the case of the Triatominae, these problems are also evident from the epidemiological requirement (e.g., are these important vectors of Chagas disease, or not?) and the increasing wealth of data offering new insights to their evolution. An important body of literature explored the phylogeny of the Triatominae, making them a monophyletic,[7-12] a polyphyletic,[13-18] or a paraphyletic group.[19,20] Today, the evidence is that the Triatominae cannot be considered anymore as a monophyletic group, yet it would make no epidemiological sense to try to reclassify them in that light.[18]

Moreover, to the sometimes confusing classification for high rank taxa of Triatominae, one has to add their evident capacity to show phenetic drift at the species or subspecies level. Their frequent morphological divergence according to geography and associated ecological variation can give rise to local variants that tempt yet more specific, or even generic, designations.[21-23]

Other problems arise from the lack of clear consensus on taxonomic concepts. Not only is the subfamily itself poorly defined, such that some predatory reduviids have been erroneously described as Triatominae,[24,25] but there is no consistent concept of features meriting tribal or generic rank, and considerable divergence on concepts of species, subspecies, and species complexes. In this chapter we summarize the current classification, and offer ways in which these concepts might be usefully reviewed.

# Subfamily: Triatominae

The Triatominae are classified as a subfamily of the Reduviidae (Hemiptera, Heteroptera) and are believed to have derived from predatory forms of the Reduviidae. They are customarily defined by their blood-sucking habit and associated morphological adaptations, particularly the straight three-segmented rostrum in which the final segment is capable of flexing upwards when the rostrum is extended for feeding. This definition is not entirely satisfactory, because although most other Reduviidae are predators on other invertebrates, several will also suck vertebrate blood on occasion.[26] Conversely, an increasing number of triatomine species have been shown to be at least facultative predators[18,27] and some particularly of the tribe Bolboderini appear to be almost entirely predaceous in habit.[28,29] Over half of the 140−148 currently recognized species of Triatominae have been shown to be naturally or experimentally infected with *Trypanosoma cruzi* (causative agent of Chagas disease) and all are suspected to have this capacity. However, although of great epidemiological relevance (and a primary stimulus to research on the group), this characteristic is not used in the definition of the subfamily because of the capacity of *T. cruzi* to infect a wide range of other arthropods[30] even though other arthropods appear to have no epidemiological significance as vectors.

For this review we refer mainly to the classification of Triatominae of Lent and Wygodzinsky[7] as updated by Schofield and Galvão[18] and Dujardin et al.[31] and Galvão and de Paula.[32] For this, the subfamily is classified into 5 tribes with 15 genera (or 18 genera according to Ref.[32] and up to 148 species (Table 6.1). The classification has a morphological basis, and has been challenged by various other arrangements based on morphology, and/or genetic characters (Tables 6.2−6.4).

**Table 6.1** **Classification of Triatominae as in Schofield and Galvão[18]**

| Tribes | Genera | Number of species |
|---|---|---|
| Alberproseniini | *Alberprosenia* | 2 |
| Bolboderini | *Belminus* | 8 |
| | *Bolbodera* | 1 |
| | *Microtriatoma* | 2 |
| | *Parabelminus* | 2 |
| Cavernicolini | *Cavernicola* | 2 |
| Rhodniini | *Psammolestes* | 3 |
| | *Rhodnius* | 19 |
| Triatomini | *Dipetalogaster* | 1 |
| | *Eratyrus* | 2 |
| | *Hermanlentia* | 1 |
| | *Linshcosteus* | 6 |
| | *Panstrongylus* | 14[a] |
| | *Paratriatoma* | 1 |
| | *Triatoma* | 84[b,c] |
| Total | *15* | 148 |

The number of species corresponds to the published works up to now, whatever the opinion we could have about their validity.
[a]This genus has a fossil species: *P. hispaniolae* Ponair Jr., 2013.
[b]Within *Triatoma* (84 species), 12 species have been assigned to 3 new genera: *Meccus* (6 species), *Mepraia* (3 species), *Nesotriatoma* (3 species).
[c]This genus has a fossil species: *T. dominicana* Ponair Jr., 2005.

## Table 6.2 Techniques most commonly used in systematics

| Techniques frequently used in molecular systematics | | |
| --- | --- | --- |
| Techniques | Strengths | Weaknesses |
| 1. **MLEE** Multilocus Enzyme Electrophoresis | Provides information on several gene loci (and individuals) simultaneously; enzyme mobility differences can be related to different alleles at the gene locus for the enzyme in question; mobility variants are called electromorphs | Samples must be fresh or frozen |
| 2. **RAPD** Random Amplification of Polymorphic DNA | Provides information on many gene loci (and individuals) simultaneously; has been used for population genetic studies similar to MLEE | Dominance may hide heterozygous forms; problems of reproducibility; little guarantee of homology between comigrant bands |
| 3. **PCR-RFLP** Polymerase Chain Reaction Restriction Fragment Length Polymorphism | Widely used for epidemiological typing of many organisms; used for population genetic studies; established marker; relatively inexpensive; codominant marker | Might reveal little polymorphism; partial digestion can lead to problems; gives information on one locus at a time |
| 4. **Cytogenetics** Chromosome analyses | Necessary for studies of genome organization and its association with chromatin; can be informative on population expansion processes; used for intraspecific variability studies and to detect cryptic species | Gonads must be fixed from live specimens |
| 5. **Microsatellites** short tandem repeats (period of 1–6 bp) | Provides information on several loci (and individuals) simultaneously; highly polymorphic; may be considered as neutral Mendelian markers; used for analysis of population genetic structure | Poor markers for phylogenetic inference; requires access to sequencer; development of primers can be time-consuming |
| 6. DNA sequencing | Highly informative; allows for studies of any taxonomic level and for comparisons between different labs through DNA data banks | Relatively expensive; access to sequencer required; labor-intensive data |

Bp, base pairs; Mya, million years ago. Gene and fragment lengths refer to published studies on Triatominae.
*Source*: Adapted from Abad-Franch F, Monteiro FA. Molecular research and control of Chagas disease vectors. *An Acad Brasil Cien* 2005; **77**:437−54.[33]

**Table 6.3 Nuclear molecular markers most commonly used in systematics**

| Markers frequently used in molecular systematics | | |
|---|---|---|
| **Markers** | **Strengths** | **Weaknesses** |
| **rDNA** Nuclear Ribosomal DNA | Generally evolves more slowly than mtDNA; follows Mendelian inheritance; special interest in studies on bisexual species; useful at different taxonomic levels and for evolutionary inference; follows a concerted evolution | Occurs in lower copy number and often is more difficult to work with it than mtDNA; sometimes more difficult to amplify by PCR; difficulties in alignments due to high number of insertions/ deletions |
| **28S** Gene 28S rRNA = Large Subunit of rRNA (LSUr-RNA); total length approx 4000 bp; region analyzed usually the D2 domain of 633 bp | Evolves faster than 18S; presents divergent domains (D1, D2, D3, etc.); can be used to distinguish between species, but mainly used for intermediate and higher taxonomic levels | Less used for phylogenetic analyses; the usefulness of the domains varies depending the organisms analyzed |
| **18S** Gene 18S = Small Subunit of rRNA (SSUrRNA); Total length 1913−1918 bp; region analyzed is usually the complete gene | Very low evolutionary rate; useful for distant species, genera and tribes; provides inferences about ancient to very ancient relationships of distantly related organisms ($\sim$ 100 Mya) | Restricted to comparisons of distant taxa |
| **ITS-1** Internal Transcribed Spacer 1; total length 573−750 bp; region analyzed is usually the complete spacer | Evolves faster than ITS-2; useful for closely related taxa that have diverged recently (¡ 50 Mya); good complement to the ITS-2 for systematic and taxonomic purposes from species to tribe levels | Presents microsatellites and minisatellites which seem specific to particular populations |
| **ITS-2** Internal Transcribed Spacer 2; Total length 470−722 bp; region analyzed is usually the complete spacer | Useful for closely related taxa that have Diverged recently ($\sim$ 50 Mya); useful in the Analysis of species, subspecies, hybrids and populations as well as for problematic taxa such as cryptic or sibling species | Not appropriate for the comparison of different tribes as no clear alignment could be obtained; microsatellites are numerous and are only population markers |

*(Continued)*

**Table 6.3 (Continued)**

| Markers frequently used in molecular systematics | | |
|---|---|---|
| **Markers** | **Strengths** | **Weaknesses** |
| **ps 5.8S + ITS-2**<br>Pseudogenic sequence of 5.8S and ITS-2 rDNA; total length 575–626 bp (592 bp) | Useful for specimen classification, phylogenetic analyses and systematic/taxonomic studies. Similar resolution power as functional ITS-2 rDNA. No longer interacts genetically with functional copies. Could be used as another completely new resource to infer phylogeny[34] | Technical problem of the risk for erroneous sequence results. Cloning and subsequent clone sequencing are needed for pseudogen verification. Specific primer sequencing for each functional and paralogous sequences are recommended |

Bp, base pairs; Mya, million years ago. Gene and fragment lengths refer to published studies on Triatominae.
*Source*: Adapted from Justi SA, Dale C, Galvão C. DNA barcoding does not separate South American Triatoma (Hemiptera: Reduviidae), Chagas disease vectors. *Parasit Vectors* 2014;7:519[23]; Bargues MD, Zuriaga MA, Mas-Coma S. Nuclear rDNA pseudogenes in Chagas disease vectors: evolutionary implications of a new 5.8S + ITS2 paralogous sequence marker in triatomines of North, Central and northern South America. *Infect Genet Evol* 2014;21:134−56[34]; Zuriaga MA, Mas-Coma S, Bargues MD. A nuclear ribosomal DNA pseudogene in triatomines opens a new research field of fundamental and applied implications in Chagas disease. *Mem Inst Oswaldo Cruz* 2015;110:353−62[35]; Mas-Coma S, Bargues M. Populations, hybrids and the systematic concepts of species and subspecies in Chagas disease triatomine vectors inferred from nuclear ribosomal and mitochondrial DNA. *Acta Trop* 2009;110:112−36[36]; Monteiro FA, Peretolchina T, Lazoski C, Harris K, Dotson EM, Abad-Franch F, et al. Phylogeographic pattern and extensive mitochondrial dna divergence disclose a species complex within the Chagas disease vector *Triatoma dimidiata*. *PLoS ONE* 2013;8:e70974[37]; Gómez-Palacio A, Triana O, Jaramillo-O N, Dotson EM, Marcet PL. Eco-geographical differentiation among Colombian populations of the Chagas disease vector *Triatoma dimidiata* (Hemiptera: Reduviidae). *Infect Genet Evol* 2013;20:352−61[38]; Gómez-Palacio A, Triana O. Molecular evidence of demographic expansion of the Chagas disease vector *Triatoma dimidiata* (Hemiptera, Reduviidae, Triatominae) in Colombia. *PLoS Negl Trop Dis* 2014;8:e2734[39]; Fernández CJ, Pérez de Rosas AR, García BA. Variation in mitochondrial NADH dehydrogenase subunit 5 and NADH dehydrogenase subunit 4 genes in the Chagas disease vector *Triatoma infestans* (Hemiptera: Reduviidae). *Am J Trop Med Hyg* 2013;88:893−96[40]; Díaz S, Panzera F, Jaramillo-O N, Pérez R, Fernández R, Vallejo G, et al. Genetic, cytogenetic and morphological trends in the evolution of the Rhodnius (Triatominae: Rhodniini) trans-andean group. *PLoS ONE* 2014;9:e87493.[41]

Difficulties in reaching a stable classification are discussed more fully by Schofield and Galvão.[18]

# Tribes and genera

## Tribe: Alberproseniini (genus Alberprosenia)

The two similar species of *Alberprosenia* forming this tribe are unusually small Triatominae (adults up to 5 mm in length) with unusually short heads, which have been little studied beyond their original descriptions. They have no known epidemiological significance. The tribal, generic, and species concepts are entirely morphological,[7] although *A. goyovargasi* has been reared in the laboratory by feeding on human blood[42] which supports inclusion in the Triatominae ("*Torrealbaia martinezi*" previously ascribed to this tribe[43] has been shown to be a Harpactorinae[24]).

### Table 6.4 **Mitochondrial molecular markers most commonly used in systematics**

| Markers frequently used in molecular systematics | | |
| --- | --- | --- |
| **Markers** | **Strengths** | **Weaknesses** |
| **mtDNA** Mitochondrial DNA; complete genome is 17,015 bp | Evolves faster than nuclear genome; clonally inherited (maternal lineage); useful for studies of closely related taxa that have diverged recently; amplification and sequencing is easier than for nuclear rDNA genes | The high substitution rate can be disadvantageous for resolving divergences of more than 5–10 Mya; saturation is a major cause of homoplasy and erases phylogenetic signal |
| **12S** Gene 12S srRNA = mitochondrial small ribosomal subunit (mt-srRNA); total length 781 bp; region analyzed is usually 339–371 bp | Shows the lowest evolutionary rate within mtDNA markers; useful up to the level of species within the same genus; can reveal differences at population level | Tends to become saturated at higher taxonomic levels; its use for comparison of species of different genera and tribes does not appear to be recommendable |
| **16S** Gene 16S rRNA = mitochondrial large ribosomal subunit (mtlrRNA); total length 1270 bp; region analyzed are usually fragments of 284 bp and from 501–510 bp | Appears to evolve in parallel with 12S, but is more variable, and so tends to reveal greater differences between species of different tribes | Differences between species of different genera can appear similar to those within the same genus; its usefulness for analyses at genus or higher levels does not appear to be recommendable |
| **COI** Cytochrome c oxidase subunit 1; total length 1534 bp; regions analyzed are fragments of 1431–1447 bp and fragments of 636–661 bp | Evolves slightly faster than NAD1 but slower than Cyt b at low level comparisons; useful for studies of closely related species; used for barcoding of various organisms | Saturation becomes a problem in comparison of distant species and at higher taxonomic levels.[36] Not applicable for identifying some Southern American *Triatoma* species which may have diverged recently[23] |
| **NAD1** NADH dehydrogenase subunit 1; total length 912–933 bp; region analyzed is usually the complete gene | Evolves faster than ITS-2 at low level comparisons; useful for studies of closely related species | Saturation is already occurring when comparing distant species of the same genus |
| **Cyt B** Cytochrome B total length 1132 bp; several different fragments are analyzed, from 313 to 682 bp | This is the fastest evolving mtDNA gene; useful for comparison of subspecies (intrapopulational, interpopulational, between morphs, and between subspecies) | Saturation may become a problem in analysis of distant species and higher taxa |

(*Continued*)

## Table 6.4 (Continued)

| Markers frequently used in molecular systematics | | |
|---|---|---|
| **Markers** | **Strengths** | **Weaknesses** |
| **NAD4** NADH dehydrogenase subunit 4; total length 1331 bp; region analyzed are usually fragments of 401–631 bp | Useful for studies of closely related species and for population genetics analyses. Similar level of resolution than Cyt b. Is one of the most variable protein-coding genes in insects in general | Low level of variation and not useful information for phylogenetic inferences in *T. infestans* |
| **NAD5** NADH dehydrogenase subunit 5; total length 1712 bp; region analyzed is complete gen | Is one of the most variable protein-coding genes in insects in general. Useful for population genetic studies | Low level of variation in *T. infestans*. Little known in other Triatominae. Only a portion of the ND5 gene, should be useful for phylogeographic studies |
| **COII** Cytochrome c oxidase subunit 2; total length 679 bp; regions analyzed are fragments of 220–364 bp and fragments of 576–649 bp | Available for many Triatomini and Rhodniini genera and species. Provides congruent phylogenies in combined analyses with other mtDNA markers | Saturation can be considered in analysis of distant species and higher taxa |

Bp, base pairs; Mya, million years ago. Gene and fragment lengths refer to published studies on Triatominae.
*Source*: Adapted from Justi SA, Dale C, Galvão C. DNA barcoding does not separate South American Triatoma (Hemiptera: Reduviidae), Chagas disease vectors. *Parasit Vectors* 2014;**7**:519[23]; Bargues MD, Zuriaga MA, Mas-Coma S. Nuclear rDNA pseudogenes in Chagas disease vectors: evolutionary implications of a new 5.8S + ITS2 paralogous sequence marker in triatomines of North, Central and northern South America. *Infect Genet Evol* 2014;**21**:134–56[34]; Zuriaga MA, Mas-Coma S, Bargues MD. A nuclear ribosomal DNA pseudogene in triatomines opens a new research field of fundamental and applied implications in Chagas disease. *Mem Inst Oswaldo Cruz* 2015;**110**:353–62[35]; Mas-Coma S, Bargues M. Populations, hybrids and the systematic concepts of species and subspecies in Chagas disease triatomine vectors inferred from nuclear ribosomal and mitochondrial DNA. *Acta Trop* 2009;**110**:112–36[36]; Monteiro FA, Peretolchina T, Lazoski C, Harris K, Dotson EM, Abad-Franch F, et al. Phylogeographic pattern and extensive mitochondrial dna divergence disclose a species complex within the Chagas disease vector *Triatoma dimidiata*. *PLoS ONE* 2013;**8**:e70974[37]; Gómez-Palacio A, Triana O, Jaramillo-O N, Dotson EM, Marcet PL. Eco-geographical differentiation among Colombian populations of the Chagas disease vector *Triatoma dimidiata* (Hemiptera: Reduviidae). *Infect Genet Evol* 2013;**20**:352–61[38]; Gómez-Palacio A, Triana O. Molecular evidence of demographic expansion of the Chagas disease vector *Triatoma dimidiata* (Hemiptera, Reduviidae, Triatominae) in Colombia. *PLoS Negl Trop Dis* 2014;**8**:e2734[39]; Fernández CJ, Pérez de Rosas AR, García BA. Variation in mitochondrial NADH dehydrogenase subunit 5 and NADH dehydrogenase subunit 4 genes in the Chagas disease vector *Triatoma infestans* (Hemiptera: Reduviidae). *Am J Trop Med Hyg* 2013;**88**:893–96[40]; Díaz S, Panzera F, Jaramillo-O N, Pérez R, Fernández R, Vallejo G, et al. Genetic, cytogenetic and morphological trends in the evolution of the Rhodnius (Triatominae: Rhodniini) trans-andean group. *PLoS ONE* 2014;**9**:e87493.[41]

## *Tribe: Bolboderini (genera: Bolbodera, Belminus, Microtriatoma, Parabelminus)*

The 13 species of Bolboderini are typically small Triatominae (adults up to 12 mm in length). *Bolbodera* is known only from Cuba, while the other genera are reported from isolated locations spanning the region from Mexico to southern Brazil. The tribal, generic, and species concepts are entirely morphological[7] and it may be that intermediate forms may be found as more natural populations are sampled.

The feeding habits of *Belminus* have been extensively studied, and suggest that these species may be at a very early stage in adaptation to hematophagy.[28,29,44] In a morphological cladogram of the four genera, Lent and Wygodzinsky[7] placed *Bolbodera* as the most primitive, with *Microtriatoma* and *Parabelminus* as the most derived. However, this is difficult to reconcile with their known geographical distribution, as *Bolbodera* is known only from Cuba. Comparison of 28S-D2 sequences placed *Microtriatoma trinidadensis* basal to the Rhodniini[45] although no other Bolboderini have yet been studied by such means.

## Tribe: Cavernicolini (genus: Cavernicola)

The two species of *Cavernicola* are small Triatominae (adults up to 11 mm in length) with unusually shaped head and neck strongly reminiscent of some Apiomerinae. They seem invariably associated with bats and bat roosts, but will feed from other vertebrates in the laboratory. The tribal, generic, and species concepts are entirely morphological.[7,46]

## Tribe: Rhodniini (genera: Psammolestes, Rhodnius)

The three species of *Psammolestes* are small Triatominae (adults up to 15 mm in length) with truncated heads. They are invariably associated with nests of woven sticks as made by dendrocolaptid or furnariid birds (irrespective of the vertebrates currently occupying the nest). Although considered a monophyletic genus by morphological and behavioral similarity, this is difficult to reconcile with their distribution: *Ps. arthuri* occurs in the llanos of Colombia and Venezuela north of the Amazon region, while *Ps. tertius* and *S. coreodes* seem to form a cline down the caatinga-cerrado-chaco corridor of open vegetation south of the Amazon region. *Ps. coreodes* has strong ecological interactions with thornbird nests in the Southern Pantanal region of Brazil[47] and has recently been reported in the Gran Chaco and La Pampa in Argentina.[48,49]

By contrast, *Rhodnius* species are distributed throughout the Amazon region, and into the llanos northwards, and the caatinga and cerrado to the south. They are primarily associated with palmtree crowns, but also occur in bird's nests and in domestic and peridomestic habitats. By morphological, behavioral, anatomical, and genetic features, they appear to form a monophyletic genus[50] with two main lineages: the "prolixus–robustus" group (*prolixus, robustus, milesi, neglectus, neivai, dalessandroi, domesticus, nasutus, barretti, zeledoni, montenegrensis*) mainly east of the Andes, and the "pictipes" group comprising one subgroup east of the Andes (*pictipes, stali, brethesi, paraensis, amazonicus*) and one subgroup west of the Andes (*pallescens, colombiensis, ecuadoriensis*).[51] *R. pictipes* may be closest to the ancestral form, since it is the most widely distributed and of more generalist habit, and shares genital characteristics with other Triatominae that are not shared with other Rhodniini except *R. stali*.[52]

The Rhodniini appear to represent a monophyletic tribe, with clear morphological, physiological, anatomical, and genetic characteristics that distinguish them from other

Triatominae. Relationships between the two genera are less clear, largely because of the paucity of studies on *Ps. arthuri*. Various phylogenetic studies based on MLEE,[53] mtDNA,[54,55] or ribosomal mtDNA[56] indicate paraphyly between *Rhodnius* and *Psammolestes*. The two genera have different morphologies and ecological habits, but both are arboricolous. They seem to represent ecological adaptations to either the tree crown (*Rhodnius*) or the bird's nests (*Psammolestes*).

## Tribe: Triatomini (genera: Dipetalogaster, Eratyrus, Hermanlentia, Linshcosteus, Panstrongylus, Paratriatoma, Triatoma)

The Triatomini is the most speciose of the tribes of Triatominae, with the widest geographical distribution covering a wide variety of ecotopes although the majority seem naturally associated with rupicoline habitats. The original tribal and generic concepts are morphological[7,57] although a number of phylogenetic studies now offer extensive support for these concepts.[56,58−60]

Phylogenetic analyses using nuclear or mitochondrial gene fragments generally indicate that the Triatomini form three main clades that are broadly consistent with their geographical distribution: the *Triatoma* of Central and North America (and the Old World species) (i.e., north of the Amazon region) with which *Dipetalogaster*, *Eratyrus*, *Linshcosteus*, *Paratriatoma*, and *Panstrongylus* are usually clustered; the *Triatoma* of South America, i.e., south and east of the Amazon region (except for *T. maculata*; and *Hermanlentia* has not yet been included); and representatives of the dispar complex that occur mainly along the Andean cordillera from Venezuela to Bolivia (i.e., west of the Amazon region). Perhaps significantly, all species of all genera so far examined that form the "northern clade" (except for *T. lecticularia*) show multiple X chromosomes, whereas those of the southern clade generally show single X chromosomes.[61] Of the exceptions, *T. tibiamaculata* and *T. vitticeps*, both Brazilian species, show two and three X chromosomes, respectively, and often cluster with the northern Triatomini in phylogenetic analyses. The other exceptions are species of the spinolai complex (*spinolai*, *gajardoi*, *eratyrusiformis*, *breyeri*) that show two or three X chromosomes[61,62] and often cluster apart from others of the southern clade of Triatomini. The morphological similarities that placed these species as the spinolai complex,[7] together with the recent karyotype studies, lend support to the concept of these species forming a separate genus: *Mepraia*.[63]

Within the northern Triatomini, several other concerns have been raised. The genus "*Meccus*" was originally proposed for some members of the phyllosoma complex, which were subsequently reduced to subspecific rank by Usinger[57]; these subspecies were then divided and raised to specific rank by Lent and Wygozinsky[7] and grouped as the phyllosoma complex. The genus was re-erected by Hypsa et al.[56] but without including all species that had been assigned to the phyllosoma complex, nor including *T. dimidiata* which appears very closely related by phylogenetic analyses.[31,64−67] The phylogenetic approach to sustain such a genus[56] might be questionable because the terminal entities are not reproductively isolated. Their interfertility has been demonstrated many times and recently confirmed by a molecular marker analysis on natural populations.[68] Thus, according to the Hennigian and to the biological type of species (see Table 6.5) the members of this genus constitute one single polytypic species. Even as evolutionary species (see below) they are not convincing. Very small genetic divergences as based on functional or pseudogenic nuclear rDNA sequences were detected between them[34,35,59,65,67,69] and the relatively higher number of nucleotide differences found in the mtDNA genes analyzed (16S, COI, and Cyt b)[17,36,56,66,67] cannot be used to support species level, as argued by Pfeiler et al.[66] Recently, the parallelism between the trees obtained with the pseudogenic 5.8S + ITS-2 and the functional ITS-2 sequences suggested that at least two derived lineages could be distinguished within this complex.[34]

Some concern is also valid for the idea of resurrecting the genus "*Nesotriatoma*" for the flavida complex of *Triatoma* (*flavida, bruneri, obscura*) which is a set of geographical populations assembled on the basis of morphological characters.[7] Phylogenetic confirmation as a monophyletic clade has not been obtained using a sample including *T. obscura* and the dimidiata/phyllosoma complex of species.

The Old World species of Triatomini have also raised concern, with the six species of *Linshcosteus* raised to tribal rank (as "Linshcosteusini") by Carcavallo et al.[70] on the basis of their uniquely Indian distribution and morphological characters not shared with most other Triatomini, especially the abbreviated rostrum that does not reach the prosternal sulcus. However, phylogenetic analyses tend to show *Linshcosteus* close to *T. rubrofasciata*[56,71] which is believed to have been spread from North America to port areas throughout the Old and New World tropics and subtropics by its association with rats on sailing ships.[71,72] The close proximity of Northern (New World) and Asiatic *Triatoma* has been recently observed also through morphometric techniques (contour of internal wing cells), as well as on the base of cytogenetics and new DNA sequence data.[73]

**Table 6.5 Most common concepts of species**

| CONCEPTOS | TYPO | BIOL | HENN | EVOL | PHG I | PHG II |
|-----------|------|------|------|------|-------|--------|
| Refs | (1) | (2,3) | (4,5) | (6,7) | (8) | (9) |
| RI | No | Yes | Yes | No | No | No |
| TD | No | No | Yes | Yes | Yes | Yes |
| ST | / | / | No | Yes | Yes | No |
| SC | / | / | Yes | / | No | Yes |
| Problems | S | A, RI | A, RI | S | M | H |

TYPO, typological concept; BIOL, biological concept; HENN, hennigian concept; EVOL, evolutionary concept; PHG I, phylogenetic concept *sensu Wheeler & Platnick*; PHG II, phylogenetic concept *sensu Mishler & Theriot*; /, not relevant; (1) Carl von Linnaeus; (2) Earl of Buffon; (3) Ref. [3]; (4,5) Refs. [4,74]; (6,7) Refs. [75,76]; (8) Ref. [6]; (9) Ref. [5]. Refs, references; RI, reproductive isolation; TD, temporal dimension; ST, stem species survival; SC, exclusive use of synapomorphic characters; A, allopatry; H, hybridism; M, exclusive use of morphological characters; S, subjectivity.

# Concept of species

Perhaps the greatest challenge for the classification of Triatominae is the lack of a unifying concept of species. To discuss some of the conflicts which arise from applying modern concepts to traditional classification, and to highlight some recurrent practices regarding the systematics of the subfamily, we needed a theoretical framework; we opted for developing our discussion in parallel with the traditional and modern concepts of species. The most important of them are shortly described below.

## Historical concept

*Morphological or Typological Concept of Species* ("morphological species," "morphospecies," see column TYPO of Table 6.5). This is the historical concept of species, the one accepted by many generations of naturalists, zoologists, and even today, by many biologists.

Most if not all the presently known species of Triatominae are morphospecies.[7] They have been described on a few,[7] very few individuals,[77] or even a single individual only.[78,79] This might be one of the most recurrent problem in morphospecies description: the lack of consideration for natural variation. When more sampling is available, it may become difficult to draw a clear demarcation line between simple geographical variation and species difference.[22] Although the idea is that morphological differences are the reflection of biological divergence, it may happen that morphology appears disconnected from other biological properties. *T. platensis* and *T. infestans* are two morphospecies, but they could appear as the same biological entities: not only do they interbreed, but they are genetically very similar.[64,80,81]

The most important objection to the TYPO concept is the existence of sibling species. Sibling (also "cryptic," or "isomorphic") species are morphologically identical or nearly identical entities recognized as different species according to other concept(s) of species. This objection to the TYPO concept is weakened by the modern possibilities of morphological comparisons, such as electron microscopy of the egg-shell,[82] biometric methods exploring the antennal phenotype (APH),[83,84] or geometric morphometrics.[85,86] Sibling species do not seem to be frequent in Triatominae.[21] Known cases are *T. sordida*[87,88] and *T. dimidiata*,[67,89] which have been split into sibling species on the basis of cytogenetic and molecular characterization techniques. However, even admitting that sibling species are infrequent in Triatominae, many morphospecies are very similar. Triatominae do not show discrete characters allowing clear-cut species differentiation, and some morphospecies are difficult to recognize without dissection of the genitalia. For morphologically very close species, the typological concept can produce confusion. For instance, *R. prolixus* and *R. robustus* are so similar that their geographical distribution is not ascertained. In their revision of the Triatominae from Guyana, the type locality of *R. robustus*,[90,91] reported *R. prolixus*, not *robustus*. To help distinguish these two entities and some other closely related species of the so-called prolixus group, geometric[92−94] and molecular tools[95] have been suggested.

## Modern concepts

The modern concepts of species make use of other criteria than simple morphological comparison, with some of them even completely free of any character examination.

They may be subdivided according to whether or not they take into account the temporal dimension of the species (see row TD, Table 6.5). Only the biological concept of species (see column BIOL, Table 6.5) (and related ones cohesion, recognition, etc.) does not consider the birth and the death of the species.

The modern concepts of species could also be subdivided according to the reproductive strategy of the organisms: biological and Hennigian concepts (Table 6.5) only consider sexually reproducing organisms, the other concepts apply to the entire range of living organisms.

*The Biological Concept of Species* ("biospecies," see column BIOL of Table 6.5). This is probably the most often used concept in entomology. Briefly, it considers as species natural interbreeding populations reproductively isolated from other such natural populations.[3,96] It has ancient roots in the texts from a contemporary of Carl von Linnaeus: the earl of Buffon (1707−88), maybe the first naturalist to consider the criterion of interfertility in the definition of species. In this concept, temporal dimension is not necessary. Indeed, the reproductive isolation criterion would be poorly contributive when considering fossils or extinct species. Other related or almost similar concepts do insist on prezygotic barriers,[97] or on gene flow within species, rather than reproductive isolation.[98,99]

The biological concept is not a character-related concept: it relies only on reproductive isolation. In addition, like the evolutionary concept but contrary to the phylogenetic concepts (see below), the biological definition of species does not contain the operation to be performed to verify its criterion. Reproductive isolation can be demonstrated in various ways, which makes the biological concept a refutable one. Thus, in spite of ignoring the time dimension of a species, i.e., ignoring evolutionary biology and phylogenetics, the concept is not an arbitrary one.

It is however difficult to reject the propensity to interbreed when natural populations are allopatric ones.[100] It might also be confusing to observe partial reproductive isolation more so between separated populations (insular regions). Such situations, not infrequent in Triatominae, may be interpreted as incipient speciation, and invite reconsideration of the use of the subspecies category.[36]

According to the biological concept of species, many well recognized species of Triatominae would become one single species. As an example, *T. platensis* and *T. infestans* are interfertile, in the laboratory as well as in nature, although the latter is not frequently detected because of ecological separation. According to the biological concept, separation, even ecological separation, does not mean reproductive isolation. *Triatoma platensis* and *T. infestans* are two morphospecies but one single biospecies. The same conclusion could be derived from the *R. prolixus*– *R. robustus* question: these morphologically close species are interfertile, but ecologically and to some extent geographically separated. Again, separation does not mean reproductive isolation in the sense of the biological concept: *R. prolixus*– *R. robustus* are one single biospecies. Similar reasoning could be applied to the members of the phyllosoma complex, some members of the brasiliensis complex (see Section 4.1.6), the dimidiata complex (see Section 4.1.8), etc.

*The Hennigian Concept of Species* ("Hennigian species," see column HENN of Table 6.5). The Hennigian Concept[74] also considers that species are reproductively isolated, but it gives them a beginning and an ending in time. The inclusion of the temporal dimension in the definition of species appears as an obvious reality, but this is exactly where discrepancies begin with other related concepts. The HENN concept considers that speciation is a splitting event (cladogenesis), which means the birth of two reproductively isolated sister species and the dissolution of the stem species.[4] Not only the survival of the stem species is not admitted, but, coherently, the idea of phyletic speciation (anagenesis) is rejected. The speciation event is the dissolution of the stem species into a reproductively isolated pair of sister species. Table 6.5 indicates which definitions agree or disagree with this point of view (see row ST, Table 6.5).

Reproductive isolation (from the sister species) is a very important component of the HENN concept, because it avoids the idea of groups linked by netlike relationships. This restriction allows clean definitions of monophyletic groups.

The HENN concept has been applied to draw hypothesized relationships within the genus *Panstrongylus*. *P. lignarius* and *P. herreri* could not be resolved,[7] suggesting one single species as supported later by their close genetic[101] and morphometric similarity (Gumiel et al., unpublished data).

However, when applied to the Rhodniini (excluding the *robustus* species since it is interfertile with *prolixus*) the cladistic tree performed on the basis of isoenzyme characters could not reveal the paraphyly between *Psammolestes* and *Rhodnius* genera,[102] as revealed later by molecular phylogenetic approaches using more sophisticated algorithms.[53–55]

*The Phylogenetic Concepts of Species* (columns PHG I and PHG II of Table 6.5). Two different positions are competing for the title of "phylogenetic" concept of species.[103] One is defining species prior to cladistic analysis on the basis of an exclusive combination of character states,[6] the other is defending the idea of using synapomorphies alone in order to define monophyletic groups of demes, hence species.[5]

1. **The phylogenetic concept sensu[6]** The phylogenetic concept of species sensu[6] (PHG I in Table 6.5) defines hypothetic species prior to any cladistic analysis, as being *"the smallest aggregation of (sexual) populations or (asexual) lineages diagnosable by a unique combination of character states."*[6] The *"unique combination of character states"* is completely independent from the circumstances of the speciation event: either a splitting into sister

species with dissolution of the stem species, a vicariance event, an allopatric or a sympatric speciation (hence with survival of the stem species). Neither synapomorphy nor monophyly, both of critical importance to cladistics, nor reproductive isolation, are prerequisites to define a phylogenetic species. A new species typically contains a fixed state of a previously polymorphic character in the ancestor species. The concept does not reject the idea of phyletic speciation (anagenesis), it thus accepts the idea of stem species survival, and relies on morphological characters. The authors of this concept recognize that it could dramatically increase the number of species in certain groups, especially in groups where many subspecies were described, which has been the case for Triatominae.[18]

This approach does not seem to have been used in the systematics of Triatominae, probably because of the paucity of discrete morphological characters.

2. **The phylogenetic concept sensu[5]** This concept of species (PHG II in Table 6.5) provides a species definition quite distinct from the previous one, but it might be considered as very close to the HENN one. It rejects the idea of stem species survival and does not accept the hypothesis of phyletic speciation. Its first criterion for a species is its monophyletic nature. The important difference with the HENN concept is about the entry groups. According to the HENN concept, the entry groups must be reproductively isolated. This is not required by the PHG II concept: terminal entities may be species, demes, or local populations. This concept makes species dependent on cladistic analysis: species are the result of phylogenetic analysis of infraspecific units, they are defined by their monophyly. The resulting criticism is that it may be difficult to correctly retrieve monophyletic groups when terminal entities are interbreeding units.

Furthermore, even the authors of the concept admit that to define a monophyletic group is not enough to raise it as a species: *"any application of fixed names to phylogenetic trees has to be arbitrary to some extent."*[5] The definition includes additional steps to rank the monophyletic group as a species (bootstrap percentage, number of synapomorphies, decay index, biological criteria, etc.). Moreover, even if they are well supported, the following monophyletic groups should not be named: groups defined only by *"selectively neutral apomorphies,"* and groups *"marked only by molecular apomorphies and thus nearly impossible to distinguish for practical use."*[5]

In Triatominae the *R. prolixus* and *R. robustus* question offers a good example of this approach. *R. prolixus* and *R. robustus*, known as interfertile taxa, appeared as different monophyletic groups in molecular cladistic analyzes, and, in a second step of the same analysis, were claimed to be different species because of relatively large mtDNA sequence divergence between groups.[55] Two different steps were (1) to recognize distinct monophyletic groups and (2) to consider them as distinct species. The first step might be considered as a rigorous application of phylogenetic rules, although even on that matter phylogeneticists may disagree because of reticulation.[104] The second one is a subjective ranking appreciation (the amount of genetic distance) which is here comparable to the "distance approach," or the "phenetic concept of species."

Thus, the phylogenetic concept sensu[5] is not free of subjective appreciation, and its main problem remains the reticulate structure of terminal entities. Interspecific or interdeme natural hybridism might be the main obstacle to the blind application of synapomorphies to define monophyletic groups. The problem is worth mentioning for Triatominae where interspecific hybridism is known to be frequent,[105-107] and the so-called *prolixus* group is far from being an exception.[108] If the relationships among the terminal taxa are reticulate rather than hierarchical, as they could be in the present concept, apparent synapomorphies might not correspond to monophyletic groups. Reticulate evolution produces confusing patterns of synapomorphy.[109,110]

The *Evolutionary Concept of Species* ("evolutionary species," see column EVOL of Table 6.5). An evolutionary species is *"an entity composed of organisms that maintain its identity from other such entities through time and over space and that has its own independent evolutionary fate and historical tendencies."*[75,76]

As for the BIOL concept, and contrary to the other modern concepts, the EVOL concept does not specify a particular operation to verify its properties. Its strength, which is unique among the various concepts presented here, is that its acceptance does not mean rejection of the other (modern) concepts. Biological and Hennigian species are "evolutionary" species, as are phylogenetic species (to the extent that they retrieve correct ancestry patterns).

Its weakness is some arbitrariness in its definition: *"historical tendencies," "evolutionary fate,"* are not easy to define or reject. However this objection is also the one making the concept potentially attractive. The definition of the evolutionary species does not dictate any rigorous system nor any kind of rigid algorithm to identify independent units. Their identification require discussion and consensus. But it is true that the phylogenetic approach does not have a preponderant place in the discussion, which is based more frequently on ecology, population genetics, geography and morphology. For instance, the *Rhodnius* genus has been discussed in terms of an assemblage of evolutionary units derived from each other, where *R. pictipes* is considered as the survival of the stem species of the genus, and where geography, vicariance, and ecological adaptation are the main forces explaining the groups observed within the genus by other approaches.[50] In this study, different criteria were considered and contrasted to evaluate the fate and destiny of each recognized member of the genus.

The example of the *T. infestans* and *T. platensis* pair is also a good model of evolutionary units where genetic and ecological criteria were applied together to reach a consensus. In spite of being naturally interbreeding and genetically similar units, their obvious ecological adaptation makes them two evolutionary species. This observation is true for the third species of the infestans subcomplex, *T. delpontei*, having partial reproductive compatibility with *T. platensis* but apparently adapted to other birds.

## Examples of specific questions

At the species level, most of the conflicts between traditional and modern concepts of species were treated using the subjective argument of "large" or "low" genetic and/or phenetic distances. Thus, in the current literature, the molecular approach to species resolution is widely inspired by the evolutionary concept of species, as well as by the subjective step of the phylogenetic (PHG 2) concept asking whether two monophyletic clades are two different species.

## R. prolixus and R. robustus

The *prolixus—robustus* pair received a phylogenetic recognition as distinct monophyletic groups,[54,55] but the problem has been treated mostly by considering the degree of genetic distances (see previous sections). The two species present the particularity of no[111,112] or very low nuclear DNA divergence,[36,55] but relatively high mitochondrial[55] genetic distances. Phenotypic distances have been found to be significant.[92,93] Thus, the recognition of monophyletic clades was not sufficient to consider them as separate species, it was the amount of sequence divergence of mitochondrial DNA and the known ecological adaptations which were the arguments to label them as distinct species. Thus far, only molecular markers may help to separate the members of this complex.[113] The morphological characters that would help discriminating them are still to be discovered, although some morphometric propositions have been made.[93,114]

## T. infestans, T. platensis, T. delpontei

In the more abundant genus *Triatoma*, many species have been revisited by using molecular tools, first by using isoenzymes,[80,88,115–117] then by DNA analyses.

The *infestans—platensis—delpontei* question has been addressed again by considering genetic distances. Contrary to the *prolixus—robustus* pair, they do not show significant mtDNA divergence,[58,64] but show a consistent, although low, genetic distance derived from MLEE,[80] or ITS-2 and ITS-1[81] as well as cytogenetic differences.[118] The genetic differences at the nuclear level were among the arguments to decide about their species status,[31] although in this case the ecological specialization also provided a very strong argument.[21,80]

## T. infestans, T. melanosoma

The *infestans—melanosoma* pair has been explored by geometric morphometrics[119] and DNA analyses. *Triatoma melanosoma* was originally described as a subspecies of *T. infestans* and later raised to species rank.[120,121] It differs only by the black color of its exoskeleton from *T. infestans*, with which it is interfertile. This melanic characteristic appears to be recessive in crossbreeds.[31,122] Analyses of Cyt b[122] and ITS-2 and ITS-1[81] considered that genetic differences were not sufficient to justify two different taxa and thus supported the synonymizing of *T. melanosoma* with *T. infestans* after morphometric comparison.[119]

## The "dark morphs" of T. infestans

The "dark morphs" of *T. infestans*[123] have been examined by RAPD,[124] by APH patterns[125] and morphometric characters.[119] Low or lack of phenotypic and genetic distances converged to the conclusion of intraspecific variation. Recently, ITS sequences showed that the dark morph haplotype (T. inf-CH5A) was identical to the majority at ITS-1 and differed from the most dispersed *T. infestans* H2 by only one transversion at ITS-2 level. In the phylogenetic reconstruction, the dark morph appeared in the branch grouping all non-Andean *T. infestans* haplotypes. These results suggested that this melanic form did not need any taxonomic distinction.[81]

## *T. sordida, T. garciabesi*

The *Triatoma sordida* species is morphologically close to *T. guasayana* and *T. patagonica*, but its variable morphology seems to cover different species. *Triatoma garciabesi* has been revalidated mainly on basis of genetic differences with *T. sordida*.[58,126] In Bolivia, the species has been shown through MLEE to contain two sibling species[88] but because of the apparent lack of morphological difference, no new name was created in this situation. This group has been revisited recently using chromosome markers and COI sequences, and more lineages (called "chromosomal taxa") have been distinguished, including a new cryptic species.[127]

## *T. brasiliensis*

*Triatoma brasiliensis* is composed of at least four geographic populations (*brasiliensis*, *melanica*, *macromelasoma*, and *juazeiro*) that have distinct chromatic, morphologic, biologic, ecologic patterns, and genetic composition. This group has been considered using different approaches, exactly in the spirit of the evolutionary concept of species. Reciprocal crosses revealed genetic incompatibility between *melanica* and *brasiliensis* samples.[100] Thus according to the biological and the Hennigian concepts of species, the group contains certainly two species. A large Cyt b study indicated that the four geographic populations of *T. brasiliensis* were genetically distinct.[128] The conclusion was reached to consider *brasiliensis-macromelasoma*, *melanica*, and *juazeiro* forms as three separate species. No taxonomic status was concluded for the *brasiliensis* and *macromelasoma* forms despite their representing distinct evolutionary lineages.[128] Geometric morphometric analyses, morphological comparisons with laboratory hybrids and ecological considerations led to suggest the hypothesis of *T. macromelasoma* as a historical hybrid (homoploid hybridization).[107,129]

## *T. eratyrusiformis*

Hypsa et al.[56] presented the Argentinian species *T. eratyrusiformis* as belonging to the same monophyletic group as *M. spinolai*, supporting its inclusion in the genus as *Mepraia eratyrusiformis*. Combined cytogenetic and nuclear rDNA and mtDNA markers indicate that populations within the *Mepraia* genus can be divided into two separate lineages with specific status supported by the level of divergence observed between their nuclear and mitochondrial sequences which correspond to recently diverged species,[130] with similar nucleotide divergence to that found between the closely related species from the infestans subcomplex.[81] This phylogenetic approach supported the recently described *M. gajardoi*[131]; unfortunately, its validity is questioned since an ingroup species, *M. eratyrusiformis*, was used as an outgroup.[130]

## T. dimidiata

Morphometric variation[132] and later chromosomal variation and genome size[89] suggested the existence of cryptic species of *Triatoma dimidiata*. The *T. dimidiata* complex of species has been suspected also thanks to a phylogenetic (PHG 2) approach.[67] According to ITS-2, *T. dimidiata* populations from Yucatan part of Guatemala and northern Honduras belong to a cryptic species (=*T.* spp. *affinis dimidiata*[67]), different from *T. dimidiata*.[67] Cyt b and ITS-2 confirmed their specific status and extended their distribution to Belize.[133] This distinction agrees with results from multidisciplinary studies using RAPD-PCR, genital structures, morphometrics,[22] APH,[134] cuticular hydrocarbons, and chromosomes[89,135] and has been confirmed by ND1 and pseudogenic sequences of 5.8S + ITS-2 analyses, and by the absence of introgressed sequences in overlapping zones.[34−36] Recently, more emphasis has been brought to the cryptic subdivision of *T. dimidiata* based on mtDNA distances and phylogeography, recognizing the previous studies but suggesting now the existence of at least four separate species.[37] Moreover, in disagreement with previous estimations, Monterio et al.[37] added *T. hegneri* as a fifth species to the *T. dimidiata* complex.

Because of the lack of clear morphological diagnostic characters, no new names have been proposed, but some possible speciation mechanisms have been explored, highlighting the possible role of geographic isolation and ecological adaptation in the process of *T. dimidiata* cryptic speciation. Evidence for niche differentiation among cryptic species was observed using the ecological niche modeling approach (ENM).[136] In Colombia, the genetic heterogeneity among Colombian populations, as observed with microsatellites, correlated with the ecoepidemiological and morphological traits observed in this species across regions.[38] The population structure, as examined through ND4, COI and ITS-2 variation, supported a significant association between genetic divergence and the ecogeographical location of Colombian population groups.[39]

## T. hegneri

*T. hegneri* is a species originally described from the Mexican island of Cozumel. Although chromatically distinguishable from most forms of *T. dimidiata*,[7] it is known to produce fertile hybrids when experimentally crossed with *T. dimidiata* (R.E. Ryckman, unpublished in Bargues et al.[67]). The two ITS-2 haplotypes of *T. hegneri* differ by only three mutations from haplotypes of *T. dimidiata* from Mexico and Guatemala. This reduced number of nucleotide differences and the location of *T. hegneri* haplotypes within the phylogenetic clade of *T. dimidiata* did not support its taxonomic status. These data suggested that it is an intraspecific morphological variation of *T. dimidiata*.[67] In contradiction with these studies, relatively high mtDNA genetic distances were disclosed by Monteiro et al.,[37] who suggested *T. hegneri* as a valid species. Thus, *T. hegneri* is another example where similar, objective genetic approaches produced different, subjective interpretations.

## Panstrongylus lignarius *and* P. herreri

*Panstrongylus lignarius* is an exclusively sylvatic species of Brazil, Guyana, Suriname, Venezuela, and perhaps Ecuador and found naturally infected by *T. cruzi. Panstrongylus herreri* from Peru and Ecuador, adapted to other habitats through its trophic link to guinea pigs and is the main domestic vector in northern Peru.[31,137] Both species are morphologically and morphometrically (Gumiel, personal communication) difficult to distinguish, and although no intermediate forms have been found,[7] they cross-fertilize giving rise to hybrids.[106] No nucleotide difference was detected between their ITS-2 sequences, suggesting that there is only one species.[101]

# Conclusions

As can be seen from the above examples, the phylogenetic concepts (mainly PHG II) have been the most efficient techniques to retrieve ancestry and discuss the validity of supraspecific levels (genera, etc.). They were less useful (or less used) to discuss the species status of various entities. For species status discussion, the biological and evolutionary definitions of the species were more helpful (or more used).

## The species level and the phylogenetic concepts

The phylogenetic concepts put evolutionary meaning to the supraspecific organization, removing the arbitrariness of taxonomists. They are less suited to decide about the species status of natural populations. To rigidly name species according to the phylogenetic concepts (HENN, PHG I, and PHG II) leads to disagreements between concepts, but also presents the risk to modify unnecessarily the number of species.

The Hennigian concept, because of its relying on reproductively isolated terminal entities, has the effect to drastically reduce the number of species, compelling the biologists to create many subspecies as the only alternative. The PHG I concepts presents the risk to dramatically amplify the number of species.[138,139] The PHG II concept, especially when relying on molecular phylogenetics, presents the risk to create unstable taxa (subject to frequent changes as more characters and taxa are discovered), trivial species in evolutionary terms (*"minor, selectively neutral apomorphies"*), as well as cryptic species impossible to distinguish for practical use.

## The species level and the nonphylogenetic concepts

*Speciation event and speciation process.* As seen above, biologists can strongly disagree about the species definition.[104] However, to the exception of possible disagreement about the speciation event itself (survival, or not, of the stem species), there is generally much less discrepancy about the likely grand mechanisms of speciation[140]: allopatry, mutation, genetic drift, disruptive selection,[22] ecological adaptation,[13] hybridization,[22,105–107] etc. Interestingly, most of these mechanisms, when considered for sexually reproducing insects, are processes tending to increase the reproductive isolation between "future" species, which is an indirect recognition to the importance of the biological concept of species.

*The biological and evolutionary concepts.* Both the biological and evolutionary definitions of species are not very useful to understand the successive steps from the past to the present state of biodiversity. However, both of them, especially the evolutionary concept, compel us to gather biological information specific to the populations under study. Their openness to various analytical approaches leads us to define species in a more informative way, in accordance with species definitions and known speciation mechanisms.

Taking into account known speciation processes to understand the species status of a population is where the evolutionary concept could be the most useful. Its receptiveness to discussion provides richer biological information on populations and their possible species status. Importantly, the evolutionary concept is also the only modern concept allowing discussion about infraspecific populations and decisions about the utility of giving them subspecific names. For instance, the partial reproductive isolation of *T. platensis* with *T. delpontei* would make them subspecies according to the biological or Hennigian concepts. Whereas the ecological adaptation of *T. delpontei* to particular bird's nests makes it a true evolutionary species.

It might be useful to mention here the existence of an Ecological Concept of Species,[141] which was progressively abandoned because of two reasons: (1) many subspecies or even simple local populations of the same species may show different ecological adaptations and (2) the rate of speciation largely exceeds the rate of ecological changes.[142]

# A consensual approach to the species

The mechanisms supposed to be at work in producing new species justify the use of phenotypic and genetic differences as an argument for species rank recognition. Indeed, in the case of an allopatric speciation, as due to genetic drift, we expect the species to show the accumulation of genetic and corresponding phenetic differences.[31] In the case of disruptive selection, we expect two optimal phenotypes to coexist.[22] In the case of ecological adaptation, we expect them to show morphological attributes related to the specific ecological niche.[13] In the case of hybridization we expect the hybrid species to occupy a different territory than the parental ones, with intermediate morphological characters and possibly some genetic evidence of introgression.[107] In the case of reproductive isolation, we expect to find biological mechanisms explaining the isolation (genitalia morphology, symbionts, pheromones, etc.).

These many aspects may be quantified in most cases, they need a multidisciplinary approach and a final consensus. They would converge to the hypothesis of an evolutionary lineage, or, conversely, to the idea of an intraspecific variation.

This information is crucial to define evolutionary species, but it is not needed by the above phylogenetic concepts of species, and even not by the biological concept. Rates of molecular (and/or morphological) divergence or acquisition of niche specializations may vary independently of the acquisition of reproductive isolation.[3] The reproductive isolation required by the biological and Hennigian concepts does not infer any amount of phenetic or genetic differences between species, nor do the two phylogenetic concepts care about any biological differences between taxa.

Thus, only the evolutionary concept would benefit from such multidisciplinary information, but this information does not exclude insights from phylogenetic studies or classical cross-breeding experiments.

## Recommendations

Such a beam of arguments should be more frequently used by entomologists to support their description of a new species. Thus morphological description, multilocus enzyme electrophoresis (MLEE), cytogenetics, DNA sequences, nuclear or mitochondrial levels of sequence divergence, as well as the amount of morphometric and APH differences, or any other approach, should not be used alone as a single argument to support species assignment.

Even in the case of multidisciplinary studies converging to the hypothesis of a separate evolutionary lineage, reaching a consensus about the idea of a new taxonomic name is not easy. A consensus indeed involves more than the use of various characterizing techniques, it requires to consider the quality of scientific communication and, for medically important insects, the epidemiological relevance of taxonomic changes.

With Schofield and Galvão[18] revising the taxonomy of Triatominae, we believe that in spite of discrepancies between typological and modern classifications, and especially for medically important insects, it is important to preserve the communication between operational teams. With Savage[139] and Wilkerson et al.[143] criticizing the too many taxonomic changes[138] required by the phylogeny of another group of vectors (the Aedinae), we recommend to entomologists to be particularly reluctant to create new genera for well-known species, suggesting them to create subgenera instead, if justified.

## Conclusion

Triatominae display a high degree of morphological plasticity,[21,22] which has been also referred to as "phenetic drift."[18] Because of that, entomologists face situations where morphological differences exist between groups (mainly size or/and color variation) without clear genetic support, and others where genetic variation seems important without morphological discriminating traits, or even without established reproductive isolation. Thus, morphological or genetic variation should not lead per se to the erection of a new species.

Consensually recognized evolutionary lineages should not be given a new name unless clear and usable morphological characters be described. Possible changes should be limited to very particular circumstances, they should be applied to morphologically diagnosable entities and should provide a benefit to the biological or to the epidemiological knowledge of the group.

## Acknowledgment

**ECLAT** http://eclat.fcien.edu.uy/.

## References

1. ICZN. International Code of Zoological Nomenclature, 4th edn. *ITZN London* 1999. 306pp. Available from: http://www.icznorg/iczn/index.jsp/.
2. Vrana P, Wheeler W. Individual organisms as terminal entities: laying the species problem to rest. *Cladistics* 1992;**8**:67−72.
3. Mayr E. The biological species concept. In: Wheeler Quenti D, Meier Rudolf, editors. *Species concepts and phylogenetic theory A debate*. New York: Columbia University Press; 2000p. 17−29.
4. Meier R, Willmann R. The Hennigian species concept. In: Wheeler Quenti D, Meier Rudolf, editors. *Species concepts and phylogenetic theory A debate*. New York: Columbia University Press; 2000. p. 30−43.
5. Mishler BD, Theriot EC. The phylogenetic species concept (*sensu* mishler and theriot): monophyly, apomorphy, and phylogenetic species concept. In: Wheeler Quenti D, Meier Rudolf, editors. *Species concepts and phylogenetic theory A debate. New York: Columbia University Press*; 2000. p. 44−54.
6. Wheeler QD, Platnick NI. The phylogenetic species concept (sensu wheeler and platnick). In: Wheeler Quenti D, Meier Rudolf, editors. *Species concepts and phylogenetic theory A debate*. New York: Columbia University Press; 2000. p. 55−69.
7. Lent H, Wygodzinsky P. Revision of the Triatominae (Hemiptera, Reduviidae), and their significance as vectors of Chagas disease. *Bull Am Museum Nat His* 1979;**163**:123−520.
8. Hypsa V, Tietz DF, Zrzavy J, Rego ROM, Galvao Cea. Phylogeny and biogeography of Triatominae (Hemiptera: Reduviidae): molecular evidence of a New World origin of the Asiatic clade. *Mol Phylogenet Evol* 2002;**23**:447−57.
9. Weirauch C. Cladistic analysis of Reduviidae (Heteroptera: Cimicomorpha) based on morphological characters. *Syst Entomol* 2008;**33**(2):229−74.
10. Weirauch C, Munro JB. Molecular phylogeny of the assassin bugs (Hemiptera: Reduviidae), based on mitochondrial and nuclear ribosomal genes. *Mol Phylogenet Evol* 2009;**53**:287−99.

11. Patterson JS, Gaunt MW. Phylogenetic multi-locus codon models and molecular clocks reveal the monophyly of haematophagous reduviid bugs and their evolution at the formation of South America. *Mol Phylogenet Evol* 2010;**56**(2):608−21.

12. Stevens L, Dorn PL, Schmidt JO, Klotz JH, Lucero D, Klotz SA. Kissing bugs. The vectors of Chagas. In: Weiss Louis M, Tanowitz Herbert B, Kirchhoff Louis V, editors. *Advances in parasitology*, Vol 75. *Burlington: Academic Press*; 2011. p. 169−92.

13. Schofield CJ. *Biosystematics of the Triatominae. Biosystematic of haematophagous insects Ed MW Service Systematics Assoc Special*, 37. *Oxford*: Clarendon Press; 1988. p. 284−312.

14. Tartarotti E, Ceron CR. Ribosomal DNA ITS-1 intergenic spacer polymorphism in triatomines (Triatominae, Heteroptera). *Biochem Genet* 2005;**43**:365−73.

15. de Paula AS, Diotaiuti L, Schofield CJ. Testing the sister-group relationship of the Rhodniini and Triatomini (Insecta: Hemiptera: Reduviidae: Triatominae). *Mol Phylogenet Evol* 2005;**35**:712−18.

16. Tartarotti E, Azeredo-Oliveira MT, Ceron CR. Phylogenetic approach to the study of triatomines (Triatominae, Heteroptera). *Braz J Biol* 2006;**66**:703−8.

17. Martinez FH, Villalobos GC, Cevallos AM, de la Torre PD, Laclette JP, Alejandre-Aguilar R, et al. Taxonomic study of the *Phyllosoma* complex and other triatomine (Insecta: Hemiptera: Reduviidae) species of epidemiological importance in the transmission of Chagas disease using ITS-2 and mtCytB sequences. *Mol Phylogenet Evol* 2006;**41**:279−87.

18. Schofield CJ, Galvão C. Classification, evolution, and species groups within the Triatominae. *Acta Trop* 2009;**110**:88−100.

19. Hwang WS, Weirauch C. Evolutionary history of assassin bugs (Insecta: Hemiptera: Reduviidae): insights from divergence dating and ancestral state reconstruction. *PLoS ONE* 2012;**7**(9):e45523. Available from: http://dx.doi.org/10.1371/journal.pone.0045523.

20. Zhang J, Gordon ER, Forthman M, Hwang WS, Walden K, Swanson D, et al. Evolution of the assassin's arms: insights from a phylogeny of combined transcriptomic and ribosomal DNA data (Heteroptera: Reduvioidea). *Sci Rep* 2016;**6**:22177.

21. Dujardin JP, Panzera P, Schofield CJ. Triatominae as a model of morphological plasticity under ecological pressure. *Mem Inst Oswaldo Cruz* 1999;**94**:223−8.

22. Dujardin JP, Costa J, Bustamante D, Jaramillo N, Catalá S. Deciphering morphology in Triatominae: the evolutionary signals. *Acta Trop* 2009;**110**:101−11.

23. Justi SA, Dale C, Galvão C. DNA barcoding does not separate South American *Triatoma* (Hemiptera: Reduviidae), Chagas disease vectors. *Parasit Vectors* 2014;**7**:519.

24. Forero D, Weirauch C, Baena M. Synonymy of the reduviid (Hemiptera: Heteroptera) genus *Torrealbaia* (Triatominae) with *Amphibolus* (Harpactorinae), with notes on *Amphibolus venator* (Klug, 1830). *Zootaxa* 2004;**670**:1−12.

25. Lent H. *Microtriatoma pratai* Sherlock & Guitton, 1982 é sinonimo do hemiptero predador *Aradomorpha championi* Lent & Wygodzinsky, 1944 (Reduviidae, Reduviinae). *Mem Inst Oswaldo Cruz* 1982;**77**:449−51.

26. Schofield CJ, Dolling WR. Bedbugs and kissing-bugs (bloodsucking Hemiptera). In: Lane RP, Crosskey RW, editors. *Medical Insects and Arachnids. London: Chapman and Hall*; 1993. p. 483−516.

27. Lorosa ES, Jurberg J, Souza AL, Vinhaes MC, Nunes I. Hemolinfa de *Dictyoptera* na manutenção do ciclo biológico silvestre de *Triatoma rubrovaria* (Blanchard, 1843) e *Triatoma circummaculata* (Stal, 1859) (Hemiptera, Reduviidae, Triatominae). *Entomol Vector* 2000;**7**:287−96.

28. Sandoval CM, Duarte R, Gutiérrez R, Rocha DS, Angulo VM, Esteban L, et al. Feeding sources and natural infection of *Belminus herreri* (Hemiptera, Reduviidae, Triatominae) from dwellings in Cesar, Colombia. *Mem Inst Oswaldo Cruz* 2004;**99**:137−40.

29. Sandoval CM, Pabon E, Jurberg J, Galvão C. *Belminus ferroae* n.sp. from the Colombian north-east, with a key to the species of the genus (Hemiptera: Reduviidae: Triatominae). *Zootaxa* 2007;**1443**:55−64.

30. Schofield CJ, Grijalva MJ, Diotaiuti L. Distribución de los vectores de la enfermedad de Chagas en pases "no endémicos": la posibilidad de transmisión vectorial fuera de América Latina. *Enfermed Emerg* 2009;**11**(Suppl. 1):20−7.

31. Dujardin JP, Schofield CJ, Panzera F. Los vectores de la enfermedad de chagas. investigaciones taxonómicas, biológicas y genéticas. *Acad R Sci Outre-Mer Class Sci Nat Méd* 2002.

32. Galvão C, de Paula S. Sistemática e evoluçao dos vectores. In: *Vetores da doença de Chagas no Brasil (Galvão, C, org) Série Zoologia Guias e manuais de identificaçao Curitiba: Sociedade Brasileira de Zoologia ISBN 978-85-98203-09-6*; 2014. p. 26−32.

33. Abad-Franch F, Monteiro FA. Molecular research and control of Chagas disease vectors. *An Acad Brasil Cien* 2005;**77**:437−54.

34. Bargues MD, Zuriaga MA, Mas-Coma S. Nuclear rDNA pseudogenes in Chagas disease vectors: evolutionary implications of a new 5.8S + ITS2 paralogous sequence marker in triatomines of North, Central and northern South America. *Infect Genet Evol* 2014;**21**:134−56.

35. Zuriaga MA, Mas-Coma S, Bargues MD. A nuclear ribosomal DNA pseudogene in triatomines opens a new research field of fundamental and applied implications in Chagas disease. *Mem Inst Oswaldo Cruz* 2015;**110**:353−62.

36. Mas-Coma S, Bargues M. Populations, hybrids and the systematic concepts of species and subspecies in Chagas disease triatomine vectors inferred from nuclear ribosomal and mitochondrial DNA. *Acta Trop* 2009;**110**:112−36.

37. Monteiro FA, Peretolchina T, Lazoski C, Harris K, Dotson EM, AbadFranch F, et al. Phylogeographic pattern and extensive mitochondrial dna divergence disclose a species complex within the Chagas disease vector *Triatoma dimidiata*. *PLoS ONE* 2013; **8**:e70974.

38. Gómez-Palacio A, Triana O, Jaramillo-O N, Dotson EM, Marcet PL. Eco-geographical differentiation among Colombian populations of the Chagas disease vector *Triatoma dimidiata* (Hemiptera: Reduviidae). *Infect Genet Evol* 2013;**20**:352−61.

39. Gómez-Palacio A, Triana O. Molecular evidence of demographic expansion of the Chagas disease vector *Triatoma dimidiata* (Hemiptera, Reduviidae, Triatominae) in Colombia. *PLoS Negl Trop Dis* 2014;**8**:e2734.

40. Fernández CJ, Pérez de Rosas AR, García BA. Variation in mitochondrial NADH dehydrogenase subunit 5 and NADH dehydrogenase subunit 4 genes in the Chagas disease vector *Triatoma infestans* (Hemiptera: Reduviidae). *Am J Trop Med Hyg* 2013;**88**:893−6.

41. Díaz S, Panzera F, Jaramillo-O N, Pérez R, Fernández R, Vallejo G, et al. Genetic, cytogenetic and morphological trends in the evolution of the *Rhodnius* (Triatominae: Rhodniini) trans-andean group. *PLoS ONE* 2014;**9**:e87493.

42. Martinez A, Carcavallo RU. Un nuevo Triatominae neotropical (Hemiptera: Reduviidae). *Fol Entomol Mexicana* 1977;**38**:109−10.

43. Carcavallo RU, Jurberg J, Lent H. *Torrealbaia martínezi*, gen. *nov. sp.n.*, da tribo Cavernicolini (Hemiptera, Reduviidae, Triatominae): uma abordagem filogenética. *Entomol Vector* 1998;**5**:143−50.

44. Sandoval CM, Joya MI, Gutierez R, Angulo VM. Cleptohaematophagy of the triatomine bug *Belminus herreri*. *Med Vet Entomol* 2000;**14**(1):100−1.

45. Patterson JS. *Comparative morphometric and molecular genetic analyses of Triatominae (Hemiptera: Reduviidae)*. PhD thesis. *University of London*; 2007.

46. Barrett TV, Arias JR. A new triatomine host of *Trypanosoma cruzi* from the central amazon of brasil: *Cavernicola lenti* n. sp. (Hemiptera, Reduviidae, Triatominae). *Mem Inst Oswaldo Cruz* 1985;**80**:91−6.

47. Santos FM, Jansen AM, Mourão GdM, Jurberg J, Nunes AP, Herrera HM. Triatominae (Hemiptera, Reduviidae) in the Pantanal region: association with *Trypanosoma cruzi*, different habitats and vertebrate hosts. *Rev Soc Bras Med Trop* 2015;**48**:532−8.

48. Marti GA, Echeverria MG, Waleckx E, Susevich ML, Balsalobre A, Gorla DE. Triatominae in furnariid nests of the Argentine Gran Chaco. *J Vector Ecol* 2014;**39**:66−71.

49. Turienzo P, Di Iorio O. Insects found in birds' nests from Argentina: *Coryphistera alaudina* Burmeister, 1860 (Aves: Furnariidae), their inquiline birds and mammals, new hosts for *Psammolestes coreodes* Bergroth, 1911 and *Triatoma platensis* Neiva, 1913 (Hemiptera: Reduviidae: Triatominae). *Zootaxa* 2014;**3811**:151−84.

50. Schofield CJ, Dujardin JP. Theories on the evolution of *Rhodnius*. *Actual Biol* 1999;**21**:183−97.

51. Abad-Franch F, Monteiro FA, Jaramillo NO, Gurgel-Gonçalves R, Dias FBS, Diotaiuti L. Ecology, evolution and the long-term surveillance of vector-borne Chagas disease: a multi-scale appraisal of the tribe rhodniini (triatominae). *Acta Trop* 2009;**110**:159−77.

52. Jurberg J. Morphology uma abordagem filogenetica entre os triatomineos baseada nas estructuras falicas. In: *Proceedings of the international workshop on population genetics and control of Triatominae Santo Domingo de los Colorados, Ecuador*; 1996. p. 43−4.

53. Monteiro FA, Lazoski C, Noireau F, Sole-Cava AM. Allozyme relationships among ten species of Rhodniini, showing paraphyly of *Rhodnius* including *Psammolestes*. *Med Vet Entomol* 2002;**16**(1):83−90.

54. Lyman DF, Monteiro FA, Escalante AA, Cordon-Rosales C, Wesson DM, Dujardin JP, et al. Mitochondrial DNA sequence variation among triatomine vectors of Chagas disease. *Am J Trop Med Hyg* 1999;**60**:377−86.

55. Monteiro FA, Wesson DM, Dotson EM, Schofield CJ, Beard CB. Phylogeny and molecular taxonomy of the Rhodniini derived from mitochondrial and nuclear DNA sequences. *Am J Trop Med Hyg* 2000;**62**(4):460−5.

56. Hypsa V, Tietz DF, Zrzavy J, Rego ROM, Galvão C, Jurberg J. Phylogeny and biogeography of Triatominae (Hemiptera : Reduviidae): molecular evidence of a New World origin of the Asiatic clade. *Mol Phylogenet Evol* 2002;**23**(3):447−57.

57. Usinger RL. The Triatominae of North and Central America and the West Indies and their public health significance. *Public Health Bulletin Washington* 1944;**288** 81pp.

58. García AG, Powell JR. Phylogeny of species of *Triatoma* (Hemiptera: Reduviidae) based on mitochondrial DNA sequences. *J Med Entomol* 1998;**3**:232−8.

59. Bargues MD, Marcilla A, Ramsey JM, Dujardin JP, Schofield CJ, Mas-Coma S. Nuclear rDNA-based molecular clock of the evolution of Triatominae (Hemiptera: Reduviidae), vectors of Chagas disease. *Mem Inst Oswaldo Cruz* 2000;**95**(4):567−74.

60. Silva de Paula A, Diotaiuti L, Schofield C. Testing the sister-group relationship of the Rhodniini and Triatomini (Insecta: Hemiptera: Reduviidae: Triatominae). *Mol Phylogenet Evol* 2005;**35**(3):712−18.

61. Panzera F, Pérez R, Panzera Y, Ferrandis I, Ferreiro MJ, Calleros L. Cytogenetics and genome evolution in the subfamily Triatominae (Hemiptera, Reduviidae). *Cytogenet Genome Res* 2010.

62. Ueshima N. Cytotaxonomy of the Triatominae (Reduviidae: Hemiptera). *Chromosoma (Berl)* 1966;**18**:97−122.

63. Lent H, Jurberg J, Galvao C. Revalidaçao do genero Mepraia, Mazza, Gajardo and Jorg, 1940 (Hemiptera, Reduviidae, Triatominae). *Mem Inst Oswaldo Cruz* 1994;**89**(3):347−52.

64. Garcia BA, Moriyama EN, Powell JR. Mitochondrial DNA sequences of triatomines (Hemiptera : Reduviidae): phylogenetic relationships. *J Med Entomol* 2001.

65. Marcilla A, Bargues MD, Ramsey JM, Magallon-Gastelum E, SalazarSchettino PM, Abad-Franch F, et al. The ITS-2 of the nuclear rDNA as a molecular marker for populations, species, and phylogenetic relationships in Triatominae (Hemiptera: Reduviidae), vectors of Chagas disease. *Mol Phylogenet Evol* 2001;**18**(1):136—42.

66. Pfeiler E, Bitler BG, Ramsey JM, Palacios-Cardiel C, Markow TA. Genetic variation, population structure, and phylogenetic relationships of *Triatoma rubida* and *T. recurva* (Hemiptera: Reduviidae: Triatominae) from the Sonoran desert, insect vectors of the Chagas' disease parasite *Trypanosoma cruzi. Mol Phylogenet Evol* 2006;**41**(1):209—21.

67. Bargues MD, Klisiowicz DR, Gonzalez-Candelas F, Ramsey JM, Monroy C, Ponce C, et al. Phylogeography and genetic variation of *Triatoma dimidiata*, the main Chagas disease vector in Central America, and its position within the genus *Triatoma. PLoS Negl Trop Dis* 2008;**2**(5):e233.

68. Martinez-Hernandez F, Martinez-Ibarra JA, Catalá S, Villalobos G, de la Torre P, Laclette JP, et al. Natural crossbreeding between sympatric species of the Phyllosoma complex (Insecta: Hemiptera: Reduviidae) indicate the existence of only one species with morphologic and genetic variations. *Am J Trop Med Hyg* 2010;**82**(1):74—82.

69. Bargues MD, Marcilla A, Dujardin JP, Mas-Coma S. Triatomine vectors of *Trypanosoma cruzi* : a molecular perspective based on nuclear ribosomal DNA markers. *Trans R Soc Trop Med Hyg* 2002;**96**(Suppl. I):159—64.

70. Carcavallo RU, Jurberg J, Lent H, Noireau F, Galvão C. Phylogeny of the Triatominae (Hemiptera, Reduviidae). Proposals for taxonomic arrangements. *Entomol Vector* 2000; **7**(Suppl. 1):1—99.

71. Patterson JS, Schofield CJ, Dujardin JP, Miles MA. Population morphometric analysis of the tropicopolitan bug *Triatoma rubrofasciata* and relationships with Old World species of *Triatoma*: evidence of New World ancestry. *Med Vet Entomol* 2001; **15**(4):443—51.

72. Gorla DE, Dujardin JP, Schofield CJ. Biosystematics of Old World Triatominae. *Acta Trop* 1997;**63**:127—40.

73. Dujardin JP, Pham Thi K, Truong Xuan L, Panzera F, Pita S, Schofield CJ. Epidemiological status of kissing-bugs in South East Asia: a preliminary assessment. *Acta Trop* 2015;**151**:142—9.

74. Hennig W. Phylogenetic systematics. *Annu Rev Entomol* 1965;**10**:97—116.

75. Wiley EO. The evolutionary species concept reconsidered. *Syst Zool* 1978;**27**:17—26.

76. Wiley EO, Mayden RL. The Evolutionary Species Concepts. In: Wheeler Quentin D, Meier Rudolf, editors. *Species concepts and phylogenetic theory A debate*. New York: Columbia University Press; 2000. p. 70—92.

77. Bérenger JM, Pluot-Sigwalt D. *Rhodnius amazonicus* Almeida, Santos & Spozina, 1973, bona species, close to *R. pictipes* Stal, 1872 (Heteroptera: Reduviidae, Triatominae). *Mem Inst Oswaldo Cruz* 2002;**97**(1):73—7.

78. Galvão AB, Palma JD. Uma nova espécie do genero *Panstrongylus* berg, 1879 (Reduviidae, Triatominae). *Rev Brasil Biol* 1968;**28**:403—5.

79. Martínez AJ, Carcavallo RU, Jurberg J. *Triatoma gomeznunezi* a new species of Triatomini from Mexico (Hemiptera, Reduviidae, Triatominae). *Entomol Vector* 1994;**1**:15—19.

80. Pereira J, Dujardin JP, Salvatella R, Tibayrenc M. Enzymatic variability and phylogenetic relatedness among *Triatoma infestans, T. platensis, T. delpontei* and *T. rubrovaria. Heredity* 1996;**77**:47—54.

81. Bargues MD, Klisiowicz DR, Panzera F, Noireau F, Marcilla A, Perez R, et al. Origin and phylogeography of the Chagas disease main vector *Triatoma infestans* based on nuclear rDNA sequences and genome size. *Infect Genet Evol* 2006;**6**:46−62.

82. Barata JMS. Eggshell architecture. In: *Proceedings of the international workshop on population genetics and control of Triatominae Santo Domingo de los Colorados, Ecuador*; 1995. p. 47−50.

83. Catalá SS. Los patrones de sensilla en Triatominae. In: *Proceedings of the international workshop on population genetics and control of Triatominae Santo Domingo de los Colorados, Ecuador*; 1995. p. 51−4.

84. Catalá SS. Sensilla associated with the rostrum of eight species of Triatominae. *J Morphol* 1996;**228**(2):195−201.

85. Baylac M, Villemant C, Simbolotti G. Combining geometric morphometrics with pattern recognition for the investigation of species complexes. *Biol J Linnean Soc* 2003;**80**(1):89−98.

86. Dujardin JP. Morphometrics applied to medical entomology. *Infect Genet Evol* 2008;**8**:875−90.

87. Panzera F, Hornos S, Pereira J, Cestau R, Canale D, Diotaiuti L, et al. Genetic variability and geographic differentiation among three species of Triatominae bugs (Hemiptera: Reduviidae). *Am J Trop Med Hyg* 1997;**57**(6):732−9.

88. Noireau F, Gutierrez T, Zegarra M, Flores R, Brenière F, Dujardin JP. Cryptic speciation in *Triatoma sordida* (Hemiptera: Reduviidae) from the Bolivian Chaco. *Trop Med Int Health* 1998;**3**(5):364−72.

89. Panzera F, Ferrandis I, Ramsey J, Ordonez R, Salazar-Schettino PM, Cabrera M, et al. Chromosomal variation and genome size support existence of cryptic species of *Triatoma dimidiata* with different epidemiological importance as Chagas disease vectors. *Trop Med Int Health* 2006;**11**:1092−103.

90. Larousse F. Etude biologique et systématique du genre *Rhodnius* Stal. *Ann Parasitol* 1927;**5**:63−88.

91. Chippaux JP, Pajot FX, Geoffroy B, Tavakilian G. Etude préliminaire sur l'écologie et la systématique des triatomes (Hemiptera, Reduviidae) de guyane française. *Cah ORSTOM Ent med Parasitol* 1985;**III**(2):75−85.

92. Matias A, De la Riva JX, Torrez M, Dujardin JP. *Rhodnius robustus* in Bolivia identified by its wings. *Mem Inst Oswaldo Cruz* 2001;**96**(7):947−50.

93. Villegas J, Feliciangeli MD, Dujardin JP. Wing shape divergence between *Rhodnius prolixus* from Cojedes (Venezuela) and *R. robustus* from Mérida (Venezuela). *Infect Genet Evol* 2002;**2**:121−8.

94. Gurgel-Gonçalves R, Abad-Franch F, Ferreira JBC, Santana DB, Cuba CAC. Is *Rhodnius prolixus* (triatominae) invading houses in central brazil ?. *Acta Trop* 2008;**107**:90−8.

95. Pavan MG, Monteiro FA. A multiplex PCR assay that separates *Rhodnius prolixus* from members of the *Rhodnius robustus* cryptic species complex (Hemiptera: Reduviidae). *Trop Med Int Health* 2007;**12**(6):751−8.

96. Mayr E. *Principles of systematic zoology. New York: McGraw-Hill*; 1969.

97. Paterson HEH. The recognition concept of species. In: Vrba ES, editor. *Species and speciation, monograph Pretoria*, 4. Transvaal Museum; 1985. p. 21−9.

98. Templeton AR. The meaning of species and speciation: a genetic perspective. In: Otte D, Endler JA, editors. *Speciation and its consequences*. Sunderland, England: Sinnauer Associates; 1989. p. 3−27.

99. Templeton AR. The role of molecular genetics in speciation studies. In: Schierwater B, et al. , editors. *Molecular Ecology and Evolution*. Basel, Switzerland: Birkhauser; 1994. p. 455−77.

100. Costa J, Almeida CE, Dujardin JP, Beard CB. Crossing exper iments detect genetic incompatibility among populations of *Triatoma brasiliensis* Neiva, 1911 (Heteroptera, Reduviidae, Triatominae). *Mem Inst Oswaldo Cruz* 2003;**98**(5):637−9.
101. Marcilla A, Bargues MD, Abad-Franch F, Panzera F, Carcavallo RU, Noireau F, et al. Nuclear rDNA ITS-2 sequences reveal polyphyly of *Panstrongylus* species (Hemiptera: Reduviidae: Triatominae), vectors of *Trypanosoma cruzi*. *Infect Genet Evol* 2002;**26**:1−11.
102. Dujardin JP, Chavez T, Moreno JM, Machane M, Noireau F, Schofield CJ. Comparison of isoenzyme electrophoresis and morphometric analysis for phylogenetic reconstruction of the Rhodniini (Hemiptera: Reduviidae: Triatominae). *J Med Entomol* 1999;**36**:653−9.
103. Cracraft J. Species concepts in theoretical and applied biology: a systematic debate with consequences. In: Wheeler Quentin D, Meier Rudolf, editors. *Species concepts and phylogenetic theory A debate*. New York: Columbia University Press; 2000p. 3−16.
104. Wheeler QD, Meier R, editors. *Species concepts and phylogenetic theory. A debate*. New York: Columbia University Press; 2000. vol. 230pp.
105. Usinger RL, Wygodzinsky P, Ryckman RE. The biosystematics of Triatominae. *Annu Rev Entomol* 1966;**11**:309−30.
106. Barrett TV. Advances in triatomine bug ecology in relation to Chagas disease. *Adv Dis Vector Res* 1991;**8**(6):142−76.
107. Costa J, Peterson AT, Dujardin JP. Indirect evidences suggest homoploid hybridization as a possible mode of speciation in Triatominae (Hemiptera, Heteroptera, Reduviidae). *Infect Genet Evol* 2008;**9**(2):263−70.
108. Barrett TV. Species interfertility and crossing experiments in triatomine systematics. In: *Proceedings of the international workshop on population genetics and control of Triatominae Santo Domingo de los Colorados, Ecuador*; 1995. p. 57−62.
109. Funk VA. Phylogenetic patterns and hybridization. *Ann Missouri Bot Garden* 1985;**72**:681−715.
110. Smith GR. Introgression in fishes: significance for paleontology, cladistics, and evolutionary rates. *Syst Biol* 1992;**41**:41−57.
111. Harry M, Galíndez I, Carriou ML. Isozyme variability and differentiation between *Rhodnius prolixus*, *R. robustus*, and *R. pictipes*, vectors of Chagas disease in Venezuela. *Med Vet Entomol* 1992;**6**:37−43.
112. Harry M. Isozymic data question the specific status of some bloodsucking bugs of the genus *Rodnius*, vectors of Chagas disease. *Trans R Soc Trop Med Hyg* 1993;**87**:492.
113. Pavan MG, Mesquita RD, Lawrence GG, Lazoski C, Dotson EM, Abubucker S, et al. A nuclear single-nucleotide polymorphism (SNP) potentially useful for the separation of *Rhodnius prolixus* from members of the *Rhodnius robustus* cryptic species complex (hemiptera: Reduviidae). *Infec Genet Evol* 2013;**14**:426−33.
114. Dujardin JP, Kaba D, Solano P, Dupraz M, McCoy KD, Jaramillo-O N. Outline-based morphometrics, an overlooked method in arthropod studies? *IGE* 2014. Available from: http://dx.doi.org/10.1016/j.meegid.2014.07.035.
115. Costa J, Freitas-Sibajev MG, Marchon-Silva V, Pires MQ, Pacheco R. Isoenzymes detect variation in populations of *Triatoma brasiliensis* (Hemiptera, Reduviidae, Triatominae). *Mem Inst Oswaldo Cruz RJ* 1997;**92**:459−64.
116. Monteiro FA, Costa J, Solé-Cava AM. Genetic confirmation of the specific status of *Triatoma petrochii* (Hemiptera: Reduviidae: Triatominae). *Ann Trop Med Parasitol* 1998;**92**(8):897−900.
117. Noireau F, Menezes dos Santos S, Gumiel M, Dujardin JP, dos Santos Soares M, Carcavallo RU, et al. Phylogenetic relationships within the oliveirai complex (Hemiptera: Reduviidae: Triatominae). *Infect Genet Evol* 2002;**2**:11−17.

118. Panzera F, Perez R, Panzera Y, Alvarez F, Scvortzoff E, Salvatella R. Karyotype evolution in holocentric chromosomes of three related species of triatomines (Hemiptera-Reduviidae). *Chromosome Res* 1995;**3**:143−50.

119. Gumiel M, Catalá S, Noireau F, de Arias AR, Garcia A, Dujardin JP. Wing geometry in *Triatoma infestans* (Klug) and *T. melanosoma* Martinez, Olmedo and Carcavallo (Hemiptera: Reduviidae). *Syst Entomol* 2003;**28**(2):173−9.

120. Lent H, Jurberg J, Galvão C, Carcavallo RU. *Triatoma melanosoma*, novo status para *Triatoma infestans melanosoma* Martinez, Olmedo and Carcavallo, 1987 (Hemiptera: Reduviidae). *Mem Inst Oswaldo Cruz* 1994;**89**(3):353−8.

121. Lent H, Jurberg J, Galvão C. Un sinónimo para *Triatoma melanosoma* Martinez, Olmedo and Carcavallo, 1987 (Hemiptera, Reduviidae). *Entomol Vector* 1995;**2**:81−2.

122. Monteiro FA, Perez R, Panzera F, Dujardin JP, Galvão C, Rocha D, et al. Mitochondrial DNA variation of *Triatoma infestans* populations and its implication on the specific status of *T. melanosoma*. *Mem Inst Oswaldo Cruz* 1999;**94**(Suppl. I):229−38.

123. Noireau F, Flores R, Gutierrez T, Dujardin JP. Detection of silvatic dark morphs of *Triatoma infestans* in the Bolivian Chaco. *Mem Inst Oswaldo Cruz RJ* 1997;**92**(5):583−4.

124. Noireau F, Bastrenta B, Catalá S, Dujardin JP, Panzera F, Torres M, et al. Sylvatic population of *Triatoma infestans* from the bolivian chaco: From field collection to characterization. *Mem Inst Oswaldo Cruz* 2000;**95**(Suppl. 1):119−22.

125. Catalá SS, Torres M. Similitude of the patterns of sensilla on the antennae of *Triatoma melanosoma* and *Triatoma infestans*. *Ann Trop Med Parasitol* 2001;**95**(3):287−95.

126. Jurberg J, Galváo C, Lent H, Monteiro F, Lopes CM, Panzera F, et al. Revalidaçáo de *Triatoma garciabesi* Carcavallo, Cichero, Martínez, Prosen and Ronderos, 1967 (Hemiptera-Reduviidae). *Entomol Vector* 1998;**5**:107−22.

127. Panzera F, Pita S, Nattero J, Panzera Y, Galvão C, Chavez T, et al. Cryptic speciation in the *Triatoma sordida* subcomplex (Hemiptera, Reduviidae) revealed by chromosomal markers. *Parasit Vectors* 2015;**8**:495.

128. Monteiro FA, Donnelly MJ, Beard C, Costa J. Nested clade and phylogeographic analyses of the Chagas disease vector *Triatoma brasiliensis* in Northeast Brazil. *Mol Phylogenet Evol* 2004;**32**:46−56.

129. Costa J, Bargues MD, Neiva VL, Lawrence GG, Gumiel M, Oliveira G, et al. Phenotypic variability confirmed by nuclear ribosomal DNA suggests a possible natural hybrid zone of *Triatoma brasiliensis* species complex. *Infect Genet Evol* 2016;**37**:77−87.

130. Calleros L, Panzera F, Bargues MD, Monteiro FA, Klisiowicz DR, Zuriaga MA, et al. Systematics of *Mepraia* (Hempitera Reduviidae): cytogenetic and molecular variation. *Infect Genet Evol* 2009. Available from: http://dx.doi.org/10.1016/j.meegid.2009.12.002.

131. Frías DA, Henry AA, Gonzalez CR. *Mepraia gajardoi*: a new species of Triatominae (Hemiptera: Reduviidae) from Chile and its comparison with *Mepraia spinolai*. *Rev Chil Hist Nat* 1998;**71**:177−88.

132. Bustamante DM, Monroy C, Menes M, Rodas A, Salazar-Schettino PM, Rojas G, et al. Metric variation among geographic populations of the Chagas vector *Triatoma dimidiata* (Hemiptera: Reduviidae: Triatominae) and related species. *J Med Entomol* 2004;**41**(3):296−301.

133. Dorn PL, Calderón C, Melgar S, Moguel B, Solorzano E, Dumonteil E, et al. Two distinct *Triatoma dimidiata* (latreille, 1811) taxa are found in sympatry in Guatemala and Mexico. *PLoS Negl Trop Dis* 2009;**3**(3):e393.

134. Catalá SS, Sachetto C, Moreno M, Rosales R, Salazar-Schettino PM, Gorla D. The antennal phenotype of *Triatoma dimidiata* populations and its relationship with species of the phyllosoma and protracta complexes. *J Med Entomol* 2005;**42**:719−25.

135. Calderón FG, Juarez MP, Ramsey J, Salazar-Schettino PM, Monroy C, Ordonez R, et al. Cuticular hydrocarbon variability among *Triatoma dimidiata* (Hemiptera: Reduviidae) populations from Mexico and Guatemala. *J Med Entomol* 2005;**42**:780−8.

136. Gómez-Palacio A, Arboleda S, Dumonteil E, Peterson AT. Ecological niche and geographic distribution of the Chagas disease vector, *Triatoma dimidiata* (Reduviidae: Triatominae): evidence for niche differentiation among cryptic species. *Infect Genet Evol* 2015;**36**:15−22.

137. Abad-Franch F, Paucar A, Carpio C, Cuba-Cuba CA, Aguilar HM, Miles MA. Biogeography of Triatominae (Hemiptera: Reduviidae) in Ecuador: implications for the design of control strategies. *Mem Inst Oswaldo Cruz* 2001;**96**:611−20.

138. Reinert JF, Harbach RE, Kitching IJ. Phylogeny and classification of *Aedini* (Diptera: Culicidae), based on morphological characters of all life stages. *Zool J Linn Soc* 2004;**142**:289−368.

139. Savage HM. Classification of mosquitoes in tribe Aedini (Diptera: Culicidae): Paraphylyphobia, and classification versus cladistic analysis. *J Med Entomol* 2005; **42**(6):923−7.

140. Schluter D. Ecology and the origin of species. *Trends Ecol Evol* 2001;**16**(7):372−80.

141. Van Valen L. Ecological species, multispecies, and oaks. *Taxon* 1976;**25**:233−9.

142. Wiley EO, Mayden RL. A defense of the Evolutionary Species Concepts. In: Wheeler Quentin D, Meier Rudolf, editors. *Species concepts and phylogenetic theory a debate*. New York: Columbia University Press; 2000. p. 198−208.

143. Wilkerson RC, Linton YM, Fonseca DM, Schultz TR, Price DC, Strickman DA. Making mosquito taxonomy useful: a stable classification of tribe Aedini that balances utility with current knowledge of evolutionary relationships. *PLoS ONE* 2015. Available from: http://dx.doi.org/10.1371/journal.pone.0133602.

# Biology of Triatominae

*S.S. Catalá[1], F. Noireau[2,†] and J.-P. Dujardin[2]*
[1]CRILAR-CONICET, Centro Regional de Investigación Científica de La Rioja, Anillaco (La Rioja), Argentina, [2]Institut de Recherche pour le Développement (IRD), UMR 177 Intertryp, Montpellier, France

**7**

## Chapter Outline

## Introduction

Of the 140 species of Triatominae currently recognized,[1] research has traditionally concentrated on those of greatest epidemiological significance as domestic vectors of *Trypanosoma cruzi*, the agent of Chagas disease. It means only a few of them, mainly *Triatoma infestans*, *Triatoma brasiliensis*, and *Panstrongylus megistus* from

---

[†] Deceased.

American Trypanosomiasis Chagas Disease. DOI: http://dx.doi.org/10.1016/B978-0-12-801029-7.00007-1

the Southern Cone countries, and *Rhodnius prolixus* and *Triatoma dimidiata* from the Andean Pact countries and parts of Central America. These five species, the main vectors of Chagas disease, represent 3 genera in 2 tribes, while the Triatominae are admittedly composed of 17 genera and 5 tribes. Our knowledge on the biology of Triatominae is thus obviously fragmentary.

Most of the Triatominae are found in the New World, a very few others in the Old World. They are hematophagous bugs living in close association with their silvatic hosts in habitats such as palm-tree crowns, bird nests, rodent burrows, opossum lodges, and rockpiles. For some genera, the classification of Triatominae reflects these associations, with for instance the *Rhodnius* adapted to the palm-trees, the *Psammolestes* living in bird nests, the *Panstrongylus* and *Paratriatoma* associated with burrows. However, with a very few exceptions, these species are opportunistic and feed on other hosts too, including the human host.

Since one of their commonly observed behaviors is to enter domestic and peridomestic structures ("intrusion," see "Intrusion" section), with some of them trying to colonize the human habitat ("domiciliation," see "Domiciliation" section), the silvatic species of Triatominae represent a possible source of infection by *T. cruzi*, so that they deserve much more interest. Due to their generally nocturnal habits and hidden refuges, they may be hard to collect in the field. In this regard, the design of a new trapping device was a welcome initiative.[2]

# General biology of vectors

The domestic vector species are generally easy to rear in the laboratory, and have provided excellent models for fundamental studies of insect physiology as well as studies related to their control. In recent years, they have also been used for studies of population genetics and basic evolutionary trends, largely linked to their process of adaptation to human dwellings which is seen as a future risk for transmission of *T. cruzi* by less well-known triatomine species.

Thus, a few species have adapted to the domestic structures ("domestication," see "Domestication" section) and represent the main providers of human Chagas disease. The biology of these species received most of the attention of the biologists, and what will follow is mainly related to them. They belong to two tribes: the Triatominii and the Rhodniini. Whether the Triatominae is a *monophyletic*,[3−7] *polyphyletic*,[1,8−12] or *paraphyletic* group,[13] these two tribes have already been proved to be very different in many aspects. Therefore, what is known in one tribe should not be generalized and applied to the other tribe. Anyway, domestic populations of Triatominae, whatever their tribal origin, tend to show a similar adapting behavior. This chapter deals mainly with domestic populations, and mentions otherwise references to silvatic species.

## *Development*

Triatominae are *exopterigote* insects. There is no pupal stage and metamorphosis is described as incomplete (hemimetabolous insects). The five successive immature stages increasingly resemble the adult, and rudimentary wings are apparent only in later stages. The cycle is composed of eggs, five nymph stages, and the male and female imagos. At temperatures between 20°C and 30°C, the development takes approximately 5–6 months, but this can vary according to species. Nymphs differ from the adults primarily by their lack of fully developed wings or genitalia, although they generally occupy the same habitat and feed on the same hosts as the adults. For Triatominae, this means that all five nymphal stages, and both sexes of adult, feed on vertebrate blood and are capable of becoming infected and transmitting *T. cruzi*.

The eggs are ellipsoid in shape and have an operculum. Most cells of the envelope are pentagonal, presenting a texture with some taxonomic importance.[14] The shape of the opercule can discriminate *Rhodnius* species.[15] Ongoing research suggests that the geometry of the eggs outline discriminates not only species, but also microhabitat or communities (Santillan et al., personal communication). The eggs are white at the oviposition, then pink, becoming darker with hardening of chitin, and finally dark when arrived at maturity. The hatching occurs generally 10–40 days after oviposition.

After a few days the hatched nymphs are able to have their first blood meal. One nymph is able to take a quantity of blood equivalent to eight to nine times its own weight. Blood taking may last 20 min for a fifth nymph (and an adult). If the quantity of blood is sufficient, the wall distension may produce a nervous stimulus to initiate molt to the next stage. At the end of the blood intake, the nymph will generally deposit urine and excreta on the host's skin. If the blood contains *T. cruzi*, it can be transmitted to the host. If blood taking is interrupted by the movements of the host or under other circumstances, there will be no defecation and the molt is not initiated.

Adult Triatominae can generally be distinguished from other reduviids by the straight, slender, three-segmented *proboscis* adpressed to the underside of the cone-shaped head, which reaches the prosternal *stridulatory sulcus* in all genera except *Cavernicola* and *Linshcosteus*.

By contrast, the proboscis of predatory reduviids is often curved, and usually more heavily chitinized. However, many predatory Reduviidae especially of the subfamily Reduviinae (around 1000 species) can appear very similar to Triatominae.

Thus, blood intake must be complete to trigger molt. Domestic bugs generally feed on sleeping hosts to reduce the likeliness of blood meal interruption. When there are many bug feeding on the same host, domestic animal or human, the host's skin will present local allergic reaction. The skin reaction has been shown to be repulsive for bugs, interrupting blood feeding or discouraging tentatives of blood taking. It is thus understandable that in the case of high population density, which is relatively common for domestic bugs (see "Density" section), many bugs will have a delay in their development, with particular consequences on population dynamics (see "Population Dynamics" section). Interrupted blood feeding also means failure to transmit the parasite if present in the intestine.

On average, the time length of a development cycle goes from a few months (*Rhodnius prolixus, Triatoma infestans*) to more than one year (*Triatoma dimidiata, Panstrongylus megistus, Dipetalogaster maximus*). This is depending on population density, as explained above, but also on external parameters such as temperature in domestic[16,17] and silvatic[18] species.

## Reproduction

Copulation lasts between 5 and 15 min, male in dorso-lateral position on female. Eggs are deposited 10–30 days after successful copulation. They can be laid individually one after the other during the whole life of the female (e.g., *T. infestans*), mainly in the burrow and saxicolous species. The eggs do not glue to the substract, except in some species and in the Rhodniini, where they also can be deposited in sets (*Psammolestes arthuri*).

The reproductive parameters of Triatominae are strongly affected by temperature, population density, and blood feeding.

Reduced or absent oviposition is very common at low temperature both in laboratory[19] and field.[16] Experiments carried out on *T. infestans* fifth-instar nymphs and adults exposed to a temperature of 12°C for 10 days showed that, in nymphs, gametic cell proliferation decreased under low temperature while spermatid production was inhibited. These effects were reversed at optimal temperature. In adults, a decrease in male accessory glands secretion was induced under low temperatures and this was directly related to blood consumption reduction. In spite of the recovery of mating behavior when temperature increased the accessory glands continued to produce inadequate quantities of secretion. Consequently, small spermatophores were produced and a diminution in fertility was observed.[20] Suboptimal temperatures are very frequent in endemic areas of *T. infestans*.

A single female of *T. infestans* oviposits around one to three hundreds of eggs during its life, but depending on density conditions it can oviposit a few times more. Under similar conditions of feeding, one female will oviposit a lot more eggs if the population density is low. Fecundity, as well as the developmental cycle, is densito-dependent (see "Density" section).

The number of eggs is also nicely correlated to the quantity of blood which has been ingested: blood availability and fecundity are tightly linked. It was shown that in *T. infestans* a minimum of 150 mg of blood consumption is necessary to start egg laying. Moreover, each laid egg means 12 mg of consumed blood.[21] Fifty percent reduction of fresh blood consumption could easily explain the lack of egg laying in females at low temperature. Looking at natural field conditions, this drastic decrease of blood consumption speed at low temperature[22] could explain the strong effect of winter upon population density.[17] Even with available food within the crop low temperatures break down blood consumption and, as in fasted insects, disrupts reproduction and the molting process.

Females can be fecundated by more than one male.[23] The use of a genetic marker allowed[24] to show that although a single mating can provide sufficient sperm for the whole reproductive life of the female *T. infestans*, multiple matings can result in balanced assortative sperm usage from the spermatheca.

## Hematophagy

As a general rule, all Triatominae are hematophagous. This character is actually the one defining the subfamily, with likely related morphological characters of the head such as a narrow and straight line rostrum with an articular membrane between second and third segment[3] but see also Ref.[25].

In the hypothesis of polyphyly, other Hemiptera should show some hematophagic habits, such as observed in *Clerada apicicornis* (Hemiptera: Lygaeidae)[26] or *Cryptophysoderes* (Physoderinae), and the characters defining the subfamily Triatominae would then be considered as an evolutionary convergence. In the alternative hypothesis of monophyly,[3−7] the ancestor should already have these characters[3]; suggesting the Physoderinae as a possible candidate. In the same hypothesis of polyphyly, some Triatominae should show also significant predatory habits; such behavior has been reported various times (see "Survival Strategy" section and Fig. 7.1).

The hematophagy is not restricted to one sex as in mosquitoes or sandflies for instance; it is obligatory for both males and females, as well as for each of the five nymphal stages. Exceptions to an exclusive hematophagy are also expected in the hypothesis of polyphyly. There are situations where nymphs, and sometimes adults, still can feed or try to feed on other invertebrates or arthropods, suggesting their remote ancestry as predators.[8] Nymphs of the silvatic *Eratyrus mucronatus* (Triatomini) or adult *T. circummaculata* may feed on other insects. The bugs may starve for more than 1 month: in our experience, some specimens of *T. infestans* could survive up to 9 months without blood meal.

In domestic Triatominae, at temperatures between 20°C and 30°C, the frequency of blood meal is around 1 meal per 4−9 days.[22] Experiments under natural conditions in experimental chicken houses indicated that one chicken may suffer no more than four bites during the winter months but over 30 bites per day during the hottest months of summer. Thus, blood consumption was strongly modified by temperature. A subsequent determination of the biting rate in an experimental system with mammals (guinea pigs) confirmed the results obtained with chickens.[22] In this experiment, the number of bug bites that each guinea pig received increased significantly during December and April, showing a strong temperature dependence.

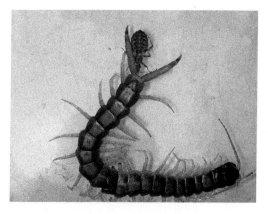

**Figure 7.1** *Triatoma brasiliensis* nymphal instar feeding on the hemolymph of an immobilized *Scolopendra*.

The same experiments allowed an estimation of the number of bites that a guinea pig required to be infected with *T. cruzi*.[27]

Adults typically take three to five times their body weight of blood at each meal if allowed to engorge. Thus during adult life, a female *T. infestans* will ingest about 10 g of blood, while larger species such as *P. megistus* may take twice this amount. In the laboratory, a female *D. maximus* has been recorded ingesting 4.5 g of blood in a single feed. From the amount of blood ingested, it is deduced that domestic infestations of Triatominae can make a significant contribution to chronic iron-deficiency anemia.[28] Calculations based on studies of *R. prolixus* in Venezuela, and *T. infestans* in Brazil, suggest that each person in a typically infested house is losing an average of about 2.5 g of blood per day due to the feeding bugs.[29]

In most Triatominae, including silvatic ones, it is worth noting a relative lack of host specificity in the feeding habits. Almost any vertebrate blood appears to be welcome, and different animals can be used in the laboratory to feed Triatominae. First instar nymphs may even feed on their older brothers or on their fathers when these latter are fully alimented (kleptohematophagy).[30] Exceptions to this lack of specificity are observed in the genus *Psammolestes* (silvatic species of Rhodniini associated with some birds), or in other silvatic bugs like *Triatoma delpontei*, associated with the parrot *Monacha* sp. or the tropicopolitan *T. rubrofasciata* found in domestic structures but feeding preferentially on rodents. Rodents are also the preferred host of the North American protracta group of bugs and *Paratriatoma hirsuta*. In the Cavernicoli tribe, *Cavernicola pilosa* also has restricted host preferences.

## Habitat

In silvatic as well as in domestic species, the behavior is generally similar: the insect seeks body contact with the elements of the habitat (wall, etc.), a feature called thygmotropism. The insect remains hidden inside its refuge (cracks, crevices, etc.) without movement during daylight hours (ataxia) so that it is not visible during the day.[31] When obscurity is coming, then it may move (walking) to look for blood.

As a general rule, and not only for domestic insects, the habitat of a Triatominae offers shelter conditions, easy access to blood, and some stability of hosts. For arboreal species it is bird nests or the crown of palm trees, but for other species with terrestrial habits it is rodent burrows or marsupial lodges. The association is not a strict one, some arboreal species may sometimes be found in other places. What seems more important than the habitat structure is the host availability.

The human habitat (and peridomestic dependencies) gives some Triatominae the best features such as stability, shelter, and blood abundance and availability. In rural areas, the domestic animals frequently are protected with wood and other natural elements which could attract some silvatic species because of some similarities with their own silvatic habitats. However, domestic species do not seem to depend on the habitat structure or composition; again, what seems important is the host availability. Human bodies provide a large amount of blood and occupy their habitat for more of the time.

## Dispersion

Studies about dispersion are important in Chagas epidemiology in order to clarify the dynamics of house invasion and colonization. However, field research in natural scenarios is not an easy task and involve some ethical problems.

In 1971 Forattini et al.[32] warned of the need to pay more attention to dispersive processes of Triatominae when they found, after a year, 2 adults and 198 nymphs of *T. infestans* in an experimental poultry house located 200 m away from any dwelling in Sao Paulo (Brazil). In a similar experiment colonization was observed by *Rhodnius neglectus* in experimental hen houses located in a palm grove and *Panstrongylus megistus* in residual vegetation surrounding homes.

It is important to distinguish in Triatominae two dispersion modes: the passive and the active ones. Passive dispersion is transportation of generally immature stages by the animal host (eggs gluing on the feathers for instance) or with the familiar objects carried or worn by the human host (even a hat). Active transportation is ensured by both walking (nymphs, but also adults) and flying.

### Active dispersion

Here is maybe one aspect of the biology of Triatominae, together with population density, where we can find clear-cut differences between domestic and silvatic species. Active dispersion is performed not only by flying,[33,34] but also, and perhaps more frequently in domestic species, by walking.

Domestic adult bugs when discovered in their hiding place do not fly, they try to escape by walking. In silvatic conditions, the same bug discovered under a stone might decide to walk away, or might remain absolutely immobile, simulating a dead body. This behavior was observed by one of us (JPD) for silvatic *T. infestans* in the Cochabamba (Bolivia) foci, probably because in silvatic situation and not in domestic places the bug is surrounded by predators and cannot beat them at running. Some silvatic species are able however to immediately take flight if disturbed, like *Parabelminus yurupucu* and *Microtriatoma trinidadensis*.[35]

The active dispersal of *T. infestans* and other *Triatoma* species was measured recently by Abrahan et al.[36] using light traps (for flying insects) and sticky dispersal barriers (for walking insects) within rural courtyards. Monthly catches were made on 30 nights in the warm season. Despite continuous and strong capture efforts a total of 8 flying adults, 6 walking nymphs, and 10 walking adults of *T. infestans* were captured, together with specimens of *T. guasayana*, *T. eratyrusiformis*, and *T. platensis*. The study demonstrated that adult *T. infestans* can disperse by walking, suggesting for females an adaptive strategy allowing them to move with eggs and/ or with blood reserves, which is unlikely when flying.

The distance of flight of *T. infestans* is around 1−2 km, however there are exceptions and some observations give *T. infestans* a much wider range.[37] The flight activity generally needs a physiological preparation.[38] It requires a previous heating during which the bug shakes its wings for a few minutes, and it is more frequent in starved specimens.[39] The flight of *T. infestans* seems to occur more often during the hot season, and at night.[40]

The factors inducing flight are many, among which are the nutritional status of the bug, external temperature and relative humidity, population density, etc. and their respective role is not easy to define.[35] Nutritional[41,42] and reproductive status,[36,43] as well as population density,[44] are known factors that modulate dispersal behavior in Triatominae. Environmental conditions as external temperature, relative humidity, and wind speed could be key factors for flight initiation.[33,41]

Flight orientation is apparently random, but it seems that during its flight the bug can be attracted by lights, as proved by the many observations of bugs either caught inside light traps set up outside villages to catch sandflies (F. Lepont, IRD, personal communication) or, in a village, observed landing on the brighten window sills during night (La Fuente, CENETROP, personal communication). Laboratory experiments have confirmed that a true attraction by white light rather than arrival by chance does exist.[45] Walking of nymphs toward a light source was reported during light trapping. It is more mysterious to understand how a silvatic habitat is left for another one. Possible but still not confirmed factors helping orientation in silvatic conditions could be a specific odor attractant[46,47] or the warmth (e.g., infra-red) emitted by animal bodies, all signals probably collected by the receptors located on antennae.[48] For some triatomine species that use flight as an important type of locomotion, such as *T. dimidiata*, light is a physical cue that might attract insects into houses, and streetlights have been associated with increased domestic infestation.[49] The removal of domestic animals in infested areas may increase vector dispersal, possibly toward nearby human sleeping spaces. Castillo-Neyra et al.[50] used a semifield system to characterize the dispersal of *T. infestans*, and compared the behavior of vector populations in the constant presence of hosts and after the removal of the hosts. The emigration rate of net insect population decline in original refuges following host removal was on average 19.7% of insects per 10 days compared to 10.2% in constant host populations. Activity of insects was significantly increased when hosts were removed.

## Passive dispersion

This mode of dispersion is the most important one to explain the territorial expansion of the main vectors.[8] Triatominae migrate with their hosts, especially the Triatominae highly adapted to their host. Dujardin[51] hypothesized that the main domestic populations of Triatominae (*T. infestans*, *R. prolixus*, *T. dimidiata*, *T. rubrofasciata*, etc.) realized a passive migration with humans because of their high adaptation to the human habitat and the hosts living there or around. *T. infestans* occupies seven countries in South America, *T. dimidiata* is found, like *R. prolixus*, in Central and South America, and *T. rubrofasciata* is a pantropicopolitan species. The large territories of these species may present discontinuities (*R. prolixus* is absent from Panama and Nicaragua, for instance) suggesting passive transportation by man, and appear as recent conquests, as suggested by their genetic structure and by historical records when available. The hypothesis is that they have been transported by their hosts (human hosts, but domestic rodents for *T. rubrofasciata*) far outside their natural ecotope, losing their contact with original silvatic foci, and increasing their dependency on human hosts.

The restricted habitat, the high dependency to humans and domestic animals, the loss of genetic resources from wild original populations, the genetic material reduction as observed by cytogenetic techniques,[52] all these factors produced a vulnerable insect, with a likely homogeneous response to control measures throughout its territory.[51] Some Triatominae increase their possibility to follow the host by producing gluing eggs. For arboreal species which may feed on birds, one can imagine the important and fast migrations possible for a small population of eggs, leading to founder effects if peripheral colonization is successful. This mechanism has been suggested to explain the colonization of Central America by *R. prolixus*,[53] but was challenged by the historical revision made by Zeledon[54] who suggested that Central America was colonized by human activities. The latter thesis was supported by genetic studies.[55]

Chickens and dogs have been suspected of being passive carriers of *T. infestans* when they enter houses and sleep in the bedrooms. However, no nymphs or adults of this or other triatomine were found in the skin of these domestic animals, in positive houses of the Argentinean arid chaco.[36,56]

## Population dynamics

Since populations are not fixed entities, the characters defining them include information about change with time, about their dynamics, and refer mainly to reproduction, density, and demography.

## Reproduction

What is meant by "reproduction" is "how many individuals will exist in a population after a given lapse of time." The lapse of time is often the generation time, and the question becomes: "what is the change in density from one generation to another?" The numeric answer to that question receives the symbol $R_0$.

Birth ($b$) and death ($d$) affect the reproduction of any population. If $r$ is the growth rate of the population, then:

$$r = b - d$$

But in a finite model, the population cannot grow indefinitely. There are some limitations, like space available, and a maximum of individuals is considered under the new variable $K$ (maximum capacity of growth). The $rN$ is modified as long as it approaches $K$. The new equation becomes:

$$dN/dt = rN[((K - N)/K)]$$

Growth depends on the population density relative to its maximum capacity ($K$). The growth of a population is a density-dependent concept. Thus, insecticides reducing population density are also modifying the growth rate.

## Density

In this aspect, striking differences are observed between domestic and silvatic species, or between the domestic and silvatic habitats of the same species. Most silvatic populations of Triatominae tend to be relatively small, composed of a few adults and nymphs. Most domestic populations show very high densities, with hundreds or thousands of adults and nymphs occupying one single house.

*Field definition.* How many individuals are there in a given unit of space? The question looks simple but the complete counting of all the individuals is generally impossible to perform in a field situation, so that an estimation is done from samples. Sampling natural populations has been suggested through various techniques.[57] The most often used approach is called "capture by effort unit": the bugs are collected during a limited amount of time and the number formulated as, for instance, in "man/hour" unit (the number of insects captured in 1 h by one man). In the frame of control interventions, only one specimen found may be enough to decide insecticide application in the house or in the village. In some cases, the following strategy may be preferred: houses are inspected during 1 h but inspection stops whenever one specimen only is found.

*Density-dependence.* Field studies of houses infested by *T. infestans* in Brazil between 1976 and 1978 showed that there was no change in density from one year to another.[58] The question was: why these populations remained at the same density level, why did they not increase their density since no active control intervention was in development. Why since it had been shown that in laboratory the bug was able to grow at a rate of 25-fold from one generation to the next?[29,59]

The search for a limiting factor considered many possibilities, among which are space availability, external temperature, the presence of predators, the availability of blood.

Space had been considered as a limiting factor.[60] A house indeed does not offer a lot of hidden places where a large population could freely grow. When no hidden places are available anymore, the bug become vulnerable because of predators (hens, dogs, etc.) and the population cannot grow further. This hypothesis was examined in a longitudinal comparative study performed in the field (Brazil) where untreated houses were compared with semitreated. In the latter, cracks and crevices in the walls were filled in half the space of the house. After treatment, the density decreased as expected. After one year, in spite of the experimentally reduced availability of space in semitreated houses, the density increased back to the values of the untreated houses.

Mortality tables have been examined to identify the possible factor able to reduce the growth rate from 25 (the laboratory observed growth rate) to 1 (the field one). It was shown that a slight increase in the time from one stage to another could considerably reduce the growth rate, and that such an increase could be the consequence of a reduction in blood quantity.[58] The same reduction in blood supply had other effects, among which the reduction of eggs number. The hypothesis became: denso-regulation would be the effect of competition for blood access; less blood meaning less fecundity as well as longer time from one stage to another.[58]

Field observations were congruent with that hypothesis. Density of *T. infestans* in a house was apparently correlated with the number of people and domestic animals living there.[61] Host availability was also demonstrated as a critical factor by laboratory[62] and experimental field populations protocols.[16,17]

An additional effect was observed: flight probability had an apparent negative correlation with blood availability. Thus, another factor modifying density, the dispersal of specimens, was dependent on nutritional factors.

However, some aspects were still obscure. For instance, there is more blood in one human than necessary for feeding a complete population of *T. infestans*. Why then exactly was there a correlation between bug density and the number of humans? Laboratory experiments provided the answer. They showed indeed that the host irritability was increasing with the number of bugs feeding[63,64]: the probability for each insect to reach complete repletion was a function of host irritability.

One obvious cause of host reaction is the saliva of the insect. It is released soon after the bite, and salivation occurs during entire feeding process. In the probing phase as observed in *R. prolixus*, saliva is pumped continuously in the host skin, including around the blood vessels.[65]

Adopting a finalist point of view, in order for the insect to feed properly, it should produce the smallest possible irritation to the host. Which could mean (1) to have small and thin mouthparts entering the skin and (2) to have a non-irritating saliva. Mouthparts entering the skin are indeed very thin, with a small 10-micron-diameter canal allowing just one blood red cell to move. This means that anticoagulating factors of the saliva must be strong to avoid obstruction of the canal. Other mechanisms controlling the contact with saliva seem related to the cibarial pump activity. It can regulate the quantity of saliva deposited in the microcirculation as necessary, and consequently minimize the host's immune response to salivary antigens.[65]

## Demography

MacArthur and Wilson[66] distinguished "*r*" and "*K*" strategies as defining populations occupying unstable or stable habitats, respectively. The first demographic strategy is typically the one of mosquitoes. They are generally relatively small insects producing a very abundant progeny, having a short developmental cycle (less than 1 month), high dispersal capacities, and an aggressive behavior to exploit at its maximum the available resources of their environment. The "*K*" strategy is the opposite one, and congruent with domestic species of Triatominae. They are relatively larger insects producing a much smaller quantity of descendants (1000 times less than what can be produced by a mosquito), they have extended developmental cycles (various months), poor active dispersal capacities, and a timorous feeding behavior. They do not try to exhaust the resources of their environment, but seem to opt for an optimum use of it. The "*r*" strategists can recover quickly after a catastrophic mortality, or they can move and disperse to other more wealthy environments, the "*K*" strategists in the same situation would probably be unable to recover or to escape.[67]

Thus, extinction would be the fate of the "*K*" strategist when confronted with an adverse environment, as observed for the domestic species of Triatominae which have been hit by international programs of vector control.[68] However, such "*K*" populations have the possibility to significantly increase their development rate and recover their previous effectives relatively quickly if a few of them could survive. Again the explanation of this recovering capacity is obtained through what we know about density regulation. In lower densities, there is no more competition to feed and each insect would take complete blood meals, which in turn would shorten the developmental cycle and increase both fecundity and fertility of females. A good control program must avoid the survival of a few insects, even a very few of them.

# Insight into the biology and ecology of Triatominae in the silvatic environment

In many areas of Latin America, the domestic intrusion of species until now considered as strictly silvatic has led to more interest in their study. The observation of a species in its natural environment supplies a basic pattern which may help to understand its process of adaptation to a new environment (for instance, when populations are displaying synanthropic behavior). However, the studies carried out in the silvatic environment are often fragmentary, principally because the field observations and collections of specimens are laborious and time-consuming.

## *Interest of a trapping device*

Searching for domestic Triatominae bugs in rural houses of Latin America is an important activity carried out by Health Services in every country affected by Chagas disease. In general, infestation by Triatominae in the domestic and peridomestic structures is recorded by active search by means of timed manual collection using a dislodging spray and a normal light torch. However, as demonstrated by Abad-Franch et al.,[69] standard vector searches used by Control Programs, had low sensitivity except in certain singular circumstances. They suggest that many infestation foci may go undetected during routine surveys, especially when vector density is low. Undetected foci can cause control failures and induce bias in entomological indices; this may confound disease risk assessment and mislead program managers into flawed decision making. A pheromone-containing infective box, was recently presented as a promising new tool to detect (and even control) indoor populations of *T. infestans*.[70] On the other hand, a new method for finding intradomestic bugs was proposed, based on the unexplored property of Triatominae feces to fluoresce when exposed to UV light.[71] Normally, a torch light is used to search for triatomines within the houses. Replacing the regular light bulb by an UV bulb could substantially improve the early detection of residual or emergent populations of domestic triatomine bugs and contribute to a successful evaluation and awareness of Chagas disease vectors.

The detection and collecting of sylvatic Triatominae in their natural environment, a necessary precondition to biological and ecological observations, would greatly benefit from the use of trapping devices.[2] In many cases, it provides the only way to detect and collect bugs in less accessible ecotopes, such as rock piles, hollow trees, or palm trees, and avoids ecological damages caused, e.g., by tree dissection or logging. Because starved bugs are preferentially attracted, the device does not allow an estimating of the accurate density of insects and population structure. Nevertheless, it allowed some interesting observations: thus, for instance, wild populations of *T. infestans*, *T. brasiliensis*, or *T. pseudomaculata* may exhibit high motivation for food search during the daylight hours (Noireau, unpublished data) whereas they are supposed to leave their refuges and make for food source during the night.[72]

## Sylvatic habitat

According to Schofield,[8] each of the three most epidemiological important genera of Triatominae is virtually associated with a type of habitat. So, species of the genus *Rhodnius* are primarily associated with palms, the genus *Panstrongylus* has predominantly evolved in burrows and tree cavities, and the genus *Triatoma* in terrestrial rocky habitats or rodent burrows. This assumption is generally true for the genera *Rhodnius* and *Panstrongylus* even though some species were found in other silvatic habitats. Thus, in the genus *Rhodnius*, *R. domesticus* has been reported in bromeliads and hollow trees in Amazonia, and *R. neglectus* in *Cereus jamacaru* (mandacaru), a cactus species characteristic of the Caatinga in north-eastern Brazil.[3,73] Although some species of the genus *Panstrongylus* can be found in palm tree crowns (e.g., *P. megistus*), all species are associated with terrestrial burrows, tree root cavities, or hollow trees.[74] On the other hand, the preference relationship of the genus *Triatoma* for terrestrial habitats is more questionable. Species can be found in arboreal as well as rocky habitat, e.g., *T. infestans*, *T. sordida*, and *T. guasayana*, of which Andean populations live in rock piles and lowland populations live in trees. Others are exclusively arboreal, found in hollow trees and/or bird nests (e.g., *T. ryckmani*, *T. pseudomaculata*, *T. platensis*, *T. delpontei*). Triatomine species may exhibit a great range of ecotopes (*P. megistus*, *T. dimidiata*) when others display a close relationship with one ecotope. *Psammolestes* species are only associated with nests of Furnariidae. Some *Rhodnius* species may be associated with particular type of palms (*R. brethesi* with *Leopoldinia piassaba*, *R. ecuadoriensis* with *Phytelephas* spp.), whereas others do not exhibit a palm preference (*R. pictipes* and *R. robustus*). A theory suggests the occurrence of rapid morphological divergence in response to different ecological factors.[75] Indeed, we observe obvious chromatic differences between arboreal *T. infestans* (*melanosoma* and dark morph populations[76,77]) and terrestrial specimens collected in rocky habitat in Bolivia (clearer morphs). Nevertheless, this model cannot be generalized when considering chromatic variation only. Also, arboreal and terrestrial wild *T. sordida* do not display chromatic differences. Similarly, the genetically closely related species *T. pseudomaculata* and *T. wygodzinkyi*, which probably come from a common ancestor and have undergone an ecological divergence (the first species is arboreal when the second is terrestrial), do not exhibit detectable morphological differences. Many triatomine species exhibit a behavioral plasticity as related to habitat selection in different environments. In silvatic environment, the habitat of *T. pseudomaculata* and *T. juazeirensis* is never shared. The first species is found in trees and bird nests, whereas the second is exclusively rupicolous. When they invade the peridomestic area, they are highly adaptable to different habitats and can occupy substrates that they do not colonize in the silvatic environment. So, *T. juazeirensis* leaves a rupicolous habitat for colonizing, in the peridomicile, wood material in more than 80% of cases.[78]

## Access to host

The host seeking classically results in the feeding. Such behavior, considered as basic in Triatominae, applies mostly to domestic/peridomestic colonies living closely with synanthropic animals or humans. It also applies to adult wild triatomines which can fly to find their feeding. This last assumption is strengthened by the uncommon capture of adult forms in traps placed in hollow trees, habitats considered as unfavorable for the permanence of feeding hosts. However, the starved nymphs which are profusely collected by trapping in such unfavorable ecotopes enjoy another type of access to host that may be called host waiting. This passive behavior is justified by the reduced locomotor activity of nymphal instars that have to wait for the intrusion of a host in order to feed. Another example of host waiting was noticed with relation to silvatic colonies of *T. guasayana* occurring in bromeliads in Bolivia. Bromeliad-beds covered no burrow and the detection of blood sources indicated the cattle as the main feeding host (Baune, personal communication).

## Survival strategy

The environmental disturbance caused by man and the consequent damage of triatomine biotopes often results in a condition of chronic distress in wild populations of insects. This was clearly demonstrated in *T. pseudomaculata* in northeastern Brazil, where the silvatic insects exhibit a great weight deficit in relation to peridomiciliary ones (Carbajal de la Fuente, personal communication). This adverse condition led the insect to apply a survival strategy related to the election of habitat, breeding behavior, and host preference and is certainly the main cause of flight dispersal and possible subsequent settlement in artificial structures. *T. pseudomaculata* is an autochthonous species of the Caatinga. In its survival strategy, this arboricolous species does not exhibit preference for any tree species. On the contrary, it can be captured in all the predominant trees of the area (more than 10 species), in hollows, or nests of Furnariidae.[73,78] The high percentage of positive trees (>50%) and the presence of small colonies of insects, rarely exceeding 10 individuals, suggest that females lay a small quantity of eggs in a large number of ecotopes to increase their chance of survival.[79] With relation to the hematophagy, some works have pointed out the occurrence of alternative feeding behavior in natural populations of Triatominae. So, wild specimens of *T. circummaculata* (Salvatella, personal communication), *T. pseudomaculata, T. sordida, T. brasiliensis,* and *Psammolestes tertius* may feed on hemolymph of invertebrates (Carbajal de la Fuente, unpublished data). The importance and consequences of this biological trait, influenced by unfavorable environmental conditions, are unknown. Relationships between hemolymphagy and population dynamics, and vector—*T. cruzi* interaction, might be contemplated. This feeding habit is derived from the predaceous behavior in other Reduviidae. Nevertheless, whilst the assassin bugs prey upon arthropods, predigesting their tissues and killing their prey, the Triatominae may only temporarily immobilize their prey and suck their fluids (Fig. 7.1).

# Vectorial capacity and domesticity

The vectorial capacity of a mosquito or a fly, be it an insect transmitting a virus or a protozoan, is often a matter of "host-parasite" specificity: the parasite is transmitted by one mosquito species, or a very few of them. The situation is very different for Chagas disease vectors, and this might be related to the mechanism of parasite transmission. The stercorarian parasite adapts to the lumen and epithelium of the bug intestine, it is evacuated with the feces dropped on the host's skin, and penetrates actively through a local wound (the one produced by the bite, for instance), or directly through the eye mucosa (Romanha's sign).

## *Adaptation to* Trypanosoma cruzi

Adaptation to the protozoan *T. cruzi* does not seem to be a critical issue in the vectorial capacity of Triatominae. Different tribes, different genera, different species are actively transmitting the diverse genetic entities assembled under the name of *T. cruzi.* Moreover, other orders of insect seem to be able to ensure the complete cycle of *T. cruzi* inside the intestine: the Diptera *Musca domestica,*[80] the *Cimex lecticularius,* and even Arachnidae were found infected by the *T. cruzi.*[81]

## *Blood feeding habits*

Hematophagy, an almost exclusive and obligatory habit in Triatominae at all their development stages and both sexes, appears as the key feature of their biology, by which much of their behavior and their microevolution is explained. Even if the transmission of the parasite is due to the contact of insect dejections on the host skin, hematophagy is a crucial feature of vectorial capacity. It allows the infection of the vector, and it ensures the regular and prolonged contact of the vector with the vertebrate host.

Since the parasite is transmitted by the feces, the presence of the feeding insect on the host must last long enough for the defecation to occur. The blood meal lasts approximately 20 min. The main vectors need less than this lapse of time to deposit their urine and dejections, but some species (like the Northern group of *Triatoma*) may defecate up to an hour after having left their host and so do not represent a high peril of transmission.

For each species, defecation also seems to be a density-dependent process. In high density populations, each insect will have less blood due to competition with others, and an incomplete engorgement can delay or cancel defecation, hence transmission. In low density conditions, however, each insect can feed without the stress of competition, and defecation will certainly occur.[82,83] The transmission of *T. cruzi* may be more likely in vector low density conditions.

## Domesticity

In the same way that hematophagy is the dominant character to consider for understanding the biology of the bugs, domesticity is the key factor to evaluate their vectorial capacity. Only the species adapted to human dwellings are actively contributing to the transmission. They are called "domestic species" in the sense of species associated with human (synanthropic species), not in the sense of species domesticated by man. These species are less than 5% of the total number of Triatominae, which means that such adaptation is not easy to obtain in spite of continuous contacts reported between man and silvatic species.

Catalá et al.[84,85] developed a *T. cruzi* risk index and demonstrated that infested Argentinean households can show a wide range of risk values (0−5 risky bites/ human). The variable showed skewed distribution, with a high frequency of lower values and few very high risk households. Of all collected *T. infestans*, 44% had had human blood meals whereas 27% had had dog or chicken blood meals. Having dogs and birds sharing a room with humans increased the risk values. Tidy and clean households contributed significantly to lower risk values as a result of low vector density. The statistical analysis showed a high correlation between current values of the entomological risk indicator and *T. cruzi* seroprevalence in children.

As observed in the literature, the frontiers between domestic, peridomestic, and domiciliary populations are not clear. The following distinction between intrusion, domiciliation, and domestication might help in defining the epidemiological importance of some populations or species of Triatominae.

## Intrusion

Many adult specimens of silvatic species are reported from inside human dwellings, probably attracted there by light or through passive carriage (marsupials, for instance). Some of them were unknown and described from the human habitat without knowing more about their biology (*T. jurbergi*, for instance). In this situation, there is no evidence of colonization (eggs, nymphs, exuviae).

## Domiciliation

What is different here is the presence inside the house of adult and of nymphs, eggs, and exuviae, which means the complete cycle of the insect was occurring inside the house. The resulting colonies are not very abundant and represent merely a tentative adaptation to the house. This situation has been described for *R. pallescens* in the North of Colombia (Moreno, personal communication), *Eratyrus mucronatus* in Bolivia[79] and in Venezuela,[86] *T. sordida,*[87] *R. stali,*[88] *Microtriatoma trinidadensis,*[89] and *P. rufotuberculatus*[90,91] in Bolivia. It is not necessarily a permanent situation. For instance, the domiciliary *R. pallescens* in the north of Colombia progressively disappeared from the houses without any control intervention (Moreno, personal communication).

## Domestication

The definition includes the aforementioned observations for domiciliation, with an additional criterion related to the type of geographic extension. It is not a local, geographically restricted observation, but a more widely extended territory with obvious arguments supporting migration by passive carriage. It is for instance a discontinuous geographic extension, with gaps apparently unexplained unless the human intervention is admitted. More research is needed to understand the factors allowing a species to reach a high level of adaptation to the domestic habitat, an adaptation which systematically reduces the size of the insect.[51,92]

It is important to recall that the label of "domestic" species does not exclude the existence of sylvatic foci. Wild populations of *T. infestans* and *R. prolixus* were recorded in Bolivia and Argentina (for *T. infestans*) and in Venezuela and Colombia (for *R. prolixus*).

# Vector control strategy

## Entomological surveillance

Domestic species have been severely hit by international programs,[68,93,94] but not all of them have been controlled in every part of their territory.[95] What we learned from their biology is that no country should allow the persistence or the development of domestic populations anymore. The entomological surveillance of Chagas disease vectors is the surveillance of the human dwellings. A serious alert should be addressed to the local health authorities in case of domiciliation, and a national alert should be raised in case of domestication, be it observed for the local "domestic" species or by another one.

## Eradication, elimination, reduction

The densito-dependent character of the delay between blood intake and defecation allows to understand why it is crucial to completely eliminate bugs from the domestic and peridomestic structures. The most dangerous bug is an infected bug allowed to feed toward complete engorgement, because it will certainly deposit its infected feces on the host's skin during the blood meal. This situation is obtained when the population density is low and no strong competition for food exists. It could be produced by poorly executed or partial vector control interventions. Because they lower the density of remaining insects, the control measures producing only the reduction of vector populations can be more dangerous than no control at all.

## Acknowledgments

This work has benefited from international collaboration through the ECLAT network. It is partly based on a chapter published by the Belgian Academy of Overseas Sciences.[81]

## Glossary

Most of the very specialized words are explained in the text; a few others are defined here.

**anemia** A deficiency of red blood cells.

**exopterygotes** Insects with incomplete metamorphosis, changing form only gradually from the immature stages to the adult; the young resemble adults but have externally-developing wings (e.g., triatomine nymph to adult).

**monophyletic group** Contains an ancestor and all of its descendants—Descending from a single, common ancestor.

**paraphyletic group** A group of organisms that includes an ancestor but not all of its descendants.

**polyphyletic group** A group of organisms having multiple origins, thus not sharing a common ancestor.

**proboscis** Long mouthpart, feeding tube of the kissing bug appearing as an elongated appendage from the head; in kissing bugs, it is an articulated appendage.

**rupicolous** Thriving among or inhabiting rocks ("saxicolous" has similar meaning).

**synanthropic** Ecologically associated with humans.

**stercorarian** Of fecal origin; said of trypanosomes passed to the recipient in the feces (an alternative mode of transmission is "salivation").

**stridulatory sulcus** A vibratory communication organ of the head playing a role in the sexual behavior of the bugs.[96]

**tropicopolitan** Inhabiting all tropical climate countries, thus covering various continents.

## References

1. Schofield CJ, Galvão C. Classification, evolution, and species groups within the Triatominae. *Acta Trop* 2009;**110**:88−100.
2. Noireau F, Menezes dos Santos S, Gumiel M, Dujardin JP, dos Santos Soares M, Carcavallo RU, et al. Phylogenetic relationships within the oliveirai complex (Hemiptera: Reduviidae: Triatominae). *Infect Genet Evol* 2002;**2**:11−17.
3. Lent H, Wygodzinsky P. Revision of the Triatominae (Hemiptera, Reduviidae), and their significance as vectors of Chagas disease. *Bull Am Museum Nat His* 1979;**163**:123−520.

4. Hypsa V, Tietz DF, Zrzavy J, Rego ROM, Galvão C. Phylogeny and biogeography of Triatominae (Hemiptera: Reduviidae): molecular evidence of a New World origin of the Asiatic clade. *Mol Phylogenet Evol* 2002;**23**:447−57.

5. Weirauch C. Cladistic analysis of Reduviidae (Heteroptera: Cimicomorpha) based on morphological characters. *Syst Entomol* 2008;**33**(2):229−74.

6. Weirauch C, Munro JB. Molecular phylogeny of the assassin bugs (Hemiptera: Reduviidae), based on mitochondrial and nuclear ribosomal genes. *Mol Phyl Evol* 2009;**53**:287−99.

7. Patterson JS, Gaunt MW. Phylogenetic multi-locus codon models and molecular clocks reveal the monophyly of haematophagous reduviid bugs and their evolution at the formation of South America. *Mol Phylogenet Evol* 2010;**56**(2):608−21.

8. Schofield CJ. *Biosystematics of the Triatominae. Biosystematic of Haematophagous Insects*, 37. MW Service Systematics Assoc Special Oxford Clarendon Press; 1988. p. 284−312.

9. Tartarotti E, Ceron CR. Ribosomal DNA ITS-1 intergenic spacer polymorphism in triatomines (Triatominae, Heteroptera). *Biochem Genet* 2005;**43**:365−73.

10. de Paula AS, Diotaiuti L, Schofield CJ. Testing the sister-group relationship of the Rhodniini and Triatomini (Insecta: Hemiptera: Reduviidae: Triatominae). *Mol Phylogenet Evol* 2005;**35**:712−18.

11. Tartarotti E, Azeredo-Oliveira MT, Ceron CR. Phylogenetic approach to the study of triatomines (Triatominae, Heteroptera). *Braz J Biol* 2006;**66**:703−8.

12. Martinez FH, Villalobos GC, Cevallos AM, de la Torre PD, Laclette JP, Alejandre-Aguilar R, et al. Taxonomic study of the *Phyllosoma* complex and other triatomine (Insecta: Hemiptera: Reduviidae) species of epidemiological importance in the transmission of Chagas disease using ITS-2 and mtCytB sequences. *Mol Phylogenet Evol* 2006;**41**:279−87.

13. Hwang WS, Weirauch C. Evolutionary history of assassin bugs (Insecta: Hemiptera: Reduviidae): insights from divergence dating and ancestral state reconstruction. *PLoS ONE* 2012;**7**(9):e45523.

14. Barata JMS. Aspectos morfológicos de ovos de Triatominae. II. Caracteristicas macroscopicas e exocoriais de dez especies do genero *Rhodnius* stal, 1859 (Hemiptera, Reduviidae). *Rev Saud Publ* 1981;**15**:490−542.

15. Páaez-Colasante X, Aldana E. Morfometria geométrica del borde borial y del collar de huevos de cinco especies del geénero *Rhodnius* Stal (Heteroptera, Reduviidae, Triatominae). *EntomoBrasilis* 2008;**1**(3):57−61.

16. Gorla DE, Schofield CJ. Analysis of egg mortality in experimental populations of *Triatoma infestans* under natural climatic conditions in Argentina. *Bull Soc Vector Ecol* 1985;**10**(2):107−17.

17. Gorla DE, Schofield CJ. Population dynamics of *Triatoma infestans* under natural climatic conditions in Argentina. *Med Vet Entomol* 1989;**3**:179−94.

18. Jimenez ML, Palacios C. Life cycle and reproductive and feeding behavior of *Dipetalogaster maximus* (Uhler) (Reduviidae : Triatominae) under laboratory conditions in Baja California Sur, Mexico. *Southwestern Entomologist* 2002;**27**(1):65−72.

19. Joerg M. Influencia de temperaturas fijas en periodos anuales sobre metamorfosis y fertilidad de *Triatoma infestans*. *Bol Chil Parasitol* 1964;**17**:17−19.

20. Giojalas L, Catalá S. Changes in male *Triatoma infestans* reproductive efficiency caused by a suboptimal temperature. *J Insect Physiol* 1993;**39**(4):297−302.

21. Catalá S. Relaciones entre consumo de sangre y ovognesis en *Triatoma infestans* (klug, 1834). *Chagas* 1989;**5**:3−10.

22. Catalá SS. The biting rate of *Triatoma infestans* in Argentina. *Med Vet Entomol* 1991;**5**:325−33.

23. Lima MM, Jurberg P, De Almeida R. Behavior of Triatomines (Hemiptera: Reduviidae) vectors of Chagas' disease. III. Influence of the number of matings on the fecundity and fertility of *Panstrongylus megistus* (Burm., 1835) in the laboratory. *Mem Inst Oswaldo Cruz RJ* 1987;**82**(1):37−41.

24. Diotaiuti L, Pires HHR, Abrao DO, Machado EMD, Schofield CJ. Eye colour as a genetic marker for fertility and fecundity of *Triatoma infestans* (Klug, 1834) Hemiptera, Reduviidae, Triatominae. *Mem Inst Oswaldo Cruz* 2002;**97**(5):675−8.

25. Schaefer CW, Coscaron MC. The status of *Linshcosteus* in the Triatominae (Hemiptera : Reduviidae). *J Med Entomol* 2001;**38**(6):862−7.

26. Torres M, Cardenas E, Perez S, Morales A. Haematophagy and cleptohaematophagy of *Clerada apicicornis* (Hemiptera: Lygaeidae), a potential biological control agent of *Rhodnius prolixus* (Hemiptera: Reduviidae). *Mem Inst Oswaldo Cruz* 2000.

27. Catalá SS, Gorla DE, Basombrio MA. Vectorial transmission of *Trypanosoma cruzi* an experimental field study with susceptible and immunized hosts. *Am J Trop Med Hyg* 1992;**47**:1.

28. Schofield C. Chagas disease, triatomine bugs, and blood loss. *Lancet* 1981;317.

29. Rabinovich J. Vital statistics of Triatominae (Hemiptera: Reduviidae) under laboratory conditions. I. *Triatoma infestans* Klug. *J Med Entomol* 1972;**9**:351−70.

30. Sandoval CM, Joya MI, Gutierez R, Angulo VM. Cleptohaematophagy of the triatomine bug *Belminus herreri*. *Med Vet Entomol* 2000;**14**(1):100−1.

31. Figueiras ANL, Lazzari CR. Temporal change of the aggregation response in *Triatoma infestans*. *Mem Inst Oswaldo Cruz* 2000;**95**(6):889−92.

32. Forattini O, Rocha E, Silva EO, Ferreira OA, Rabello EX, Pattoli DGB. Aspectos ecolgicos da tripanossomose americana. III Dispersão local de triatomíneos, com especial referência ao *Triatoma sordida*. *Rev Saúde Públ, S Paulo* 1971;**5**:193−205.

33. Schofield CJ, Lehane MJ, McEwan P, Catalá SS, Gorla DE. Dispersive flight by *Triatoma sordida*. *Trans R Soc Trop Med Hyg* 1991;**85**:676−8.

34. Noireau F, Dujardin JP. Flight and nutritional status of sylvatic *Triatoma sordida* and *Triatoma guasayana*. *Mem Inst Oswaldo Cruz RJ* 2001;**96**(3):385−9.

35. Barrett TV. Advances in triatomine bug ecology in relation to Chagas disease. *Adv Dis Vector Res* 1991;**8**(6):142−76.

36. Abrahan L, Gorla D, Catalá S. Dispersal of *Triatoma infestans* and other Triatominae species in the arid Chaco of Argentina. Flying, walking or passive carriage? the importance of walking females. *Mem Inst Oswaldo Cruz RJ* 2011;**106**(2):232−9.

37. Schweigmann N, Vallve S, Muscio O, Ghillini M, Alberti A, WisniveskyColli C. Dispersal flight by *Triatoma infestans* in an arid area of Argentina. *Med Vet Entomol* 1988;**2**:401−4.

38. Lehane MJ, Schofield CJ. Preliminary report on flight some Triatominae bugs. *Trans R Soc Trop Med Hyg* 1976;**70**(5/6):526.

39. Lehane MJ, Schofield CJ. Flight initiation in *Triatoma infestans* (Klug) (Hemiptera: Reduviidae). *Bull Entomol Res* 1982;**72**:497−510.

40. Lehane MJ, Schofield CJ. Field experiments of dispersive flight by *Triatoma infestans*. *Trans R Soc Trop Med Hyg* 1981;**75**(3):399−400.

41. Lehane MJ, McEwen PK, Whitaker CJ, Schofield CJ. The role of temperature and nutritional status in flight initiation by *Triatoma infestans*. *Acta Trop* 1992;**52**:27−38.

42. McEwen PK, Lehane MJ. Factors influencing flight initiation in the triatomine bug *Triatoma sordida* (Hemiptera: Reduviidae). *Insect Sci Appl* 1993;**14**:461−4.

43. McEwen PK, Lehane MJ. Relationships between flight initiation and oviposition in *Triatoma infestans* (Klug) (Hemiptera: Reduviidae). *J Appl Entomol* 1994;**117**:217−23.

44. McEwen PK, Lehane MJ, Whitaker CJ. The effect of adult population density on flight initiation in *Triatoma infestans* (Klug) (Hemiptera: Reduviidae). *J Appl Entomol* 1993;**116**:321−5.

45. Minoli SA, Lazzari CR. Take-off activity and orientation of triatomines (Heteroptera: Reduviidae) in relation to the presence of artificial lights. *Acta Trop* 2006;**97**:324−30.

46. Pires HHR, Lorenzo MG, Diotaiuti L, Lazzari CR, Figueiras ANL. Aggregation behaviour in *Panstrongylus megistus* and *Triatoma infestans*: inter and intraspecific responses. *Acta Trop* 2002;**81**(1):47−52.

47. Vitta ACR, Figueiras AN, Lazzari CR, Diotaiuti L, Lorenzo MG. Aggregation mediated by faeces and footprints in *Triatoma pseudomaculata* (Heteroptera : Reduviidae), a Chagas disease vector. *Mem Inst Oswaldo Cruz* 2002;**97**(6):865−7.

48. de la Fuente ALC, Catalá SS. Relationship between antennal sensilla pattern and habitat in six species of Triatominae. *Mem Inst Oswaldo Cruz* 2002;**97**(8):1121−5.

49. Pacheco-Tucuch FS, Ramirez-Sierra MJ, Gourbière S, Dumonteil E. Public street lights increase house infestation by the Chagas disease vector *Triatoma dimidiata*. *PLoS ONE* 2012;**7**:e36207. Available from: http://dx.doi.org/10.1371/journal.pone.0036207.

50. Castillo-Neyra R, Barbu CM, Salazar R, Borrini K, Naquira C, Levy MZ. Host-seeking behavior and dispersal of *Triatoma infestans*, a vector of Chagas disease, under semi-field conditions. *PLoS NTD* 2015. Available from: http://dx.doi.org/10.1371/journal.pntd.0003433.

51. Dujardin JP. Population genetics and the natural history of domestication in Triatominae. *Mem Inst Oswaldo Cruz* 1998;**93**:34−6.

52. Panzera F, Dujardin JP, Nicolini P, Caraccio MN, Rose V, Tellez T, et al. Genomic changes of Chagas disease vector, South America. *Emerg Infect Dis* 2004;**10**:438−46.

53. Gamboa CJ. Dispersión de Rhodnius prolixus en Venezuela. *Bol Dir Malariol Saneamiento Ambiental* 1962;**3**:262−72.

54. Zeledon R. Enfermedad de Chagas en Centro America. In: Schofield CJ, Dujardin JP, Jurberg J (editors) Proceedings of the international workshop on population genetics and control of Triatominae Santo Domingo de los Colorados, Ecuador INDRE, Ciudad de Méjico, 116 pp; 1996. p. 31.

55. Dujardin JP, Muñoz M, Chavez T, Ponce C, Moreno J, Schofield CJ. The origin of *Rhodnius prolixus* in Central America. *Med Vet Entomol* 1998;**12**:113−15.

56. Abrahan LB. Dispersión de Triatoma infestans (Hemiptera:Reduviidae) en áreas rurales de los Llanos riojanos. Tesis Doctoral, Universidad Nacional de Córdoba, Argentina; 2013. 122pp.

57. Schofield CJ. A comparison of sampling techniques for domestic populations of Triatominae. *Trans R Soc Trop Med Hyg* 1978;**72**:449−55.

58. Schofield CJ. Density regulation of domestic populations of *Triatoma infestans* in Brazil. *Trans R Soc Trop Med Hyg* 1980;**74**(6):761−9.

59. Feliciangeli MD, Rabinovich J. Vital statistics of Triatominae (Hemiptera: Reduviidae) under laboratory conditions. II. Triatoma maculata. *J Med Entomol* 1985;**22**(1):43−8.

60. Gomez-Nunez JC. Desarrollo de un nuevo método para evaluar la infestación intradomiciliaria por *Rhodnius prolixus*. *Acta Cientif Venezol* 1965;**16**:26−31.

61. Piesman J, Sherlock IA, Christensen HA. Host availability limits population density of *Panstrongylus megistus*. *Am J Trop Med Hyg* 1983;**32**:1445−50.

62. Schofield CJ. The role of blood intake in density regulation of populations of *Triatoma infestans* (Klug) (Hemiptera: Reduviidae). *Bull Entomol Res* 1982;**72**:617−29.

63. Wier Lopez EH. Estado alimentario y regulación poblacional en Rhodnius prolixus (Hemiptera: Reduviidae). Tesis, Universidad Simón Bolivar, Venezuela; 1982. 285pp.
64. Schofield CJ, Williams NG, Marshall C. Density-dependent perception of triatominae bug bites. *Ann Trop Med Parasitol* 1986;**80**(3):351−8.
65. Soares AC, Carvalho-Tavares J, de Figueiredo Gontijo N, dos Santos VC, Teixeira MM, Pereira MH. Salivation pattern of *Rhodnius prolixus* (Reduviidae; Triatominae) in mouse skin. *J Insect Physiol* 2006;**52**(5):468−72.
66. Mac Arthur RH, Wilson EO. *The Theory of Island* Biogeography. Princeton: Princeton University Press; 1967.
67. Rabinovich JE. Demographic strategies in animal populations: a regression analysis. In: Golloy FB, Medina E, editors. *Tropical Ecological Systems*. New York: Springer Verlag; 1974. p. 19−40.
68. Schofield CJ, Dias JCP. The Southern Cone initiative against Chagas disease. *Adv Parasitol* 1999;**42**:1−27.
69. Abad-Franch F, Valença-Barbosa C, Sarquis O, Lima MM. All that glisters is not gold: sampling-process uncertainty in disease-vector surveys with false-negative and false-positive detections. *PLoS NTD* 2014;**8**(9):e3187. Available from: http://dx.doi.org/10.1371/journal.pntd.0003187.
70. Forlani L, Pedrini N, Girotti JR, Mijailovsky SJ, Cardozo RM, Gentile AG, et al. Biological control of the Chagas disease vector *Triatoma infestans* with the entomo-pathogenic fungus *Beauveria bassiana* combined with an aggregation cue: field, laboratory and mathematical modeling assessment. *PLoS NTD* 2015;**9**(5). Available from: http://dx.doi.org/10.1371/journal.pntd.0003778.
71. Catalá S. Searching for triatomines. a new method for field search using UV light. *Acta Trop* 2010;**116**(1):111−14. Available from: http://dx.doi.org/10.1016/j.actatropica.2010.04.017.
72. Guerenstein PG, Lazzari CR. Host-seeking: how triatomines acquire and make use of information to find blood. *Acta Trop* 2009;**110**:148−58.
73. Dias-Lima AG, Menezes D, Sherlock I, Noireau F. Wild habitat and related fauna of *Panstrongylus lutzi* (Reduviidae, Triatominae). *J Med Entomol* 2003;**40**:989−90.
74. Galvão C, Patterson JS, Rocha DD, Jurberg J, Carcavallo R, Rajen K, et al. A new species of Triatominae from Tamil Nadu, India. *Med Vet Entomol* 2002;**16**(1):75−82.
75. Dujardin JP, Panzera P, Schofield CJ. Triatominae as a model of morphological plasticity under ecological pressure. *Mem Inst Oswaldo Cruz* 1999;**94**:223−8.
76. Martinez A, Olmedo RA, Carcavallo RU. Una nueva subespecie argentina de *Triatoma infestans*. *Chagas* 1987;**4**:479−80.
77. Noireau F, Flores R, Gutierrez T, Dujardin JP. Detection of silvatic dark morphs of *Triatoma infestans* in the Bolivian Chaco. *Mem Inst Oswaldo Cruz RJ* 1997;**92**(5):583−4.
78. Carbajal de la Fuente AL, Dias-Lima A, Lopes CM, Emperaire L, Walter A, Ferreira A, et al. Behavioural plasticity of Triatominae related to habitat selection in North-East Brazil. *J Med Entomol* 2008;**45**:14−19.
79. Noireau F, Bosseno MF, Carrasco R, Telleria J, Vargas F, Camacho C, et al. Sylvatic triatomines (Hemiptera: Reduviidae) in Bolivia : trends toward domesticity and possible infection with *Trypanosoma cruzi* (Kinetoplastida: Trypanosomatidae). *J Med Entomol* 1995;**32**(5):594−8.
80. Diaz-Ungria. Transmission du *Trypanosoma cruzi* chez les Mammifères. *Ann Parasitol (Paris)* 1966;**41**(6):549−71.

81. Dujardin JP, Schofield CJ, Panzera F. Les vecteurs de la maladie de Chagas. Recherches taxinomiques, biologiques et génétiques. *Acad R Sci Class Sci Nat Méd NS* 2000;**24**(5). 162pp.
82. Kirk ML, Schofield CJ. Density-dependent timing of defaecation by *Rhodnius prolixus*, and its implications for the transmission of *Trypanosoma cruzi*. *Trans R Soc Trop Med Hyg* 1987;**81**:348−9.
83. Trumper EV, Gorla DE. Density-dependent timing of defaecation by *Triatoma infestans*. *Trans R Soc Trop Med Hyg* 1991;**85**:800−2.
84. Catalá S, Crocco L, Morales G. *Trypanosoma cruzi* transmission risk index (TcTRI): an entomological indicator of Chagas disease vectorial transmission to human. *Acta Trop* 1997;**68**(3):285−95.
85. Catalá S, Crocco L, Muñoz A, Morales G, Paulone I, Giraldez E, et al. Entomological aspects of *Trypanosoma cruzi* vectorial transmission in the domestic habitat of Argentina. *J Public Health* 2004;**38**(2):216−22.
86. Viva AS, Barazarte H, Fernandez DM. Primer registro de *Eratyrus mucronatus* Stahl, 1959 (Hemiptera: Reduviidae) en el ambiente domiciliario en Venezuela. *Entomotropica* 2001;**16**(3):215−17.
87. Noireau F, Brenière F, Ordonez J, Cardozo L, Morochi W, Gutierrez T, et al. Low probability of transmission of *Trypanosoma cruzi* to humans by domiciliary *Triatoma sordida* in Bolivia. *Trans R Soc Trop Med Hyg* 1997;**91**:653−6.
88. Matías A, De la Riva JX, Martinez E, Dujardin JP. Domiciliation process of *Rhodnius stali* (Hemiptera: Reduviidae) in the Alto Beni (La Paz, Bolivia). *Trop Med Int Health* 2002;**8**(3):264−8.
89. De la Riva J, Matías A, Torrez M, Martínez E, Dujardin JP. Adults and nymphs of *Microtriatoma trinidadensis* (Lent, 1951) (Hemiptera: Reduviidae) caught from peridomestic environment in Bolivia. *Mem Inst Oswaldo Cruz* 2001;**96**(7):889−94.
90. Noireau F, Bosseno MF, Vargas F, Brenière SF. Apparent trend to domesticity observed in *Panstrongylus rufotuberculatus* Champion, 1899 (Hemiptera: Reduviidae) in Bolivia. *Res Rev Parasitol* 1994;**54**:263−4.
91. Dujardin JP, Forgues G, Torrez M, Martínez E, Cordoba C, Gianella A. Morphometrics of domestic *Panstrongylus rufotuberculatus* in Bolivia. *Ann Trop Med Parasitol* 1998;**92**(2):219−28.
92. Caro-Riaño H, Jaramillo N, Dujardin JP. Growth changes in *Rhodnius pallescens* under simulated domestic and sylvatic conditions. *Inf Genet Evol* 2009;**9**(2):162−8.
93. WHO. Andean countries initiative launched in Colombia. *TDR News* 1997;53.
94. Schofield CJ, Dujardin JP. Chagas disease vector control in Central America. *Parasitol Today* 1997;**13**:141−4.
95. Dias JCP, Silveira AC, Schofield CJ. The impact of Chagas disease control in Latin America. *Mem Inst Oswaldo Cruz* 2002;**97**:603−12.
96. Manrique G, Lazzari CR. Sexual behaviour and stridulation during mating in *Triatoma infestans* (Hemiptera: Reduviidae). *Mem Inst Oswaldo Cruz* 1994;**89**(4):629−33.

# Population genetics of Triatominae

L. Stevens[1] and P.L. Dorn[2]
[1]University of Vermont, Burlington, VT, United States, [2]Loyola University New Orleans, New Orleans, LA, United States

## Chapter Outline

## Introduction

### The importance of population genetics in Chagas disease epidemiology and control

Launched in 1991, the "Southern Cone Initiative" was the first multicountry control program designed to eliminate domestic populations of *Triatoma infestans*, arguably the main vector of Chagas disease worldwide at the time and certainly in the Southern Cone of South America. This initiative was followed by Andean and Central American initiatives in 1997. Although implementation of control activities in the Andean subregion has been slow and coverage incomplete,[1] these three initiatives have been highly successful in eliminating domestic vector populations, thus interrupting disease transmission throughout much of Latin America.[2,3] However,

American Trypanosomiasis Chagas Disease. DOI: http://dx.doi.org/10.1016/B978-0-12-801029-7.00008-3

less success has been realized in the Gran Chaco region (northern Argentina, Bolivia, and Paraguay), partially due to high levels of insect reinfestation after spraying.[4] A key question is whether recurrent infestations are due to residual domestic populations that survive insecticide spraying, or to reinvasion of insects from external sources (either from unsprayed communities or from sylvatic [wild] foci).

In the Southern Cone, 10 years of coordinated control actions reduced disease incidence by 94%.[5] Nonetheless, recent estimates show that infection prevalence remains at 6 million, with 12,000 deaths annually.[6] What epidemiological factors contribute to new cases? Current hypotheses include: residual insects—perhaps from inadequate insecticide application or insecticide resistance; reinfestation from nearby houses or villages; and invasion of sylvatic vectors. Historically passive transport by humans expanded the geographic range of many vector species including two major vectors, *Triatoma infestans* and Rhodnius *prolixus*. In many cases, the vector species were exclusively domestic in the extended range and once eliminated, disease transmission was greatly reduced. However, over their native range, species are distributed across extensive sylvatic ecotopes, making the recolonization of treated villages a recurrent problem. In their own respective "home" areas in the Bolivian highlands and Venezuelan plains, *T. infestans* and *R. prolixus* reinfestation from sylvatic foci requires continued vigilance.[7,8] New epidemiological scenarios are also a matter of concern. For example, in Amazonia, foci of relatively intense transmission related to large-scale harvesting or consumption of forest products (such as açaí fruits and piaçava fibers) are overlaid onto a background of low-intensity, widespread, continuous vector-borne transmission.[9] Insecticide resistance is also an increasing problem.[10]

## *Why study the population genetics of insect disease vectors?*

Population genetics can provide insight into ecological and evolutionary processes (i.e., mutation, genetic drift, natural selection, and migration) relevant to vector-borne disease transmission by examining spatial and temporal patterns of genetic variation in insect vectors (Fig. 8.1). How much migration and interbreeding occur among nearby

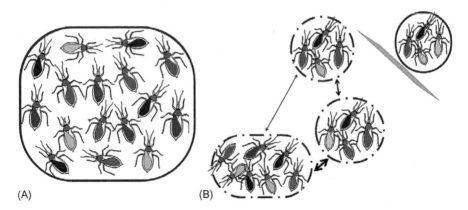

(A)   (B)

**Figure 8.1** Examples of (A) random population genetic structure and (B) distinct subpopulations with different amounts of gene flow (migration) among them.

populations? What barriers limit gene flow (e.g., deforestation, mountain ranges, biogeographical limits)? When insects reappear following insecticide treatment, do they represent recrudescent domestic populations, sylvatic colonizers, or migrants from nearby houses or villages? Do genetically different subpopulations also differ in vectorial competence or capacity? How fast might insecticide-resistance alleles spread throughout a population? The answers to these population genetics questions are of fundamental importance to the epidemiology and control of vector-borne diseases.

## Vector population structure directs Chagas disease epidemiology and control

A central tenant of population genetics is a hypothetical population with random genetic variation; that is, variation in alleles are randomly distributed with respect to space, time, ecological conditions, or any other factor. Ecological and evolutionary processes result in deviations from a random distribution. A textbook definition of population is a collection of interbreeding organisms of a particular species, but in practical terms populations are usually defined according to operational criteria (e.g., geographic proximity, sample availability, or even geopolitical limits). Genetic variation can be observed over multiple spatial and temporal scales, for example, within individuals as heterozygosity, within populations as deviations from HWE, and as genetic distance between populations. Human Chagas infection is endemic throughout Latin America, where its associated burden is larger than the combined burden of malaria, leprosy, leishmaniasis, filariasis, schistosomiasis, dengue, and the major intestinal nematode infections.[11] Although the etiological agent, *Trypanosoma cruzi*, is most often transmitted by insect vectors, recently Chagas is a concern in nonendemic areas, including the United States and Europe, due to immigration of infected individuals act as blood or organ donors or transmit the parasite congenitally.

There is no vaccine against *T. cruzi*, and the troublesome side effects of the medications make large-scale disease treatment difficult. As a consequence, disease control relies heavily on the elimination of domestic vector populations by house improvements combined with the spraying of residual insecticides and serological screening of blood donations. The importance of vector transmission results in a constant need for the development and optimization of vector control strategies to keep pace with the ever-changing epidemiological scenarios.[12] This is why furthering knowledge of triatomine population structure and gene flow, along with detection of cryptic (morphologically similar but genetically different) taxa that could exhibit different vectorial capabilities is so important.

## Genetic variation, population structure, and implications for vector control

### Evolutionary forces and genetic variation

Mutation increases genetic diversity in a population. These new alleles are then subject to natural selection whereby deleterious alleles are removed by purifying selection and advantageous alleles increase through directional selection. For example, directional selection from insecticide application removes susceptible alleles and over time an insecticide resistance allele can become "fixed" in the population. Directional and purifying selection reduce genetic variability; however, heterozygote advantage and changes in selection (e.g., movement between environments selecting for different alleles) can increase genetic variation.

The variability of a region of the genome depends on the mutation rate and the degree of functional constraint by natural selection. Protein coding genes are usually quite conserved due to purifying selection, but often show more variability in third position codons. Because of the critical role that ribosomes play in protein synthesis, and the three-dimensional structure needed to carry out this role, most regions of ribosomal DNA are even more conserved than protein coding genes. Noncoding regions including the mitochondrial control region, and nuclear repetitive DNA (e.g., microsatellites) and intergenic regions (e.g., ribosomal Internal Transcribed Spacers, ITS), are usually the most variable regions of genomes.

In addition to the effects of mutation and selection, genetic variation can be reduced simply due to chance alone, a process known as genetic drift. Genetic drift is the change in allele frequencies that occur due to finite population size and is especially important in smaller populations. Migration is a counteracting force to genetic drift. By mixing alleles among populations, migration distributes and homogenizes genetic variation among populations. In the absence of mutation, selection, and migration, genetic drift leads to the random fixation and loss of alleles. The pattern of reduced variation from drift is distinct from that caused by selection because the whole genome is affected, not just a particular locus. Inbreeding is also more prevalent in smaller populations and, in the absence of selection on inbred genotypes, does not change allele frequencies but reduces the frequency of heterozygotes.

## Microsatellites

The study of microsatellite loci has been instrumental in understanding fine scale population structure including estimating movement between ecotopes and identifying potential sources of reinfestation following insecticide application (Table 8.1). Microsatellites (2−5 tandemly repeated nucleotides, Fig. 8.2) have a relatively high mutation rate, are presumably not under selection and heterozygotes are easily distinguished from homozygotes.

## DNA sequence

DNA sequences or haplotypes are favored because of their objectivity and resolution. The differences between the mitochondrial and nuclear genomes, and a wide range of variability due to different mutation rates and functional constraints among regions of DNA facilitate addressing many population genetics questions.[22]

**Table 8.1 Microsatellite estimates of population subdivision for major triatomine species**

| Species | No. of loci | No. insects per population | Geographic distance (km) | $F_{ST}$ | Ref. |
|---|---|---|---|---|---|
| **Among villages** | | | | | |
| Triatoma dimidiata[a] | 4 | 11−36 | <280 | 0−0.553 | 13 |
| T. dimidiata | 7 | 28−30 | <13 | 0.05 | 14 |
| T. dimidiata | 10 | 10−25 | <600 | 0.3−0.522 | 15 |
| Triatoma infestans | 10 | 19−74 | <1464 | 0.135[b] | 16 |
| T. infestans | 10 | 12−99 | <31 | 0.018−0.192 | 17 |
| T. infestans | 10 | 18−70 | <220 | 0.169 | 18 |
| T. infestans | 10 | 1−78 | <100 | 0.06 | 19 |
| **Among ecotopes** | | | | | |
| T. dimidiata | 4 | 21−36 | Within villages, sylvan/ domestic/ peridomestic | 0.010−0.046 | 13 |
| Rhodnius prolixus | 9−10 | 10−39 | Varied, sylvan/ domestic | 0.002−0.2 | 8 |
| T. infestans | 9 | 6−32 | <1.1 km sylvan/ sylvan; sylvan/ domestic | 0.002−0.110; 0.026−0.072 | 20 |

[a]May include a cryptic species.
[b]$\theta_{ST}$.

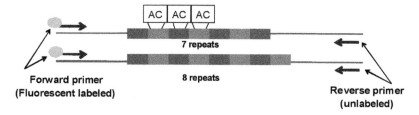

**Figure 8.2** Schematic representation of an AC microsatellite repeat. DNA polymerase slippage during replication results in alleles with different numbers of repeats that show different-sized bands after amplification using primers flanking the repeat region. Mutations in the primer binding sites can prevent primer annealing and amplification, resulting in a null allele and underestimates of heterozygosity.[21]

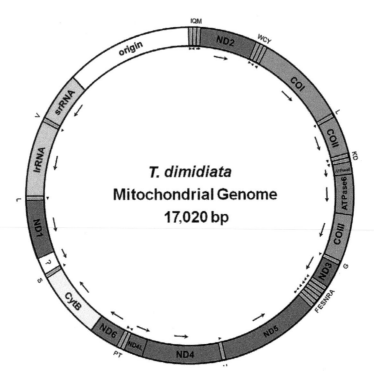

**Figure 8.3** Schematic representation of the mitochondrial genome of *T. dimidiat*.
*Source*: From Dotson EM, Beard CB. Sequence and organization of the mitochondrial
genome of the Chagas disease vector, *Triatoma dimidiata. Insect Mol Biol*
2001;**10**:205−15.[23]

Mitochondrial DNA (Fig. 8.3), especially cytochrome b (*cyt* b), cytochrome oxidase I (*co*I), and NADH ubiquinone oxidoreductase core subunit 4 (*ND4*), has been very important in understanding the geographic origin and movement of Triatominae.[24] It is highly variable, evolving approximately 10 times faster than the nuclear genome. This haploid genome eliminates complications due to crossing-over and heterozygosity. However, as mitochondria are maternally inherited, inferences about variation and gene flow are based on females only.

Ribosomal DNA (rDNA) sequences have also been useful in Chagas vector control studies and the more variable internal transcribed spacers, ITS-1 and ITS-2 (Fig. 8.4) and less variable 18S, 5.8S, and 28S (in that order) regions, are useful at different taxonomic scales. As a tandemly-repeated array, mutations within individual repeat units are usually homogenized by concerted evolution. The high copy number makes it an abundant PCR target, however, pseudogenes sometimes can confound the analysis. Although nuclear single copy genes (e.g., protein coding genes) have many advantages over ribosomal genes, to date, a sufficiently variable

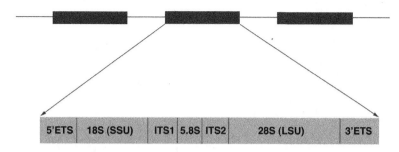

**Figure 8.4** Schematic representation of the tandemly repeated nuclear rDNA cistron unit (blue (black in print versions) boxes, above) and its primary transcript (below).

gene has not been identified. ITS-2 is the rDNA region most often used in population level studies in triatomines (Table 8.2), and has led to the discovery of hybridization,[36] and introgression. Recent multigene studies have revealed that several Chagas vector species actually are complexes including cryptic species, often with different epidemiological properties.[27,30,36−39]

## Hardy−Weinberg equilibrium

Hardy−Weinberg Equilibrium (HWE) is a null model of the relationship between allele and genotype frequencies, both within and between generations, under assumptions of no mutation, no migration, no selection, random mating, and infinite population size. Population geneticists often use SNPs or microsatellite data to test if observed genotype frequencies are significantly different from those expected based on HWE. If the population is not in HWE one or more assumption(s) of the model is incorrect.

Analysis starts by estimating allele frequencies from a sample of organisms ($N$) and calculating the expected genotype frequencies under HWE. For example, for a SNP, the frequencies of allele A (Adenine), $p_A$, and G (Guanine), $p_G$, would be

$$p_A = (N_{AA} + N_{AG})/2N$$

$$p_G = (2N_{GG} + N_{AG})/2N$$

where $N_{AA}$, $N_{AG}$, and $N_{GG}$ are the number of individuals of each genotype. Expected genotype frequencies are: $f_{AA} = p_A^2$, $f_{AG} = 2p_Ap_G$, and $f_{GG} = p_G^2$.

The following example is based on high throughput sequencing data from a SNP of Triatoma *dimidiata* ($N = 32$) collected from Guatemala to Nicaragua (Stevens and Dorn, unpublished data) with $N_{AA} = 19$, $N_{AG} = 2$, and $N_{GG} = 11$:

$$p_A = (2 \times 19 + 2)/2 \times 32 = 0.625$$

$$p_G = 1 - p_A = 0.235$$

## Table 8.2 Mitochondrial and nuclear DNA sequence diversity of major triatomine species

| | Gene | No. populations | $n$ | No. haplotypes | $H_d$ | $F_{ST}$ | Reference |
|---|---|---|---|---|---|---|---|
| **Mexico and Central America** | | | | | | | |
| *Triatoma dimidiata*[a] | cyt b | 12 | 24 | 21 | 0.960 | | 25 |
| *T. dimidiata* s.s. | cyt b | 7 | 58 | 15 | 0.901 | | 26 |
| *T. dimidiata*[a] | ITS-2 | 93 | 190 | 39 | 0.918 | | 25,27 |
| *T. dimidiata* s.s. | ITS-2 | 7 | 58 | 1 | 0 | | 26 |
| *T. dimidiata* s.s. | coI | 12 | 82 | 63 | 0.985 | 0.225 | 15 |
| *T. dimidiata* s.s. | ND4 | 3 | 40 | | 0.863 | 0.761 | 28 |
| *T. dimidiata* s.s. | ND4 | 22 | 228 | 155 | 0.991 | 0.482 | 29 |
| *Rhodnius prolixus* | cyt b | 34 | 551 | 15 | 0.518 | | 8 |
| **South America** | | | | | | | |
| *Triatoma brasiliensis* s.s. | cyt b | 4 | 361 | 29 | 0.905 | | 24 |
| *T. brasiliensis*[b] | cyt b | 17 | 136 | 35 | 0.920 | | 30 |
| *Panstrongylus megistus* | ITS-1-5.8-ITS-2 | 26 | 90 | 26 | 0.946 | | 31 |
| *Triatoma infestans* | cyt b | 43 | 98 | 11 | 0.737 | | 32,33 |
| *T. infestans* | coI | 45 | 207 | 32 | 0.812 | | 34 |
| *T. infestans* | ITS-2 | 31 | 35 | 5 | 0.591 | | 35 |

$H_d = \frac{n}{(n-1)}\left(1 - \sum \hat{x}_i^2\right); n =$ sample size, $x_i =$ haplotype frequency.

s.s. = senso stricto.

[a]May include a cryptic species.

[b]Includes proposed species *T. brasiliensis/macromelasoma, T. juazeiro, T. melanica.*

and the expected numbers of each genotype under HWE:

$$N_{AA} = N^* p_A{}^2 = 12.5 \text{ individuals}$$

$$N_{AG} = N^* 2 p_A p_G = 15.0 \text{ individuals}$$

$$N_{GG} = N^* p_G{}^2 = 4.5 \text{ individuals}$$

Comparison of expected with the observed numbers using a Chi-squared statistic gives $\chi^2 = 7.922$, $P < 0.015$, so we reject the null hypothesis and start looking for possible ecological processes that might cause the deviation. One likely contributing factor is nonrandom mating across the geographic range. It is probable that nearby *T. dimidiata* are more likely to mate and reproduce than are geographically distant individuals. Other possibilities are different migration rates across the landscape, variation in mutation rates, or natural selection.

The expected number of heterozygotes ($H_O = N_{AG}$) for this example is 15, but the observed number of heterozygotes ($H_E$) could range from 0 to 32. When there are multiple subpopulations, we can quantify the deviation of the actual from the expected heterozygosity with Wright's $F$ statistics[40] measuring the ratio of observed to expected heterozygosity:

$$F_{ST} = 1 - \frac{H_O}{H_E}$$

For a population in HWE $H_O = H_E$ and $F_{ST} = 0$, the greater the deviation from HWE the higher $F_{ST}$ to a maximum with no heterozygotes ($F_{ST} = 1$). In our example $F_{ST} = (1 - 0.063/0.468) = 0.867$, i.e., the heterozygosity is 87% less than expected. Wright suggested an $F_{ST}$ of 0–0.05 indicates little genetic differentiation, 0.05–0.15 moderate, 0.15–0.25 great, and >0.25 very great differentiation. Regardless of the magnitude of $F_{ST}$, only $F_{ST}$ values that are significantly different from zero are amenable to biological interpretation. Our $F_{ST} = 0.867$ indicates >80% loss in heterozygosity and "very great genetic differentiation" for our sample of *T. dimidiata*.

Additional analyses based on deviations from expected heterozygosity include estimating migration, testing for clinal variation, Bayesian clustering, and analysis of molecular variance. Under certain assumptions,[41] the number of mating migrants per generation, $N_e m$, between subpopulations is estimated with: $N_e m = \frac{1 - F_{ST}}{4 F_{ST}}$, where $N_e$ = effective population size (i.e., breeding adults) and $m$ = migration rate between populations (proportion of alleles replaced by alleles from migrants each generation). Clinal variation (replacement of one allele by another along the cline) can be tested with the Isolation by Distance model.[42] Bayesian clustering can identify genetic clusters and detect first generation hybrids.[43,44] Population genetic structure at multiple geographic scales can be partitioned through a hierarchical analysis of molecular variance[45] to determine the contribution of each geographic level (region, community, house) to the total variability. With biallelic data such as SNPs, analysis of molecular variance is expressed as $F_{ST}$. Modified versions of the statistic have been developed for multiallelic microsatellite data, $R_{ST}$,[46] and mitochondrial sequence data, $\Phi_{ST}$.[45] $R_{ST}$ is based on the stepwise mutation model that assumes alleles of similar size are more closely related. Population genetic data is commonly analyzed using freely available software including Arlequin,[47] Structure,[43] and DnaSP.[48]

## *The neutral theory and statistical tests*

The surprising amount of DNA sequence variation discovered as increasing data became available led to a more sophisticated model to infer ecological processes from population genetic data: the neutral theory. The theory states that most genetic variants are neutral with respect to natural selection and thus genetic variation can be modeled as a mutation-drift equilibrium resulting from finite population size. To determine if genetic variation in a sample fits the predictions of the neutral theory, one would calculate the expected genetic diversity for a set of DNA sequences under the assumptions of the neutral theory and compare it to the observed diversity in DNA sequence. One well known test for neutrality is Tajima's $D$ based on the difference between two parameters, the number of SNPs, $S$, and the average number of pairwise differences, $\pi = \frac{2*\sum_{i<j} d_{ij}}{n(n-1)}$. Under the neutral theory, $\pi$ and $S/a$ are expected to be equal, where $a$ is a scaling factor (for a full explanation, the reader is referred to any population genetics textbook[41]). The difference, normalized by the standard deviation, $\sqrt{V}$, is Tajima's $D$:

$$D = \frac{\pi - s/a}{\sqrt{V}}$$

If the sample reflects mutation-drift equilibrium as predicted by the neutral theory, $D = 0$. Under purifying selection, mutations will accumulate at third position codons, but are not likely to be common resulting in multiple low frequency SNPs, and $D < 0$. After a recent population expansion a similar pattern is expected. New mutations occur and because the population is expanding such mutations will persist, but will not be very common. In contrast, for a population bottleneck or either heterozygote advantage (for diploid nuclear genes) or balancing selection (for nuclear or mitochondrial genes), $D > 0$.

Statistical significance of $D$ is determined by a $\beta$-distribution.[49] Online interfaces (http://wwwabi.snv.jussieu.fr/achaz/neutralitytest.html) as well as software such as DnaSP[48] are available for calculating Tajima's $D$ and its statistical significance, as well as other tests of the neutral theory.

We briefly outline how DNA sequence data can be used to infer evolutionary and ecological processes with a subset of the data from the *T. infestans* mitochondrial *cyt* b gene.[32] The data, seven sequences from Yamperez, Bolivia with two haplotypes and three SNPs (Table 8.3), address the questions: Is the observed variation different from that expected by the neutral theory? If so, what might be causing the difference?

## Table 8.3 **The three SNPs in 411 nucleotides of** *cyt* **b in** *T. infestans* **from Yamparez, Bolivia**

| Nucleotide position relative to 1131 nucleotide *cyt* b gene | 537 | 741 | 789 | No. haplotypes in Yamperez |
|---|---|---|---|---|
| Haplotype A | C | G | G | 6 |
| Haplotype B | T | A | A | 1 |

The number of segregating sites, $S = 3$, the scaling factor, $a = \sum_{i=1}^{n-1} \frac{1}{i} = \frac{1}{1} + \frac{1}{2} + \frac{1}{3} + \frac{1}{4} + \frac{1}{5} + \frac{1}{6} = 2.450$, and $\frac{S}{a} = 1.224$. To calculate $\pi$ we compare all possible pairs of the seven sequences ($(7/2) = \frac{7!}{5!2!} = 21$ possible comparisons). For the 15 comparisons of a haplotype A with another haplotype A, there are no differences, $d_{ij} = 0$, and for the six comparisons of haplotype A with haplotype B with three SNPs, $d_{ij} = 3$, therefore:

$$\pi = \frac{2 * \sum_{i<j} d_{ij}}{n(n-1)}$$

$$= \frac{2*(0+0+0+0+0+0+0+0+0+0+0+0+0+0+0+3+3+3+3+3+3)}{(7*6)/2}$$

$$= 1.7143.$$

Using the online interface, $\sqrt{V} = 0.270$, $D = 1.812$, and $0.10 > P > 0.05$. The small, almost significant value of $D$ hints at balancing selection or a population bottleneck.

Using DNA sequence data to test the neutral theory expanded the field of theoretical population genetics, which now includes the use of mathematical, statistical, and computational models investigating and predicting quantities and patterns of genetic variation resulting from mutation, changes in population size, migration, selection, and nonrandom mating acting either individually or in combination.

### Spatial scale

The question posed determines the sampling strategy. At the large-scale, e.g., "Are there any cryptic species within the nominal species?" requires collections over a large geographic area, perhaps the entire range of the species; whereas the smaller, regional scale, e.g., "Are insects from sylvatic sites reinfesting treated houses?" requires insects from houses, perhaps multiple villages and the surrounding forest. The even smaller, locality scale question, "Are animal corrals, wood piles and other peridomestic structures the source of reinfesting insects?" requires insects from houses and surrounding peridomestic areas.

It is important to compare the amount of genetic variation only between different studies that cover similar geographic scales and sampling schemes. Likewise, results of studies based on DNA sequence are not directly comparable with studies based on differences in numbers of microsatellite repeats. Finally, for population genetics studies in which small differences in allele frequencies are important, a large enough sample size is needed to accurately represent the diversity in the subpopulation.

## Genetic variation and population structure of *T. infestans*, *T. dimidiata*, *R. prolixus* and other significant vectors of human Chagas disease

### T. infestans

*T. infestans* is the most important Chagas vector in South America (Fig. 8.5) and arguably the main vector of Chagas disease worldwide. There is strong evidence for two major evolutionary groups of *T. infestans*: one in the Andean regions of Bolivia and Peru and a second, non-Andean group. Currently restricted to the Andes as well as in the dry Chaco of Bolivia, Argentina, and Chile where domestic/peridomestic and sylvatic populations occur, it was once widespread throughout southern Brazil, much of Paraguay and northern Chile, Argentina, and Ecuador.

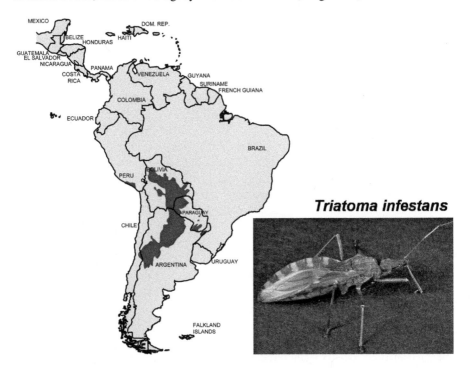

**Figure 8.5** Approximate current distribution of *T. infestans*.
*Source*: Data from Schofield CJ, Jannin J, Salvatella R. The future of Chagas disease control. *Trends Parasitol* 2006;**22(12)**:583−8.[50] Artist: Linda Waller; Photographer: James Gathany (Centers for Disease Control and Prevention).

## The hypothesized origin of T. infestans

A key hypothesis for the lack of success with control efforts in the Andes was rein-festation from sylvatic foci. Because sylvatic populations were first found in the Andes it was thought to be the geographic origin of the species. Discovery of sylvatic populations including dark morphs in non-Andean regions (Fig. 8.5), led to an alternative hypothesis that the Chaco was the origin.[51]

Genetic divergence of the Andean and non-Andean *T. infestans* is evident by differences in chromosomes and DNA content,[52] as well as nuclear[35,53] and mito-chondrial sequence data.[32,34] The chromosome studies show Andean *T. infestans* have about 30% more DNA than non-Andean populations,[52] reduced DNA content is often the derived state, supporting an Andean origin. Chromosomal evidence also suggested a hybrid zone associated with resistance to pyrethroid insecticides. The location of the hybrid zone in the non-Andean, Chaco area[54,55] suggests regional hybridization by secondary contact of Andean with non-Andean insects.[54,56]

The largest study of sylvatic specimens to date, perhaps for any Triatominae species, was a comparison of nuclear ITS-2 and mitochondrial *cyt* b based on 223 sylvatic Andean and non-Andean specimens.[53] Combined with data for domestic specimens,[35] the data show an ITS-2 dichotomy between Andean and non-Andean specimens, but do not indicate which group might be older.

The *cyt* b sequences from numerous *T. infestans* studies show possible ancient isolation and a population bottleneck in the Northern Andes[32,53] as well as strong structuring among most of the sylvatic populations.[53] However, a non-Andean origin cannot be excluded because of the high diversity among the non-Andean spe-cimens.[53] Study of *co*I also found reduced diversity in the Andes.[34] The pattern of *co*I sequence variation gives a positive, although nonsignificant, value for Tajima's $D_T$, suggesting the lower genetic diversity in the Andes could be the result of bottle-necks due to persistent insecticide spraying in that region and suggests multiple domestication events in both Andean and non-Andean areas.

## Population genetic studies to examine the sylvatic—domestic interface

Sylvatic populations are important because they represent a source for recoloniza-tion following insecticide treatment. Researchers recognize two groups of sylvatic *T. infestans*—those with normal coloration and "wild" melanic forms.

The first melanic *T. infestans* were discovered in peridomestic trees in the Argentine Chaco.[57] Subsequent reports describe a "dark morph" in the Bolivian Andes[51] and the non-Andean "*T. melanosoma*" in Argentina.[58] Several unique *co*I mutations in the dark morph lineage[34] indicate strong isolation between the non-Andean sylvatic dark morph and all other domestic and sylvatic Andean *T. infestans* populations as well as non-Andean domestic populations. However, there is yet no final agreement on whether the non-Andean darker populations are a result of migration from domestic to sylvatic ecotopes[35,52] or recurrent expansion from the Andean populations.[34] Recently, nonmelanic sylvatic *T. infestans* have been found to be much more widespread and common than originally thought including a wider geographic range in the Andes, as well as non-Andean specimens in Brazil, Chile, Argentina, Bolivia, and Paraguay.[53,59]

Statistical analysis of patterns of variation in DNA sequences indicates Argentinian populations of *T. infestans* likely represent a two-wave dispersal of *T. infestans* into Argentina along with either a recent population expansion or recent selection, population fragmentation, and Isolation by Distance.[34] Another study from the Argentina Chaco examining *co*I, ITS-1, and microsatellites reported significant differentiation between sylvatic and peridomestic specimens with limited asymmetric gene flow from the peridomestic to the sylvatic ecotope based on analysis of molecular variance and Bayesian assignment tests.[60]

In the Bolivian Andes, a study from three locations examining microsatellite loci in 277 domestic/peridomestic and sylvatic specimens found three lines of evidence suggesting significant mixing between the sylvatic and domestic ecotopes but not among locations. First, analysis of molecular variance found no difference between sylvatic and domestic populations, yet significant differentiation among locations. Second, Bayesian assignment tests gave very similar assignment to sylvatic and domestic ecotopes in each locality. And third, Bayesian analysis suggested first-generation migrants between sylvatic and domestic ecotopes within each location.[7]

## Effects of insecticide treatments on T. infestans *populations*

Domestic *T. infestans* populations subjected to vector control actions repeatedly go through bottleneck events or are locally eliminated; however, surprisingly high levels of genetic variability were observed in populations from the Great Chaco and Bolivia despite intensive insecticide application.[16,17,32,34,61]

Two studies based on 10 microsatellite loci addressed the influence of insecticide treatment on population genetic variability. The studies were conducted at the macrogeographical scale, involving samples from several provinces in Argentina,[16] and at the microgeographic (house) scale in Santiago del Estero, Argentina.[17] In both cases there were no significant differences in allelic richness (*aRich*) and genetic diversity ($H_e$) between recently (1−5 years) insecticide-treated populations (*aRich* = 3.8; $H_e$ = 0.6) and those not previously treated, or that had not been treated for more than 9 years previous (*aRich* = 3.8; $H_e$ = 0.7).

Results based on mitochondrial DNA sequence were similar to those for microsatellites. High levels of haplotype diversity ($H_d$) for the *cyt* b gene were found for four locations in Bolivia[32] that had not been sprayed for at least 3 years ($H_d$ = 0.29−0.67). Consistently, results of the 12S and 16S genes[61] in four provinces of Argentina showed the highest haplotype diversity and private haplotypes in the insecticide treated locations of El Jardín and Chancaní (La Rioja province) compared with untreated areas.

However, although variability seems not to have been severely affected by the insecticide control measures the pattern of variation is affected. Genetic structure of villages under long term control and surveillance was compared with villages randomly treated and not subject to surveillance. Strong genetic structure was observed in the area with high vector control pressure, represented in significant differentiation among most houses ($F_{ST} = 0.04–0.235$; $P < 0.0005$) and among all villages ($F_{ST} = 0.03–0.14$; $P < 0.001$) and Bayesian clustering methods supported eight significant genetic clusters within this area. On the other hand, in the randomly treated area, with populations from houses located 2–60 km apart, 31% of the houses were not significantly differentiated, variation on the village level was not significant, and all samples from this area fell within a single genetic cluster.[17]

A plausible explanation for this pattern is that the genetic structure of *T. infestans* subpopulations recovering from heavy insecticide spraying is molded by recrudescent subpopulations. Such "founder effects" would randomly preserve in each surviving subpopulation subsets of the variability originally detected, but each subpopulation would be independently subjected to the effects of genetic drift, promoting genetic differentiation.[16,17]

Population genetic analysis after insecticide treatments can detect not only effects on genetic variation within populations, but can also help recognize sources of reinfestation. Recolonization by the sylvatic ecotope after insecticide treatment[59,62] has been examined in several studies. A study from northwest Argentina comparing 20 sylvatic insects to domestic/peridomestic insects collected after spraying reported unrestricted gene flow between ecotopes. Further, mitochondrial DNA and microsatellite sibship analyses showed that the largest sylvatic colony had progeny from five females.[63]

Non-Andean specimens from four villages in the Bolivian Chaco collected before and after spraying showed strong differences in *cyt* b sequence among villages before insecticide spraying. Specimens collected after spraying showed that two villages were recolonized by local insects, and new Andean haplotypes appeared, suggesting passive transport from the Andes to the Chaco.[64]

## Genetic structure among domestic and peridomestic T. infestans populations

Several microsatellite based studies at the microgeographic (household) found high levels of population substructure within a locality, including differentiation among neighboring households well as between domestic and peridomestic sites.[16–20]

Support for an Isolation by Distance model of genetic differentiation varies among studies. Lack of fit was observed in *T. infestans* populations at the microgeographic, e.g., household or rocky outcrop, scale based on microsatellite markers.[17,19,20] However, support for the model was found at different geographic scales (houses, villages, provinces, or countries) based on mitochondrial DNA and microsatellites in Argentina.[16,34] The contradiction between results is likely due to the variation in geographic scales, differences in definition of a population, as well as geographic diversity in ecology.

## Promising areas for future studies

While challenges to vector control to reduce human disease incidence are indicated by data showing multiple events of domestication in both Andean and non-Andean areas, new genomic level studies could determine if the multiple events have a similar underlying genetic basis. Vector control efforts can be enhanced by studying the evolutionary history of insecticide resistance including possible recombination suppression or a reduction in hybrid vitality or fertility associated with the chromosomal hybrids between Andean and non-Andean lineages.

The evidence of local processes of genetic diversification calls for microgeographic scale studies characterizing local patterns of genetic variation. Follow-up studies are needed to identify sources of reinfestation and monitor insecticide resistance. High variability in sampling design, lack of a precise definition of "populations" being studied, and the diversity of analytical tools used complicates comparison between studies. The development of standard research strategies to address specific vector control questions is needed.

The process of reinfestation likely includes local survivors, migrants from nearby, and occasional importation by passive dispersal and would gradually mix genetic variants. The speed of this process depends on vector movement which can be assessed from population studies using $F_{ST}$, analysis of molecular variance, Bayesian genetic clusters, and testing for deviation from the neutral theory. Population genetic analysis must incorporate the epidemiological history of the populations being studied. Estimates of genetic structure, variability patterns, and other genetic parameters should be discussed and interpreted depending on the scale of the populations being investigated and insecticide spraying history.

## T. dimidiata

*T. dimidiata* is the most important Chagas vector in southern Mexico, Central America, and a secondary vector, after *R. prolixus*, in northern South America (Fig. 8.6). The diversity of this species across its geographic range in morphologic, behavioral, phenotypic, and genetic characteristics has resulted in its being split and merged many times into various species and subspecies (reviewed in Ref 38). Many variable attributes have significant implications for the epidemiological importance of particular populations (e.g., domestic or sylvan habitat, blood source preference). This diversity across a large geographic range and presence in multiple ecotopes make it quite challenging to control, and local approaches are needed for the different local conditions.

### *Cryptic species within* T. dimidiata

Cross breeding studies[66] combined with genetic data including nuclear, mitochondrial, and cytogenetic data[27,38,67,68] identify the geographic range of cryptic species to include Yucatan, Mexico; Belize; Peten, Guatemala; and Yoro, Honduras. However, since the various studies were done on different individuals, it is not clear if there is one or more cryptic species.

The most comprehensive *T. dimidiata* phylogeny to date, combining both nuclear and mitochondrial DNA markers on the same individuals, shows there is likely at

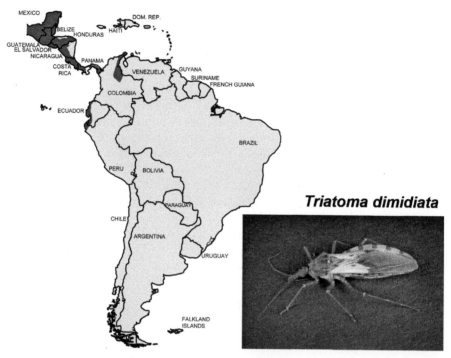

**Figure 8.6** Approximate current distribution of *T. dimidiata*.
*Source*: Data from World Health Organization. Geographical distribution of arthropod-borne diseases and their principal vectors. WHO/VBC/89.967, Geneva; 1989.[65] Artist: Linda Waller; Photographer: James Gathany (Centers for Disease Control and Prevention).

least two cryptic species and a large diverse clade, *T. dimidiata* s.s.[69]. This result indicates that population genetic studies conducted in areas with cryptic species must be interpreted with caution. Specimens from areas without reported cryptic species will be referred to as *T. dimidiata* s.s. below.

Unlike the mostly domestic nature of *T. infestans*, *T. dimidiata* occupies domestic, peridomestic, and sylvatic ecotopes over its geographic range. Interestingly, the distribution among ecotopes is quite different among geographic populations. *T. dimidiata* is nearly exclusively domestic and peridomestic over most of its range, from southern Mexico (except the Yucatan peninsula), southern Guatemala to Costa Rica and Ecuador, as well as the central Andean region of Colombia. However, it is largely sylvatic with occasional or seasonal entry into houses in northern Guatemala, the Yucatan peninsula in Mexico, and in the Caribbean plains and Sierra Nevada de Santa Marta mountains in Colombia.[13,29,38,70] The distinct habitats occupied, the degree of migration among habitats, as well as the underlying demographic history have been implicated in shaping the current patterns of genetic diversity for *T. dimidiata* across its geographic range.

## Genetic variation and structure in T. dimidiata *populations*

In spite of the distribution of *T. dimidiata* populations among different ecotopes, and with limited studies to date, a consistent pattern emerges of *T. dimidiata* as a highly mobile species migrating between sylvan and domestic/peridomestic ecotopes[13] or simply between domestic ecotopes (among houses and villages) in regions where it is largely domestic and there is little remnant forest.[14] *T. dimidiata* shows high genetic diversity, perhaps as a result of different selective pressures in the different ecotopes and genetic mixing between populations. Populations tend to show limited genetic structure at small distances (the evidence for high migration), and greater subdivision over larger geographic areas. In Central America, across large geographic distances there is support for the Isolation by Distance model of population subdivision[42]; whereas demographic history appears to play a larger role than Isolation by Distance in Colombia (described later).

Studies using both nuclear and mitochondrial DNA sequence show high diversity across large geographic regions in Central America. In Costa Rica, *T. dimidiata* s.s. populations from seven localities including both domestic/peridomestic and sylvan ecotopes were surprisingly monomorphic for the nuclear ITS-2 gene but genetically differentiated based on mitochondrial *cyt* b sequences[26] (Table 8.2) ($H_d = 0.901$). The $\sim 200$ km between the two regions which shared only one of 15 haplotypes, likely contributes to the genetic diversity.

Although with too few samples for statistical analysis, high genetic variation was also observed in mitochondrial ND4 and *cyt* b genes among 15 *T. dimidiata* sampled across central and southern Guatemala ($H_d = 0.924$).[71]

In Colombia, three studies comparing *T. dimidiata* from domestic/peridomestic and sylvan ecotopes across three ecogeographic regions (northern Caribbean plains, Sierra Nevada de Santa Marta mountain, and central Inter-Andean valleys) using mitochondrial and microsatellite markers show high genetic diversity and population subdivision. The first study, with limited sampling and using the mitochondrial marker *ND4*, shows high haplotype diversity ($H_d = 0.863$) and significant population subdivision ($\Phi_{ST} = 0.761$), that weakly correlates with Isolation by Distance.[28] The second study, with a broader sampling and using mitochondrial *coI* also shows high genetic diversity ($H_d = 0.985$) and strong genetic structure ($F_{ST} = 0.225$),[15] results supported by microsatellite markers in the same study. Haplotypes clustered geographically with evidence of rare gene flow between the mountain and plains (the two nearest regions), and some subdivision within Caribbean plains. Again, results weakly supported Isolation by Distance. The third study with extensive sampling and again using the mitochondrial gene *ND4* showed high genetic diversity and genetic differentiation within and among regions (overall $H_d = 0.991$) and strong structure ($F_{ST} = 0.482$), which could not be explained by Isolation by Distance.[29] With this larger sampling population, subdivision appears to be due to recent ($> \sim 4.5$ mya) population expansion after the joining of the continents with the formation of the Isthmus of Panama and differentiation influenced by isolation and drift of the populations with the upwelling of the Andes. Demographic history may be more important in Colombia rather than Isolation by Distance, better explaining the population structure.

In the Yucatan Peninsula, Mexico, microsatellites revealed weak population structure where *T. dimidiata* enters houses seasonally but does not establish domestic colonies, migrating between sylvan and domestic/peridomestic ecotopes. Analysis of only three microsatellites in and around 14 villages indicated high migration among nearby houses ($F_{ST} = 0.037$), more distant houses ($F_{ST} = 0.055$, <250 km), and between forest and houses ($F_{ST} = 0.01-0.03$, <280 km).[13] Longer distance migration could be due to passive transport. High migration was also indicated by 10–22% of domestic insects being more similar to those from peridomestic or sylvatic habitats. However, the recently described cryptic species occurs in this area (along with putative hybrids),[36] so these results must be interpreted with caution.

In Guatemala, microsatellite studies among domestic populations from six nearby villages (<27 km) showed small but significant differentiation ($F_{ST} = 0.05$) among populations; shared genetic clusters indicated some limited migration.[14] Although apparently *T. dimidiata* s.s. in Central America is moving less than in Yucatan, Mexico, the finding that in nearly all houses insects were half-sibs to completely unrelated suggests frequent migration is occurring, in this case among houses and villages rather than between ecotopes.

## *Implications for control and future studies for* T. dimidiata

From the data to date, *T. dimidiata* s.l. appears to have generally higher diversity and movement than *T. infestans*. In localities where it is exclusively domestic and peridomestic, *T. dimidiata* moves readily among houses within villages and among nearby villages. Where sylvatic populations exist, insects transiently enter homes. Evidence suggests long-distance, passive dispersal in human belongings or agricultural products. Broad geographic sampling shows Isolation by Distance occurs in Central America but not in Colombia.

Because of the extensive peridomestic and sylvatic populations and high migration, simply spraying insecticide in houses is unlikely to be effective for vector control. Ecohealth strategies, including house improvements, community participation, and control strategies designed for local situations will be more effective and sustainable.[72] Areas in need of further research include population genetics studies to determine the geographic range of differentiated subpopulations and their epidemiological importance. In addition, it will be important to determine the geographic, environmental, and anthropogenic factors keeping subpopulations apart, as well as the effects of Ecohealth interventions compared to traditional spraying on the population genetics of *T. dimidiata*.

## R. prolixus

*R. prolixus* is the primary Chagas disease vector in Venezuela and Colombia (Fig. 8.7), and was responsible for significant numbers of human infections before its recent eradication in Central America.[3] Its epidemiological importance is due to its high degree of adaptability for living in human habitations, where it can build up very large colonies.[73]

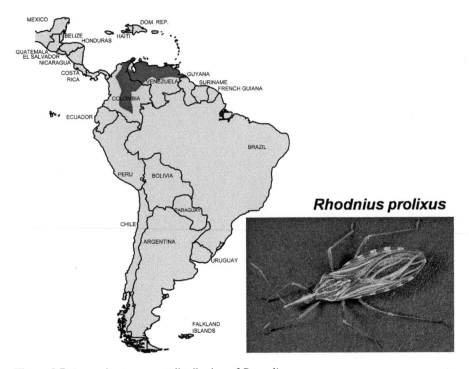

**Figure 8.7** Approximate current distribution of *R. prolixus*.
*Source*: Data updated from World Health Organization. Geographical distribution of arthropod-borne diseases and their principal vectors. WHO/VBC/89.967, Geneva; 1989.[65] Artist: Linda Waller; Photographer: James Gathany (Centers for Disease Control and Prevention).

## A single or multiple species?

As with *T. infestans* and *T. dimidiata*, there is uncertainty about *R. prolixus* being a single or multiple species, and whether the morphologically indistinguishable *R. robustus* is a sister taxa or subspecies. Slight morphological differences[74] combined with the observation that the smaller *R. prolixus* often forms large domestic colonies, whereas *R. robustus* seems to be exclusively sylvatic, led to the use of "smaller size and domesticity" versus "larger size and nondomesticity" as a practical means to separate *R. robustus* from *R. prolixus*.[75] Most importantly, it was also believed that domestication occurred only once and that all *R. prolixus* populations became reproductively isolated from their sylvatic counterparts.[76]

Mitochondrial DNA sequence analyses were crucial to confirming that *R. prolixus* and *R. robustus* are separate species, and that *R. robustus* comprises a species complex.[77] However, the confirmation of *R. prolixus* and *R. robustus* as separate taxa does not remove the challenge to household level insecticide-based vector control efforts. Control efforts against *R. prolixus*, although quite successful in Central America, have been hampered in Venezuela and Colombia where sylvatic populations co-occur. In Venezuela challenges to vector control efforts were indicated by a study combining *cyt* b and microsatellite data finding no difference between domestic and nearby sylvatic populations; however, there was evidence of past hybridization and introgression.[8] In Colombia, one study of four populations, three domestic and one sylvatic, reported genetic differentiation among all the populations, leaving the question of differentiation between geographically close domestic and sylvatic unresolved.[78]

## Implications for control and future studies for R. prolixus

These findings indicate sylvatic *R. prolixus* populations are a perennial source of migrants to recolonize insecticide-treated area constituting real challenge to vector control. In light of the ease with which *R. prolixus* colonizes houses, suitable habitat inside houses through Ecohealth strategies, is the best option to diminish domestic populations.[79]

Further knowledge on the genetic structure of natural populations is likely to advance quickly, with 20 newly described microsatellite loci of *R. prolixus*.[80] Another important scientific accomplishment that will certainly revolutionize the field is publication of the *R. prolixus* genome,[81] which at the very least will allow for the identification of many new nuclear markers.

## Other species of Triatoma

### Panstrongylus megistus

Since eradication of major vector species in large geographic regions, species that rarely invaded houses previously are being reported within houses and peridomestic areas more frequently, are perhaps becoming domesticated, and are an increasing concern for disease transmission. *P. megistus* occurs across the eastern coast of Brazil and is the most important vector of Chagas disease in Brazil since *T. infestans* eradication. Network analysis of ITS-1, 5.8S, ITS-2 sequences from 90 specimens from 26 localities along the eastern coast, identified Sao Paulo as a source of geographic spread.[31]

### Triatoma sanguisuga

*Triatoma sanguisuga* occurs in 23 states of the United States and at least two in Mexico. A study from a single location in Louisiana found amazing high diversity using the *cyt* b ($H_d = 0.978$) and 16S genes ($H_d = 0.713$). There were 37 haplotypes among 54 specimens from a single location. Fu's $F_S$ test[82] suggested a recent population expansion, rejecting the null hypothesis of selective neutrality and population equilibrium. The study was 1 year after significant environmental event, hurricane Katrina in 2005, and perhaps conditions after the storm led to population expansion.

A second study examined the *co*II gene of 33 insects collected inside and outside of houses from seven sites across two islands ~50 km apart off the east coast of Georgia.[83] No estimates of diversity were provided or tests of neutrality; however, there were 12 haplotypes with a maximum difference of 6% between haplotypes. Each island had distinct haplotypes and a haplotype network showing two groups, one of which was only on one island, the other of which was on both islands.

With respect to disease transmission, *T. sanguisuga* is not a very efficient vector,[84] however, the finding from Louisiana of many haplotypes among adults from a single location and the haplotypes occurring at additional locations >100 km away suggests *T. sanguisuga* is quite mobile. Such mobility would make the vector difficult to control were it an efficient vector.

## Perspective and future directions

Population genetics studies have provided important contributions to developing control strategies for Chagas vectors. We have learned about the identity of the epidemiologically important species, the origins of triatomine populations, and the adequacy of control strategies, among other findings. Certainly, there are many interesting questions to be addressed with new and emerging tools. With the advances in geographic information system technology, it is now possible to combine genetic with geographic and environmental data to predict the potential distribution of the vector populations and how such distributions might be affected by global climate change.

The origin and evolutionary history of several species has begun to be studied. What are the historical, geological, ecological, and demographical conditions that resulted in the current distribution of species and differentiated subpopulations? Have populations undergone bottlenecks, population expansions, or introductions into new localities? How has this affected their epidemiological importance? The issue of hybridization and introgression, observed in many triatomine species, is very intriguing. Where distinct taxa are sympatric (occur in the same area), are there differences that keep species reproductively isolated? What will be the effect of human activities such as deforestation and climate change? What will be the results of the ongoing control efforts?

Comparative genomics and proteomics can help to identify genes and proteins involved in colonization of human dwellings, hematophagy, and insecticide resistance. These approaches can also help to unravel vector/parasite interactions (e.g., does parasite infection result in changes in vector behavior in ways that increase transmission, and what genes are involved in vector competence and capacity?).

While DNA-based molecular markers provided population geneticists with dramatically increased resolution over previous approaches, development of new tools such as SNP assays and whole-genome sequencing will provide a new leap in resolution over current molecular methods used in triatomines.

## Acknowledgments

The authors wish to acknowledge the contributions to an earlier version by Paula Marcet and Fernando Monteiro, and technical assistance from Silvia Justi and Adrienne Woods. This work was made possible in part by support from National Science Foundation (NSF) grant BCS-1216193 as part of the joint NSF-NIH-USDA Ecology and Evolution of Infectious Diseases program.

# References

1. Guhl F. Chagas disease in Andean countries. *Mem Inst Oswaldo Cruz* 2007; **102**(Suppl. 1):29−38.
2. Dias JC, Silveira AC, Schofield CJ. The impact of Chagas disease control in Latin America: a review. *Mem Inst Oswaldo Cruz* 2002;**97**(5):603−12.
3. Hashimoto K, Schofield CJ. Elimination of *Rhodnius prolixus* in Central America. *Parasit Vectors* 2012;**5**:45.
4. Gürtler RE, Kitron U, Cecere MC, Segura EL, Cohen JE. Sustainable vector control and management of Chagas disease in the Gran Chaco, Argentina. *Proc Natl Acad Sci USA* 2007;**104**(41):16194−9.
5. World Health Organization. Control of Chagas disease (Second Report). In: WHO, editor. *WHO Technical Report Series 905*. Geneva: World Health Organization; 2002. p. 109.
6. World Health Organization. Weekly Epidemiology Report: Chagas disease in Latin America: an epidemiological update based on 2010 estimates, Switzerland; 2015.
7. Breniere SF, Salas R, Buitrago R, Bremond P, Sosa V, Bosseno MF, et al. Wild populations of *Triatoma infestans* are highly connected to intra-peridomestic conspecific populations in the Bolivian Andes. *PLoS ONE* 2013;**8**(11):e80786.
8. Fitzpatrick S, Feliciangeli MD, Sanchez-Martin MJ, Monteiro FA, Miles MA. Molecular genetics reveal that silvatic *Rhodnius prolixus* do colonise rural houses. *PLoS NTD* 2008;**2**(4):e210.
9. Aguilar HM, Abad-Franch F, Dias JC, Junqueira AC, Coura JR. Chagas disease in the Amazon region. *Mem Inst Oswaldo Cruz* 2007;**102**(Suppl. 1):47−56.
10. Germano MD, Picollo MI, Mougabure-Cueto GA. Microgeographical study of insecticide resistance in *Triatoma infestans* from Argentina. *Acta Trop* 2013;**128**(3):561−5.
11. Mathers CD, Lopez AD, Murray CJL. The burden of disease and mortality by condition: data, methods, and results for 2001. In: Lopez AD, Mathers CD, Ezzati M, Murray CJL, Jamison DT, editors. *Global Burden of Disease and Risk Factors*. New York: Oxford University Press-World Bank; 2006. p. 45−234.
12. Abad-Franch F, Monteiro FA, Jaramillo ON, Gurgel-Goncalves R, Dias FB, Diotaiuti L. Ecology, evolution, and the long-term surveillance of vector-borne Chagas disease: a multi-scale appraisal of the tribe Rhodniini (Triatominae). *Acta Trop* 2009; **110**(2-3):159−77.
13. Dumonteil E, Tripet F, Ramirez-Sierra MJ, Payet V, Lanzaro G, Menu F. Assessment of *Triatoma dimidiata* dispersal in the Yucatan Peninsula of Mexico by morphometry and microsatellite markers. *Am J Trop Med Hyg* 2007;**76**(5):930−7.
14. Stevens L, Monroy MC, Rodas AG, Hicks RM, Lucero DE, Lyons LA, et al. Migration and gene flow among domestic populations of the Chagas insect vector *Triatoma dimidiata* (Hemiptera: Reduviidae) detected by microsatellite loci. *J Med Entomol* 2015;**52**(3):419−28.
15. Gomez-Palacio A, Triana O, Jaramillo ON, Dotson EM, Marcet PL. Eco-geographical differentiation among Colombian populations of the Chagas disease vector *Triatoma dimidiata* (Hemiptera: Reduviidae). *Infect Genet Evol* 2013;**20**:352−61.
16. Pérez de Rosas AR, Segura EL, García BA. Microsatellite analysis of genetic structure in natural *Triatoma infestans* (Hemiptera: Reduviidae) populations from Argentina: its implication in assessing the effectiveness of Chagas' disease vector control programmes. *Mol Ecol* 2007;**16**(7):1401−12.

17. Marcet PL, Mora MS, Cutrera AP, Jones L, Gürtler RE, Kitron U, et al. Genetic structure of *Triatoma infestans* populations in rural communities of Santiago Del Estero, northern Argentina. *Infect Genet Evol* 2008;**8**:835—46.

18. Pérez de Rosas AR, Segura EL, Fichera L, Garcia BA. Macrogeographic and microgeographic genetic structure of the Chagas' disease vector *Triatoma infestans* (Hemiptera: Reduviidae) from Catamarca, Argentina. *Genetica* 2008;**133**(3):247—60.

19. Pizarro JC, Gilligan LM, Stevens L. Microsatellites reveal a high population structure in *Triatoma infestans* from Chuquisaca, Bolivia. *PLoS NTD* 2008;**2**(3):e202.

20. Richer W, Kengne P, Cortez MR, Perrineau MM, Cohuet A, Fontenille D, et al. Active dispersal by wild *Triatoma infestans* in the Bolivian Andes. *Trop Med Int Health* 2007;**12**(6):759—64.

21. Lehmann T, Licht M, Elissa N, Maega BT, Chimumbwa JM, Watsenga FT, et al. Population structure of *Anopheles gambiae* in Africa. *J Hered* 2003;**94**(2):133—47.

22. Mas-Coma S, Bargues MD. Populations, hybrids and the systematic concepts of species and subspecies in Chagas disease triatomine vectors inferred from nuclear ribosomal and mitochondrial DNA. *Acta Trop* 2009;**110**(2-3):112—36.

23. Dotson EM, Beard CB. Sequence and organization of the mitochondrial genome of the Chagas disease vector, *Triatoma dimidiata*. *Insect Mol Biol* 2001;**10**:205—15.

24. Almeida CE, Pacheco RS, Haag K, Dupas S, Dotson EM, Costa J. Inferring from the Cyt B gene the *Triatoma brasiliensis* Neiva, 1911 (Hemiptera: Reduviidae: Triatominae) genetic structure and domiciliary infestation in the state of Paraiba, Brazil. *Am J Trop Med Hyg* 2008;**78**(5):791—802.

25. Dorn PL, Calderon C, Melgar S, Moguel B, Solorzano E, Dumonteil E, et al. Two distinct *Triatoma dimidiata* (Latreille, 1811) taxa are found in sympatry in Guatemala and Mexico. *PLoS NTD* 2009;**3**(3):e393.

26. Blandon-Naranjo M, Zuriaga MA, Azofeifa G, Zeledon R, Bargues MD. Molecular evidence of intraspecific variability in different habitat-related populations of *Triatoma dimidiata* (Hemiptera: Reduviidae) from Costa Rica. *Parasitol Res* 2010;**106**(4):895—905.

27. Bargues MD, Klisiowicz DR, Gonzalez-Candelas F, Ramsey JM, Monroy C, Ponce C, et al. Phylogeography and genetic variation of *Triatoma dimidiata*, the main Chagas disease vector in Central America, and its position within the genus *Triatoma*. *PLoS NTD* 2008;**2**(5):e233.

28. Grisales N, Triana O, Angulo V, Jaramillo N, Parra-Henao G, Panzera F, et al. Genetic differentiation of three Colombian populations of *Triatoma dimidiata* (Heteroptera: Reduviidae) by ND4 mitochondrial gene molecular analysis. *Biomed Rev Inst Nacl Salud* 2010;**30**(2):207—14.

29. Gomez-Palacio A, Triana O. Molecular evidence of demographic expansion of the Chagas disease vector *Triatoma dimidiata* (Hemiptera, Reduviidae, Triatominae) in Colombia. *PLoS NTD* 2014;**8**(3):e2734.

30. Monteiro FA, Donnelly MJ, Beard CB, Costa J. Nested clade and phylogeographic analyses of the Chagas disease vector *Triatoma brasiliensis* in Northeast Brazil. *Mol Phylogenet Evol* 2004;**32**(1):46—56.

31. Cavassin FB, Kuehn CC, Kopp RL, Thomaz-Soccol V, Da Rosa JA, Luz E, et al. Genetic variability and geographical diversity of the main Chagas' disease vector *Panstrongylus megistus* (Hemiptera: Triatominae) in Brazil based on ribosomal DNA intergenic sequences. *J Med Entomol* 2014;**51**(3):616—28.

32. Giordano R, Cortez JC, Paulk S, Stevens L. Genetic diversity of *Triatoma infestans* (Hemiptera: Reduviidae) in Chuquisaca, Bolivia based on the mitochondrial cytochrome b gene. *Mem Inst Oswaldo Cruz* 2005;**100**(7):753—60.

33. Monteiro FA, Perez R, Panzera F, Dujardin JP, Galvao C, Rocha D, et al. Mitochondrial DNA variation of *Triatoma infestans* populations and its implication on the specific status of *T. melanosoma*. *Mem Inst Oswaldo Cruz* 1999;**94**(Suppl. 1):229−38.
34. Piccinali RV, Marcet PL, Noireau F, Kitron U, Gürtler RE, Dotson EM. Molecular population genetics and phylogeography of the Chagas disease vector *Triatoma infestans* in South America. *J Med Entomol* 2009;**46**(4):796−809.
35. Bargues MD, Klisiowicz DR, Panzera F, Noireau F, Marcilla A, Perez R, et al. Origin and phylogeography of the Chagas disease main vector *Triatoma infestans* based on nuclear rDNA sequences and genome size. *Infect Genet Evol* 2006;**6**(1):46−62.
36. Herrera-Aguilar M, Be-Barragan LA, Ramirez-Sierra MJ, Tripet F, Dorn P, Dumonteil E. Identification of a large hybrid zone between sympatric sibling species of *Triatoma dimidiata* in the Yucatan peninsula, Mexico, and its epidemiological importance. *Infect Genet Evol* 2009;**9**(6):1345−51.
37. Monteiro FA, Barrett TV, Fitzpatrick S, Cordon-Rosales C, Feliciangeli D, Beard CB. Molecular phylogeography of the Amazonian Chagas disease vectors *Rhodnius prolixus* and *R. robustus*. *Mol Ecol* 2003;**12**(4):997−1006.
38. Dorn PL, Monroy C, Curtis A. *Triatoma dimidiata* (Latreille, 1811): a review of its diversity across its geographic range and the relationship among populations. *Infect Genet Evol.* 2007;**7**(2):343−52.
39. Martinez-Hernandez F, Martinez-Ibarra JA, Catala S, Villalobos G, de la Torre P, Laclette JP, et al. Natural crossbreeding between sympatric species of the phyllosoma complex (Insecta: Hemiptera: Reduviidae) indicate the existence of only one species with morphologic and genetic variations. *Am J Trop Med Hyg* 2010;**82**(1):74−82.
40. Wright S. *Variability within and among natural populations*. Chicago: University of Chicago Press; 1978.
41. Nielsen R, Slatkin M. *An introduction to population genetics: theory and applications*. Sinauer Associates, Inc; 2013.
42. Mantel N. The detection of disease clustering and a generalized regression approach. *Cancer Res* 1967;**27**(2):209−20.
43. Pritchard JK, Stephens M, Donnelly P. Inference of population structure using multilocus genotype data. *Genetics* 2000;**155**(2):945−59.
44. Falush D, Stephens M, Pritchard JK. Inference of population structure using multilocus genotype data: dominant markers and null alleles. *Mol Ecol Notes* 2007;**7**(4):574−8.
45. Excoffier L, Smouse PE, Quattro JM. Analysis of molecular variance inferred from metric distances among DNA haplotypes: application to human mitochondrial DNA restriction data. *Genetics* 1992;**131**(2):479−91.
46. Slatkin M. A measure of population subdivision based on microsatellite allele frequencies. *Genetics* 1995;**139**(1):457−62.
47. Excoffier L, Lischer HE. Arlequin suite ver 3.5: a new series of programs to perform population genetics analyses under Linux and Windows. *Mol Ecol Res* 2010;**10**(3):564−7.
48. Librado P, Rozas J. DnaSP v5: a software for comprehensive analysis of DNA polymorphism data. *Bioinformatics (Oxford, England)* 2009;**25**:1451−2.
49. Tajima F. Statistical method for testing the neutral mutation hypothesis by DNA polymorphism. *Genetics* 1989;**123**(3):585−95.
50. Schofield CJ, Jannin J, Salvatella R. The future of Chagas disease control. *Trends Parasitol* 2006;**22**(12):583−8.
51. Noireau F, Flores R, Gutierrez T, Dujardin JP. Detection of sylvatic dark morphs of *Triatoma infestans* in the Bolivian Chaco. *Mem Inst Oswaldo Cruz* 1997;**92**(5):583−4.

52. Panzera F, Dujardin JP, Nicolini P, Caraccio MN, Rose V, Tellez T, et al. Genomic changes of Chagas disease vector, South America. *Emerg Infect Dis* 2004;**10**(3): 438−46.

53. Waleckx E, Salas R, Huaman N, Buitrago R, Bosseno MF, Aliaga C, et al. New insights on the Chagas disease main vector *Triatoma infestans* (Reduviidae, Triatominae) brought by the genetic analysis of Bolivian sylvatic populations. *Infect Genet Evol* 2011; **11**(5):1045−57.

54. Panzera F, Ferrandis I, Ramsey J, Salazar-Schettino PM, Cabrera M, Monroy C, et al. Genome size determination in Chagas disease transmitting bugs (Hemiptera: Triatominae) by flow cytometry. *Am J Trop Med Hyg* 2007;**76**(3):516−21.

55. Noireau F. Wild *Triatoma infestans*, a potential threat that needs to be monitored. *Mem Inst Oswaldo Cruz* 2009;**104**(Suppl. 1):60−4.

56. Panzera F, Ferreiro MJ, Pita S, Calleros L, Perez R, Basmadjian Y, et al. Evolutionary and dispersal history of *Triatoma infestans*, main vector of Chagas disease, by chromosomal markers. *Infect Genet Evol* 2014;**27**:105−13.

57. Martinez A, Olmedo R, Carcavallo RU. Una nueva subespecie Argentina de *Triatoma infestans*. *Chagas* 1987;**4**(1):7−8.

58. Ceballos LA, Piccinali RV, Berkunsky I, Kitron U, Gurtler RE. First finding of melanic sylvatic *Triatoma infestans* (Hemiptera: Reduviidae) colonies in the Argentine Chaco. *J Med Entomol.* 2009;**46**(5):1195−202.

59. Bacigalupo A, Segura JA, Garcia A, Hidalgo J, Galuppo S, Cattan PE. First finding of Chagas disease vectors associated with wild bushes in the Metropolitan Region of Chile. *Rev Med Chile* 2006;**134**(10):1230−6.

60. Piccinali RV, Marcet PL, Ceballos LA, Kitron U, Guertler RE, Dotson EM. Genetic variability, phylogenetic relationships and gene flow in *Triatoma infestans* dark morphs from the Argentinean Chaco. *Infect Genet Evol* 2011;**11**(5):895−903.

61. Garcia BA, Manfredi C, Fichera L, Segura EL. Short report: variation in mitochondrial 12S and 16S ribosomal DNA sequences in natural populations of *Triatoma infestans* (Hemiptera: Reduviidae). *Am J Trop Med Hyg* 2003;**68**(6):692−4.

62. Noireau F, Cortez MG, Monteiro FA, Jansen AM, Torrico F. Can wild *Triatoma infestans* foci in Bolivia jeopardize Chagas disease control efforts? *Trends Parasitol* 2005;**21**(1):7−10.

63. Ceballos LA, Piccinali RV, Marcet PL, Vazquez-Prokopec GM, Cardinal MV, Schachter-Broide J, et al. Hidden sylvatic foci of the main vector of Chagas disease *Triatoma infestans*: threats to the vector elimination campaign? *PLoS NTD* 2011;**5**(10).

64. Quisberth S, Waleckx E, Monje M, Chang B, Noireau F, Breniere SF. "Andean" and "non-Andean" ITS-2 and mtCytB haplotypes of *Triatoma infestans* are observed in the Gran Chaco (Bolivia): population genetics and the origin of reinfestation. *Infect Genet Evol* 2011;**11**(5):1006−14.

65. World Health Organization. *Geographical distribution of arthropod-borne diseases and their principal vectors*. Geneva: WHO/VBC/89.967; 1989.

66. Garcia M, Menes M, Dorn PL, Monroy C, Richards B, Panzera F, et al. Reproductive isolation revealed in preliminary crossbreeding experiments using field collected *Triatoma dimidiata* (Hemiptera: Reduviidae) from three ITS-2 defined groups. *Acta Trop* 2013;**128**(3):714−18.

67. Panzera F, Ferrandis I, Ramsey J, Ordonez R, Salazar-Schettino PM, Cabrera M, et al. Chromosomal variation and genome size support existence of cryptic species of

*Triatoma dimidiata* with different epidemiological importance as Chagas disease vectors. *Trop Med Int Health* 2006;**11**(7):1092—103.

68. Monteiro FA, Peretolchina T, Lazoski C, Harris K, Dotson EM, Abad-Franch F, et al. Phylogeographic pattern and extensive mitochondrial DNA divergence disclose a species complex within the Chagas disease vector *Triatoma dimidiata*. *PLoS ONE* 2013;**8**(8): e70974.

69. Dorn PL, de la Rúa NM, Axen H, Smith N, Richards BR, Charabati J, et al. Hypothesis testing clarifies the systematics of the main Central American Chagas disease vector, Triatoma dimidiata (Latreille, 1811), across its geographic range. *Infect Genet Evol* 2016;**44**.

70. Monroy MC, Bustamante DM, Rodas AG, Enriquez ME, Rosales RG. Habitats, dispersion and invasion of sylvatic *Triatoma dimidiata* (Hemiptera: Reduviidae: Triatominae) in Peten, Guatemala. *J Med Entomol* 2003;**40**(6):800—6.

71. Pennington PM, Messenger LA, Reina J, Juarez JG, Lawrence GG, Dotson EM, et al. The Chagas disease domestic transmission cycle in Guatemala: parasite-vector switches and lack of mitochondrial co-diversification between *Triatoma dimidiata* and *Trypanosoma cruzi* subpopulations suggest non-vectorial parasite dispersal across the Motagua valley. *Acta Trop* 2015;**151**:80—7.

72. Monroy C, Castro X, Bustamante DM, Pineda SS, Rodas A, Moguel B, et al. An ecosystem approach for the prevention of Chagas disease in rural Guatemala. In: Charron DF, editor. *Ecohealth research in practice: innovative applications of an ecosystem approach to health, insight and innovation in international development*. Dordrecht: Springer; 2012.

73. Sandoval CM, Gutierrez R, Luna S, Amaya M, Esteban L, Ariza H, et al. High density of *Rhodnius prolixus* in a rural house in Colombia. *Trans R Soc Trop Med Hyg* 2000;**94**(4):372—3.

74. Lent H, Wygodzinsky P. Revision of the Triatominae (Hemiptera, Reduviidae) and their significance as vectors of Chagas disease. *Bull Am Mus Nat Hist* 1979;**163**:123—520.

75. Pavan MG, Monteiro FA. A multiplex PCR assay that separates *Rhodnius prolixus* from members of the *Rhodnius robustus* cryptic species complex (Hemiptera: Reduviidae). *Trop Med Int Health* 2007;**12**(6):751—8.

76. Dujardin JP, Munoz M, Chavez T, Ponce C, Moreno J, Schofield CJ, et al. The origin of *Rhodnius prolixus* in Central America. *Med Vet Entomol* 1998;**12**:113—15.

77. Pavan MG, Mesquita RD, Lawrence GG, Lazoski C, Dotson EM, Abubucker S, et al. A nuclear single-nucleotide polymorphism (SNP) potentially useful for the separation of *Rhodnius prolixus* from members of the *Rhodnius robustus* cryptic species complex (Hemiptera: Reduviidae). *Infect Genet Evol* 2013;**14**:426—33.

78. Lopez DC, Jaramillo C, Guhl F. Population structure and genetic variability of *Rhodnius prolikus* (Hemiptera : Reduviidae) from different geographic areas of Colombia. *Biomed Rev Inst Nacl Salud* 2007;**27**:28—39.

79. Feliciangeli MD, Campbell-Lendrum D, Martinez C, Gonzalez D, Coleman P, Davies C. Chagas disease control in Venezuela: lessons for the Andean region and beyond. *Trends Parasitol* 2003;**19**(1):44—9.

80. Fitzpatrick S, Watts PC, Feliciangeli MD, Miles MA, Kemp SJ. A panel of ten microsatellite loci for the Chagas disease vector *Rhodnius prolixus* (Hemiptera: Reduviidae). *Infect Genet Evol* 2009;**9**(2):206—9.

81. Mesquita RD, Vionette-Amaral RJ, Lowenberger C, Rivera-Pomar R, Monteiro FA, Minx P, et al. Genome of *Rhodnius prolixus*, an insect vector of Chagas disease, reveals unique adaptations to hematophagy and parasite infection. *Proc Natl Acad Sci USA* 2015;**112**(48):14936−41.

82. Fu YX. New statistical tests of neutrality for DNA samples from a population. *Genetics* 1996;**143**(1):557−70.

83. Roden AE, Champagne DE, Forschler BT. Biogeography of *Triatoma sanguisuga* (Hemiptera: Reduviidae) on two barrier islands off the coast of Georgia, United States. *J Med Entomol* 2011;**48**(4):806−12.

84. Dorn PL, Perniciaro L, Yabsley MJ, Roellig DM, Balsamo G, Diaz J, et al. Autochthonous transmission of *Trypanosoma cruzi*, Louisiana. *Emerg Infect Dis* 2007;**13**(4):605−7.

# Geographic distribution of Triatominae vectors in America

D. Gorla[1] and F. Noireau[2]

[1]Consejo Nacional de Investigaciones Científicas y Técnicas, Universidad Nacional de Córdoba, Argentina, [2]Institute de Recherche pour le Ddéveloppement (IRD), UMR 177 Intertryp, Montpellier, France

## Chapter Outline

## Introduction

At present, some 150 species are grouped in the subfamily Triatominae. The number of valid species in this subfamily is mainly based on the revision by Lent and Wygodzinsky,[1] later updated by Galvão et al.[2] and has increased afterwards by the description of new taxa since 2010, including *Belminus corredori, Belminus ferroae, Panstrongylus mitarakaensis, Triatoma boliviana, Triatoma juazeirensis, Triatoma jatai, Triatoma pintodiasi, Rhodnius barretti, Rhodnius montenegrensis.*[3−10] Most triatomine species (∼135) occur exclusively in the New World, between latitude 42°N (northeast of the United States) and 46°S (Argentine Patagonia).[11] One species (*Triatoma rubrofasciata*) is widespread according to reports from port areas, both in the New World (mainly northeast Brazil) and in many tropical regions of Asia and Africa.[12] Seven species of *Triatoma* and six species of the genus *Linshcosteus* are known to exist only in Asia and India, respectively.[1,2] Some authors suggest that the

American Trypanosomiasis Chagas Disease. DOI: http://dx.doi.org/10.1016/B978-0-12-801029-7.00009-5

Old World species are derived from *T. rubrofasciata* and transported from North America, associated with rats on sailing ships.[12-15]

The Triatominae occurring in the Americas are customarily classified into 5 tribes and 15 genera,[1] including Alberproseniini (genus *Alberprosenia*), Bolboderini (genera *Belminus*, *Bolbodera*, *Microtriatoma*, and *Parabelminus*), Cavernicolini (*Cavernicola*), Rhodniini (*Psammolestes* and *Rhodnius*), and Triatomini (*Dipetalogaster*, *Eratyrus*, *Hermanlentia*, *Mepraia*, *Panstrongylus*, *Paratriatoma*, and *Triatoma*). Extensive information exists on their geographic distribution, and as a general review of the group we suggest the reading of a few studies.[1,2,11] A recent open access bibliographic database BIBTRI, compiled under the coordination of Dr. J. Rabinovich, offers 7000 + references with pdf support (www.bibtri.com.ar).

The present review on the geographic distribution of Triatominae considers the species of epidemiological importance or the groups of species in which at least one species has an epidemiological significance as a vector of *Trypanosoma cruzi* to humans. All the species considered belong to the tribes Rhodniini and Triatomini.

## Limitation of sampling methods to estimate the geographic distribution of Triatominae

Data on the distribution of triatomine species are usually obtained from the detection of peridomestic/domestic colonies, focal sampling of sylvatic populations, and information on the domestic intrusion of wild adult forms. Consequently, the more the synanthropic process of a Chagas disease vector is advanced, the more its geographic range may be precisely known. Thus, the past and recent changes in the geographic range of the most efficient vectors of *T. cruzi* to humans (*T. infestans* and *R. prolixus*) are well known. However, an incomplete knowledge of species distribution exists when these organisms are restricted to sylvatic environments. It is unfeasible to systematically sample over wide areas (wild populations are usually focally sampled) because it is difficult to access certain types of ecotopes, thus making it difficult to investigate these areas. Moreover, in the case of exclusively sylvatic species, the sampling is generally random and, consequently, often unproductive. The sampled subsets are considered isolated species when they may represent components of an unknown continuous population.[12] With regard to triatomine species that exhibit a certain level of domestic incursion, their easy detection will depend on some behavioral traits, such as flight ability and attraction to light. The live-baited trap and light trap are the tools currently available to collect wild Triatominae. Unfortunately, both trapping systems only catch starved triatomines and, in the case of the light trap, only adult forms. Thus, the number of bugs a trap would be able to capture in a defined area would be inversely correlated to the nutritional status of the population.[16]

The decrease of the relative importance of the main domestic triatomine species, accompanied by the demographic transition of populations from rural areas to large urban centers that frequently results in a disordered occupation of forest remnants and the expansion of agricultural lands (led by soy fields) and cattle ranching, increased the relative importance of the once called "secondary" species. The increased attention of these secondary species is reflected by an increasing number of articles studying the process of house invasion by wild species of Triatominae.[17–22]

# Pattern of species richness in the New World Triatominae

Of the five tribes within the Triatominae subfamily, Triatomini and Rhodniini include 88% of the recognized 150 species. Within the two most numerous tribes, the genera *Rhodnius*, *Panstrongylus*, and *Triatoma* constitute 86.5% of the species found in the Americas. Controversies about the evolution of the Triatominae still exist, although there is ample evidence supporting its polyphyletic constitution. The *Rhodnius* species are generally associated with palm tree species found in the geographic range from southern Amazonia to Central America. The majority of the 13 *Panstrongylus* species are exclusively sylvatic with a wide variety of habitats and wild animals. *Triatoma* is the most numerous genus, including 80+ species distributed as far as the extreme northern and southern latitudes. Recent evidence suggests that *Triatoma* species of Central and North America constitute a group that evolved independently from the *Triatoma* species of South America.[12]

A study considering 118 Triatominae species of the New World showed that groups analyzed at the continental scale had patterns of species richness that showed a significant linear latitudinal gradient with low values at the extreme latitudes and highest values near the equator (precisely on the 5–10° southern latitudinal band). The study also showed that species richness is significantly associated with habitable geographic area and temperature in the Southern hemisphere; in this hemisphere, there is a significant longitudinal gradient given by the Andes range, an element that influences the increase of species richness toward the east of South America.[23]

We expanded the analysis of the data used by Rodriguero and Gorla[23] and used a similar methodology to analyze the latitudinal range for the species (difference between maximum and minimum latitude of the species geographic distribution). The results showed a significant linear increase of the latitudinal range of the species from the equator (i.e., narrower near the equator, wider toward higher latitudes), as predicted by the Rapoport's rule (Fig. 9.1). When considering the species richness across the latitudinal regions of the most numerous Triatominae genus, it is clear that individual genera do not follow the same pattern shown by the complete set of Triatominae species. For instance, *Triatoma* shows a bimodal pattern of species richness with low frequency at low latitudes and modal maxima at around 23° north or south. *Rhodnius* shows an unimodal species richness distribution but strongly skewed with modal number of species located on the Northern Hemisphere at low latitudes and a few species on the Southern Hemisphere, some of them reaching the 30° southern latitude. *Panstrongylus* also shows a unimodal species richness distribution with the majority of species located on the Southern Hemisphere (Fig. 9.2).

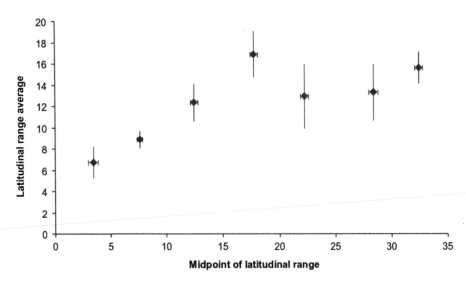

**Figure 9.1** Relationship between the average latitudinal range and the midpoint of the latitudinal range for Triatominae species in the Americas. Vertical and horizontal lines over the points indicate standard errors.

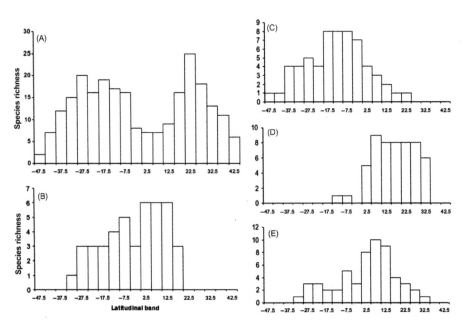

**Figure 9.2** Species richness of Triatominae per 10° latitudinal band. (A) *Triatoma* species; (B) *Rhodnius* species and *Psammolestes* species; (C) *Panstrongylus* species; (D) Old World Triatominae; (E) *Dipetalogaster*, *Eratyrus*, *Hermanlentia*, Alberproseniini, Bolboderini, and Cavernicolini. Negative latitudinal bands are in the Southern Hemisphere.

In a more recent analysis, the geographical ranges and richness patterns of Triatominae richness in Latin America was analyzed,[24] using spatial eigenvector mapping, multiple regressions, and generalized linear models. They found that richness and species ranges show high correlation and identified an important role for temperature and temperature seasonality in explaining richness and distributions.

# Distribution of Triatominae in the Americas

## *Genus* Rhodnius

At the moment, the genus *Rhodnius* consists of 18 valid species (16 from Galvão et al.[2] plus two additional recent additions). All *Rhodnius* species have been primarily associated with palm trees even though some species were found in other sylvatic habitats. Thus, *R. domesticus* has been reported as colonizing bromeliads and hollow trees in Amazonia, and specimens of *Rhodnius* species have been found in the cactus mandacaru (*Cereus jamacaru*) in the Caatinga of northeastern Brazil.[1,25,26] Some *Rhodnius* species may be associated with particular types of palms, such as *Rhodnius brethesi* with *Leopoldinia piassaba* and *Rhodnius ecuadoriensis* with *Phytelephas* species. Consequently, the distribution of sylvatic *Rhodnius* broadly coincides with the distribution of palm trees.[25] Recent work suggests that deforestation and the associated loss of habitat and host diversity might increase the frequency of *Rhodnius*–human contact.[22,27]

The genus *Rhodnius* encompasses a variety of species, including one primary domestic vector (*R. prolixus*), various synanthropic species that invade and sporadically colonize man-made ecotopes (*R. pallescens, R. neglectus, R. nasutus, R. stali,* and *R. ecuadoriensis*), species that invade but do not colonize houses (*R. robustus, R. pictipes,* and *R. brethesi*), and strictly sylvatic species.[27] *Rhodnius* naturally occurs from Central America to northern Argentina, and species richness is highest in Amazonia.

*R. prolixus* is a domestic vector of *T. cruzi* to humans in Venezuela, Colombia. It was an important vector in some countries of Central America, but national control programs successfully interrupted *T. cruzi* transmission by *R. prolixus*, and even eliminated the species in several regions.[28] *R. prolixus* was likely erroneously recorded from Bolivia, Brazil, Ecuador, French Guiana, Guiana, Panama, and Suriname due to confusion with *R. robustus* (all countries) and *R. neglectus* (Central Brazil). *R. prolixus* is no longer found in its previously reported collection areas in Mexico (Oaxaca and Chiapas), Guatemala, El Salvador, and most of Honduras. Sylvatic populations have been captured in palm trees in Venezuela and the Orinoco region in Colombia but they have never been found in Central America.[29–31] Moreover, neither sylvatic nor domestic populations have ever been collected in Panama or south of Costa Rica. The discontinuity of the distribution area combined with the genetic homogeneity of *R. prolixus* in Central America suggest that domestic vectors from the South American populations have invaded several countries of Central America.[32] Two explanations have been put forward. One explanation suggests that these vectors have been dispersed through passive carriage of eggs and young nymphs in the plumage of storks (*Mycteria americana*), which are known to migrate between the two regions and nest in palm trees.[33] The second explanation suggests that these vectors have spread due to an accidental escape of laboratory-bred insects.[34]

The species forming the *prolixus* group (*R. prolixus, R. robustus, R. neglectus,* and *R. nasutus*) are particularly difficult to distinguish. The specific status of *R. robustus,* which is virtually indistinguishable from *R. prolixus* using morphological characters, has been clarified by the use of modern techniques of species characterization, such as the sequence analysis for a fragment of the mitochondrial cytochrome b. *R. robustus* currently includes four cryptic species. *R. robustus* I, which occurs in Venezuela (Orinoco region), is more closely related to *R. prolixus* than to the other three cryptic species found in the Amazon region.[35] The near-sibling *R. neglectus* and *R. nasutus* are Brazilian species. The geographic distribution of *R. nasutus* is restricted to the northeastern region, particularly to the semiarid Caatinga. *R. neglectus* has a wider distribution across the Cerrado and the adjacent regions of Central Brazil.[2,11] Recent studies show that both species are sympatric in the northern Bahia State.[27]

*R. pallescens* has been reported in Belize, Nicaragua, Costa Rica, Panama, and Colombia, where it inhabits sylvatic environments and it is often found in human dwellings although without building intradomestic colonies.[36] The palm tree *Attalea butyracea* is its primary biotope. This species is characterized by its sporadic presence inside dwellings in Panama, where it is the only vector of *T. cruzi* to humans.[37] *R. stali* is a fairly unknown Bolivian species that has been historically confused with *R. pictipes*. The distribution of Rhodnius *stali* closely matches that of *Attalea phalerata* palms in the southwestern fringe of the Amazon biome. *R. stali* is able to establish colonies in domestic and peridomestic habitats, and the observation of Chagas disease seropositivity in the indigenous population of the Alto Beni region strongly suggests the presence of an ongoing anthropozoonotic disease transmission cycle.[38]

*R. ecuadoriensis* survives under a wide range of climatic conditions in Ecuador and northern Peru.[27] Sylvatic populations of this species have been mainly found living in the *Phytelephas aequatorialis* palm trees in northern Ecuador.[1,27] The strong synanthropic behavior of *R. ecuadoriensis* and the absence of palm trees in southern Ecuador and northern Peru suggested that this species might have spread to the region through association with humans.[39,40] The recent detection of *R. ecuadoriensis* in sylvatic habitat (squirrel nests) in the southern Highlands of Ecuador contradicts this hypothesis.[41]

*R. brethesi* is a species occurring in the Brazilian Amazon that seems to be tightly associated with *L. piassaba* palm trees. *T. cruzi* transmission in the Negro River region (Amazonas, Brazil) is caused by invasion of human dwellings by the vectors. Other observations attribute the attack of wild triatomines to the collectors of fronds from the piassaba palm.[42] *R. pictipes* has a wide geographic distribution throughout the Amazon basin (north and northwest South America) in association with various species of palm trees.[11] The sporadic invasion of houses by light-attracted adult *R. pictipes* may be promoted by the presence of palm trees near households. The ingestion of palm fruit juices contaminated with crushed vectors was documented in some outbreaks of acute oral Chagas disease, which is the main transmission mechanism of *T. cruzi* in the Amazon region.[43]

## *Genus* Panstrongylus

There are 13 recognized species within the genus *Panstrongylus* that have a wide geographic distribution throughout the Neotropical region, extending from Mexico to Argentina.[44] Among these species, some appear to be involved in a process of domiciliation, showing the ability of the species to colonize human dwellings (*P. geniculatus, P. rufotuberculatus, P. lutzi,* and *P. chinai*). Other species are more opportunistic and occasionally fly from the sylvatic environment to houses without colonizing (e.g., *P. lignarius* in the Amazon basin). The phylogeny of the group is currently under discussion, although there is evidence suggesting the existence of a northern and a southern clade that are parallel to the northern and southern clade of *Triatoma* species; *Panstrongylus* species are considered to be evolved from this latter clade.[45]

Although some species can be found in palm tree crowns (e.g., *P. megistus*), all species are associated with terrestrial burrows, tree-root cavities, or hollow trees.[25] *P. geniculatus* and *P. rufotuberculatus* have the widest geographic distribution, extending from Mexico to Argentina, including the Caribbean Islands (found in 18 and 10 countries, respectively). *P. lignarius* is the third most widely dispersed and it is found in seven South American countries. *P. megistus* is restricted to eastern and central South America. The remainder of the species have more limited or undetermined geographic distributions. *P. geniculatus* has been considered a eurythermic species, meaning that it is adapted to several dry as well as humid ecotopes, and it is found in a great variety of sylvatic habitats (very dry forests or savannahs, dry, wet, moist, and rainy forests). This species is frequently captured in peridomestic environments and its occurrence inside houses has been cited in several countries.[25,46−48] This species has epidemiological importance because of the high incidence of blood-fed specimens on humans concomitantly infected with *T. cruzi* I in Venezuela.[48] The ingestion of fruit juice accidentally contaminated by *P. geniculatus* is thought to have caused an outbreak of infections in 2007 in Caracas possibly via oral transmission.

*P. rufotuberculatus* is generally considered to be a sylvatic species ranging from Mexico to Argentina. This species has been found in palms, hollow trees, and the refuges of wild mammals.[1,49,50] Adult insects frequently invade human dwellings as they are attracted by electric light.[1,51,52] Breeding colonies have been found inside dwellings in Bolivia, Ecuador, and Peru.[39,53,54] *P. rufotuberculatus* has been incriminated as a vector of Chagas disease in Andean and coastal foci of Ecuador. In the municipality of Amalfi (Antioquia, Colombia), the presence of *P. rufotuberculatus* is an epidemiological risk factor.[55] Several characteristics that could be linked to high vectorial capacity were observed for this species, including longevity, rapid response to the presence of a host, large volumes of blood ingested, and frequent defecation during the feeding process.[56]

*P. megistus* has a wide geographic distribution, ecological valence, and great potential for the colonization of artificial ecotopes. This species occurs in all varieties of Brazilian forests, including dry and moist humid forests in the Cerrado and Caatinga. The species is usually associated with humid forests from where adults can invade houses,[57] especially during the rainy season.[58] In other countries, such as Argentina, Bolivia, Paraguay, and Uruguay, *P. megistus* is almost entirely sylvatic.[59] On the occasions when this species is found in domestic habitats, it is usually associated with synanthropic hosts, especially opossums.[60] *P. megistus* was considered the main domestic vector in Brazil until it was progressively replaced by *T. infestans*, probably since 1930.[58,61] Following the success of the Southern Cone Chagas Disease Control Programme (INCOSUR) that achieved the elimination of *T. infestans* in many areas,[62] *P. megistus* reinitiated house invasion and is once again domiciliated in several states of Brazil. Thus, *P. megistus* is currently considered to be the main autochthonous vector of Chagas disease in the central, eastern, and southeastern regions of Brazil. The most strongly synanthropic species, *P. lignarius* (formerly *P. herreri*), is considered to be the principal vector of Chagas disease in Peru.[54]

Transmission of sylvatic *T. cruzi* to humans has also been associated with *P. lignarius*. In the Amazon basin, this species was observed flying from palm trees (*A. phalerata*) to houses.[63] In Colombia, this species has been found in bird nests and it is not considered of epidemiological importance.[64]

*P. lutzi* is one of the most important secondary vectors in Brazil. It has great capacity for invading houses through flight and shows high rates of natural infection with *T. cruzi*, likely due to the close vector association with armadillos.[26] *P. chinai* may act as the vector of *T. cruzi* in sylvatic cycles in arid areas of northern and eastern Peru (Vazquez-Prokopec et al., 2005) as well as southeastern Ecuador.[65] *P. howardi* is considered to be a potential vector of *T. cruzi* in the coastal region of Ecuador.[65] The remaining *Panstrongylus* species (*P. diasi*, *P. guentheri*, *P. humeralis*, *P. lenti*, *P. mitarakaensis*, and *P. tupynambai*) have not been described as vectors of *T. cruzi* to humans, but most of them are probably involved in sylvatic *T. cruzi* cycles.[45]

## Genus Triatoma

*Triatoma* is the most numerous genus of Triatominae, with 80 + formally recognized species (Schofield and Galvão[12] and latter additions). Species of the genus occupy a wide array of habitats that are mainly associated with mammals and birds.[66] According to Gaunt and Miles,[25] the genus *Triatoma* has predominantly evolved in terrestrial, rocky habitats. However, many *Triatoma* species are specifically or preferentially arboreal and found in bird nests, palm trees, hollow trees, and under the barks of trees. This is the case for *T. delpontei*, *T. platensis*, *T. infestans* "dark morph," *T. pseudomaculata*, *T. sordida*, *T. guasayana* (except for the Andean populations that live among stones), *T. nigromaculata*, *T. maculata*, *T. ryckmani*, and *T. tibiamaculata*. The review dedicated to the geographic distribution of the genus *Triatoma* only addresses species of epidemiological importance, namely those that establish domestic colonies or occasionally infest houses by intrusion from peridomestic or sylvatic habitats. These invasions require innovative control strategies to disrupt *T. cruzi* transmission and represent an important challenge for public health.

## Triatoma infestans subcomplex (sensu Schofield and Galvão[12])

This subcomplex includes the species *infestans*, *delpontei*, and *platensis*. The latter two species are closely associated with bird nests and have never been found colonizing intradomestic habitats. These three species are very closely related and have the same diploid chromosome number 2n 5 22 (20 autosomes 1 XX/XY). They also have several cytogenetic traits that differ from all other triatomines, including large autosomes, C-heterochromatic blocks, and meiotic heteropycnotic chromocenters formed by autosomes and sex chromosomes.[67] *T. infestans* remains the most important and widespread vector of Chagas disease in South America. *T. platensis* is a species almost exclusively present in nests of Furnariidae (*Anumbius* species, *Coryphistera alaudina*, *Pseudoseisura lophotes*) in northern Argentina, Paraguay, Uruguay, and southern Brazil.[66] This species has been occasionally found in chicken coops, where it is able to crossbreed with *T. infestans*,[68] and also on furnariid nests, as recently reported.[69] All evidence indicates that within this subcomplex, *T. platensis* is the closest relative to *T. infestans*.[70] The status of *T. infestans* and *T. platensis* as two distinct species is almost entirely based upon their ecological niche separation. *T. delpontei* is another ornithophilic arboreal species and has a marked preference for woven stick nests of colonial monk parrots (*Myopsitta monachus*).[66] It is distributed in Bolivia, Paraguay, Uruguay, and Argentina. Despite the bird specificity, *T. delpontei* females are able to crossbreed with *T. platensis* males under laboratory conditions.[71] Their morphological similarity would be the consequence of a convergence related to a highly specialized adaptation to bird nests rather than having a common ancestry.[68] Both species have no role in the transmission of *T. cruzi* because of their specific association with birds that are not susceptible to the parasite infection.

## Triatoma dimidiata

This species is a major Chagas disease vector found in Central Mexico, the Yucatan peninsula, Central America, northern Colombia, Venezuela, and Ecuador.[2] *T. dimidiata* is becoming the most important vector of Chagas disease in this region because the control activities to eliminate *R. prolixus* have made substantial progress.[28] This species has extensive phenotypic, genotypic, and behavioral diversity in sylvatic, peridomestic, and domestic habitats across its geographic range. Thus, it is a domiciliated vector in most of Central America and Central Mexico where sylvatic and peridomestic populations also occur. This species may also act as vector of intrusion in the southeast of Mexico, Belize, and some parts of Guatemala. In Ecuador, where no sylvatic populations have been reported, it is an exclusively domestic vector. Across their geographic range, sylvatic populations of *T. dimidiata* have been found in a great variety of microhabitats, such as in the bark of dead trees and hollow trees, palm trees, rock piles, Mayan ruins, caves occupied by bats, and nests of several mammals (e.g., opossums and armadillos).[72] Recent studies strongly suggest that *T. dimidiata*, which has been historically regarded as a single species, includes several cryptic species distributed in specific geographic areas with different epidemiological importance.[73–75] More than 60 years ago, *T. dimidiata* represented an assemblage of morphologically variable populations, and Usinger[76] had given subspecific status for some populations, namely *T. d. dimidiata* (Central American forms), *T. d. capitata* (Colombian forms), and *T. d. maculipennis* (some Mexican forms). Cytogenetics and molecular tools have confirmed this diversity[73,75] and the taxonomy adopted by Usinger[76] has been reused.[74] Currently, Central American populations in Honduras, Nicaragua, and southern Guatemala correspond to subspecies *T. d. dimidiata*. A southern spread into Panama and Colombia gave the *T. d. capitata* form. A northwestern spread rising from Guatemala into Mexico gave the *T. d. maculipennis* form. *Triatoma hegneri* appears as a subspecific insular form (Cozumel Island). A cryptic species is confined to the Yucatan Peninsula and northern parts of Chiapas State (Mexico), Guatemala, and Honduras. Finally, the population introduced in Ecuador derives from Central America and corresponds to *T. d. dimidiata*.[74] The large intraspecific genetic variability found in *T. dimidiata* s.l. and subsequent distinction between the five different taxa have major implications for transmission capacity and vector control.

## Other Triatoma of epidemiological importance

Some autochthonous species of the genus *Triatoma* that were originally restricted to the wild environment are increasingly found as domiciliated colonies. Studies of these species are relevant because such species may act as vectors of *T. cruzi* to humans and are generally not targets of control actions. In the Southern Cone of South America, four species may be considered as emerging vectors; these species include *T. brasiliensis*, *T. pseudomaculata*, *T. sordida*, and *T. guasayana*.

*T. brasiliensis* is a species complex consisting of two subspecies (*T. b. brasiliensis* and *T. b. macromelasoma*) and two other taxa recently identified as different species (*T. melanica* and *T. juazeirensis*). This species complex is found under large piles of rocks in the sylvatic environment and is native of the Caatinga, a xerophytic region in northeastern Brazil.[77] The four members of this complex present varying rates, of epidemiological importance. The most significant is *T. b. brasiliensis*, given its geographic range covering five states in Brazil, high *T. cruzi* infection rate, and ability to form abundant domestic colonies.[78] *T. pseudomaculata* is another species native to xerophytic ecosystems in northeastern Brazil. Its geographic range covers 13 states in Brazil in the Caatinga and the Cerrado. In the sylvatic environment, *T. pseudomaculata* is strictly arboricolous, found in hollow trees and bird nests. It often invades peridomestic structures but does not display a significant ability to colonize human dwellings.[79]

*T. sordida* and *T. guasayana* are considered potential substitutes for *T. infestans* in some areas of the Southern Cone, where they are particularly prevalent in peridomestic habitats and frequently found to be infected by *T. cruzi*. They occasionally invade human habitations and feed on humans and synanthropic animals.

Nevertheless, there is still no evidence of vector transmission of *T. cruzi* to humans by these vectors.[80,81] Both species may be occasionally found in the Andean valleys of Bolivia at altitudes as high as 2800 m above sea level for *T. sordida* and 1800 m above sea level for *T. guasayana*. However, the two species are more prevalent in the lowlands. *T. sordida* occurs in the Cerrado and Chaco ecoregions whereas *T. guasayana* is restricted to the Chaco. In addition to some Andean valleys of Bolivia, their distributions overlap throughout northern Argentina and parts of the Chaco region in Bolivia and Paraguay. In the highlands, both species can be collected in rupicolous ecotopes or hollow trees. In the lowlands, *T. sordida* is arboricolous, found in hollow trees and bird nests, whereas *T. guasayana* is mainly found in dry cacti, bromeliads, and fallen logs.[82]

*T. maculata* and *T. venosa* may be considered as emerging vectors in the northern Andean countries (Venezuela and Colombia). In some areas of Venezuela and Colombia, *T. maculata* has the capacity to colonize human dwellings and may be involved in Chagas disease transmission.[64,83] In the sylvatic environment, this species has been found in palm trees of the *Attalea* complex (genera *Attalea* and *Scheelea*), bird nests, bromeliads, and dead trunks.[66] Wild and peridomestic *T. maculata* is also found in Brazil (Roraima state). In Guiana, French Guiana, and Suriname, this species has a distribution in only the sylvatic environment.[2] *T. venosa*, which occurs in Costa Rica, Ecuador, and Colombia, is considered as a secondary vector of Chagas disease in Colombia where it is frequently found in houses and peridomestic structures in active *T. cruzi* vectorial transmission areas. However, its sylvatic habitat is unknown.[84]

Some *Triatoma* species, such as *T. barberi* and species of the *Phyllosoma* complex, are restricted to Mexico and are regarded as locally important vectors.[85] Currently, *T. barberi* is considered to be the most important vector in Mexico. This insect is confined to the central valleys that are south of the Tropic of Cancer. This species has only been observed in domestic and peridomestic habitats, but it is assumed to have wild habitats in rock piles. Domestic population density is generally low.[85] The *Phyllosoma* complex is composed of nine species, including several of epidemiological importance in Mexico: *T. longipennis*, *T. mazzotti*, *T. mexicana*, *T. pallidipennis*, *T. phyllosoma*, and *T. picturata*. These species dominate the central and northwestern part of the country in both tropical and subtropical areas. They additionally display different degrees of synanthropism, showing a behavioral gradient from household occasional invasion by adult triatomines to the stable colonization of artificial structures.[85,86]

# Environmental variables as indicators of Triatominae geographic distribution

Because of their hematophagous habit, Triatominae species are generally associated either with their blood sources and/or specific habitats where there is a significant chance of finding a blood meal. Some species are host-specific and others are habitat-specific. As an example, *T. delpontei* is exclusively found in *M. monachus* colonial nests. The nest is occupied over several years, and individual nests are added every year to the colonial structure. During this time, the triatomine population has a relatively stable population of *M. monachus* to feed upon. A closely related species to *T. delpontei*, *T. platensis*, is associated with nests of various species of furnariid birds, which are only occupied during the breeding season when the species has the opportunity to feed on brooding adults and chicks. During the nonbreeding season, birds abandon the nest, and this nest is eventually occupied by other birds and/or mammals (especially rodents) that will become hosts for the triatomines. *Rhodnius* species are well-known generalists among the triatomines that occupy palm tree crowns. Different *Rhodnius* species are associated specifically (or preferentially) with a palm species, where the triatomines will feed on the rich fauna of birds and mammals nesting in the crown (e.g., *R. brethesi* with *L. piassaba*). Habitat availability for sylvatic populations of particular triatomine species strongly depends on the community structure and environmental conditions. Given this close association between habitat and Triatomine species, a number of studies have used sets of environmental variables at continental and subcontinental scales to analyze the geographic distribution of Triatominae species. The basic hypothesis of these studies investigates if places with similar environmental conditions would potentially represent places of additional occurrence of the species based on other areas with known occurrence of a particular Triatominae species. The idea is mainly applicable to studies on the geographic distribution of species at regional scales, where extrinsic factors of the studied populations are more important than intrinsic factors (i.e., climate variables and vegetation versus intra/interspecific competition and predation). For these types of studies, discriminant analysis and ecological niche modeling were used. The distribution of Triatominae species was studied using climate variables data that were collected at the ground level by meteorological stations available at continental scales (i.e., Worldclim database) and land cover and climate variables data recorded by earth observation satellites. Studies showed that environmental variables are good indicators of the geographic distributions of sylvatic, peridomestic, and domestic species of Triatominae.

## *Environmental variables and the distribution of* T. infestans

Gorla[87] described the maximum potential expansion of the geographic distribution of *T. infestans* using a 20-year time series of satellite imagery produced by the advanced very high resolution radiometer (AVHRR). From these images, statistics of a temporal Fourier analysis (amplitude and phase of 1-, 2-, 3-annual cycles, maximum, minimum, average, variance) of the normalized difference vegetation index (NDVI), estimations of land surface temperature (LST), air temperature (AT), vapor pressure deficit (VPD), and a measure of middle infrared radiation (MIR) were estimated. The maximum potential distribution was derived from a multivariate discriminant analysis and then compared with the *T. infestans* distribution determined using data collected by field teams of vector control programs of the Southern Cone countries and academic reports. This analysis resulted in an overall 90% correct classification of either presence or absence of *T. infestans*. The model identified the variability of the AT, air temperature average, and amplitude of the AT annual cycle as the main variables defining the geographic distribution of *T. infestans*.

The maximum expansion of *T. infestans* geographic distribution probably occurred between 1970 and 1980 when the presence of the species was first reported to have crossed the São Francisco River in northeastern Brazil.[88,89] Although some discussions remain, current knowledge of the species distribution originated from studies using different methodological approaches (i.e., population genetics, morphometric geometry, cytogenetics, antennal phenotypes) supports the hypothesis that the Andean valleys in Bolivia were the center of origin and expansion of *T. infestans* throughout the southern countries of South America, along the trade routes of the Incas first, and then along the trade routes of the new European empires of Spain and Portugal.[70,90,91] The present geographic distribution of domestic populations significantly decreased their habitat ranges compared with the maximum geographic distribution of the species,[87,92] and they are patchily distributed over the arid Chaco and the inter-Andean valleys of Bolivia. This reduction was caused by concerted actions of the vector control programs of the Southern Cone countries, living conditions improvement of previously affected communities and the generalized migration from rural to urban settings in many areas.

Because of *T. infestans* importance as vector of *T. cruzi*, the biology and population ecology of their domestic and peridomestic populations have been studied intensively from the 1970s. Although frequently debated during the 1980s, the existence of sylvatic populations were minimized (sylvatic populations were underreported during the period, e.g., findings of *T. infestans* adults in bird nests up to 1.2 km from the nearest house,[93] but their relative importance was increased during the last 15 years). Recent studies showed sylvatic populations of *T. infestans* occurring more frequently than previously expected in the Andean and the Chaco regions of Bolivia and Argentina.[94,95]

Taking into account the existence of the Andean and non-Andean (Chaco) cytotypes described by Panzera,[91] Gorla and Noireau[96] analyzed the distribution of Andean and Chaco sylvatic populations of *T. infestans*, using field-collected data and environmental variables to identify potential areas of the geographic distribution of both types of sylvatic populations. The derived geographic distribution models showed that the Andean population of sylvatic *T. infestans* is restricted mainly to the southern part of La Paz department, southern Cochabamba, and the boundary between the departments of Chuquisaca and Tarija with Potosi. The Chaco populations of sylvatic *T. infestans* have a wider area of potential distribution around the Chaco region of Argentina, Bolivia, and Paraguay (Fig. 9.3).

Population genetics, geometric morphometry, and cytogenetics data show that *T. infestans* is a heterogeneous entity that can colonize domestic, peridomestic, and sylvatic ecotopes. In the domestic and/or peridomestic ecotopes, the species is able to constitute highly frequent and abundant populations, but in the sylvatic ecotopes, the populations are rare and always constituted by a few individuals. The entity we call *T. infestans* includes an Andean form, living in the Bolivian Montane Dry Forests, mainly associated with rodents and a non-Andean form[97] and later discovered in several other places of the arid Gran Chaco and also in colonies near

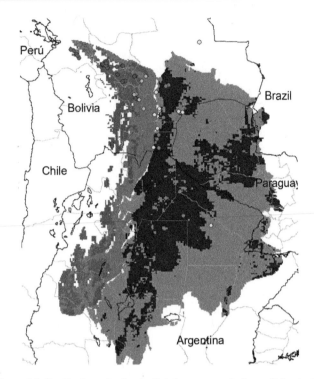

**Figure 9.3** Potential distribution of sylvatic *T. infestans* populations of the Andean and Chaco regions. In the print version: Dark and light grey shades to the left of the map are predictions of presence and absence of Andean populations, respectively. Dark and light grey shades to the right of the map are predictions of presence and absence of Chaco populations of *T. infestans*, respectively.

Santiago city in Chile,[98] frequently found associated with bird nests. Where the non-Andean form constitutes peridomestic populations, it frequently constitutes abundant populations associated with chicken nests. It is still under debate whether all these sylvatic populations are of truly sylvatic origin, or they are in fact domestic populations that migrated to the sylvatic ecotopes. Panzera et al.[99] described a hybrid *T. infestans* population group geographical restricted to the border between Argentina and Bolivia, that was recently associated with the highest resistant populations to pyrethroid insecticides.[100]

## *Environmental variables and the distribution of other Triatominae*

Costa et al.[78] described the geographic distribution of *T. brasiliensis* in the northeast of Brazil. These authors used 22 environmental variables, including climate data (temperature, precipitation, vapor pressure, etc.), terrain elevation, and land cover data, which were analyzed with the genetic algorithm for rule-set production (GARP) tool. The results showed the allopatric and parapatric distribution of four

*T. brasiliensis* populations. *T. b. brasiliensis* occupies regions at 16.5−22.5°C that experienced 10−35 mm of precipitation. *T. b. juazeirensis* was similar but had a narrower ecologic altitude. *T. b. macromelasoma* was found at the highest altitude, occupying two potentially disjunct ecological zones where annual mean temperature ranges from 11.0°C to 23.5°C and annual mean precipitation of 10−45 mm. *T. b. melanica* appears restricted to a narrow ecological zone with annual temperatures between 18°C and 19°C and precipitation of 20−35 mm.

Studying *T. brasiliensis* and *T. melanica*, two species occupying the northern and southern extremes of the geographic distribution of the *brasiliensis* species complex, Souza et al.[77] analyzed the ecological niche overlap between them. They compared the geographic distribution of the species using generalized linear models fitted to elevation and current data on land surface temperature, vegetation cover, and rainfall recorded by Earth observation satellites for northeastern Brazil. The ecological niche models show that the environmental spaces currently occupied by *T. brasiliensis* and *T. melanica* are similar although not equivalent, and associated with the caatinga ecosystem.

Carbajal de la Fuente et al.[101] showed that the sylvatic triatomine species of eastern Brazil, *T. pseudomaculata* and *T. wygodsinskyi*, have allopatric but not partially sympatric populations as previously accepted. This was discovered after studying their geographic distributions characterized by temperature, VPD, vegetation, and altitude estimated from information provided by the satellite remote sensors AVHRR and moderate-resolution imaging spectroradiometer (MODIS). In this study, the 8 × 8 km spatial resolution of the AVHRR imagery more accurately described the species distributions compared to the MODIS imagery. Both satellites were able to produce a >85.7% correct classification for presence and absence from point data.

Peterson et al.[102] studied the joint distribution of *Triatoma* species of the *Protracta* complex with packrat species (*Neotoma* species) using terrain elevation, hydrological, and climate data, which were analyzed with the ecological niche modeling GARP tool. This study showed a close association between the distribution of *T. barberi* (one of the main vector species for *T. cruzi* transmission in Mexico) and *N. mexicana*, a finding that led these authors to suggest a specific interaction between the species.

Gurgel-Goncalves and Cuba[103] studied the distribution of *R. neglectus* in Central Brazil, using data on biophysical variables (altitude, temperature, vegetation, and rainfall) obtained from the Worldclim database with information about the distribution of palm tree and bird species. This study showed that this *Rhodnius* species is closely associated with dry areas of the Cerrado-Caatinga corridor and partially overlaps with the considered palm tree and birds species. In a more recent article and using a similar methodology, Gurgel-Goncalves et al.[104] later reported the distribution of 16 triatomine species among the most frequent and synanthopic in Brazil and showed a strong association between species distribution and the biome in which they are distributed.

Arboleda et al.[36] studied the geographic distribution of *R. pallescens* using the 1982−2000 monthly time series of AVHRR imagery at the 8 × 8 km spatial resolution mentioned above. The analysis showed that the minimum VPD is the most important variable for determining the geographic distribution of the species, along with its stenohydric status. The study also showed the potential distribution of most species of *Rhodnius*, except *R. domesticus*, *R. neglectus*, and *R. nasutus*, a result probably derived from the evolution of common ancestors among the species groups. Using correlation analysis and logistic regression, the distribution of domestic Triatominae species in Guatemala was studied.[105] Results of this study showed that the distribution of *T. nitida* is positively associated with places of lower average minimum temperature, whereas the past distribution of *R. prolixus* corresponded with areas of maximum absolute temperature and relative humidity.

## Global warming and expansion of geographic range of *T. infestans*

The Intergovernmental Panel on Climate Change (IPCC) synthesis report of 2007 concluded that local maximum temperatures will only modestly increase while minimum temperatures will increase dramatically under climate change scenarios.[106] Because of the predicted increase in temperature and the known effect of temperature on insect development and reproduction, a number of authors have predicted a global increase in the transmission of vector-borne diseases (VBDs).[107,108] However, not all experts agree on these predictions because of the simplistic linear relationship that underlies the former argument. In the latter case, authors argue that the epidemiology of each VBD is a system-specific product of complex, commonly nonlinear interactions between many disparate environmental factors. These factors include climate and other abiotic conditions (e.g., land cover), the physical structure of the environment, host abundance and diversity, socioeconomic factors driving human living conditions and behavior that determines the degree of exposure to vectorial transmission risk, and the nutritional status and concomitant immunity that determine resistance to infection.[109] In addition to the complexity argument, these authors state that there is no single infectious disease with increased incidence over recent decades that can be reliably attributed to climate change.[110] For the case of Chagas disease vectors, there are no specific studies on their relationship with the expected climate change, except for an early article by Gorla et al.[111] which discussed the potential changes in the geographic distribution of *T. infestans* and Chagas disease transmission under a global temperature increase scenario. Based on 3-year field data on the population ecology of *T. infestans* under the natural climate conditions of the southern Gran Chaco (reported by Gorla[112]), Gorla et al.[111] estimated the effect of a generalized temperature increase on the maximum potential population growth rate (r) of *T. infestans* and *T. cruzi* transmission risk (based on the relationship between temperature and *T. infestans* biting frequency) over the Argentinian territory. At a hypothesized 2°C or 4°C temperature increase, the vector populations may potentially expand the southern limit of the geographic distribution and have a greater capacity to increase its population abundance in the Gran Chaco region, which corresponds with a parallel increase in the *T. cruzi* transmission risk. The authors stated that the distribution and abundance of *T. infestans* and the vectorial transmission of *T. cruzi* depend on factors other than just temperature. Although the study predicts the species-potential expansion of the southern limit and an eventually increased transmission risk, the vector control activities and the improved living conditions of rural communities in previously infested areas were able to eliminate domestic infestations by *T. infestans*. Additionally, interruption of the vectorial transmission of *T. cruzi* in several provinces outside the Gran Chaco region by 2001, as certified by the Pan American Health Organization,[113] has significantly contributed to a decrease in disease prevalence.

A recent study of the impact of climate change on the geographic distribution and its influence on the force of *T. cruzi* infection by *T. infestans* and *R. prolixus* was published.[114] The authors assessed the implications of climatic projections for 2050 on the geographical distribution of the two vector species. They estimated the epidemiological implications of current to future transitions in the climatic niche in terms of changes in the force of infection (FOI) on the rural population of Venezuela (tropical) and Argentina (temperate). They report a decreasing trend of suitability of areas that are currently at high-to-moderate transmission risk. As the analysis is based exclusively on temperature and rainfall (from the Worldclim database), the projection for 2050 produces a spurious result in central Argentina, where in spite of the climatic suitability for *T. infestans*, *T. cruzi* transmission no longer occurs because of the change in the lifestyle of rural communities after the land use change promoted by the advance of soy bean production. As the authors mention, the effect of other factors, besides climate, should be considered in a modeling effort to reliable project the epidemiological scenario for *T. cruzi* transmission.

# Glossary

Some of the specialized words are explained in the text; others are defined here.

**Allopatric** geographically isolated and thus unable to crossbreed

**Anthropozoonotic** transmissible from animals to humans

**Arboreal** living in trees

**Autosome** chromosome that is not a sex chromosome

**Biotope** area of uniform environmental conditions providing a living place for a specific assemblage of plants and animals

**C-heterochromatic blocks** densely staining chromosomal material that appears as nodules and contains relatively few genes

**Caatinga** dry forest region in the northeastern part of Brazil

**Cerrado** extensive woodland savannah in Central Brazil

**Clade** group of biological taxa (as species) that includes all descendants of one common ancestor

**Cryptic species** species that appear morphologically identical but are genetically isolated from each other

**Cytochrome b** mitochondrial gene

**Cytogenetics** study of the structure and function of the chromosomes
**Diploid** having a pair of each type of chromosome
**Ecological niche** multidimensional space defined by biotic and abiotic variables occupied by a species
**Furnariidae** family of ovenbirds
**Genotypic** relating to the genetic makeup of an individual
**Ornithophilic** that feeds on bird
**Parapatric** having contiguous geographic ranges
**Phenotypic** relating to the observable traits of an organism
**Phylogeny** evolutionary relationships within and between groups
**Polyphyletic** derived from two or more distinct ancestral lineages; the alternative is "monophyletic"
**Rapoport's rule** relationship between the average latitudinal range and the midpoint of the latitudinal range
**Stenohydric** tolerant of a narrow range of humidity
**Sympatric** occupying the same or overlapping geographic areas without interbreeding
**Synanthropic** ecologically associated with humans
**Taxon (pl. taxa)** taxonomic category or group such as a phylum, order, family, genus, or species
**Xerophytic** adapted to a dry environment

# References

1. Lent H, Wygodzinsky P. Revision of the Triatominae (Hemiptera, Reduviidae), and their significance as vectors of Chagas disease. *Bull Am Mus Nat Hist* 1979;**163**:127−520.
2. Galvão C, Carcavallo R, Rocha DS, Jurberg J. A checklist of the current valid species of the subfamily Triatominae Jeannel, 1919 (Hemiptera, Reduviidae) and their geographic distribution, with nomenclature and taxonomic notes. *Zootaxa* 2003;**202**:1−36.
3. Galvão C, Angulo VM. *Belminus corredori*, a new species of Bolboderini (Hemiptera: Reduviidae: Triatominae) from Santander, Colombia. *Zootaxa* 2006;**1241**:61−8.
4. Bérenger JM, Blanchet D. A new species of the genus *Panstrongylus* from French Guiana (Heteroptera; Reduviidae; Triatominae). *Mem Inst Oswaldo Cruz* 2007;**102**:733−6.
5. Costa J, Felix M. *Triatoma juazeirensis* sp. nov. from the state of Bahia, Northeastern Brazil (Hemiptera: Reduviidae: Triatominae). *Mem Inst Oswaldo Cruz* 2007;**102**:87−90.
6. Martinez E, Chavez T, Sossa D, Aranda R, Vargas B, Vidaurre P. *Triatoma boliviana* sp. n. de los valles subandinos de La Paz, Bolivia (Hemiptera; Reduviidae; Triatominae), similar a *Triatoma nigromaculata* Stal, 1859. *Bol Inst Inv Salud Des (UMSS)* 2007;**3**:1−11.
7. Sandoval CM, Pabon E, Jurberg J, Galvão C. *Belminus ferroae* n. sp. from the Colombian north-east, with a key to the species of the genus (Hemiptera: Reduviidae: Triatominae). *Zootaxa* 2007;**1443**:55−64.
8. Rosa JA, Rocha CS, Gardim S, Pinto MC, Mendonça VJ, Ferreira Filho JCR, et al. Description of *Rhodnius montenegrensis* n. sp. (Hemiptera: Reduviidae: Triatominae) from the state of Rondônia, Brazil. *Zootaxa* 2012;**3478**:62−76.
9. Abad-Franch F, Pavan MG, Jaramillo-O N, Palomeque FS, Dale C, Chaverra D, et al. *Rhodnius barretti*, a new species of Triatominae (Hemiptera: Reduviidae) from western Amazonia. *Mem Inst Oswaldo Cruz* 2013;**108**(Suppl. 1):92−9.

10. Jurberg J, Cunha V, Cailleaux S, Raigorodschi R, Lima MS, Rocha DS, et al. *Triatoma pintodiasi* sp. nov. do subcomplexo *T. rubrovaria* (Hemiptera, Reduviidae, Triatominae). *Rev Pan-Amazón Saúd* 2013;**4**(1):43−56.

11. Carcavallo RU, Curto de Casas SI, Sherlock IA, Galíndez Girón I, Jurberg J, Galvão C, et al. Geographic distribution and alti-latitudinal dispersion. In: Carcavallo RU, Galindez Girón I, Jurberg J, Lent H, editors. *Atlas of Chagas Disease Vectors in the Americas*, vol. II. Rio de Janeiro, Brazil: Fiocruz; 1999. p. 747−92.

12. Schofield CJ, Galvão C. Classification, evolution, and species groups within the Triatominae. *Acta Trop* 2009;**110**:88−100.

13. Gorla DE, Dujardin JP, Schofield CJ. Biosystematics of Old World Triatominae. *Acta Trop* 1997;**63**:127−40.

14. Patterson JS, Schofield CJ, Dujardin JP, Miles MA. Population morphometric analysis of the tropicopolitan bug *Triatoma rubrofasciata* and relationships with Old World species of *Triatoma*: evidence of New World ancestry. *Med Vet Entomol* 2001;**15**:443−51.

15. Hypsa V, Tietz DF, Zrzavy J, Rego ROM, Galvão C, Jurberg J. Phylogeny and biogeography of Triatominae (Hemiptera: Reduviidae): molecular evidence of a New World origin of the Asiatic clade. *Mol Phylogenet Evol* 2002;**23**:447−57.

16. Noireau F, Abad-Franch F, Valente SAS, Dias-Lima A, Lopes CM, Cunha V, et al. Trapping Triatominae in sylvatic habitats. *Mem Inst Oswaldo Cruz* 2002;**97**:61−3.

17. Ribeiro G, Gurgel-Goncalves R, Reis RB, dos Santos CGS, Amorim A, Andrade SG, et al. Frequent house invasion of *Trypanosoma cruzi*-infected triatomines in a suburban area of Brazil. *PLoS NTD* 2015;**9**(4):e0003678. Available from: http://dx.doi.org/10.1371/journal.pntd.0003678.

18. Cavallo MJ, Amelotti I, Gorla DE. Invasion of rural houses by wild Triatominae in the arid Chaco. *J Vector Ecol* 2016;**41**(1):97−102.

19. Dias JVL, Mota Queiroz DM, Rodrigues Martins H, Gorla DE, Rocha Pires HH, Diotaiuti L. Spatial distribution of triatomines in domiciles in an urban area of Brazilian Southeast. *Mem Inst Oswaldo Cruz* 2016;**111**:43−50.

20. Waleckx E, Goubiere S, Dumonteil E. Intrusive versus domiciliated triatomines and the challenge of adapting vector control practices against Chagas disease. *Mem Inst Oswaldo Cruz* 2015;**110**:324−38.

21. Brito RN., 2015. Avaliaçao dos eventos de invasao no Estado de Tocantins, Brasil. Tesis Mestrado. Ministério da Saúde, Fundação Oswaldo Cruz, Centro de Pesquisas René Rachou, Programa de Pós-Graduação em Ciência da Saúde, 176 pp.

22. Abad-Franch F, Lima MM, Sarqui O, Gurgel-Goncalves R, Sanchez-Martin M, Calzada J, et al. On palms, bugs, and Chagas disease in the Americas. *Acta Trop* 2015;**151**:126−41.

23. Rodriguero M, Gorla DE. Latitudinal gradient of species richness in the New World Triatominae (Reduviidae). *Global Ecol Biogeo* 2004;**13**:75−84.

24. Diniz-Filho JA, Ceccarelli S, Hasperue W, Rabinovich J. Geographical patterns of Triatominae (Heteroptera: Reduviidae) richness and distribution in the Western Hemisphere. *Insect Conserv Divers* 2013;**6**:704−14.

25. Gaunt M, Miles M. The ecotopes and evolution of triatomine bugs (Triatominae) and their associated trypanosomes. *Mem Inst Oswaldo Cruz* 2000;**95**:557−65.

26. Dias-Lima AG, Menezes D, Sherlock I, Noireau F. Wild habitat and related fauna of *Panstrongylus lutzi* (Reduviidae, Triatominae). *J Med Entomol* 2003;**40**:989−90.

27. Abad-Franch F, Monteiro FA, Jaramillo N, Gurgel-Gonçalves R, Dias FB, Diotaiuti L. Ecology, evolution, and the long-term surveillance of vector-borne Chagas disease: a multi-scale appraisal of the tribe Rhodniini (Triatominae). *Acta Trop* 2009;**110**:159−77.

28. Hashimoto K, Schofield CJ. Review: elimination of *Rhodnius prolixus* in Central America. *Parasit Vectors* 2012;**5**:45.

29. Guhl F. Chagas disease in Andean countries. *Mem Inst Oswaldo Cruz* 2007;**102** (Suppl. I):29–37.

30. Guhl F, Pinto N, Aguilera G. Sylvatic Triatominae: a new challenge in vector control transmission. *Mem Inst Oswaldo Cruz* 2009;**104**(Suppl. I):71–5.

31. Fitzpatrick S, Feliciangeli MD, Sanchez-Martin MJ, Monteiro FA, Miles MA. Molecular genetics reveal that sylvatic *Rhodnius prolixus* do colonise rural houses. *PLoS NTD* 2008;**2**:e210.

32. Dujardin JP, Muñoz M, Chavez T, Ponce C, Moreno J, Schofield CJ. The origin of *Rhodnius prolixus* in Central America. *Med Vet Entomol* 1998;**12**:113–15.

33. Gamboa CJ. Comprobación de *Rhodnius prolixus* extradomiciliario en Venezuela. *Bol Of San Panam* 1963;**54**:18–25.

34. Zeledon R., 1996. Enfermedad de Chagas en Centro America. In: Schofield, C.J., Dujardin, J.P., Jurberg, J. (Eds.), Proceedings of the International Workshop on Population Genetics and Control of Triatominae, Santo Domingo de los Colorados, Ecuador, INDRE, Ciudad de Méjico, p. 40.

35. Monteiro FA, Barrett TV, Fitzpatrick S, Cordon-Rosales C, Feliciangeli D, Beard CB. Molecular phylogeography of the Amazonian Chagas disease vectors *Rhodnius prolixus* and *R. robustus*. *Mol Ecol* 2003;**12**:997–1006.

36. Arboleda S, Gorla DE, Porcasi X, Saldaña A, Calzada J, Jaramillo N. Development of a geographic distribution model of *Rhodnius pallescens* Barber, 1932 using environmental data recorded by remote sensing. *Infect Gen Evol* 2009;**9**:441–8.

37. Calzada JE, Pineda V, Montalvo E, Alvarez D, Santamaria AM, Samudio F, et al. Human trypanosome infection and the presence of intradomicile *Rhodnius pallescens* in the western border of the Panama canal, Panama. *Am J Trop Med Hyg* 2006;**74**:762–5.

38. Matias A, de la Riva J, Martinez E, Torrez M, Dujardin JP. Domiciliation process of *Rhodnius stali* (Hemiptera: Reduviidae) in Alto Beni, La Paz, Bolivia. *Trop. Med. Int. Health* 2003;**8**:264–8.

39. Abad-Franch F, Paucar A, Carpio C, Cuba CA, Aguilar HM, Miles MA. Biogeography of Triatominae (Hemiptera: Reduviidae) in Ecuador: implications for the design of control strategies. *Mem Inst Oswaldo Cruz* 2001;**96**:611–20.

40. Vargas F, Paz Soldan C, Marin C, Rosales MJ, Sanchez-Gutierrez R, Sanchez-Moreno M. Epidemiology of American trypanosomiasis in northern Peru. *Ann Trop Med Parasitol* 2007;**101**:643–8.

41. Grijalva MJ, Villacis AG. Presence of *Rhodnius ecuadoriensis* in sylvatic habitats in the southern highlands (Loja Province) of Ecuador. *J Med Entomol* 2009;**46**:708–11.

42. Coura JR, Junqueira ACV, Fernández O, Valente SAS, Miles MA. Emerging Chagas disease in amazonian Brazil. *Trends Parasitol* 2002;**18**:171–6.

43. Aguilar HM, Abad-Franch F, Dias JCP, Junqueira ACV, Coura JR. Chagas disease in the Amazon region. *Mem Inst Oswaldo Cruz* 2007;**102**(Suppl. I):47–55.

44. Curto de Casas SI, Carcavallo RU, Galíndez GI, Burgos JJ. Bioclimatic factors and zones of life. In: Carcavallo RU, Galíndez Girón I, Jurberg J, Lent H, editors. *Atlas of Chagas' Disease Vectors in the Americas*, vol. III. Rio de Janeiro: Fiocruz; 1999. p. 793–838.

45. Patterson JS, Barbosa SS, Feliciangeli MD. On the genus *Panstrongylus* Berg 1879: evolution, ecology and epidemiological significance. *Acta Trop* 2009;**110**:187–99.

46. Valente VC, Valente SAS, Noireau F, Carrasco HJ, Miles MA. Chagas disease in the Amazon basin: association of *Panstrongylus geniculatus* (Hemiptera: Reduviidae) with domestic pigs. *J Med Entomol* 1998;**35**:99–103.

47. Feliciangeli MD, Carrasco H, Patterson JS, Suarez B, Martínez C, Medina M. Mixed domestic infestation by *Rhodnius prolixus* Stal 1859 and *Panstrongylus geniculatus* Latreille 1811 vector incrimination, and seroprevalence for *Trypanosoma cruzi* among inhabitants in El Guamito, Lara state, Venezuela. *Am J Trop Med Hyg* 2004;**71**:501–5.

48. Carrasco HJ, Torellas A, García C, Segovia M, Feliciangeli MD. Risk of *Trypanosoma cruzi* I (Kinetoplastida: Trypanosomatidae) transmission by *Panstrongylus geniculatus* (Hemiptera: Reduviidae) in Caracas (Metropolitan District) and neighboring States, Venezuela. *Int J Parasitol* 2005;**35**:1379–84.

49. D'Alessandro A, Barreto P, Thomas M. Nuevos registros de triatominos domiciliarios y extradomiciliarios en Colombia. *Colomb Méd* 1981;**12**:75–85.

50. Miles MA, de Souza AA, Povoa M. Chagas disease in the Amazon basin. III. Ecotopes of ten triatomine bug species (Hemiptera: Reduviidae) from vicinity of Belem, Para state, Brazil. *J Med Entomol* 1981;**18**:266–78.

51. Salomón OD, Ripoll CM, Rivetti E, Carcavallo RU. Presence of *Panstrongylus rufotuberculatus* (Champion 1899) (Hemiptera: Reduviidae: Triatominae) in Argentina. *Mem Inst Oswaldo Cruz* 1999;**94**:285–8.

52. Erazo D, Cordobez J. The role of light in Chagas disease infection risk in Colombia. *Parasit Vectors* 2016;**9**:9. Available from: http://dx.doi.org/10.1186/s13071-015-1240-4.

53. Noireau F, Vargas F, Bosseno MF, Breniére SF. Apparent trend to domesticity observed in *Panstrongylus rufotuberculatus* (Hemiptera: Reduviidae) in Bolivia. *Res Rev Parasitol* 1994;**54**:249–50.

54. Cuba CA, Abad-Franch F, Roldán Rodríguez J, Vargas Vásquez F, Pollack Velásquez L, Miles MA. The triatomine of Northern Peru, with emphasis on the ecology and infection by trypanosomes of *Rhodnius ecuadoriensis* (Triatominae). *Mem Inst Oswaldo Cruz* 2002;**97**:175–83.

55. Wolff M, Castillo D, Uribe J, Arboleda JJ. *Tripanosomiasis americana*: determinación de riesgo epidemiológico de transmisión en el municipio de Amalfi, Antioquia. *Iatreia* 2001;**14**:111–21.

56. Wolff M, Cuartas E, Velásquez C, Jaramillo N. Development cycle of *Panstrongylus rufotuberculatus* (Hemiptera: Reduviidae) under laboratory conditions. *J Med Entomol* 2004;**41**:1010–14.

57. Forattini OP, Ferreira OA, Rocha e Silva EO, Rabello EX. Aspectos ecológicos da tripanossomíase Americana. VIII-Domiciliacão de *Panstrongylus megistus* e sua presença extradomiciliar. *Rev Saúde Públ* 1977;**11**:73–86.

58. Dias JCP, Dias E. Variações mensais da incidência das formas evolutivas do *Triatoma infestans* e *Panstrongylus megistus* no município de Bambuí estado de Minas Gerais. iia nota: 1951–1964. *Mem Inst Oswaldo Cruz* 1968;**66**:209–26.

59. Salvatella R. Triatomíneos del Uruguay. *Rev Méd Uruguay* 1986;**2**:106–13.

60. Steindel M, Toma HK, Carvalho-Pinto CJ, Grisard EC, Schlemper BR. Colonization of artificial ecotopes by *Panstrongylus megistus* in Santa Catarina Island, Florianópolis, Santa Catarina, Brazil. *Rev Inst Méd Trop São Paulo* 1994;**36**:43–50.

61. Dias JCP. *Doença de Chagas em Bambuí, Minas Gerais, Brasil. Estudo Clínico-Epidemiológico a Partir da Fase Aguda, Entre 1940 e 1982*. MG: Tese de Doutorado, Faculdade de Medicina, Universidade Federal de Minas Gerais; 1982. p. 375.

62. Dias JCP, Schofield CJ. The evolution of Chagas disease (American trypanosomiasis) control after 90 years since Carlos Chagas discovery. *Mem Inst Oswaldo Cruz* 1999;**94** (Suppl. I):103−21.

63. Teixeira ARL, Monteiro PS, Rebelo JM, Argañaraz HR, Vieira D, Lauria-Pires, et al. Emerging Chagas disease: trophic network and cycle of transmission of *Trypanosoma cruzi* from palm trees in the Amazon. *Emerg Infect Dis* 2001;**7**:100−12.

64. Guhl F, Aguilera G, Pinto N, Vergara D. Actualización de la distribución geográfica y ecoepidemiología de la fauna de triatominos (Reduviidae: Triatominae) en Colombia. *Biomédica* 2007;**27**(Suppl. 1):143−62.

65. Abad-Franch F, Aguilar HM. *Control de la enfermeded de Chagas en el Ecuador. OPS/OMS—Ministerio de Salud Pública del Ecuador.* Resumen Ejecutivo; 2003. p. 70.

66. Carcavallo RU, Rodríguez MEF, Salvatella R, Curto de Casas SI, Sherlock IS, Galvão C, et al. Habitats and related fauna. In: Carcavallo RU, Galíndez Girón I, Jurberg J, Lent H, editors. *Atlas of Chagas' Disease Vectors in the Americas*, vol. II. Rio de Janeiro: Fiocruz; 1998. p. 561−600.

67. Panzera F, Perez R, Panzera Y, Alvarez F, Scvortzoff E, Salvatella R. Karyotype evolution in holocentric chromosomes of three related species of triatomines (Hemiptera−Reduviidae). *Chromosome Res* 1995;**3**:143−50.

68. Pereira J, Dujardin JP, Salvatella R, Tibayrenc M. Enzymatic variability and phylogenic relatedness among *Triatoma infestans, T. platensis, T. delpontei* and *T. rubrovaria. Heredity* 1996;**77**:47−54.

69. Martí GA, Echeverría MG, Waleckx E, Susevich ML, Balsalobre A, Gorla DE. Triatominae in furnariid nests in the Argentine Gran Chaco. *J Vector Ecol* 2014; **39**:66−71.

70. Bargues MD, Klisiowicz DR, Panzera F, Noireau F, Marcilla A, Perez R, et al. Origin and phylogeography of the Chagas disease main vector *Triatoma infestans* based on nuclear rDNA sequences and genome size. *Infect Gen Evol* 2006;**6**:46−62.

71. Usinger RL, Wygodzinsky P, Ryckman RE. The biosystematics of Triatominae. *Ann Rev Entomol* 1966;**11**:309−30.

72. Dorn PL, Monroy C, Curtis A. *Triatoma dimidiata* (Latreille, 1811): a review of its diversity across its geographic range and the relationship among populations. *Infect Gen Evol* 2007;**7**:343−52.

73. Panzera F, Ferrandis I, Ramsey J, Ordoñez R, Salazar-Schettino PM, Cabrera M, et al. Chromosomal variation and genome size support existence of cryptic species of *Triatoma dimidiata* with different epidemiological importance as Chagas disease vectors. *Trop Med Int Health* 2006;**11**:1092−103.

74. Bargues MD, Klisiowicz DR, Gonzalez-Candelas F, Ramsey JM, Monroy C, Ponce C, et al. Phylogeography and genetic variation of *Triatoma dimidiata*, the main Chagas disease vector in Central America, and its position within the genus *Triatoma. PLoS NTD* 2008;**2**:e233.

75. Dorn PL, Calderon C, Melgar S, Moguel B, Solorzano E, Dumonteil E, et al. Two distinct *Triatoma dimidiata* (Latreille, 1811) taxa are found in sympatry in Guatemala and Mexico. *PLoS NTD* 2009;**3**:e393.

76. Usinger RL. The Triatomine of North and Central America and the West Indies and their public health significance. *Publ Health Bull* 1944;**288**:1−83.

77. Souza RC, Campolina-Silva GH, Mendonca Bezerra C, Diotaiuti L, Gorla DE. Does *Triatoma brasiliensis* and *T. melanica* share the same environmental niche space? *Parasit Vectors* 2015;**8**:361. Available from: http://dx.doi.org/10.1186/s13071-015-0973-4.

78. Costa J, Peterson AT, Beard CB. Ecological niche modeling and differentiation of populations of *Triatoma brasiliensis* Neiva, 1911, the most important Chagas disease vector in northeastern Brazil (Hemiptera, Reduviidae, Triatominae). *Am J Trop Med Hyg* 2002; **67**:516−20.

79. Carbajal de la Fuente AL, Dias-Lima A, Lopes CM, Emperaire L, Walter A, Ferreira A, et al. Behavioural plasticity of Triatominae related to habitat selection in Northeast Brazil. *J Med Entomol* 2008;**45**:14−19.

80. Noireau F, Breniére F, Ordoñez J, Cardozo L, Morochi W, Gutierrez T, et al. Low probability of transmission of *Trypanosoma cruzi* to man by domestic *Triatoma sordida* in Santa Cruz department, Bolivia. *Trans R Soc Trop Med Hyg* 1997;**91**:653−6.

81. Vazquez-Prokopec GM, Cecere MC, Canale DM, Gürtler RE, Kitron U. Spatiotemporal patterns of reinfestation by *Triatoma guasayana* (Hemiptera: Reduviidae) in a rural community of northwestern Argentina. *J Med Entomol* 2005;**42**:571−81.

82. Carcavallo RU, Martinez A. Biología, ecología y distribución geográfica de los triatominos americanos (excepto *R. prolixus, P. megistus, T. dimidiata* y *T. infestans*). In: Carcavallo RU, Rabinovich JE, Tonn RJ, editors. *Factores Biológicos y Ecológicos en la Enfermedad de Chagas*, vol. I. Buenos Aires, Argentina: Ministerio de Salud y Acción Social de Argentina; 1985. p. 149−208.

83. Feliciangeli MD, Campbell-Lendrum D, Martinez C, Gonzalez D, Coleman P, Davies C. Chagas disease control in Venezuela: lessons for the Andean region and beyond. *Trends Parasitol* 2003;**19**:44−9.

84. Vargas E, Espitia C, Patiño C, Pinto N, Aguilera G, Jaramillo C, et al. Genetic structure of *Triatoma venosa* (Hemiptera: Reduviidae): molecular and morphometric evidence. *Mem Inst Oswaldo Cruz* 2006;**101**:39−45.

85. Guzman-Bracho C. Epidemiology of Chagas disease in Mexico: an update. *Trends Parasitol* 2001;**17**:372−6.

86. Ramsey JM, Ordoñez R, Cruz-Celis A, Alvear AL, Chavez V, Lopez R, et al. Distribution of domestic Triatominae and stratification of Chagas disease transmission in Oaxaca, Mexico. *Med Vet Entomol* 2000;**14**:19−30.

87. Gorla DE. Variables ambientales registradas por sensores remotos como indicadores de la distribución geográfica de *Triatoma infestans*. *Ecol Austr* 2002;**12**:117−27.

88. Barrett TV, Hoff R, Mott KE, Guedes F, Sherlock IA. An outbreak of acute Chagas disease in the Sao Francisco valley region of Bahia, Brazil: triatomine vectors and animal reservoirs of *Trypanosoma cruzi*. *Trans R Soc Trop Med Hyg* 1979;**73**:703−9.

89. Silveira AC, Feitosa VR, Borges R. Distribução de Triatomíneos capturados no ambiente domiciliar, no período 1975/83, Brasil. *Rev Brasil Malariol D Trop* 1984;**36**: 15−312.

90. Schofield CJ. Biosystematics of the Triatominae. In: Service MW, editor. *Biosystematics of Haematophagous Insects. Systematic Associations Special*, vol 37. Oxford: Clarendon; 1988. p. 284−312.

91. Panzera F, Dujardin JP, Nicolini P, Caraccio MN, Rose V, Tellez T, et al. Genomic changes of Chagas disease vector, South America. *Emerg Infect Dis* 2004;**10**:438−46.

92. Schofield CJ, Jannin J, Salvatella R. The future of Chagas disease control. *Trends Parasit* 2006;**22**:583−8.

93. Brewer M, Arguello N, Delfino M, Gorla DE. Parasitismo natural de *Telenomus fariai* Costa Lima 1927 (Hym.: Scelionidae) en monte y presencia de *Proanastatus excavatus* De Santis 1952 (Hym.: Eupelmidae) parasitoides oófagos de Triatominae en Cruz del Eje, Córdoba Argentina. *Anais Soc Entomol do Brasil* 1978;**7**:141−54.

94. Noireau F, Cortez MGR, Monteiro FA, Jansen AM, Torrico F. Can wild *Triatoma infestans* foci in Bolívia jeopardize Chagas disease control efforts? *Trends Parasitol* 2005;**21**:7−10.

95. Noireau F. Wild *Triatoma infestans*, a potential threat that needs to be monitored. *Mem Inst Oswaldo Cruz* 2009;**104**(Suppl. 1):60−4.

96. Gorla DE, Noireau F. Chapter 9. Geographic distribution of Triatominae vectors in America. In: Tybairenc M, editor. *American Trypanosomiasis: Chagas Disease*. J. Wiley & Sons; 2010. p. 209−31.

97. Noireau F, Flores R, Gutierrez T, Dujardin JP. Detection of sylvatic dark morphs of Triatoma infestans in the Bolivian Chaco. *Mem Inst Oswaldo Cruz* 1997;**92**:583−4.

98. Bacigalupo A, Torres-Perez F, Segovia V, García A, Correa JP, Moreno L, et al. Sylvatic foci of the Chagas disease vector *Triatoma infestans* in Chile: description of a new focus and challenges for control programs. *Mem Inst Oswaldo Cruz* 2010;**105**: 633−41.

99. Panzera F, Ferreiro MJ, Pita S, Calleros L, Pérez R, Basmadjián Y, et al. Evolutionary and dispersal history of *Triatoma infestans*, main vector of Chagas disease, by chromosomal markers. *Infect Genet Evol* 2014;**27**:105−13.

100. Bustamante Gomez M, Gonçalves Diotaiuti L, Gorla DE. Distribution of pyrethroid resistance in Triatoma infestans populations. *PLoS NTD* 2016;**10**(3):e004561.

101. Carbajal de la Fuente AL, Porcasi X, Noireau F, Diotaiuti L, Gorla DE. The association between the geographic distribution of *Triatoma pseudomaculata* and *Triatoma wygodzinskyi* (Hemiptera: Reduviidae) with environmental variables recorded by remote sensors. *Infect Gen Evol* 2009;**9**:54−61.

102. Peterson AT, Sánchez-Cordero V, Beard CB, Ramsey JM. Ecologic niche modeling and potential reservoirs for Chagas disease, Mexico. *Emerg Infect Dis* 2002;**8**:662−7.

103. Gurgel-Gonçalvez R, Cuba CA. Predicting the potential geographic distribution of *Rhodnius neglectus* (Hemiptera, Reduviidae) based on ecological niche modeling. *J Med Entomol* 2009;**46**:952−60.

104. Gurgel-Goncalves R, Galvão C, Costa J, Peterson AT. Geographic distribution of Chagas disease vectors in Brazil based on ecological niche modelling. *J Trop Med* 2012;**2012**:15. Article ID 705326. Available from: http://dx.doi.org/10.1155/2012/705326.

105. Bustamante DM, Monroy MM, Rodas AG, Juarez JA, Malone JB. Environmental determinants of the distribution of Chagas disease vectors in south-eastern Guatemala. *Geospat. Health* 2007;**2**:199−211.

106. Ostfeld RS. Climate change and the distribution and intensity of infectious diseases. *Ecology* 2009;**90**:903−5.

107. Epstein PR. Is global warming harmful to health? *Sci. Am* 2000;**283**:50−7.

108. Campbell-Lendrum D, Pruss-Ustun A, Corvalan C. How much disease could climate change cause? In: McMichael AJ, Campbell-Lendrum D, Corvalan C, Ebi KL, Githeko AK, Scheraga JS, Woodward A, editors. *Climate Change and Health: Risks and Responses*. Geneva, Switzerland: World Health Organization; 2003. p. 133−58.

109. Randolph SE. Perspectives on climate change impacts on infectious diseases. *Ecology* 2009;**90**:927−31.

110. Lafferty KD. The ecology of climate change and infectious diseases. *Ecology* 2009;**90**: 888−900.

111. Gorla DE, Catalá SS, Grilli MP. Efecto de la temperatura sobre la distribución de *Triatoma infestans* y el riesgo de transmisión vectorial de la enfermedad de Chagas en Argentina. *Acta Toxicol Arg* 1997;**5**:36−9.

112. Gorla DE. Population dynamics and control of *Triatoma infestans*. *Med Vet Entomol* 1992;**6**:91−7.
113. INCOSUR, 2002. XIth Meeting of the Southern Cone Intergovernmental Commision to Eliminate *Triatoma infestans* and interrupt the Transmission of Transfusional Trypanosomiasis. http://www.paho.org/Spanish/AD/DPC/CD/xi-incosur-3-arg.pdf [accessed 27.01.10].
114. Medone P, Ceccarelli S, Parham PE, Figuera A, Rabinovich JE. The impact of climate change on the geographical distribution of two vectors of Chagas disease: implication for the force of infection. *Philos Trans R Soc B* 2015;**370**:20130560. Available from: http://dx.doi.org/10.1098/rstb.2013.0560.

# Control strategies against Triatominae

*D. Gorla[1] and K. Hashimoto[2]*

[1]Consejo Nacional de Investigaciones Científicas y Técnicas, Universidad Nacional de Córdoba, Argentina, [2]Freelance Global Health Consultant, Japan

## Introduction

Control of Triatominae (Hemiptera, Reduviidae) is a primary component of strategies to halt the transmission of Chagas disease, along with serological screening of blood donors to reduce the likelihood of transmission through infected blood transfusions. In the early 1990s, an estimated 80% of Chagas disease cases were attributed to transmission from triatomine vectors.[1] Since 1991, a series of multinational initiatives have focused on elimination of the domestic vector populations throughout the endemic areas of Latin America. Largely as a result of these initiatives, transmission rates have been steadily reduced, with corresponding reductions in infection prevalence. Current estimates suggest that around 7 million people are infected, down from the 1984 estimate of 24 million[2]; annual transmission rates are probably fewer than 50,000 new cases per year.[3,4] The geographical distribution of domestic vector populations has been drastically reduced, especially *Triatoma infestans* in Southern Cone countries and *Rhodnius prolixus* in Central America. Uruguay, Chile, and Brazil, together with several provinces and departments of Argentina, Bolivia, and Paraguay, have been formally declared free of transmission due to *T. infestans*. Costa Rica, El Salvador, Honduras, Guatemala, and Nicaragua

American Trypanosomiasis Chagas Disease. DOI: http://dx.doi.org/10.1016/B978-0-12-801029-7.00010-1

have recently been declared free of transmission due to *R. prolixus* and/or its elimination. In addition, there has been steady progress in blood donor screening, with coverage now approaching 100% in most of the endemic countries.[5]

But this is not to say that the task of controlling Chagas disease is concluded. Rates of transmission due to domestic vectors remain high in several regions, most notably the Gran Chaco region of Argentina, Bolivia, and Paraguay, as well as parts of the Andean Pact countries and Mexico. Even in those regions where the main domestic vector populations have been eliminated, there is a consistent requirement to maintain surveillance with focal interventions against potential new domestic infestations.

There is not only a risk of repopulation by the main vector species but also a risk of other species invading domestic habitats and either establishing new domestic colonies or provoking "accidental" transmission (e.g., through contamination of food or drink) without necessarily establishing new colonies. This, in conjunction with declining public health interest in Chagas disease as the apparent control successes become more widely discussed, imposes a need for additional strategies in vector surveillance and control that can be sustained as a matter of routine over the long term. Current strategies, based on large-scale campaigns of indoor residual spraying (IRS) against established vector populations, are still required in many areas, but will need to become progressively more focal and guided by a sustainable surveillance system integrated with routine public health vigilance. Such techniques are available, and the strategies are being developed.[6]

# Elimination of domestic populations of Triatominae

Since the pioneering work of Carlos Chagas and colleagues in Brazil, and Salvador Mazza and colleagues in Argentina, a very wide range of vector control methods has been trialed with a view to eliminating domestic infestations of Triatominae, including biological control and insect pathogens, as well as a range of physical and chemical methods. The resulting experience accumulated from experiments and field trials in most countries of Latin America has led to a basic vector control approach with three main components: (1) IRS by trained professionals; (2) householder and community participation in monitoring and surveillance; and (3) rural house improvement and health education.

In general, a well-applied IRS campaign is sufficient to eliminate existing domestic bug populations, although repeat treatments are sometimes given after 3–6 months[7] and, in regions like the Gran Chaco, elimination of peridomestic populations is unlikely.[8,9] Since the 1980s, wettable powder (WP) or suspension concentrate (SC) formulations of pyrethroids have been the products of choice; other classes of insecticide are not generally used except when donated (or against some recently reported foci of pyrethroid-resistant *T. infestans* in southern Bolivia and northwestern Argentina).[10] Throughout Latin America, IRS campaigns followed by long-term surveillance have been the primary component of Chagas disease control programs, together with improved blood bank screening to reduce the likelihood of transfusional transmission from infected blood donors, and improved patient care, counseling, and treatment for those already infected.

By itself, rural house improvement seems insufficient to eliminate an established domestic bug population[11] and it tends to be a relatively slow process that rarely reaches all the poorest householders. In addition, house improvement programs need not be guided by the presence or absence of a particular vector, nor do they necessarily rely on health sector professionals. By contrast, well-managed IRS programs can reach all domiciles and can usually treat 2–10 houses per worker per day, depending on terrain, size, and distribution of houses and the extension of peridomestic structures that are included in the treatment.

However, community agreement and householder participation are essential, both to assist in preparing the premises for spraying and to participate in postcontrol monitoring and surveillance to ensure that the domestic bug population has indeed been eliminated and to provide early warning if any subsequent infestations are found.

Education is seen not only as a way of motivating people to make better efforts to avoid the presence of triatomines within a house in the long term, but also as a way of encouraging schoolchildren, teachers, and the community to participate actively in the vector surveillance activities after the insecticide application in the endemic areas.[12]

Although difficult to achieve because of the inherent complexities, the more integrated the vector control and vigilance program (vector control, community education, house improvement, productivity of domestic animals), the more efficient and long-lasting would be the eventual elimination of intradomestic infestations. Integration of vector surveillance activities with the primary educational system is also seen as a crucial component for long-term sustainability. The essential difficulty for dedicated Chagas disease control programs is that the more successful they are in reducing the epidemiological indices, the less the perceived demand for their expertise. Consequently, successful Chagas disease control programs become essentially self-limiting—the so-called "punishment of success"—and must therefore adapt the surveillance and control strategy in accordance with the changing epidemiological patterns.[13] An effective way to do this involves a routine program of interview and serological surveillance of schoolchildren; for example, as part of a routine program of school health care such that absence of reports of domestic Triatominae, combined with absence of serologically positive children, can be used as evidence that there is no currently active transmission within the school catchment area. Similarly, the presence of serologically positive children can guide both specific treatment for those children and entomological inspection of their houses with selective insecticidal treatment where necessary.[6]

# Multinational initiatives

Following a great many trials during the postwar decades and national control campaigns in Venezuela, Argentina, and Brazil, the enlightened response to the geographical scale of Chagas disease control came as a series of multinational initiatives, beginning with the Southern Cone countries in 1991, followed by initiatives of the Andean Pact (IPA) and Central American countries (IPCA) launched in 1997 and the Amazon Initiative (AMCHA) launched in 2002. The Southern Cone Initiative (INCOSUR) involved six countries (Argentina, Bolivia, Brazil, Chile, Paraguay, and Uruguay) which, with southern Peru, was designed to cover the entire distribution of the main vector, *T. infestans*. At the time, it was believed that *T. infestans* was almost entirely domestic throughout its range (except for small sylvatic foci in the Cochabamba-Sucre region of central Bolivia); the aim of the INCOSUR program was to halt Chagas disease transmission by eliminating all domestic populations of *T. infestans* (with concurrent elimination of any other domestic vector populations in the same area) and by improving screening of blood donors to reduce the risk of transfusional transmission. The idea was that simultaneous vector control programs throughout the area would prevent reinfestation of treated premises by *T. infestans* being accidentally transported from nontreated regions. In addition, the multinational nature of the program—coordinated by the Pan American Health Organization (PAHO)—should give political continuity to the interventions, making it less likely that a country would suddenly divert resources away from the Chagas disease control program.[14]

The Andean Pact and Central American Initiatives had similar aims and rationale, focusing on the elimination of domestic populations of their main vector, *Rhodnius prolixus*, together with control of other vectors in the region, particularly *Triatoma dimidiata*. There was strong evidence that *R. prolixus* had been accidentally imported from Venezuela into Central America at the turn of the last century[15,16]; consequently, it appeared that *R. prolixus* could be completely eliminated in Central America. Similarly, there was evidence that *T. dimidiata* had been accidentally transported from Central America to Ecuador and northern Peru during pre-Colombian times[17] so that it could potentially be eliminated from there even if not from Central America, where it retains extensive sylvatic populations.

The INCOSUR, IPA, and IPCA initiatives were designed primarily as vector elimination programs and, at the time of writing, Brazil, Chile, and Uruguay in the Southern Cone of South America and Guatemala, El Salvador, Honduras, and Nicaragua have been formally declared free of Chagas disease transmission due to their main vectors.[18,19] Similar declarations have been made for various provinces and departments of Argentina, Bolivia, and Paraguay.

The distribution of *T. infestans* has been reduced from its predicted maximum of 6.28 million km$^2$ [20] to well under 1 million km$^2$,[4,6,21] while *R. prolixus* appears to have disappeared from Central America.[18] In all countries of Latin America, screening of blood donors has been improved, with a coverage now close to 100% in most countries.[22]

Costs averaged around US$30 million per year for the Southern Cone, and around US$4 million to $7 million per year for the Central American countries, but studies in Argentina and Brazil indicate economic returns equivalent to over US$7 for every dollar invested in the Chagas disease control programs.[23,24] Benefits have also accrued to those already infected, as clinicians throughout the intervened regions report reductions in the severity of the chronic lesions,[21] which, from studies in mouse models, seems to be largely due to lack of reinfection once the domestic vectors have been eliminated.[25,26]

By contrast, the Amazon Initiative (AMCHA), which includes parts of nine countries, was designed primarily as a surveillance program because domestic vector populations are rare in most of the Amazon region (except for *Triatoma maculata* in parts of Roraima and southern Venezuela).[27] Instead, vector-borne transmission in the Amazon region is attributed primarily to adventitious sylvatic bugs (mainly species of *Rhodnius* and *Panstrongylus*) flying into houses and contaminating food and drink.[28] Such transmission is often described as "oral-route transmission" and has resulted in a series of so-called family microepidemics of acute Chagas disease in various parts of the Amazon region (and elsewhere). In such circumstances, there is little role for vector control programs; instead emphasis is given to detection and treatment of those occasional outbreaks of acute disease, a task in which malaria slide microscopists are playing an increasing role by identifying trypanosomes in the peripheral blood smears of febrile patients originally suspected of malaria. In a sense, the Amazon Initiative may also be revealing aspects of how the future of Chagas disease control could proceed throughout the Americas once the existing domestic vector populations have been eliminated.

# The beginning of the end?

With these apparent successes, a much-debated question then becomes "can Chagas disease be eliminated?" We must be clear on terminology: The causative agent, *Trypanosoma cruzi*, will not be eliminated—it is a widespread parasite of small mammals and marsupials throughout the Americas; the vectors, Triatominae, will not be eliminated—there are over 140 species distributed in the Americas (and some also in India and Southeast Asia). As a consequence, the disease will not be eliminated, in the sense that the ubiquity of parasites and vectors in Latin America will always pose a risk of occasional transmission to humans. These, without prompt diagnosis and treatment, can in turn pose a risk of onward transmission through nonvectorial routes, such as blood transfusion, organ transplant, and occasional congenital cases.

But some vector populations can be eliminated: domestic *T. infestans* over most of its original distribution in Argentina, Bolivia, Brazil, Chile, Paraguay, Uruguay, and southern Peru; the central American form of *R. prolixus* and the South American form—at least from the central valleys of Colombia; *R. ecuadoriensis* from northern Peru; and *T. dimidiata* from Ecuador. All these populations appear to have been imported as domestic variants from elsewhere, mainly by accidental carriage by humans, and mostly within the last 150 years. In a sense, their presence outside their original foci is aberrant, due to human accidents that should (and could) be corrected.

These populations have probably accounted for over 80% of Chagas disease transmission, but they are not the only vectors. All populations of all species of

Triatominae should be considered at least as potential vectors, although without human contact they can play no epidemiological role. Perhaps the focus should be to minimize that contact, and then to minimize the risk of that contact. With this perspective, outline strategies become clear. All existing domestic populations of Triatominae, of whatever species, should be eliminated, and experience accumulated from control trials and programs throughout Latin America shows that this is possible. But then how do we sustain this absence of domestic Triatominae, knowing that the previously infested houses may remain susceptible to reinvasion?

Promotion of rural house improvements may help, but for reasons already mentioned, this is unlikely to reach all communities that may merit such development. Land use change and rural–urban migration was associated with the reduction of house infestation by triatomines, although it is sometimes difficult to tell apart the contribution of these socioeconomic changes and the vector control activities.[29] The other technical response is to improve insecticide formulations, in an attempt to give longer protection to the treated premises. But recognizing that no treatment can last for ever, the strategic response, as illustrated by the multinational initiatives, is to try to remove source populations to make reinfestation unlikely.

Successful when dealing with an imported domestic variant (such as *R. prolixus* in Central America), this strategy is much less successful when dealing with domestic populations that also occupy extensive peridomestic habitats (such as *T. infestans* in the Chaco region of northwest Argentina and southern Bolivia) or that retain local sylvatic ecotopes (such as *T. dimidiata* in parts of Central America).

The control of peridomestic populations of Triatominae is seen as a major technical challenge. Conventional spraying with WP or SC pyrethroids, such as those used inside houses, tends to have reduced impact as the superficial deposits can be degraded by sunlight or quickly covered with dust or animal dejections. Some authors report better results using a double spray[30] or using slow-release polymer formulations.[31–33] Others prefer physical modifications to the peridomestic habitat, for example, by using higher standard fencing materials instead of piled brushwood for goat corrals in the Argentine Chaco, which can greatly reduce the habitat available for peridomestic *Triatoma infestans* and *Triatoma guasayana*.[34,35] Other approaches involve the concept of "xenointoxication," or treating domestic animals with a pour-on or powder formulation of insecticide, in order to kill any bugs that may attempt to feed on them.[36–40] Insecticide-impregnated dog collars have been used for a similar purpose[41,42] and it seems likely that further technical developments will lead to improvements in the ways to control peridomestic Triatominae. But perhaps a strategic response needs also to be considered. The importance of peridomestic Triatominae is primarily as a potential source for reinfesting the domestic habitat. Domestic reinfestation from peridomestic populations after 1–4 years of insecticide application is a well-established concept, based on long-term studies mainly in Santiago del Estero (Argentina) carried out by Gürtler et al.[43] Studies based on population genetics and morphometry suggest that populations are highly structured, even at the habitat level.[44,45] The latest studies, showing spatial structure at the habitat level (i.e., habitat-specific populations that do not show evidence for little movement of individuals flow between populations), raise questions about the speed at which peridomestic populations actually reinfest intradomestic structures. The latest questioning is supported by a 10-year observation on house infestation in the Department Castro Barros (La Rioja) and field data collected from the region of Los Llanos by the Chagas vector control program of La Rioja.

During the last 12 years, house infestation by *T. infestans* in the Department of Castro Barros (north of La Rioja-Argentina, 743 houses distributed in 10 villages) was periodically evaluated either by research teams or provincial or national Chagas vector control programs.[46] Repeatedly, evaluations of peridomestic infestation ranged between 25% and 30% and intradomestic infestation between 0% and 4%. But in spite of the relatively high infestation of peridomestic structures, intradomestic infestation remained low, with very small vector populations. The virtual absence of vectors inside the rooms, where the parasite transmission by vectors usually takes place, was associated with zero infection in children younger than 15 years of age evaluated three times between 1998 and 2011 (except four cases associated with *T. cruzi*-infected mothers, which were identified as congenital cases and treated accordingly).

House infestation in the Department San Martin (south of La Rioja, within the highly endemic region of Los Llanos) was 34.4% and 48.4% (intradomestic and peridomestic, respectively) on average until 2004.[47] After systematic vector control interventions during the last 9 years, intradomestic infestation dropped to 3%, although peridomestic infestation averages 30%. In spite of the relatively high peridomestic infestation, no children below 6 years of age were found to be infected with *T. cruzi*, except for a few congenital cases (Programa Chagas La Rioja, unpublished data).

*T. cruzi* vectorial transmission seems to be interrupted in the Departments of Castro Barros and San Martin, even though there has been a sustained 25–30% peridomestic infestation during the last decade. So, in at least these two departments of La Rioja, the sustained interruption of vectorial transmission of *T. cruzi* did not require the elimination of peridomestic infestations of *T. infestans*.

Although it would be risky to make extrapolations, it seems that there is at least some heterogeneity about the speed at which the intradomestic infestation from peridomestic populations of *T. infestans* takes place (faster in Santiago del Estero, slower in La Rioja). One possibility that has to be considered is the origin of the individuals that produce the intradomestic colonization. Because of the imperfect methods to detect intradomestic infestation, the origin of the population producing the intradomestic colonization after a vector control intervention with residual insecticide (individuals coming from peridomestic structures or intradomestic survivors reconstituting the original population) has not been routinely analyzed. If the newly apparent intradomestic colonization in fact results from survivors of the original intradomestic residual population, then improved evaluation of the quality of spraying is crucial.

Where possible, peridomestic populations of Triatominae should be reduced or eliminated (not least, for their effects on the productivity of peridomestic animals), but from a public health standpoint they can also be viewed as akin to sylvatic populations, some of which are also potential sources for reinfesting the domestic habitat. Seen in this light, the strategy changes. It is both impractical and ecologically unacceptable to contemplate large-scale interventions against sylvatic populations of Triatominae. It is also irrelevant in terms of transmission control. Only by coming into contact with humans, e.g., by entering a house, does a sylvatic bug assume possible epidemiological significance, either by causing direct transmission or by establishing a new domestic colony. But a newly established domestic colony can be eliminated, and a transmission event can be treated, which is the basis of the Amazon surveillance strategy. Perhaps even elsewhere, peridomestic and sylvatic populations should be considered similarly, focusing on the vectors only when incipient domestic colonization is apparent, but otherwise focusing only on diagnosis and treatment of possible new cases of infection.

## Criteria for stratification of vector control priorities

Often, the available resources for the vector control interventions do not allow the coverage of all the endemic areas. In these cases, some sort of prioritization is needed, and knowledge to build priorities under these circumstances has been accumulated from a number of operational research studies. Two cases, with different approaches, are presented below showing possibilities to carry out the interventions under tight budgets.

The first case is the control of Chagas disease vectors in Central America (CA) within the context of the Initiative of the Central American Countries (IPCA). Since establishment of the IPCA in 1997, Chagas disease vector control in Central America shifted in three dimensions: the main target from *R. prolixus* to *T. dimidiata*; operational phase from attack to surveillance; and management focus from impact to sustainability. From 2000, efforts to eliminate *R. prolixus* and to reduce *T. dimidiata* were intensified in Guatemala, El Salvador, Honduras, and Nicaragua. Vector control activities received assistance from several sources, particularly the Pan American Health Organization (PAHO), Japan International Cooperation Agency (JICA), NGOs, and local universities. Through this assistance, the Ministries of Health of the IPCA government obtained IRS equipment, insecticides, and vehicles, and developed management capacity to administer vector control and surveillance activities at the national and local levels through projects with JICA. The projects reinforced the communication between the National Programs and local health services, which had been debilitated during the process of decentralization of the health systems, and consequently improved the operational performance. As the vector control activities were scaled up, villages with *R. prolixus* were identified and treated by IRS. The number of villages identified with *R. prolixus* reached 317 in Guatemala during 2000−8, 228 in Honduras during 2003−10 and 9 in Nicaragua during 2002−13.[18,48] As of February 2016, there have been no further reports of this vector species in Central America since the last finding in a village in Matagalpa in Nicaragua 2013. As a result of the coordinated effort the IPCA and PAHO certified Guatemala in 2008, Nicaragua and Honduras in 2011 for interruption of Chagas disease transmission by *R. prolixus*, and El Salvador in 2010 and Costa Rica in 2011 for elimination of the vector. Along with the advance in elimination of *R. prolixus*, indoor infestation rates with *T. dimidiata* have also declined from 14.5% in 2000 to 3.6% in 2012 in Guatemala, from 20.9% in 1999−2000 to 2.0% in 2012 in El Salvador, and from 21.9% in 2004 to 3.1% in 2012 in Honduras.[19]

As the vector infestation decreased substantially, the operational phase shifted from attack to surveillance and so did the management focus from impact to sustainability. Considering the need to sustain vector surveillance extensively and indefinitely in particular for *T. dimidiata*, a strategy had to be cost-effective and practical, that is, community-based and embedded in local health systems. To this end, Guatemala, El Salvador, Honduras, and Nicaragua installed Chagas disease vector surveillance mostly at the health facilities closest to the community. It was aimed to facilitate optimization of locally available resources and opportunities, efficient response to vector notification from the community and therefore efforts to sustain the surveillance systems. Having divided vector surveillance into five core components (1. health promotion, 2. vector detection, 3. vector notification, 4. data analysis and action planning, 5. response to vector notification), the activities became customizable, distributable, and sharable among different stakeholders, including physicians, nurses, operational technicians, community health volunteers, community sprayers, and the population.[49,50] In Guatemala, while vector control specialists of departmental health offices continued promoting vector notification, analyzing data, and providing response for sporadic notifications, these tasks were delegated to municipal vector control teams in endemic areas. In El Salvador where a limited number of vector control specialists were stationed at the departmental health office, the surveillance tasks were shifted to health promotors of health centers who visit communities monthly or bimonthly. The departmental vector control specialists became trainers, supervisors, and supporters to provide technical assistance, maintain equipment, and supply materials. In Honduras, where operational functions were more decentralized and incorporated into primary health care, the surveillance responsibilities were assigned to the health centers in which activities are organized among clinical and operational staff, community heath volunteers, and community sprayers. In Nicaragua, the surveillance responsibilities were also assigned to the health centers, where the tasks are mostly carried out by the community family health team consisting of physicians, nurses, and auxiliary nurses during their regular visits and by vector control technicians during their occasional visits to communities. In addition to the surveillance models, response criteria varied slightly between countries. Although the countries agreed to spray all houses in villages infested with *R. prolixus*, for *T. dimidiata* Guatemala and Honduras responded with IRS only when nymphs or numerous adults were found inside houses as possible indication of colonization and for other vector notifications provided educational advice for house improvement. El Salvador applied IRS to all houses notified with nymphs or adults of *T. dimidiata* and all houses within a radius of 100 m where vector-borne Chagas transmission occurred. Nicaragua implemented a strategy to accumulate the vector notifications for 6 months and spray all houses in the village if more than 20% of houses were infested with *T. dimidiata*, spray all infested houses in villages with 5−20% of indoor infestation rates, and visit all infested houses where less than 5% of houses in the community notified the vector. Because of heterogeneous vector distribution, notification patterns, involved actors and response criteria between and within countries, monitoring of community-based surveillance focused on the number of houses found infested by vector notifications and the rate of infested houses with response. Despite the lack of statistical representativeness and standardized quality, these indicators were sufficient to approximate vector distributions and functionality of community-based surveillance, to take further actions such as entomological surveys, close monitoring, and specific training. Further, response to vector notification was the most important yet challenging task, in particular in resource limited settings, to minimize the infection risks and sustain the surveillance systems. The key to maintain a high response rate to vector notification was constant monitoring of surveillance systems by the departmental health office, regardless of the number of vector notifications, the number of operational technicians or community health volunteers, the degree of decentralization of response to vector report, interval between vector notification and response, and presence of aid agencies.[51]

Community-based surveillance once embedded in local health systems may be sustained with minimum resources and efforts, however, it can also relax and languish—potentially leading to unreported reinfestation of vectors. To reactivate surveillance activities, bug search campaigns were found to be effective. In the Department of Jalapa in Guatemala where *R. prolixus* had previously been found in 15 out of 64 villages but apparently absent since 2002, according to community-based vector surveillance, the departmental health office organized a Chagas bug hunting campaign in 2007 involving local health services, primary schools, NGOs, community health volunteers, media, and private companies. As a result, two villages were found infested with *R. prolixus*. The number of notifications of *T. dimidiata* also rose sharply from an annual average of 36 during 2004–2006 to 205 in 2007.[52] Similar effects of such campaigns were found in the department of Intibucá in Honduras, where a bug hunting campaign involving schoolchildren, community health volunteers, and media led to discovery of a new village infested with *R. prolixus* in 2010. To augment the sensitivity of vector detection, the Central American countries have also investigated houses at risk of infestation and reinfestation in villages with a history of presence of *R. prolixus* and in areas previously endemic to *T. dimidiata*. However, countries are yet to implement systematic serological evaluation mechanisms, which could be facilitated by a regional policy and leadership, to analyze the disease transmission levels over time under community-based surveillance. Currently long-term consequence of surveillance is to be observed through seroprevalence of screening at blood banks.

The second case refers to vector control activities in La Rioja province (Argentina)—historically highly endemic for Chagas disease with active vectorial transmission.[53] From 2004, a new structure for the vector control program of the province was organized. The new vector control activities, besides the normal entomological evaluation and insecticide application, included the individual coding of rural houses and geolocation using a global positioning system device and the organization of a regularly maintained information system. After 6–12 months, the vector control field teams returned to the previously reported intradomestic infested houses to carry out a new entomological evaluation and respray the houses (intra- and peridomestic application) if still infested. In parallel, using the geographic information collected in the field, a spatial analysis was carried out of house infes- tation to identify spatial aggregates, where the activities of the field teams could be reinforced. Using this simple strategy, with a modest number of personnel and field vehicles during 5 years of uninterrupted activities, the intradomestic infestation rates by *T. infestans* dropped from 25% to less than 1%, and no acute cases of Chagas disease were reported. Peridomestic infestation is still relatively high in some provincial departments (>20%), and continued efforts integrating other vec- tor control methods (e.g., modification of peridomestic structures for animal shel- ters) are currently under way in the affected areas.[9,34,35,47]

# Insecticide resistance

During 2000, a control failure after a pyrethroid application for *T. infestans* control was reported for the region of Salvador Mazza (Salta, Argentina), which was attributed to pyrethroid resistance.[54] Subsequent studies have shown the occurrence of other con- trol failure events of *T. infestans* populations, that were shown resistant to pyrethroids in the interandean valleys and Chaco region of Bolivia[54,55] and more recently in several places in the Chaco province in Argentina.[10] Studies showed the existence of several mechanisms of insecticide resistance (including penetrability of the insect cuti- cle, KDR genes,[56] suggesting independent development of resistance appearance), and geographical distribution of highly resistant populations (producing pyrethroid-based control failures) limited to the Argentinian-Bolivian border.[10] Studies reported so far on the *T. infestans* populations of the Bolivian Chaco and S. Mazza indicate a resis- tance rate to deltamethrin higher than 1000 in some places, with some cross-resistance to other pyrethroids and to fipronil, but generally susceptible to organophosphates and carbamates. Organophosphate and carbamate compounds have been sprayed by professional field teams of Argentina and Bolivia to control domestic and peridomestic populations of *T. infestans* in S. Mazza and various localities in Bolivia. Although postspraying reports indicate a decrease of vector abundance and house infestation, the resistant *T. infestans* populations are still present in the area.

A recent meta-analysis of insecticide resistance of *T. infestans* populations showed that although the phenomenon is widespread, control failure due to insecti- cide resistance is limited to the Argentinian-Bolivian border, it is associated with a particular combination of environmental variables values[10] and with the occurrence of the intermediate cytogenetic phenotype (*sensu*[57]).

# New technologies for vector control

Suspension concentrate formulations of synthetic pyrethroid insecticides were the basic tool that allowed the successful elimination of domestic triatomines over several Latino American regions. In the Southern Cone countries of South America, the area affected by *T. infestans* was reduced by over 90%. The success in the elimination of the domestic infestation contrasts with the difficulty of obtaining the same result in vast areas of the arid Gran Chaco. This difficulty comes from the low efficacy of the residual spray of current suspension concentrate formulations over the peridomestic structures (goat corrals, chicken nests, deposits, etc.). The low efficacy is caused by the rapid degradation of the active ingredient, as shown in several studies.[58]

A number of studies evaluated two different ways of using chemical control (*xenointoxication, microencapsulated formulations*) and one nonchemical control intervention alternatives (*environmental management*) to overcome the limitation of the low-efficacy pyrethroid formulations when applied to peridomestic structures. The idea of xenointoxication was to lay the active ingredient not over all the house unit (domestic and peridomestic structures), but only over the domestic vertebrate hosts of *T. infestans*. A series of articles by Amelotti and colleagues[36–39] showed that current pour-on formulations already registered in Argentina for veterinary use produced high *T. infestans* mortality when applied on chickens during 45 days, but lower and shorter mortality when applied on goats. A pour-on formulation of fipronil produced low mortality during 15 days when applied on dogs. Similar positive and negative results on xenointoxication using pyrethroids and fipronil were also obtained.[8,41,42] The second different approach to chemical control was to lay the active ingredient over the house unit, but with a formulation that protects the active ingredient inside a polymeric microcapsule. This formulation showed longer lasting effect than the traditional suspension concentrate formulation, under both experimental[32] and field conditions.[33,59]

The nonchemical control evaluated under the arid Chaco conditions was environmental management, changing the structure and construction materials of the goat corrals. By doing this with the participation of the productive community, the corrals that had been highly infested with abundant *T. infestans* populations, showed decreased infestation prevalence and vector abundance, as well as offering a substrate surface that improved the efficacy of the suspension concentrate pyrethroid formulations and improving the goat productivity, through 15% increased goat fecundity + decreased calf mortality + shorter calf development time.[35]

A different intervention type, using insecticidal paints based on organophosphate compounds, was applied to domestic and peridomestic structures in southern localities of Santa Cruz in Bolivia (intervention applied to over 2000 houses), where *T. infestans* is resistant to pyrethroids. In this case, houses show no infestation by *T. infestans*, either intradomestic or peridomestic populations, even 3 years after the application of the insecticidal paint.[31,33]

A number of recent published studies has shown the usefulness of mobile phone technology applied for vector surveillance and control, particularly malaria.[60] A few projects testing the support that computer and information technology within the context of Chagas disease control were carried out during the last decade. A project coordinated from the University of Cordoba by 2009 developed an application for hand held devices to collect data on household inhabitants during the routine visits of primary health-care workers.[61] After completing the round, data was downloaded into a desktop computer installed in the regional hospital, connected to a data server. The project confronted a number of technical problems, but was able to show the potentiality of the approach. One session was enough to train the field personnel of the primary health-care system on the use of the technology. Data collected through the application showed the distribution of infected children and pregnant women over an endemic area of Córdoba province (central Argentina). A comparison of two groups followed with the use of the application or not, showed that data from the group studied using the mobile application was better covered and patient follow up was higher than data collected from the group studied without the mobile application. The popularization of mobile phones using high level operative systems (i.e., Android) and the improvement of the communication infrastructure make easier than a few years back the implementation of a surveillance system over vector control, infection detection and treatment. Unfortunately, in spite of the advantages shown for the disease surveillance and control, the technology was never inserted within the health system of the Córdoba province.

Unpublished results of a public—private collaboration in Argentina (CRILAR-VARSTAT) explored the feasibility of developing a citizen information system for vector detection based on the combined use of SMS sent from mobile phones, through emails, or online forms. The development used the advances of the information system of the vector control programs installed in some provinces (e.g., La Rioja), that identified individually an recorded the geographic coordinates of all houses located in the endemic area (about 12,000 in La Rioja). Using a nonsmartphone to inform the house code number or a smartphone with GPS about the potential presence of triatomine vectors in the house was shown a perfectly feasible within the area with improved infrastructure of mobile communications (for the SMS management). In areas outside the mobile communication grid, the system could use synchronically or asynchronically the network of millions of personal netbooks that were distributed to primary and secondary school children through a federal funded program. The system could not only receive text data, but also pictures of the insects. The data could be received by a server installed in a federal and/or provincial health office that would eventually trigger a request the entomological evaluation of the house by the local health agency and carry out an IRS would the infestation by a domestic colony was confirmed. Technically, this development could be scaled up, provided there is the political commitment to fund and sustain such development. More importantly perhaps, is the need to organize and sustain a local health system that is alert and capable of responding promptly to such a request of a house infestation event, either to carry out the evaluation and eventually the vector control intervention.

At the national level, national programs of Chagas disease control have been trying to implement information systems to help improve the evaluation of the disease control activities. The case of Chile is the only example of a working information system for the vector control component, that provides regularly updated information to evaluate the ongoing activities. The system currently offers public access detailed public access information (based on an information transparency law) of house by house infestation by *T. infestans* and *Mepraia spinolai* and vector control interventions. Although the technical solutions and local knowledge are in place, no Chagas disease control program in Latin America was able to install such an information system. In spite of the very important advances made in the control of Chagas disease during the last decades, the road still to be traveled is probably the hardest. Although we have better knowledge and technical facilities than decades before, the lack of political commitment refrain further advances.

## The political commitment

Maintenance of the political commitment is critical for the control of Chagas disease. The case of the Central American countries allows the delineation of lessons to sustain such political commitment. Along the road of the IPCA activities, three strategies have been implemented: (1) establishment of the Chagas Day at the regional and national level; (2) constitution of a national roundtable for Chagas; and (3) strengthening of information and monitoring systems.

Political and public interest in Chagas disease need to be activated on a regular basis, because the less visible the vectors become as a result of successful interventions the more likely the health agencies relax or even languish in surveillance activities. Political commitment is a key drive to maintain the interest, but this is only sustainable and effective when built into governmental systems with key policies, active stakeholders, and good evidence.

An effective policy, which strategically attracts social attention, is the regulation to celebrate a national day to recognize the importance of Chagas disease once a year. In 2008, the IPCA countries proposed and agreed to establish the Central American Chagas Day, the 9th of July, the birthdate of the discoverer of the disease, Carlos Chagas. This proposal was also agreed as a resolution in a meeting of the Council of Ministers of Health of Central America (COMISCA) later in the same year. Since then, Guatemala, El Salvador, Honduras, and Nicaragua began celebrating the annual Chagas day at the national level to raise awareness through media and at the local level to promote vector surveillance and prevention of Chagas disease infection. In El Salvador in 2010, the Ministry of Health established an official agreement with the Ministry of Education to celebrate the National Chagas Day. As a result of these initiatives, the number of participating schools incremented from 668 in 2008 to 1647 in 2012. These campaigns also augmented the number of villages notified with vectors from 306 in 2008 to 1471 in 2011.

Involvement of different stakeholders can contribute to maintain the undervalued and underbudgeted disease control interventions, especially by supporting the National Programs. The National Chagas Program in Guatemala, El Salvador and Honduras constituted a national roundtable, involving officials of other programs (e.g., Epidemiology, Blood Bank, National Reference Laboratory, and Health Promotion) of the Ministry of Health, scholars from local universities, staff of international cooperation agencies and NGOs involved in activities related to Chagas disease. Members of the roundtable supported production and monitoring of national strategic plans of the National Chagas Program, and also provided information including progress, plans and challenges of their own activities and feedback to activities of others during regular meetings held every few months. In sustaining the momentum of disease control efforts, e.g., the roundtable members supported orientation of a new coordinator of the National Chagas Program after personnel changes and provided ideas for alternative cost-effective approaches such as house improvement methods[62] and bug search campaigns,[52] which could also be used to transform and vitalize disease control approaches. Such external support can empower the National Program in terms of management, leadership and political economy.

Evidence is crucial because lack of data can cause not only misunderstanding but the end of budgets and activities. Good evidence derives from systematic data collection and analysis. The national information and monitoring systems play vital roles in understanding the vector distribution patterns. In Guatemala, El Salvador, Honduras, and Nicaragua, where native vector, *T. dimidiata*, is found in almost all departments, regular reporting projected a rough national map signaling the degree of infection risks and apparent coverage of surveillance activities. To analyze the situation and progress, the National Chagas Program held biannual evaluation meetings, where the departmental health offices presented data including vector notification, response coverage and absence of data every 6 months in the presence of members of other departments and the roundtable.[19] Although budget constraints may change styles of evaluation meetings, the National Programs and departmental health offices would benefit from such opportunities to present and discuss ongoing activities, and to continue improving interventions. At the regional level, consolidated data of each country became more understandable and comparable at the annual IPCA meetings through a standardized presentation format. Spatial projection of surveillance data at the regional level, if carried out annually, may also encourage political commitment.

The experience accumulated over the last decades—illustrated by the examples given earlier—seems to suggest that control of Chagas disease vectors is feasible, and results in strikingly reduced rates of infection incidence and prevalence. The end point for elimination of Chagas disease as a public health problem can be then described when all existing domestic infestations of Triatominae have been eliminated, and local health authorities are structured and equipped to diagnose and treat occasional new infections, and to eliminate—perhaps through contracts with local pest control operators—any incipient domestic vector infestation. Epidemiologically, the situation might then resemble that of Lyme disease in Europe—the vector ticks (*Ixodes ricinus*) are present in gardens (which may be said to comprise both peridomestic and sylvatic habitats), and there is a risk of *Borrelia* transmission; however, the ticks do not enter houses (and if they did, would be rapidly dealt with), and if a new infection occurs, it is relatively simple to diagnose and can be treated.

Although Chagas disease will not be eliminated in the sense of ceasing to exist as a human disease, we believe that it could be eliminated as a serious public health problem—when all existing domestic vector populations have been eliminated, and all aspects of current control programs are adequately incorporated into routine local health programs. The products, equipment, and experience are available for this, and strategies have been developed both for the initial campaigns and their consolidation through active vigilance, and for subsequent integration of the surveillance activities into routine public health activities.[6] But all comes to nought without political commitment and leadership, which in turn liberates the required resources. In a few countries, there is still no coherent national program; in others the national program is in disarray, with spraymen and vehicles idle as they lack the minimum resources to mobilize. Perhaps the initial successes of the multinational initiatives were too widely hailed, but relieving some 60 million people from the molestation of Triatominae and risk of disease (as some have claimed) still leaves some 40 million with little protection—which is both inappropriate and unethical, given the demonstrated feasibility of the large-scale control interventions. Paradoxically perhaps, a renewed urgency to complete the control interventions may come from the previously nonendemic countries now receiving migrants from Latin America—some of whom require treatment for their chronic Chagas infection, and some of whom pose a new risk for onward transmission by blood transfusion or organ transplant (cf. Ref. [22]). It is to be hoped that the domestic Latin American vectors can be eliminated before they too begin to arrive in Europe and elsewhere.[63]

## Acknowledgments

This work has benefited from international collaboration through the ECLAT network. The text represents an edited update of the chapter previously published as Gorla et al. (2010) (Gorla DE, Ponce C, Dujardin JP, Schofield CJ. Control strategies against Triatominae. In: Telleria J, Tibayrenc M, editors. *American Trypanosomiasis Chagas Disease: one hundred years of research.* Elsevier; 2010. p. 234—45). David E. Gorla is a researcher of the Consejo Nacional de Investigaciones Científicas y Técnicas of Argentina (CONICET).

## References

1. Schofield CJ. *Triatominae: biology & control.* West Sussex: Eurocommunica Publications; 1994, 80 p.
2. Walsh JA. Estimating the burden of illness in the tropics. In: Warren KS, Mahmoud AAF, editors. *Tropical and geographical medicine.* USA: McGraw-Hill; 1984. p. 1073—85.
3. Jannin J, Salvatella R. *Estimación Cuantitativa de la Enfermedad de Chagas en las Americas.* Washington, DC: Organización Panamericana de la Salud; 2006. OPS/HDM/CD/425-06, 27 p.
4. Schofield CJ, Kabayo JP. Trypanosomiasis vector control in Africa and Latin America. *Parasit Vectors* 2008;**1**:24 http://www.parasitesandvectors.com/content/pdf/1756-3305-1-24.pdf [accessed March 2016].

5. Schmunis GA, Cruz JR. Safety of the blood supply in Latin America. *Clin Microbiol Rev* 2005;**18**:12−29.
6. Schofield CJ, Jannin J, Salvatella R. The future of Chagas disease control. *Trends Parasitol* 2006;**21** 583−8.
7. Hashimoto K, Cordon-Rosales C, Trampe R, Kawabata M. Impact of single and multiple residual sprayings of pyrethroid insecticides against *Triatoma dimidiata* (Reduviidae; Triatominae), the principal vector of Chagas disease in Jutiapa, Guatemala. *Am J Trop Med Hyg* 2006;**75**:226−30.
8. Gürtler RE, Ceballos LA, Stariolo R, Kitron U, Reithinger R. Effects of topical application of fipronil spot-on on dogs against Chagas disease vector *Triatoma infestans*. *Trans R Soc Trop Med Hyg* 2009;**103**:298−304.
9. Porcasi X, Catalá SS, Hrellac H, Scavuzzo MC, Gorla DE. Infestation of rural houses by *Triatoma infestans* (Hemipera: Reduviidae) in the southern area of the Gran Chaco in Argentina. *J Med Entomol* 2006;**43**(5):1060−7.
10. Bustamante Gomez M., Gonçalves Diotaiuti L., Gorla D.E. Distribution of pyrethroid resistance in *Triatoma infestans* populations. *PLoS NTD* 10(3). e0004561, 1−15.
11. Guillén G, Diaz R, Jemio A, Alfred Cassab J, Teixeira Pinto C, Schofield CJ. Chagas disease vector control in Tupiza, southern Bolivia. *Mem Inst Oswaldo Cruz* 1997;**92**:1−8.
12. Sanmartino M, Crocco L. Conocimientos sobre la enfermedad de Chagas y factores de riesgo en comunidades epidemiológicamente diferentes de Argentina. *Rev Panam Salud Publ/Pan Am J Pub Health* 2000;**7**:173−8.
13 Wanderley DMV. *Perspectivas de Controle da Doença de Chagas no Estado de Sao Paulo. Thesis*. Brazil: Universidade de Sao Paulo; 1994, 161 p.
14. Schofield CJ, Dias JCP. The Southern Cone Initiative against Chagas disease. *Adv Parasitol* 1999;**42**:1−27.
15. Dujardin JP, Muñoz M, Chavez T, Ponce C, Moreno J, Schofield CJ. The origin of *Rhodnius prolixus* in Central America. *Med Vet Entomol* 1998;**12**:113−15.
16. Zeledón RA. Some historical facts and recent issues related to the presence of *Rhodnius prolixus* (Stal, 1859) (Hemiptera, Reduviidae) in Central America. *Entomol Vectores* 2004;**11**:233−46.
17. Abad-Franch F, Paucar A, Carpio C, Cuba CA, Aguilar HM, Miles MA. Biogeography of Triatominae (Hemiptera: Reduviidae) in Ecuador: implications for the design of control strategies. *Mem Inst Oswaldo Cruz* 2001;**96**:611−20.
18. Hashimoto K, Schofield JC. Review: Elimination of *Rhodnius prolixus* in Central America. *Parasit Vectors* 2012;**5**:45.
19. JICA, 2014. Best practices from the Chagas disease control in Guatemala, El Salvador, Honduras and Nicaragua 2000−2014. 285 pp. Edited by K. Hashimoto. s, Honduras [Original in Spanish, Summary in English].
20. Gorla DE. Variables ambientales registradas por sensores remotos como indicadores de la distribución geográfica de *Triatoma infestans*. *Ecol Aust* 2002;**12**:117−27.
21. Dias JCP, Silveira AC, Schofield CJ. The impact of Chagas disease control in Latin America. *Mem Inst Oswaldo Cruz* 2002;**97**:603−12.
22. Schmunis GA. Epidemiology of Chagas disease in non-endemic countries: the role of international migration. *Mem Inst Oswaldo Cruz* 2007;**102**(Suppl. 1):75−85.
23. Basombrio MA, Schofield CJ, Rojas CL, Del Rey EC. A cost−benefit analysis of Chagas disease control in northwest Argentina. *Trans R Soc Trop Med Hyg* 1998;**92**:137−43.

24. Akhavan D. *Análise de Custo-Efetividade do Programa de Controle da Doença de Chagas no Brazil*. Brazilia: Organização PanAmericana da Saude; 2000, 271 p.

25. Bustamante JM, Rivarola HW, Fernandez AR, Enders JE, Fretes R, Palma JA, et al. *Trypanosoma cruzi* reinfections in mice determine the severity of cardiac damage. *Int J Parasitol* 2002;**32**:889−96.

26. Bustamante JM, Novarese M, Rivarola HW, Lo Presti MS, Fernández AR, Enders JE, et al. Reinfections and *Trypanosoma cruzi* strains can determine the prognosis of the chronic chagasic cardiopathy in mice. *Parasitol Res* 2007;**100**:1407−10.

27. Proceedings of the ECLAT-AMCHA International Workshop on Chagas disease surveillance in the Amazon Region, Palmari, BrazilIn: Guhl F, Schofield CJ, editors. Bogota: Universidad de Los Andes; 2004, 174 p.

28. Coura JR, Junqueira AC, Fernandes O, Valente SA, Miles MA. Emerging Chagas disease in Amazonian Brazil. *Trends Parasitol* 2002;**18**:171−6.

29. Moreno M, Hoyos L, Cabido M, Catalá SS, Gorla DE. Exploring the association between *Trypanosoma cruzi* infection in rural communities and environmental changes in the southern Gran Chaco. *Mem Inst Oswaldo Cruz* 2012;**107**(2):231−7.

30. Cecere MC, Vazquez-Prokopec GM, Ceballos LA, Gurevitz JM, Zarate JE, Zaidenberg M, et al. Comparative trial of effectiveness of pyrethroid insecticides against peridomestic populations of *Triatoma infestans* in northwestern Argentina. *J Med Entomol* 2006;**43**:902−9.

31. Dias JCP, Jemio A. Sobre uma pintura inseticida para o controle de *Triatoma infestans*, na Bolívia. *Rev Soc Braz Med Trop* 2008;**41**:79−81.

32. Amelotti I, Catalá SS, Gorla DE. Experimental evaluation of insecticidal paints against *Triatoma infestans* (Hemiptera: Reduviidae), under natural climatic conditions. *Parasit Vectors* 2009;**2**:30. Available from: http://dx.doi.org/10.1186/1756-3305-2-30.

33. Gorla DE, Vargas R, Catalá SS. Control of rural house infestation by *Triatoma infestans* in the Bolivian chaco using a microencapsulated insecticide formulation. *Parasit Vectors* 2015;**8**(1):255.

34. Gorla DE, Porcasi X, Hrellac H, Catalá SS. Spatial stratification of house infestation by *Triatoma infestans* in La Rioja (Argentina). *Am J Trop Med Hyg* 2009;405−9, 80-3.

35. Gorla DE, Abrahan L, Hernández ML, Porcasi X, Hrellac HA, Carrizo H, et al. New structures for goat corrals as an environmental management tool for the control of peridomestic populations of *Triatoma infestans* in the Gran Chaco of Argentina. *Mem Inst Oswaldo Cruz* 2013;**108**(3):352−8.

36. Amelotti I, Catalá SS, Gorla DE. Response of *Triatoma infestans* to pour-on cypermethrin applied to chickens under laboratory conditions. *Mem Inst Oswaldo Cruz* 2009;**104**:481−5.

37. Amelotti I, Catalá SS, Gorla DE. The effects of Cypermethrin *Pour-on* and piperonyl butoxide on *Triatoma infestans* under laboratory conditions. *J Med Entomol* 2010;**47**:1135−40.

38. Amelotti I, Catalá SS, Gorla DE. Effects of fipronil on dogs over *Triatoma infestans*, the main vector of *Trypanosoma cruzi*, causative agent of Chagas disease. *Parasitol Res* 2012;**111**:1457−62.

39. Amelotti I, Catalá SS, Gorla DE. Mortality and blood intake in *Triatoma infestans* fed on goats treated with *pour-on* formulation of cypermethrin. *Mem Inst Oswaldo Cruz* 2012;**107**(8):1011−15.

40. Amelotti I, Catalá SS, Gorla DE. Control of experimental *Triatoma infestans* populations: effect of pour-on cypermethrin applied to chickens under natural conditions in the Argentinean Chaco region. *Med Vet Entomol* 2014;**28**(2):210−16.

41. Reithinger R, Ceballos L, Stariolo R, Davies CR, Gürtler RE. Chagas disease control: deltamethrin-treated collars reduce *Triatoma infestans* feeding success on dogs. *Trans R Soc Trop Med Hyg* 2005;**99**:502−8.

42. Reithinger R, Ceballos L, Stariolo R, Davies CR, Gürtler RE. Extinction of experimental *Triatoma infestans* populations following continuous exposure to dogs wearing deltamethrin-treated collars. *Am J Trop Med Hyg* 2006;**74**:766−71.

43. Gürtler RE, Kitron U, Cecere MC, Segura EL, Cohen JE. Sustainable vector control and management of Chagas disease in the Gran Chaco, Argentina. *Proc Natl. Acad Sci* 2007;**104**:16194−9.

44. Schachter-Broide J, Gürtler RE, Kitron U, Dujardin JP. Temporal variations of wing size and shape of *Triatoma infestans* (Hemiptera: Reduviidae) populations from northwestern Argentina using geometric morphometry. *J Med Entomol* 2009;**46**:994−1000.

45. Hernandez ML, Abrahan LB, Dujardin JP, Gorla DE, Catalá SS. Phenotypic variability and population structure in peridomestic *Triatoma infestans* (Hemiptera, Reduviidae): influence of macro and micro habitat. *Vector Borne Zoonot Dis* 2010;**11**(5):503−13.

46. Zerpa M, Catalá SS. Evaluación del riesgo de transmisión de *Trypanosoma cruzi* en peridomicilios del Departamento Castro Barros (La Rioja). *UNLaR Ciencia* 2001;**2**:9−13.

47. Porcasi X, Hrellac H, Catalá S, Moreno M, Abrahan L, Hernandez L, et al. Infestation of rural houses by *Triatoma infestans* in the region of Los Llanos (La Rioja, Argentina). *Mem Inst Oswaldo Cruz* 2007;**102**(1):63−8.

48. Yoshioka K, Tercero D, Pérez B, Lugo E. *Rhodnius prolixus* en Nicaragua: distribución geográfica, control y vigilancia entre 1998 y 2009. *Rev Panam Salud Publ* 2011;**30** (5):439−44.

49. Hashimoto K, Yoshioka K. Review: surveillance of Chagas disease. *Adv Parasitol* 2012;**79**:375−428.

50. Hashimoto K, Zúniga C, Nakamura J, Hanada K. Integrating an infectious disease programme into the primary health care service: a retrospective analysis of Chagas disease community-based surveillance in Honduras. *BMC Health Services Res* 2015;**15**:116.

51. Hashimoto K, Zúniga C, Romero E, Morales Z, Maguire JH. Determinants of health service responsiveness in community-based vector surveillance for Chagas disease in Guatemala, El Salvador, and Honduras. *PLoS NTD* 2015;**9**(8):e0003974.

52. Yoshioka K. Impact of a community-based bug-hunting campaign on Chagas disease control: a case study in the department of Jalapa, Guatemala. *Mem Inst Oswaldo Cruz* 2013;**108**(2):205−11.

53. Segura EL. El control de la enfermedad de Chagas en la República Argentina. In: Silveira AC, editor. *El Control de la Enfermedad de Chagas en los Países del Cono Sur de América. Historia de una iniciativa internacional 1991/2001*. Uberaba: Faculdade de Medicina do Triangulo Mineiro; 2002. p. 45−108.

54. Picollo MI, Vassena C, Santo Orihuela P, Barrios S, Zaidemberg M, Zerba EN. High resistance to pyrethroid insecticides associated with ineffective field treatments in *Triatoma infestans* (Hemiptera: Reduviidae) from northern Argentina. *J Med Entomol* 2005;**42**:367−642.

55. Santo Orihuela PL, Vassena CV, Zerba EN, Picollo MI. Relative contribution of monooxygenase and esterase to pyrethroid resistance in *Triatoma infestans* (Hemiptera: Reduviidae) from Argentina and Bolivia. *J Med Entomol* 2008;**45**:298−306.

56. Mougabure-Cueto G, Picollo MI. Insecticide resistance in vector Chagas disease: evolution, mechanisms and management. *Acta Trop.* 2015;**149**:70−85.

57. Panzera F, Ferreiro MJ, Pita S, Calleros L, Pérez R, Basmadjián Y, et al. Evolutionary and dispersal history of *Triatoma infestans*, main vector of Chagas disease, by chromosomal markers. *Infect Genet Evol.* 2014;**27**:105−13.
58. Gürtler RE, Canale DM, Spillmann C, Stariolo R, Salomón OD, Blanco S, et al. Effectiveness of residual spraying of peridomestic ecotopes with deltamethrin and permethrin on *Triatoma infestans* in rural western Argentina: a district-wide randomized trial. *Bull. WHO* 2004;**82**:196−205.
59. Gemio A, Romero N, Hernandez ML, Alberto X, Franz X, Catalá SS, et al. Residual effect of microencapsulated organophosphate insecticides on the mortality of *Triatoma infestans* in the bolivian Chaco region. *Mem Inst Oswaldo Cruz* 2010;**105**:752−6.
60. Buckee CO, Wesolowski A, Eagle NN, Hansen E, Snow RW. Mobile phones and malaria: modeling human and parasite travel. *Travel Med Infect Dis* 2013;**11**:15−22.
61. Cravero C, Brunazzo F, Willington A, Burrone S, Fernández AR. Sistema de vigilancia en Chagas facilitado por tecnologías de información y comunicación. *Rev Salud Públ (XV)* 2011;**2**:56−69.
62. Monroy C, Bustamante DM, Pineda S, Rodas A, Castro X, Ayala V, et al. House improvements and community participation in the control of *Triatoma dimidiata* reinfestation in Jutiapa, Guatemala. *Cad Saúd Públ* 2009;**25**(Suppl. 1):S168−78.
63. Schofield CJ, Grijalva MJ, Diotaiuti L. Distribución de los vectores de la Enfermedad de Chagas en países "no endémicos": la posibilidad de transmisión vectorial fuera de América Latina. *Enfermed Emerg* 2009;**11**(Suppl. 1):20−7.

# Ecological aspects of *Trypanosoma cruzi*: wild hosts and reservoirs

*A.M. Jansen, S.C.C. Xavier and A.L.R. Roque*
Oswaldo Cruz Institute, Rio de Janeiro, Brazil

## Chapter Outline

## Introduction

It has been classically admitted that *Trypanosoma cruzi* originated around 80 million years ago (mya) in the Southern Supercontinent comprised of South America, Antarctica, and Australia, which remained connected after its separation from Africa. In this scenario, marsupials and xenarthrans, which represented the extant autochthonous mammalian fauna, were accepted as *T. cruzi*'s very first hosts.[1−3] This hypothesis resulted in a conflict represented by the absence of hematophagous insects at that time. Thus, authors proposed a parasite transmission independent of a vector that occurred most probably by (1) predation of infected mammals; (2) material from anal glands of infected opossums (by ingestion and/or contact with mucosal and injured skin), since these glands can maintain the extracellular multiplication cycle of *T. cruzi* and eliminate infective metacyclic forms[4,5]; and/or (3) congenital route. In this scenery, the enzooty in South America remained unchanged up to the arrival of caviomorph rodents and primates from Africa (35 mya), which represented the first of several mammal migration waves that occurred up to 5 mya and resulted in the subsequent diversification of the fauna observed nowadays in the whole continent.[6] Carnivores and others including man, the last *T. cruzi* mammal host, were then included in the parasite transmission as soon as they arrived the continent in subsequent waves of migration cycles. More recently, Hamilton et al.[7] proposed a fascinating and quite different evolutionary scenario for the origin of *T. cruzi*. These authors proposed that this

*American Trypanosomiasis Chagas Disease.* DOI: http://dx.doi.org/10.1016/B978-0-12-801029-7.00011-3

trypanosomatid has emerged much more recently, within the clade of *Schizotrypanum* trypanosomes of bats when these flying mammals arrived in Americas. From the bats, the parasite has successfully dispersed and adapted to its hundreds species of mammals that act as its hosts in all forest strata. Authors elegantly coined their hypothesis as the "bat seeding hypothesis." Although there is no archeological record of Old World bats in the Americas to support this hypothesis, molecular analysis that followed has made the "bat seeding hypothesis" even more robust.[8–10] As a consequence, the origin of *T. cruzi* is much more recent than proposed by the classical hypothesis. Moreover, the exact geographical origin and migration pattern of Chiroptera lineages are far from being known, and the finding and analysis of archaeological material of this taxon will be extremely enlightening.

Regardless of its primary host, the diversity of mammalian host species that have been introduced subsequently in the *T. cruzi* transmission cycle provided different selective pressures that were certainly one of the factors that drove the emergence of the huge variety of parasite subpopulations observed today. These subpopulations that display distinct biological and molecular patterns still constitute an ecological challenge. These differences are discussed in a specific chapter in this book (see chapter: Classification and Phylogeny of *Trypanosoma cruzi*).

The acquisition of a hematophagic habit by the triatomine vectors is relatively recent.[11] Although the origin of their Reduviidae ancestors date from about 230 mya, the vast majority of its subfamilies consist of predatory insects and so far, only one supposedly hematophagic fossil species was found.[12] Thus, the digenetic cycle observed today, which involves Triatominae vectors and mammalian hosts, seems to have started only after the acquisition of hematophagic habits by triatomines, which is supposed to have occurred approximately 5 mya, and after the adaptation of the parasite to the gut of these vectors.[5,13] Before that, the transmission of *T. cruzi* occurred through other routes, mainly the oral route.

Since the majority of studies on wild *T. cruzi* reservoirs were performed before knowledge leading to the current separation of the parasites subpopulations based on DTUs (discrete typing units),[14] besides the new terminology,[15] here we also considered the previous consensus proposed by experts in 1999 that recognized two major genotypes, TCI and TCII, and a group of subpopulations of parasites that do not fall within these two genotypes and continued to be known as Z3 (zymodeme 3).[16] This is the context in which we present some of the mammalian species that during our 20-year-long study in Brazilian biomes demonstrated to act as the main reservoirs of *T. cruzi*.

# Order Didelphimorphia

Representative of American autochthonous fauna, the order Didelphimorphia displays its greatest diversity of species in the Australian continent, while only one family is recognized in the Americas, the Didelphidae, regarded as one of the oldest and most important reservoirs of *T. cruzi*.[17,18] The genus *Didelphis* (Fig. 11.1) is

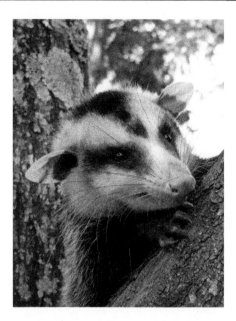

**Figure 11.1** Opossum *Didelphis albiventris* from São Borja, Brazil.
*Photo*: Ana Maria Jansen.

the largest representative of the family Didelphidae besides being the most spread genus on the continent, occurring from southeastern Canada to southern Argentina. Our experience confirms that didelphids are indeed very important reservoirs of *T. cruzi* highlighting the genera *Didelphis* and *Philander*.[19] *Didelphis* spp. display a wide distribution that is mainly due to their remarkable adaptability to different ecological niches, including environments with a high degree of human action.[20] *Didephis* spp. may be considered as biomarkers of degraded environments and their association with humans seems to be very old. On the one hand *Didelphis* spp. benefits from human food remains, whilst on the other hand, humans have in *Didelphis* a food source.[21] Besides, these animals also use human dwellings as they can colonize ceilings of houses and other shelters in domestic and peridomestic areas. *Didelphis* spp. are nomadic, solitary (especially males), excellent climbers, and their main refuges are holes and the foliage of trees. As observed for all other mammalian species their importance as a reservoir varies in time and space, as observed in the infection rates of *Didelphis aurita*, which range between 11% and 90% among animals collected in different localities in the state of Rio de Janeiro, Brazil.[22] Besides vector transmission, its omnivorous habits favor the oral acquisition of infection by predation of infected bugs or small mammals.

When infected by *T. cruzi*, these marsupials exhibit some characteristics that make them unique when compared to other hosts of the parasite. Thus, in experimentally infected *Didelphis* spp., *T. cruzi* DTU TcI (but not TcII) may reach the scent gland's lumen where the bloodstream trypomastigotes differentiate into epimastigotes which multiply by binary division, then differentiate into metacyclic trypomastigotes that are the infective forms, which are released with the secretion of this gland.[4] This stage simulates the multiplication cycle of the parasite observed in the digestive tract of the bugs and occurs simultaneously with the intracellular multiplicative cycle that is driven by amastigote forms in various tissues of the marsupial. The transmission competence of these glands and, therefore, their epidemiological importance, remains unknown, regardless of the elevated rate of metacyclogenesis (50%) that points to this way being an efficient route of spreading the parasite. Notwithstanding, monogenetic trypanosomatids (*Leptomonas*, *Crithidia*, and *Herpetomonas*) may also efficiently colonize the scent glands of *Didelphis aurita* under experimental conditions when the axenic culture forms are directly inoculated into these glands.[23] Besides *Didelphis* spp., the *Trypanosoma cruzi* multiplication cycle in scent glands has also been demonstrated in experimentally infected *Lutreolina crassicaudata*.[24] Another remarkable point is that the metacyclogenesis occurs without depending on the adhesion of the parasite to any cellular debris or host epithelium as is the case in the intestinal lumen of triatomine and in axenic medium.

Experimental studies showed the absence of neonatal transmission of the parasite in *D. aurita* and that they are able to maintain stable infections by subpopulations of the DTU TcI and control to subpatent levels or even elimination of subpopulations of DTU TcII. However, these studies were performed with a small number of reference strains that are not representative of the heterogeneity observed among parasite subpopulations of the DTU TcII.[25] In fact, although these animals are most commonly associated to DTU TcI, the DTUs TcII, TcIII, and TcIV have also been isolated.[19,26] Although often associated with the arboreal strata, *Didelphis* spp. move among all ecological strata and may act as a bridge of transmission cycles, since they can become infected at soil level and be a source of infection for another bug in the crown of a tree (and vice versa).[27,28] Despite the numerous studies on the interaction of Didelphidae with *T. cruzi*, there is still much to clarify as nothing is known about the interaction of Didelphidae with the DTUs TcIII to TcVI. In our experience *Didelphis* spp. demonstrated up to 41% of positive hemocultures.[19]

In nature, *Philander frenatus* and Philander opossum may also play an important role in the transmission of the parasite, since they are found displaying a prevalence of positive hemocultures that can reach 80%. Distinct from *D. aurita*, the experimental infection of *P. frenatus* resulted in high parasitemia and elevated antibody titers when infected by both TcI and TcII DTUs of the parasite. Once more, we have to consider that the authors conducted their study with the reference Y strain, which is in fact a DTU TcII, but there is no study on experimental infection with other TcII strains.[29] The patterns of experimental infections of *D. aurita* and *P. frenatus* showed that these species exert different selective pressures for distinct *T. cruzi* subpopulations, and thus probably play different roles in the transmission of the parasite in nature. Both *Philander* spp. species are mainly associated to gallery forests and do not show the synanthropic behavior observed in *Didelphis* spp., which may indicate a more limited importance as bridge host between the natural and domestic environment.

Apparently *Didelphis* spp. and *Philander* spp. are competent bioaccumulators of *T. cruzi* DTUs in the wild environment. There are no reports of Tcbat or hybrid DTUs (TcV and TcVI) infecting these two taxa but mixed or single infections with all other DTUs have been observed.[19] TcI/TcII (which in general is the most common mixed infection in nature) was observed in *Didelphis* spp. from Santa Catarina State, Brazil. These marsupial species may also maintain mixed infection by respectively, TcI and TcIII, and TcII and TcV/TcVI. It is worth mentioning that *Didelphis* spp. was the only genus in which we found this combination of mixed DTU infection. This only confirms their role as bioaccumulators of *T. cruzi* DTUs.

*Monodelphis domestica* is a terrestrial marsupial species commonly found infected with *Trypanosoma cruzi* and that was identified as the main reservoir of the parasite in an outbreak of orally transmitted Chagas disease in northeastern Brazil.[30] Mixed infection by DTU TcI and TcIV was detected in this species from the Amazon region, exactly the same DTUs that infect humans in that area. *M. domestica* acting as the main reservoir of *T. cruzi* (in an area where several *D. albiventris* were also collected) was a unique and quite unexpected finding and confirms the temporal and space differences concerning reservoir species. In fact, in other areas this small marsupial species (around 80 g weight) did not display significant biomass. *Caluromys lanatus*, *Marmosops parvidens*, *Lutreolina crassicaudata*, *Marmosa* sp., *Marmosops* sp., *Metachirus nudicaudatus*, *Micoreus demerarae*, *Marmosa paraguayanus*, *Monodelphis brevicaudata*, *Thylamys* sp. are other species of Didelphid marsupials already found naturally infected by *T. cruzi*.[19,31−33]

Tissue lesions of experimental *T. cruzi* infections in *D. aurita* are characterized by mild inflammatory infiltrates mainly composed by lymphocytes and macrophages; more severe infiltrates by the same cell type have been described in naturally infected *D. aurita*. Moreover, in both cases, these lesions were demonstrated to be significantly milder in comparison to Swiss mice. In fact, mortality was observed only in 24-day-old still pouch-dependent experimentally infected opossums.[34]

Opossums are fascinating mammals due to their unique reproduction strategy: a new born opossum is in fact still a fetus and still unable to control body temperature; it does not produce immunoglobulins, does not reject allografts; its eyes and ears are sealed; hind limbs are still not differentiated and its mouth displays a small aperture, sufficient only to allow the attachment to the nipple, that after attachment almost reaches the stomach of this newborn. Struggle for life starts at the very beginning of the opossum's life, since there are generally more newborn than available nipples. Moreover, newborns must literally crawl with the aid of their forelimbs on their mothers belly toward the maternal pouch and attach to a nipple where it will remain until around 45 days of age without detaching. Total independence from the mother opossum will be reached by 100−120 days after birth. Neonatal or vertical transmission was not observed in experimentally infected opossums, even during the acute phase.

# Superorder Xenarthra

Xenarthrans were previously classified in an order termed Edentata, found to be polyphyletic and that also included ant-eating Pangolins. With the reclassification of the latter to the Pholidota order, the orders Cingulata (armadillos) and Pilosa (anteaters and sloths) were classified together in the superorder Xenarthra (odd joints). Xenarthra display fascinating biological peculiarities such as fused pelvic bones, spine reinforcing bones, and a peculiar blood vessel structure that allows energy sparing by an extremely low metabolic rate. These adaptations did not prevent a massive extinction of a huge number of representatives of this taxon so that the current extant genera represent only a minor part of those found in the Tertiary. In modern times the specific niche destruction due to human action certainly contributed, but the overall causes of this massive extinction are still under debate.

Armadillos, sloths, and anteaters, currently the main representatives of this superorder, have a long coevolutionary history with trypanosomatids. So, besides the bizarre genus *Endotrypanum*, sloths may harbor several *Leishmania* and *Trypanosoma* species.[35] These mammals represent, beside marsupials, ancient hosts of *T. cruzi*. The first description of a wild reservoir of this parasite was made by Carlos Chagas, in 1912, when he found tripomastigote forms similar to *Trypanosoma cruzi* in the wild nine-banded armadillo *Dasypus novemcinctus*, which he classified as a "depository of the agent of Brazilian trypanosomiasis in the outside world."[36] This definition of Carlos Chagas shows clearly what was understood at that time as a reservoir. The term "depository" means preservation and not a living dynamic system that exerts and undergoes selective pressures all the time. In its underground refuges, armadillos are usually associated with triatomines from the *Panstrongylus* genus and some studies suggest an association between this mammalian host and the parasite DTU TcII−TcVI (currently nomenclature).[18] Nevertheless, these animals have also been found infected with DTU TcI, showing its putative importance in the maintenance of distinct transmission cycles in nature.[33,37]

Armadillos are widely distributed and found infected by *T. cruzi* in a prevalence of infection that ranges from 4% to 50%, from the southern United States to Uruguay. In Louisiana, USA, infection by *T. cruzi* was detected in 26% of 80 armadillos.[38] In the same state, but in another region, only 3.9% of 415 *D. novemcinctus* were infected.[39] In a retrospective study conducted in French Guiana, *Dasypus novemcinctus* were identified as an important reservoir of *Trypanosoma cruzi*, following *Didelphis marsupialis*.[40] Other species found to be infected by *Trypanosoma cruzi* are *Cabassous unicinctus*, *Chaetophractus vellorosous*, *Tolypeutes matacus*, and *Euphractus sexcinctus*[41] (Fig. 11.2). It is worth mentioning that, in rural areas, *E. sexcinctus* regularly invade chicken facilities to prey on eggs and/or chicks. This behavior favors the nearness of this armadillo species with peridomestic areas, where it can be a source of infection for triatomine bugs that nest there.

Concerning the arboreal xenarthrans, sloths are usually associated to triatomines from the genera *Belminus*, *Panstrongylus*, and *Rhodnius*[42] and some sloth species, such as the three-toed sloth (*Bradypus torquatus*) have been found naturally infected.[22] Two different species of anteaters, the lesser anteater (*Tamandua tetradactyla*) and the silky anteater (*Cyclops didactylus*) have also been considered natural hosts of *Trypanosoma cruzi*.[18,43] It is worth mentioning that one *Tamandua tetradactyla* found infected by *Trypanosoma cruzi* in Pará State, Brazil, showed a mixed infection with two other trypanosomatids, *Trypanosoma rangeli* and *Leishmania infantum*.[44]

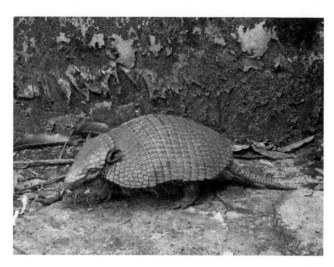

**Figure 11.2** Armadillo *Euphractus sexcinctus* from Axixá, Brazil.
*Photo*: Ana Maria Jansen.

The epidemiological importance of these mammalian species is enhanced as sloths, anteaters, and armadillos are hunted and eaten in some areas of South America, such as the Amazon region. The careless handling of the carcass or the ingestion of undercooked meat from infected animals can be a source of *T. cruzi* infection for humans.

# Order Rodentia

Rodents represent perhaps the most diverse and widespread mammalian taxa. A common point of rodents is the continuously growing single incisor tooth pair that does not present enamel on its posterior face. The morphological diversity in the taxon is exemplified by the contrast between a tiny 5 g pigmy mouse and the huge capybara that may reach 70 kg in weight. Rodents may be found in desert areas, adapted to aquatic media, digging long and interconnected tunnels, as well as on forest canopies. In spite of being so diverse, there are several groups whose systematic position is still under debate and that may only be separated by karyotyping.[45] Reproduction strategies are also quite distinct, thus, reproduction seasonality, gestation time, and number of offspring may differ significantly among the genera of this order.[46]

Rodents are not autochthonous in the Americas and the first animals (Hystricognathi-caviomorphs) arrived along with the first primates, originating from Africa about 45 mya. The second great migration wave of rodents to the Americas (Sciurognathi-cricetids) is much more recent and appears to be related to the diversification of murids and cricets in Africa with arrival by a migration route that included an initial establishment in North America. Since their arrival, rodents have adapted well and diversified into a large number of species in the Americas. They colonized

various types of habitats, from rainforests to deserts, high altitude plateaus to flood-
plains, wild to urban environments; moreover, they colonize the diverse vegetation
strata, being classified from fossorial up to arboreal and semiaquatic rodents.[46]

In nature, rodents are ubiquitous mammalian species and their diverse microhabitats are often shared with bugs from genus *Triatoma* (associated with rocky terrestrial refuges) and *Panstrongylus* (associated with holes in the ground).[42] Among
mammalian species, rodents are the main targets of predation and this is an important feature since it enables the transmission of *T. cruzi* by the oral route. Their
epidemiological importance is even more evident when we consider that many
rodent species, although predominantly wild, can frequent human dwellings and
participate in the *T. cruzi* transmission cycle in peridomestic areas.[30,47]

Despite being a widespread mammalian order, the natural infection of wild rodents
by *T. cruzi* is poorly reported, which may be the result of the limited methodology
employed for animal sampling in several studies, frequently restricted to peridomestic
areas. This is confirmed by the fact that the most common rodent species found
infected by *T. cruzi* is the rat *Rattus rattus*, a synanthropic species highly abundant
in most urbanized cities in South America, but rare inside rainforests. Although
abundant in experimental studies, natural *Trypanosoma cruzi* infection in the mouse
*Mus musculus* is little reported. Other rodent species already found naturally infected
by *Trypanosoma cruzi* are: *Agouti paca, Akodon montensis, Akodon toba, Baiomys
musculus, Calomys expulsus, Calomys callosus, Cavia* sp., *Cerradomys subflavus,
Clyomys laticeps, Dasyprocta* sp., *Echymis chrysurus, E. dasytrix, Galea
spixii, Graomys chacoensis, Holochilus brasiliensis, Hylaeamys* sp., *Kerodon rupes-
tris, Necromys lasiurus, Nectomys squamipes, Neotoma floridana, Neotoma
mexicana, Neotoma micropus, Octodon degus, Octodontomys* sp., *Oecomys mamorae,
Oligoryzomys chacoensis, Oligoryzomys nigripes, Oligoryzomys stramineus,
Oryzomys capito, Oryzomys scotti, Peromyscus gossypinus, Peromyscus
levipes, Proechimys* spp., *Rhiphidomys macrurus, Sigmodon hispidus, Thrichomys*
spp., and *Tylomys mirae*.[18,19,30,32,48–53]

Another aspect that deserves to be highlighted is the overall low *T. cruzi* infection rates observed in the Rodentia order. These animals, that are highly susceptible
to experimental infection with *T. cruzi*, seem to play a secondary role as reservoirs.
This is especially striking in the Brazilian Cerrado biome, as expressed by their low
infection rates (5% of positive serological tests and 2% of positive hemocultures).[19]
Two hypotheses may explain these findings: (1) either the infected animals do not
resist the infection and die or (2) rodents are not exposed to infection in the studied
Cerrado regions. Finally, these findings are similar to what was observed in the
Pantanal biome[54] and support the hypothesis that, in fact, wild rodents only exceptionally play an important role as *T. cruzi* reservoirs. Overall, in the Atlantic Forest,
only 0.4% of the rodents displayed positive blood cultures.[19]

Apart from this, a wild rodent species whose participation in the transmission
cycles of *Trypanosoma cruzi* is more empirically proven are the caviomorphs from
*Thrichomys* spp. This genus comprises at least five sibling species distributed in the
Pantanal/Chaco (marshlands), Cerrado (savannah), and Caatinga (white shrub)
biomes.[55] *Thrichomys laurentius* (Fig. 11.3) was found displaying high infective

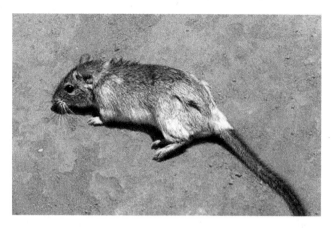

**Figure 11.3** Punare rodent *Thrichomys laurentius* from São Raimundo Nonato, Brazil. *Photo*: Ana Maria Jansen.

potential for *Trypanosoma cruzi* as demonstrated by 44% (positive hemocultures) in some localities surrounding the Serra da Capivara National Park in Brazil.[32] In the Caatinga (White Shrub), this caviomorph rodent species displayed the highest relative abundance and competence to keep DTUs TcI, TcII, TcIV, and TcV in simple or mixed infections with *T. rangeli*.[19,48,56] Caviomorph rodent species were also found infected in an area of orally transmitted Chagas disease in an outbreak in the Ceará state, Brazil.[30] *T. fosteri* and *T. apereoides* are other species from the same genus also found infected by *T. cruzi*.

Experimental studies have shown that *T. apereoides* are able to maintain stable infections by both DTUs TcI and TcII of the parasite.[57] Two other *Thrichomys* species (*T. laurentius* and *T. fosteri*) were also able to maintain a controlled experimental infection with *Trypanosoma cruzi*, displaying patent parasitemia, effective humoral immune response, and important tissue damage.[58] In the latter study, the differences observed in *Trypanosoma cruzi* infection patterns showed that *Thrichomys laurentius* was more resistant to infection than *Thrichomys fosteri*, as expressed by lower parasitemia and less tissue damage. The differences observed in these experimental infections may probably reflect the distinct competences of these two rodent species to act as *T. cruzi* reservoirs in their respective biomes.[32]

Taken together the results from the experimental infection, the wide distribution of *Thrichomys* spp. in nature and the prevalence of natural infection by *Trypanosoma cruzi*, these rodents can act as (1) maintenance hosts, due to the ability to maintain long-lasting subpatent parasitemias and (2) amplifier hosts, demonstrated by the long period of patent parasitemia in experimental conditions and positive hemocultures in natural infections.[48,57,58]

Finally, studies involving *T. cruzi* and caviomorphs showed that a long historic host–parasite relationship does not necessarily evolve into a harmonic interaction; but may evolve into one that favors the transmission of the parasite. In *Thrichomys* sp., experimentally infected rodents presented significant heart damage, which is certainly reflected in its ability to provide tissue oxygenation. This means that an infected rodent would have a diminished ability to avoid predators, predisposing them to transmit the parasite to other mammalian species.

## Order Primata

A marmoset *Callithrix penicillata* was the first host identified by Carlos Chagas when he discovered a new trypanosome species in Lassance (Minas Gerais state, Brazil), which he named *Trypanosoma minasense*. Later, investigating the local triatomines, Chagas found flagellates that he inferred to be the intermediate forms of the trypanosomes diagnosed in marmosets. To confirm this hypothesis, Chagas sent some infected bugs to be used to infect groups of *Callithrix jacchus* that were kept in captivity. Performed by Oswaldo Cruz, this resulted in the visualization of flagellates in the peripheral blood of marmosets displaying morphology quite distinct from *T. minansensis*: it was the discovery of *T. cruzi*.[59]

Since then, different species of Neotropical primates included in Cebidae (monkeys) and Callitrichidae (marmosets) families are commonly found naturally infected by *T. cruzi*.[19] Widespread in the Americas, these primates occupy different forest strata and have varied feeding habits, including species that feed on invertebrates and small mammals, which facilitate *T. cruzi* transmission by the oral route. Their nightly refuges in hollow trees are often shared with triatomine bugs, which allows (or propitiates) vectorial contaminative transmission of the parasite to these mammalian species.[42]

The infection prevalence in primates varies between 4% and 88% and can be quite elevated in tamarins.[60,61] Both the prevalence of infection and the transmissibility potential of the parasite by the host (attested by positive hemocultures) may vary according to gender, age, species, coinfection with other parasites and general health, ecological characteristics, and origin of the studied population. Even as an important point in parasitism phenomenon, the effects of concomitant parasitic infections on the host are attracting the attention. A positive association between the presence of trichostrongilid nematode infection and positive hemocultures, has already been described in lion tamarins *Leontophitecus rosalia* and *Leontophitecus chrysomelas* that are endangered callitrichidae species endemic to the Atlantic forest.[62]

In the Poço das Antas National Reserve (Rio de Janeiro, Brazil), the Golden lion tamarin (*Leontophitecus rosalia*) (Fig. 11.4) acts as an important *Trypanosoma cruzi* reservoir since it displays a high prevalence of seropositive animals and high rates of positive hemoculture (46%). Tamarins live in quite stable social groups and are extremely territorial. The members of the groups share tasks like carrying the newborns. The *T. cruzi* infection prevalence is not homogeneously distributed among the Tamarin social groups and, in fact, the prevalence of infection varies among the different social groups from the Poço das Antas National Reserve. The aggregated character of the *T. cruzi* infection among the tamarin groups is probably due to microenvironmental peculiarities, since these tamarins display no expressive

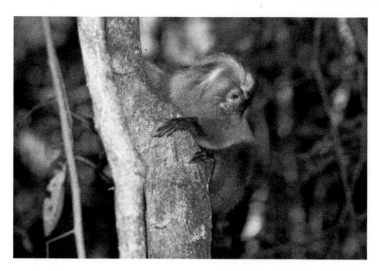

**Figure 11.4** Golden lion tamarin *Leonthopitecus rosalia* from Silva Jardim, Brazil. *Photo*: Rodrigo Mexas.

genetic heterogeneity.[63] This prevalence of infection was found to be quite distinct from other areas, adjacent to the reserve, where the same species *L. rosalia* presents low prevalence of *T. cruzi* infection, reinforcing the nidal characteristic of the parasite maintenance in nature. This tamarin population could be monitored annually for 10 years and has proved to be the more conspicuous focus of *T. cruzi* DTU TcII transmission and maintenance in this wild environment. Indeed *L. rosalia* demonstrated to be able to maintain long-lasting infections with significant rates of positive hemocultures by this DTU formerly associated to the domestic transmission cycle. An interesting aspect is that the authors observed 3-year variations in rates of blood cultures of the tamarin of the Biological reserve of Poço das Antas.[61]

High positive hemoculture prevalence was also observed in the sibling tamarin species *Leontopithecus chrisomellas* in a biological reserve located in Una, Bahia state in a Brazilian northeastern fragment of the Atlantic coastal rain forest. The absolute majority of the *T. cruzi* isolates derived from both tamarin species were characterized as DTU TcII. The DTU TcI was observed in other species of nonprimate mammals from the Poço das Antas and in a dozen tamarins of both biological reserves.[61]

The infection of primates is not primordially by the DTU TcII of the parasite, but many other primate species, besides *Leontophitecus* spp. have been found naturally infected with *T. cruzi* DTU TcII in different regions of Brazil, from the Atlantic to the Amazon region.[19] The DTUs TcIII/IV described as genotype Z3 of the parasite has also been found in primates, but this finding is still restricted to the Amazon region.[64]

An important feature that has to be taken in consideration is that several Neotropical primates are threatened species submitted to conservation programs, as is the case of the Golden lion tamarin. These programs often include exchange, translocation, and reintroduction of animals, without considering the prevalence and pattern of infection by parasites such as *T. cruzi*. Such programs can lead to an introduction of infected mammals in untouched areas and trigger the establishment of new transmission cycles in other areas. Also, the concentration of primate groups of different origin in the same preservation reserve will increase the probability of infection of the threatened species.

Experimental studies in Neotropical (*Cebus* sp., *Callithrix* sp., and *Saimiri* sp.) and African (*Macaca mulatta*) primates show that infection by *Trypanosoma cruzi* in these mammalian species presents some similarities with Chagas disease, such as a low frequency of cardiac abnormalities and the rare occurrence of mega-syndromes and systemic changes. Electrocardiographic alterations observed were the low voltage of T- and R-waves and high voltage of V3 wave, all of them in DII.[65]

# Order Carnivora

Carnivores are also a very heterogeneous group that includes meat eaters, as diverse as the grizzly bear, the skunks, weasels, coatis, and wild and domestic dogs and cats. Besides predating other vertebrates, carnivores complete their diet feeding also on plant, fruits, and insects, among others food items. In fact, many representatives of the carnivores are opportunistic feeders. Their common trait is the presence of five finger feet presenting claws and a typical denture comprising teeth adapted to tear. Highly persecuted due to their livestock predation potential and human atavistic fear, among other reasons, this has resulted in many of the big carnivore species being near to extinction. Wild carnivores such as the ocelot (*Leopardus pardalis*), the coati (*Nasua nasua*), the raccoon (*Procyon lotor*), the weasel (*Eira barbara*), and crab-eating fox (*Cerdocyon thous*) have been found naturally infected with *Trypanosoma cruzi*.[18,31,66]

Some of them, like the coati and the weasel, are found both on the ground and in the canopy of trees, acting as bridge hosts, favoring parasite spread among the different forest strata. Coatis, in particular, build their nests in treetops that can be 20 m from ground. Carnivores have important body mass and large life areas that are important traits that enhance acquisition and spreading of parasites, resulting in their potential competence as amplifier reservoirs. Large and medium sized carnivores are known to be top predators of their food chain that usually include smaller mammals that may be infected by *T. cruzi*.[66] Thus, although the contaminative vectorial transmission also occurs, the most common way of infection for these mammalian species, as for any other predator in nature, seems to be the oral route through ingestion of infected mammals or triatomine since several carnivore species are avid insect consumers.[66,67]

In the Brazilian Pantanal/Chaco region (marshland), the coati species *Nasua nasua* (Fig. 11.5) was demonstrated to be the main *Trypanosoma cruzi* reservoir.

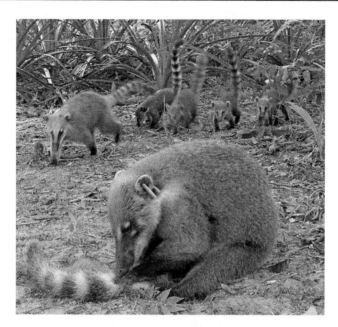

**Figure 11.5** Coatis *Nasua nasua* from Brazilian Pantanal.
*Photo*: Rita de Cassia Bianchi.

Actually, 86 of 235 examined animals (36.6%) displayed positive *T. cruzi* hemocultures.[19] Besides, coatis were demonstrated to be infected by and maintain DTUs TcI, TcII, and TcIII/TcIV in single or mixed infections.[19,68] The monitoring of recaptured mammals showed that *T. cruzi*-infected coatis can present high and long-lasting parasitemias by TcI and TcII. Due to their high biomass and high relative abundance among mammalian species, coatis certainly play a role in the amplification and dispersal of the main *T. cruzi* subpopulations in this region, demonstrating that predator−prey links may be excellent mechanisms for *T. cruzi* transmission and perpetuation in the wild.[66−68] In the Pantanal the presence of *Didelphis* spp., considered as the main reservoir host of *Trypanosoma cruzi* was only negligible. In fact in this area, coatis were acting as the main reservoir hosts. This finding reinforces the importance of not electing a priori any target species as a reservoir.

Domestic and wild felines are animals that are especially difficult to handle. Maybe that's why studies of *T. cruzi* infection of this taxon are less frequent and that their role in the transmission cycle of *T. cruzi* is still a matter of debate. Moreover, felines have a combination of ecological characteristics that favor them to get infected by *T. cruzi*: they are predatory animals, use large life areas, and have abilities to explore the arboreal and terrestrial strata of various habitats. We examined by hemocultures and serological methods free ranging *Leopardus pardalis* ($N = 33$), *Leopardus tigrinus* ($N = 2$), *Leopardus geoffroyi* ($N = 1$), *Felis yagouaroundi* ($N = 2$), *Puma concolor* ($N = 2$), and wild *Felis catus* ($N = 3$), from

Cerrado, Atlantic Forest, Pampa, and Pantanal biomes. From these, seven (16%) were positive and displayed serological titers that ranged from 1/40 to 1/160. Two *L. pardalis* with serological title 1/160, from the Cerrado, had positive blood cultures that were characterized as DTU TcI.[66] The felines participate in the *T. cruzi* transmission cycle, both near the houses and in the wild environment. Nevertheless, one of the points that still needs to be observed is the duration of the competence infective; i.e., the period of high parasitemia that is expressed by positive parasitological tests.

Species diet could be associated with *T. cruzi* infection rates, showing the importance of predator−prey links as an important mechanism for *T. cruzi* dispersion in the wild. Also, it became clear that the distinct Carnivore taxa play distinct roles in the ecology of *T. cruzi*. Musteloidea species demonstrated high infectivity competence since they consistently exhibit high parasitemias as expressed by positive hemocultures.[66] The DTU TcIII was isolated from a ferret (*Galictis vitatta*) in the Atlantic Forest of Rio de Janeiro, Brazil.[19] Moreover, the isolation of *Trypanosoma cruzi* Z3 (that includes TcIII and TcIV) was achieved from skunks (*Conepatus chinga*) from Argentina,[69] and gray foxes (*Urocyon cinereoargenteus*) in Central America and southern United States.[70]

One of the little known aspects concerning wild mammal and parasite interaction refers to the evaluation of their health status. Such clinical evaluation of an animal that was just captured and is at the peak of its stress is probably misleading. Besides, very probably, wild mammals are parasitized by several other species of parasites that interact and result in distinct outcomes, in addition to the physiological changes such as the case of the physiological immunosuppression during pregnancy and distinct susceptibility according to age and stress during the breeding season. Very little is known about the energetic costs for an animal that can result in a pattern of infection that could characterize it as an amplifier or maintenance host. Actually, a promising approach to better understand the outcome of parasite−host interactions in free living specimens is the evaluation of hematological parameters.[71]

# Order Chiroptera

Bats are the only flying mammalian species and besides birds, the only animals that perform seasonal migration, a trait that is suggested to have evolved several times and independently in the distinct bat lineages. These nocturnal mammalian species perform true flapping flight, an attribute that probably was inherited from their gliding ancestors and that also apparently evolved in several distinct times within the lineages of this taxon. Excepting Old World fruit bats, Chiroptera display a sophisticated echolocation system that allows them to identify the environment. Both, the flight and this sensitive orientation system resulted in their high dispersion capacity. In spite of their high diversity, currently bats are considered as a monophyletic group.[72−74]

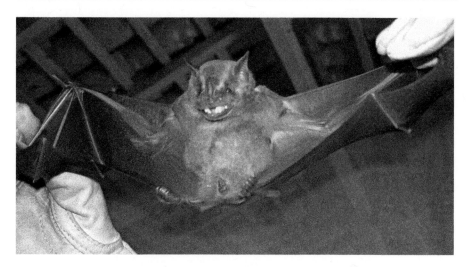

**Figure 11.6** Bat *Artibeus planirostris* from Cachoeira do Arari, Brazil.
*Photo*: Ana Maria Jansen.

Besides *Trypanosoma cruzi*, bats are commonly found infected with several other *Schyzotrypanum* species, even outside the Americas.[8,10,75] These parasites are morphologically similar and cannot be separated only based on the size of DNA fragments after molecular reactions, as is the case of other trypanosomatid species. In this case, the *Schizotrypanum* species identification is assured by the analysis of the DNA sequences after PCR with some targets being the 18S, gGAPDH, and Cyt1.[10]

The bat's refuges include hollow trees, canopy of palm trees, and ceilings of human houses and other rural buildings, which can be shared with triatomine bugs, vectors of *T. cruzi*. These mammalian species may be important reservoirs of the parasite, since they are abundant, well-adapted to anthropoid environments, and may display a high prevalence of infection in certain areas.

*T. cruzi* infection of bats occurs by different ways, but oral transmission due to ingestion of infected bugs certainly plays an important role. Bats from the genus *Carollia*, *Artibeus*, and *Molossus* became infected after experimental feeding on infected *Rhodnius prolixus*.[75] Furthermore, the omnivorous species *Phyllostomus hastatus* became experimentally infected after preying on infected mice.[76] Even predominantly frugivorous bats such as *Artibeus* sp. (Fig. 11.6), *Carollia* sp., and *Glossophaga* sp. often feed on insects and can become infected in this way.[77] Although feeding on mammalian blood that may contain infective forms of the parasite occurs, *T. cruzi* infection in hematophagic bats is rarely documented. This feature can be explained by the fact that these bats feed preferentially on cattle and horses, two groups of mammalian species almost never associated with infection by *T. cruzi*.

Among the triatomines that share refuges with bats are bugs from the genus *Cavernicola* (*C. lenti* and *C. pilosa*), often found in caves, and genera *Rhodnius* and *Panstrongylus*, found in hollow trees.[42] *Rhodnius prolixus* kept in contact with

*Carollia perspicillata, Glossophaga soricina*, and *Desmodus rotundus* were able to perform a complete blood meal, suggesting that this vector route may also be effective for the transmission of the parasite in nature.[76] *Trypanosoma cruzi* congenital transmission was already described in *Molossus molossus*, and was pointed to as another important way of parasite spread,[78] which contrasts with the observations made in primates and marsupials[60,79] that did not evidence congenital transmission. These data, apparently contradictory, reinforce the extreme complexity of the transmission cycle of *T. cruzi* among wild mammals.

In our experience, the highest variety of bat species has been found in the Amazon, followed by those of the Atlantic forest.[19] Characterization of the *Trypanosoma* spp. Isolates by 18S targets showed single and mixed infections with *T. marinkellei*, *T. dionisii*, *T. rangeli*, and *T. cruzi* TcI (Jansen et al., unpublished data). An interesting aspect was the distribution pattern of the *Trypanosoma* species. Thus, in the northern region of the country (Amazon), 13 isolates of *Trypanosoma* spp. included *T. cruzi* TcI ($n = 3$), *T. dionisii* ($n = 2$) and *T. marinkellei* ($n = 8$). In the Northeast, we found two bats infected by *T. cruzi* TcI. In the Southeast, the predominant species was *T. dionisii* ($n = 12$), besides *T. marinkellei* ($n = 2$), *T. cruzi* TcIII ($n = 2$), and *T. rangeli* ($n = 1$). Single infections by *T. rangeli* and *T. marinkellei* were observed in respectively one bat specimen for each *Trypanosoma* species.

The majority of the isolates derived from generalist species from genera *Carollia*, *Artibeus*, and *Phyllostomus*, which can become infected by eating infected bugs or small mammals.[19] The Phyllostomidae family is the most prevalent in Brazil (57% of bat species) and their high prevalence of infection points to the putative importance of these mammalian species in the parasite dispersal. *M. molossus*, found in different environments and usually associated with human settlements, is another bat species frequently found infected by *T. cruzi*. No firm associations between bats and *T. cruzi* subpopulations has been established yet as DTUs TcI, TcII, TcIII, and TcIV, besides Tcbat, have already been described in these mammalian species. In fact, there is still much to learn of trypanosomes from bats trypanosomes and we still have numerous isolates that could not be characterized at species level and are currently being studied.

# Order Artiodactyla

Mammals from this order are rarely studied in the wild concerning their putative role played on the transmission cycle of *T. cruzi*. Despite that, a study conducted in the Pantanal region of Brazil observed an interesting situation represented by the feral pig (Fig. 11.7), which are domestic pigs (*Sus scrofa*) that returned to the wild environment in the Brazilian Pantanal: these animals were infected with the DTU TcI genotype of *Trypanosoma cruzi* and described as important maintenance reservoir hosts of the parasite in nature.[80] In the same study, two sympatric species of wild boar (*Tayassu tajacu* and *Tayassu pecari*) were also found infected, as demonstrated by the presence of anti-*T. cruzi* antibodies in their serum.

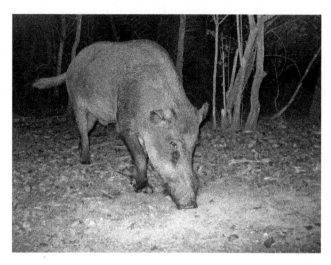

**Figure 11.7** Feral pig *Sus scrofa* from Brazilian Pantanal.
*Photo*: Rita de Cassia Bianchi.

# References

1. Briones MR, Souto RP, Stolf BS, Zingales B. The evolution of two *Trypanosoma cruzi* subgroups inferred from rRNA genes can be correlated with the interchange of American mammalian faunas in the Cenozoic and has implications to pathogenicity and host specificity. *Mol Biochem Parasitol* 1999;**104**:219−32.
2. Stothard JR, Frame IA, Miles MA. Genetic diversity and genetic exchange in *Trypanosoma cruzi*: dual drug-resistant "progeny" from episomal transformants. *Mem Inst Oswaldo Cruz* 1999;**94**(Suppl. 1):189−93.
3. Buscaglia CA, Di Noia JM. *Trypanosoma cruzi* clonal diversity and the epidemiology of Chagas' disease. *Microbes Infect* 2003;**5**:419−27.
4. Deane MP, Lenzi HL, Jansen AM. *Trypanosoma cruzi*: vertebrate and invertebrate cycles in the same mammal host, the opossum *Didelphis marsupialis*. *Mem Inst Oswaldo Cruz* 1984;**79**:513−15.
5. Schofield CJ. *Trypanosoma cruzi*−the vector-parasite paradox. *Mem Inst Oswaldo Cruz* 2000;**95**:535−44.
6. Flynn JJ, Wyss AR. Recent advances in South American mammalian paleontology. *Tree* 1998;**13**:449−54.
7. Hamilton PB, Teixeira MM, Stevens JR. The evolution of *Trypanosoma cruzi*: the "bat seeding" hypothesis. *Trends Parasitol* 2012;**28**(4):136−41. Available from: http://dx.doi.org/10.1016/j.pt.2012.01.006.
8. Lima L, Silva FM, Neves L, Attias M, Takata CS, Campaner M, et al. Evolutionary insights from bat trypanosomes: morphological, developmental and phylogenetic evidence of a new species, *Trypanosoma (Schizotrypanum) erneyi* sp. nov, in African bats closely related to *Trypanosoma (Schizotrypanum) cruzi* and allied species. *Protist* 2012;**163**:856−72.
9. Lima L, Espinosa-Álvarez O, Hamilton PB, Neves L, Takata CSA, Campaner M, et al. *Trypanosoma livingstonei*: a new species from African bats supports the bat seeding hypothesis for the *Trypanosoma cruzi* clade. *Parasit Vectors* 2013;**6**:221.

10. Lima L, Espinosa-Álvarez O, Ortiz PA, Trejo-Varón JA, Carranza JC, Pinto CM, et al. Genetic diversity of *Trypanosoma cruzi* in bats, and multilocus phylogenetic and phylogeographical analyses supporting Tcbat as an independent DTU (discrete typing unit). *Acta Trop* 2015;**151**:166−77. Available from: http://dx.doi.org/10.1016/j.actatropica. 2015.07.015.

11. Schofield CJ, Galvão C. Classification, evolution, and species groups within the Triatominae. *Acta Trop.* 2009;**110**:88−100.

12. Poinar Jr GO. *Triatoma dominicana* sp. n. (Hemiptera: Reduviidae: Triatominae) and *Trypanosoma antiquus* sp. n. (Stercoraria: Trypanosomatidae): the first fossil evidence of a Triatomine-Trypanosomatid vector association. *Vector Borne Zoonotic Dis* 2005;**5**:72−81.

13. Carcavallo RU, Jurberg J, Lent H. Filogenia dos triatomíneos. In: Carcavallo RU, Galíndez Girón I, Jurberg J, Lent H, editors. *Atlas dos vetores da doença de Chagas nas Américas*, Vol III. Rio de Janeiro: Fiocruz; 1999. p. 925−80.

14. Brisse S, Barnabé C, Tibayrenc M. Identification of six *Trypanosoma cruzi* phylogenetic lineages by random ampliyed polymorphic DNA and multilocus enzyme electrophoresis. *Int J Parasitol* 2000;**30**:35−44.

15. Zingales B, Miles MA, Campbell DA, Tibayrenc M, Macedo AM, Teixeira MM, et al. The revised *Trypanosoma cruzi* subspecific nomenclature: rationale, epidemiological relevance and research applications. *Infect Genet Evol* 2012;**12**(2):240−53. Available from: http://dx.doi.org/10.1016/j.meegid.2011.12.009.

16. Anonymous. Recommendations from a satellite meeting. *Mem Inst Oswaldo Cruz* 1999;**94**:429−32.

17. World Health Organization (WHO). Control of Chagas Disease. *Tech Rep Series* 1991;**811**. 95pp.

18. Yeo M, Acosta N, Llewellyn M, Sanchez H, Adamson S, Miles GA, et al. Origins of Chagas disease: *Didelphis* species are natural hosts of *Trypanosoma cruzi* I and armadillos hosts of *Trypanosoma cruzi* II, including hybrids. *Int J Parasitol* 2005;**35**:225−33.

19. Jansen AM, Xavier SC, Roque AL. The multiple and complex and changeable scenarios of the *Trypanosoma cruzi* transmission cycle in the sylvatic environment. *Acta Trop* 2015. pii: S0001-706X(15)30066-8. http://dx.doi.org/10.1016/j.actatropica.2015.07.018.

20. Olifiers N, Gentile R, Fiszon JT. Relation between small-mammal species composition and anthropic variables in the Brazilian Atlantic Forest. *Braz J Biol* 2005;**65**:495−501.

21. Austad NS. The adaptable opossum. *Sci Am* 1988;**258**(2):98−104.

22. Fernandes O, Mangia RH, Lisboa CV, Pinho AP, Morel CM, Zingales B, et al. The complexity of the complexity of the sylvatic cycle of *Trypanosoma cruzi* in Rio de Janeiro State revealed by non-transcribed spacer of the mini exon gene. *Parasitology* 1999;**118**:161−6.

23. Jansen AM, Carreira JC, Deane MP. Infection of a mammal by monogenetic insect trypanosomatids (Kinetoplastida, Trypanosomatidae). *Mem Inst Oswaldo Cruz* 1988;**83**: 271−2.

24. Steindel M, Pinto CJ. *Trypanosoma cruzi* development in the anal glands of experimentally infected *Lutreolina crassicaudata* (Marsupialia, Didelphidae). *Mem Inst Oswaldo Cruz* 1988;**83**:397.

25 Jansen AM, Leon LL, Machado GM, da Silva MH, Souza-Leão SM, Deane MP. *Trypanosoma cruzi* in *Didelphis marsupialis*: an parasitological and serological follow up of the acute phase. *Exp Parasitol* 1991;**73**:249−59.

26. Pinho AP, Cupolillo E, Mangia RH, Fernandes O, Jansen AM. *Trypanosoma cruzi* in the sylvatic environment: distinct transmission cycles involving two sympatric marsupials. *Trans R Soc Trop Med Hyg* 2000;**94**:1−6.

27. PAHO – Pan-American Health Organization. Doença de Chagas—guia para vigilância, prevenção, controle e manejo clínico da doença de Chagas aguda transmitida por alimentos. 2009; 92pp. Available from: http://bvs.panalimentos.org/local/File/Guia_Doenca_Chagas_2009.pdf.

28. Jansen AM, Pinho APS, Lisboa CV, Cupolillo E, Mangia RH, Fernandes O. The sylvatic cycle of *Trypanosoma cruzi*: a still unsolved puzzle. *Mem Inst Oswaldo Cruz* 1999;**94** (Suppl. I):203–4.

29. Legey AP, Pinho AP, Xavier SCC, Leon L, Jansen AM. Humoral immune response kinetics in *Philander opossum* and *Didelphis marsupialis* infected and immunized by *Trypanosoma cruzi*. *Mem Inst Oswaldo Cruz* 1999;**94**:371–3.

30. Roque ALR, Xavier SCC, da Rocha MG, Duarte AC, D'Andrea PS, Jansen AM. *Trypanosoma cruzi* transmission cycle among wild and domestic mammals in three areas of orally transmitted Chagas disease outbreaks. *Am J Trop Med Hyg* 2008;**79**: 742–9.

31. Barretto MP, Ribeiro RD. Reservatórios silvestres do *Trypanosoma* (*Schizotrypanum*) *cruzi*, Chagas 1909. *Rev Inst Adolfo Lutz* 1979;**39**:25–36.

32. Herrera L, D'Andrea PS, Xavier SC, Mangia RH, Fernandes O, Jansen AM. Trypanosoma cruzi infection in wild mammals of the National Park 'Serra da Capivara' and its surroundings (Piaui, Brazil), an area endemic for Chagas disease. *Trans R Soc Trop Med Hyg* 2005;**99**:379–88.

33. Marcili A, Lima L, Valente VC, Valente SA, Batista JS, Junqueira AC, et al. Comparative phylogeography of *Trypanosoma cruzi* TCIIc: new hosts, association with terrestrial ecotopes, and spatial clustering. *Infect Genet Evol* 2009;**9**:1265–74.

34. Carreira JCA, Jansen AM, Deane MP, Lenzi H. Histopathological study of experimental and natural infections by *Trypanosoma cruzi* in *Didelphis marsupialis*. *Mem Inst Oswaldo Cruz* 1996;**91**:609–18.

35. Rotureau B. Trypanosomatid (Protozoa, Kinetoplastida) parasites of sloths (Mammalia, Xenarthra). *Bull Soc Pathol Exot* 2006;**99**:171–5.

36. Chagas C. Sobre um trypanosomo do tatú *Tatusia novemcincta*, transmitido pela *Triatoma geniculata* Latr. (1811): Possibilidade de ser o tatu um depositário do *Trypanosoma cruzi* no mundo exterior (Nota Prévia. *Brazil-Médico* 1912;**26**:305–6.

37. Acosta N, Samudio M, López E, Vargas F, Yaksic N, Brenière SF, et al. Isoenzyme profiles of *Trypanosoma cruzi* stocks from different areas of Paraguay. *Mem Inst Oswaldo Cruz* 2001;**96**:527–33.

38. Yaeger RG. The prevalence of *Trypanosoma cruzi* infection in armadillos collected at a site near New Orleans, Louisiana. *Am J Trop Med Hyg* 1988;**38**:323–6.

39. Paige CF, Scholl DT, Truman RW. Prevalence and incidence density of *Mycobacterium leprae* and *Trypanosoma cruzi* infections within a population of wild nine-banded armadillos. *Am J Trop Med Hyg* 2002;**67**:528–32.

40. Raccurt CP. *Trypanosoma cruzi* in French Guiana: review of accumulated data since 1940. *Med Trop* 1996;**56**:79–87.

41. Orozco MM, Enriquez GF, Alvarado-Otegui JA, Cardinal MV, Schijman AG, Kitron U, et al. New sylvatic hosts of *Trypanosoma cruzi* and their reservoir competence in the humid Chaco of Argentina: a longitudinal study. *Am J Trop Med Hyg* 2013;**88** (5):872–82.

42. Carcavallo RU, Franca-Rodríguez ME, Salvatella R, Curto de Casas SI, Sherlock I, Galvão C, et al. Habitats e fauna relacionada. In: Carcavallo RU, Galíndez Girón I, Jurberg J, Lent H, editors. *Atlas dos vetores da doença de Chagas nas Américas*, Vol II. Rio de Janeiro: Fiocruz; 1998. p. 561–600.

43. Bento DN, Farias LM, Godoy MF, Araújo JF. The epidemiology of Chagas' disease in a rural area of the city of Teresina, Piauí, Brazil. *Rev Soc Bras Med Trop* 1992;**25**:51−8.

44. Araújo VA, Boité MC, Cupolillo E, Jansen AM, Roque AL. Mixed infection in the anteater *Tamandua tetradactyla* (Mammalia: Pilosa) from Pará State, Brazil: *Trypanosoma cruzi*, *T. rangeli* and *Leishmania infantum*. *Parasitology* 2013;**140**(4): 455−60. Available from: http://dx.doi.org/10.1017/S0031182012001886.

45. Bonvicino CR, Oliveira JA, D'Andrea PS Guia dos Roedores do Brasil, com chaves para gêneros baseadas em caracteres externos/Rio de Janeiro: Centro Pan-Americano de Febre Aftosa—OPAS/OMS; 2008:120 p.: il. (Série de Manuais Técnicos, ISSN 0101-6970).

46. Wilson DE, Reeder DM. *Mammal species of the World: a taxonomic and geographic reference*. 3rd ed. Baltimore, MD: Johns Hopkins University Press; 2005. p. 2142.

47. Mills JN, Childs JE. Ecologic studies of rodent reservoirs: their relevance of human health. *Emerg Infect Dis* 1998;**4**:529−37.

48. Herrera HM, Rademaker V, Abreu UG, D'Andrea PS, Jansen AM. Variables that modulate the spatial distribution of *Trypanosoma cruzi* and *Trypanosoma evansi* in the Brazilian Pantanal. *Acta Trop* 2007;**102**:55−62.

49. Vaz VC, D'Andrea PS, Jansen AM. Effects of habitat fragmentation on wild mammal infection by *Trypanosoma cruzi*. *Parasitology* 2007;**134**:1785−93.

50. Ramsey JM, Gutiérrez-Cabrera AE, Salgado-Ramírez L, Peterson AT, Sánchez-Cordero V, et al. Ecological connectivity of *Trypanosoma cruzi* reservoirs and *Triatoma pallidipennis* hosts in an anthropogenic landscape with endemic Chagas disease. *PLoS ONE* 2012;**7**(9): e46013.

51. Charles RA, Kjos S, Ellis AE, Barnes JC, Yabsley MJ. Southern plains woodrats (*Neotoma micropus*) from southern Texas are important reservoirs of two genotypes of *Trypanosoma cruzi* and host of a putative novel *Trypanosoma* species. *Vector Borne Zoonotic Dis* 2013;**13**(1):22−30.

52. Orozco MM, Piccinali RV, Mora MS, Enriquez GF, Cardinal MV, Gürtler RE. The role of sigmodontine rodents as sylvatic hosts of *Trypanosoma cruzi* in the Argentinean Chaco. *Infect Genet Evol* 2014;**22**:12−22.

53. Herrera CP, Licon MH, Nation CS, Jameson SB, Wesson DM. Genotype diversity of *Trypanosoma cruzi* in small rodents and *Triatoma sanguisuga* from a rural area in New Orleans, Louisiana. *Parasit. Vectors* 2015;**8**:123.

54. Rademaker V, Herrera HM, Raffel TR, D'Andrea PS, Freitas TP, Abreu UG, et al. What is the role of small rodents in the transmission cycle of *Trypanosoma cruzi* and *Trypanosoma evansi* (Kinetoplastida Trypanosomatidae)? A study case in the Brazilian Pantanal. *Acta Trop* 2009;**111**(2):102−7.

55. Bonvicino CR, Otazu IB, D'Andrea PS. Karyologic evidence of diversification of the genus *Thrichomys* (Rodentia, Echimyidae). *Cytogenet Genome Res* 2002;**97**:200−4.

56. Araújo CAC, Waniek PJ, Xavie SCC, Jansen AM. Genotype variation of *Trypanosoma cruzi* isolates from different Brazilian biomes. *Exp Parasitol* 2011;**127**:308−12.

57. Herrera L, Xavier SCC, Viegas C, Martinez C, Cotias PM, Carrasco H, et al. *Trypanosoma cruzi* in a caviomorph rodent: parasitological and pathological features of the experimental infection of *Trichomys apereoides* (Rodentia, Echimyidae). *Exp Parasitol* 2004;**107**:78−88.

58. Roque ALR, D'Andrea PS, de Andrade GB, Jansen AM. *Trypanosoma cruzi*: distinct patterns of infection in the sibling caviomorph rodent species *Thrichomys apereoides laurentius* and *Thrichomys pachyurus* (Rodentia, Echimyidae). *Exp Parasitol* 2005;**111**: 37−46.

59. Dias JCP, Coura JR. Comments on Carlos Chagas, 1909—Nova tripanosomíase humana: estudos sobre a morfologia e ciclo evolutivo do *Schizotrypanum* n. gen., n.sp., agente etiológico de nova entidade mórbida do homem. In: Carvalheiro JR, Azevedo N, Araújo-Jorge TC, Lannes-Vieira J, Soeiro MNC, Klein L, editors. *Clássicos em doença de Chagas—história e perspectivas no centenário da descoberta.* Rio de Janeiro: Fiocruz; 2009. p. 51–130.

60. Lisboa CV, Mangia RH, Rubião E, de Lima NR, das Chagas Xavier SC, Picinatti A, et al. *Trypanosoma cruzi* transmission in a captive primate unit, Rio de Janeiro, Brazil. *Acta Trop* 2004;**90**:97–106.

61. Lisboa CV, Monteiro RV, Martins AF, Xavier SC, Lima VD, Jansen AM. Infection with *Trypanosoma cruzi* TcII and TcI in free-ranging population of lion tamarins (*Leontopithecus* spp): an 11-year follow-up. *Mem Inst Oswaldo Cruz* 2015;**110**(3): 394–402.

62. Monteiro RV, Dietz JM, Raboy B, Beck B, De Vleeschouwer K, Baker A, et al. Parasite community interactions: *Trypanosoma cruzi* and intestinal helminths infecting wild golden lion tamarins *Leontopithecus rosalia* and golden-headed lion tamarins *L. chrysomelas* (Callitrichidae, L., 1766). *Parasitol Res* 2007;**101**:1689–98.

63. Lisboa CV, Dietz J, Baker AJ, Russel NN, Jansen AM. *Trypanosoma cruzi* infection in *Leontopithecus rosalia* at the Reserva Biologica de Poco das Antas, Rio de Janeiro, Brazil. *Mem Inst Oswaldo Cruz* 2000;**95**:445–52.

64. Marcili A, Valente VC, Valente SA, Junqueira AC, da Silva FM, Pinto AY. *Trypanosoma cruzi* in Brazilian Amazonia: Lineages TCI and TCIIa in wild primates, *Rhodnius* spp. and in humans with Chagas disease associated with oral transmission. *Int J Parasitol* 2009;**39**:615–23.

65. Monteiro RV, Baldez J, Dietz J, Baker A, Lisboa CV, Jansen AM. Clinical, biochemical, and electrocardiographic aspects of *Trypanosoma cruzi* infection in free-ranging golden lion tamarins (*Leontopithecus rosalia*). *J Med Primatol* 2006;**35**:48–55.

66. Rocha FL, Roque AL, de Lima JS, Cheida CC, Lemos FG, de Azevedo FC, et al. *Trypanosoma cruzi* infection in neotropical wild carnivores (Mammalia: Carnivora): at the top of the *T. cruzi* transmission chain. *PLoS ONE* 2013;**4;8**(7):e67463. Available from: http://dx.doi.org/10.1371/journal.pone.0067463.

67. Herrera HM, Rocha FL, Lisboa CV, Rademaker V, Mourão GM, Jansen AM. Food web connections and the transmission cycles of *Trypanosoma cruzi* and *Trypanosoma evansi* (Kinetoplastida, Trypanosomatidae) in the Pantanal Region, Brazil. *Trans R Soc Trop Med Hyg* 2011;**105**(7):380–7. Available from: http://dx.doi.org/10.1016/j.trstmh.2011.04.008.

68. Herrera HM, Lisboa CV, Pinho AP, Olifiers N, Bianchi RC, Rocha FL, et al. The coati (*Nasua nasua*, Carnivora, Procyonidae) as a reservoir host for the main lineages of *Trypanosoma cruzi* in the Pantanal region, Brazil. *Trans R Soc Trop Med Hyg* 2008;**102**:1133–9.

69. Pietrokovsky SM, Schweigmann NJ, Riarte A, Alberti A, Conti O, Montoya S, et al. The skunk *Conepatus chinga* as new host of *Trypanosoma cruzi* in Argentina. *J Parasitol* 1991;**77**:643–5.

70. Rosypal AC, Tidwell RR, Lindsay DS. Prevalence of antibodies to *Leishmania infantum* and *Trypanosoma cruzi* in wild canids from South Carolina. *J Parasitol* 2007;**93**:955–7.

71. Olifiers N, Jansen AM, Herrera HM, Bianchi Rde C, D'Andrea PS, Mourão Gde M, et al. Co-infection and wild animal health: effects of trypanosomatids and gastrointestinal parasites on coatis of the Brazilian pantanal. *PLoS ONE* 2015;**14;10**(12):e0143997. Available from: http://dx.doi.org/10.1371/journal.pone.0143997.

72. Jones G, Teeling EC. The evolution of echolocation in bats. *Trends Ecol Evol* 2006;**21**: 149−56.

73. Bishop KL. The evolution of flight in bats: narrowing the field of plausible hypotheses. *Q Rev Biol* 2008;**83**:153−69.

74. Bisson IA, Safi K, Holland LA. Evidence for repeated independent evolution of migration in the largest family of bats. *PLoS ONE*. 2009;**21**:e7504.

75. Pinto CM, Ocaña-Mayorga S, Tapia EE, Lobos SE, Zurita AP, Aguirre-Villacís F, et al. Bats, Trypanosomes, and Triatomines in Ecuador: new insights into the diversity, transmission, and origins of *Trypanosoma cruzi* and Chagas disease. *PLoS ONE* 2015;**10**(10): e0139999.

76. Thomas ME, Rasweiler JJ, D'Alessandro A. Experimental transmission of the parasitic flagellates *Trypanosoma cruzi* and *Trypanosoma rangeli* between triatomine bugs or mice and captive neotropical bats. *Mem Inst Oswaldo Cruz* 2007;**102**:559−65.

77. Gardner AL. Feeding habitats. In: Baker, RJ, Jones, JK, Carter, DC, editors. *Biology of bats of the New World family Phillostomatidae, Part III, Spec. Publ. Mus. Texas Tech. Univ.*, vol. 13. 1977;13:293−350.

78. Añez N, Crisante G, Soriano PJ. *Trypanosoma cruzi* congenital transmission in wild bats. *Acta Trop* 2009;**109**:78−80.

79. Jansen AM, Madeira FB, Deane MP. *Trypanosoma cruzi* infection in the opossum *Didelphis marsupialis*: absence of neonatal transmission and protection by maternal antibodies in experimental infections. *Mem Inst Oswaldo Cruz* 1994;**89**:41−5.

80. Herrera HM, Abreu UG, Keuroghlian A, Freitas TP, Jansen AM. The role played by sympatric collared peccary (*Tayassu tajacu*), white-lipped peccary (*Tayassu pecari*), and feral pig (*Sus scrofa*) as maintenance hosts for *Trypanosoma evansi* and *Trypanosoma cruzi* in a sylvatic area of Brazil. *Parasitol Res* 2008;**103**:619−24.

# Trypanosoma cruzi enzootic cycle: general aspects, domestic and synanthropic hosts and reservoirs

**12**

*A.M. Jansen, A.L.R. Roque and S.C.C. Xavier*
Oswaldo Cruz Institute, Rio de Janeiro, Brazil

## Chapter Outline

## The complex *Trypanosoma cruzi* transmission cycle

*T. cruzi* is a successful parasite that is transmitted among more than 100 mammalian species dispersed in 7 different orders and dozens of species of insect vectors, bugs of the Reduviidae family.[1,2] Actually, birds and cold-blooded vertebrates are refractory to the parasite but may act as a feeding source for triatomine enhancing their survival chances, contributing in this way, indirectly, to the maintenance of the parasite. *T. cruzi* transmission cycles occur in all phytogeographical regions in the Americas, from northern Argentina to southern United States. The diverse environments (habitats and niches) where the parasite can be found consist of numerous microfoci of transmission that display peculiar epidemiological profiles. *T. cruzi* is able to colonize almost all tissues in its many mammalian hosts, including unconventional sites, such as the scent glands of *Didelphis* spp.[3] and *Lutreolina crassicaudata*,[4] as well as the cornea of *Thrichomys apereoides*.[5] The multiplicity of host—parasite interactions in the wild, constitute transmission cycles that can be characterized as complex and multivariable systems.[2]

Triatomines transmit the parasite only if infected, which occurs when they feed on an infected mammalian host and ingest, with their blood, the trypomastigote forms of the parasite. In the digestive tract of triatomines, the parasites differentiate into epimastigotes (multiplicative form) and then to metacyclic trypomastigotes in

American Trypanosomiasis Chagas Disease. DOI: http://dx.doi.org/10.1016/B978-0-12-801029-7.00012-5

the final portion of the intestine. Infection of mammals occurs when they come into contact with the infective metacyclic forms of the parasite that are eliminated with the feces of triatomines after feeding. This contact occurs through the mucosa or through injury, preexistent or resulting from the bite of the bug. The oral route, i.e., ingestion of infective forms of the parasite, occurs when the animal scratches with his mouth the place of its body where the bugs' feces were deposited, eats food contaminated with the parasite, or preys on bugs or other infected mammals. Very probably the oral route is the main infection route of wild free ranging mammals. Actually, the contaminative infection route is quite unlikely[6] mainly if we consider the dense fur of the animals that certainly acts as a barrier to the infective metacyclic forms. The oral route has proven to be highly efficient for the establishment of *T. cruzi* infection.[7,8] In fact, the chances of animals to acquire the infection orally, by predation of infected triatomine bugs was estimated[9] as superior to that of humans acquiring the infection by the contaminative route.[6]

Even having already been studied for over a century, there are still epidemiological challenges that need to be faced: (1) the epidemiological importance of congenital transmission for reservoirs and humans; (2) prophylactic measures to prevent the recurrent outbreaks of Chagas disease due to the oral route; and (3) the ecology of the distinct *T. cruzi* discrete typing units (DTUs). Mother to child *T. cruzi* transmission, a rather rare event[10] represents a major public health problem in Bolivia, a highly endemic country. Additionally, due to migration of people from endemic areas, congenital Chagas disease is also becoming a problem in nonendemic countries.[11] Among the still open questions are the role played by the distinct DTUs in the establishment of congenital infections as well as the mother's immune response, genetic background, and even microbiome.[10] This issue is discussed in a specific chapter in this book (see Chapter 23, Maternal–fetal transmission of *Trypanosoma cruzi*). Regarding the congenital transmission in free ranging animals, almost nothing is known. Thus, a great effort is presently needed to clarify what variables (host- and parasite-related) determine vertical transmission.

## What are the *Trypanosoma cruzi* reservoirs?

Defining a reservoir is a challenging theoretical and practical task and this difficulty is not different regarding *T. cruzi*. Since its description more than a century ago, several researchers have tried to determine which mammalian species were the main sources of infection for the triatomines and, hence, to man. Numerous species of wild mammals were found to be infected by *T. cruzi* and named "natural reservoirs" of the parasite.[12] Subsequent studies showed that, for multihost parasites such as *T. cruzi*, several mammalian species may act as the bugs' source of infection in a given place. The researchers started to understand that these mammalian species differ in their importance as source of infection for the triatomine vector, and that the same mammalian species can play different roles in the maintenance and transmission of the parasite in different regions and time schedules. Under this focus, we now consider a reservoir not as a single mammal species found infected in a given locality, but a complex biological system that includes one or more species of mammals that are involved in the maintenance of the parasite in nature. In each ecological system, the mammalian species may play different roles in the maintenance of the parasite, which means that the reservoir system varies and should be considered as unique within a certain spatiotemporal scale. As in any other host−parasite system, the *T. cruzi* infection patterns in a given mammalian host species, is determined by host traits (species, sex, age, and behavioral patterns), parasite traits (generation time, dispersion strategies, molecular and biochemical characteristics of its subpopulations), and by the environmental conditions (stress, host coinfections, and availability of natural resources) where the host−parasite interaction takes place. A nice review of these concepts may be found in Ref. [13].

In our casuistry, which includes the examination of 7285 free-living wild mammals, we observed that infectivity (high parasitemia expressed by positive blood cultures) was found in only 8% of the animals.[2] Obviously, due to the complexity of the transmission cycle of *T. cruzi* and the aggregated distribution of the parasite, the standard deviation is extremely high. The overall rate of *T. cruzi* infection as demonstrated by serological tests is around 20%, nothing extraordinary considering the wide distribution of this parasite.

We consider as maintenance reservoirs those mammal species that are able to get infected and retain the infection of a given parasite. Amplifier reservoirs are those animals that display a pattern of infection that favors the transmission of this parasite (i.e., high transmissibility potential or high infective competence). It is worth mentioning that these characteristics are interchangeable—therefore, maintenance reservoirs may act as amplifier reservoirs according to, among others, health conditions including immune suppression, concomitant parasitic infections, and subpopulation of the parasite. Regarding *T. cruzi*, the transmissibility from a given mammalian species to the triatominae vector is guaranteed if this host displays high parasitemia. This feature is demonstrated by the detection of parasites in the mammalian's blood by parasitological techniques that include fresh blood sample examination, hemoculture, or xenodiagnosis. In contrast, transmission of parasites between two mammalian species (predator−prey) can be attained even in the absence of circulating infective forms in blood, since amastigotes present in the tissues of the preyed mammalian host can also be a source of infection.[14] Molecular diagnosis by polymerase chain reaction (PCR) can be considered an enriched direct parasitological assay, since it detects constitutive parts of the parasites, in this case fragments of DNA.

This technique can be applied to diagnose *T. cruzi* in the blood, but an important feature should be taken into account: the inhibitor property of the iron ions present in the mammal's blood during PCR reaction, which can induce false-negative results.[15,16] Even for the *T. cruzi* infected ones, we have to consider that this test indicates the presence of DNA fragments, and its high sensitivity does not allow us to conclude whether the parasite load detected would be sufficient to ensure the transmissibility of that parasite.[17,18] Alternatively, a quantitative reaction (real-time

PCR) is a promising tool to indicate the minimum parasite load capable to ensure transmissibility to the vectors.[18,19]

The diagnosis of *T. cruzi* infection obtained by indirect tests, such as the serological ones, show the exposure of those mammalian specimens to the parasite, but also does not reflect its transmissibility competence to the bugs or other mammals. Serum-positive mammals demonstrate that they have been exposed to *T. cruzi* infection (are indeed hosts of this parasite), but are not necessarily important for the maintenance of that parasite in nature, i.e., are not necessarily reservoirs of the parasite, but in some cases act as *dead-end* hosts.

In this sense, an epidemiological investigation on *T. cruzi* wild hosts should include, essentially, a representative sampling of the most abundant mammalian species in the area and a broad methodological approach that includes the diagnosis of infection by direct and indirect parasitological tests.[20] Nevertheless, most studies are geographically restricted and do not include data on the overall environmental conditions, for instance local fauna diversity, relative abundance of infected and uninfected mammalian species or their population structure. The restriction of studies to some specific mammalian taxa or habitats, such as the peridomestic ones (which are not representative of the whole area), results in misinterpretation of data and description of the most common species in a given habitat as the main (or even the unique) reservoirs of the parasite. Some mammalian species such as the synanthropic *Rattus rattus*, *Mus musculus*, and *Didelphis* spp. are described infected in several studies, but do not always represent the most important species implicated in the maintenance of the parasite in the area.[21] Additionally, due to the difficulties inherent to the conduct of field work, long-term studies of wild mammalian fauna are very rare even though it is known that they are extremely important. Actually, important seasonal differences of the parasite transmission pattern occur and must be taken into account. This is specially the case for small mammals that display a short life span and that display high population turnover rates. As pointed out before, a reservoir host must be able to maintain the transmission cycle of the parasite and for that, this mammalian species should display a high relative abundance in the area. If this species represents only a negligible relative abundance of the local mammalian species, its importance in the transmission cycle of the parasite is lower than the importance of a second mammalian species that displays a lower prevalence of infection but is much more abundant in the area. Likewise, in some scenarios, an infected species that displays a high relative abundance is more competent as reservoir host in a given area than in another, where its abundance and total biomass are not very significant.[20,22] Very important, but unfortunately rarely considered during field work are the kinds of connections and encounters that occur between the components of the fauna of a target study area. Actually the mere isolation of a given DTU of *T. cruzi* of an infected animal species still does not mean that this is important as a reservoir of this DTU. In fact each habitat displays its landscape peculiarities which, in turn, shapes the local fauna composition, their interactions and consequently the *T. cruzi* transmission network. This is clearly exemplified by the sequential use of the same shelter by different mammalian species or individuals of the same species but of different social groups. This may be the case of mammal species that may display high *T. cruzi* infective competence. Thus, in the central Brazil region termed Cerrado (Savannah) the little fox *Lycalopex vetulus* uses tunnels previously dug and abandoned by armadillos, as their abode to give birth and raise their pups during their first months of life. Other wild mammals also use these tunnels: ocelots, coatis, and tamanduas, among others, have been reported.[23] Of course the succession of animals seeking shelter in these places supply the nutritional needs of any triatomine colony that may perhaps may be there. Also coati nests may act as simultaneous shelter to both triatomine bugs and wild mammals. The emblematic description of *Thrichomys fosteri*, a kind of exclusively terrestrial caviomorph rodent inside a coati nest that was in the canopy of a 30 m high tree, clearly shows the complexity of the wild transmission cycle of *T. cruzi*.[24] In the same coati nest *T. cruzi*-infected *Rhodnius stali* and *Triatoma sordida* were also found.[25]

Due to this complex epidemiology, it is clear that unlike linear systems, the transmission cycles of *T. cruzi* in nature have to be understood as dynamic webs, with parasite transmission by different routes in transmission cycles in the forest floor, understory, or canopy that may or not overlap.[26] In these transmission networks are included different species of mammals and bugs, which display peculiarities of their interaction with *T. cruzi* that result in their higher or lower infectivity competence. It is worth mentioning that one of the most interesting features of this extremely successful parasite is its remarkable diversity already noticed by the seminal researchers. It is hard to say what is cause and what is consequence but what seems certain is that the diversity of *T. cruzi* is associated with its amazing ecological plasticity.

*T. cruzi* diversity has become more evident after the increase of the analytical power of the tools that emerged from the 1960s onward. At the moment the *T. cruzi* subpopulations are grouped into seven DTUs, but some authors seriously question this structuring, proposing the classification into three clusters based on mitochondrial typing: mTcI, mTcII, and mTcIII, the latter including the DTUs TcIII to TcVI.[27] Independent of the classification that is considered, one of the biggest challenges is to understand their ecology and their eventual association to the different manifestations of human disease. We dare propose that an association of a *T. cruzi* DTU with a specific kind of clinical manifestation in infected humans or animals will be unlikely to be proven, as is it known that the outcome of a parasite−host interaction is multifactorial, idiosyncratic, and changeable in the spatial and temporal scales.

# Importance of wild and synanthropic mammals in public health—Brazil

Since June 2006, Brazil is considered free from Chagas disease transmission due to *Triatoma infestans*.[28] This statement means that the maintenance of a domiciliary *Trypanosoma cruzi* transmission solely by infected men and domiciliary bugs are not encountered in the country anymore. Human infection nowadays occurs due to vectorial transmission outside the houses, nondomiciliated bugs that invade the houses, or by ingestion of food contaminated with feces of infected bugs.[29] In all of these cases, infected wild and synanthropic mammals play a crucial role in the maintenance of parasite circulation.

In a given environment, several mammalian species frequent different forest strata, which favor the parasite exchange among them. Opossums, for example, are habitat generalists and excellent climbers that may be found on the top of trees, although they can also easily be found also on the ground. Opossum species of the genus *Didelphis* are rather generalist mammals. They can be found dwelling in tree holes and other natural refugees in the forest but they are also highly associated to humans. It is easy to find *Didelphis* spp. nesting in garbage cans, or even the attic of the houses. Actually, this marsupial genus that is currently considered as a synanthropic animal may act as a very important *T. cruzi* reservoir and also as a link between the sylvatic and the domestic transmission cycle of *T. cruzi*.

Several carnivores, such as coatis and weasels, are terrestrial mammalian species that can use tree trunks as refuges. Moreover, coatis construct resting reproduction nests on trees. That means that a given mammal infected through the ingestion of an infected bug on the ground may be later a source of infection for other triatomine species in a hollow tree refuge or in the canopy. In fact, the multiplicity of mammalian host species and possibilities of parasite transmission is probably the main responsible factor for the extremely well-succeeded dissemination of the parasite in the Americas. It is difficult to find a forest fragment in South America where triatomines and potential mammalian hosts cohabit absolutely free from *T. cruzi* infection. For this reason, human exposure to the wild environment, during extractive activities for example, common in several areas, but especially in the Amazon basin, should always be considered as a risk of coming into contact with infected triatomines and in acquiring *T cruzi* infection. Human cases of the disease, as a consequence of this kind of exposure, are very common in the northern part of Brazil (Pará State), inside the Brazilian Amazon. These cases occur as outbreaks involving familiar groups and are due to the ingestion of Açaí juice contaminated with infected triatomine.[20,30–32] Besides, these outbreaks are clearly seasonal, linked to the Açaí harvest time.[33]

In nature, *T. cruzi* transmission cycles assume different profiles that are mostly dependent on the local mammalian fauna, their encounter pattern, and ability to disseminate the parasite, i.e., their infective competence. Since these vary according to parasite DTU and the different conditions of the environment in which they are inserted, it is not possible to predict the intensity of the enzootic cycle before examining the local fauna. Moreover, due to the dynamic character of the *T. cruzi* transmission network, even surveillance like this, should be considered as restricted to a given period of time. Modifications of local fauna and dynamics of *T. cruzi* infection may result in higher or lesser prevalence of infection in the local fauna, in a process that is called "amplifier or dilution effect."[34] These kinds of effects were first described for Lyme disease, and since then, applied to other parasitic interactions: Cutaneous Leishmaniasis,[35] Hantaviroses,[36] West Nile Fever,[37] and also Chagas disease.[20,38,39]

The dilution effect occurs when the number of infected and competent *T. cruzi* reservoirs (those that display a pattern of infection that favors the parasite transmissibility to the vectors) is low when compared to other possible sources of blood meal for triatomines. As a result, the probability of an encounter between one infected and competent reservoir and the triatomine bug is limited, resulting in an overall low prevalence of infection in the local triatomine fauna. Conversely, the amplifier effect is observed when some modification of the environment results in a positive selection of infected mammalian hosts that are competent *T. cruzi* reservoirs. In this case, the probability of an encounter between infected mammals and triatomine bugs is enhanced, resulting in a higher prevalence of *T. cruzi* infection in the local triatomine fauna. When such modifications are trigged by men who colonize adjacent forest areas, synanthropic mammalian species—especially marsupials, rodents, and bats—can start to frequent peridomestic areas where they can be a source of a blood meal, i.e., of infection, for triatomines. Hence, environmental modifications imposed by men on areas adjacent to their dwellings, besides all the ecological consequences, could also result in a higher risk of infection by *T. cruzi*. Infected triatomines are attracted by light and invade the houses where human infection can take place both during the bug's blood meal or accidentally by the ingestion of food contaminated with feces of infected triatomines. In fact, the latter process seems to be involved in recent outbreaks of Chagas disease in Brazil.[20,32]

# Domestic mammalian species

Dogs, cats, pigs, and goats are the main domestic mammalian species investigated for the *T. cruzi* infection. Dogs and cats represent the first domestic *T. cruzi* hosts studied by Carlos Chagas: a cat in Lassance (Minas Gerais state, Brazil) was the first mammalian host in which he found trypomastigote forms of the parasite in the blood, while dogs were among the first experimental models used by him. Since then, several studies have shown that dogs and cats can be competent *T. cruzi* reservoirs, but as described for the other taxa of mammals (see chapter: Ecological aspects of *Trypanosoma cruzi*: wild hosts and reservoirs), their importance in the transmission cycle of the parasite varies between different regions and local characteristics.

In the Argentinean Gran Chaco, both dogs and cats are epidemiologically important and described as highly infective to the triatomine vectors.[13,40] A similar profile was found in Venezuela, where DTUs TcI and TcII have already been described in dogs.[41] The DTUs TcIII and TcIV (formerly Z3) were described in infected dogs from Paraguay,[42] Argentina,[43,44] Colombia,[45] and Brazil.[46] Also hybrid DTUs (TcV and TcVI) were already found infecting dogs in Argentina,[44] Colombia,[45] and Brazil.[47] Active transmission, which includes symptomatic dogs, was also observed in the southern United States.[48] An opposite scenario is observed in Brazil where, despite being exposed to parasite infection (as evidenced by the high infection rates of dogs displaying positive serological tests; IFAT and ELISA)

*T. cruzi* isolation of parasites from dogs is rarely documented, whether by hemoculture or xenodiagnosis.[1,39,49] Our experience includes more than 2589 dogs examined in different regions of the country, from the Amazon region to Southern Brazil, including several states from the northeast and southeast regions of the country, and the pattern of infection in dogs in all of these areas were quite similarly subpatent.

The search for an animal model that mimics Chagas disease resulted in that some mammal species were tested, and domestic dogs have been one of the most exploited species. In general the primary infection of domestic dogs results in patent parasitemia that appears around 3 days after inoculation and fades away after 3 or 4 weeks.[50–52] A second inoculum does not result in a second parasitemic peak as has been observed in mice.[50] The course of infection depends obviously on all the variables related to the host and the parasite DTU as already mentioned above. Also in natural conditions, dogs display a short patent parasitemia, or even parasitemia detectable by hemocultures, period.[20,39] That means that the infectiousness of dogs in Brazil is not comparable to that of other mammal hosts species that have demonstrated to be able to maintain long lasting parasitemia, as is the case of *Didelphis* spp., *Philander* spp., *Leontopithecus* spp., and *Nasua nasua* (Jansen et al., unpublished data). However, dogs may act as efficient sentinel animals. Actually, Xavier et al.[39] observed a positive association between serologically positive dogs and: (1) lower diversity of small mammal fauna and (2) high rates of small mammal fauna with high infective competence as expressed by positive hemocultures.

Studying the role of dogs in the *T. cruzi* transmission cycle in Brazilian biomes, a country of continental dimensions, we concluded after sampling 2589 dogs that these play just a negligible role in the transmission cycle of *T. cruzi* on the grounds that only 29 (2.2%) of these animals had positive hemocultures; i.e., high infective potential. Additionally, dogs with positive blood culture were aggregated into two very distant locations from one another, namely Monte Alegre, a small village of the Pará state in the Amazon, where there was not even a single human case and in the Urucum massive, of the Pantanal biome where there are also no reports of human cases[47] (Jansen et al., unpublished data). Moreover, the short period of only 3–4 weeks of high parasitemia observed under experimental conditions seems to be repeated in natural infections. Only once did we achieve two sequential isolations from a dog from Abaetetuba (Pará State, Brazil) in an interval of 6 months.[53] Actually, when we went back to Monte Alegre to reassess the animals we could no longer obtain positive blood cultures. It is worth mentioning that the epidemiological picture of Argentina is rather distinct since dogs represent an important transmission risk factor for man in areas where there is housing infested by *Triatoma infestans* and *Triatoma dimidiata*.[13]

In the Argentine Chaco, cats are described as important reservoirs since high rates of positive xenodiagnoses (up to 65%), indicating high competence infective, have been described.[13,54] Our experience with Brazilian cats included 281 animals that have been examined by serological methods from one Brazilian biome, the Caatinga. Despite the fact that this is obviously not representative, we observed positive serological tests ranging between 20% and 65% (Jansen et al., unpublished data). *T. cruzi* parasites were isolated only twice in Brazilian cats, one from Bahia State, characterized as DTU TcI,[55] and another from São Paulo State.[56]

Concerning domestic pigs, these animals are attractive to bugs, especially for species from the genus *Panstrongylus*, as observed in some parts of the Amazon region.[57] Despite being exposed to the *T. cruzi* transmission cycle, there are few reports on isolation of parasites from domestic pigs[57,58] and their role as reservoir still needs to be further studied. Their exposure to the parasite's transmission cycles in peridomestic areas and the possibility of diagnosing the infection by serological tests points to the importance of these mammalian hosts as sentinels in surveillance and control programs.[49]

The low number of studies in goats suggests that the role played by these mammalian species in the peridomestic transmission of *T. cruzi* is of minor importance, although they are frequently found to be exposed to the parasite.[1] High parasitemias in naturally infected goats have never been reported and the diagnosis of infection was only performed with highly sensitive molecular methods (PCR) or indirect serological methods (indirect immunofluorescence assay).[59,60] Isolation of *T. cruzi* from goats by xenodiagnosis or hemoculture has been achieved only from experimentally infected animals.[61] This is probably also the case of bovines, equines, and rabbits.

## Domestic nonmammalian species

Amphibians, reptiles, and birds are refractory to *T. cruzi* infection since they are capable of destroying the trypomastigote forms of the parasite due to a complement-mediated lytic effect of their blood.[62] Despite that and concerning specially the birds, these domestic animals may play an indirect but considerable role in the transmission cycle of *T. cruzi* in both wild and peridomestic areas since they represent important feeding sources for the triatominae vectors. It is known that the amount and frequency of blood intake by infected bugs influences the *T. cruzi* development. Hence, blood ingestion in shorter intervals due to availability results in an increase of the total parasite population, while starvation reduces the density of this population and percentage of trypomastigotes in the bug's digestive tract.[63]

In peridomestic areas, poultry shelters may be very attractive to triatomines and are frequently constructed close to human dwellings. This practice certainly results in an increase of the local bug population, but the consequences for the *T. cruzi* transmission may be completely antagonistic. The availability of blood sources to triatomines may prevent their evasion of chicken coops while searching for other blood sources, acting as a barrier against domiciliary invasion by the bugs. Without taking a blood meal on an infected mammalian host, these insects will never come into contact with *T. cruzi*. In this case, even accidental contact of these insects with men would not result in human infection. However, the continuously offered blood sources for triatomines may result in an overpopulation of insects, which in a given moment may evade this poultry and start to colonize other adjacent rural buildings.

In this second situation, the increase of the local bug population enhances the chances of contact between the triatomine vectors, domestic and synanthropic mammalian species (that may be infected), and humans. Also, the introduction of resistant vertebrate species may result in the increase of the infected triatomine population if this environment is shared by infected mammals.[13] The higher the abundance and prevalence of *T. cruzi* infection in the triatomine bugs and mammals that live in peridomestic and domestic areas, the higher the probability of transmission of the parasite to humans.[13] These findings make any attempt of zooprophylactic measures of control rather reckless.

## Importance of infected domestic mammals on public health in Brazil

The detection of *T. cruzi* infection in domestic mammalian species reveals the presence of transmission cycles of the parasite in areas used by these animals. The main objectives of the surveillance of *T. cruzi* infection in domestic animals are: (1) identify mammalian species that can act as amplifiers of parasite populations and (2) identify mammalian species that can act as bioindicators (sentinels) of *T. cruzi* transmission risk to humans. It is known that, similar to what occurs in *Leishmania* sp. infection, in areas that present a high prevalence of *T. cruzi* infection in wild mammalian and triatomine hosts, domestic and peridomestic mammalian species are exposed to infection and this infection usually precedes the establishment of human disease in that area.[39]

The characteristics of the domestic mammalian species management differ in distinct localities, which means in that different mammalian species have greater or lesser importance in surveillance programs, depending on the area. In Cachoeira do Arari (Pará State, Brazil), dogs are the main responsible for house protection, and thus these animals are more restricted to domestic areas. In the same area, pigs are managed in a semiextensive manner, which results in these mammals being on their own and freely foraging in the wild environment. For this reason, in this locality, pigs were more exposed to the *T. cruzi* wild transmission cycles and, therefore, displayed the highest prevalence of infection in comparison to other localities.[20,49]

An opposite scenario was observed on the periphery of Abaetetuba, in the same Pará State. Here, pigs were raised in confined pigsties while dogs move freely between the houses (almost all without external walls) and the remaining forest fragments. In this area, the infection rates of *T. cruzi* infection were higher in dogs, as a consequence of their higher exposure to the wild transmission cycles.[53] The differences of rates of *T. cruzi* infection in domestic mammalian species that display different behavior signals the parasite transmission focuses. *T. cruzi* infection in pigs from Cachoeira do Arari and dogs from Abaetetuba points to the presence of wild transmission cycles near peridomestic areas. In a reverse situation, dogs from Cachoeira do Arari and pigs from Abaetetuba points to *T. cruzi* transmission in peridomestic areas and, therefore, a greater risk of *T. cruzi* transmission to humans. The results obtained in our studies of acute Chagas disease outbreaks areas in Brazil,[20,33,39,49,53] as well as others,[59,64] show that in areas where an effective *T. cruzi* wild transmission cycle occurs (with mammals presenting high rates of positive hemocultures), domestic mammalian species are exposed to infection and their infection usually precedes the cases of human Chagas disease.[39] In this scenario, these animals serve as biological barriers (or "shields") since they are exposed to the transmission cycle, but with no role in the amplification of parasite populations, since they almost never show parasites in their blood (low percentage of positive hemocultures). This means that these mammalian species have come into contact with *T. cruzi*, are most probably still infected, but are not sources of infection for the bug vectors.

A proposal from our group that has received increasing attention from the Brazilian Health Authorities is the longitudinal serological survey of domestic and peridomestic mammalian species to determine the prevalence and/or incidence of *T. cruzi* infection.[21,49] This is because areas that present a high prevalence of infection among these mammalian species are probably those that display the highest rates of infection among wild and synanthropic mammalian species and vectors and, therefore, are at elevated risk for the emergence of human cases. Xavier et al.[39] later confirmed by geospatial analysis by interpolation and map algebra methods, as well as the Generalized Linear Model, that species richness and positive hemocultures in wild mammals were associated with *T. cruzi* infection in dogs.

The use of domestic mammals as sentinels was already proposed and applied in Argentina,[40] Venezuela,[41] Mexico,[65] and the United States.[66] Among them, the importance of dogs in such investigations is greater, since dogs are easy to handle and their movements may be monitored most of the time. Blood collection and the subsequent serological assay (or sending of serum samples to governmental central laboratories for diagnosis) does not require great cost and/or structure. Moreover, in Brazil, collection of dog's blood samples is routinely performed for diagnosis of *Leishmania* sp. infection in many areas of the country, and this serum could also be used for the diagnosis of *T. cruzi* infection. Alternatively, vaccination campaigns against rabies occur once a year in the whole country and provide a good opportunity to collect blood samples from a representative amount of dogs in a given area.[49]

Whichever strategy is employed, the pivotal importance is that seropositive dogs reflect exposure to *T. cruzi* and indicate the presence of parasites in areas where these animals roam. The knowledge of the prevalence of *T. cruzi* infection in these hosts may direct epidemiological measures to risk areas even before the occurrence of human cases. Once this measure is implemented, health authorities will have an important indicator for the selection of areas that present a higher risk of *T. cruzi* transmission to humans and, therefore, need more urgently the implementation of epidemiological control measures and health education to present the situation and correctly inform the residents from that area.[39,49]

# Mixed infection

Rarely if ever is a living being parasitized only by one species of parasite. This also applies to coinfections by different subpopulations of a single parasite species. Still, parasitologists only recently began to consider more closely parasitic disease/infection of humans and animals at a population level.[67]

Parasite interactions in the same individual may result either in increasing of the fitness of one of the parasite species or even of both, but it can also result in a decrease in fitness of the parasites that interact. In nature, both free ranging and domestic animals are often parasitized by several species of parasites, which makes the outcome of these interactions much more complex. Additionally, there are other variables that modulate the result of concomitant infections, such as the sequence in which they occur, animal age, gender, and inocula sizes. All of these factors together will result in an almost infinite number of combinations and impact possibilities to the host.

There are some classical examples: Wolbachia, an insect symbiont, when introduced in *Aedes aegypti* is able not only to decrease the life span of this mosquito species, but also directly decrease the competence of other parasite species that infect it. Actually, Moreira et al.[68] observed that, in experimental conditions, Wolbachia-infected *A. aegypti* were able to control Dengue and Chikungunya Virus, as well as *Plasmodium gallinaceum*, two absolutely unrelated group of parasite species. Also more related species may interfere with one another when in concomitant infections. In fact, an expressive decrease of the frequencies and strength of the response of malaria-specific Th1 and Th17 T cells in individuals presenting concomitant infection by two distinct filariae species (*Wuchereria bancrofti* and *Mansonella perstans*) was observed by Metenou et al.[69] Concomitant infections is a matter within parasitology that is gaining importance and there are already authors who warn against mistaken conclusions as a result of not considering parasite communities but studying parasite species in isolation.[70]

*T. cruzi*'s huge heterogeneity is still a matter of debate. Since its description, scholars have been trying to establish an association between the different manifestations of the disease and epidemiological profiles with given parasite subpopulations, currently DTU. The possibility that, at least partially, the result of the *T. cruzi* infection in humans and animals is due to concomitant infections of two or more DTUs only recently started to be considered.[67] At least, in the intestine of *Rhodnius prolixus* a distinct infection pattern was already recognized in mixed DTUs TcI and TcII infections. Both the distribution and population density displayed differences if in single or mixed infections.[71]

Regarding concomitant *T. cruzi* DTU infections, it is more frequently observed in wild mammals. In these hosts, we observed that the most frequent combination was TcI and TcII—they also are the most frequently isolated DTUs. Didelphidae marsupials, as well as Procyonidae, Phyllostomidae, and Cebidae have been demonstrated to harbor the largest diversity of *T cruzi* DTUs in mixed infections (Jansen et al., unpublished data). Moreover, *Nasua* spp. and *Didelphis* spp. were the mammalians that displayed the highest rate of mixed DTU infection[2] (Fig. 12.1).

The study of the consequences of mixed infections in wild and domestic animals is a methodological challenge, but in experimental conditions, studies have proven a change of the infection profile in concomitant infection by *T. cruzi* isolates with distinct biological characteristics,[72] as well as the interaction of different genotypes molecular level.[73]

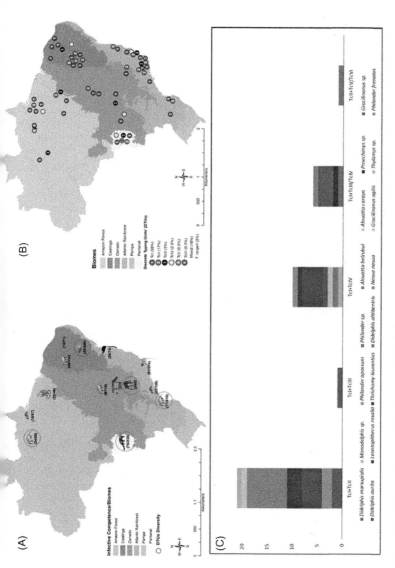

**Figure 12.1** (A) Map of the *T. cruzi* mammalian hosts with higher infective competence, showing the ones that displayed the higher DTU diversity in the wild environment from Brazilian biomes: Amazon Forest, Atlantic Forest, Caatinga, Cerrado, and Pantanal; (B) Spatial distribution of *T. cruzi* DTUs in the Brazilian biomes: Amazon Forest, Atlantic Forest, Caatinga, Cerrado, and Pantanal; (C) The distribution of the *T. cruzi* mixed DTU infections among naturally infected hosts in wild environments from Brazil.

*Source:* Adapted from Jansen AM, Xavier SC, Roque AL. The multiple and complex and changeable scenarios of the *Trypanosoma cruzi* transmission cycle in the sylvatic environment. Acta Trop 2015; pii: S0001-706X(15)30066-8. http://dx.doi.org/10.1016/j.actatropica.2015.07.018.

Evidently, we are underestimating the rate of mixed DTU infections. Actually, we are showing just what we could isolate through blood culture, a low sensitive and selective testing method. Even so, we found mixed infections in 16% of mammals with positive blood cultures[2] and Martinez-Perez et al.[67] found up to 22% of mixed infections among Latin America migrants in Spain. Probably these rates are much higher, especially considering that the absolute majority of the examined mammals displayed a subpatent infection by *T. cruzi*, demonstrated only by serological tests, as is the case of most of the dogs and cats examined in Brazil.[2]

# References

1. Noireau F, Diosque P, Jansen AM. *Trypanosoma cruzi*: adaptation to its vectors and its hosts. *Vet Res* 2009;**40**:26.
2. Jansen AM, Xavier SC, Roque AL. The multiple and complex and changeable scenarios of the *Trypanosoma cruzi* transmission cycle in the sylvatic environment. *Acta Trop* 2015. pii: S0001-706X(15)30066-8. Available from: http://dx.doi.org/10.1016/j.actatropica.2015.07.018.
3. Deane MP, Lenzi HL, Jansen AM. *Trypanosoma cruzi*: vertebrate and invertebrate cycles in the same mammal host, the opossum *Didelphis marsupialis*. *Mem Inst Oswaldo Cruz* 1984;**79**:513−15.
4. Steindel M, Pinto CJ. *Trypanosoma cruzi* development in the anal glands of experimentally infected *Lutreolina crassicaudata* (Marsupialia, Didelphidae). *Mem Inst Oswaldo Cruz* 1988;**83**:397.
5. Herrera L, Martinez C, Carrasco H, Jansen AM, Urdaneta-Morales S. Cornea as a tissue reservoir of *Trypanosoma cruzi*. *Parasitol Res* 2007;**100**:1395−9.
6. Nouvellet P, Dumonteil E, Gourbire S. The improbable transmission of *Trypanosoma cruzi* to human: the missing link in the dynamics and control of Chagas disease. *PLoS Negl Trop Dis* 2013;**7**(11):e2505.
7. Yoshida N. *Trypanosoma* cruzi infection by oral route: how the interplay between parasite and host components modulates infectivity. *Parasitol Int* 2008;**57**(2):105−9.
8. Yoshida N. Molecular mechanisms of *Trypanosoma cruzi* infection by oral route. *Mem Inst Oswaldo Cruz* 2009;**104**(Suppl. 1):101−7.
9. Kribs-Zaleta CM. Alternative transmission modes for *Trypanosoma cruzi*. *Math Biosci Eng* 2010;**7**(3):657−73. Available from: http://dx.doi.org/10.3934/mbe.2010.7.657.
10. Carlier Y, Truyens C. Congenital Chagas disease as an ecological model of interactions between *Trypanosoma cruzi* parasites, pregnant women, placenta and fetuses. *Acta Trop* 2015;**151**:103−15. Available from: http://dx.doi.org/10.1016/j.actatropica.2015.07.016.
11. Dias JCP. Elimination of Chagas disease transmission: perspectives. *Mem Inst Oswaldo Cruz* 2009;**104**(Suppl. 1):41−5.
12. Barretto MP, Ribeiro RD. Reservatórios silvestres do *Trypanosoma* (*Schizotrypanum*) *cruzi*, Chagas 1909. *Rev Inst Adolfo Lutz* 1979;**39**:25−36.
13. Gürtler RE, Cardinal MV. Reservoir host competence and the role of domestic and commensal hosts in the transmission of *Trypanosoma cruzi*. *Acta Trop* 2015;**151**:32−50. Available from: http://dx.doi.org/10.1016/j.actatropica.2015.05.029.
14. Mortara RA, Andreoli WK, Fernandes MC, da Silva CV, Fernandes AB, L'Abbate C, et al. Host cell actin remodeling in response to *Trypanosoma cruzi*: trypomastigote versus amastigote entry. *Subcell Biochem* 2008;**47**:101−9.

15. Lachaud L, Marchergui-Hammami S, Chabbert E, Dereure J, Dedet JP, Bastien P. Comparison of six PCR methods using peripheral blood for detection of canine visceral leishmaniasis. *J Clin Microbiol* 2002;**40**:210−15.

16. Piron M, Fisa R, Casamitjana N, López-Chejade P, Puig L, Vergés M, et al. Development of a real-time PCR assay for *Trypanosoma cruzi* detection in blood samples. *Acta Trop* 2007;**103**:195−200.

17. Castro AM, Luquetti AO, Rassi A, Rassi GG, Chiari E, Galvão LMC. Blood culture and polymerase chain reaction for the diagnosis of the chronic phase of human infection with *Trypanosoma cruzi*. *Parasitol Res* 2002;**88**:894−900.

18. Britto CC. Usefulness of PCR-based assays to assess drug efficacy in Chagas disease chemotherapy: value and limitations. *Mem Inst Oswaldo Cruz* 2009;**104**(S1):122−35.

19. Ramírez JC, Cura CI, da Cruz Moreira O, Lages-Silva E, Juiz N, Velázquez E, et al. Analytical validation of quantitative real-time PCR methods for quantification of *Trypanosoma cruzi* DNA in blood samples from Chagas disease patients. *J Mol Diagn* 2015;**17**(5):605−15.

20. Roque ALR, Xavier SCC, da Rocha MG, Duarte AC, D'Andrea PS, Jansen AM. *Trypanosoma cruzi* transmission cycle among wild and domestic mammals in three areas of orally transmitted Chagas disease outbreaks. *Am J Trop Med Hyg* 2008;**79**:742−9.

21. PAHO—Pan-American Health Organization. Doença de Chagas—guia para vigilância, prevenção, controle e manejo clínico da doença de Chagas aguda transmitida por alimentos. 2009. p. 92. Available in: http://bvs.panalimentos.org/local/File/Guia_Doenca_Chagas_2009.pdf.

22. Ashford RW. What it takes to be a reservoir host. *Bel J Zool* 1997;**127**:85−90.

23. Desbiez ALJ, Kluyber D. The role of giant armadillos (*Priodontes maximus*) as physical ecosystem engineers. *Biotropica* 2013;**45**(5):537−40.

24. Cássia-Pires R, Boité MC, D'Andrea PS, Herrera HM, Cupolillo E, Jansen AM, et al. Distinct *Leishmania* species infecting wild caviomorph rodents (Rodentia: Hystricognathi) from Brazil. *PLoS Negl Trop Dis* 2014;**11**;**8**(12):e3389. Available from: http://dx.doi.org/10.1371/journal.pntd.0003389.

25. de Lima JS, Rocha FL, Alves FM, Lorosa ES, Jansen AM, de Miranda Mourão G. Infestation of arboreal nests of coatis by triatomine species, vectors of *Trypanosoma cruzi*, in a large Neotropical wetland. *J Vector Ecol* 2015;**40**(2):379−85.

26. Herrera HM, Rocha FL, Lisboa CV, Rademaker V, Mourão GM, Jansen AM. Food web connections and the transmission cycles of *Trypanosoma cruzi* and *Trypanosoma evansi* (Kinetoplastida, Trypanosomatidae) in the Pantanal Region, Brazil. *Trans R Soc Trop Med Hyg* 2011;**105**(7):380−7. Available from: http://dx.doi.org/10.1016/j.trstmh.2011.04.008.

27. Barnabé C, Mobarec HI, Jurado MR, Cortez JA, Brenière SF. Reconsideration of the seven discrete typing units within the species *Trypanosoma cruzi*, a new proposal of three reliable mitochondrial clades. *Infect Genet Evol* 2016;**39**:176−86.

28. Shofield CJ, Janin J, Salvatella R. The future of Chagas disease control. *Trends Parasitol* 2006;**22**:583−8.

29. Dias JCP. Southern Cone Initiative for the elimination of domestic populations of *Triatoma infestans* and the interruption of transfusional Chagas disease. Historical aspects, present situation, and perspectives. *Mem Inst Oswaldo Cruz* 2007;**102**:11−18.

30. Coura JR, Barrett TV, Naranjo MA. Human populations attacked by wild Triatominae in the Amazonas: a new form of transmission of Chagas disease? *Rev Soc Bras Med Trop* 1994;**27**(4):251−4.

31. Coura JR, Junqueira AC, Fernandes O, Valente SA, Miles MA. Emerging Chagas disease in Amazonian Brazil. *Trends Parasitol* 2002;**4**:171—6.
32. Coura JR, Viñas PA, Junqueira AC. Ecoepidemiology, short history and control of Chagas disease in the endemic countries and the new challenge for non-endemic countries. *Mem Inst Oswaldo Cruz* 2014;**109**(7):856—62.
33. Xavier SCC, Roque ALR, Bilac D, de Araújo VAL, Neto SFC, Lorosa ES, et al. *Distantiae* transmission of *Trypanosoma cruzi*: a new epidemiological feature of acute Chagas disease in Brazil. *PLoS Negl Trop Dis* 2014;**8**(5):e2878. Available from: http://dx.doi.org/10.1371/journal.pntd.0002878.
34. Ostfeld RS, Keesing F. Biodiversity and disease risk: the case of Lyme disease. *Conserv Biol* 2000;**14**:722—8.
35. Chaves LF, Hernandez MJ. Mathematical modeling of American cutaneous leishmaniasis: incidental hosts and threshold conditions for infection persistence. *Acta Trop* 2004;**92**:245—52.
36. Dobson A, Cattadori I, Holt RD, Ostfeld RS, Keesing F, Krichbaum K, et al. Sacred cows and sympathetic squirrels: the importance of biological diversity to human health. *PLoS Med* 2006;**3**:e231.
37. Kilpatrick AM, Kramer LD, Jones MJ, Marra PP, Daszak P. West Nile virus epidemics in North America are driven by shifts in mosquito feeding behavior. *PLoS Biol* 2006;**4**:e82.
38. Vaz VC, D'Andrea PS, Jansen AM. Effects of habitat fragmentation on wild mammal infection by *Trypanosoma cruzi*. *Parasitology* 2007;**134**:1785—93.
39. Xavier SC, Roque AL, Lima Vdos S, Monteiro KJ, Otaviano JC, et al. Lower richness of small wild mammal species and Chagas disease risk. *PLoS Negl Trop Dis* 2012;**6**(5): e1647. Available from: http://dx.doi.org/10.1371/journal.pntd.0001647.
40. Gurtler RE, Cecere MC, Lauricella MA, Cardinal MV, Kitron U, Cohen JE. Domestic dogs and cats as sources of *Trypanosoma cruzi* infection in rural northwestern Argentina. *Parasitol* 2007;**134**:69—82.
41. Crisante G, Rojas A, Teixeira MM, Añez N. Infected dogs as a risk factor in the transmission of human *Trypanosoma cruzi* infection in western Venezuela. *Acta Trop* 2006;**98**:247—54.
42. Chapman MD, Baggaley RC, Godfrey-Faussett PF, Malpas TJ, White G, Canese J, et al. *Trypanosoma cruzi* from the Paraguay Chaco: isoenzyme profiles of strains isolated at Makthlawaiya. *J Protozool* 1984;**31**:482—6.
43. Cardinal MV, Lauricella MA, Ceballos LA, Lanati L, Marcet PL, Levin MJ, et al. Molecular epidemiology of domestic and sylvatic *Trypanosoma cruzi* infection in rural northwestern Argentina. *Int J Parasitol* 2008;**38**:1533—43.
44. Monje-Rumi MM, Brandán CP, Ragone PG, Tomasini N, Lauthier JJ, Alberti D'Amato AM, et al. *Trypanosoma cruzi* diversity in the Gran Chaco: mixed infections and differential host distribution of TcV and TcVI. *Infect Genet Evol* 2015;**29**:53—9.
45. Ramírez JD, Turriago B, Tapia-Calle G, Guhl F. Understanding the role of dogs (*Canis lupus familiaris*) in the transmission dynamics of *Trypanosoma cruzi* genotypes in Colombia. *Vet Parasitol* 2013;**196**:216—19.
46. Marcili A, Valente VC, Valente SA, Junqueira AC, da Silva FM, Pinto AY. *Trypanosoma cruzi* in Brazilian Amazonia: Lineages TCI and TCIIa in wild primates, *Rhodnius* spp. and in humans with Chagas disease associated with oral transmission. *Int J Parasitol* 2009;**39**:615—23.
47. Lima VS, Xavier SCC, Maldonado IFR, Roque ALR, Vicente ACP, Jansen AM. Expanding the knowledge of the geographic distribution of *Trypanosoma cruzi* TcII and TcV/TcVI genotypes in the Brazilian Amazon. *PLoS One* 2014;**9**(12):e116137. Available from: http://dx.doi.org/10.1371/journal.pone.0116137.

48. Kjos SA, Snowden KF, Craig TM, Lewis B, Ronald N, Olson JK. Distribution and characterization of canine Chagas disease in Texas. *Vet Parasitol* 2008;**15**:249−56.
49. Roque ALR, Jansen AM. Importância dos animais domésticos sentinelas na identificação de áreas de risco de emergência de doença de Chagas. *Rev Soc Bras Med Trop* 2008;**41**(Sup. III):191−3.
50. Andrade SG, Campos RF, Sobral KS, Magalhães JB, Guedes RS, Guerreiro ML. Reinfections with strains of *Trypanosoma cruzi* of different biodemes as a factor of aggravation of myocarditis and myositis in mice. *Rev Soc Bras Med Trop* 2006;**39**(1):1−8.
51. Lauricella MA, Riarte A, Lazzari JO, Barousse AP, Segura EL. Chagas' disease in dogs experimentally infected with *Trypanosoma cruzi*. *Medicina (B Aires)* 1986;**46** (2):195−200.
52. Machado EM, Fernandes AJ, Murta SM, Vitor RW, Camilo DJ Jr, Pinheiro SW, et al. A study of experimental reinfection by *Trypanosoma cruzi* in dogs. *Am J Trop Med Hyg* 2001;**65**:958−65.
53. Roque ALR, Xavier SCC, Gerhardt M, Silva MFO, Lima VS, D'Andrea PS, et al. *Trypanosoma cruzi* among wild and domestic mammals in different areas of the Abaetetuba municipality (Pará State, Brazil), an endemic Chagas disease transmission area. *Vet Parasitol* 2013;**193**:71−7.
54. Enriquez GF, Cardinal MV, Orozco MM, Schijman AG, Gürtler RE. Detection of *Trypanosoma cruzi* infection in naturally-infected dogs and cats using serological, parasitological and molecular methods. *Acta Trop* 2013;**126**(3):211−17.
55. Rimoldi A, Tomé Alves R, Ambrósio DL, Fernandes MZ, Martinez I, De Araújo RF, et al. Morphological, biological and molecular characterization of three strains of *Trypanosoma cruzi* Chagas, 1909 (Kinetoplastida, Trypanosomatidae) isolated from *Triatoma sordida* (Stal) 1859 (Hemiptera, Reduviidae) and a domestic cat. *Parasitology* 2012;**139**(1):37−44.
56. Eloy LJ, Lucheis SB. Hemoculture and polymerase chain reaction using primers TCZ1/ TCZ2 for the diagnosis of canine and feline trypanosomiasis. *ISRN Vet Sci* 2012;419378.
57. Valente VC, Valente SA, Noireau F, Carrasco HJ, Miles MA. Chagas disease in Amazon basin: association of *Panstrongylus geniculatus* (Hemiptera: Reduviidae) with domestic pigs. *J Med Entomol* 1998;**35**:99−103.
58. Salazar-Schettino PM, Bucio MI, Cabrera M, Bautista J. First case of natural infection in pigs. Review of *Trypanosoma cruzi* reservoirs in Mexico. *Mem Inst Oswaldo Cruz* 1997;**92**:499−502.
59. Herrera L, D'Andrea PS, Xavier SC, Mangia RH, Fernandes O, Jansen AM. *Trypanosoma cruzi* infection in wild mammals of the National Park 'Serra da Capivara' and its surroundings (Piaui, Brazil), an area endemic for Chagas disease. *Trans R Soc Trop Med Hyg* 2005;**99**:379−88.
60. Rozas M, Botto-Mahan C, Coronado X, Ortiz S, Cattan PE, Solari A. Coexistence of *Trypanosoma cruzi* genotypes in wild and peridomestic mammals in Chile. *Am J Trop Med Hyg* 2007;**77**:647−53.
61. Fernandes AJ, Vitor RW, Dias JC. Parasitologic and serologic evaluation of caprines experimentally inoculated with *Trypanosoma cruzi*. *Rev Inst Med Trop São Paulo* 1994;**36**:11−17.
62. Kierszenbaum F, Gottilieb CA, Budzko DB. Antibody-independent, natural resistance of birds to *Trypanosoma cruzi* infection. *J Parasitol* 1981;**67**:656−60.
63. Kollien AH, Schaub GA. The development of *Trypanosoma cruzi* in triatominae. *Parasitol Today* 2000;**16**:381−7.

64. Herrera HM, Rademaker V, Abreu UG, D'Andrea PS, Jansen AM. Variables that modulate the spatial distribution of *Trypanosoma cruzi* and *Trypanosoma evansi* in the Brazilian Pantanal. *Acta Trop* 2007;**102**:55−62.

65. Estrada-Franco JG, Bhatia V, Az-Albiter H, Ochoa-Garcia L, Barbosa A, Vazquez-Chagoyan JC, et al. Human *Trypanosoma cruzi* infection and seropositivity in dogs, Mexico. *Emerg Infect Dis* 2006;**12**:624−30.

66. Shadomy SV, Waring SC, Martins-Filho OA, Oliveira RC, Chappell CL. Combined use of enzyme-linked immunosorbent assay and flow cytometry to detect antibodies to *Trypanosoma cruzi* in domestic canines in Texas. *Clin Diagn Lab Immunol* 2004;**11**:313−19.

67. Martinez-Perez A, Poveda C, Ramírez JD, Norman F, Gironés N, Guhl F, et al. Prevalence of *Trypanosoma cruzi*'s discrete typing units in a cohort of Latin American migrants in Spain. *Acta Trop* 2016;**157**:145−50.

68. Moreira LA, Iturbe-Ormaetxe I, Jeffery JA, Lu G, Pyke AT, Hedges LM, et al. A Wolbachia symbiont in *Aedes aegypti* limits infection with dengue, Chikungunya, and *Plasmodium*. *Cell* 2009;**139**:1268−78.

69. Metenou S, Dembele B, Konate S, Dolo H, Coulibaly YI, Diallo AA, et al. Filarial infection suppresses malaria-specific multifunctional Th1 and Th17 responses in malaria and filarial coinfections. *J Immunol* 2011;**186**:4725−33.

70. Telfer S, Lambin X, Birtles R, Beldomenico P, Burthe S, Paterson S, et al. Species interaction in a parasite community drive infection risk in a wildlife population. *Science* 2010;**330**:243−6.

71. Araújo CA, Waniek PJ, Jansen AM. TcI/TcII co-infection can enhance *Trypanosoma cruzi* growth in *Rhodnius prolixus*. *Parasit Vectors* 2014;**7**:94. Available from: http://dx.doi.org/10.1186/1756-3305-7-94.

72. Ragone PG, Prez Brandn C, Monje Rumi M, Tomasini N, Lauthier JJ, Cimino RO, et al. Experimental evidence of biological interactions among different isolates of *Trypanosoma cruzi* from the Chaco region. *PLoS One* 2015;**10**(3):e0119866.

73. Machin A, Telleria J, Brizard JP, Demettre E, Sveno M, Ayala F, et al. *Trypanosoma cruzi*: gene expression surveyed by proteomic analysis reveals interaction between different genotypes in mixed in vitro cultures. *PLoS One* 2014;**9**(4):e95442.

# Veterinary aspects

*M. Desquesnes[1,2]*
[1]CIRAD-Bios, UMR177-Trypanosomes, Montpellier, France,
[2]Kasetsart University, Bangkok, Thailand

**13**

## Chapter Outline

## Introduction

*Trypanosoma cruzi* is a parasite in man but it is also a parasite in many other animal species both wild and domestic; human infection can occur in rural as well as in urban areas, which reveals various roles of insects and other mammals in its epidemiology.[1] Even if the main mammalian hosts and/or reservoirs are considered to be humans, marsupials, dogs, and cats,[2] a nonexhaustive list of 150−200 wild animals (including the vampire bat *Desmodus rotundus*) and some 10 domestic or peridomestic animals, which are found to be infected, has been compiled.[3,4] In particular, *T. cruzi* can be naturally found in dogs, cats, cattle, goats, sheep, rabbits, and equines.[3,5−7] Among susceptible domestic animals, guinea pigs may play an important epidemiological role, particularly in Peru where they are bred for meat. In Paraguay, it was suggested that cattle, pigs, dogs, and cats provide reservoirs for *T. cruzi*.[7] In French Guiana, the studies have shown that *Didelphis marsupialis* and *Philander opossum* are frequently infected,[8] as well as domestic dogs,[9] however, *T. cruzi* was not reported in livestock and humans.[10] Indeed, *T. cruzi* is rarely reported in livestock, but is it due to a lack of presence or a lack of investigation and a lack of an efficient diagnosis method?

From a veterinary point of view, it is difficult to classify these various categories of animals since their role is variable from one situation to another, and, in some instance, may be underestimated. As a first attempt to gather animals into categories, we can consider (1) animal species which are known to have a potential role in the epidemiology of the disease; they may be wild (opossum, armadillo, raccoons, rats, mice, etc.)

American Trypanosomiasis Chagas Disease. DOI: http://dx.doi.org/10.1016/B978-0-12-801029-7.00013-7

or domestic (dog, cat, guinea pig etc.); and (2) animals that are receptive but are not known to be reservoirs, although they may have a role in the epidemiology; they may be wild animals such as monkeys, deer, and wild pigs or domestic and/or livestock such as equidae, bovines, ovines, caprines, and suidae. A third category would be the experimental model animals which have been very useful to study the human disease, such as mice, rats, guinea pigs, hamsters, rabbits, dogs, and monkeys.

Wild animals as reservoir, domestic animals as reservoir, and animals as experimental models are studied respectively in three specific chapters, so the present chapter will focus on livestock infections. Due to the lack of knowledge on this latter part, it is important to overview the potential ways of infection of livestock and the difficulties encountered to establish a reliable diagnosis in these animal species. Indeed, a study aiming at establishing the seroprevalence of *T. cruzi* infection in livestock (or dogs) would meet the problem of species specificity due to the interference of *Trypanosoma vivax* and/or *Trypanosoma evansi* in the detection of *T. cruzi* infection, as well as *Leishmania* infections which are known to cross-react with trypanosomes antigens[11]; conversely, *T. cruzi* can interfere with the diagnosis of trypanosomoses in livestock, in particular serological diagnosis of *T. vivax* in ruminants and *T. evansi* in equines.[10]

In rodents, monkey, and dog—infections which have been observed under natural and experimental conditions—information on the pathogenicity and evolution of the infection is available; on the contrary, the information on the livestock aspects of *T. cruzi* infection is very limited, probably due to the following reasons: (1) *T. cruzi* infection is not suspected to be of medical and economical significance in livestock; (2) some of the symptoms are greatly delayed from the infection, far beyond the duration of most of the experimental designs in livestock species; (3) the lack of specificity of the diagnosis tools; (4) the existence of a high risk of human infection when handling experimentally infected animals, especially large animals such as horses and bovines; and (5) the existence of a great number of other obviously more important hosts and reservoirs of the parasite.

This chapter will present the scarce information on *T. cruzi*'s natural and experimental infections in livestock, but it will also focus on the specific natural way of infection of these animals and the potential and possible risks and way back of the infection from these animals toward other animals including humans. A part of it will be speculative due to the very poor information available on the real status and role of livestock in the epidemiology of the infection.

## The various ways of infection of animals (and humans)

*T. cruzi* is not a livestock trypanosome as such, but it is sometimes found in domestic ruminants, pigs, and horses. However, the ways of infection of livestock have not been studied; hypotheses can then be suggested based on the various ways of transmission of the parasite already known and briefly reminded here.

In humans, the transmission of *T. cruzi* is mainly due to the triatomine, or reduviid bugs, of the genera *Rhodnius*, *Panstrongylus*, and *Triatoma*.

The metacyclic trypomastigote infective form (metatrypanosome) present in the excrement of the bugs contaminates bite skin wounds or mucous membranes, particularly the eye; in this cycle, the best vectors are the bugs that defecate soon after having their blood meal. This transcutaneous or transconjunctival way of contamination to livestock and pets is possible, but might not be predominant.

Being a blood parasite, *T. cruzi* can be transmitted with blood by a number of ways with variable probability and consequences, depending on the host considered: laboratory accidents, blood transfusion, and organ transplants (humans)[12]; congenital transplacental (in utero) or perinatal infection[13]; surgery or any other iatrogenic transmission (human and animals); and mechanical transmission by tabanids and stomoxes (animals), but also by some other vectors should also be considered, such as lice which is a potential vector in monkeys,[14] etc.

However the most important secondary way of transmission of *T. cruzi* is by peroral route[15]: in humans and animals (1) by ingestion of infected flesh or blood, or (2) by ingestion of food infected by triatomine feces or opossum feces, and, in animals, (3) by ingestion of infected triatomine bugs themselves.

Indeed, the transmission of the infective forms found in the feces of the bugs can take the peroral route.[15] Recent work indicates that, in mice ingesting infected bugs or their excreta, the parasite gains an entry through the gastric mucosae and produces local immunity.[16] This may explain how a number of family infections arise from food contaminated by the excreta of the bugs.[17] Ingestion of infected bugs is also thought to be a significant cause of contamination of dogs, cats, and livestock. The peroral infection may have a significant role in the epidemiology of *T. cruzi* disease, especially in livestock, but also in humans as shown by the recent outbreaks in Brazil and Venezuela where humans were contaminated when ingesting fruit juice of either sugar cane in the Catarina State,[18] palm fruit in Pará and Amapá States,[19] or guava in a school in Caracas, Venezuela.[20] Experimental work proved that *T. cruzi* can survive at least 24 h in the sugar cane juice.[19] In an epidemic outbreak described and analyzed in Venezuela, in 2009, with *Panstrongylus geniculatus* as vector, 89 persons had a peroral contamination.[21] Additionally, it was recently demonstrated that nonsteroidal anti-inflammatory drugs such as aspirin may favor the peroral infection by *T. cruzi*, by the gastric mucosae.[22] Based on the increasing incidence of oral acute cases of Chagas disease, it appears that food is becoming one of the most important modes of transmission in the Amazon, Caribbean, and Andes regions of America.[21]

Similarly, if failing conventional transcutaneous transmission via reduviid bugs feces, livestock may be contaminated by ingesting these insects themselves or their *excreta* with feed contaminated by the bugs or by *D. marsupialis* feces. Cattle and horses rarely share the same habitat as reduviid bugs; for this reason and except in very unusual circumstances, contamination of cattle and horses by bugs would seem to be limited. However, small ruminants and pigs are more likely to share the same habitat as these vectors, in particular under conventional stock-farming conditions. The opossum (see below) is perhaps another important link in the chain of contamination, from the bugs to the livestock.

Carnivores and omnivores are exposed to a specific risk of peroral infection. Just as with *T. evansi*,[23] it was clear, from a very early stage, that the bloodstream form of *T. cruzi* was transmissible peroral,[24] even if the amastigote form is not infective.[25] Dias was able to achieve contamination of a cat by ingestion of infected rats. It can therefore be concluded that ingestion of the fresh raw flesh of infected animals can cause infections in humans and animals, in particular dogs (orodigestive transmission). Although this observation was not possible in raccoons fed with amastigote infected tissues, they were susceptible to trypomastigote ingestion; consequently, ingestion of infected fresh flesh should still be considered in the epidemiology of *T. cruzi* in carnivores but also in livestock such as pigs known to be able to eat flesh, notably that of rodents. Even horses should be considered here; indeed, one should be reminded of the origin of some important outbreaks of trichinellosis in Europe, where horses were thought to be infected by ingestion of infected mice broiled in their feed.[26]

As a stercorarian parasite, *T. cruzi* is cyclically transmitted by biting bugs, however, Triatomine insects are not the only cyclical vectors of *T. cruzi*. Indeed, the life cycle described in the gut of triatomines has also been observed in the lumen of the anal scent glands of *D. marsupialis* (southern opossum) in which the parasite multiplies as epimastigote and differentiates into metacyclic.[27] The parasites extracted from the scent glands have the same features as the metacyclic forms in insects and are infective via the subcutaneous, intraperitoneal, peroral, and transconjunctival routes.[28] Because infective forms of *T. cruzi* are present in the excreta of marsupials, contamination between marsupials is highly likely, making the opossum a true reservoir of the parasite. It also means that the parasite can be transmitted in the absence of insect vectors, e.g., in urban areas or in wild, through the contamination of food by opossum feces. All mammals can be contaminated via this way by the oral route.

On the basis of these observations, *D. marsupialis* can be classified amongst the biological reservoirs/hosts/vectors for cyclical transmission of *T. cruzi*; it is remarkable that the typical stercorarian cycle described for insects occurs in an analogue way in the distal portion of a mammal's gut.[10] Finally, triatomines and opossums may both contaminate the human and animal food making of Chagas disease not only a vector-borne but also a food-borne disease.

The role of opossum suggests that the extension of *T. cruzi* infection may even emancipate from the triatomine bug, and would be possible via the marsupials alone.

## The problem of diagnosis in animals

If the diagnosis of a pathogen in its favorite host is generally made easy by a natural high proliferation of the pathogen in this host and/or a strong immune response of the latter, this diagnosis is of lower efficacy (sensitivity especially) in hosts of lower susceptibility, due to the fact that the pathogenemia and/or the immune response can be low. In the case of *T. cruzi*, the diagnosis is already not easy in humans, but is considerably more difficult in animals in terms of sensitivity, due to very low and transient parasitemia, as well as in terms of specificity. Indeed, Latin

America is nowadays an endemic region for a number of *Trypanosoma* species which some of them can interfere in this detection, such as *T. rangeli, T. vivax, T. evansi, T. equiperdum,* and *T. theileri.*

In the early stage of the infection, *T. cruzi* is classically found in the host in circulating bloodstream forms. Its characteristics are: total length 16−22 μm, morphology of the parasite is C- or S-shaped; kinetoplast of large size (1.2 μm) and sometimes forms a "stain" that overlaps over the edge of the body; an undulating stunted membrane and a nucleus located in the central or front portion of the body (NI: 0.9−1.9 or more). In fresh samples, slender forms move rapidly while stumpy forms move slowly. Rather than replicating, this form invades the tissues and gives rise to an intracellular form of the Leishmania type that replicates in the amastigote, epimastigote, and trypomastigote forms located in the reticuloendothelial cells, muscles (including the heart), liver, nervous system, etc.[29]; bloodstream and tissue forms alternate periodically. From that stage, in terms of routine parasitological diagnosis, it becomes almost undetectable.

During the early stage, detection of the blood forms of *T. cruzi* in animals can be achieved by direct examination of blood, preferably after enrichment by centrifugation (Hematocrit Centrifuge Technique) as used for African animal trypanosomes.[30] Using this method, positive cases in livestock are rarely reported,[7] most probably because the parasitemia is low and transient. Mini anion column techniques are generally considered as too expensive for veterinary studies. More sensitive methods can be applied, such as mouse inoculation, but they are no longer popular since they are using living animal and present a risk of handling highly infective material for humans. The uses of xenodiagnosis and hemoculture are also limited in animals.

Nowadays, DNA detection is the most sensitive and specific method for diagnosis of active infection. Since the first specific primers for the detection of *T. cruzi* were described (TCZ1 and TCZ2),[31] a number of primers with variable levels of specificity have been published.[32] However, very few studies report their use for demonstrating the presence of the parasite in livestock. In fact, as indicated earlier, very few studies focus on *T. cruzi* in livestock.

Serological tests such as immuno-fluorescent assay (IFA) or enzyme linked immuno-sorbent assay (ELISA) can be used for detection of antibodies directed against *T. cruzi* in livestock; however the species specificity of these tests is not high. With African trypanosomes, the evaluation demonstrated a strong cross-reactivity between the various species (*T. brucei, T. vivax,* and *T. congolense*) which could even allow using heterologous antigens for diagnosis.[33] Complement Fixation Test (CFT), indirect hemagglutination test or the Card Agglutination Test for Trypanosome, CATT test-*T. evansi,* which cross-react with other trypanosomes, such as *T. congolense* and *T. vivax,* would most probably not be species-specific, but a few have been evaluated for their specificity toward *T. cruzi.* For example with IFA, animals infected with *T. vivax* or *T. congolense* produce up to 85% positive results using IFA for *T. brucei.* Cross-reactions between *T. evansi* and *T. cruzi* have been reported in horses[34−36] and between *T. evansi* and *T. vivax* in cattle.[37] In ELISA, using *T. evansi* antigens, it was demonstrated to have the same level of sensitivity and specificity as when using *T. cruzi* antigen for detection of *T. cruzi* infection in humans.[11] *T. evansi* is antigenically a very rich parasite—in Latin America, indirect-ELISA *T. evansi* is probably able to detect infections induced by *T. vivax*, *T. evansi*, *T. equiperdum*, and/or *T. cruzi* with almost equal effectiveness.

In fact cross-reactivity amongst salivarian and stercorarian have been recorded with all serological methods evaluated so far, and it should finally be concluded that none of them is able to detect specifically the pathogenic trypanosomes. With studies on *T. cruzi* being scarce in livestock, there are very few positive reference samples from livestock experimentally infected by *T. cruzi*. This obviously limits the evaluation of cross-reactions and the value of serological findings, but based on the experience of African trypanosomes and on what has been achieved so far by Monzon et al.[34,36] it can be speculated that the species specificity of *T. cruzi* serological tests would be very low in endemic areas of *T. evansi* and *T. vivax*.

*Trypanosoma vivax*, *T. evansi*, *T. cruzi*, and *T. equiperdum* have been reported in practically all Latin American countries. With all of the serological tools being unable to discriminate these species, knowledge on the distribution, prevalence, and medical and economic impact of *T. cruzi* in livestock is therefore very limited. Improving the diagnostic tools is a priority if better knowledge of livestock trypanosomoses in this region of the world is to be achieved.

Serological studies carried out with *T. cruzi* antigens would be very risky to analyze in areas potentially infected by other *Trypanosoma* species, especially *T. evansi* and especially if the latter is highly endemic while the status of the former one is really unknown and unsuspected. Interpretation of such surveys should be made with high care. Moreover and reciprocally, leishmaniosis could also strongly interfere in such serological studies.[38,39]

Finally, little can be concluded from studies strictly conducted with serological tools in potentially mixed infected hosts and areas (other *Trypanosoma* and *Leishmania* species), unless they are completed by DNA tools specific for *T. cruzi*.

## Natural infections in domestic animals and livestock

The role of animals in the epidemiology of Chagas disease is variable, depending on the type of the 200 species found infected.[4] Thus we can globally divide them into three categories which may be involved in the three mammalian cycles (domestic, peridomestic, and wild).

Domestic species are dogs, cats, guinea pigs, hamsters, and rabbits. *T. cruzi* is markedly pathogenic in dogs (and to a lesser extend in cats) in which it produces cardiac signs with a potentially fatal outcome. It is speculated that dogs and cat can get the infection by the bug's bite, but also by eating infected bugs, or, by eating fresh infected preys (especially mice for cats), and may have an important role in the epidemiology of the human disease in some circumstances, like in Argentina[40] or in newly settled human populations of Amazon.[41] The prevalence of infection in domestic carnivores is around 10% in Chile, 9−24% in Mexico,[42] 20% in Brazil, 37% in dogs and cats in Paraguay,[7] and 42% in Argentina,[40] and up to 50% in dogs in some areas of Venezuela. An expert report published by WHO on Chagas disease[3] mentions that the studies conducted in Argentina, Brazil, Chile, Bolivia, and Venezuela yield highly variable rates of infection by *T. cruzi* that range, in humans, from 0.5% to 2% in large cities, to between 20% and 63% in highly endemic areas; in dogs, from 4.5% to 100% and, in cats, from 0.5% to 60.9%. In Chile, serological studies in the provinces of Elqui, Limari, and Choapa revealed the presence of antibodies for 12−24% of dogs, 0−15% of cats, and 4−26% of rabbits.[6] In guinea pigs in Bolivia, prevalence ranges from 10% to 60%.[43] In the United States, dogs are sometimes found infected and are most often related to human cases[44]; sporting and working breeds account for the majority of the cases, presumably due to greater exposure to infected vectors and mammalian tissues.[45]

Domestic but living in the peridomestic area are the livestock species such as cattle, buffaloes, horses, sheep, goats, and pigs. None of them is considered to be highly susceptible to the infection by *T. cruzi*. In Chile, serological studies in the provinces of Elqui, Limari, and Choapa revealed the presence of antibodies in 5−12% of goats and 4.8% of sheep.[6] In another study in Chile, the seroprevalence by IFA and ELISA in goats ranged from 6.5% to 38.3%.[46] In Paraguay, a survey demonstrated that antibodies raised against *T. cruzi* were found in 8% of cattle and 10% of pigs.[7] Ox and pigs were found to be naturally infected in Mexico.[5] In the other countries, very little, if any, information is available. In some instances, *T. cruzi* could be isolated from these animals, but in serological surveys conducted in areas endemic for other *Trypanosoma* species, the seroprevalence observed cannot be attributed to *T. cruzi* with certainty. Because appropriate diagnostic tools are lacking, the prevalences in livestock cannot really be determined. Putting aside *Trypanosoma theileri*, which does not induce serological cross-reaction with other *Trypanosoma* species, there is a reciprocal interference of all trypanosomes potentially present in livestock: *T cruzi*, *T. equiperdum*, and *T. evansi* in equids, and *T. cruzi*, *T. evansi*, and *T. vivax* in others. For example, in 1995 although there were no clinical signs, positive antibody serologies (CFT) for *T. equiperdum* were found in the state of Chihuahua (Mexico) on horses and mules intended for export to the United States. The same samples tested for *T. cruzi* with hemagglutination inhibition also turned out positive. The positive animals were slaughtered but infection was never demonstrated. Furthermore, investigations conducted on 3000 equidae in that state were never able to isolate the pathogen or discover clinical signs of dourine. Interference from *T. cruzi* or *T. evansi* may be the cause of serological cross-reactions. *T. cruzi* has been found in circulation in Mexico even in urban areas; a recent serological survey has shown that 8.8−24.2% of dogs are infected.[42] Another example is in Argentina, where diagnosis in horses cannot distinguish *T. evansi* from *T. cruzi* infection, both of them being equally probable.[34−36] Hence, it would seem that the incidence of *T. cruzi* infection of livestock is by no means negligible. Little research has been conducted either in the field, where no specific diagnostic tools are available, or under experimental conditions owing to the limited risk of human infection and/or a lack of interest in this work because its pathogenicity is presumed to be low and because of the short economic life expectancy of farm animals. However the recent case of a 10-year-old Texan Quarter horse found to be infected brings a new light on the potential for horse infection by *T. cruzi*[47]; this animal exhibited ataxia and lameness in the hind limbs for 6 months and was finally euthanized after its condition worsened. Amastigote trypanosomes morphologically similar to *T. cruzi*, were detected within segments of the thoracic spinal cord, with mild lymphoplasmacytic inflammation. Identification was confirmed by *T. cruzi* satellite DNA polymerase chain reaction (PCR) and sequencing. Such a case might easily remain undetected if the authors were not be so cautious. *T. cruzi* should now be considered as a differential diagnosis in horses with similar neurologic clinical signs and lesions.[47] Horses and other livestock infections might occur and remain undetected if accurate diagnosis procedures are not employed.

Synanthropic species, which may be peridomestic or sylvatic, are mice, rats, armadillos, raccoons, coyotes, and marsupials; the latter are considered to be the oldest and most important reservoir of the parasite.[48] In a review made in Mexico in 1997, 12 peridomestic mice, rats, squirrel, armadillo, bat, and marsupials were found to be infected. A huge number of species have been found to be infected but few studies indicate the prevalence of the infection; it ranges from 13% in octodon (*Octodon degus*) to 28% in rats (*Rattus rattus*) in Chile,[49] and from 6% in *P. opossum* to 43% in *D. marsupialis* in French Guiana.[8] Complex epidemiological features may include marsupials, armadillo, monkeys, and raccoons as reservoirs, bugs as active or passive vectors toward same or other host species, including mice and rats, which may be responsible for the infection of cats and dogs. The epidemiological studies carried out in diverse circumstances tend to show how complex and unique the situations can be, therefore no generalization or prediction should be made and each ecotope should be considered as an unique system.[48] In a sylvatic area Brazil, collared peccary (*Tayassu tajacu*), white-lipped peccary (*Tayassu pecari*), and feral pig (*Sus scrofa*) are maintenance hosts for *Trypanosoma cruzi* and *Trypanosoma evansi*.[50] In wild rabbits, prevalence reaches 38% in Chile.[51] In Bolivia, wild populations of *Triatoma infestans* were shown to create a link between humans and domestic and peridomestic hosts, including cat, donkey, and wild rodents.[52] In the United States, *T. cruzi* is frequently found in raccoons; in Tennessee, a higher seroprevalence is observed in rural habitats (35%) than in suburban habitats (23%) with an average of 29%,[53] but it can reach 63% in Oklahoma[54]; however autochtonous human cases seem to be related to both raccoons and dogs.[44]

# Experimental infections in livestock

Most of the experimental work done in *T. cruzi* was carried out in rats and mice, monkeys or dogs.[55−57] In some instances other models have been used, such as rabbit or even the stripped skunk[58] which appear to be also a natural host of *T. cruzi* in Argentina[59] but very little of the experimental studies concern livestock.

Young pigs, lambs, kids, and calves were proved to be susceptible to *T. cruzi* infection in experimental conditions in the United states,[60] but little is known about the pathogenicity since no clinical signs were detected; however 10% of the animals had tissue stages, suggesting a possible role in the epidemiology of the disease. The infection persisted at least 21 days in calves, 38 days in kids, 53 days in lambs, and 57 days in pigs.

In experimentally infected kids, no symptoms were visible although a ventricular hypertrophy was detected using electrocardiography.[46] The long-term effects of the infection deserve more thorough investigation.

In experimental infection of four English pigs challenged with a virulent Peruvian strain of *T. cruzi*, only three became infected. The course of the infection in the pigs was mild and the parasitemia too low to be detected except by mouse inoculation.[61]

In all cases, pathogenicity, but also role of livestock appeared to be fairly low according to the few experimental findings available, but certainly, duration of the observation under these experimental designs are too short to observe a complete range of pathogenicity of this slow developing disease.

Recent studies have emphasized the importance of two types of peridomestic reservoirs for *T. cruzi* that had so far been underestimated: pets (dogs, cats, guinea pigs, and other rodents) but also farm bred animals (horses, cattle, sheep, goats, pigs, rabbits, and guinea pigs).[5] Indeed, the peridomestic cycles are precisely those that present the highest risk of human contamination.[62] The effective involvement of livestock in the epidemiology of Chagas disease is very difficult to estimate because of the (sometimes high) prevalence of true livestock trypanosomes (*T. vivax*, *T. evansi*, and *T. equiperdum*). Since receptivity and susceptibility of livestock appeared to be low in these scarce experimental studies, with low and transient parasitemia, livestock infections probably play only a minor role in the epidemiology of the human disease, and, livestock is probably an epidemiological dead end. However, in disadvantaged rural populations, close cohabitation between species might foster peridomestic zoonotic spread of the parasite. Disease control relies essentially on hygiene and education of the populations at risk. Veterinary practitioners who deal with pets and livestock in endemic areas and veterinarians that work in the disadvantaged areas where there is little separation between human and animal habitats should be warned. A positive diagnosis in an animal may be an indication of risk for humans.

Pathogenicity of *T. cruzi* in livestock is assumed to be low but it requires further investigation to determine the potential role of these animals in the epidemiology of the disease.

## New cycles establish in the United States

Although Chagas disease in humans is generally considered to be present in Latin America from 38°S up to the southern part of Mexico (25°N), *T. cruzi* is present from Argentina and Chile (43°S) up to the southern part of the United States (42°N), as high as in Missouri, occasionally in humans, and regularly in domestic animals, particularly dogs and cats,[62] but also in a large range of wild animals, such as opossums, wood rats, racoons, striped skunks, armadillos, antelope squirrels, gray foxes, and coyotes,[2,63] with some high prevalences such as 33% in opossum and 63% in raccoons.[4]

*T. cruzi* is known to be present in the following states: California, Arizona, Texas, Oklahoma, Tennessee, Missouri, Louisiana, Florida, Georgia, Virginia, South Carolina, and North Carolina.[53,63–68] In humans in Texas, blood donor screenings have shown prevalence of antibodies to *T. cruzi* as high as 1/6500, and a strong link was drawn with poverty,[69] however, the rate of possibly autochtonous cases was not determined.

Several vectors have been reported in the United States: *Triatoma gersaecheri* in Texas; *Triatoma sanguisuga* and *T. lecticularia* in South Carolina and Georgia, etc.[66] The very few cases of native Chagas disease were recorded in California, Texas, and Tennessee, most often by means of postmortem PCR.[70,71] Many wild and domestic animals were found to be infected, sometimes with high prevalence, such as in armadillos, badgers, and coyotes, as well as cattle and sheep which were found to be carriers of antibodies in Texas and Louisiana; in South Carolina and Georgia, nearly 50% of raccoons (*Procyon lotor*) were serologically positive as well as some opossums (*Didelphis virginiana*).[66]

The isolation of *T. cruzi* in dogs in Virginia[72] showed that a new epidemiological pattern is being established by the spread of the parasite; in this case, the mother Walker hound and seven of its eight pups were found to be infected. This pattern relies on a wild host/bug/carnivore cycle in which wild host or rodents probably act as reservoir (direct transmission from rodent to rodent is also possible by biting) whereas dogs are thought to be an epidemiological cul-de-sac.

In Tennessee, five autochtonous human cases were reported so far; in the last case, a child was infected without significant clinical signs and would not have been detected if the bugs had not been noticed by the mother; in this case *Triatoma sanguisuga* were caught and found to be infected as well as three raccoons which were trapped in the vicinity of the house.[71]

Another autochtonous case was reported from California[73] and the strain isolated could develop in two species of triatominae native to California: *Triatoma protracta* and *T. rubida*.

The way of infection of autochtonous human cases have not been identified yet. Several hypotheses remain, including vectorial transmission, transconjunctival or peroral infection by bug feces or contaminated food, or another unidentified way.

These cases where the origin and way of infection are not clearly elucidated do not preclude the possible cyclical transmission of the parasite by a vicariant vector that the parasite might be found on its way toward the North.

One must remember that cyclical transmission of *T. cruzi* has been described in opossums (*D. marsupialis*).[28] Hence, in the United States, *T. cruzi* has a huge wild and domestic reservoir together with two cyclical vectors (bugs and opossum) and other potential vectors (louse). Infections in dogs are seen more and more often. It is presumed that the main cycle occurs in bugs and wild animals (raccoons and opossums). Domestic animals are infected by ingesting bugs and/or, in the case of carnivores, by ingesting infected wild prey. Although infected bugs may be found in the vicinity of human habitat, there are very few reports of human contamination and this is thought to be attributable to the long interval that elapses in the United States between the time when the vectors take their meals and the time when they defecate, making it unlikely for a bite wound to be contaminated, i.e., the most common mode of human contamination in South America. Furthermore, living and hygiene conditions in the United States are far less likely to foster contact between humans and vectors than those that prevail in Latin America. However, dogs and cats may be a potential link between wild reservoir and humans, since they attract and/or maintain bugs in the vicinity of human habitat, thus making possible the contamination of human's food by bug's feces.

Progression in the distribution and establishment of *T. cruzi* should be taken very seriously. *T. cruzi* is already capable of transmitting cyclically in the United States, by ingestion of food contaminated by opossum or bugs excreta and by entry of the metatrypanosomes present in the feces of bugs (or opossum) through bite wounds or mucosal membranes. Thus, infection focus in humans can already occur in the United States by a similar way as in Brazil where numerous people have been infected when drinking fruit juice, further to the contamination of the fruit stock or utensils by bugs or opossum's feces. Eloquent is the recent case detected in a Texan horse, indicating that horse, and possibly other domestic animals such as livestock, may already act potential links between wild fauna and humans.[47] The geographical extension of *T. cruzi* in wild and peridomestic fauna is currently spreading. Furthermore, *T. cruzi* may be able to find vicarious vectors in the course of its progression, possibly establishing a new epidemiological link to humans.


# Conclusions

The data brought by the veterinary aspects of *T. cruzi* are of various types.

The data based on the observation of the parasite in insects and wild animals as well as in domestic animals such as dogs and cats allowed to evaluate the geographical distribution of *T. cruzi* (especially toward its northern limit if any) and then to estimate the existence of a potential risk for human exposure outside the endemic area of typical Chagas disease.

*T. cruzi* occurs in livestock but its incidence is poorly known because no adequate diagnostic tools exist. In view of its epidemiology, it can be assumed that livestock is not highly exposed to infection. However, according to recent investigations, prevalence is not insignificant. Its occurrence in livestock deserves special attention and further investigation.

Although the human disease is typically South American ($25°N-38°S$), the parasite is spreading northward in the United States to Texas, California, and Virginia where the main epidemiological vehicles would appear to be dogs and wild animals (opossums, raccoons, etc.), but also occurring in horse. It is likely that *T. cruzi* in North America fulfils its complete cycle in *D. virginiana*[66] in much the same way as has already been described for South America in *D. marsupialis*.[28] In view of the parasite's huge domestic and wild reservoir and its various transmission modes (including the peroral route), it is reasonable to predict that *T. cruzi* will maintain and extend its area of establishment northwards. In addition, the long incubation period for Chagas disease and its weak obvious clinical incidence makes it a covert scourge that tends to be underestimated and belatedly discovered. Finally, just like *T. evansi* in vampire bats, it could be that *T. cruzi* is able to call on new vectors in North America and thereby renew its geographical progression, and possibly eventually find a new epidemiological link leading to human infections. It is advisable to call the attention of the US sanitary authorities to this threat. The spreading of *T. cruzi* would most probably lead, at some time if not already, to the extension of Chagas disease.

Finally, it must also be emphasized that new cycles could just as well be established in other countries where potential vectors of *Trypanosoma cruzi* are endemic, such as in Asia, Thailand for example, where *Triatoma rubrofasciata* seems to be well established. Travel of Latin American carriers to such areas could lead to the establishment of new endemic areas. Diagnosis of such infection in Asia for instance would of course not be early, due to epidemiological and geographical considerations. Serological surveillance in humans could be one of the ways to ensure free status of such countries.

# References

1. Medrano-Mercado N, Ugarte-Fernandez R, Butron V, Uber-Busek S, Guerra HL, Araujo-Jorge TC, et al. Urban transmission of Chagas disease in Cochabamba, Bolivia. *Mem Inst Oswaldo Cruz* 2008;**103**(5):423−30.
2. Woo P, Soltys M. Animals as reservoir hosts of human trypanosomes. *J Wildl Dis* 1970; **6**:313−22.
3. Anonyme. Lutte contre la maladie de Chagas. *OMS Serie de rapports techniques, Genève* 1991;**811**:106.
4. Roellig DM, Ellis AE, Yabsley MJ. Genetically different isolates of *Trypanosoma cruzi* elicit different infection dynamics in raccoons (*Procyon lotor*) and Virginia opossums (*Didelphis virginiana*). *Int J Parasitol* 2009;**39**(14):1603−10.
5. Salazar-Schettino PM, Bucio MI, Cabrera M, Bautista J. First case of natural infection in pigs. Review of *Trypanosoma cruzi* reservoirs in Mexico. *Mem Inst Oswaldo Cruz* 1997;**92**(4):499−502.
6. Correa V, Briceno J, Zuniga J, Aranda JC, Valdes J, Contreras C,M, et al. Infeccion por *Trypanosoma cruzi* en animales domesticos de sectores rurales de la IV region Chile. *Bol, Chile Parasit* 1982;**37**:27−8.
7. Fujita O, Sanabria L, Inschaustti A, De Arias A, Tomizawa Y, Oku Y. Animal reservoirs for *Trypanosoma cruzi* infection in an endemic area in Paraguay. *J Vet Med Sci* 1994;**56**:305−8.
8. Dedet JP, Chippaux JP, Goyot FX, Tibayrenc M, Geoffroy B, Gosselin H, et al. Les hôtes naturels de *Trypanosoma cruzi* en Guyane Française. *Ann Parasitol Hum Comp* 1985;**60**:111−17.
9. Raccurt CP. *Trypanosoma cruzi* en Guyane Française: revue des données accumulées depuis 1940. *Med Trop* 1996;**56**:79−87.
10. Desquesnes M. *Livestock trypanosomoses and their vectors in Latin America*. Paris: CIRAD-EMVT Publication, OIE; 2004. p. 174, ISBN 92-9044-634-X. http://www.oie.int/doc/ged/D9818.PDF.

11. Desquesnes M, Bosseno MF, Breniere SF. Detection of Chagas infections using *Trypanosoma evansi* crude antigen demonstrates high cross-reactions with *Trypanosoma cruzi*. *Infect Genet Evol* 2007;**7**(4):457−62.

12. Monteon-Padilla VM, Hernandez-Becerril N, Guzman-Bracho C, Rosales-Encina JL, Reyes-Lopez PA. American trypanosomiasis (Chagas' disease) and blood banking in Mexico City: seroprevalence and its potential transfusional transmission risk. *Arch Med Res* 1999;**30**(5):393−8.

13. Myriam HL, Bahamonde MI, Garcia A, Tassara R, Urarte E, Contreras Mdel C, et al. *Trypanosoma cruzi* transplacental infection in Chile: diagnosis, treatment and control. *Rev Soc Bras Med Trop* 2005;**38**(Suppl. 2):46−8.

14. Arganaraz ER, Hubbard GB, Ramos LA, Ford AL, Nitz N, Leland MM, et al. Blood-sucking lice may disseminate *Trypanosoma cruzi* infection in baboons. *Rev Inst Med Trop Sao Paulo* 2001;**43**(5):271−6.

15. Coura JR. Transmission of chagasic infection by oral route in the natural history of Chagas disease. *Rev Soc Bras Med Trop* 2006;**39**(Suppl. 3):113−17.

16. Hoft DH, Farrar PL, Kraz-Owens K, Shaffer D. Gastric invasion by *Trypanosoma cruzi* and induction of protective mucosal immune responses. *Infect Immun* 1996;**64**:3800−10.

17. Lainson R, Shaw JJ, Naiff RD. Chagas' disease in the Amazon basin: speculations on transmission per os. *Rev Inst Trop Sao Paulo* 1980;**22**:294−7.

18. Steindel M, Kramer Pacheco L, Scholl D, Soares M, de Moraes MH, Eger I, et al. Characterization of *Trypanosoma cruzi* isolated from humans, vectors, and animal reservoirs following an outbreak of acute human Chagas disease in Santa Catarina State, Brazil. *Diagn Microbiol Infect Dis* 2008;**60**(1):25−32.

19. Cardoso AV, Lescano SA, Amato Neto V, Gakiya E, Santos SV. Survival of *Trypanosoma cruzi* in sugar cane used to prepare juice. *Rev Inst Med Trop Sao Paulo* 2006;**48**(5):287−9.

20. Alarcon de Noya B, Diaz-Bello Z, Colmenares C, Ruiz-Guevara R, Mauriello L, Zavala-Jaspe R, et al. Large urban outbreak of orally acquired acute Chagas disease at a school in Caracas, Venezuela. *J Infect Dis* 2010;**201**(9):1308−15.

21. Alarcon de Noyan B, Colmenares C, Diaz-Bello Z, Ruiz-Guevara R, Medina K, Munoz-Calderon A, et al. Orally-transmitted Chagas disease: epidemiological, clinical, serological and molecular outcomes of a school microepidemic in chichiriviche de la costa, Venezuela. *Parasite Epidemiol Control* 2016;**1**(2):188−98.

22. Cossentini L, Da Silva R, Yamada-Ogatta S, Yamauchi L, De Almeida Araújo E, Pinge-Filho P. Aspirin treatment exacerbates oral infections by *Trypanosoma cruzi*. *Exp Parasitol* 2016;**164**:64−70.

23. Raina AK, Rakesh-Kumar, Rajora VS, Sridhar, Singh RP. Oral transmission of *Trypanosoma evansi* infection in dogs and mice. *Vet Parasitol* 1985;**18**:67−9.

24. Dias E. Transmissao do *Schizotrypanum cruzi* entre vertebrados por via digestiva. *Brasil Medico* 1940;**54**:775.

25. Roellig DM, Ellis AE, Yabsley MJ. Oral transmission of *Trypanosoma cruzi* with opposing evidence for the theory of carnivory. *J Parasitol* 2009;**95**(2):360−4.

26. Murrell K, Djordjevic M, Cuperlovic K, Sofronic L, Savic M, Djordjevic M, et al. Epidemiology of *Trichinella* infection in the horse: the risk from animal product feeding practices. *Vet Parasitol* 2004;**123**:223−33.

27. Deane MP, Lenzi HL, Jansen A. *Trypanosoma cruzi*: vertebrate and invertebrate cycles in the same mammal host, the opossum *Didelphis marsupialis*. *Mem Inst Oswaldo Cruz* 1984;**79**(4):513−15.

28. Urdaneta-Morales S, Nironi I. *Trypanosoma cruzi* in the anal glands of urban opossums. I. Isolation and experimental infections. *Mem Inst Oswaldo Cruz* 1996;**91**:399–403.

29. Hoare CA. *The trypanosomes of mammals. A zoological monograph.* Oxford, UK: Blackwell Scientific Publications; 1972, 749 p.

30. Woo PTK. The haematocrit centrifuge technique for the detection of trypanosomes in blood. *Can J Zool* 1969;**47**:921–3.

31. Moser DR, Kirchhof LV, Donelson JE. Detection of *Trypanosoma cruzi* by DNA amplification using the polymerase chain reaction. *J Clin Microbiol* 1989;**27**:1477–82.

32. Desquesnes M, Dávila AMR. Applications of PCR-based tools for detection and identification of animal trypanosomes: a review and perspectives. *Vet Parasitol* 2002;**109**(3-4): 213–31.

33. Desquesnes M, Bengaly Z, Millogo L, Meme Y, Sakande H. The analysis of the cross-reactions occurring in antibody-ELISA for the detection of trypanosomes can improve identification of the parasite species involved. *Ann Trop Med Parasitol* 2001;**95**(2): 141–55.

34. Monzón CM. Estudio serológico de equinos infectados com *Trypanosoma equinum*, utilizando la hemaglutinación indirecta con antígeno homólogo y de *Trypanosoma cruzi*. *Rev Med Vet (Bs. As.)* 1986;**67**(6):193–298.

35. Bakos E. Epidemiología de la enfermedad de Chagas en la Província del Chaco y Prevalenia en el Noreste Argentino. *Gac Vet B Aires* 1982;**44**(367):69–73.

36. Monzon CM, Colman OLR. Estudio seroepidemiologique de la tripanosomiasis equina (O. Mal de Caderas) mediante la prueba de immunofluorescencia indirecta en la Provincia de Formosa (Argentina) Anos 1983 à 1987. *Arq Bras Med Vet Zoot* 1988; **40**:279–85.

37. Ferenc SA, Stopinski V, Courteney CH. The development of an enzyme-linked immunosorbent assay for *Trypanosoma vivax* and its use in a seroepidemiological survey in the eastern Caribbean Basin. *Int J Parasitol* 1990;**20**:51–6.

38. Savani ES, Nunes VL, Galati EA, Castilho TM, Araujo FS, Ilha IM, et al. Occurrence of co-infection by *Leishmania (Leishmania) chagasi* and *Trypanosoma (Trypanozoon) evansi* in a dog in the state of Mato Grosso do Sul, Brazil. *Mem Inst Oswaldo Cruz* 2005;**100**(7):739–41.

39. Grosjean NL, Vrable RA, Murphy AJ, Mansfield LS. Seroprevalence of antibodies against *Leishmania* spp among dogs in the United States. *J Am Vet Med Assoc* 2003;**222** (5):603–6.

40. Gurtler RE, Cecere MC, Lauricella MA, Cardinal MV, Kitron U, Cohen JE. Domestic dogs and cats as sources of *Trypanosoma cruzi* infection in rural northwestern Argentina. *Parasitology* 2007;**134**(Pt 1):69–82.

41. Briceno-Leon R. Chagas disease and globalization of the Amazon. *Cad Saude Publica* 2007;**23**(Suppl. 1):S33–40.

42. Garcia-Vazquez Z, Rosaria-Cruz R, Miranda-Miranda E, Dominguez-Marquez A. A serological survey of *Trypanosoma cruzi* infection in dogs of two urban areas of Mexico. *Prev Vet Med* 1995;**25**:1–6.

43. Acha P, Szyfres B. *Zoonoses et maladies transmissibles à l'homme et aux animaux.* 3rd ed. Paris: OIE; 2005. p. 406.

44. Newsome A, McGhee C. *Trypanosoma cruzi* in triatomes from an urban and a domestic setting in middle Tennessee. *J Tenn Acad Sci* 2006.

45. Bern C, Kjos S, Yabsley MJ, Montgomery SP. *Trypanosoma cruzi* and Chagas' disease in the United States. *Clin Microbiol Rev* 2011;**24**(4):655–81.

46. Alcaino TV, Lorca M, Nunez F, Issota A, Gorman T. Chagas' disease in goats from the Metropolitan region (Chile): seroepidemiological survey and experimental infection. *Parasitologia al Dia* 1995;**19**:30−6.

47. Bryan LK, Hamer SA, Shaw S, Curtis-Robles R, Auckland LD, Hodo CL, et al. Chagas disease in a Texan horse with neurologic deficits. *Vet Parasitol* 2016;**216**:13−17.

48. Jansen AM, Santos de Pinho AP, Lisboa CV, Cupolillo E, Mangia RH, Fernandes O. The sylvatic cycle of *Trypanosoma cruzi*: a still unsolved puzzle. *Mem Inst Oswaldo Cruz* 1999;**94**(Suppl. 1):203−4.

49. Galuppo S, Bacigalupo A, Garcia A, Ortiz S, Coronado X, Cattan PE, et al. Predominance of *Trypanosoma cruzi* genotypes in two reservoirs infected by sylvatic *Triatoma infestans* of an endemic area of Chile. *Acta Trop* 2009;**111**(1):90−3.

50. Herrera HM, Abreu UG, Keuroghlian A, Freitas TP, Jansen AM. The role played by sympatric collared peccary (*Tayassu tajacu*), white-lipped peccary (*Tayassu pecari*), and feral pig (*Sus scrofa*) as maintenance hosts for *Trypanosoma evansi* and *Trypanosoma cruzi* in a sylvatic area of Brazil. *Parasitol Res* 2008;**103**(3):619−24.

51. Botto-Mahan C, Acuna-Retamar M, Campos R, Cattan PE, Solari A. European rabbits (*Oryctolagus cuniculus*) are naturally infected with different *Trypanosoma cruzi* genotypes. *Am J Trop Med Hyg* 2009;**80**(6):944−6.

52. Buitrago R, Bosseno MF, Depickere S, Waleckx E, Salas R, Aliaga C, et al. Blood meal sources of wild and domestic *Triatoma infestans* (Hemiptera: Reduviidae) in Bolivia: connectivity between cycles of transmission of *Trypanosoma cruzi*. *Parasit Vectors* 2016;**9**(1):214.

53. Maloney J, Newsome A, Huang J, Kirby J, Kranz M, Wateska A, et al. Seroprevalence of *Trypanosoma cruzi* in raccoons from Tennessee. *J Parasitol* 2009;1.

54. John DT, Hoppe KL. *Trypanosoma cruzi* from wild raccoons in Oklahoma. *Am J Vet Res* 1986;**47**(5):1056−9.

55. Andersson J, Englund P, Sunnemark D, Dahlstedt A, Westerblad H, Nennesmo I, et al. CBA/J mice infected with *Trypanosoma cruzi*: an experimental model for inflammatory myopathies. *Muscle Nerve* 2003;**27**(4):442−8.

56. Guedes PM, Veloso VM, Afonso LC, Caliari MV, Carneiro CM, Diniz LF, et al. Development of chronic cardiomyopathy in canine Chagas disease correlates with high IFN-gamma, TNF-alpha, and low IL-10 production during the acute infection phase. *Vet Immunol Immunopathol* 2009;**130**(1-2):43−52.

57. Guedes PM, Veloso VM, Tafuri WL, Galvao LM, Carneiro CM, Lana M, et al. The dog as model for chemotherapy of the Chagas' disease. *Acta Trop* 2002;**84**(1):9−17.

58. Davis DS, Russell LH, Adams LG, Yaeger RG, Robinson RM. An experimental infection of *Trypanosoma cruzi* in striped skunks (*Mephitis mephitis*). *J Wildl Dis* 1980;**16**(3):403−6.

59. Pietrokovsky SM, Schweigmann NJ, Riarte A, Alberti A, Conti O, Montoya S, et al. The skunk *Conepatus chinga* as new host of *Trypanosoma cruzi* in Argentina. *J Parasitol* 1991;**77**(4):643−5.

60. Diamond LS, Rubin R. Experimental infection of certain farm mammals with a North American strain of *Trypanosoma cruzi* from the raccoon. *Exp Parasitol* 1958;**7**(4):383−90.

61. Marsden PD, Blackie EJ, Rosenberg ME, Ridley DS, Hagstrom JW. Experimental *Trypanosoma cruzi* infections in domestic pigs (*Sus scrofa domestica*). *Trans R Soc Trop Med Hyg* 1970;**64**(1):156−8.

62. Rodhain F, Perez C. Précis d'entomologie médicale et vétérinaire. *Eds Maloines, Paris* 1985. 458p.

63. Kjos SA, Snowden KF, Craig TM, Lewis B, Ronald N, Olson JK. Distribution and characterization of canine Chagas disease in Texas. *Vet Parasitol* 2008;**152**(3-4):249−56.

64. Brown EL, Roellig DM, Gompper ME, Monello RJ, Wenning KM, Gabriel MW, et al. Seroprevalence of *Trypanosoma cruzi* among eleven potential reservoir species from six states across the southern United States. *Vector Borne Zoonotic Dis* 2009.

65. Karsten V, Davis C, Kuhn R. *Trypanosoma cruzi* in wild raccoons and opossums in North Carolina. *J Parasitol* 1992;**78**:547−9.

66. Yabsley MJ, Noblet GP. Seroprevalence of *Trypanosoma cruzi* in raccoons from South Carolina and Georgia. *J Wildl Dis* 2002;**38**(1):75−83.

67. Diaz JH. Chagas disease in the United States: a cause for concern in Louisiana? *J La State Med Soc* 2007;**159**(1). 21−3, 5−9.

68. Dorn PL, Perniciaro L, Yabsley MJ, Roellig DM, Balsamo G, Diaz J, et al. Autochthonous transmission of *Trypanosoma cruzi*, Louisiana. *Emerg Infect Dis* 2007;**13** (4):605−7.

69. Garcia M, Woc-Colburn L, Rossmann S, Townsend R, Stramer S, Bravo M, et al. *Trypanosoma cruzi* screening in Texas blood donors, 2008−2012. *Epidemiol Infect* 2016;**144**(5):1010−13.

70. Ochs DE, Hnilica VS, Moser DR, Smith JH, Kirchhoff LV. Postmortem diagnosis of autochtonous acute chagasic myocarditis by polymerase chain reaction amplification of a species-specific DNA sequence of *Trypanosoma cruzi*. *Am J Trop Med Hyg* 1996;**54**: 526−9.

71. Herwaldt BL, Grijalva MJ, Newsome AL, McGhee CR, Powell MR, Nemec DG, et al. Use of polymerase chain reaction to diagnose the fifth reported U.S. case of autochtonous transmission of *Trypanosoma cruzi*—Tennessee, 1998. *J Infect Dis* 2000;**181**(1): 395−9.

72. Barr SC, Van Beek O, Carlise-Nowak MS, Kirchoff LV, Allison N, Zajac A, et al. *Trypanosoma cruzi* infection in Walker Hounds from Virginia. *Am J Vet Res* 1995; **56**:1037−44.

73. Deneris J, Marshall NA. Biological characterization of a strain of *Trypanosoma cruzi* chagas isolated from a human case of trypanosomiasis in California. *Am J Trop Med Hyg* 1989;**41**(4):422−8.

# Experimental studies of Chagas disease in animal models

*M. de Lana*
Federal University of Ouro Preto, Minas Gerais, Brazil

## Chapter Outline

## Introduction

An important requisite to study any disease and the mechanisms involved in its pathogenic process is the choice of a good experimental model that reproduces the different phases and clinical forms observed in humans. In this context, several experimental models have been used to study Chagas disease. Since the beginning of these studies the first isolate of *Trypanosoma cruzi* was sent to Oswaldo Cruz Institute to be used to infect several animal species such as dogs, cats, monkeys, rabbits, guinea pigs, and some rodents to try to reproduce the disease.[1]

The requisites of a good experimental model to study Chagas disease established by the Chagas Disease Committee of Training Special Program and Research of Parasitic Disease from the World Health Organization[2] are:

- to allow the isolation of the parasite throughout the course of the infection;
- to present positive serological reactions indicative of the infection;
- to present the diverse clinical manifestations of chronic Chagas disease;
- to develop myocarditis, myosite, and other pathological alterations characteristic of the disease;
- to induce the immune response against the host tissue;
- to be of easy maintenance and of accessible price.

American Trypanosomiasis Chagas Disease. DOI: http://dx.doi.org/10.1016/B978-0-12-801029-7.00014-9

# Animal species used as experimental model in Chagas disease

## *Mice*

Mice have been more frequently used as experimental models to study Chagas disease for several reasons. They are easily reproduced, of low cost, easier to handle, and easy to be experimentally infected and maintained in experimental conditions. The existence of a great number of strains and isogenic species, appropriated to study different aspects of the disease make this species the most commonly used in experimental studies. Different strains of mice present distinct patterns of susceptibility to *T. cruzi* infection. Moreover, the existence of several knockout lineages has facilitated particularly the study of different immunological aspects of *T. cruzi* infection.

The acute phase is easily reproduced in this model[3,4] making this species very useful to isolate and also to maintain the parasite in the laboratory through blood successive passages because young mice are very susceptible to infection. Different aspects of acute disease are reproduced in mice including symptoms (anorexia, increase of temperature, loss of weight, decrease of general activity, patent parasitemia, general edema, and mortality) and histopathological lesions (diffuse myocarditis, myosite, lymphadenopathy, and congestion with infiltrate of mononuclear cells). Some authors[5–7] studied lesions of the autonomous nervous system of mice infected with different *T. cruzi* strains verifying their presence in celiac, sympathetic, lumbar, cardiac superficial, and myoenteric ganglion with the lesions being irregular and dependent of the parasite strain with the inflammatory process having an important role in this origin.[8] The neuronal changes are observed in ganglia of the myoenteric plexus as well as intracardiac parasympathic, celiac, and sympathic. Using electronic microscopy are observed tumefaction and vacuolization of mitochondrias, hypertrophy of Golgi complex, dilatation of the endoplasmic reticular system, chromatolysis and vacuolization of a great number of lysosomes, and neuronal osmiophilic granulations.[9] Recently, a novel murine model of long-term infection[10] infected with Y *T. cruzi* was developed to elucidate the pathogenesis of megacolon and neuromuscular intestinal changes. It was observed that there was significant lower parasitism, decrease in the number of neurons, and in the density of intramuscular nerve bundles. Also it was verified that there was increased thickness of the colon wall, diffuse muscle cell hypertrophy, and increased collagen deposition, interpreted as a demonstration of early fibrosis in the damaged areas.

Apparently the neuronal destruction occurs in the presence of a great concentration of tissue parasitism during the acute phase. Autoimmune mechanisms probably participate in this process, being responsible for the inflammation that involves sympathic and parasympathic ganglia. The use of polymerase chain reaction (PCR) technique in tissue identified the presence of parasite kDNA in fragments of biopsy from chagasic patients with megaesophagus suggesting that presence of the parasite, or its DNA, are important in the genesis of the inflammatory process triggering also the autoimmune process present in Chagas disease.[11] The role of the parasite strain on denervation was suggested when 138 *T. cruzi* strains of three Brazilian regions were characterized by isoenzimatic profile and the association between the presence of "megas" and Zymodema II of *T. cruzi* was observed.[12] The evaluation of hematologic alterations in mice infected with different *T. cruzi* strains[13] verified anemia, decrease of platelets, and leucopenia being the hematological changes more intense in mice with higher parasitemia.

The chronic phase is also reproduced in mice especially regarding myocardiopathy. A study of mice infected with 12 different *T. cruzi* strains isolated from Virgem da Lapa, MG, evaluating the infectivity, parasitemia, and tissue parasitism during the acute and chronic phases of the infection was carried out.[14] Except for the fibrosis, lesion stability was observed during the evolution of the infection. Arteritis with necrosis was observed in skeletal and heart muscles. In the study of the morphology of the heart conduction system in C3H mice[15] infected with Tulahuen strain the evolution of the lesions during the infection was not verified. No correlation with the morphological aspects and electrocardiogram (ECG) alterations were observed with the human chronic chagasic cardiopathy. On the other hand, in this same lineage of mice infected with a Colombian strain,[16] cardiomegaly with hypertrophy, ventricular dilatation, ventricular aneurysm, necrosis in myofibrils myocardium degeneration, inflammatory reaction with predominance of mononuclear cells, interstitial fibrosis, and the occasional presence of pseudocysts were verified. These authors demonstrated the involvement of microcirculation and ischemia on chronic chagasic cardiopathy. The mechanisms of cardiac fibrosis in mice[17] infected with highly virulent and pathogenic *T. cruzi* strains was studied. The ultrastructural analysis revealed predominance of monocytes, activated macrophages, fibroblasts, myofibroblasts, and intense deposition of collagen, suggestive of the association of the inflammatory process and fibrogenesis with chronic chagasic cardiopathy. The immunotyping revealed different types of collagen during the infection evolution and the possibility of fibrosis reversion during the later infection.

IgG2a was more associated with protection. In a similar study with the same *T. cruzi* strains in six different strains of mice similar results were verified.[18] No correlation was observed between the level of antibodies and the protection to infection. Later it was discovered that IgG1 and IgG2 are the most important IgG isotypes with participation in the phenomenon of lyses mediated by complement, the most important humoral process of protection in chronic chagasic infection.[19]

The digestive forms of Chagas disease named "megas" have not yet been observed and/or reproduced in mice. An exception is the study of Campos et al.[10] So, the related data described in the literature until now are controversial. Fig. 14.1 illustrates several aspects of experimental Chagas disease in mice during the acute and chronic phases of the infection.

Besides all these aspects, the murine model has been used for the biological characterization of *T. cruzi* strains and the results are correlated with the genetic classification of the parasite characterized by isoenzymatic profiles or other molecular markers.[20] The association between biological aspects observed in mice and the genetic characterization of *T. cruzi* has been confirmed by several authors even using different genetic markers.

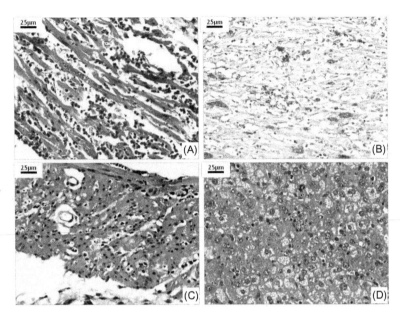

**Figure 14.1** Several aspects of experimental Chagas disease in murine model during the acute phase of the infection (A, C, and D: hematoxylin and eosin counterstained). (A) Acute myocarditis with presence of amastigotes nest and mononuclear cells dissociating the cardiac fibers. (B) Immunohistochemistry showing acute myocarditis and intense presence of amastigotes. (C) Muscular layer of the intestine with presence of diffuse inflammatory infiltrate and amastigotes. (D) Liver showing amastigotes nest in Kupffer cells and diffuse inflammatory infiltrate.
*Source*: Photographs by de Lana and colleagues.

It was verified that C3H was the most susceptible lineage of mice, BALB/c of intermediary susceptibility, while B10 was the most resistant to infection.[21] It was also verified in mice of different isogenic lineages (AKR, A/J, CBA, BALB/c, C3H, and B10)[18] infected with three *T. cruzi* strains typical of the three Biodemes of Andrade and Magalhaes[20] that the parasitemia and mortality index were different among the lineages. It was verified that the same lineage may be more resistant or susceptible in function of the *T. cruzi* strain considered. In general CBA and B10 mice were more resistant and A/J and AKR more susceptible.

The existence of different knock-out lineages of mice have allowed better studies about different humoral and cellular immunological process during the acute and chronic phases of *T. cruzi* infection and its genetic regulation.[22–24] Although the immune response had an important role in the resistance, the survival is more related to the genetic pattern of the mice than with the H-2 locus (mice histocompatibility system). It means that the resistance of mice to acute infection is regulated by multiple genetic components present in the H-2 locus and that the final resultant infection and evolution depends on the parasite characteristics and the allele's combination of each mouse lineage, including immunological and nonimmunological factors. According to Minoprio et al.[24] the consequence of acute infection by *T. cruzi* is the intense and polyclonal lymphocyte activation with the majority not driven to *T. cruzi* antigens, leading to a fast blastic activation and proliferative activity of CD4[+], CD8[+], and LyB. The infection evolution is dependent on the lymphocyte response and the patterns of cytokines able to modify this response with the predominance of Th1 or Th2 response.

Recently, the use of a highly sensitive in vivo imaging system based on bioluminescent of *T. cruzi* capable of expressing luciferase was explored to monitor parasite burden in real time throughout the chronic phase of the infection.[25] The authors demonstrated benznidazole treatment efficacy in the acute and chronic phases in mice infected with CL Brener strain, as well as the distribution of the parasite in different organs and tissue. The gastrointestinal tract was identified as the major niche of long-term infection, and that chagasic heart disease can be developed in the absence persistent parasites.

A new therapeutic option for Chagas disease employing cardiac mesenchymal stem cells (CMSCs) was used[26] in the chronic infection (6 months) of C57BL/6 mice model infected with Colombian strain, resistant to treatment. Cells were injected into the left ventricle wall of the animals, which were submitted to cardiac histopathological analysis of heart sections. Results revealed that treated mice showed significant reduction of inflammatory cells, but not of the fibrotic area. The CMSCs treatment had a protective effect in chronic chagasic cardiomyopathy mainly through immunomodulation based on the analysis of some inflammatory cytokines and this option of treatment must be further explored in other experimental models used in Chagas disease study.

Finally it is considered that mice reproduce with relative facility several aspects of the acute and chronic phases of Chagas disease. One of the principal limitations of the mouse model is the short life span of this species (approximately 2 years), which probably makes impossible the reproduction of the later clinical forms of the disease such as intense fibrosis, dilated myocardiopathy, aneurysm, and the digestive clinical forms, especially megaesophagus and megacolon, all of later evolution.

Another limitation of mice is the noncorrespondence between electrocardiographic alterations with the typical patterns verified in humans. However, the recent advances obtained in the study of several aspects of Chagas disease immunology in this animal, as well as the use of the murine model for testing of new drugs associated with the facility of handling, fully justify the use of this model in the study of different aspects of experimental Chagas disease.

## Rats

Although easy to handle and maintain in the laboratory, rats have not been very much used as experimental model for the studies of Chagas disease, especially because they are more resistant to *T. cruzi* infection with the acute phase generally showing very low parasitemia or subpatent, which makes the evaluation of the infection difficult. On the other hand, this limitation makes this species useful for studies of the chronic phase of the infection since the mortality during the acute phase is not so frequent.

Considering the unpredictability of the disease evolution in this model as well as the difficulty for demonstration of the parasite persistency throughout long-term infection, other authors have reproduced the acute phase of the infection in rats with several *T. cruzi* strains of higher virulence and using great inoculum. A study of the course of the infection of five strains[27] demonstrated that the acute phase is later (around 3 weeks), with higher or low parasitemias followed by chronic infection or mortality dependent on the pathogenicity of the strain. The studies of several viscera of Wistar rats in the chronic infection with Y strain[28,29] showed that the cardiopathy was very frequent, with the occurrence of "megas" of colon, bladder, seminal vesicle, and uterus. Neurons of the Meissner complex of the stomach, transverse and descendent colon were reduced, as well as those of the Auerbach plexus from the stomach to rectum. The evaluation of the sympathetic denervation in rats infected with Y strain[30] verified that this process begins very early (6 days after infection) in parallel with intense parasitism and myocardial inflammation. The evaluation of the ECG changes in Wistar rats infected with the Colombian strain[31] detected some alterations similar to those observed in human except more severe in the right block of the His branch. Discrete ECG alterations of later occurrence in rats infected with Y, 12SF, and Colombian strains were verified.[32] On the other hand, chronic myocarditis with fibrosis in 15% of the animals was verified in histopathological evaluations of these same animals,[33] recommending this model for the cardiac study of Chagas disease.

To better understand the immunological resistance of the rats to acute *T. cruzi* infection the contribution of mononuclear phagocytes was studied in animals inoculated with *T. cruzi*, Y strain.[34] Acute *T. cruzi* infection triggered a dramatic increase (93.7%) in peripheral blood monocyte number at day 12 of infection. At this point, histological analysis of the heart showed high parasitism and diffuse and moderate to intense mononuclear inflammatory process. Clusters of macrophages exhibited different morphological phenotypes, with evident signs of activation. The present findings indicate that the early phase of infection with *T. cruzi* induces rapid production, maturation, and activation of the monocyte/macrophage system so as to control *T. cruzi* replication, emphasizing the crucial role of macrophages in the rat resistance to Chagas disease. Immunological studies verified in rats infected with Sylvio X10/7 strain during the acute phase[35] that 1.5 days postinfection, when no parasite or immune cell infiltration could be detected, the myocardium expressed high levels of nitric oxide synthase and nitric oxide metabolites, although not sufficient to clear the parasites.

Taking together the results here mentioned shows that the rat model, despite the relative resistance to *T. cruzi* infection, has important applicability to study certain aspects, especially of the chronic infection of Chagas disease. Furthermore, rats are easily reproduced, relatively low cost, and easy to handle.

## Dogs

Young dogs, different from older dogs, are highly susceptible to infection, and reproduce with great facility the acute phase of the disease when usually the mortality is very high. The high mortality observed during this phase disables the systematized studies of the chronic phase in young dogs. The survival of the animals to the acute phase is very dependent on the parasite virulence, source and size of the inoculum, route of infection, and animal age.

One of the most important advantages of the dog in relation to other animal models is the advanced knowledge and the similarity of the cardiac morphology and physiology of the heart conduction system with man.[36,37] Another advantage is the long life span of this animal (15−25 years), which naturally allows the evolution of the later clinical forms of the disease, as well as dogs' easy reproduction and handling.

The first reproduction of the "chagoma" of inoculation, one of the signals of parasite entry in the vertebrate host, was demonstrated in dogs,[38] as well as neurological symptoms, such as paraplegia including lesions on the brain and cerebellum of the animals. Other signals of acute infection were also reproduced in dogs, such as ascites, neurological symptoms, and congestive cardiac insufficiency.[39,40] The neurological symptoms and lesions were also observed.[41,42] Young dogs were infected with various inocula of metacyclic and blood trypomastigotes by subcutaneous and conjunctival routes, simulating with this last inoculation the natural mechanisms of infection.[43] The authors verified intense infection and parasites were observed in blood, urine, and saliva, suggesting that probably the conjunctival route facilitated the brain parasitism observed in animals inoculated by this last route. A comparative study in dogs infected with metacyclic and blood trypomastigotes from the Be-62 and Be-78 strains via intraperitoneal and conjunctival[44] also verified that all dogs inoculated intraperitoneally became infected independently of the *T. cruzi* strain and source of trypomastigotes. However, when blood trypomastigotes of both strains were inoculated by conjunctival route the percentages of infectivity were significantly lower. The results suggested that the source of the inoculum and the route of inoculation remarkably influenced the evolution of the infection even when the same strain of the parasite is used.

In the acute phase dogs developed intense myocarditis with accentuated parasitism of myocytes and necrotic lesions of cardiac cells associated with parasites, disintegrated or not, in parallel with an intense inflammatory process. These lesions begin in the atria, especially the right, and migrate to the ventricles. The sinoatrial nodule and atriaventricular nodules as well as the branches of the His branch are reached.[45] The ultrastructural aspects of cellular infiltrate with granular and agranular lymphocytes adhere to the cardiac cells leading to myocytolysis, separation of intercellular junctions, and the presence of necrosis and apoptosis are suggestive of cytotoxic and cytolytic mechanisms mediated by immune cells.[46] Microangiopathy with adherent granular lymphocytes to endothelium of the capillaries was observed. ECG alterations were normally discrete (ischemic, intraventricular blocks, hemiblock of the left branch of the His bundle) and reversible, being important only when lesions of the heart conduction system were associated to necrosis of the myocells, a sign of a bad prognosis.

The electrocardiographic changes in dogs included, since the decrease of the QRS complex, enlargement of P wave, changes of T wave and ST T segment, disturbance of ventricular repolarization, arrhythmia, partial and total AV blocks, and the typical ECG changes of chagasic patients, such as total block of the right branch of His bundle, associated or not with the anterior or posterior block of the left branch as well as extrasystoles or inactive zone. The three last alterations are associated with the occurrence of sudden death, the most shocking event in Chagas disease. The authors[47–49] verified correlation between the histopathologic lesions and the ECG alterations, especially in the acute phase.

The cardiac lesions of nine dogs infected with the *T. cruzi* strains 12SF and Colombian[50] were very discrete. All animals presented the indeterminate phase of the infection and were considered a good model to reproduce this clinical form of the disease. The cardiac dilatation, when it occurred, was minimal and the histopathology revealed the presence of mononuclear cells and focal fibrosis, especially in the right atria, without the presence of parasites, with these lesions being considered probably sequels of the acute phase. Afterward it was observed that these dogs with the indeterminate phase of the infection[51] presented evolution of the myocarditis and fibrosis only when they received minimum doses of cyclosphosphamide.

The occurrence of dilatation of hollow organs and the characterization of the typical "megas" especially of esophagus and colon in dog model is rare, but already described in dogs.[52] However others authors never reproduced these findings, independent of the *T. cruzi* strain and experimental protocol used.

Andrade and Andrade[53] highlighted the importance of the reproduction of the indeterminate phase of the infection and the unpredictability and later evolution of the typical cardiac form of the disease, including the absence of the experimental digestive form of the disease in dogs, considering this fact as a serious limitation of this model taking into account the requisites established by WHO.[2] However, Lana et al.[54] believe that apparently the reproduction of the characteristic cardiac lesions of the chronic phase in dogs is very dependent of the *T. cruzi* strains. These authors succeeded in developing in dogs the diffuse and fibrosing chronic chagasic cardiopathy in several animals infected with the Be-78 strain despite the source and inoculum, route of inoculation, and time of infection. The inflammatory process was diffuse and followed by dissociation and substitution of the cardiac cells by intense deposition of collagen, not associated with the parasite presence, highly suggestive of participation of auto-immune mechanisms on the pathogenesis of the heart lesions. The cellular infiltrate was predominantly lymphocytic with aggregation of plasmocytes and macrophages. The authors[55] demonstrated parasitemia during the acute phase and chronic phases of the infection with several histopathological lesions, electrocardiographic alterations and symptoms very similar to those observed in man involving, either some cases of sudden death in different periods or the chronic infection of the severe cardiac lesions observed only in dogs infected with Be-78 strain.[54,55] In parallel[56] the humoral immune response (IgM and IgG profiles) was registered from the first week of the infection up to 36 months. A later evaluation of the same animals that survived the infection (5−12 years)[57] and studied by Lana et al.[55] using PCR in comparison with parasitological and serological methods was performed. PCR analyses were 100% positive, demonstrating the presence of parasite kDNA in all infected dogs. These data validate once more the dog as a model for Chagas' disease because it demonstrated the permanence of infection by PCR, hemoculture/xenodiagnosis, and serological methods, relevant requisites for an ideal model to study this disease. Several aspects of the experimental infection in dog model during the acute and chronic phase of the disease are showed in Fig. 14.2.

The qualitative and quantitative neurological lesions as well the mechanisms involved in this process in dogs experimentally infected with Be-62 and Be-78 *T. cruzi* strains were studied.[58−60] The evaluation of *beagle* dogs infected with Be-78 and Y strains[61] demonstrated the occurrence of myoenteric plexus denervation during the acute phase of infection in animals infected by both strains, but persistent in the chronic infection only in dogs infected with Be-78 strain.

The authors[62,63] studied the immunopathologic phenomena that participate in the cardiac lesions in the acute phase and the participation of different types of lymphocytes during the evolution of the disease. The apoptosis was observed in myocytes, endothelial cells, macrophages, lymphocytes, interstitial dendritic cells, and intra- and

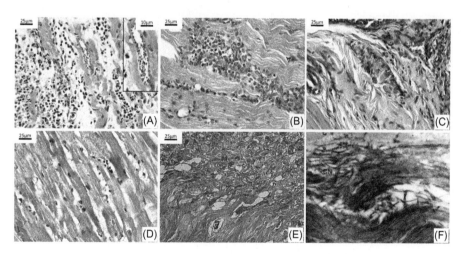

**Figure 14.2** Several aspects of experimental Chagas disease in dog model during the acute and chronic phases of the infection (A−E: hematoxylin and eosin counterstained). (A) Acute myocarditis with presence of mononuclear cells dissociating the muscle cells (inset-amastigotes nest). (B) Muscle layer of esophagus showing focal inflammatory infiltrate. (C) Ganglionitis and inflammatory cells in muscular layer of intestine. (D) Indeterminate chronic phase of the infection with discrete infiltrate of inflammatory cells. (E) Cardiac muscle with intense fibrosis during the chronic phase of the disease. (F) Collagen fibers in the heart during the chronic phase of the infection (electron microscopy).
*Source*: Photographs by de Lana and colleagues.

extracellular parasites. The results reinforce the participation of parasite antigens on the maintenance of cellular immune response in infected dogs and confirm the importance of the later hypersensitivity phenomena on the development of lesions with the demonstration of antigens retained in the dendritic cells. Other authors[64] studying immunological aspects of the disease in dogs during the chronic phase in animals infected by the Be-78 strain also verified an intense myocarditis and higher level of caCD8$^+$ cells, even without evidence of tissue parasitism, in contrast with animals infected by Be-62 strain, which suggests the involvement of other mechanisms in the genesis of the inflammatory process (Fig. 14.3).

The role of reinfection in the evolution of Chagas' disease in dogs alternately infected five times with two *T. cruzi* strains was evaluated.[65] Animals presented a brief oligosymptomatic acute phase. The level of parasitemia decreased progressively with the number of reinfections. All parasite samples isolated during the follow-up were zymodeme B, corresponding to one of the strains, independent of the strain used in the first inoculum. The PCR of a segment of the *T. cruzi* mini-exon gene showed the simultaneous presence of both strains in three of the eight animals. Antibody titers were higher among the dogs successively infected than those infected only once. All animals developed the indeterminate form of the disease.

The dog model has been used in chemotherapy studies. The results of posttreatment evaluations were similar to those reported in clinical trials in human in both phases of the disease.[66] Important result show the demonstration of the positive impact of treatment on lesions and electrocardiographic changes in dogs infected with *T. cruzi* strains both sensitive and resistant to drugs and treated during the acute phase with benznidazole.[67] The results illustrated one example of the benefit of early etiological treatment even in animals not cured.

In conclusion, the principal advantage of the dog model is the reproduction of the distinct phases of the disease. Several clinical aspects of the disease similar to those verified in humans have been observed in dogs, giving the possibility of electrocardiographic monitoring of the infected animal and verified correlations between these alterations with the cardiac excitoconduction system lesions, offering a very good interpretation of the results. The disadvantage of the dog model is that, in the majority of the cases dogs need a very long time to develop the cardiac chronic clinical form of the disease which is rare and apparently *T. cruzi* strain-dependent.

## Rabbits

Of all the experimental models used to study Chagas disease rabbits are considered the model with the most contradictory results in the literature, the reason why they are not very often used for this purpose. Agosin and Badinez[68] were the first authors that isolated *T. cruzi* from the peripheral blood and verified tissue lesions and parasites in muscular fibers of rabbits experimentally infected with *T. cruzi*. In the infection of rabbits with metacyclical trypomastigotes[69] it was verified low parasitemia, detected only by xenodiagnosis, and humoral immune response similar to that observed in human. On the other hand, in rabbits infected with Ernestina

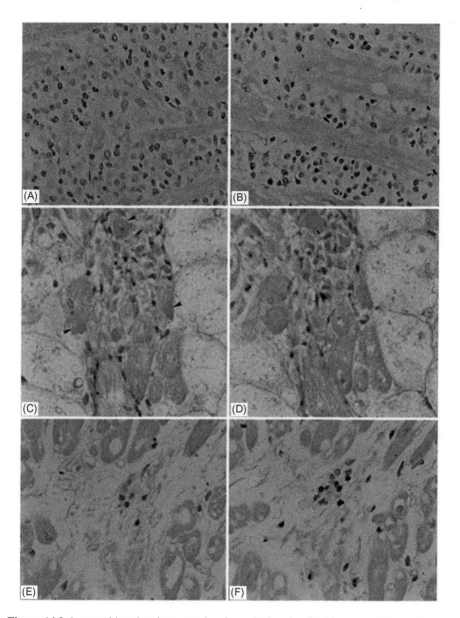

**Figure 14.3** Immunohistochemistry reaction for caCD8 and caCD4 in myocardium of dogs necropsied during acute and chronic phases. (A) Acute myocarditis with large number of labeled caCD8$^+$ T cells. (B) Myocardium of the same dog showing large number of stained caCD4$^+$ T cells. (C) Chronic myocarditis of dog infected with Be-78 strain showing a focus of caCD8$^+$ T cells, close to damaged myocardiocytes (*arrowheads*) and without parasitism. (D) The same region contains a similar number of caCD4$^+$ T cells. (E) Chronic myocarditis with Be-62 strain showing absence of caCD8$^+$ T cells. (F) caCD4$^+$ T cells in the same region. Hematoxylin and eosin counterstained $\times$ 440.
*Source*: From Caliari et al.[64]

strain,[70] which is considered highly virulent, the acute phase with patent parasitemia and also the chronic phase of the infection were reproduced. The animals survived the acute phase, four died with myocarditis, two presented megacolon, the majority remained asymptomatic, and the lesions observed were considered similar to those observed in human. In rabbits infected with Y, Colombian, and 12 SF strains[71] it was also observed subpatent parasitemia and in general discrete lesions in both phases of the infection. These results were also confirmed when rabbits and mice were infected in parallel with Y, MR, and CL strains.[72] However, in a systematized study with Ernestina and Albuquerque strains[73] important results were achieved in the acute and chronic phase of the infections concerning the parasitological, serological, histopathological, and clinical (ECG) aspects of the disease similar to human disease. Similar results to these[73] were reproduced when rabbits were infected with Y, CL, and Ernani strains,[74] with the occurrence of cardiac fibrosis, aneurysm, and several ECG changes being verified. However, the cardiac electrophysiology of rabbits is not very well known, which makes the interpretation of the electrocardiographic changes in this animal model difficult. The authors[75] concluded that advanced fibrosis occurred only in the later chronic phase in rabbits infected with different parasite's strains. Tissue parasitism occurred only in the acute phase and in the digestive tract. Skeletal muscles showed mild and occasional lesions which indicate that rabbits experimentally infected with *T. cruzi* reproduce some lesions similar to that of human chagasic patients, in the indeterminate form of the disease. However, the development of megasyndromes were not effectively demonstrated in this model.[71] Finally the authors concluded that rabbits may be a useful, but not an ideal model for studying Chagas disease.

## Guinea pig

This animal develops the acute phase of the disease with patent parasitemia in the first days of infection followed by mortality or spontaneously evolves for the chronic phase. However, studies that have evaluated the chronic phase of the infection in this animal model are rare. The evaluation of the humoral immune response of guinea pigs experimentally infected was carried out using three serological tests.[76] The study[77] considered the histopathological findings of the chronic phase in this model as suggestive of participation of autoimmune mechanisms in the myocarditis independent of the parasite's presence. The authors[78] demonstrated that guinea pig was a good model to study the experimental cardiac lesions in immunological and ultra-structural aspects. The study[79] verified that during the first months of infection the association of parasite's antigens and interstitial inflammatory reactions are independent of the parasite's presence in guinea pig. In *Cavia porcelus* species, a natural reservoir of *T. cruzi* rarely used as experimental model for Chagas disease studies, animals infected with Y strain[80] presented patent parasitemia during the acute phase, positive IgM and IgG in Western blots technique, vasculitis, necrosis, moderate to severe inflammation, and abundant amastigote nests. Few amastigote nests were present in kidney, brain, and other organs. During the early chronic phase the parasitemia became subpatent and anti-*T. cruzi* IgG antibodies were present. In cardiac tissue the number of amastigote nests and the level of inflammatory process decreased. In the later chronic phase (365 days), the cardiac tissue showed vasculitis and fibrosis and the presence of the parasite detectable by the presence of parasite DNA was associated with higher levels of inflammation. Thus, the authors demonstrated that this guinea pig species also shows biological and pathological changes similar to those found in human disease.

Although guinea pig is very susceptible to *T. cruzi* infections this animal model has always been substituted by other models such as mice, rats, and dogs that better reproduce the different aspects of acute and chronic infections of Chagas disease similar to those observed in humans.

## Hamster

The Syrian hamster has been used as experimental model for Chagas disease. The species *Mesocricetus auratus* is considered to generally have low immune resistance to several infections. This is one of the reasons why they have not been often used as model for Chagas disease studies. However, a detailed evaluation of *M. auratus* as a model[81] studying the acute and chronic phases of the infection demonstrated that both phases of the disease were reproduced in animals infected with Y and Benedito *T. cruzi* strains. A careful follow-up of the acute phase demonstrated easy recovery of the parasites by hemoculture or xenodiagnosis in all animals. Inflammatory reaction characterized by mononuclear and polymorphous leukocyte infiltration in the majority of tissues and organs, was observed, especially in the connective loose and fatty tissues, smooth muscle myocardium, and skeletal muscle. In the chronic phase animals were evaluated periodically from 3rd to 10th month with the lesions observed in the same tissues and organs. The inflammatory response of the chronic phase was less severe and characterized by mononuclear infiltration mainly with focal or zonal fibrosis in the myocardium. Parasites were detected in 50% of infected animals in the myocardium and recovered from pericardic, peritoneal, and ascitic fluids in some animals. Signs of heart failure, sudden death, and enlargement of bowel were observed regularly. The authors concluded that the hamster is a useful model for Chagas' disease studies.

Persisting in the study of these same animals the behavior of the cardiac nervous system in the chronic phase of the infection in hamster was investigated.[82] The counting of neuronal cells of the cardiac autonomic nervous plexus in the 5th, 8th, and 10th month after infection revealed for the first time severe neuronal destruction with characteristics similar to those observed in human Chagas disease. The influence of reinfections in this animal model with VIC *T. cruzi* strain was evaluated[83] and it was verified that important changes were not observed. The use of Syrian hamster as a model for the study of chronic cardiopathy in animals infected with the Y strain was also investigated.[84] Animals were evaluated by histopathology, morphometry, and echocardiography. More intense changes and mortality were observed in animals with higher inocula and interstitial fibrosis. Finally, the Syrian hamster developed a cardiomyopathy which resembles human Chagas' disease.

However, hamsters like guinea pigs are not currently used as experimental model for the studies of Chagas disease, in comparison to other more traditional models.

## Monkeys

The experimental studies of Chagas disease are not so frequent in monkeys due to the great difficulties in obtaining, maintaining, and handling these animals in confinement situations for long periods of time in experimental conditions. However, even considering all these difficulties the phylogenetic proximity of these animals with humans make these models more appropriate than others particularly in the immunological and pathological studies of Chagas disease or in the development of the immunological methods for the diagnosis of this disease.

## Primates autochthonous from the American continent

Chagas[1] was the first to infect primates from *Callithrix* genus (*C. penicillata*) with blood trypomastigotes isolated from Berenice patient, the first human case of the disease. The acute phase of the infection with the first reproduction of the Romaña signal in this species was demonstrated when the animals were inoculated by conjunctival route with feces of infected triatomines.[85] *Cebus* monkeys were infected with blood and metacyclic trypomastigotes by oral mucosa, skin, and conjunctival routes.[86] The authors tried to verify the influence of repeated infections in the anatomopathological pictures of these animals. The mortality of the animals occurred between 75 and 243 days and the diffuse cardiac fibrosis observed was distinct from that verified in human. In two exemplars of this same genus[87] that were infected the symptoms of the acute phase were not verified. However, 9 months later they developed cardiac symptomatology with important anatomopathological and ECG alterations. When these animals were necropsied megaesophagous, fibrosis, and inflammatory infiltrates were found in the myocardium. This same author, infecting another group of 3-year-old animals, verified only discrete infection with decreasing serological titles throughout the infection.

The little primates *Saimiri*, naturally infected in nature, offer relatively easier handling and maintenance in experimental conditions. Trying to use this model for the study of Chagas disease infected with metacyclic trypomastigotes of the Brazil strain,[88] the reproduction of the acute infection was obtained with patent parasitemia, ECG, and hematological alterations, specific anti-*T. cruzi* antibodies, and intense lymphoproliferative response to parasite's antigens.

In a group of 18 *Cebus apella*, named "prego" monkey, 15 months old, infected with repeated inoculations in each animal using three different *T. cruzi* strains[89] a discrete and asymptomatic acute phase was shown. Only one animal infected with the Tulahuen strain presented patent parasitemia. The antibody level increased with each reinoculation. One case of megacolon and one of dolichocolon were reproduced. Various ECG and echocardiographic changes similar to the observed in man were recorded, but the histopathological lesions and fibrosis were discrete. Survived animals that were sacrificed 20−25 months later presented myocytolysis and leukocytes infiltrates between the muscular fibers.[90] In animals with 36–47 months of infection interstitial diffuse or focal fibrosis with discrete infiltrate of leukocytes were present predominantly in the cardiac ventricle wall or septum. This evolutionary character of the histopathological lesions suggests that this model could be more appropriate for the experimental studies of the natural evolution of Chagas disease than other primates models nonautochthonous from the American Continent. Other authors[91] studied the immune response in animals of this species infected with Y strain. Parasitological, serological, and clinical parameters were monitored during a 19-month follow-up, and systemic cytokine responses were assessed sequentially. Elevated expression of interleukin (IL)-4 was observed throughout the study in monkeys that had persistent and higher parasitemias, whereas a high level of interferon (IFN)-gamma was seen in monkeys that controlled parasitemia soon after infection.

## Primates nonautochthonous from the Americas/American continent

*Macacus rhesus* is one of the species of primates not autochthonous from the Americas used as model for Chagas disease studies. This species is phylogenetically considered more similar to the human genome (98% of homology) in relation to the species present in the American Continent.

*M. rhesus* were infected by the conjunctival route with metacyclic trypomastigotes from triatomines naturally infected[92] in parallel with other animals infected with another strain isolated from human. The infection with the wild strain was verified in all animals. Romaña signal was observed in some monkeys as well as chronic myocarditis with tissue parasitism. One case of megaesophagus[93] with the presence of parasites in the muscular fibers in monkeys of this species with 10 years of infection was reproduced. One of the animals that survived for 29 years revealed discrete electrocardiographic changes, discrete increase of the cardiac area, and several indicators of autoimmune response, such as antibody antiendothelium, vases, interstice, and antiperipherical nerves.[94] Other authors[95] also reproduced the infection in three exemplars of rhesus monkeys inoculated with the Peru strain by the conjunctival route. Several signs of the acute phase of the infection were observed, such as patent parasitemia, ocular edema, decrease of red cells and hemoglobin, presence of IgM and IgG antibodies, tissue parasitism in several organs and tissues, and presence of parasites in ocular secretion.

An ultrastructural and cytochemical study of peroxidase and acid phosphatase in skin, lymph node, and heart muscle of rhesus monkeys was performed,[96] providing evidence that these animals could be used as a reliable model to develop histopathological alterations of the human disease.

The evaluation over 3 years of the acute and chronic infection in rhesus monkeys 4- and 10-years-old, inoculated by subcutaneous route with low inoculum of Colombian strain was carried out.[97] Several clinical symptoms typical of acute phase were observed. IgM and IgG anti-*T. cruzi* were observed from the third and fourth weeks of infection, respectively. Antibodies IgM disappeared in the ninth month of infection and IgG increased during all period of study. Myocarditis and myositis were observed only in the acute and subacute phases. However all animals that were autopsied in the later phase presented characteristics of the indeterminate clinical form of the disease without any signal of evolutionary chronic chagasic cardiopathy.

Although primates have been the animals model that develop the acute phase of the infection most similar to that observed in human disease, the difficulty of obtaining, maintaining, and handling of these animals model in experimental conditions associated with the scarcity/rarity of data about the cardiac lesions of the chronic phase discourages the use of this animal model for the experimental study of Chagas disease.

## Conclusions

Although a great variety of animal models could be used as experimental models for the study of Chagas disease, the reproducibility in experimental conditions of all histopathological and clinical manifestations of Chagas disease observed in humans is not possible in all species. Unfortunately, the studies are not performed in standardized conditions even when the same animal species is considered, with regards to race; genetic background; T. cruzi strain; source of the inoculum; inoculum; number of inoculations; route of inoculation; age, sex, and weight of the animal; parameters of evaluation; and length of infection. Moreover, when studies using the same T. cruzi strains in similar conditions in different animal species show that the results observed are not similar, it suggests that it is not possible to extrapolate experimental results from one animal model to another.

Thus, the choice of an experimental model is dependent on the subject to be investigated and the previous knowledge acquired throughout time after one century of research related with this theme. A new system based on a highly sensitive in vivo imaging system of genetically modified T. cruzi bioluminescent may be capable of expressing luciferase open perspectives for both better comprehension of the pathogenesis of Chagas disease in distinct animal models as well as evaluation of therapeutic efficacy of current and new drugs.

## References

1. Chagas C. Nova tripanosomiase humana. Estudos sobre a morfologia e ciclo evolutivo do Schizotrypanum cruzi n. gen., n. sp., agente etiologico de nova entidade morbida do homem. *Mem Inst Oswaldo Cruz* 1909;**1**(59):159−218.
2. World Health Organization. Report of the Scientific Working Group on the development and evaluation of animal models for Chagas' disease. Geneva: 1984.
3. Collier HOJ, Fulton JD, Innes JRM. The oedema of mice infected with *Trypanosoma cruzi* and the accompanying pathological lesions. *Ann Trop Med Parasitol* 1942;**36**: 137−50.

4. Federici EE, Abelmann WH, Neva FA. Chronic and progressive myocarditis and myositis in C3H mice infected with *Trypanosoma cruzi*. *Am J Trop Med* 1964;**13**:272−80.
5. Tafuri WL, Brener Z. Lesões no plexo de Meissner e de Auerbach no intestino do camundongo albino na fase crônica da tripanosomíase cruzi experimental. *Rev Inst Med Trop São Paulo* 1967;**9**:149−54.
6. Tafuri WL, Brener Z. Lesões no sistema nervoso autônomo do camundongo albino na tripanosomíase cruzi experimental, na fase aguda. *O Hospital* 1966;**69**:179−91.
7. Andrade SG, Andrade ZA. Patologia da doença de Chagas experimental de longa duração. *Rev Inst Med Trop São Paulo* 1968;**10**:180−7.
8. Andrade SG, Andrade ZA. Doença de Chagas e alterações neuronais no plexo de Aurebach (estudo experimental em camundongos). *Rev Inst Med Trop São Paulo* 1966;**8**:219−24.
9. Tafuri WL. Light and electron microscope studies of the autonomic nervous system in experimental and human American trypanosomiasis. *Virchows Arch Adt A Pathol Anat* 1971;**3549**:136−49.
10. Campos C, Cangussú S, Duz A, Cartelle C, Noviello Mde L, Veloso V, et al. Enteric neuronal damage, intramuscular denervation and smooth muscle phenotype changes as mechanisms of chagasic megacolon: evidence from a long-term murine model of *Tripanosoma cruzi* infection. *PLoS One* 2016;**5**(11):e0153038.
11. Vago AR, Macedo AM, Adad SJ, Reis DD, Correa-Oliveira R. PCR detection of *Trypanosoma cruzi* DNA in oesophageal tissues of patients with chronic digestive Chagas' disease. *Lancet* 1996;**28**(348):891−2.
12. Luquetti AO, Miles MA, Rassi A, de Rezende JM, de Souza AA, Póvoa MM, et al. *Trypanosoma cruzi*: zymodemes associated with acute and chronic Chagas' disease in central Brazil. *Trans R Soc Trop Med Hyg* 1986;**80**:462−70.
13. Cardoso JE, Brener Z. Hematological change in mice experimentally infected with *Trypanosoma cruzi*. *Mem Inst Oswaldo Cruz* 1980;**75**:97−104.
14. Schlemper Jr BR, Avila CM, Coura JR, Brener Z. Course of infection and histopathological lesions in mice infected with seventeen *Trypanosoma cruzi* strains isolated from chronic patients. *Rev Soc Bras Med Trop* 1983;**16**:23−30.
15. Molina HA, Milei J, Rimoldi MT, Gonzalez Cappa SM, Storino RA. Histopathology of the heart conducting system in experimental Chagas' disease in mice. *Trans R Soc Trop. Med Hyg* 1988;**82**:241−6.
16. Rossi MA, Gonçalves S, Ribeiro dos Santos R. Experimental *Trypanosoma cruzi* cardiomyopathy in Balb/c mice. The potential hole of intravascular platelet aggregation in its genesis. *Am J Pathol* 1984;**114**:209−16.
17. Andrade SG, Grimaldi JA. Chronic murine myocarditis due to *Trypanosoma cruzi*—an ultrastructural study and immunochemical characterization of cardiac interstitial matrix. *Mem Inst Oswaldo Cruz* 1986;**81**:29−41.
18. Andrade V, Barral Neto M, Andrade SG, Magalhães JB. Aspectos imunológicos da infecção de seis linhagens isogênicas de camundongos por três diferentes cepas de *Trypanosoma cruzi*. *Mem Inst Oswaldo Cruz* 1985;**80**:203−11.
19. Krettli AU, Cançado JR, Brener Z. Criterion of cure of human Chagas disease after specific chemotherapy: recent advances. *Mem Inst Oswaldo Cruz* 1984;**79**:157−64.
20. Andrade SG, Magalhães JB. Biodemes and zimodemes of *Trypanosoma cruzi* strains: correlations with clinical data and experimental pathology. *Rev Soc Bras Med Trop* 1996;**30**:27−35.
21. Trischmann TM. *Trypanosoma cruzi*: early parasite proliferation and host resistance in inbred strains of mice. *Exp Parasitol* 1986;**62**:194−201.

22. Minoprio P, Coutinho A, Spinella S, Hontebeyrie-Joskowicz M. Xid immunodeficiency imparts increased parasite clearance and resistance to pathology in experimental Chagas' disease. *Int Immunol* 1991;**3**:427−33.

23. Minoprio P, El Cheikh MC, Murphy E, Hontebeyrie-Joskowicz M, Coffman R, Coutinho A, et al. Xid-associated resistance to experimental Chagas' disease is IFN-gamma dependent. *J Immunol* 1993;**151**:4200−8.

24. Minoprio P, Itohara S, Heusser C, Tonegawa S, Coutinho A. Immunobiology of murine *Trypanosoma cruzi* infection: the predominance of parasite-nonspecific responses and the activation of TCRI T cells. *Immunol Rev* 1989;**112**:183−207.

25. Lewis M, Francisco A, Taylor M, Kelly J. A new experimental model for assessing drug efficacy against *Trypanosoma cruzi* infection based on highly sensitive in vivo imaging. *J Biomol Screen* 2015;**20**:36−43.

26. Silva D, Souza B, Azevedo C, Vasconcelos J, Carvalho R, Soares M, et al. Intramyocardial transplantation of cardiac mesenchymal stem cells reduces myocarditis in a model of chronic Chagas disease cardiomyopathy. *Stem Cell Res Ther* 2014;**5**(4):81.

27. Brand T, Tobie EJ, Kissling RE, Adans G. Physiological and pathological observations on four strains of *Trypanosoma cruzi*. *J Infect Dis.* 1949;**85**:5−16.

28. Alcântara FG, Oliveira JAM. Fase crônica da moléstia de Chagas em ratos Wistar. Pesquisas quantitativas dos neurônios no plexo de Meissner. *Rev Inst Med Trop São Paulo* 1964;**6**:204−6.

29. Alcântara FG, Oliveira JAM. Destruição neuronal do plexo de Auerbach em ratos chagá-sicos crônicos. *Rev Inst Med Trop São Paulo* 1964;**6**:207−10.

30. Machado CR, Ribeiro AL. Experimental American trypanomiasis in rats: sympathetic denervation, parasitism and inflammatory process. *Mem Inst Oswaldo Cruz* 1989;**84**:549−56.

31. Bestetti RB, Soares EG, Sales-Neto VN, Araujo RC, Oliveira SM. The resting electro-cardiogram of *Trypanosoma cruzi* infected rats. *Rev Inst Med Trop São Paulo* 1987;**29**:224−9.

32. Junqueira Jr LF. Modelos experimentais da doença de Chagas: considerações críticas, dados obtidos e contribuições. O modelo representado pelo rato. *Rev Soc Bras Med Trop* 1991;**24**(Suppl 1):53−4.

33. Chapadeiro E, Beraldo PSS, Jesus PC, Oliveira Jr WP, Junqueira Jr LF. Lesões cardíacas em ratos wistar inoculados com diferentes cepas do *Trypanosoma cruzi*. *Rev Soc Bras Med Trop* 1988;**21**:95−108.

34. Melo RC, Machado CR. *Trypanosoma cruzi*: peripheral blood monocytes and heart macrophages in the resistance to acute experimental infection in rats. *Exp Parasitol* 2001;**97**:15−23.

35. Chandrasekar B, Melby PC, Troyer DA, Freeman GL. Differential regulation of nitric oxide synthase isoforms in experimental acute chagasic cardiomyopathy. *Clin Exp Immunol* 2000;**121**:112−19.

36. Lumb G, Shacklett RS, Dawkins WA. The cardiac conduction tissue and its blood supply in the dog. *Am J Pathol* 1959;**35**:467−87.

37. Mirowski M, Lau SA, Bobb GA, Steiner C, Damato AM. Studies on left atrial automa-ticity in dogs. *Circ Res* 1970;**26**:317−25.

38. Goble FC. Observations on experimental Chagas' disease in dogs. *Am J Trop Med Hyg* 1952;**1**:189−204.

39. Pellegrino J. O eletrocardiograma na fase crônica da doença de Chagas experimental no cão. *Mem Inst Oswaldo Cruz* 1946;**44**:615−47.

40. Laranja FS. Aspectos clínicos da moléstia de Chagas. *Rev Bras Med* 1953;**10**:482−91.

41. Campos ES. Estudos sobre uma raça neurotrópica de *Trypanosoma cruzi*. *An Fac Med São Paulo* 1927;**2**:197−201.

42. Koberle F. Cardiopatia chagásica. *O Hospital* 1958;**53**:9−50.

43. Marsden PD, Hagstrom JWC. Experimental *Trypanosoma cruzi* infection in *beagle* puppies. The effect of variations in the dose and source of infecting trypanosomes and the route of inoculation on the course of the infection. *Trans R Soc Trop Med Hyg* 1968;**62**:816−24.

44. Bahia MT, Tafuri WL, Caliari MV, Veloso VM, Carneiro CM, Machado-Coelho GLL, et al. Comparison of *Trypanosoma cruzi* infection in dogs inoculated with blood or metacyclic trypomastigotes of Berenice-62 and Berenice-78 strains via intraperitoneal and conjunctival routes. *Rev Soc Bras Med Trop* 2002;**35**:339−45.

45. Andrade ZA. Patologia do sistema excito-condutor do coração na cardiopatia chagásica. *Rev Pat Trop* 1974;367−428.

46. Andrade ZA, Andrade SG, Correa R, Sadigursky M, Ferrans UJ. Myocardial changes in acute *Trypanosoma cruzi* infection. Ultrastructural evidence of immune damage and the role of microangiopathy. *Am J Pathol* 1994;**144**:1403−11.

47. Anselmi A, Moleiro F, Suarez R, Suarez JA, Ruesta V. Ventricular aneurysms in acute experimental Chagas' myocardiopathy. *Chest* 1971;**59**:654−8.

48. Anselmi A, Gurdiel Q, Suarez JA, Anselmi G. Disturbances in the A-V conduction system in Chagas' myocarditis in the dog. *Circ Res* 1967;**20**:56−64.

49. Andrade ZA, Andrade SG, Sadigursky M. Damage and healing in the conducting tissue of the heart. *J Pathol* 1984;**143**:93−101.

50. Andrade ZA, Andrade SG, Sadigursky M, Maguire JH. Experimental Chagas' disease in dogs. A pathologic and ECG study of the chronic indeterminate phase of the infection. *Arch Pathol Lab Med* 1981;**105**:460−4.

51. Andrade ZA, Andrade SG, Sadigursky M. Enhancement of chronic *Trypanosoma cruzi* myocarditis in dogs treated with low doses of cyclophosphamide. *Am J Pathol* 1987;**127**:467−73.

52. Correa V, Briceno J, Zuniga J, Aranda JC, Valdes JJ, Contreras C, et al. Infeccion por *Trypanosoma cruzi* en animales domesticos de sectores rurales de la IV region Chile. *Bol Chil Parasit* 1982;**37**:27−8.

53. Andrade ZA, Andrade SG. A patologia da doença de Chagas experimental no cão. *Mem Inst Oswaldo Cruz* 1980;**75**:77−95.

54. Lana M, Tafuri WL, Caliari MV, Bambirra EA, Chiari CA, Rios Leite VH, et al. Fase crônica cardíaca fibrosante da tripanosomíase *cruzi* experimental no cão. *Rev Soc Bras Med Trop* 1988;**21**:113−21.

55. Lana M, Chiari E, Tafuri WL. Experimental Chagas' disease in dogs. *Mem Inst Oswaldo Cruz* 1992;**87**:59−71.

56. Lana M, Vieira LM, Machado-Coelho GL, Chiari E, Veloso VM, Tafuri WL. Humoral immune response in dogs experimentally infected with *Trypanosoma cruzi*. *Mem Inst Oswaldo Cruz* 1991;**86**(4):471−3.

57. Araújo FM, Bahia M, Magalhães NM, Martins-Filho OA, Veloso VM, Carneiro CM, et al. Follow-up of experimental chronic Chagas' disease in dogs: use of polymerase chain reaction (PCR) compared with parasitological and serological methods. *Acta Trop* 2002;**81**:21−31.

58. Caliari MV, Lana M, Caliari ER, Tafuri WL. Cardiac plexus of dogs experimentally infected with *Trypanosoma cruzi*: inflammatory lesions and quantitative studies. *Rev Soc Bras Med Trop* 1995;**28**:13−17.

59. Caliari ER, Caliari MV, Lana M, Tafuri WL. Quantitative and qualitative studies of the Auerbach and Meissner plexuses of the esophagus in dogs inoculated with *Trypanosoma cruzi*. *Rev Soc Bras Med Trop* 1996;**29**:17—20.

60. Machado CR, Caliari MV, Lana M, Tafuri WL. Heart autonomic innervation during the acute phase of experimental American trypanosomiasis in the dog. *Am J Trop Med Hyg* 1998;**59**:492—6.

61. Nogueira-Paiva N, Fonseca Kda S, Vieira PM, Diniz L, Caldas I, et al. Myenteric plexus is differentially affected by infection with distinct *Trypanosoma cruzi* strains in *Beagle* dogs. *Mem Inst Oswaldo Cruz* 2014;**109**:51—60.

62. Andrade S, Rassi A, Magalhães J, Ferriollli F, Luquetti A. Specific chemotherapy of Chagas disease: a comparison between the response in patients and experimental animals inoculated with the same strains. *Trans R Soc Trop Med Hyg* 1992;**86**:624—6.

63. Zhang J, Andrade Z, Andrade S, Takeda K, Sadigursky M, Ferrans V. Apoptosis in a canine model of acute chagasic myocarditis. *J Mol Cell Cardiol* 1999;**31**:581—96.

64. Caliari MV, Lana M, Cajá RAF, Carneiro CM, Bahia MT, Santos CAB, et al. Immunohistochemical studies in acute and chronic canine chagasic cardiomyopathy. *Virchows Arch* 2002;**441**:69—76.

65. Machado EM, Fernandes AJ, Murta SM, Vitor RW, Camilo DJR, Pinheiro SW, et al. A study of experimental reinfection by *Trypanosoma cruzi* in dogs. *Am J Trop Med Hyg* 2001;**65**:958—65.

66. Guedes PM, Veloso VM, Tafuri WL, Galvão LM, Carneiro CM, Lana M, et al. The dog as model for chemotherapy of the Chagas' disease. *Acta Trop* 2002;**84**(1):9—17.

67. Caldas I, da Matta Guedes P, dos Santos F, de Figueiredo Diniz L, Martins TA, da Silva do Nascimento AF, et al. Myocardial scars correlate with eletrocardiographic changes in chronic *Trypanosoma cruzi* infection for dogs treated with Benznidazole. *Trop Med Int Health* 2013;**18**:75—84.

68. Agosin M, Badinez O. Algumas características de la infección experimental em conejos. *Infor Parasitol Chilenas* 1948;**4**:6—7.

69. Katzin AM, Bronzina A, Casanova M, Cossio PM, Segura EL, Arana RM, et al. Infeccion experimental del conejo con *Trypanosoma cruzi*. I Estudos parasitologicos y serologicos. *Medicina* 1977;**37**:507.

70. Teixeira ARL, Texeira ML, Santos—Buch CA. The immunology of experimental Chagas' disease. IV The production of lesions in rabbits similar to those of chronic Chagas' disease in man. *Am J Pathol* 1975;**80**:163—78.

71. Andrade ZA, Andrade SG. Patologia. In: Brener Z, Andrade Z, editors. *Trypanosoma cruzi e doença de Chagas*. Rio de Janeiro: Guanabara Koogan; 1979. p. 199—248.

72. Chiari E, Tafuri WL, Bambirra EA, Rezende MM, Ribeiro TO, Castro LP, et al. The rabbit as laboratory animal for studies on Chagas' disease. *Rev Inst Med Trop São Paulo* 1980;**22**:207—8.

73. Teixeira ARL, Figueiredo F, Resende-Filho J, Macedo V. Chagas disease: a clinical parasitological, immunological and pathological study in rabbits. *Am J Trop Med Hyg* 1983;**32**:258—72.

74. Ramirez LE, Brener Z. Evaluation of the rabbit as a model for Chagas disease. I. Parasitological studies. *Mem Inst Oswaldo Cruz* 1987;**82**:531—6.

75. Da Silva AM, Eduardo Ramirez L, Vargas M, Chapadeiro E, Brener Z. Evaluation of the rabbit as a model for Chagas disease-II. Histopathologic studies of the heart, digestive tract and skeletal muscle. *Mem Inst Oswaldo Cruz* 1996;**91**:199—206.

76. Knierim F. Estudio serologico en animales experimentalmente infectados por *Trypanosoma cruzi*. *Bol Chileno Parasitol* 1954;**9**:2—6.

77. Kozma C, Jaffe R, Jaffe W. Experimental study of the pathogenesis of myocarditis. *Arq Bras Cardiol* 1960;**13**:155—61.

78. Lopes EA, Pileggi F, Decourt LV. Ultrastructural aspects of acute experimental Chagas' heart disease in the *guinea-pig*. *Arq Bras Cardiol* 1969;**22**:161—74.

79. Franco MF. Cardite experimental no cobaio pela cepa Y do *Trypanosoma cruzi*. Correlação entre histopatologia e a presença de antígenos parasitários identificados por imunofluorescência indireta. *Rev Soc Bras Med Trop* 1990;**23**:187—9.

80. Castro-Sesquen Y, Gilman R, Yauri V, Angulo N, Verastegui M, Velásquez D, et al. *Cavia porcellus* as a model for experimental infection by *Trypanosoma cruzi*. *Am J Pathol* 2011;**179**:281—8.

81. Ramirez LE, Lages-Silva E, Soares Jr JM, Chapadeiro E. The hamster (*Mesocricetus auratus*) as experimental model in Chagas' disease: parasitological and histopathological studies in acute and chronic phases of *Trypanosoma cruzi* infection. *Rev Soc Bras Med Trop* 1994;**27**:163—9.

82. Chapadeiro E, Silva EL, Silva AC, Fernandes P, Ramirez LE. Cardiac neuronal de population in hamsters (*Mesocricetus auratus*) chronically infected with *Trypanosoma cruzi*. *Rev Soc Bras Med Trop* 1999;**32**:35—9.

83. Cabrine-Santos M, Lages-Silva E, Chapadeiro E, Ramirez LE. Trypanosoma cruzi: characterization of reinfection and search for tissue tropism in hamsters (*Mesocricetus auratus*). *Exp Parasitol* 2001;**99**:160—7.

84. Bilate AM, Salemi VM, Ramires FJ, De Brito T, Silva AM, Umezawa ES, et al. The *Syrian* hamster as a model for the dilated cardiomyopathy of Chagas' disease: a quantitative echocardiographical and histopathological analysis. *Microbes Infect* 2003;**5**: 1116—24.

85. Romaña C. Reproduction chez le singe de la "conjonctivite schizotrypanosomienne unilaterale." *Bull Soc Path Exot* 1939;**4**:390—4.

86. Torres CM, Tavares BM. Miocardite no macaco *Cebus* após inoculações repetidas com *Schizotrypanum cruzi*. *Mem Inst Oswaldo Cruz* 1958;**56**:85—152.

87. Bolomo N, Milei J, Cossuo PM, Segura E, Laguens RP, Fernandez LM, et al. Experimental Chagas' disease in a South American primate (*Cebus* sp). *Medicina (Buenos Aires)* 1980;**40**:667—72.

88. Pung OJ, Hulsebos LH, Kuhn RE. Experimental American leishmaniasis and Chagas' disease in the Brazilian squirrel monkey: cross immunity and electrocardiographic studies of monkeys infected with *Leishmania braziliensis* and *Trypanosoma cruzi*. *Int J Parasitol* 1988;**18**:1053—9.

89. Falasca A, Grana D, Buccolo J, Gilli M, Merlo A, Zoppi J, et al. Susceptibility of the *Cebus apella* monkey to different strains of *Trypanosoma cruzi* after single or repeated inoculations. *PAHO Bulletin* 1986;**20**:117—37.

90. Falasca CA, Gili M, Grana D, Gomez H, Zoppi J, Mareso E. Chronic myocardial damage in experimental *Trypanosoma cruzi* infection of a new world primate *Cebus* sp. monkey. *Rev Inst Med Trop São Paulo* 1990;**32**:151—61.

91. Samudio M, Montenegro-James S, Kasamatsu E, Cabral M, Schinini A, Rojas De Arias A, et al. Local and systemic cytokine expression during experimental chronic *Trypanosoma cruzi* infection in a *Cebus* monkey model. *Parasite Immunol* 1999;**21**:451—60.

92. Dorland JD. Infection in monkeys with strains of *Trypanosoma cruzi* isolated in the United States. *Public Health Rep* 1943;**58**:1006—10.

93. Guimarães J.P., Miranda A. Megaesôfago em macacos rhesus com 10 anos de infecção chagásica. In: Anais Congresso Internacional sobre doença de Chagas. Rio de Janeiro: 1961. p. 567—71.

94. Szarfman A, Gerecht D, Drapper CC, Marsden PD. Tissue-eacting immunoglobulins on rhesus monkeys infected with *Trypanosoma cruzi*: a follow-up study. *Trans R Soc Trop Med Hyg* 1978;**75**:114—16.
95. Marsden PD, Voller A, Seah SKK, Hawkey C, Green D. Behaviour of a Peru strain of *Trypanosoma cruzi* in *rhesus* monkeys. *Rev Soc Bras Med Trop* 1970;**4**(3):177—82.
96. De Meirelles Mde N, Bonecini-Almeida Mda G, Pessoa MH, Galvão-Castro B. *Trypanosoma cruzi*: experimental Chagas' disease in *rhesus* monkeys. II. Ultrastructural and cytochemical studies of peroxidase and acid phosphatase activities. *Mem Inst Oswaldo Cruz* 1990;**85**:173—81.
97. Bonecini-Almeida MG, Galvão-Castro B, Pessoa MHR, Pirmez C, Laranja F. Experimental Chagas' disease in *rhesus* monkeys. I. Clinical, parasitological hematological and anatomopathological studies in the acute and indeterminate phase of the disease. *Mem Inst Oswaldo Cruz* 1990;**85**:163—71.

# Classification and phylogeny of *Trypanosoma cruzi*

*P.B. Hamilton and J.R. Stevens*
University of Exeter, Exeter, United Kingdom

## Chapter Outline

## Application of molecular phylogenetics to trypanosome taxonomy and understanding evolution

All trypanosomes (genus *Trypanosoma*) are vertebrate parasites and have a characteristic morphology in the vertebrate bloodstream. Trypanosomes are diverse and successful, being found in all classes of vertebrate—fish, amphibians, birds, reptiles, and mammals (monotremes, marsupial, and placental)[1]—and in all continents. The vast majority of trypanosome species are transmitted by leeches and arthropods (mostly insects), although a few species can be passed directly between vertebrates. There are no free-living stages. Although several species are associated with important diseases of humans and domestic livestock, there is little evidence for health impacts on their wild vertebrate hosts, with the exception of some Australian trypanosomes which have been linked to poor health of marsupials.[2,3]

There has been considerable interest in the evolutionary origin of trypanosomes (genus *Trypanosoma*) and the relationships of species within the genus since the early 1900s.[1,4–6] In particular, the relationship between the two human pathogens, *Trypanosoma cruzi* and *Trypanosoma brucei* has received considerable attention.[7–12] However, due to the absence of a fossil record, and with few morphological features,

*American Trypanosomiasis Chagas Disease.* DOI: http://dx.doi.org/10.1016/B978-0-12-801029-7.00015-0

testing evolutionary hypotheses has only become possible since the late 1980s/early 1990s with the advent of molecular phylogenetics. Molecular phylogenetic trees (phylogenies) are constructed through comparisons of DNA sequences (or amino acid sequences inferred from them) from a range of organisms. Phylogenies can be used to trace the evolutionary history of a group of organisms, thus providing robust frameworks for testing evolutionary hypotheses.

It is now relatively straightforward to sequence short (100–2000 bp) stretches of DNA from trypanosomes. First the chosen gene is amplified using the polymerase chain reaction (PCR), followed by sequencing of purified PCR products. Computer programs can then be used to align sequences from different taxa (e.g., species) and for subsequent construction of evolutionary trees. Increased computing power has allowed advanced computer-intensive tree building methods, such as maximum-likelihood and Bayesian methods, to be applied to sequences from many organisms, and even sequence data from whole genomes.[11] Although the first studies of this nature relied on DNA isolated from cultured parasites, many more recent studies have used DNA extracted directly from the host tissue, such as blood, or from insect guts. The development of such methods led the way to larger-scale surveys of parasite diversity, which have transformed our understanding of the diversity of trypanosome species and their host ranges.

A range of genes have been used for phylogenetic and taxonomic studies. The majority of early studies that examined relationships between species used nuclear ribosomal DNA markers, in particular, 18S rDNA (also known as the small subunit (SSU) rDNA), and to a lesser extent 28S rDNA (also known as the large subunit (LSU) rDNA). The 18S rRNA gene has both conserved regions, suitable for primer design and for resolving relationships between distantly related species, and faster-evolving regions, suitable for deducing evolutionary relationships between closely related species and at the subspecies level. The V7–V8 region of 18S rDNA is the most variable and is often called the "barcoding" region, because it is useful for species identification. It has also been used to develop species-specific PCR primers. The noncoding internal transcribed spacer (ITS) regions, ITS1 and ITS2, also have fast evolutionary rates, and have proved useful for studying within-species diversity. Protein-coding genes have also been used; in particular, glycosomal glyceraldehyde phosphate dehydrogenase (*gGAPDH*) for phylogenetic placement of newly described species and for resolving some "difficult" relationships within the genus. Due to the ease of alignment of sequences from distantly related species, and because it is often possible to amplify the majority of the gene in a single PCR using DNA from uncultured parasites, *gGAPDH* has sometimes been used in preference to 18S rDNA. The faster-evolving kinetoplast (mitochondrial) cytochrome b (*Cyt b*) gene has also been used for examining within-species diversity.[13,14]

Phylogenies based on *gGAPDH* and 18S rDNA sequences both separately and combined have resolved many of the relationships within the genus and in most cases are sufficient for taxonomic placement of new trypanosomes. However, relationships between some of the major groups remain poorly resolved. This is likely to change in the near future as it has become relatively straightforward to sequence complete genomes of trypanosome species using next generation sequencing technologies.[15] The use of such data enables phylogenies to be constructed using vastly more information than using just one or two genes, providing greater resolution. For instance, analysis of the full genome sequence of *T. grayi*, a tsetse-fly transmitted trypanosome of African crocodiles demonstrated unequivocally that it is more closely related to *T. cruzi* than to *T. brucei*, indicating separate origins of tsetse-fly transmission in Africa for this crocodile trypanosome and the *T. brucei* group.[15] Previously, in *gGAPDH* and 18S rDNA trees, the relationship of this crocodile parasite to other trypanosomes of terrestrial mammals had been only poorly resolved.

Molecular phylogenetics has also informed taxonomy.[16] Taxonomic groups should have evolutionary relevance, and arguably names should only be applied to monophyletic groups. Molecular studies have questioned the validity of some species that were previously described using only morphological and lifecycle data. Molecular methods have also raised new questions, such as whether new species should be named on the basis of sequence information alone, and the degree of genetic divergence necessary to classify lineages as the same or different species.[17] At the same time, surveys of trypanosomatid diversity that use rapid methods for species identification based on sequencing[18,19] or length differences within regions of ribosomal DNA[3,20−24] have led to the description of new species. While many of these new species were found in previously unstudied hosts, such as Australian marsupials,[25−29] some potentially pathogenic species have also been found in well-studied groups, such as the African tsetse fly-transmitted group of trypanosomes.[19,20,30] Analysis of DNA from Giemsa-stained microscope slides revealed that one of the "new" trypanomes described recently using molecular methods from tsetse flies in Tanzania[20] and the Central African Republic[19] was *T. suis*. This pig pathogen was first described in the 1950s but was subsequently largely forgotten.[31] It is clear that much trypanosomatid diversity is yet to be discovered.

# Origin of trypanosomes and the relationship between *T. cruzi* and *T. brucei*

Trypanosomes are kinetoplastids, which include both free-living and parasitic groups. There has been considerable interest in the transitional steps between the free-living ancestor and trypanosomes which are parasitic at all life cycle stages. Two groups of theories have dominated debate. Vertebrate-first theories proposed that the ancestral trypanosome evolved from a gut parasite of vertebrates,[4] while invertebrate-first theories proposed that it evolved from a single-host (monogenetic) invertebrate parasite, similar to the trypanosomatids now found in insect guts.[1,5,6]

Resolving the relationships between trypanosomes, other trypanosomatids (family Trypanosomatidae) and bodonids is the key to understanding the origin of the genus. Bodonids are mostly free living. All trypanosomatids are parasitic at all stages of their lifecycles. Most trypanosomatid genera (e.g., *Blastocrithidia*, *Crithidia*, *Herpetomonas*, *Leptomonas*, *Sergeia*, *Wallaceina*) are single-host (monogenetic) parasites of insects. Recent studies using molecular methods have led to significant changes to the taxonomy of trypanosomatids and have revealed a large diversity among these insect parasites. Several new genera have been recently described by investigating less-studied insect host groups,[32,33] including *Sergeia* from a biting midge,[34] *Blechomonas* from fleas,[35] and *Paratrypanosoma* from a mosquito.[36] Nonetheless, *Trypanosoma* and *Leishmania* remain the only two-host (digenetic) vertebrate parasites. The existence of another digenetic vertebrate parasite, *Endotrypanum*, has not been verified using molecular techniques, as the isolates of this genus examined to date have turned out to be *Leishmania*.[37,38] A few other trypanosomatid genera have been isolated from humans that are either immuno-compromised,[39] or coinfected with *Leishmania* [40], but these are thought not to infect healthy vertebrates. *Phytomonas* (another digenetic genus) is a parasite of plants, which is also transmitted by insects.[41,42]

A central question that has been the source of considerable debate is whether trypanosomes are monophyletic. A monophyletic group is a collection of organisms, which form a single clade comprising an ancestor and all its descendants. Monophyly of trypanosomes would indicate that all described taxa within the genus had a single common origin and did not gave rise to other trypanosomatid groups, by for example losing dependence on the vertebrate lifecycle stage. If this had occurred we may expect some of the insect-only trypanosomatids would fall among trypanosomes in the evolutionary tree. The monophyly debate has also been central to resolving whether the two trypanosome groups that include the human pathogens *T. brucei* and *T. cruzi* evolved vertebrate parasitism independently.

In several early phylogenetic trees, based on comparisons of genes encoding ribosomal RNAs, trypanosomes appeared paraphyletic.[43–45] Often the evolutionary trees obtained from these studies suggested that the clade including *T. brucei* and related parasites (the "*T. brucei*" clade) diverged early in trypanosomatid evolution and evolved vertebrate parasitism independently to the other trypanosomes that include *T. cruzi*. On the other hand, most later studies, also using ribosomal RNA genes, but with substan-tially increased taxon-sampling, supported monophyly of trypanosomes,[8,10,28,46] although several supported paraphyly.[9] The issue was resolved using taxon-rich trees based on protein-coding genes, which strongly supported monophyly of the genus,[10,47–49] confirming earlier studies using protein-coding genes that had included fewer taxa.[50–53] This question was subsequently addressed using whole-genome phylogenetic analyses including *Trypanosoma brucei*, *Trypanosoma cruzi*, *Leishmania major*, and two outgroup taxa, *Euglena gracilis* and *Naegleria gruberi*; almost all of the analyzed gene markers shared between the genomes of *T. brucei*, *T. cruzi*, and *L. major* supported the hypothesis that these trypanosomes form a monophyletic group.[11] This analysis demonstrated the power of using whole genome sequences to resolve deep trypanosomatid relationships. Significantly, trypanosome monophyly indicates that trypanosome species might share some common, ancestral adaptations for survival in vertebrates. Understanding such ancestral adaptations could aid the rational design of therapeutics that target a broad range of pathogenic trypanosome species.

Recent phylogenetic studies suggest that trypanosomes and *Leishmania* evolved from different insect parasites, supporting the "invertebrate first" hypothesis.[1,5,6] In support of this hypothesis, a newly described trypanosomatid genus, *Paratrypanosoma*, fell at the base of all trypanosomatids in a multigene phylogenetic analysis, suggesting that the first trypanosomatids were parasites of insects.[36] Trypanosomes and all other trypanosomatids are sister groups in this tree, as is the case in most 18S rDNA trees (but differing from some *gGAPDH* gene trees), indicating that trypanosomes likely emerged relatively early in trypanosomatid evolution.[10] Strong evidence that *Leishmania* acquired vertebrate parasitism independently from trypanosomes comes from the discovery of *Leptomonas costaricensis*, an insect-only trypanosomatid that is closely related to *Leishmania*,[54] and studies that have resolved relationships between the genus and other insect trypanosomatids.[32,36] *Leishmania* appears to have evolved considerably more recently than *Trypanosoma*, which may partially explain its comparatively narrow vertebrate (mammals, reptiles) and invertebrate (sandflies) host range. Thus, *T. cruzi* and other trypanosomes will not share common, ancestral adaptations to vertebrate parasitism with *Leishmania* spp.

The evolution of trypanosomes from a monogenetic insect parasite indicates that the first trypanosomes were insect-transmitted parasites of amphibious or terrestrial vertebrates. In this scenario, trypanosomes of fish that are transmitted by leeches must have evolved later. This hypothesis receives some support as, while the deepest split within genus *Trypanosoma* is between the Aquatic clade (that includes the fish trypanosomes) and the Terrestrial clade (Fig. 15.1A), both clades contain insect-transmitted parasites. The position of leech-transmitted trypanosomes of freshwater and marine fish in phylogenetic trees provides further support for this scenario[7]; they all fall in one of the two major subclades of the Aquatic clade,[8] indicating that they were not the first to evolve, as had previously been hypothesized.[55] Trypanosomes of marine fish form a monophyletic subclade within the fish clade, further indicating that these were not the first to evolve, as may have been expected if trypanosomes first evolved in early vertebrates (marine fish). It therefore appears that adaptation to transmission by aquatic leeches, perhaps by leeches feeding on infected amphibious vertebrates, enabled trypanosomes to colonize many aquatic vertebrates, including both freshwater and marine fish.

## Relationships within the genus *Trypanosoma*

Studies have also examined relationships within the genus *Trypanosoma*. The composition of the clade that includes *T. cruzi* (the "*T. cruzi*" clade) has provided valuable clues to the origin of *T. cruzi*. The most taxon rich phylogenetic trees are based on alignments of 18S rDNA and *gGAPDH* genes.[7–10,28,47,56–59] From these studies, it is clear that *T. brucei* and *T. cruzi* are in different clades and acquired human parasitism independently.[8] While *T. brucei* falls in the *T. brucei* clade with other tsetse-fly transmitted trypanosomes from Africa, indicating a long history largely confined to Africa,[8] the *T. cruzi* clade is associated with South American and Australian mammalian hosts, and with bats (see "The *T. cruzi* Clade" section).

There are now approximately 10 well-established clades within the genus *Trypanosoma* (Fig. 15.1A), all of which are found on more than one continent. Although newly described trypanosomes tend to fall within one of these clades, it is

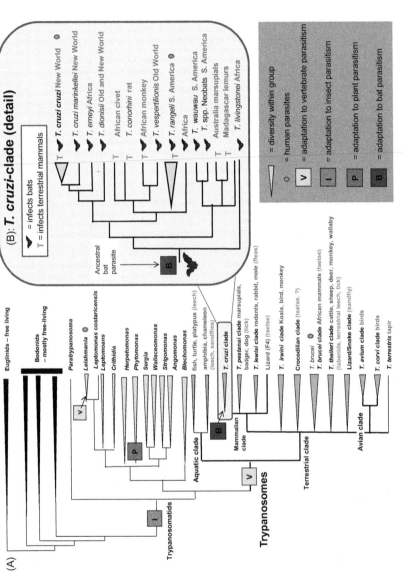

**Figure 15.1** (A) Phylogenetic relationships of kinetoplastids, showing the relationships between the main trypanosomatid lineages. Groups connected by horizontal lines are descended from a common ancestor. I, origin of single-host (monogenetic) insect parasitism; V, origins of two-host (digenetic) vertebrate parasitism; P, origin of digenetic plant parasitism. (B) Detail of relationships within the *T. cruzi* clade. *Source:* Refs. 8,10.27–29,47,49,54,60–62 Relationships of trypanosomatids other than trypanosomes are from Refs. 32,36,63–65 Taxa in gray are vertebrate hosts. Taxa in parentheses are invertebrate hosts (vectors).

likely that other distinct groups are yet to be discovered. Mapping the hosts of trypanosomes onto a phylogenetic tree has revealed some highly informative associations between clades and certain types of vertebrate and invertebrate host.[47] For example, two groups are restricted to birds, one to crocodilians, and there are several distinct mammalian clades. Other clades appear to be largely restricted to a particular type of invertebrate, such as the *T. brucei* clade, in which most species are transmitted by tsetse flies. Overall, cospeciation with either vertebrates or invertebrates appears to have played little role in trypanosome evolution. Instead, adaptations to host types and opportunities appear to have played a more important role in determining the host range of trypanosome clades.[47] Analyses based on combined datasets of 18S rDNA and *gGAPDH* gene sequences have provided increased resolution, combining some of these clades into "superclades". These analyses have resolved the deepest split within the genus which is between the Aquatic clade and the Terrestrial clade, which includes all the other clades. Importantly, both *T. cruzi* and *T. brucei* are in the Terrestrial Clade. Another of these "superclades", the Mammalian clade, includes the *T. cruzi* clade and two other mammalian clades (Fig. 15.1A).

# Molecular phylogenetics and traditional taxonomy of mammalian trypanosomes

Prior to the advent of molecular methods, taxonomy of trypanosomes relied on comparisons of morphology, lifecycle and disease data. The most commonly used taxonomy of Hoare[1] divides mammalian trypanosomes into two sections. The section Salivaria comprises trypanosomes in which the infective forms are passed in the saliva of the insect. The section Stercoraria comprises species in which the developmental cycle in the insect vector is completed in the hindgut, and transmission is through contact with infective forms in the feces. In this taxonomy, *Trypanosoma cruzi* was placed within the subgenus *Schizotrypanum* within the section Stercoraria. This taxonomy is given below; type species of each subgenus are in parentheses:

| | |
|---|---|
| Section: Stercoraria | |
| Subgenera: | *Herpetosoma* (*T. lewisi*) |
| | *Megatrypanum* (*T. theileri*) |
| | *Schizotrypanum* (*T. cruzi*) |
| Section: Salivaria | |
| Subgenera: | *Duttonella* (*T. vivax*) |
| | *Nannomonas* (*T. congolense*) |
| | *Pycnomonas* (*T. suis*) |
| | *Trypanozoon* (*T. brucei*) |

Molecular phylogenetic studies have largely supported recognition of the Salivaria and its subgenera. In contrast, the Stercoraria, and its subgenera have generally not received consistent support. This is perhaps not surprising as subgenera within this section are less well defined, e.g., Hoare,[1] while classifying *T. rangeli* in subgenus *Herpetosoma*, noted its "aberrant or atypical" developmental characteristics and status, and the defining characteristic of trypanosomes within *Megatrypanum* is their large size. More recently, based on phylogenetic evidence, Stevens et al.[66] proposed that use of the names *Herpetosoma* and *Megatrypanum* be discontinued because these groupings are polyphyletic and so lack taxonomic and evolutionary relevance, while *Schizotrypanum* be expanded to include all trypanosomes that fall in the *T. cruzi* clade (see "*T. cruzi* Clade" section, Fig. 15.1). All trypanosomes originally placed within the subgenus *Schizotrypanum* fall within this suggested clade, and the clade now also includes species originally placed within *Herpetosoma* (*T. lewisi*, *T. rangeli*) and *Megatrypanum* (*T. conorhini*). Subsequently, however, the name *Schizotrypanum* has been more commonly applied to a subclade within the *T. cruzi* clade that contains trypanosomes with typical *Schizotrypanum* morphology, i.e., *T. cruzi*, *T. c. marinkellei*, *T. dionisii*, and *T. erneyi*.[67]

The use of *Herpetosoma* continues and is applied to trypanosomes related to *T. lewisi*, while *Megatrypanum* continues to be applied to trypanosomes related to *T. theileri*. Most trypanosomes, however, do not fall within these categories. Recently Votýpka et al.[17] proposed practicality over rigid taxonomic codes or a blind phylogenetic approach for trypanosomatid taxonomy. For example, they suggest that existing names should be kept whenever possible, especially for medically or veterinary important species.

# The main groups of trypanosomes recognized in molecular phylogenetic analyses

A brief description of the main trypanosome clades follows (Fig. 15.1A):

- **The Aquatic clade**: This clade comprises trypanosomes of mainly aquatic and amphibious vertebrates, including all species from fish and several from amphibia. The vertebrate hosts also include reptiles (caiman, chameleon, turtle) and a mammal (platypus).[25,27,28,68–70] Many of these species are transmitted by proboscid leeches.[71–77] The platypus trypanosome has also been found in a leech, possibly implicating it as a vector.[78] There is evidence that some of the trypanosomes from amphibious vertebrates are transmitted by insects,[76] and the chameleon trypanosome presumably also has an insect vector. Considerable diversity within this clade has been found in amphibians and sandflies in South America.[79]
- **The *T. cruzi* clade**: See "*T. cruzi* Clade" section.
- **The *T. pestanai* clade**: This clade contains trypanosomes from the Eurasian badger (*T. pestanai*),[8,80] ticks from Japan,[81] Australian marsupials, *T. copemani*, *T. gilletti* and *T. vegrandis*,[8,25,26,62,82,83] and Brazilian dogs, *T. caninum*.[84] There is some evidence implicating fleas in the transmission of *T. pestanai*[80] and evidence implicating ticks in the transmission of these Australian marsupial trypanosomes.[85]
- **The *T. lewisi* clade**: This clade contains trypanosomes from a wide range of rodents. It also contains trypanosomes from a lagomorph and insectivores.[86–88] Each trypanosome species in this clade is thought to be specific to its vertebrate host. The vast majority of the vectors of these trypanosomes are fleas, although the lifecycles of some species are

not completely known.[1] One exception is *T. talpae*, from a mole, that is believed to be transmitted by mites.[89] The clade contains *T. lewisi*, the type species of the subgenus *Herpetosoma*, thus the name *Herpetosoma* is occasionally used for this clade.[16]

- **The *T. irwnini* clade**: This clade contains *T. irwnini* from an Australian marsupial (koala), *T. bennetti* from an American kestrel,[26] and *T. minasense* from a South American primate (red-handed tamarind, *Saguinus midas*), imported into Japan[90]; see "*T. cruzi* Clade" section— *T. rangeli* for further discussion on this species. The presence of both mammalian and avian trypanosomes within this clade demonstrates that host-switching between different vertebrate classes has occurred, which is unusual among trypanosomes of terrestrial vertebrates.

- **The crocodilian clade**: This clade comprises crocodilian trypanosomes from Africa and South America and includes *T. grayi*, transmitted by tsetse flies in Africa.[60,91] A recent analysis found some strains in South America and Africa to be closely related, suggesting dispersal after continental separation.[92] This clade is more closely related to *T. cruzi* than to the other trypanosomes transmitted by tsetse flies in the *T. brucei* group.[15]

- **The *T. brucei* clade**: This clade contains mostly trypanosomes of African mammals. Two subspecies of *T. brucei*—*T. b. gambiense* and *T. b. rhodesiense*—are also human pathogens. Many of these species are pathogens of domestic livestock (*T. brucei*, *T. congolense*, *T. evansi*, *T. godfreyi*, *T. simiae*, *T. suis*, and *T. vivax*). The majority of trypanosomes in the *T. brucei* clade are transmitted by tsetse flies (genus *Glossina*) via the saliva when the fly takes a blood meal. *T. congolense* and *T. simiae* are further split into "types" that are, arguably, sufficiently different to warrant species status. *gGAPDH* sequences from tsetse flies in East Africa suggest the existence of two further species related to *T. vivax*,[30] and 18S rDNA sequences from tsetse flies in Central Africa demonstrate the existence of a further undescribed species.[19] Two trypanosomes in the clade, *T. evansi* and *T. vivax*, are known from South America, and are believed to have been accidentally introduced into the continent by humans in domestic animals.[1,93] DNA microsatellite data support a single introduction of *T. vivax* into South America from West Africa.[94]

- **The *T. theileri* clade**: This clade contains trypanosomes from marsupial and placental mammals (deer, cattle, primates). It includes *T. theileri*, the type species for the subgenus, that is commonly found in domestic cattle across the world.[56,95] There are two distinct subgroups of *Megatrypanum*, TthI and TthII, which are arguably different species, with considerable genetic diversity in each.[95] *Megatrypanum* in both subclades, when found in cattle is generally referred to as *T. theileri*[17] even though each subclade includes isolates from various other hosts including deer and duikers. *T. (Megatrypanum) melophagium* a parasite of sheep transmitted by the sheep ked (*Melophagus ovinus*) is in one of the subgroups and appears to be host specific.[96,97] *T. theileri* is known from South American cattle and buffalo, with distinct strains in each.[95] Tabanid flies act as the principal vectors of *T. theileri*, although ticks also have the capacity to transmit this trypanosome,[1,95,98–100] and a high prevalence in tsetse flies raises the question of whether they also act as vectors.[19] Stevens et al.[12] found a monkey trypanosome, *T. cyclops* from Southeast Asia, to be related to *T. theileri*, but fell outside the *Megatrypanum* group. Subsequently this trypanosome formed a distinct subclade with trypanosomes from Australian marsupials (wallabies) and terrestrial bloodsucking leeches (Haemadipsidae). These leeches are common in tropical forests across Asia and Australia implicating them in the transmission of this trypanosome subgroup.[56] The name *Megatrypanum* has been used for the *T. theileri* clade [16,95] but is now more commonly used for the two subclades that contain *T. theileri*.[17]

- **The lizard/snake clade**: This clade contains trypanosomes of lizards and snakes.[61] Sandflies are the only known vectors of trypanosomes in this clade.[91,101]
- **The avian clade**: The two main subclades of avian trypanosome, the *T. avium* and the *T. corvi* clades,[102,103] first grouped together in this clade in a tree produced from combined data from *gGAPDH* and 18S DNA sequences.[47] A wide range of insect vectors transmit the trypanosomes in this clade, including black flies,[104,105] hippoboscid flies, and mosquitoes.[106,107] Both subclades have a wide distribution, e.g., the *T. corvi* clade is found in both Australia and Europe.[56]

## The *T. cruzi* clade

This clade contains trypanosomes that are parasitic in a diverse range of mammals, including two human-infective parasites: *T. cruzi* and *T. rangeli*, both of which are restricted to the New World. It also contains trypanosomes from Chiropteran (bat) hosts from both the Old and New Worlds (*T. erneyi*, *T. cruzi T. marinkellei*, *T. dionisii*, *T. livingstonei*, *T. vespertilionis*, and several unnamed species). Other trypanosomes within the clade are *T. conorhini*, a rat parasite, and trypanosomes from African terrestrial mammals (monkey, civet)[62,108] and Australian marsupials.[8,23,25,27,28,83] The majority of known invertebrate vectors of these trypanosomes are bugs (suborder Heteroptera; order Hemiptera). Three species are transmitted by triatomine bugs: *Trypanosoma rangeli* and *Trypanosoma cruzi* by a wide range of species, and *Trypanosoma conorhini* by *Triatoma rubrofasciata*. The bat trypanosomes are also thought to be transmitted by bat-feeding bugs. For instance, infections of *T. cruzi marinkellei* have been described in the bat-feeding triatomine bugs of genus *Cavernicola*,[109] while cimicid bugs in the genus *Cimex* are frequently found infected with trypanosomes and have been implicated in the transmission of three species of bat trypanosome: *T. dionisii*, *T. incertum*, and *T. vespertilionis*.[110–112] An exception to bug-mediated transmission may be the Australian marsupial group trypanosomes, which have been identified in tabanid flies, potentially implicating them as vectors.[113] The vectors of the trypanosomes from the African terrestrial mammals and other bats are as yet unknown. Interestingly, Salazar et al.[114] found that the common bed bug, *Cimex lectularius*, has the capacity to transmit *Trypanosoma cruzi*, although the epidemiological importance of this finding is not known.

The *T. cruzi* clade contains several trypanosomes originally placed within the subgenus *Schizotrypanum* on the basis of their morphology and lifecycles, prior to phylogenetic evidence. The close relationship between trypanosome species originally classified in subgenus *Schizotrypanum* is not surprising, as the subgenus has well defined morphology and development within the vertebrate host. The subgenus comprises small trypanosomes that are very difficult to distinguish morphologically from the type species, *T. cruzi*. They have a voluminous kinetoplast and, typically, curved bloodstream forms in the shape of a C or S, with a short pointed posterior end, which constitute distinctive morphological characters.[1] Within the vertebrate host, multiplication occurs within various tissues and organs, rather than in the blood (like many other trypanosome species). Several *T. cruzi*-like trypanosomes from non-bat South American wild mammals have been described using traditional parasitological techniques: *T. (S.) lesourdi* Leger and Porry, 1918 from a Spider monkey; *T. (S.) prowazeki* Berenberg-Gossler, 1908 from a Uakari (a species of New World monkey); and *T. (S.) sanmartini* Garnham and Gonzales-Mugaburur, 1962 from a Squirrel monkey. It is also possible that several (and perhaps all) of the morphologically described *Schizotrypanum* species in South American terrestrial mammals represent synonyms of *T. cruzi* (see next section of this chapter). Likewise, a range of bat trypanosomes have been classified within the subgenus *Schizotrypanum* using parasitological techniques, including two from Australia, *T. (S.) pteropi* Breinl, 1921 and *T. (S.) hipposideri* Mackerras, 1959; and *T. (S.) hedricki*, *T. (S.) myoti* and *T. (S.) dionisii* from elsewhere in the Old World. Morphological similarities between these bat trypanosomes have made it difficult to delineate species and to match molecular data with old parasitological descriptions.

Trypanosomes within the *T. cruzi*-clade are listed below (Fig. 15.1B):

- **T. cruzi cruzi**: Also called *T. cruzi* sensu stricto.
- **T. cruzi marinkellei**: This bat trypanosome is apparently restricted to South America and was sufficiently divergent to warrant subspecies status.[115] Its close relationship to *T. cruzi cruzi* has been verified using 18S rDNA,[8] *gGAPDH* gene,[10,47] and kinetoplast *Cyt* b gene[13] sequences. The genome of this species has been sequenced and analyzed.[116]
- **T. dionisii**: This bat trypanosome was first described from Europe.[117,118] A strain of this species has been found in South America[13,119] and is closely related to one of the two known European strains.[62]
- **T. erneyi**: This bat trypanosome was described from Molossidae bats captured in Mozambique, Africa and is the closest known living relative to *T. cruzi*.[67]
- **T. sp. (civet) and T. sp. (monkey)**: These trypanosomes were isolated in a study that examined trypanosome diversity in a wide range of wild vertebrates in Cameroon, West Africa.[108] In that study they remained unidentified, but later characterization, by sequence analysis of their 18S rDNA and *gGAPDH* genes, demonstrated—for the first time—the presence of the *T. cruzi* clade in non-bat hosts in Africa.[62]
- **T. conorhini**: A trypanosome found worldwide in rats and transmitted by the triatomine bug *T. rubrofasciata*.[1] The origin of *T. conorhini* is far from clear, but evidence suggests an Old World origin for this species. Its vector, *T. rubrofasciata*, is part of a group with very close affinity to an Old World genus, *Linshcosteus*.[120] Interestingly, trypanosome species that resemble *T. conorhini* have been described in Indonesian primates[121]; under laboratory conditions, they developed in a triatomine bug, *T. rubrofasciata*,[122] a natural vector of *T. conorhini*. This led Hoare[1] to argue that these Indonesian trypanosomes were primate-adapted strains of *T. conorhini*. On the other hand, Weinman[122] argued that Indonesian monkey trypanosomes are unlikely to be *T. conorhini*, as *T. rubrofasciata* is rat-specific and, while it has been found in cities, it has never been found in the tropical rainforests of Asia.
- **T. livingstonei**: This trypanosome was described from bats (*Rhinolophus landeri* and *Hipposideros caffer*) captured in Mozambique in Africa and is the most divergent member of the *Trypanosoma cruzi* clade.[123]

- **T. vespertilionis**: This is a widely distributed trypanosome of bats. The single isolate included in phylogenetic trees is from Europe.[8,10,47] There is some debate as to whether the isolate used to obtain sequences for phylogenetic trees represents the originally described species on the basis of morphology.[124]

- **T. rangeli**: This trypanosome is restricted to South America and has a wide mammalian host range including humans, although it is not pathogenic to human hosts. A high prevalence of *T. rangeli* in humans has been reported in Central America and northwestern South America.[125] The only known vectors are triatomine bugs of the genus *Rhodnius*. The inclusion of this species within the *T. cruzi* clade[66] resolved the debate regarding the classification of this species; its ability to develop in salivary glands and be transmitted through saliva of triatomine bugs (although it is also transmitted via feces), had led to it being classified within the Salivaria, while resemblance of the bloodstream forms to *T. lewisi* led to classification within the subgenus *Herpetosoma*.[1] Comparisons of a wide range of isolates of this species using sequences of the spliced-leader gene, 18S rDNA and ITS regions, and fluorescent fragment length barcoding (FFLB)[22] have revealed four lineages in terrestrial mammals (Lineages A, B, C, and D) and Lineage E, which is apparently restricted to bats.[126,127] Lineage divergence appears to be associated with species of *Rhodnius*, without any clear association of trypanosome lineages with particular vertebrate hosts.

- **An unnamed bat trypanosome**: This trypanosome was isolated from a fruit bat *Rousettus aegyptiacus* from Gabon in West Africa. Sequence analysis based on 18S rDNA indicated that it was only distantly related to the other bat trypanosomes in the clade.[28,66]

- **Australian mammal group**: A trypanosome from a kangaroo was isolated in Australia.[25] Analysis by Stevens et al.[8] provided strong support for placing this taxon within, but at the extremity of, the *T. cruzi* clade; as such, this taxon played a major part in hypothesizing the origin of the *T. cruzi* clade (see next section). Related trypanosomes that are sufficiently different to warrant being classified as separate species have subsequently been found in a native Australian rodent, *Rattus fuscipes*,[128] possums,[23] and quokka (*Setonix brachyurus*)[83]; see Thompson and Thompson[113] for a full listing of trypanosomes identified from Australian mammals. Related trypanosomes have also been identified in tabanid flies in Australia, potentially implicating them as vectors.[113]

- **Madagascar group**: Trypanosome 18S rDNA sequences were recently identified in transcriptomes produced from the blood of two endangered wild lemurs (*Indri indri* and *Propithecus diadema*) in Madagascar.[63] These sequences are most similar to those of the Australian group, differing by only 1.7%.[63]

- **T. spp. Neobats**: This group of three closely related bat trypanosomes was first described in bats from the Panamá Canal Zone. In this study phylogenetic analysis placed the group near the base of the *T. cruzi* clade, although resolution within the clade was insufficient to determine its exact relationship with *T. livingstonei*.[129] Later this group was named *T. spp. Neobats*.[64]

- **T. wauawu**: This recently described trypanosome has, as yet, only been found in *Pteronotus* bats (Mormoopidae) in South America from Guatemala to the Brazilian Atlantic Coast. *T. wauwau* is a sister taxon to *T. spp. Neobats*.[64] Together these are related to the Australian mammal group in this clade, providing additional support for the bat origin of the *T. cruzi* clade.

# The origin of the *T. cruzi* clade

Two main hypotheses have been proposed for the origin of the *T. cruzi* clade and *T. cruzi cruzi* itself.[8,29,62] The first proposal based on phylogenetic evidence placed the origin of the *T. cruzi* clade in the southern supercontinent of Gondwana, comprising present day Antarctica, Australia, and South America, when marsupials were the dominant mammalian fauna, more than 45 million years ago.[8] This hypothesis was supported by the existence of two species that are restricted to terrestrial mammals in South and Central America, *T. cruzi* and *T. rangeli*, and the placement of a trypanosome from an Australian kangaroo within, but on the periphery of the clade[8]; Stevens et al.[8] termed this group the "*T. cruzi* clade." As both *T. cruzi* and *T. rangeli* are genetically diverse, they are likely to have had a long history within the New World. Additionally, other *Schizotrypanum* trypanosomes had been described from other South American terrestrial vertebrates[1] suggesting a diversity of related species existed in the continent. According to this hypothesis, the ability of bats to disperse by flying is responsible for spreading bat-trypanosome lineages within the clade to the Old World.[8,70]

Barnabe et al.[130] proposed an alternative, in which *T. cruzi* evolved from a trypanosome of bats and adaptation of *T. cruzi* to other mammalian hosts is a derived character that was acquired from a bat-restricted ancestor. This scenario was inferred from evidence of a close relationship between *T. cruzi* and a range of bat trypanosomes in an analysis of isoenzymes, random amplified polymorphic DNA, and cytochrome b nucleotide sequences. Later this hypothesis gained further support through surveys of bat trypanosomes and phylogenetic studies based on 18S rDNA and *gGAPDH* sequences. These increased the known diversity of bat trypanosomes within the *T. cruzi* clade and resolved relationships in the group. Indeed, the closest living relative of *T. c. cruzi* is *T. c. marinkellei* (from South American bats), followed by *T. erneyi*, from bats in Mozambique, Africa,[67] and *T. dionisii*, from both Old and New World bats.[8,13,47,66,131] Explaining the distribution of bat trypanosomes in the clade at the time using the southern supercontinent hypothesis would have required at least seven independent host switches from terrestrial mammals into bats.[124] The existence of several terrestrial lineages interspersed with bat trypanosomes in different branches of the *T. cruzi* clade led to the "bat seeding hypothesis".[124] In this scenario bats were the original hosts of the *T. cruzi* clade. These trypanosomes then diversified and dispersed in bats, achieving a transcontinental distribution. Several jumps into terrestrial mammals occurred, including one that led to *T. cruzi* in South American terrestrial mammals. Other jumps into terrestrial mammals led to *T. rangeli* in South America, the Australian mammal group, the African monkey and civet trypanosomes [62] and the recently described Madagascar lemur group.[63]

Recent studies have added further support to a probable bat origin of the group. In particular, a number of surveys of trypanosomes of bats in Africa and South America has considerably increased the known genetic diversity of bat trypanosomes within the *T. cruzi* clade.[64,123,129] Notably, *T. livingstonei*, a trypanosome described in African bats, falls basal to the Australian kangaroo group within the *T. cruzi* clade.[123] Likewise, *T. wauawu*, and *T.* spp. *Neobats*, recently described from South American bats, formed a sister group to the Australian marsupial group.[64] A comparison of the nucleotide diversity of cytochrome b (*cytb*) in *T. cruzi marinkellei*, the subspecies restricted to bats, revealed higher diversity within this subspecies than any other *T. cruzi* subgroup, suggesting it to be the oldest *T. cruzi* subgroup.[132]

These findings raise the question of whether further host switches of bat trypanosomes in the *T. cruzi* clade into terrestrial mammals have occurred. Interestingly, a trypanosome morphologically resembling *T. cruzi* has been described in the slow loris (a primate) in Malaysia[133]; to date, all trypanosomes morphologically similar (typical *Schizotrypanum* morphology) to *T. cruzi* have demonstrated a close relationship with *T. cruzi*. Unfortunately, however, the molecular data required to test this are not currently available.

It is also notable that, despite an increasing number of studies that have characterized trypanosomes from a wide range of South American terrestrial mammals using molecular techniques, no further *bona fide* species within the *T. cruzi* clade have been discovered in terrestrial mammals from this continent. This apparent low level of diversity does not accord with what might be expected if *T. cruzi*-group trypanosomes had been present in the continent for at least 40 million years, a key aspect of the southern supercontinent hypothesis. For example, some parasite cultures identified as *Trypanosoma leeuwenhoeki* (from a sloth, *Choloepus hoffmanni*) and *Trypanosoma minasense* (from a neotropical primate, the squirrel monkey, *Saimiri boliviensis*) on the basis of morphology turned out to be *Trypanosoma rangeli* when classified in 18S rDNA genes trees.[66] Other recently described parasites from the region have also fallen outside the *T. cruzi* clade including the "real" *T. minasense* from primates,[90] *T. caninum* from dogs,[134] *T. terrestris* from a lowland tapir,[61] and *T. lewisi*-like trypanosomes from captive south American primates.[135]

Several attempts have been made to date the origin of *T. cruzi* using gene sequence data. Most have relied on the calibration points provided by the southern supercontinent hypothesis. For instance, the separation of Africa and South America, which occurred approximately 100 million years ago, has been used to date the split between the *T. brucei* and *T. cruzi* clades.[8,29] Similarly, the separation of Australia from Antarctica/South America, which occurred approximately 80−45 million years ago, has been used to date the spilt between the kangaroo trypanosome from the rest in the *T. cruzi* clade. [28] Under the alternative bat seeding hypothesis,[124] the bat origin of *T. cruzi* clade trypanosomes necessitates that the parasites evolved after the diversification of bats. The fossil record for bats is poor, but molecular dating places the first major split approximately 55 million years ago, and not more than 70 million years ago.[136] However, there is no guarantee that parasite evolution and diversification of the *T. cruzi* clade trypanosomes proceeded at the same rate as the diversification of their bat hosts, and we might expect that the radiation/evolution of the trypanosomes lagged behind that of their hosts. The timing of host−parasite coevolutionary relationships has been the focus of much research,[137,138] but *bona fide* examples from nature that are uncomplicated by host switching, lineage extinction events, etc. are surprisingly hard to find.[139] Nonetheless, we might still anticipate that some species within the *T. cruzi* clade are "younger" than their bat hosts.

# Outlook

Molecular phylogenetic studies provide a useful framework for understanding many aspects of trypanosome biology and evolution. In addition, this research can be of direct relevance in applied studies, e.g., research into diseases of humans and livestock. For instance, one goal of the trypanosomatid genome sequencing projects[140,141] is to identify genes involved in pathogenicity, so comparisons with closely related, but nonpathogenic species can be informative[116]; molecular-taxonomic studies have been instrumental in identifying such species. Knowledge of trypanosome diversity also aids the development of diagnostic tools, e.g., to distinguish pathogenic and nonpathogenic species. Recently discovered trypanosomes of Australian marsupials have now been linked with disease[2] and the application of molecular methods recently led to the rediscovery of *T. suis*, a pig pathogen in Africa.[31] There is also now recognition that introducing nonnative trypanosomes in translocated hosts could have major conservation implications.[142] Finally, an improved understanding of the origins of the trypanosomes that cause diseases of humans and domestic animals provides insights into the likely sources of new and emerging pathogens. For instance, we now know that four primate-infective species are closely related to trypanosome species found in bats and thus bats may be regarded as (at least) potential sources of novel human parasites in the future. Thus, understanding the evolution and diversity of trypanosomes has the potential to deliver real benefits in applied science, epidemiology and medicine.

# Glossary

**Clade** A group of biological taxa or species that comprises a common ancestor and all its descendents (if the placement of all taxa within a clade is robust and no unrelated taxa are included within the clade, then the group can be referred to as monophyletic).

**Digenetic** A parasitic lifecycle involving hosts of two different species. The two host species are essential for the completion of a particular parasite's life cycle.

**Monogenetic** A parasitic lifecycle involving only a single species of host.

**Monophyletic group** A group of taxa that derive from a single common ancestor; specifically, the group includes all the descendants of a common ancestor and **no** unrelated taxa (see also "Clade").

**Paraphyletic group** A group of taxa that derive from a single common ancestor; the group includes **all** the descendants of a common ancestor, plus additional apparently unrelated taxa.

**PCR (polymerase chain reaction)** A method used in molecular biology to amplify a region of DNA, generating large quantities of a particular DNA region using oligonucleotide primers and a thermostable DNA polymerase.

**Phylogenetic tree (phylogeny)** A diagram (often referred to as a "tree") illustrating relationships of evolutionary lineages among organisms (taxa).

**Polyphyletic group** A collection of taxa derived from more than one ancestor, i.e., taxa do not share a single common ancestor.

**Primer** A short oligonucleotide from which DNA replication can initiate. Primers used for PCR are synthetically made and are designed to anneal to the template DNA.

**rDNA (ribosomal DNA)** DNA sequences encoding ribosomal RNA molecules that form subunits that together form the structure of a ribosome.

**Systematics** The rules, principles and practice underlying formal biological classification.

**Taxon (pl. taxa)** Any grouping within the classification of organisms such as species, genus, family, and order.

**Taxonomy** The science and methodology of classifying and naming organisms based on morphological and/or molecular similarities.

**Type species** The first recorded described specimen of a species; the specimen to which the binomial name of the species (genus name and species name) is permanently attached.

# References

1. Hoare CA. *The trypanosomes of mammals.* Oxford and Edinburgh: Blackwell Scientific Publications; 1972.
2. McInnes LM, Gillett A, Hanger J, Reid SA, Ryan UM. The potential impact of native Australian trypanosome infections on the health of koalas (*Phascolarctos cinereus*). *Parasitology* 2011;**138**(7):873–83.
3. Smith A, Clark P, Averis S, Lymbery AJ, Wayne AF, Morris KD, et al. Trypanosomes in a declining species of threatened Australian marsupial, the brush-tailed bettong *Bettongia penicillata* (Marsupialia: Potoroidae). *Parasitology* 2008;**135**(11):1329–35.
4. Minchin EA. Investigations on the development of trypanosomes in the tsetse flies and other Diptera. *Quart J Microsc Sci* 1908;**52**:159–260.
5. Léger L. Sur les affinites de l'*Herpetomonas subulata* et la phylogene des trypanosomes. *Comp Rend Seances Soc Biol Ses Fil* 1904;**56**:615–17.
6. Vickerman K. The evolutionary expansion of the trypanosomatid flagellates. *Int J Parasit* 1994;**24**(8):1317–31.
7. Haag J, O'hUigin C, Overath P. The molecular phylogeny of trypanosomes: evidence for an early divergence of the Salivaria. *Mol Biochem Parasitol* 1998;**91**(1):37–49.
8. Stevens JR, Noyes HA, Dover GA, Gibson WC. The ancient and divergent origins of the human pathogenic trypanosomes, *Trypanosoma brucei* and *T. cruzi. Parasitology* 1999;**118**(1):107–16.
9. Hughes AL, Piontkivska H. Phylogeny of Trypanosomatidae and Bodonidae (Kinetoplastida) based on 18S rRNA: evidence for paraphyly of *Trypanosoma* and six other genera. *Mol Biol Evol* 2003;**20**(4):644–52.
10. Hamilton PB, Stevens JR, Gaunt MW, Gidley J, Gibson WC. Trypanosomes are monophyletic: evidence from genes for glyceraldehyde phosphate dehydrogenase and small subunit ribosomal RNA. *Int J Parasit* 2004;**34**:1393–404.
11. Leonard G, Soanes DM, Stevens JR. Resolving the question of trypanosome monophyly: a comparative genomics approach using whole genome data sets with low taxon sampling. *Infect Genet Evol* 2011;**11**(5):955–9.

12. Stevens JR, Noyes H, Gibson WC. The evolution of trypanosomes infecting humans and primates. *Mem Inst Oswaldo Cruz* 1998;**93**(5):669−76.

13. Cavazzana Jr M, Marcili A, Lima L, da Silva FM, Junqueira ÂCV, Veludo HH, et al. Phylogeographical, ecological and biological patterns shown by nuclear (ssrRNA and gGAPDH) and mitochondrial (Cyt b) genes of trypanosomes of the subgenus *Schizotrypanum* parasitic in Brazilian bats. *Int J Parasit* 2010;**40**(3):345−55.

14. Ramirez JD, Duque MC, Montilla M, Cucunuba Z, Guhl F. Natural and emergent *Trypanosoma cruzi* I genotypes revealed by mitochondrial (Cytb) and nuclear (SSU rDNA) genetic markers. *Exp Parasitol* 2012;**132**(4):487−94.

15. Kelly S, Ivens A, Manna PT, Gibson W, Field MC. A draft genome for the African crocodilian trypanosome *Trypanosoma grayi*. *Sci Data* 2014;**1** 140024.

16. Stevens JR, Brisse S. The systematics of trypanosomes of medical and veterinary importance. In: Maudlin I, Holmes PH, Miles M, editors. *Trypanosomiasis*. Oxford: CABI Publishing; 2005. p. 1−23.

17. Votýpka J, d'Avila-Levy CM, Grellier P, Maslov DA, Lukeš J, Yurchenko V. New approaches to systematics of Trypanosomatidae: criteria for taxonomic (re)description. *Trends Parasitol* 2015;**31**(10):460−9.

18. Votypka J, Maslov DA, Yurchenko V, Jirku M, Kment P, Lun Z-R, et al. Probing into the diversity of trypanosomatid flagellates parasitizing insect hosts in South-West China reveals both endemism and global dispersal. *Mol Phylogenet Evol* 2010;**54**(1):243−53.

19. Votýpka J, Rádrová J, Skalický T, Jirků M, Jirsová D, Mihalca AD, et al. A tsetse and tabanid fly survey of African great apes habitats reveals the presence of a novel trypanosome lineage but the absence of *Trypanosoma brucei*. *Int J Parasit* 2015;**45** (12):741−8.

20. Hamilton PB, Adams ER, Malele II, Gibson WC. A novel, high throughput technique for species identification reveals a new species of tsetse-transmitted trypanosome related to the *Trypanosoma brucei* subgenus, *Trypanozoon*. *Infect Genet Evol* 2008;**8**: 26−33.

21. Adams ER, Hamilton PB. New molecular tools for the identification of trypanosome species. *Future Microbiol* 2008;**3**(2):167−76.

22. Hamilton PB, Lewis MD, Gaunt MW, Cruickshank C, Yeo M, Llewellyn MS, et al. Identification and lineage genotyping of South American trypanosomes using fluorescent fragment length barcoding. *Infect Genet Evol* 2011;**11**:44−51.

23. Paparini A, Irwin PJ, Warren K, McInnes LM, de Tores P, Ryan UM. Identification of novel trypanosome genotypes in native Australian marsupials. *Vet Parasitol* 2011;**183** (1−2):21−30.

24. Austen JM, Jefferies R, Friend JA, Ryan U, Adams P, Reid SA. Morphological and molecular characterization of *Trypanosoma copemani* n. sp (Trypanosomatidae) isolated from Gilbert's potoroo (*Potorous gilbertii*) and quokka (*Setonix brachyurus*). *Parasitology* 2009;**136**(7):783−92.

25. Noyes H, Stevens JR, Teixeira M, Phelan J, Holz P. A nested PCR for the ssrRNA gene detects *Trypanosoma binneyi* in the platypus and *Trypanosoma* sp. in wombats and kangaroos in Australia. *Int J Parasit* 1999;**29**(2):331−9.

26. McInnes LM, Gillett A, Ryan UM, Austen J, Campbell RSF, Hanger J, et al. *Trypanosoma irwini* n. sp (Sarcomastigophora: Trypanosomatidae) from the koala (*Phascolarctos cinereus*). *Parasitology* 2009;**136**(8):875−85.

27. Jakes KA, O'Donoghue PJ, Adlard RD. Phylogenetic relationships of *Trypanosoma chelodina* and *Trypanosoma binneyi* from Australian tortoises and platypuses inferred from small subunit rRNA analyses. *Parasitology* 2001;**123**(5):483−7.

28. Stevens JR, Noyes HA, Schofield CJ, Gibson WC. The molecular evolution of Trypanosomatidae. *Adv Parasit* 2001;**48**:1−56.
29. Stevens JR, Rambaut A. Evolutionary rate differences in trypanosomes. *Infect Genet Evol* 2001;**1**:143−50.
30. Adams ER, Hamilton PB, Rodrigues AC, Malele II, Delespaux V, Teixeira MMG, et al. New *Trypanosoma* (*Duttonella*) *vivax* genotypes from tsetse flies in East Africa. *Parasitology*. 2010;**137**(04):641−50.
31. Hutchinson R, Gibson W. Rediscovery of *Trypanosoma* (*Pycnomonas*) *suis*, a tsetse-transmitted trypanosome closely related to *T. brucei*. *Infect Genet Evol* 2015;**36**:381−8.
32. Yurchenko V, Votypka J, Tesarova M, Klepetkova H, Kraeva N, Jirku M, et al. Ultrastructure and molecular phylogeny of four new species of monoxenous trypanosomatids from flies (Diptera: Brachycera) with redefinition of the genus Wallaceina. *Folia Parasitol* 2014;**61**(2):97−112.
33. Yurchenko V, Kostygov A, Havlová J, Grybchuk-Ieremenko A, Ševčíková T, Lukeš J, et al. Diversity of trypanosomatids in cockroaches and the description of *Herpetomonas tarakana* sp. n. *J Eukaryot Microbiol* 2015;**63**(2):198−209.
34. Svobodova M, Zidkova L, Cepicka I, Obornik M, Lukes J, Votypka J. *Sergeia podlipaevi* gen. nov., sp nov (Trypanosomatidae, Kinetoplastida), a parasite of biting midges (Ceratopogonidae, Diptera). *Int J Syst Evol Micr* 2007;**57**:423−32.
35. Votypka J, Sukova E, Kraeva N, Ishemgulova A, Duzi I, Lukes J, et al. Diversity of trypanosomatids (Kinetoplastea: Trypanosomatidae) parasitizing fleas (Insecta: Siphonaptera) and description of a new genus *Blechomonas* gen. n. *Protist* 2013;**164**(6):763−81.
36. Flegontov P, Votypka J, Skalicky T, Logacheva MD, Penin AA, Tanifuji G, et al. *Paratrypanosoma* is a novel early-branching trypanosomatid. *Curr Biol.* 2013;**23**(18):1787−93.
37. Cupolillo E, Medina-Acosta E, Noyes H, Momen H, Grimaldi G. A revised classification for *Leishmania* and *Endotrypanum*. *Parasitol Today* 2000;**16**(4):142−4.
38. Noyes H, Pratlong F, Chance M, Ellis J, Lanotte G, Dedet JP. A previously unclassified trypanosomatid responsible for human cutaneous lesions in Martinique (French West Indies) is the most divergent member of the genus *Leishmania* ss. *Parasitology* 2002;**124**(1):17−24.
39. Morio F, Reynes J, Dollet M, Pratlong F, Dedet JP, Ravel C. Isolation of a protozoan parasite genetically related to the insect trypanosomatid *Herpetomonas samuelpessoai* from a human immunodeficiency virus-positive patient. *J Clin Microbiol* 2008;**46**(11):3845−7.
40. Kraeva N, Butenko A, Hlavacova J, Kostygov A, Myskova J, Grybchuk D, et al. *Leptomonas seymouri*: adaptations to the dixenous life cycle analyzed by genome sequencing, transcriptome profiling and co-infection with *Leishmania donovani*. *PLoS Pathogens* 2015;**11**(8).
41. McGhee RB, Hanson WL. Comparison of life cycle of *Leptomonas oncopelti* and *Phytomonas elmassiani*. *J Protozool* 1964;**11**:555−62.
42. Muller E, Gargani D, Schaeffer V, Stevens J, Fernandezbecerra C, Sanchezmoreno M, et al. Variability in the phloem restricted plant trypanosomes (*Phytomonas* spp.) associated with wilts of cultivated crops—isoenzyme comparison with the tower trypanosomatids. *Eur J Plant Pathol* 1994;**100**(6):425−34.
43. Gomez E, Valdes AM, Pinero D, Hernandez R. What is a genus in the Trypanosomatidae family? Phylogenetic analysis of two small rRNA sequences. *Mol Biol Evol* 1991;**8**:254−9.

44. Fernandes AP, Nelson K, Beverley SM. Evolution of nuclear ribosomal RNAs in kinetoplastid protozoa: perspectives on the age and origins of parasitism. *Proc Natl Acad Sci USA* 1993;**90** (24):11608−12.

45. Landweber LF, Gilbert W. Phylogenetic analysis of RNA editing: a primitive genetic phenomenon. *Proc Natl Acad Sci USA* 1994;**91**(3):918−21.

46. Lukes J, Jirku M, Dolezel D, Kral'ova I, Hollar L, Maslov DA. Analysis of ribosomal RNA genes suggests that trypanosomes are monophyletic. *J Mol Evol* 1997;**44** (5):521−7.

47. Hamilton PB, Gibson WC, Stevens JR. Patterns of co-evolution between trypanosomes and their hosts deduced from ribosomal RNA and protein-coding gene phylogenies. *Mol Phylogenet Evol* 2007;**43**(1):15−25.

48. Simpson AG, Roger AJ. Protein phylogenies robustly resolve the deep-level relationships within Euglenozoa. *Mol Phylogenet Evol* 2004;**30**(1):201−12.

49. Simpson AGB, Stevens JR, Lukes J. The evolution and diversity of kinetoplastid flagellates. *Trends Parasitol* 2006;**22**:168−74.

50. Hannaert V, Opperdoes FR, Michels PA. Comparison and evolutionary analysis of the glycosomal glyceraldehyde-3-phosphate dehydrogenase from different Kinetoplastida. *J Mol Evol* 1998;**47**(6):728−38.

51. Simpson AGB, Lukes J, Roger AJ. The evolutionary history of kinetoplastids and their kinetoplasts. *Mol Biol Evol* 2002;**19**(12):2071−83.

52. Adjé CA, Opperdoes FR, Michels PA. Molecular analysis of phosphoglycerate kinase in *Trypanoplasma borreli* and the evolution of this enzyme in kinetoplastida. *Gene* 1998;**217**(1−2):91−9.

53. Wiemer EA, Hannaert V, van den IPR, Van Roy J, Opperdoes FR, Michels PA. Molecular analysis of glyceraldehyde-3-phosphate dehydrogenase in *Trypanoplasma borelli*: an evolutionary scenario of subcellular compartmentation in kinetoplastida. *J Mol Evol* 1995;**40**(4):443−54.

54. Yurchenko VY, Lukes J, Jirku M, Zeledon R, Maslov DA. *Leptomonas costaricensis* sp n. (Kinetoplastea : Trypanosomatidae), a member of the novel phylogenetic group of insect trypanosomatids closely related to the genus *Leishmania*. *Parasitology* 2006;**133**:537−46.

55. Vickerman K. The diversity of the kinetoplastid flagellates. In: Lumsden WHR, Evans DA, editors. Biology of the Kinetoplastida. *1*. London: Academic Press; 1976. p. 1−34.

56. Hamilton PB, Stevens JR, Gidley J, Holz P, Gibson WC. A new lineage of trypanosomes from Australian vertebrates and terrestrial bloodsucking leeches (Haemadipsidae). *Int J Parasit* 2005;**35**(4):431−43.

57. Wright AD, Li S, Feng S, Martin DS, Lynn DH. Phylogenetic position of the kinetoplastids, *Cryptobia bullocki*, *Cryptobia catostomi*, and *Cryptobia salmositica* and monophyly of the genus *Trypanosoma* inferred from small subunit ribosomal RNA sequences. *Mol Biochem Parasitol* 1999;**99**(1):69−76.

58. Martin DS, Wright AD, Barta JR, Desser SS. Phylogenetic position of the giant anuran trypanosomes *Trypanosoma chattoni*, *Trypanosoma fallisi*, *Trypanosoma mega*, *Trypanosoma neveulemairei*, and *Trypanosoma ranarum* inferred from 18S rRNA gene sequences. *J Parasitol* 2002;**88**(3):566−71.

59. Overath P, Haag J, Lischke A, O'HUigin C. The surface structure of trypanosomes in relation to their molecular phylogeny. *Int J Parasit* 2001;**31**(5−6):468−71.

60. Viola LB, Almeida RS, Ferreira RC, Campaner M, Takata CSA, Rodrigues AC, et al. Evolutionary history of trypanosomes from South American caiman (*Caiman yacare*)

and African crocodiles inferred by phylogenetic analyses using SSU rDNA and gGAPDH genes. *Parasitology* 2009;**136**(1):55−65.

61. Viola LB, Attias M, Takata CSA, Campaner M, De Souza W, Camargo EP, et al. Phylogenetic analyses based on small subunit rRNA and glycosomal glyceraldehyde-3-phosphate dehydrogenase genes and ultrastructural characterization of two snake trypanosomes: *Trypanosoma serpentis* n. sp from *Pseudoboa nigra* and *Trypanosoma cascavelli* from *Crotalus durissus terrificus. J Eukaryot Microbiol* 2009;**56**(6):594−602.

62. Hamilton PB, Adams ER, Njiokou F, Gibson WC, Cuny G, Herder S. Phylogenetic analysis reveals the presence of the *Trypanosoma cruzi* clade in African terrestrial mammals. *Infect Genet Evol* 2009;**9**:81−6.

63. Larsen PA, Hayes CE, Williams CV, Junge RE, Razafindramanana J, Mass V, et al. Blood transcriptomes reveal novel parasitic zoonoses circulating in Madagascar's lemurs. *Biol Lett* 2016;**12**(1).

64. Lima L, Espinosa-Álvarez O, Pinto CM, Manzelio CJ, Pavan AC, Carranza JC, et al. New insights into the evolutionary history of the clade *Trypanosoma cruzi* provided by a new trypanosome species tightly linked to the Neotropical *Pteronotus* (Mormoopidae) bats connected to Australian trypanosomes. *Parasit Vector* 2015; **8**:657.

65. Acosta IdCL, da Costa A, Nunes P, Gondim MF, Gatti A, Rossi Jr J, et al. Morphological and molecular characterization and phylogenetic relationships of a new species of trypanosome in *Tapirus terrestris* (lowland tapir), *Trypanosoma terrestris* sp. nov., from Atlantic Rainforest of southeastern Brazi. *Parasit Vector* 2013;**6**(1):349.

66. Stevens JR, Teixeira MM, Bingle LE, Gibson WC. The taxonomic position and evolutionary relationships of *Trypanosoma rangeli. Int J Parasit* 1999;**29**(5):749−57.

67. Lima L, da Silva FM, Neves L, Attias M, Takata CSA, Campaner M, et al. Evolutionary insights from bat trypanosomes: morphological, developmental and phylogenetic evidence of a new species, *Trypanosoma (Schizotrypanum) erneyi* sp nov., in African bats closely related to *Trypanosoma (Schizotrypanum) cruzi* and allied species. *Protist* 2012;**163**(6):856−72.

68. Fermino BR, Paiva F, Soares P, Tavares LER, Viola LB, Ferreira RC, et al. Field and experimental evidence of a new caiman trypanosome species closely phylogenetically related to fish trypanosomes and transmitted by leeches. *Int J Parasitol Parasites Wildlife* 2015;**4**(3):368−78.

69. Dvořáková N, Čepička I, Qablan MA, Gibson W, Blažek R, Široký P. Phylogeny and morphological variability of trypanosomes from African pelomedusid turtles with redescription of *Trypanosoma mocambicum* Pienaar. *Protist* 1962.

70. Stevens J, Gibson W. The molecular evolution of trypanosomes. *Parasitol Today* 1999;**15**(11):432−7.

71. Bardsley JE, Harmsen R. The trypanosomes of anura. *Adv Parasit* 1973;**11**:1−73.

72. Jones SRM, Woo PTK. Development and infectivity of *Trypanosoma phaleri* in leech and fish hosts. *Can J Zoolog* 1991;**69**(6):1522−9.

73. Khan RA. The life cycle of *Trypanosoma murmanensis* Niktin. *Can J Zoolog* 1976;**54** (11):1840−9.

74. Karlsbakk E. A trypanosome of Atlantic cod, *Gadus morhua* L., transmitted by the marine leech *Calliobdella nodulifera* (Malm, 1863) (Piscicolidae). *Parasitol Res* 2004;**93**(2):155−8.

75. Siddall ME, Desser SS. Alternative leech vectors for frog and turtle trypanosomes. *J Parasitol* 1992;**78**(3):562−3.

76. Desser SS, McIver SB, Ryckman A. *Culex territans* as a potential vector of *Trypanosoma rotatorium*. I. Development of the flagellate in the mosquito. *J Parasitol* 1973;**59**(2):353–8.

77. Martin DS, Desser SS. A light and electron microscopic study of *Trypanosoma fallisi* N. Sp. in toads (*Bufo americanus*) from Algonquin Park, Ontario. *J Protozool* 1990;**37**(3):199–206.

78. Paparini A, Macgregor J, Irwin PJ, Warren K, Ryan UM. Novel genotypes of *Trypanosoma binneyi* from wild platypuses (*Ornithorhynchus anatinus*) and identification of a leech as a potential vector. *Exp Parasitol* 2014;**145**:42–50.

79. da S, Ferreira JIG, da Costa AP, Ramirez D, Roldan JAM, Saraiva D, et al. Anuran trypanosomes: phylogenetic evidence for new clades in Brazil. *Syst Parasitol* 2015;**91**(1):63–70.

80. Lizundia R, Newman C, Buesching CD, Ngugi D, Blake D, Sin YW, et al. Evidence for a role of the host-specific flea *Paraceras melis* in the transmission of *Trypanosoma* (*Megatrypanum*) *pestanai* to the European badger. *PLoS ONE* 2011;**6**(2):e16977.

81. Thekisoe OMM, Honda T, Fujita H, Battsetseg B, Hatta T, Fujisaki K, et al. A trypanosome species isolated from naturally infected *Haemaphysalis hystricis* ticks in Kagoshima Prefecture, Japan. *Parasitology* 2007;**134**:967–74.

82. McInnes LM, Hanger J, Simmons G, Reid SA, Ryan UM. Novel trypanosome *Trypanosoma gilletti* sp. (Euglenozoa: Trypanosomatidae) and the extension of the host range of *Trypanosoma copemani* to include the koala (*Phascolarctos cinereus*). *Parasitology* 2011;**138**(1):59–70.

83. Austen JM, Paparini A, Reid SA, Friend JA, Ditcham WGF, Ryan U. Molecular characterization of native Australian trypanosomes in quokka (*Setonix brachyurus*) populations from Western Australia. *Parasitol Int* 2016;**65**(3):205–8.

84. Barros JS, Toma H, de Fatima Madeira M. Molecular study of *Trypanosoma caninum* isolates based on different genetic markers. *Parasitol Res* 2015;**114**(2):777–83.

85. Austen JM, Ryan UM, Friend JA, Ditcham WGF, Reid SA. Vector of *Trypanosoma copemani* identified as *Ixodes* sp. *Parasitology* 2011;**138**(7):866–72.

86. Hamilton PB, Stevens JR, Holz P, Boag B, Cooke B, Gibson WC. The inadvertent introduction into Australia of *Trypanosoma nabiasi*, the trypanosome of the European rabbit (*Oryctolagus cuniculus*), and its potential for biocontrol. *Mol Ecol* 2005;**14**(10):3167–75.

87. Sato H, Osanai A, Kamiya H, Obara Y, Jiang W, Zhen Q, et al. Characterization of SSU and LSU rRNA genes of three *Trypanosoma* (*Herpetosoma*) *grosi* isolates maintained in Mongolian jirds. *Parasitology* 2005;**130**:157–67.

88. Bray DP, Bown KJ, Stockley P, Hurst JL, Bennett M, Birtles RJ. Haemoparasites of common shrews (*Sorex araneus*) in Northwest England. *Parasitology* 2007;**134**:819–26.

89. Mohamed HA, Molyneux DH, Wallbanks KR. On *Trypanosoma* (*Megatrypanum*) *talpe* from *Talpa europaea:* method of division and evidence of haemogamasinae as vectors. *J Parasitol* 1987;**73**(5):1050–2.

90. Sato H, Leo N, Katakai Y, Takano J, Akari H, Nakamura S, et al. Prevalence and molecular phylogenetic characterization of *Trypanosoma* (*Megatrypanum*) *minasense* in the peripheral blood of small neotropical primates after a quarantine period. *J Parasitol* 2008;**94**(5):1128–38.

91. Minter-Goedbloed E, Leake CJ, Minter DM, McNamara J, Kimber C, Bastien P, et al. *Trypanosoma varani* and *T. grayi*-like trypanosomes: development in vitro and in insect hosts. *Parasitol Res* 1993;**79**:329–33.

92. Fermino BR, Viola LB, Paiva F, Garcia HA, de Paula CD, Botero-Arias R, et al. The phylogeography of trypanosomes from South American alligatorids and African crocodilids is consistent with the geological history of South American river basins and the transoceanic dispersal of Crocodylus at the Miocene. *Parasit Vector* 2013;**6**.

93. Cortez AP, Ventura RM, Rodrigues AC, Batista JS, Paiva F, Anez N, et al. The taxonomic and phylogenetic relationships of *Trypanosoma vivax* from South America and Africa. *Parasitology* 2006;**133**:159−69.

94. Garcia HA, Rodrigues AC, Rodrigues CMF, Bengaly Z, Minervino AHH, Riet-Correa F, et al. Microsatellite analysis supports clonal propagation and reduced divergence of *Trypanosoma vivax* from asymptomatic to fatally infected livestock in South America compared to West Africa. *Parasit Vector* 2014;**7**.

95. Rodrigues AC, Paiva F, Campaner M, Stevens JR, Noyes HA, Teixeira MM. Phylogeny of *Trypanosoma* (*Megatrypanum*) *theileri* and related trypanosomes reveals lineages of isolates associated with artiodactyl hosts diverging on SSU and ITS ribosomal sequences. *Parasitology* 2005;**132**:215−24.

96. Gibson W, Pilkington JG, Pemberton JM. *Trypanosoma melophagium* from the sheep ked *Melophagus ovinus* on the island of St Kilda. *Parasitology* 2010;**137**(12): 1799−804.

97. Martinkovic F, Matanovic K, Rodrigues AC, Garcia HA, Teixeira MMG. *Trypanosoma* (*Megatrypanum*) *melophagium* in the sheep ked *Melophagus ovinus* from organic farms in Croatia: phylogenetic inferences support restriction to sheep and sheep keds and close relationship with trypanosomes from other ruminant species. *J Eukaryot Microbiol* 2012;**59**(2):134−44.

98. Bose R, Friedhoff KT, Olbrich S. Transmission of *Megatrypanum* trypanosomes to *Cervus dama* by Tabanidae. *J Protozool* 1987;**34**(1):110−13.

99. Bose R, Friedhoff KT, Olbrich S, Buscher G, Domeyer I. Transmission of *Trypanosoma theileri* to cattle by Tabanidae. *Parasitol Res* 1987;**73**(5):421−4.

100. Burgdorfer W, Schmidt ML, Hoogstraal H. Detection of *Trypanosoma theileri* in Ethiopian cattle ticks. *Acta Tropica* 1973;**30**(4):340−6.

101. Ayala SC. Two new trypanosomes from California toads and lizards. *J Eukaryot Microbiol* 1970;**17**(3):370−3.

102. Votypka J, Lukes J, Obornik M. Phylogenetic relationship of *Trypanosoma corvi* with other avian trypanosomes. *Acta Protozool* 2004;**43**:225−31.

103. Votypka J, Obornik M, Volf P, Svobodova M, Lukes J. *Trypanosoma avium* of raptors (Falconiformes): phylogeny and identification of vectors. *Parasitology* 2002;**125**: 253−63.

104. Votypka J, Svobodova M. *Trypanosoma avium*: experimental transmission from black flies to canaries. *Parasitol Res* 2004;**92**:147−51.

105. Desser SS, McIver SB, Jez D. Observations on the role of simuliids and culicids in the transmisssion of avian and anuran trypanosomes. *Int J Parasit* 1975;**5**:507−9.

106. Baker JR. Studies on *Trypanosoma avium* Danilewsky 1885 II. Transmission by *Ornighomyia avicularia* L. *Parasitology* 1956;**46**:321−33.

107. Votypka J, Szabova J, Radrova J, Zidkova L, Svobodova M. *Trypanosoma culicavium* sp nov., an avian trypanosome transmitted by *Culex* mosquitoes. *Int J Syst Evol Micr* 2012;**62**:745−54.

108. Njiokou F, Simo G, Nkinin SW, Laveissiere C, Herder S. Infection rate of *Trypanosoma brucei* s.l., *T. vivax*, *T. congolense* "forest type," and *T. simiae* in small wild vertebrates in South Cameroon. *Acta Tropica* 2004;**92**(2):139−46.

109. Marinkelle CJ. Developmental stages of *Trypanosoma cruzi*-like flagellates in *Cavernicola pilosa*. *Rev Biol Trop* 1982;**30**(2):107–11.

110. Paterson WB, Woo PTK. The development of the culture and blood-stream forms of 3 *Trypanosoma* (*Schizotrypanum*) spp (Protista, Zoomastigophorea) from bats in *Cimex lectularius* (Hemiptera, Cimicidae). *Can J Zool* 1984;**62**(8):1581–7.

111. Gardner RA, Molyneux DH. *Schizotrypanum* in British bats. *Parasitology* 1988;**97**: 43–50.

112. Gardner RA, Molyneux DH. *Trypanosoma* (*Megatrypanum*) *incertum* from *Pipistrellus pipistrellus*: development and transmission by cimicid bugs. *Parasitology* 1988;**96**(Pt 3): 433–47.

113. Thompson CK, Thompson RCA. Trypanosomes of Australian mammals: knowledge gaps regarding transmission and biosecurity. *Trends Parasitol* 2015;**31**(11):553–62.

114. Salazar R, Castillo-Neyra R, Tustin AW, Borrini-Mayorí K, Náquira C, Levy MZ. Bed bugs (*Cimex lectularius*) as vectors of *Trypanosoma cruzi*. *Am J Trop Med Hyg* 2015; **92**(2):331–5.

115. Baker JR, Miles MA, Godfrey DG, Barrett TV. Biochemical characterization of some species of *Trypanosoma* (*Schizotrypanum*) from bats (Microchiroptera). *Am J Trop Med Hyg* 1978;**27**:483–91.

116. Franzen O, Talavera-Lopez C, Ochaya S, Butler CE, Messenger LA, Lewis MD, et al. Comparative genomic analysis of human infective *Trypanosoma cruzi* lineages with the bat-restricted subspecies *T. cruzi marinkellei*. *BMC Genomics* 2012;**13**.

117. Baker JR, Green SM, Chaloner LA, Gaborak M. *Trypanosoma* (*Schizotrypanum*) *dionisii* of *Pipistrellus pipistrellus* (Chiroptera): intra- and extracellular development *in vitro*. *Parasitology* 1972;**65**:251–63.

118. Bettencourt A, França C. Sur un trypanosome de la chauve-souris. *Comp Rend Séan Soc Biol* 1905;**59**:305–7.

119. Maia da Silva F, Marcili A, Lima L, Cavazzana Jr M, Ortiz PA, Campaner M, et al. *Trypanosoma rangeli* isolates of bats from Central Brazil: genotyping and phylogenetic analysis enable description of a new lineage using spliced-leader gene sequences. *Acta Tropica* 2009;**109**(3):199.

120. Hypsa V, Tietz DF, Zrzavy J, Rego RO, Galvao C, Jurberg J. Phylogeny and biogeography of Triatominae (Hemiptera: Reduviidae): molecular evidence of a New World origin of the Asiatic clade. *Mol Phylogenet Evol* 2002;**23**(3):447–57.

121. Weinman D. Trypanosomiases of man and macaques in South Asia. In: Kreier JP, editor. Parasitic Protozoa. *1*. New York: Academic Press; 1977. p. 329–55.

122. Weinman D, Wallis RC, Cheong WH, Mahadevan S. Triatomines as experimental vectors of trypanosomes of Asian monkeys. *Am J Trop Med Hyg* 1978;**27**(2 Pt 1):232–7.

123. Lima L, Espinosa-Alvarez O, Hamilton PB, Neves L, Takata CSA, Campaner M, et al. *Trypanosoma livingstonei*: a new species from African bats supports the bat seeding hypothesis for the *Trypanosoma cruzi* clade. *Parasit Vector* 2013;**6**:221.

124. Hamilton PB, Teixeira MMG, Stevens JR. The evolution of *Trypanosoma cruzi*: the "bat seeding" hypothesis. *Trends Parasitol* 2012;**28**(4):136–41.

125. D'Alessandro A, Saravia NG. Trypanosoma rangeli. In: Kreier JP, Baker JR, editors. *Parasitic Protozoa*. San Diego: Academic Press; 1992. p. 1–54.

126. Maia da Silva FM, Junqueira ACV, Campaner M, Rodrigues AC, Crisante G, Ramirez LE, et al. Comparative phylogeography of *Trypanosoma rangeli* and Rhodnius (Hemiptera: Reduviidae) supports a long coexistence of parasite lineages and their sympatric vectors. *Mol Ecol* 2007;**16**(16):3361–73.

127. Maia da Silva FM, Noyes H, Campaner M, Junqueira AC, Coura JR, Anez N, et al. Phylogeny, taxonomy and grouping of *Trypanosoma rangeli* isolates from man, triatomines and sylvatic mammals from widespread geographical origin based on SSU and ITS ribosomal sequences. *Parasitology* 2004;**129**(Pt 5):549–61.

128. Averis S, Thompson RCA, Lymbery AJ, Wayne AF, Morris KD, Smith A. The diversity, distribution and host–parasite associations of trypanosomes in Western Australian wildlife. *Parasitology*. 2009;**136**(11):1269–79.

129. Cottontail VM, Kalko EKV, Cottontail I, Wellinghausen N, Tschapka M, Perkins SL, et al. High local diversity *of Trypanosoma* in a common bat species, and implications for the biogeography and taxonomy of the *T. cruzi* clade. *PLoS ONE* 2014;**9**(9):e108603.

130. Barnabe C, Brisse S, Tibayrenc M. Phylogenetic diversity of bat trypanosomes of subgenus *Schizotrypanum* based on multilocus enzyme electrophoresis, random amplified polymorphic DNA, and cytochrome b nucleotide sequence analyses. *Infect Genet Evol* 2003;**2**(3):201–8.

131. Hamilton PB, Cruickshank C, Stevens JR, Teixeira MMG, Mathews F. Parasites reveal movement of bats between the New and Old Worlds. *Mol Phylogenet Evol* 2012;**63**(2):521–6.

132. Pinto CM, Ocaña-Mayorga S, Tapia EE, Lobos SE, Zurita AP, Aguirre-Villacís F, et al. Bats, trypanosomes, and triatomines in ecuador: new insights into the diversity, transmission, and origins of *Trypanosoma cruzi* and Chagas disease. *PLoS ONE* 2015;**10**(10):e0139999.

133. Kuntz RE, Myers BJ, McMurray TS. *Trypanosoma cruzi*-like parasites in the slow loris (*Nycticebus coucang*) from Malaysia. *T Am Microsc Soc* 1970;**89**(2):304–7.

134. Madeira MF, Sousa MA, Barros JHS, Figueiredo FB, Fagundes A, Schubach A, et al. *Trypanosoma caninum* n. sp (Protozoa: Kinetoplastida) isolated from intact skin of a domestic dog (*Canis familiaris*) captured in Rio de Janeiro, Brazil. *Parasitology* 2009; **136**(4):411–23.

135. Maia da Silva F, Marcili A, Ortiz PA, Epiphanio S, Campaner M, Catão-Dias JL, et al. Phylogenetic, morphological and behavioural analyses support host switching of *Trypanosoma* (*Herpetosoma*) *lewisi* from domestic rats to primates. *Infect Genet Evol*. 2010;**10**(4):522–9.

136. Teeling EC, Springer MS, Madsen O, Bates P, O'Brien SJ, Murphy WJ. A molecular phylogeny for bats illuminates biogeography and the fossil record. *Science* 2005;**307** (5709):580–4.

137. Hafner MS, Nadler SA. Phylogenetic trees support the coevolution of parasites and their hosts. *Nature* 1988;**332**:258–9.

138. Hafner MS, Sudman PD, Villablanca FX, Spradling TA, Demastes JW, Nadler SA. Disparate rates of molecular evolution in cospeciating hosts and parasites. *Science* 1994;**265**:1087–90.

139. Stevens JR. Computational aspects of host-parasite phylogenies. *Brief Bioinform* 2004;**5**:339–49.

140. Berriman M, Ghedin E, Hertz-Fowler C, Blandin G, Renauld H, Bartholomeu DC, et al. The genome of the African trypanosome *Trypanosoma brucei*. *Science* 2005;**309** (5733):416–22.

141. El-Sayed NM, Myler PJ, Bartholomeu DC, Nilsson D, Aggarwal G, Tran AN, et al. The genome sequence of *Trypanosoma cruzi*, etiologic agent of Chagas disease. *Science* 2005;**309**(5733):409–15.

142. Wyatt KB, Campos PF, Gilbert MTP, Kolokotronis S-O, Hynes WH, DeSalle R, et al. Historical mammal extinction on Christmas Island (Indian Ocean) correlates with introduced infectious disease. *PLoS ONE* 2008;**3**(11):e3602.

# Biology of *Trypanosoma cruzi* and biological diversity

# 16

*M. de Lana and E.M. de Menezes Machado*
Federal University of Ouro Preto, Minas Gerais, Brazil

## Chapter Outline

## Taxonomy

Kingdom: Protista
Subkingdom: Protozoa
Phylum: Sarcomastigophora
Subphylum: Mastigophora
Class: Zoomastigophora
Order: Kinetoplastida
Suborder: Trypanosomatina
Family: Trypanosomatidae
Genus: *Trypanosoma*
Subgenus: *Schyzotrypanum*
Species: *Trypanosoma (Schyzotrypanum) cruzi*

American Trypanosomiasis Chagas Disease. DOI: http://dx.doi.org/10.1016/B978-0-12-801029-7.00016-2

# Introduction

*Trypanosoma cruzi*, the etiological agent of Chagas disease, or American trypanosomiasis, is a flagellate of the Kinetoplastida order, family Trypanosomatidae, characterized by the presence of one flagellum and a single mitochondrion in which the kinetoplast, a specialized DNA-containing organelle, is situated. This protozoa was discovered by Carlos Ribeiro Justiniano das Chagas, a Brazilian physician, in 1909[1] when he was a member of the Instituto Oswaldo Cruz, Rio de Janeiro, Brazil. The genius of the still very young Carlos Chagas enabled him to describe the etiological agent, the vectors, the principal reservoirs, and mechanisms of infection, as well as several clinical stages of the disease with heart, gastrointestinal, and neurological manifestations.

The consensual genetic characterization of *T. cruzi* divides this species into six genetic groups, named TcI to TcVI,[2] and an additional DTU was more recently described named TcBat.[3,4] Apparently this genetic variability may be associated to parasite virulence as well as pathogenicity and the clinical manifestations of the disease that is also variable.[5] Chagas disease is endemic only on the American continent, especially Latin America, with its vectors present from the south of United States to Argentina. Today, due to immigration, the infection is also present in nonendemic countries like Australia, Canada, Spain, United States, and some Asiatic countries.[6] Chagas disease is considered to be responsible for the greatest socioeconomic impact in Latin America due to the loss of productivity with an estimated cost of US$ 1.2 billion annually. In addition the medical costs for treatment of the affected individuals by cardiac and/or digestive pathologies are several times more expensive.[7]

# Evolutionary stages

*T. cruzi* undergoes three distinct morphological and physiological evolutionary stages during its cycle, which are identified by the relative position of the kinetoplast in relation to the cell nucleus and the flagellum's emergence.[8] All these evolutive forms can be identified in microscopy in Giemsa-stained preparations (Figs. 16.1−16.3).

1. Amastigotes (Fig. 16.1) are round intracellular stages in mammalian cells, displaying a short inconspicuous flagellum that is not free from the cell body[9] when they are observed on electron microscopy. These forms multiply by longitudinal binary fission. This stage can be reproduced in cellular culture of different types of mammalian cells; they are approximately 25 mm in length and 2 mm in diameter and are infective for mammals.

2. Epimastigotes (Fig. 16.2) are 20−40 mm long and are present in the intestinal tract and urine of the insect vector, where they multiply by longitudinal binary fission and present a free flagellum which originates in the anterior position of the nucleus.[9] This stage can be reproduced in liquid culture media and is not infective for mammals.

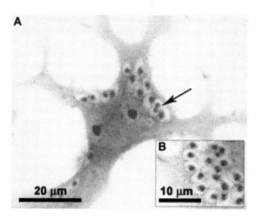

**Figure 16.1** Amastigote form of *Trypanosoma cruzi* in cell culture stained by Giemsa.[10]

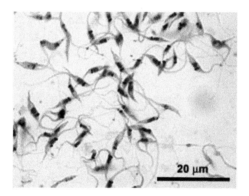

**Figure 16.2** Epimastigote forms of *Trypanosoma cruzi* in axenic culture.[10]

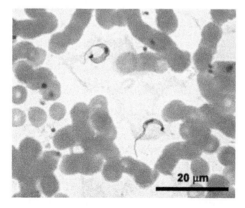

**Figure 16.3** Trypomastigote forms of *Trypanosoma cruzi* from blood stained by Giemsa showing differential morphological aspects,[10] according to the Andrade[79] classification.

3. Trypomastigotes (Fig. 16.3) present a large free flagellum which originates after the nucleus.[9] This stage is the most important, classically known as infective form, and trypomastigotes are present in the blood of mammalian hosts (called blood trypomastigotes), and infect triatomine vectors during blood sucking. This stage is also present in the feces and urine of the triatomine vectors (called metacyclic trypomastigotes) where it is eliminated during blood feeding onto the skin or mucous of the feeding source. They originate from the epimastigote forms by a process of metacyclogenesis, during the stationary phase of growth in axenic cultures or from amastigotes of cell cultures (Fig. 16.3). These forms do not multiply.

# Biological cycle

The entire cycle of *T. cruzi* develops in two types of hosts, the mammalians of seven different orders including humans (vertebrate hosts) and several species of triatomine vectors (invertebrate host) from the Hemiptera order, Reduviidae family.

# Biology in the vertebrate host

## Cellular adhesion

All *T. cruzi* stages are able to interact with vertebrate cells (Fig. 16.4A). However, only some parasites remain adherent to the cells and the level of adhesion is strain-dependent. Several studies show that each infective form, but also the strain and parasite phylogeny, will determine the outcome of this interaction.[11,12] The establishment of the infection depends on a series of events involving interactions of diverse parasite' molecules with host cell components. In this process, several glycoproteins, proteins with lectin activities present in both parasites and cells, are involved.

Yoshida[13] showed that the penetration into the cell is particularly facilitated when the parasite presents surface glycoproteins with a higher gp82-kDa concentration, as observed with trypomastigotes of the CL strain. It has been observed that parasites with a predominance of gp90 and low levels of gp82 (G strain) show a very low ability to invade mammalian cells, whereas those with gp45 and gp50 display a moderate ability to infect these cells. More recently it was demonstrated that gp82-kDa of metacyclic forms has an essential role in host cell invasion and in the establishment of infection by oral route, whereas Tc85-11, which has affinity for laminin, would facilitate the parasite dissemination through diverse organs and tissues of the vertebrate host.[14,15]

With the metacyclic trypomastigotes, derivative forms of cellular culture, the internalization signal transduction pathways are activated both in parasite and host cells, leading to $Ca^{2+}$ mobilization.[16,17] Some important differences are observed among the different sources of the parasite (trypomastigotes of tissue culture, metacyclic trypomastigotes of acellular culture) or even with different *T. cruzi* strains.

Another important factor that participates in this interaction is sialic acid, also present in both parasite and host cells. In *T. cruzi*−macrophage interaction, the presence of sialic acid in the membrane of the trypomastigote hinders

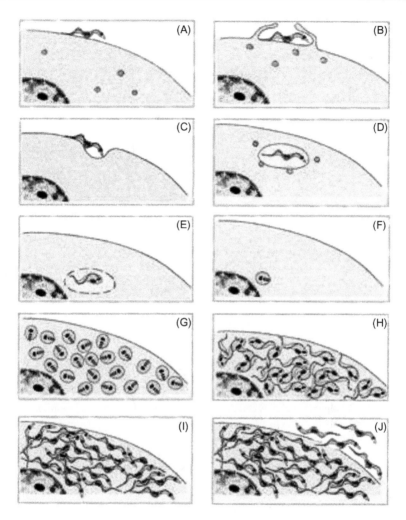

**Figure 16.4** Schematic view of the various phases of the interaction of *Trypanosoma cruzi* with vertebrate cells. (A) The parasite adheres to the host cell membrane; (B) internalization of the parasite via pseudopods or depression (C) of the cell surface; (D) parasite inside the parasitophorous vacuole and fusion with the lysosomes; (E) change in trypomastigote morphology and disintegration of the parasitophorous vacuole membrane; (F) amastigote free in the cytoplasm of the host cell; (G) multiplication of the amastigotes; (H) amastigote−trypomastigote differentiation process passing through the intermediate epimastigote stage; (I) trypomastigotes in the cytoplasm of the host cell; and (J) rupture of the host cell and release of trypomastigotes into the intercellular space[9].

the interaction process, which is facilitated when parasites are treated to remove or block this component.[18] The trypomastigote normally presents transialidase and neuramidase in its membrane, which facilitates its interaction with vertebrate cells. Parasites that have a higher concentration of these enzymes are more invasive for the mammalian cells. Curiously, the epimastigote form, the noninfective stage, presents low levels of sialic acid. In contrast, it was demonstrated that the presence of sialic acid in the host cell membrane is also important for its interaction with *T. cruzi*. More recently it was demonstrated that the level of active transialidase (aTS) or inactive transialidase (iTS) in the parasite is associated with the phylogenetic divergence of the parasite or different DTUs.[19]

## Cellular invasion and formation of the parasitophorous vacuole

Trypomastigotes enter host cells by three distinct mechanisms (Fig. 16.4B and C), two of them involving an early interaction with host cell lysosomes.

1. **The first mechanism** is mediated by a direct fusion of lysosomes with the plasma membrane at the parasite's attachment site, a process that originates the parasitophorous vacuole (PV)[20] (Fig. 16.4D), which may comprise the host cell plasma membrane, either endosomal or lysosomal components.
2. **The second mechanism** observed is the invagination of the plasma membrane, without participation of the host cell actin cytoskeleton. In this case, the PV contains plasma membrane markers that rapidly mature by fusing with lysosomes (Fig. 16.4D). This early fusion of the vacuole with the lysosome is critical for retaining the trypomastigotes inside host cells, further transformations, and replication. An important event during the first and second mechanism of cellular invasion is the release of $Ca^{2+}$ ions from the parasite and host cells, which, together with lysosomes, migrate closer to the PV membrane.[21,22] Thus, the process of cellular invasion by *T. cruzi* is considered a particular type of endocytosis for the epimastigote or phagocytosis for the trypomastigotes. Thus, the invasion of macrophages by epimastigotes involves the polymerization of actin and formation of pseudopodes. This process is strongly blocked when the parasites or macrophages are treated with cytochalasin, which is not observed with nonphagocytic cells.
3. **The third mechanism** of parasite cell interaction that occurs with the nonphagocytic cells in contrast, undergo a process of proteins phosphorylation with participation of phosphoinositide 3-kinase[23] from the parasite and host cell. This last mechanism is a lysosome-independent pathway.

Subsequently to all these mechanisms of parasite—cell interaction and with the parasite in the PV, it maturates and acquires the early endossomic and lysosomic markers.

## Trypomastigote—amastigote differentiation

The parasite's time of residence inside the PV varies between infective forms, ranging from 1 to 2 h for amastigotes and trypomastigotes derived from tissue culture to several hours for metacyclic trypomastigotes.[24] Once inside the host cells, trypo-mastigotes and amastigotes secrete Tc-Tox protein, a complement 9 (C9) factor-related molecule that, at low pH, destroys the PV membrane, releasing parasites into the cytosol[25] (Fig. 16.4E). When the infective forms are metacyclic trypomasti-gotes, this process is not the same and still has not been completely studied. When the interaction is between macrophages and epimastigotes or opsonized trypomasti-gotes, the activation of NAD(P)H enzyme occurs, leading to the formation of free radicals of $O_2$ and $H_2O_2$ that lyse the parasite membrane with its consequent digestion.[26]

Once free in the cytoplasm, trypomastigotes differentiate into amastigotes that remain quiescent for 24−35 h (Fig. 16.4F), then begin to grow by binary fission for up to nine cycles.[27] Some authors believe that a limiting factor for parasite multipli-cation is the cytoplasmic area of the host cell. During amastigote division, several transformations occur, such as growth of the parasite, duplication of the basal cor-puscle, initial kinetoplast division, modification of the nuclear chromatin, and for-mation of a new flagellum. During the interphase, the nuclear chromatin is condensed in the nuclear membrane or sometimes in the central region of the nucleus with the nucleoli in a central position. With the beginning of the division process, the nucleus becomes less electrodense with branches of intranuclear micro-tubules and electrodense plates. Afterward the mitotic fuse is formed. Gradually the nucleus acquires an oval and later a long shape followed by a central constriction producing a new cell with two nucleoli. At this time, the new cell has two kineto-plasts, the cell body is lengthened, the cytoplasm constricts, and two new indepen-dent amastigotes are formed. Then new successive divisions of amastigotes occur (Fig. 16.4G) with a doubling time around 14 h depending on the characteristics of the parasite strain and culture conditions.[8]

## Amastigote−trypomastigote differentiation

After successive amastigote divisions, these cells begin a differentiation process into trypomastigotes, the infective stage for vertebrate and invertebrate hosts, first going through an intermediary stage like epimastigotes[28] (Fig. 16.4H). The crucial stimulus that triggers the amastigote to the trypomastigote transformation process, which is not synchronous, is not clear. When the cell becomes filled with trypomas-tigotes, the plasma membrane ruptures and significant degenerative processes can be observed, probably due to the intense movement of the parasites[24] that are released outside the host cell (Fig. 16.4J).

Amastigote stages are also infective in vitro and in vivo. In laboratory condi-tions, it is possible to infect different lineages and cell types as well as laboratory animals with amastigote forms of *T. cruzi*.[29] Moreover, the transmission of Chagas disease with transplants is an additional clear evidence of this possibility of infec-tion.[30] The interaction of trypomastigotes with the host cells as well as the amasti-gote stages on the cytoplasm are illustrated in Fig. 16.5.

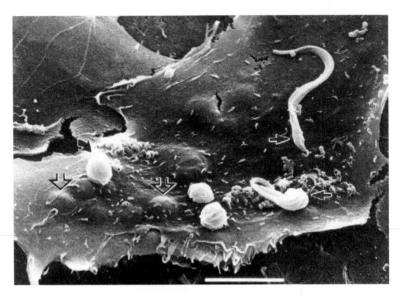

**Figure 16.5** Scanning electron micrograph showing *Trypanosoma cruzi* trypomastigotes (black arrows) and extracellular amastigotes (curved black arrow) invading Vero cells. Open downward arrows show surface protrusions compatible in size with internalized amastigotes. Bar = 5 μm[31].

## Biology in the invertebrate host

The Triatominae are defined as Reduviidae (Hemiptera, Heteroptera) that suck vertebrate blood,[32] several of which are vectors or potential vectors of *T. cruzi*, in contrast to the other Reduviidae subfamilies that prey on invertebrates.[33] There are more than 130 species classified in this Reduviidae subfamily.[34,35] Most of them are widespread in the Americas and maintain an enzootic cycle involving wild mammals in a variety of biotopes.[36] According to these authors, several triatomine species have adapted to human dwellings, becoming vectors of Chagas disease. Studies on orientation mechanisms and dispersal activity, could greatly assist the understanding of the process of triatomine domestication. Similarly, studies on the vectorial potential of these species in the process of domestication are very important.

In the invertebrate host, the development of the parasite has been known since the original work by Carlos Chagas[1] and has been studied by different authors.[37–40] The biological cycle in the vector initiates when the insect feeds on the mammalian host by sucking blood contaminated with trypomastigotes. A few days after feeding the trypomastigotes form from the infected vertebrate host blood transform into epimastigotes or spheromastigotes in the midgut of the insect vector. Then these epimastigotes divide by longitudinal binary fission and can attach to the perimicrovillar membranes, which are secreted by midgut epithelial cells,[41,42] to continue their establishment and development.[43–45] In the rectum a proportion of epimastigotes differentiate into

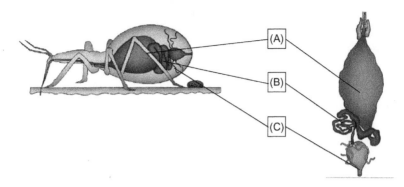

**Figure 16.6** Scheme of the digestive tract of the Triatominae. The insect feeds on blood infected with trypomastigote forms of *Trypanosoma cruzi* that transform into epimastigotes and some spheromastigotes in the stomach (A). In the intestine, the epimastigotes multiply by longitudinal binary fission (B), increasing the population of parasites. In the rectum, the epimastigotes transform into metacyclic trypomastigotes (C), which are eliminated with the feces and urine[46].

metacyclic trypomastigotes (metacyclogenesis), which eventually are eliminated together with feces and urine, and thus are able to complete the biological cycle through contact of the infected Triatominae feces with the skin or mucosal tissues of the vertebrate host.[47]

Apparently, *T. cruzi* and the triatomine insect probably have not coevolved to facilitate parasite transmission.[33,48] Changes in the disease vectorial transmission is dependent to a high degree on insect vector−parasite interaction.[47] Several reports on vector gut and the aggressive hemocoelic reactions that follow the establishment of *T. cruzi* infections in vectors have been described as preventing the development of parasites inside the invertebrate host, potentially making their transmission difficult[47] (Fig. 16.6A and B).

The establishment of *T. cruzi* infection in the gut of the insect vector may depend on, and is possibly regulated by, a range of complex biochemical and physiological factors involved in the mechanism of the *T. cruzi*−vector interaction.[49] Phillips and Bertran[50] suggested that the vector's genetic factors may be involved in the *T. cruzi* cycle in the invertebrate. They reported that the experimental infection rate of the progeny of a group of vectors that failed to become infected after ingesting *T. cruzi* was significantly lower than that obtained for the whole vector population.

After being ingested by the vector, the parasites encounter the components of the insect midgut and the products of blood digestion (hemolytic factor, proteolytic enzymes, peptides derived from aD-globin and lectins), bacterial symbionts, and other resident bacteria in the gut. Similarly, components of the vector's humoral immune system, such as defensin molecules, may also modulate the dynamics of establishment of *T. cruzi* transformation in the triatomine vector gut, illustrating the complexity of the mechanisms involved.[40,45,51−56]

Kollien and Schaub[53] showed that diuresis rather than factors from the hemolymph or digestive products induced the development of metacyclic trypomastigotes of *T. cruzi*. Kollien and Schaub[40] also demonstrated that there is competition of *T. cruzi* with the vector's nutrients, showing that feeding affects not only the parasite population density, but also changes the percentages of different evolutionary stages observed in the rectum.

In contrast with dipteran vectors that have trypsin for the digestion of blood proteins, triatomines use cathepsins that require acid pH in the intestinal contents. Borges et al.[56] showed that in insects experimentally infected with *T. cruzi*, the level of cathepsin D activity increased 1 and 3 days after the blood meal.

Kollien et al.[57] described and characterized cDNA encoding for a lysozyme from the gut of *Triatoma infestans* that was expressed differentially in the various regions of the digestive tract. Kollien et al.[58] characterized two cysteine proteases in the digestive tract of *T. infestans* and Aruajo et al.[59] reported the sequence and expression patterns of defensins (def1 and def2), antibacterial peptides, and lysozyme (lys1) encoding genes from the gut of *T. brasiliensis*. The importance of these enzymes in the *T. cruzi*—insect interaction is unknown.

A hemolytic factor has been shown to be present in the stomach of *Rhodnius prolixus*[60] which has effect on trypanosomatids.[61] These authors also verified that different *T. cruzi* strains present distinct susceptibility to the hemolytic factor, which suggests a selective advantage for the development of certain *T. cruzi* strains over others in the insect vector.

Parasite attachment in the gut of the insect vector is an important point to be considered in the *T. cruzi*—vector interaction. One process of *T. cruzi*—insect interaction involves attachment of the parasite to the gut's epithelial surfaces. On the anterior midgut surface, epimastigotes bound through the cell body or flagellum and on the posterior midgut occur only as flagellar attachment to perimicrovillar membranes. *T. cruzi* epimastigotes adhere to the luminal surface of the triatomid vector's digestive tract by molecular mechanisms that are not completely understood to date. Nogueira et al.[62] demonstrated that *T. cruzi* epimastigote GIPLs (glycoinositolphospholipids, formerly collectively known as lipopeptidophosphoglycan—LPPG) are the major cell surface glycoconjugates of the epimastigote forms of *T. cruzi*[63−65] involved in parasite attachment to the midgut and, somehow, are able to modulate the development of the parasite infection in *R. prolixus*, suggesting that glycoproteins from phosphomannomutase (PMM) and hydrophobic proteins from epimastigotes are important for parasite adhesion to the vector's posterior midgut cells.

It is known that not only the kinetics of *T. cruzi* epimastigote division but also the metacyclogenesis process is dependent on the strains and clones of the infecting parasites.[45,66−68] In vivo and in vitro metacyclogenesis experiments with the Y and Berenice *T. cruzi* strains using different Triatominae species resulted in a higher percentage of metacyclics for both strains in *Rhodnius neglectus* gut than in *Triatoma maculate*.[69] Considering the high genetic variability of *T. cruzi*, some authors point out that an interaction and cooperation effect among the different parasite subpopulations in the insect gut should be considered.[66−68,70]

# Biological diversity of *T. cruzi*

## In the vertebrate host

*T. cruzi* displays great polymorphism or biological diversity in several aspects, which may be correlated with the morphology of this parasite in the bloodstream. Since the early studies of Chagas disease discovery,[1] blood polymorphism has been interpreted by some authors as indicative of sexual dimorphism of the parasite.[71] Although the clonal theory of *T. cruzi* structure and evolution is accepted,[72] the hypothesis of *T. cruzi* sexuality remains an open question for some authors.[73]

Some evidence suggests that the morphological variations of *T. cruzi* are related to the parasites' physiological variations. Studying different *T. cruzi* populations, Brener[74] and Brener and Chiari[75] verified that in some strains the slender forms (Fig. 16.7A) are present throughout the course of infection, whereas in others the slender parasites are present only in the first days of infection and are gradually replaced by the broad forms (Fig. 16.7B) that become predominant in the later days of the acute infection. Therefore, when blood trypomastigotes are inoculated via the intravenous route in normal mice, the slender forms quickly disappear from the circulation to reproduce within the cell. Moreover, the broad forms remain in the circulation without interacting and infecting the host cells.[76] Additionally, it has been demonstrated that naturally surviving animals previously infected with *T. cruzi* and intravenously inoculated with slender trypomastigotes, are rapidly destroyed, while the broad ones are resistant and remain in the circulation for a long time. Afterward, Howells and Chiari[77] demonstrated that broad trypomastigotes present greater ability to infect the triatomine vectors than the slender parasites, which degenerate without carrying out metacyclogenesis. Interestingly, blood trypomastigotes are antigenically different from trypomastigotes obtained in cellular culture.[75] Moreover, blood trypomastigotes have a different ability to infect vertebrate and invertebrate hosts.[79,80]

This dual behavior in strains with predominantly slender (Fig. 16.7A) or intermediate (Fig. 16.7D) versus large or stout trypomastigotes (Figs. 16.7B and 16.7C) led[8] to purposing the term "polar strains" for the Y and CL strains. Striking differences are observed in the parasitemia curves induced by the two strains in experimental hosts such as mice, dogs, and rabbits. The Y strain infects mice more efficiently and higher parasitemia is observed early in the course of infection followed by early mortality, whereas in animals infected with the CL strain, infection, increase of parasitemia and mortality are observed later. In addition, the Y strain exhibits tropism for cells from the mononuclear phagocytic system as demonstrated by the peculiar parasitism of macrophages from the spleen, liver, and bone marrow; in contrast, the CL strain induces a negligible parasitism in these cells. As both strains infect muscle cells, the concept of macrophagotropic and nonmacrophagotropic strains has been suggested to characterize these distinct tropisms. In vitro experiments with mouse peritoneal resident macrophages confirmed the in vivo findings. In addition, blood forms of the Y strain (but not the CL strain) collected

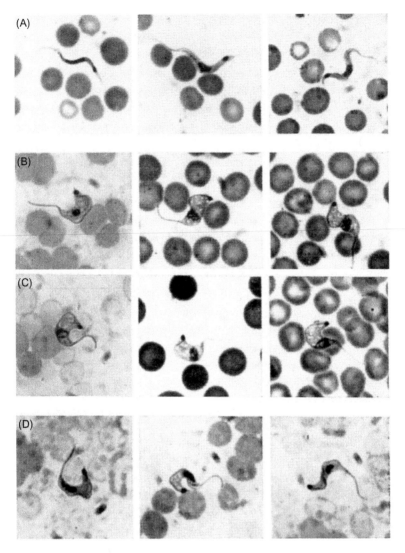

**Figure 16.7** Morphological variation of blood trypomastigotes in *Trypanosoma cruzi*. (A) slender; (B) broad; (C) stout; and (D) intermediate.[74]

from infected mice in the acute phase are readily lysed by complement via membrane-bound specific immunoglobulins. The resistance of the CL strain to the complement-mediated lyses strongly suggests that broad blood forms are equipped with evasion mechanisms that are lacking in the Y population.

The observation that different tissue tropism (cardiotropism or myotropism) of *T. cruzi* is verified in individuals infected with parasites with distinct genetic characteristics[81] led Macedo et al.[5] to propose the "clonal histiotropic model theory" for this parasite since the correlation between *T. cruzi* genetic and tissue tropism could be associated with the different clinical manifestations of the disease (cardiopathy, megaesophagus, and megacolon), alone or in combination.

These variations in *T. cruzi* morphology are correlated with several other aspects of its infection in the murine model such as parasitemia curves, tissue tropism, mortality and resistance or susceptibility to treatment. These associations led Andrade[82] to propose the subdivision of *T. cruzi* populations into types I, II, and III. Type I includes the Y and Peruvian strains, which present predominance of slender trypomastigotes, rapid multiplication in mice, a higher and early parasitemia peak (Fig. 16.8A), higher and early mortality, and particularly tropism for macrophagic cells during the acute phase of infection, and are susceptible or partially resistant to benznidazole and nifurtimox. Type II includes the strains typical of "Recôncavo baiano," Bahia state, Brazil, which presents a predominance of broad trypomastigotes but with slender forms at the beginning of infection, slow multiplication in mice (Fig. 16.8B), irregular peaks of parasitemia between 12 and 20 days, null mortality in the acute phase, myocardial tropism, and is partially resistant or resistant to treatment. Type III includes, e.g., the Colombian strain, which presents a predominance of broad trypomastigotes throughout infection, slow multiplication in mice, higher peaks of parasitemia between 20 and 30 days of infection (Fig. 16.8C), lower rates of mortality occurring slowly throughout acute infection, tropism for the skeletal musculature, and resistance to treatment. Types I, II, and III correspond to Biodemes I, II, and III, respectively,[83] since these associations were observed with the isoenzymatic profile of the parasites. Several other authors observed similar associations between the parasite genetics and its biological properties when comparatively studying clonal stocks in acellular culture,[84] cellular culture,[85] and mice[86] of the three principal *T. cruzi* genotypes,[87] such as principal genotypes 19 and 20, or *T. cruzi* I, principal genotype 32 or *T. cruzi* II, and principal genotype 39 or *T. cruzi* hybrid genotype, currently called *T. cruzi* I, *T. cruzi* II, and *T. cruzi* V groups, respectively, according to the recent genetic *T. cruzi* classification.[2] They are equivalent to Biodemes I, II, and III,[83] respectively. These authors demonstrated higher values for the growth and metacyclogenesis variables in acellular culture,[84] infectivity and differentiation in trypomastigotes in cellular culture,[85] virulence, and parasitemia in mice[86] for the *T. cruzi* I group in relation to *T. cruzi* II group, differently from the published data about TcI *T. cruzi* strains isolated from the Occidental Amazonia in Brazil[88]; whereas *T. cruzi* V presented intermediate values for these same variables. With the same group of clonal stocks, Revollo et al.[85] and Toledo et al.[89] also demonstrated that *T. cruzi* I was more resistant to benznidazole and nifurtimox (in vitro) and benznidazole and itraconazole (in mice), whereas *T. cruzi* II was the most susceptible, and the hybrid stocks (*T. cruzi* V) presented intermediate results. Moreover, all stocks belonging to the principal genotype 20 were 100% resistant to treatment with all the compounds assayed in vitro and in vivo. These results may explain the regional differences observed in human chemotherapy, which differs from region to region, and explains why it is easier to cure patients from Argentina and Chile, where *T. cruzi* II is predominant, than in the north of the Americas, where *T. cruzi* I is more widespread.[90,91]

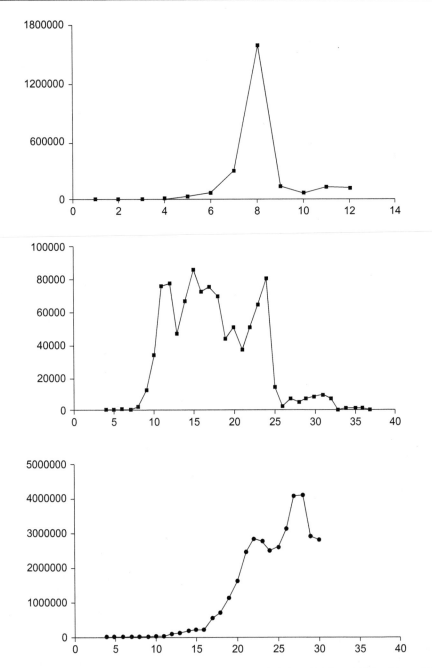

**Figure 16.8** Parasitemia curves in mice infected with Y (A), Be-78 (B) and Colombiana (C) strains of *Trypanosoma cruzi* corresponding to Types I, II, and III, respectively, according to the Andrade (1974)[79] classification.

The genetic polymorphism in *T. cruzi* is also related to trypomastigote small surface antigen (TSSA) sequences, a highly antigenic surface glycosylphosphatidyl inositol (GPI)-anchored mucin-like protein. Thus, Di Noia et al.[92] described the first immunological marker in *T. cruzi* that discriminated the two *T. cruzi* lineage groups (*T. cruzi* I and *T. cruzi* II).

### In the invertebrate vector

The genetic structure of *T. cruzi* is predominantly clonal, with restricted recombination. Various strains persist as stable genotypes that can spread through large geographic regions.[72,73] The clonal model does not totally exclude recombination, but is compatible with occasional genetic recombination events[93–95] which on the evolutionary scale have an important impact on the adaptation of *T. cruzi* to new environments, including new vectors.

The role of triatomines in the selective transmission of *T. cruzi* has been studied by some authors, but some factors involved in the mechanisms and processes of parasite–vector interaction remain unknown. The number of parasites that develop into epimastigotes in the invertebrate host is apparently proportional to the number of broad forms in the ingested blood.[96,97] Pereira da Silva[96] suggested that only broad forms of the parasite would be able to survive in the vector, while the slender forms would degenerate. On the other hand, there is no evidence that only broad forms evolve in vectors. The fact is that the same dual behavior observed between Y and CL strains in mice is also verified in vectors.[97]

In experimental infections, it is known that not all *T. cruzi* strains developed in the same way in all species of triatomines.[69,98–100] Few studies have been undertaken using genetically characterized *T. cruzi* clones in triatomine infections. Lana et al.[66] and Pinto et al.[68] confirmed that *T. infestans* does not always present the same efficiency in the transmission of different *T. cruzi* genotypes. In a recent investigation, the sylvatic species *Mepraia* (=*Triatoma*) *spinolai* transmitted a greater number of subpopulations (TcI, TcIIb, TcIId, and TcIIe) than *T. infestans*.[101]

## Maintaining *T. cruzi* in the laboratory

*T. cruzi* can be cultivated and maintained in the laboratory in several conditions: acellular/axenic cultures, cellular cultures, successive passages in different laboratory animal models (especially mice), alternative passages through vertebrate (mice or other experimental models) and invertebrate hosts (triatomine vectors), and cryopreservation.

### Acellular culture

Acellular culture reproduces the biological cycle of *T. cruzi* developed in triatomine vectors. The first cultures of *T. cruzi* were in acellular biphasic or monophasic medium. The monophasic medium offers advantages because the parasite can be obtained with less contaminant and parasite growth can be assessed by cell counting using an electronic device. The most important and most widely used were liver infusion-tryptose (LIT) and Warren media. Camargo[102] was the first to describe the cellular transformations of *T. cruzi* and growth in LIT medium, the most useful monophasic medium used in the laboratory. Several important studies on metacyclogenesis in LIT media have been described. It was also demonstrated that in the medium called M16, nutrient-poor with low pH, a higher percentage of metacyclogenesis is obtained, although the type of *T. cruzi* strain considered is also important.

The semidefined and defined media for trypanosomes were described byYoshida[103] and Roitman et al.[104] Chemically defined TAUP[104] or TAU3GAA[106] media using components similar to vector urine were used for better differentiation in vitro. The existence of culture media free of macromolecules, especially the chemically defined medium, provides the large quantity of parasite cells necessary for antigen preparations, biochemical studies on nutritional requirements, metabolic pathways, and molecular characterization. Using the semidefined medium 4 as overlay and a monophasic medium using blood of different animal species, high rates of *T. cruzi* and *Leishmania donovani* growth were obtained by Perlewitz and Koch,[107] which improves the chance of obtaining isolations of these parasites.

Bonaldo et al.[108] verified that nutritionally poor medium promotes the metacyclogenesis of *T. cruzi*. The results of Duschak et al.[109] indicate the presence of a novel cysteine proteinase secreted by metacyclic trypomastigotes and reinforces the important role played by these enzymes in *T. cruzi* metacyclogenesis. Interestingly, biological changes in the parasite's infectivity and metacyclogenesis have been observed after successive passages in acellular culture, which can be restored after maintenance by successive passages in triatomines.[110] De Lima et al.[111] verified that cultivation of *T. cruzi* epimastigotes in low-glucose axenic media shifts its competence to differentiate at metacyclic trypomastigotes. Differential gene expression for different periods (6 and 24 h) of *T. cruzi* metacyclogenesis was observed by Krieger et al.[112] and a proteomic analysis[113] identified relevant proteins involved in the metacyclogenesis process. Their identification and molecular characterization is highly important in understanding the steps of parasite differentiation into the infective form.

## *Cellular culture*

In cellular media, the entire biological cycle of *T. cruzi* in the vertebrate host is reproduced. The first culture experiments were with tissue fragments absorbed with coagulated plasma or pendant drop.[114,115] Further monolayer culture of cell lineages regularly maintained in the laboratory was used. Cells of various tissues and organs such as heart, kidney, lung, skin, and skeletal muscle can be used. Metacyclic trypomastigotes originating from culture and vector, as well as bloodstream forms of the parasite are able to infect cells in culture although it has been demonstrated that vector trypomastigotes are more infective than the metacyclic forms of culture.[116,117] Inside these cells, the parasite transforms into amastigotes, which after some time or several cell generations differentiate into new trypomastigotes that will be released in the extracellular medium and be able to invade new cells. With the cultivation of the cells in liquid medium containing mammal sera, several lineages of cells were adapted for *T. cruzi* culture. Today several different cell lineages are used for *T. cruzi* cultivation.

## Cryopreservation

*T. cruzi*, as well as other microorganisms, can be preserved for long periods of time in liquid nitrogen ($-196°C$) without changing its original characteristics. Filardi and Brener[118] were the first to systematically study *T. cruzi* cryopreservation and verifying its effect on several biological characteristics of the parasite (infectivity to vertebrate and invertebrate hosts; morphology, parasitemia, and mortality in mice). These authors verified that initially blood trypomastigotes and epimastigotes obtained from artificial cultures need to be mixed with an equal volume of glycerin 10% and maintained at $-73°C$ for $16-20$ h before cryopreservation in nitrogen. Later these same authors[119] verified that exemplars of triatomine vectors infected with *T. cruzi* can also be cryopreserved with preservation of parasite characteristics including its infectivity to vectors. Dimethyl-sulfoxide (DMSO) $5-10\%$ is also used as a cryoprotective agent for trypanosomes. However, it was demonstrated later[120] that cryopreservation and thawing of *T. cruzi* may lead to severe damage of the mitochondrial apparatus and thus to severe disorders of metabolic function, exhaustion of the metabolic pool, and finally to death of the damaged trypanosomes, despite the use of DMSO as a cryoprotective agent. Yager[121] demonstrated that tissue homogenates containing *T. cruzi* amastigotes or *Leishmania* spp. were also rapidly frozen with 10% glycerol as cryoprotectant and the viability and pathogenicity of the parasites maintained for several years.

Cryopreservation made it possible to create banks of *T. cruzi* strains with parasites from around the world, which was very important to several studies on various aspects of this parasite and provided a better idea of its polymorphism. Moreover, cryopreservation avoids biological changes in its original characteristics induced by selection throughout long-term maintenance in the laboratory in different conditions, such as successive passages in mice, the risk of accidental infections in the laboratory, and the comparative study of a large number of parasite populations of distinct origins.

## Successive and alternative passages in animals and vectors

These alternatives are very frequently used in the laboratory to maintain the parasite for experimental studies. Murine models were the most widely used models for this purpose because they are very susceptible to infection and easy to reproduce and maintain in the laboratory. Parasite populations are maintained in this animal model by successive reproduction of the acute phase of the infection. Moreover, *T. cruzi* can also be maintained by successive passages in triatomines and alternative passages through triatomine vectors and laboratory animals. This type of maintenance has been considered to be very important to prevent the biological behavior of the parasite observed in the laboratory after long-term successive passages in animal models or culture.

# Glossary

**Biological diversity of *T. cruzi*** The polymorphism that *T. cruzi* presents in several parameters used for its biological characterization such as antigenicity, infectivity for vertebrate and invertebrate hosts, metacyclogenesis, virulence and pathogenicity for vertebrate hosts, susceptibility or resistance to drugs, and others.

**Blood polymorphism of *T. cruzi*** The different morphological aspects observed in the blood trypomastigote stages of different *T. cruzi* stocks or strains or even during the acute phase of infection of the same *T. cruzi* strain. The morphological aspects can vary from slender, intermediate, broad, and stout forms.

**Cytoskeleton** A heavily microtubule-based skeleton, containing many interesting protein structures which involves and sustain the parasite shape. For details see Refs. [9,122].

**Flagellum** An organelle usually attached to the cell body that emerges from an invagination called the flagellar pocket present in all trypanosomatids responsible for cell movement. It emerges at the anterior tip or somewhere along the side of the cell depending on the evolutive form or developmental stage. Its length also varies with their developmental stage. It has a basic structure similar to other flagella, showing a 9 + 2 pattern of axonemal microtubules. For details see Refs. [9,122].

**Kinetoplast** An important structure in the recognition of the order Kinetoplastida that includes the family Trypanosomatidae comprising a mass of circular DNA inside the trypanosome's mitochondrion attached to the basal bodies of the flagellum. Division of the kinetoplast is a reliable marker of a certain point in the cell cycle, making it important in cell cycle studies. Electron microscopy shows that the kinetoplast consists of a network of minicircle molecules associated with each other and with long linear molecules concatenated to the maxicircles. Restriction enzyme analysis has shown that the minicircles are heterogeneous and their study has been used for the genetic characterization of the parasite. It is believed that the maxicircles contain genetic information. For details see Refs. [9,122].

**Lysosome** An organelle present in the cytoplasm of the parasite rich in digestive substances and $Ca^{2+}$ ions that approximates from the phagocytic vacuoles during parasite penetration in the vertebrate cells.

**Parasitophorous vacuole** Resultant of the transformations that the host mammalian membrane cell and the *T. cruzi* membrane surface suffer after interaction, which results in the parasite offering temporary conditions of its survival before further transformation into amastigote stages. Inside this vacuole the transformation of trypomastigote into amastigotes occurs after passage by an intermediate epimastigote stage. For details see Refs. [9,122].

**Plasma membrane** An organelle strongly associated with microtubules and microfilaments that cover the trypanosome surface with hundreds of important receptors. A large number of proteins are associated with the plasma membrane. Recent studies have characterized some details of the biosynthesis of the GPI anchor, which involves several important biochemical steps for this parasite. The surface receptors are involved in the uptake of all the necessary host resources for the parasite. For details see Refs. [9,122].

**Spheromastigote** The first *T. cruzi* evolutionary stage present in the prior intestine (midgut) of the invertebrate host (triatomine vectors) that initiates the epimastigote stage of the parasite in the vector described by Brack.[38]

**Tc-Tox protein (Tc85 kDa)** A complement 9 (C9) factor-related molecule or hemolysin that, at low pH, destroys the parasitophorous vacuole membrane releasing the parasite in the cytosol of the host cell[25] where the biological cycle of *T. cruzi* continues.

# References

1. Chagas C. Nova tripanozomiase humana. Estudos sobre a morfologia e o ciclo evolutivo do *Schizotrypanum cruzi*. n. gen., n. sp. agente etiológico de nova entidade mórbida do homem. *Mem Inst Oswaldo Cruz* 1909;**1**:159−218.
2. Zingales B, Andrade SG, Briones MRS, Campbell DA, Chiari E, Fernandes O, et al. A new consensus for *Trypanosoma cruzi* intraspecific nomenclature: second revision meeting recommends TcI to TcVI. *Mem Inst Oswaldo Cruz* 2009;**104**:1051−4.
3. Zingales B, Miles MA, Campbell DA, Tibayrenc M, Macedo AM, Teixeira MM, et al. The revised *Trypanosoma cruzi* subspecific nomenclature: Rationale, epidemiological relevance and research applications. *Infect Genet Evol* 2012;**12**:240−53.
4. Consentino RO, Aguerro F. A simple typing assay for *Trypanosoma cruzi*: discrimination of major evolutionary lineages from a single amplification product. *PLoS NTD* 2012;**6**(7):e1777.
5. Macedo AM, Machado CR, Oliveira RP, Pena SDJ. *Trypanosoma cruzi*: genetic structure of populations and relevance of genetic variability to the pathogenesis of Chagas disease. *Mem Inst Oswaldo Cruz* 2004;**99**(1):1−2.
6. Schmunis GA, Yadon ZE. Chagas disease: a Latin American health problem becoming a world health problem. *Acta Trop* 2010;**115**(1-2):14−21.
7. WHO. Chagas disease (American trypanosomiasis). *Fact sheet N 340* [updated March 2015].
8. Brener Z. Biology of *Trypanosoma cruzi*. *Annu Rev Microbiol* 1973;**27**:347−82.
9. De Souza W. Special organelles of some pathogenic protozoa. *Parasitol Res* 2002;**88** (12):1013−25.
10. De Souza W, de Carvalho TM, Barrias ES. Review on Trypanosoma cruzi: Host Cell Interaction. *Int J Cell Biol* 2010. 2010. pii: 295394. Available from: http://dx.doi.org/ 10.1155/2010/295394.
11. Ley V, Robbins ES, Nussenzweig V, Andrews NW. The exit of *Trypanosoma cruzi* from the phagosome is inhibited by raising the pH of acidic compartments. *J Exp Med* 1990;**171**(2):401−13.
12. Fernandes MC, Cortez M, Geraldo Yoneyama KA, Straus AH, Yoshida N, Mortara RA. Novel strategy in *Trypanosoma cruzi* cell invasion: implication of cholesterol and host cell microdomains. *Int J Parasitol* 2007;**37**(13):1431−41.
13. Yoshida NA. Molecular basis of mammalian cell invasion by *Trypanosoma cruzi*. *An Acad Bras Cienc* 2006;**78**(1):87−111.
14. Cortez C, Yoshida N, Bahia D, Sobreira TJ. Structural basis of the interaction of a *Trypanosoma cruzi* surface molecule implicated in oral infection with host cells and gastric mucin. *PLoS ONE* 2012;**7**(7):e42153.
15. Cortez C, Sobreira TJ, Maeda FY, Yoshida N. The gp82 surface molecule of *Trypanosoma cruzi* metacyclic forms. *Subcell Biochem* 2014;**74**:137−50.
16. Tardieux I, Webster P, Ravesloot J, Boron W, Lunn JA, Heuser JE, et al. Lysosome recruitment and fusion are early events required for trypanosome invasion of mammalian cells. *Cell* 1992;**71**(7):1117−30.
17. Andrews NW. Lysosomes and the plasma membrane: trypanosomes reveal a secret relationship. *J Cell Biol* 2002;**158**(3):389−94.
18. Meirelles MN, Juliano L, Carmona E, Siva SG, Costa EM, Murta AC, et al. Inhibitors of the major cysteinyl proteinase (GP57/51) impair host cell invasion and arrest the intracellular development of *Trypanosoma cruzi in vitro*. *Mol Biochem Parasitol* 1992;**52**(2):175−84.

19. Burgos JM, Risso MG, Breniére SF, Barnabé C, Campetella O, Leguizamo MS. Differential distribution of genes encoding the virulence factor Trans-Sialidase along *Trypanosoma cruzi* discrete typing units. *PLoS ONE* 2013;**8**(3):e58967.

20. Andrade LO, Andrews NW. Lysosomal fusion is essential for the retention of *Trypanosoma cruzi* inside host cells. *J Exp Med* 2004;**200**(9):1135−43.

21. Moreno SN, Sillva J, Vercesi AE, Docampo R. Cytosilic-free calcium elevation in *Trypanosoma cruzi* is required for cell invasion. *J Exp Med* 1994;**180**(4):1536−40.

22. Andrews NW. From lysosomes into the cytosol: the intracellular pathway of *Trypanosoma cruzi*. *Braz J Med Biol Res* 1994;**27**(2):471−5.

23. Woolsey AM, Sunwoo L, Petersen CA, Brachmann SM, Cantley LC, Burleigh BA. Novel PI 3-kinase-dependent mechanisms of trypanosome invasion and vacuole maturation. *J Cell Sci* 2003;**116**(Pt 17):3611−22.

24. Alves MJ, Mortara RA. A century of research: what have we learned about the interaction of *Trypanosoma cruzi* with host cells? *Mem Inst Oswaldo Cruz* 2009;**104**(Suppl. I):76−88.

25. Andrews NW. The acid-active hemolysin of *Trypanosoma cruzi*. *Exp Parasitol* 1990;**71**(2):241−4.

26. De Carvalho TU, De Souza W. Study of mitochondrial organization in living resident and activated macrophages using the laser dye rhodamine 123. *J Leukoc Biol* 1989;**45**(6):498−502.

27. Dvorak JA, Hyde TP. *Trypanosoma cruzi*: interaction with vertebrate cells *in vitro*. 1. Individual interactions at the cellular and subcellular levels. *Exp Parasitol* 1973;**34**(2):268−83.

28. Low HP, Paulin JJ, Keith CH. *Trypanosoma cruzi* infection of BSC-1 fibroblast cells causes cytoskeletal disruption and changes in intracellular calcium levels. *J Protozool* 1992;**39**(4):463−70.

29. Carvalho TU, De Souza W. Infectivity of amastigotes of *Trypanosoma cruzi*. *Rev Inst Med Trop São Paulo* 1986;**28**(4):205−12.

30. Dobarro D, Gomez-Rubin C, Sanchez-Recalde A, Olias F, Bret-Zurita M, Cuesta-Lopez E, et al. Chagas' heart disease in Europe: an emergent disease? *J Cardiovasc Med (Hagerstown)* 2008;**9**(12):1263−7.

31. Procópio DO, da Silva S, Cunningham CC, Mortara RA. *Trypanosoma cruzi*: effect of protein kinase inhibitors and cytoskeletal protein organization and expression on host cell invasion by amastigotes and metacyclic trypomastigotes. *Exp Parasitol* 1998;**90**(1):1−3.

32. Lent H, Wygodzinsky P. Revision of the triatominae (Hemiptera: Reduviidae), and their significance as vectors of Chagas' disease. *Bull Am Mus Nat Hist* 163:123−520.

33. Schofield CJ. Biosystematics and evolution of the Triatominae. *Cad Saúde Pública* 2000;**16**(Suppl. 2):89−92.

34. Galvão C, Carcavallo R, Rocha DS, Jurberg J. A checklist of the current valid species of the subfamily Triatominae Jeannel, 1919 (Hemíptera, Reduviidae) and their geographical distribution, with nomenclatural and taxonomic notes. *Zootaxa* 2003;**202**:1−36.

35. Schofield CJ, Galvão C. Classification, evolution and species groups within the Triatominae. *Acta Trop* 2009;**110**(2−3):88−100.

36. Noireau F, Carbajal-De-La-Fuente AL, Lopes CM, Diotaiuti L. Some considerations about the ecology of Triatominae. *An Acad Bras Ciênc* 2005;**77**(3):431−6.

37. Dias E. Estudos sobre o *Schizotrypanum cruzi*. *Mem Inst Oswaldo Cruz* 1934;**28**(8):1−15.

38. Brack C. Elektronmikopische undersuchungen zum lebenszyklus von *Trypanosoma cruzi*. Unterbesonderes berucksichtigung der entwicklungsformen in ubertrager *Rhodnius prolixus*. *Acta Trop* 1968;**25**(4):289–356.

39. Brener Z, Alvarenga NJ. *Life cycle of* Trypanosoma cruzi *in the vector. New approaches of American Trypanosomiasis Research. Sci Publ, 318*. Washington, DC: Pan American Healthe Organization; 1976. p. 83–8.

40. Kollien AH, Schaub GA. The development of *Trypanosoma cruzi* in Triatominae. *Parasitol Today* 2000;**16**(9):381–7.

41. Billingsley PF, Downe AE. The surface morphology of the midgut cells of *Rhodnius prolixus* Stal (Hemiptera: Reduviidae) during blood digestion. *Acta Trop* 1986;**43**(4):355–66.

42. Billingsley PF. The posterior midgut ultrastructure of hematophagous insect. *Ann Rev Entomol* 1990;**35**:219–48.

43. Zeledon R. Infection of the insect host by *Trypanosoma cruzi*. In: Carcavallo RU, Galindez I, Jurberg J, Lent H, editors. *Atlas of Chagas' Disease Vectors in the Americas*, vol. 1. Rio de Janeiro: Fiocruz; 1997. p. 271–87.

44. Gonzalez MS, Nogueira NF, Mello CB, de Souza W, Schaub GA, Azambuja P, et al. Influence of brain and azadirachtin on *Trypanosoma cruzi* development in the vector, *Rhodnius prolixus*. *Exp Parasitol* 1999;**92**(2):100–8.

45. Azambuja P, Ratcliffe NA, Garcia ES. Towards an understanding of the interactions of *Trypanosoma cruzi* and *Trypanosoma rangeli* within the reduviid insect host *Rhodnius prolixus*. *An Acad Bras Cienc* 2005;**77**(3):397–404.

46. Garcia ES, Ratcliffe NA, Whitten MM, Gonzalez MS, Azambuja P. Exploring the role of insect host factors in the dynamics of *Trypanosoma cruzi-Rhodnius prolixus* interactions. *J Insect Physiol* 2007;**53**(1):11–21 122.

47. Garcia ES, Ratcliffe NA, Whitten MM, Gonzalez MS, Azambuja P. Exploring the role of insect host factors in the dynamics of *Trypanosoma cruzi−Rhodnius prolixus* interactions. *J Insect Physiol* 2007;**53**(1):11–21.

48. Takano-Lee M, Edman JD. Lack of manipulation of *Rhodnius prolixus* (Hemiptera: Reduviidae) vector competence by *Trypanosoma cruzi*. *J Med Entomol* 2002;**39**(1):44–51.

49. Garcia ES. The digestion of Triatominae. In: Brenner RR, Stoka A, editors. *Chagas' disease vector II. Anatomic and physiological aspects*. Florida: CRC Press; 1987. p. 47–59.

50. Phillips NR, Bertram DS. Laboratory studies of *Trypanosoma cruzi* infections in: *Rhodnius prolixus*-larvae and adults in: *Triatoma infestans, T. protracta* and *T. maculata*-adults. *J Med Entomol* 1967;**4**:68–74.

51. Garcia ES, Azambuja P. Development and interactions of *Trypanosoma cruzi* within the insect vector. *Parasitol Today* 1991;**7**(9):240–4.

52. Garcia E, Gonzalez M, Azambuja P. Biological factors involving *Trypanosoma cruzi* life cycle in the invertebrate vector, *Rhodnius prolixus*. *Mem Inst Oswaldo Cruz* 1999;**94**(Suppl. 1):213–16.

53. Kollien AH, Schaub GA. *Trypanosoma cruzi* in the rectum of the bug *Triatoma infestans*: effects of blood ingestion of the vector and artificial dieresis. *Parasitol Res* 1997;**83**(8):781–8.

54. Lopez L, Morales G, Ursic R, Wolff M, Lowenberger C. Isolation and characterization of a novel insect defensin from *Rhodnius prolixus*, a vector of Chagas disease. *Insect Biochem Mol Biol* 2003;**33**(4):439–47.

55. Azambuja P, Feder D, Garcia ES. Isolation of *Serratia marcescens* in the midgut of *Rhodnius prolixus*: impact on the establishment of the parasite, *Trypanosoma cruzi*, in the vector. *Exp Parasitol* 2004;**107**(1−2):89−96.

56. Borges EC, Machado EM, Garcia ES, Azambuja P. *Trypanosoma cruzi*: effects of infection on cathepsin D activity in the midgut of *Rhodnius prolixus*. *Exp Parasitol* 2006;**112** (2):130−3.

57. Kollien AH, Fechner S, Waniek PJ, Schaub GA. Isolation and characterization of a cDNA encoding for a lysozyme from the gut of the reduviid bug *Triatoma infestans*. *Arch Insect Biochem Physiol* 2003;**53**(3):134−45.

58. Kollien AH, Waniek PJ, Nisbet AJ, Billingsley PF, Schaub GA. Activity and sequence characterization of two cysteine proteases in the digestive tract of the reduviid bug *Triatoma infestans*. *Insect Mol Biol* 2004;**13**(6):569−79.

59. Araújo CA, Waniek PJ, Stock P, Mayer C, Jansen AM, Schaub GA. Sequence characterization and expression patterns of defensin and lysozyme encoding genes from the gut of the reduviid bug *Triatoma brasiliensis*. *Insect Biochem Mol Biol* 2006;**36**(7):547−60.

60. Azambuja P, Guimarães JA, Garcia ES. Hemolytic factor from the stomach of *Rhodnius prolixus*: evidence and partial characterization. *J Insect Physiol* 1983;**11**:833−7.

61. Azambuja P, Mello CB, D'Escoffier LN, Garcia ES. In vitro cytotoxicity of *Rhodnius prolixus* hemolytic factor and mellitin towards different trypanosomatids. *Braz J Med Biol Res* 1989;**22**(5):597−9.

62. Nogueira NF, Gonzalez MS, Gomes JE, de Souza W, Garcia ES, Azambuja P, et al. *Trypanosoma cruzi*: involvement of glycoinositolphospholipids in the attachment to the luminal midgut surface of *Rhodnius prolixus*. *Exp Parasitol* 2007;**116**(2):120−8.

63. Alves MJ, Colli W. Glycoproteins from *Trypanosoma cruzi*: partial purification by gel chromatography. *FEBS Lett* 1975;**52**(2):188−90.

64. Colli W, Alves MJ. Relevant glycoconjugates on the surface of *Trypanosoma cruzi*. *Mem Inst Oswaldo Cruz* 1999;**94**(Suppl. 1):37−49.

65. Zingales B, Martin NF, Lederkremer RM, Colli W. Endogenous and surface labeling of glycoconjugates from the three differentiation stages of *Trypanosoma cruzi*. *FEBS Lett* 1982;**142**(2):238−42.

66. Lana M, Pinto AS, Barnabé C, Quesney V, Noel S, Tibayrenc M. *Trypanosoma cruzi*: compared vectorial transmissibility of three major clonal genotypes by *Triatoma infestans*. *Exp Parasitol* 1998;**90**(1):20−5.

67. Pinto AS, Lana M, Bastrenta B, Barnabé C, Quesney V, Noel S, et al. Compared vectorial transmissibility of pure and mixed clonal genotypes of *Trypanosoma cruzi* in Triatoma infestans. *Parasitol Res* 1998;**84**(5):348−53.

68. Pinto AS, Lana M, Britto C, Bastrenta B, Tibayrenc M. Experimental *Trypanosoma cruzi* biclonal infection in *Triatoma infestans*: detection of distinct clonal genotypes using kinetoplast DNA probes. *Int J Parasitol* 2000;**30**(7):843−8.

69. Carvalho-Moreira CJ, Spata MC, Coura JR, Garcia ES, Azambuja P, Gonzalez MS, et al. *In vivo* and *in vitro* metacyclogenesis tests of two strains of *Trypanosoma cruzi* in the triatomines vectors *Triatoma pseudomaculata* and *Rhodnius neglectus*: short/long-term and comparative study. *Exp Parasitol* 2003;**103**(3−4):102−11.

70. Lima VS, Mangia RH, Carreira JC, Marchewski RS, Jansen AM. *Trypanosoma cruzi*: correlations of biological aspects of the life cycle in mice and triatomines. *Mem Inst Oswaldo Cruz* 1999;**94**(3):397−402.

71. Brumpt E. *Shizotrypanum cruzi*—differentes phases de son cycle evolutif. *Bull Soc Pathol Exot* 1912;**5**:261−2.

72. Tibayrenc M, Ayala FJ. Isoenzyme variability of *Trypanosoma cruzi*, the agent of Chagas' disease. *Evolution* 1988;**42**(2):277–92.
73. Tibayrenc M, Ward P, Moya A, Ayala FJ. Natural populations of *Trypanosoma cruzi*, the agent of Chagas disease, have a complex multiclonal structure. *Proc Natl Acad Sci USA* 1986;**83**(1):115–19.
74. Brener Z, Chiari E. Variações morfológicas observadas em diferentes amostras de *Trypanosoma cruzi*. *Rev Inst Med Trop São Paulo* 1963;**5**:220–4.
75. Brener Z. Comparative studies of different strains of *Trypanosoma cruzi*. *Ann Trop Med Parasitol* 1965;**59**:19–26.
76. Brener Z. The behavior of slender and stout forms of *Trypanosoma cruzi* in the bloodstream of normal and immune mice. *Ann Trop Med Parasitol* 1969;**63**(2):215–20.
77. Howells RE, Chiari CA. Observations on two strains of *Trypanosoma cruzi* in laboratory mice. *Ann Trop Med Parasitol* 1975;**69**(4):435–48.
78. Da Silva AM, Brodskyn CI, Takehara HA, Mota I. Comparison between the antigenic composition of bloodstream and cell culture-derived trypomastigotes of *Trypanosoma cruzi*. *Braz J Med Biol Res* 1988;**21**(5):991–3.
79. Bahia MT, Tafuri WL, Caliari MV, Veloso VM, Carneiro CM, Coelho GL, et al. Comparison of *Trypanosoma cruzi* infection in dogs inoculated with blood or metacyclic trypomastigotes of Berenice-62 and Berenice-78 strains via intraperitoneal and conjunctival routes. *Rev Soc Bras Med Trop* 2002;**35**(4):339–45.
80. McHardy N, Neal RA. A comparison of challenge with *Trypanosoma cruzi* bloodstream trypomastigotes and metacyclic trypomastigotes from *Rhodnius prolixus* in mice immunized with killed antigens. *Trans R Soc Trop Med Hyg* 1979;**73**(4):409–14.
81. Vago AR, Andrade LO, Leite AA, D'Avila RD, Macedo AM, Adad SJ, et al. Genetic characterization of *Trypanosoma cruzi* directly from tissues of patients with chronic Chagas disease: *differential distribution of genetic types into diverse organs*. *Am J Pathol* 2000;**156**(5):1805–9.
82. Andrade SG. Caracterização de cepas de *Trypanosoma cruzi* isoladas no Recôncavo Baiano. *Rev Pat Trop* 1974;**1**:65–121.
83. Andrade SG, Magalhães JB. Biodemes and zimodemes of *Trypanosoma cruzi* strains: correlations with clinical data and experimental pathology. *Rev Soc Bras Med Trop* 1996;**30**(1):27–35.
84. Laurent JP, Barnabé C, Quesney V, Noel S, Tibayrenc M. Impact of clonal evolution on the biological diversity of *Trypanosoma cruzi*. *Parasitology* 1997;**114**(Pt3):213–18.
85. Revollo S, Oury B, Laurent JP, Barnabé C, Quesney V, Carrière V, et al. *Trypanosoma cruzi*: impact of clonal evolution of the parasite on its biological and medical properties. *Exp Parasitol* 1998;**89**(1):30–9.
86. Toledo MJ, Lana M, Carneiro CM, Bahia MT, Machado-Coelho GL, Veloso VM, et al. Impact of *Trypanosoma cruzi* clonal evolution on its biological properties in mice. *Exp Parasitol* 2002;**100**(3):161–72.
87. Tibayrenc M, Brenière SF. *Trypanosoma cruzi*: major clones rather than principal zymodemes. *Mem Inst Oswaldo Cruz* 1988;**83**(Suppl. 1):249–55.
88. Teston AP, Monteiro WM, Reis D, Bossolani GD, Gomes ML, de Araújo SM, et al. In vivo susceptibility to benznidazole of *Trypanosoma cruzi* strains from the western Brazilian Amazon. *Trop Med Int Health* 2013;**18**:85–95.
89. Toledo MJ, Bahia MT, Carneiro CM, Martins-Filho OA, Tibayrenc M, Barnabé C, et al. Chemotherapy with benznidazole and itraconazole for mice infected with different *Trypanosoma cruzi* clonal genotypes. *Antimicrob Agents Chemother* 2003;**47**(1):223–30.

90. Zingales B, Souto RP, Mangia RH, Lisboa CV, Campbell DA, Coura JR, et al. Molecular epidemiology of American trypanosomiasis in Brazil based on dimorphisms of rRNA and mini-exon gene sequences. *Int J Parasitol* 1998;**28**(1):105−12.

91. Briones RSM, Souto RP, Stolf BS, Zingales B. The evolution of two *Trypanosoma cruzi* subgroups inferred from rRNA genes can be correlated with the interchange of American mammalian faunas in the Cenozoic and had implications to pathogenicity and host specificity. *Mol Biochem Parasitol* 1999;**104**(2):219−32.

92. Di Noia JM, Buscaglia CA, De Marchi CR, Almeida IC, Frasch ACA. *Trypanosoma cruzi* small surface molecule provides the first immunological evidence that Chagas' disease is due to a single parasite lineage. *J Exp Med* 2002;**195**(4):401−13.

93. Tibayrenc M, Kjelberg F, Ayala FJ. A clonal theory of parasitic protozoa: the population structure of *Entamoeba*, *Giardia*, *Leishmania*, *Naegleria*, *Plasmodium*, *Trichomonas* and *Trypanosoma* and their medical and taxonomical consequences. *Proc Natl Acad Sci USA* 1990;**87**(7):2414−18.

94. Machado CA, Ayala FJ. Nucleotide sequences provide evidence of genetic exchange among distantly related lineages of *Trypanosoma cruzi*. *Proc Natl Acad Sci USA* 2001;**98**(13):7396−401.

95. Brisse S, Henriksson J, Barnabé C, Douzery EJ, Berkvens D, Serrano M, et al. Evidence of genetic exchange and hybridization in *Trypanosoma cruzi* based on nucleotide sequences and molecular karyotype. *Infect Genet Evol* 2003;**2**(3):173−83.

96. Pereira da Silva LH. Observacões sobre o ciclo evolutivo do *Trypanosoma cruzi*. *Inst Med Trop São Paulo* 1959;**1**:99−118.

97. Brener Z. Life cycle of *Trypanosoma cruzi*. *Rev Inst Med Trop São Paulo* 1971;**13**(3):171−8.

98. Kollien AH, Goncalves TC, Azambuja P, Garcia ES, Schaub GA. The effect of azadirachtin on fresh isolates of *Trypanosoma cruzi* in different species of triatomines. *Parasitol Res* 1998;**84**(4):286−90.

99. Perlowagora-Szumlewicz A, Müller CA. Studies in search of a suitable experimental insect model for xenodiagnosis of hosts with Chagas' disease. 1. Comparative xenodiagnosis with nine triatomine species of animals with acute infections by *Trypanosoma cruzi*. *Mem Inst Oswaldo Cruz* 1982;**77**(1):37−53.

100. Cortez MG, Gonzalez MS, Cabral MM, Garcia ES, Azambuja A. Dynamic development of *Trypanosoma cruzi* in *Rhodnius prolixus*: role of decapitation and ecdysone therapy. *Parasitol Res* 2002;**88**(7):697−703.

101. Campos R, Acuña-Retamar M, Botto-Mahan C, Ortiz S, Cattan PE, Solari A. Susceptibility of *Mepraia spinolai* and *Triatoma infestans* to different *Trypanosoma cruzi* strains from naturally infected rodent hosts. *Acta Trop* 2007;**104**(1):25−9.

102. Camargo EP. Growth and differentiation in *Trypanosoma cruzi*. I. Origin of metacyclic trypanosomes in liquid media. *Rev Inst Med Trop São Paulo* 1964;**6**:93−100.

103. Yoshida NA. Macromolecule-free partially defined medium for *Trypanosoma cruzi*. *J Protozool* 1975;**22**(1):128−30.

104. Roitman C, Roitman I, De Azevedo HP. Growth of an insect Trypanosomatid at 37°C in a defined medium. *J Protozool* 1972;**19**(2):346−9.

105. Contreras VT, Morel CM, Goldenberg S. Stage specific gene expression precedes morphological changes during *Trypanosoma cruzi* metacyclogenesis. *Mol Biochem Parasitol* 1985;**14**(1):83−96.

106. Goldenberg S, Contreras VT, Salles JM, Bonaldo MC, Lima-Franco MPA, Laffaile JJ, et al. In vitro differentiation systems for the study of differential gene expression during *Trypanosoma cruzi* development. In: Agabian N, Goldman H, Nogueira, editors. *Molecular strategies of parsitic invasion. UCLA Symp Molec Cell Biology, New Series*, vol 42. New York: Alan R. Liss Inc; 1987. p. 203–12.

107. Perlewitz J, Koch A. Trials for optimization of the culture conditions of human pathogenic trypanosomas and leishmania. *Angew Parasitol* 1985;**26**(4):185–91.

108. Bonaldo MC, Souto-Padron T, Souza W, Goldenberg S. Cell-substrate adhesion during *Trypanosoma cruzi* differentiation. *J Cell Biol* 1988;**106**(4):1349–58.

109. Duschak VG, Barboza M, García GA, Lammel EM, Couto AS, Isola EL. Novel cysteine proteinase in *Trypanosoma cruzi* metacyclogenesis. *Parasitology* 2006;**132** (Pt3):345–55.

110. Contreras VT, Araque W, Delgado VS. *Trypanosoma cruzi*: metacyclogenesis in vitro. I. Changes in the properties of metacyclic trypomastigotes maintained in the laboratory by different methods. *Mem Inst Oswaldo Cruz* 1994;**89**(2):253–9.

111. De Lima AR, Navarro MC, Arteaga RY, Contrerasb VT. Cultivation of *Trypanosoma cruzi* epimastigotes in low glucose axenic media shifts its competence to differentiate at metacyclic trypomastigotes. *Exp Parasitol* 2008;**119**(3):336–42.

112. Krieger MA, Ávila AR, Ogatta SF, Plazanet-Menut C, Goldenberg S. Differential gene expression during *Trypanosoma cruzi* metacyclogenesis. *Mem Inst Oswaldo Cruz* 1999;**94**(Suppl. 1):165–8.

113. Parodi-Talice A, Monteiro-Goes V, Arrambide N, Avila AR, Duran R, Correa A, et al. Proteomic analysis of metacyclic trypomastigotes undergoing *Trypanosoma cruzi* metacyclogenesis. *J Mass Spectrom* 2007;**42**(11):1422–32.

114. Kofoid CA, Wood FD, Mcneil E. The cycle of *Trypanosoma cruzi* in tissue culture of embryonic heart muscle. *Univ California Publ Zool* 1935;**41**(3):23–4.

115. Meyer H, Oliveira MX. Cultivation of *Trypanosoma cruzi* in tissue cultures: a four-year study. *Parasitology* 1948;**39**(1–2):91–4.

116. Bertelli MS, Golgher RR, Brener Z. Intraspecific variation in *Trypanosoma cruzi*: effect of temperature on the intracellular differentiation in tissue culture. *J Parasitol* 1977;**63**(3):434–7.

117. Dvorak JA, Schmunis GA. *Trypanosoma cruzi*: interaction with mouse peritoneal macrophages. *Exp Parasitol* 1972;**32**(2):289–300.

118. Filardi LS. Cryopreservation of *Trypanosoma cruzi* bloodstream forms. *J Protozool* 1975;**22**(3):398–401.

119. Filardi LS, Brener Z. Cryopreservation of *Trypanosoma cruzi* in examples of *Triatoma infestans* experimentally infected. *Rev Inst Med Trop São Paulo* 1976;**18**(5):301–5.

120. Raether W, Michel R, Uphoff M. Effects of dimethylsulfoxide and the deep-freezing process on the infectivity, motility, and ultrastructure of *Trypanosoma cruzi*. *Parasitol Res* 1988;**74**(4):307–13.

121. Yaeger RG. Long term cryopreservation of the amastigote stages of hemoflagellates. *J Protozool* 1988;**35**(1):114–15.

122. De Souza W, Sant'Anna C, Cunha-e-Silva NL. Electron microscopy and cytochemistry analysis of the endocytic pathway of pathogenic protozoa. *Prog Histochem Cytochem* 2009;**44**(2):67–124. Available from: http://dx.doi.org/10.1016/j.proghi.2009.01.001.

# Biochemistry of *Trypanosoma cruzi*

R. Docampo and S.N.J. Moreno
University of Georgia, Athens, GA, United States

## Introduction

Completion of the *Trypanosoma cruzi* genome project[1] and proteomic studies of the different stages of the parasite[2–11] as well as their subcellular fractions[5,7,12,13] has provided a wealth of information about their biochemistry and metabolic pathways. This is especially important because most metabolic studies were done before using the culture or epimastigote form of the parasite, and not the more clinically relevant mammalian stages. The analysis and validation of these pathways will considerably increase our knowledge of the biology of *T. cruzi*. In addition, the rational development of new drugs against *T. cruzi* depends on the identification of differences between human metabolism and that of the parasite.

American Trypanosomiasis Chagas Disease. DOI: http://dx.doi.org/10.1016/B978-0-12-801029-7.00017-4

Developments in the study of the basic biochemistry of the parasite have allowed the identification of peculiar metabolic pathways in *T. cruzi* that provide or could provide novel targets for chemotherapy. Redox metabolism is involved in the mechanism of action of the drugs currently in use against Chagas disease. The study of the isoprenoid pathway has resulted in drugs that are being used in clinical trials against the disease, and other potent agents that are active in vitro and vivo against *T. cruzi* such as bisphosphonates and prenyl transferase inhibitors. Acidocalcisome metabolism has a number of characteristics that make these organelles potential targets for trypanocidal drugs. These metabolic pathways are the subjects of this chapter.

## Chemotherapy of Chagas disease

Chemotherapy against Chagas disease[14–21] depends on the use of two drugs, nifurtimox and benznidazole (Fig. 17.1). These drugs can cure at least 50% of recent infections as shown by disappearance of symptoms and negativization of parasitemia and serology.[14,22–24] However, results of treatment trials for acute infections have not been uniform in different countries,[14,24] probably as a consequence of the different drug sensitivity of different *T. cruzi* strains. Both drugs have side effects, which are more common in adults than in children, although they disappear when treatment is discontinued.[14,22,24] Another drawback of these drugs is the need for an extensive treatment period. Nifurtimox is given for 30–120 days,[14] while benznidazole is given for at least 30 days.[14]

The use of these drugs in the indeterminate or chronic stage of the infections has been less frequent; after treatment, serology in most cases remains positive even when parasitemia is absent.[22,24,25] It has been shown that antiparasite treatment of chronic Chagasic patients with benznidazole results in fewer electrocardiographic changes and a lower frequency of deterioration in their clinical condition.[26] Lack of progress in the myocardiopathy correlated well with negativization of serology.[26,27]

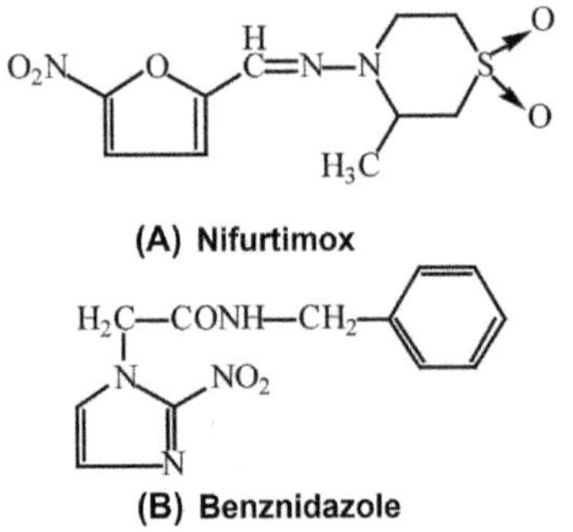

**(A) Nifurtimox**

**(B) Benznidazole**

**Figure 17.1** Structures of nifurtimox (A) and benznidazole (B), drugs currently used against Chagas disease.

Moreover, even when asymptomatic, some children aged 12 years or less, could be parasitologically cured when treated with benznidazole.[28] Side effects were mild and fewer children in the benznidazole-treated group showed myocardiopathy.[28,29] These findings match well with the fact that benznidazole treatment of *T. cruzi*-infected mice induces a late regression of lesions in the myocardium and skeletal muscle,[30] and that parasitization of heart tissue is both necessary and sufficient for the induction of tissue damage in *T. cruzi* infection.[31,32] These findings stress the need for chemotherapeutic agents that are effective against all strains of *T. cruzi*, and with fewer or no side effects than those currently available.[33]

# Metabolic pathways in *T. cruzi* that could provide targets for drugs against Chagas disease

## Isoprenoid pathway

One pathway that has been particularly useful for the identification of new targets against *T. cruzi* is the isoprenoid pathway (Fig. 17.2). Several enzymes of this pathway, involved in the synthesis of farnesyl diphosphate[34] and sterols,[20] and in protein prenylation,[35] have been reported to be excellent drug targets against these parasites.

Isoprenoids are the most diverse and abundant compounds occurring in nature. Isoprenoids such as steroids, cholesterol, retinoids, carotenoids, ubiquinones, and prenyl proteins are essential components of the cells of all organisms due to their roles in different biological processes. Despite their structural and functional variety, all isoprenoids derive from a common precursor: isopentenyl diphosphate (IPP), and its isomer, dimethylallyl diphosphate (DMAPP). In *T. cruzi*, IPP is synthesized exclusively via the so-called mevalonate pathway, which has the 3-hydroxy-3-methylglutaryl-CoA (HMG-CoA) reductase as the key regulatory enzyme[36,37] (Fig. 17.2). Mevalonate is then converted to IPP with two continuous phosphorylation steps and one decarboxylation step. Isomerization of IPP by IPP isomerase yields DMAPP.

## Polyprenyl diphosphate synthases

Once IPP is formed polyprenyl diphosphate synthases are responsible for chain elongation and catalyze the sequential condensation of IPP with allylic prenyl diphosphates.[36] So far, only the genes encoding farnesyl diphosphate synthase (FPPS),[38] and solanesyl diphosphate synthase (SPPS)[39] have been cloned from *T. cruzi*. Both of these genes are single copy. While the FPP synthase is localized in the cytosol,[40] the SPP synthase is localized in the glycosomes.[39] Glycosomes are specialized peroxisomes that, like them, contain several enzymes in pathways of ether lipid synthesis, fatty acid β-oxidation, and peroxide metabolism, and, in addition, contain the Embden-Meyerhof segment of glycolysis.[41]

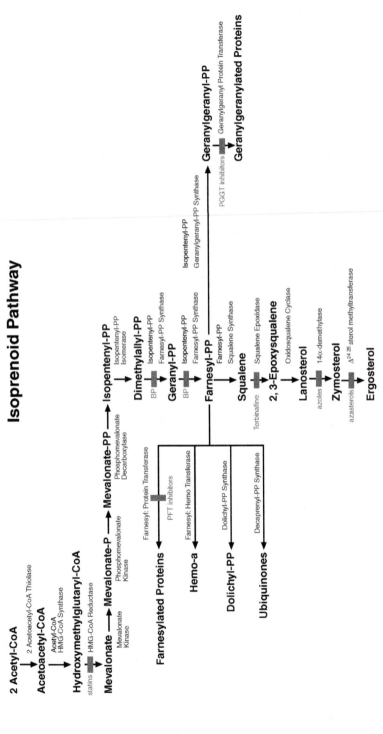

**Figure 17.2** Isoprenoid pathway in *T. cruzi*. Enzyme names are in gray (blue in web version), products in black, and inhibitors in light gray (red in web version).

T. *cruzi* farnesyl diphosphate synthase (TcFPPS) catalyzes the consecutive condensation of IPP with DMAPP and with geranyl diphosphate (GPP) to form the 15-carbon isoprenoid compound, farnesyl diphosphate (FPP) (Fig. 17.2). FPP is the substrate for enzymes catalyzing the first committed step for biosynthesis of sterols (which in *T. cruzi* is mainly ergosterol[42]), ubiquinones (which in *T. cruzi* is mainly ubiquinone-9[39]), dolichols (which are required for the synthesis of complex carbohydrates and are present in *T. cruzi*[43]), heme A (a component of the cytochrome oxidase, also present in *T. cruzi*[44]), and prenylated proteins (also present in *T. cruzi*[45−48]). FPP could be condensed with an additional molecule of IPP by the geranylgeranyl diphosphate synthase (GGPPS) to form the 20-carbon isoprenoid GGPP (Fig. 17.2), although this enzyme has not been studied in *T. cruzi*. The FPPS gene appears to be essential in all organisms.[49,50] As most FPPSs that have been characterized, *T. cruzi* FPPS is an homodimeric enzyme, and requires divalent metal ions such as $Mg^{2+}$ or $Mn^{2+}$ for activity.[38] The 3D structure of TcFPPS has been solved in complex with different substrates and inhibitors.[51−53]

TcFPPS is the main target of bisphosphonates in *T. cruzi*.[34,38] Bisphosphonates are pyrophosphate analogues in which a carbon atom replaces the oxygen atom bridge between the two phosphorus atoms of the pyrophosphate. The substitution of carbon with different side chains has generated a large family of compounds (Fig. 17.3). Several bisphosphonates are potent inhibitors of bone resorption and are in clinical use for the treatment and prevention of osteoporosis, Paget's disease, hypercalcemia, tumor bone metastases, and other bone diseases.[54] Selective action

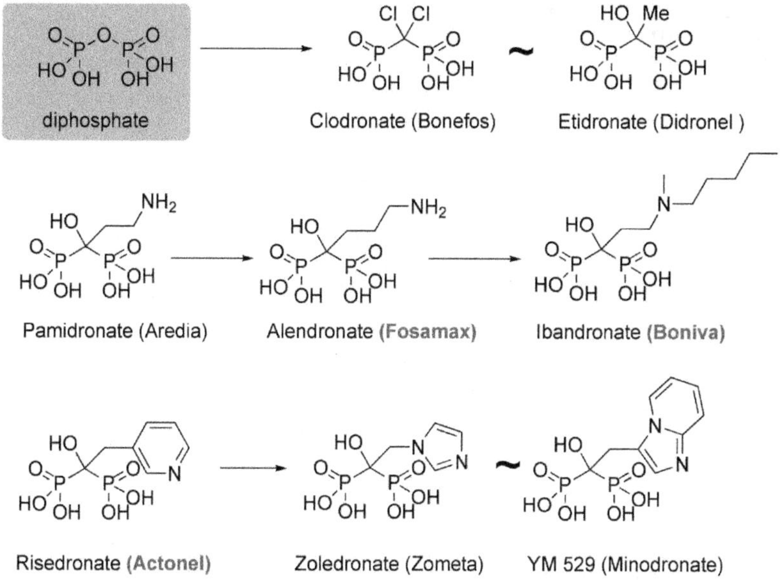

**Figure 17.3** Structure of pyrophosphate (diphosphate) and selected bisphosphonates. First- (clodronate and etidronate), second- (pamidronate, alendronate, and ibandronate), and third- (risedronate, zolendronate, and YM 529) generation bisphosphonates are shown.

on bone is based on the binding of the bisphosphonate to the bone mineral.[54] It has been postulated that the acidocalcisomes, organelles rich in phosphorus and calcium in trypanosomes, are equivalent in composition to the bone mineral and that accumulation of bisphosphonates in these organelles, as they do in bone mineral, facilitates their antiparasitic action.[55] Nitrogen-containing bisphosphonates were first found to be effective in the inhibition of *T. cruzi* in vitro and in vivo without toxicity to the host cell.[56,57] In vivo testing of bisphosphonates against *T. cruzi* in mice has shown that risedronate can significantly increase the survival of mice infected by *T. cruzi*.[58,59] All these results indicate that bisphosphonates are promising candidate drugs to treat infections by *T. cruzi*.

*T. cruzi* solanesyl diphosphate synthase (TcSPPS) catalyzes the formation of the 45-carbon compound solanesyl diphosphate (SPP), which is an intermediate in the synthesis of ubiquinone-9. Ubiquinone is synthesized de novo in both prokaryotes and eukaryotes. The two parts of the molecule, the benzoquinone ring and the isoprene chain, are synthesized independently and assembled in a reaction catalyzed by a prenyl-4-hydroxybenzoate-transferase.[60] 4-Hydroxybenzoate originates from tyrosine or phenylalanine in eukaryotes.[61] In *T. cruzi* it was shown that epimastigotes synthesize and keep mainly UQ9 in their membranes.[39] Human tissues have mostly UQ10 while rat tissues have UQ9. Valuable functions have been adjudicated to this molecule, including acting as a component of the mitochondrial electron transfer system, as the only lipid-soluble antioxidant that is endogenously synthesized in both unicellular and multicellular organisms, and as an acceptor of electrons from sulfide.[62] Two genes with homology to the yeast[63] and human[64] prenyl-4-hydroxybenzoate-transferases are present in the genome of *T. cruzi* differing in only two amino acids and possessing a mitochondrial targeting signal (TcCLB.510903.60 and TcCBL.505965.30). The protein has a putative polyprenyl diphosphate-binding domain similar to those found in other enzymes known to bind isoprenoid substrates. Bisphosphonates can also inhibit the activity of TcSPPS and amastigote growth in culture cells.[65]

## Protein prenylation

The occurrence of protein prenylation in *T. cruzi* has been demonstrated.[47] Protein prenylation in mammals and yeast involves the attachment of 15-carbon farnesyl or 20-carbon geranylgeranyl groups to a conserved cysteine residue in a CaaX motif of a subset of cellular proteins (Fig. 17.2). Many of these prenylated proteins are small GTPases, including Ras, Rac, Rab, and Rho, that have roles in cellular signal transduction and intracellular vesicle trafficking.[66,67] The known functions of prenyl groups attached to cellular proteins is to anchor proteins to membranes and to serve as molecular handles for mediating protein—protein interactions.[68] Three enzymes have been identified in eukaryotic cells including those from mammals and plants and in yeast that attach prenyl groups to proteins: protein farnesyl transferase (PFT); protein geranylgeranyl transferase I (PGGT-I); and protein geranylgeranyl transferase II (PGGT-II).[68,69] Different studies have detected the presence of prenylated proteins and a farnesyl transferase activity in *T. cruzi*.[45−48] Over the past several years, hundreds of potent PFT inhibitors have been synthesized with the primary goal of developing anticancer drugs.[70] Some of these compounds have been shown to inhibit the growth of *T. cruzi*[47] and are potential chemotherapeutic agents.

## Ergosterol synthesis

Squalene synthase (SQS) catalyzes the first step committed to the biosynthesis of sterols within the isoprenoid pathway, and several quinuclidine inhibitors of the enzyme were shown to have selective anti-*T. cruzi* activity both in vitro and in vivo.[71] SQ-109, which is in clinical trials against drug-sensitive and drug-resistant tuberculosis,[72] and a variety of aryloxyethyl thiocyanates[73] also inhibit the enzyme. The enzyme is membrane-bound, and was expressed in truncated form in *Escherichia coli* and biochemically characterized.[71] Its X-ray crystallographic structure in the presence of inhibitors has been reported.[74] The following step in the synthesis of ergosterol is catalyzed by the squalene epoxidase, which is the target of terbinafine, a drug that is active in vitro and in vivo against *T. cruzi*.[20] Lanosterol is then synthesized by a reaction catalyzed by the lanosterol synthase or oxidosqualene cyclase (Fig. 17.2). Several inhibitors of the enzyme showed activity in vitro against *T. cruzi*.[75] Interestingly, the antiarrhythmic bis-aryl-ketone amiodarone, which is used in chronic Chagas patients with heart problems, also inhibits this enzyme and has activity in vitro and in vivo against *T. cruzi*.[76] Lanosterol is converted into zymosterol by a series of reactions started by the sterol 14a-demethylase, a target of azole (imidazole and triazole) derivatives.[20] This enzyme is a member of the cytochrome P450 superfamily (CYP51), and catalyzes the oxidative removal of the 14$\alpha$-methyl group from postsqualene sterol precursors. The gene encoding this enzyme was cloned and expressed and its substrate preferences studied.[77] The crystal structure of *T. cruzi* CYP51 bound to inhibitors has also been reported.[78−80]

Azole compounds were first detected to have activity against *T. cruzi* in 1981.[42] Miconazole and econazole showed a potent growth inhibitory action parallel to a decrease in its 5,7-diene sterol content.[42] Later studies showed that ketoconazole, and other potent antimycotic azoles were also active in protecting mice against lethal infections with *T. cruzi*,[81,82] in inhibiting intracellular multiplication of the parasites,[83−85] and in blocking their biosynthesis of fungal-type sterols.[83,84] More recent work on a number of inhibitors of this enzyme has been reviewed recently.[20] Although the enzyme is present in mammalian cells, it is much less sensitive to the drugs than that present in fungi and trypanosomatids. Several of these azole compounds have undergone clinical trials against Chagas disease.[21]

Ergosterol differs from cholesterol, the predominant mammalian sterol, by the presence of a 24-methyl group and $\Delta^7$ and $\Delta^{22}$ double bonds. The enzymatic reactions that introduce the extra methyl group and the $\Delta^{22}$ double bond of ergosterol have no counterpart in mammalian sterol biosynthesis, and may be regarded as targets for new antiparasitic agents. In agreement with this hypothesis it has been shown that azasterols, which are $\Delta^{24(25)}$ sterol methyl transferase inhibitors, have a potent antiproliferative effect on *T. cruzi* in vitro and in vivo.[86]

# Redox metabolism

## Deficient metabolic utilization of $H_2O_2$ in T. cruzi

Almost four decades ago *T. cruzi* was reported to be deficient in enzyme systems necessary for the removal of hydrogen peroxide ($H_2O_2$).[15,17,33,87−90] Despite extensive studies on the antioxidant defenses of this and other trypanosomatids over subsequent years, this characterization appears to be still valid. *T. cruzi* lacks genes for catalase, selenocysteine-dependent glutathione peroxidases, glutathione reductase, and thioredoxin reductase.[91,92] The two cysteine-dependent glutathione peroxidases that have been described are not able to hydrolyze $H_2O_2$[91,92]. One enzyme able to catalyze this reaction is the ascorbate peroxidase (TcAPx), first described in 1976 in *T. cruzi*.[93] The recombinant enzyme was studied more recently.[94] The activity of this enzyme in epimastigote homogenates is only $6−15$ nmol $H_2O_2$/min × mg protein.[95] In addition, expression of the enzyme is not correlated to virulence or metacyclogenesis,[96] the enzyme is not essential for parasite viability within the mammalian host, and does not have a significant role in establishment and maintenance of chronic infections.[97] However, *null* mutants of TcAPx have decreased ability to infect mammalian cells in vitro and an increased sensitivity to exogenous $H_2O_2$.[97] TcAPx expression is enhanced in *T. cruzi* strains resistant to benznidazole.[98] The trypanothione-dependent peroxidase activity with $H_2O_2$ as substrate in extracts of epimastigotes (which include the activities of tryparedoxin peroxidases and any other NADPH-dependent peroxidases, i.e., peroxidases dependent on the reduction of T(SH)$_2$), is only $1.86 \pm 0.54$ nmol NADPH oxidized/min × mg protein.[99] It has been pointed out that these trypanothione-dependent peroxidase activities are quite low in comparison with approximately 150 nmol/min × mg protein found in lung mitochondria.[100] Assuming that $10^8$ epimastigotes are approximately equivalent to 1 mg protein[100] it seems that ascorbate peroxidase and other trypanothione-dependent peroxidases are approximately 10 and 80 times less active, respectively, than the equivalent activities in mammalian tissues on a mg protein basis. In other words, trypanosomatids may be protected for dealing with a slow endogenous rate of $H_2O_2$ generation but they are probably quite sensitive to an increased steady state concentration of $H_2O_2$.[100] The reason for this deficiency is probably that there is little need for decomposing $H_2O_2$ in the conditions under which the parasite, a facultative aerobe, develops, either in the intestine of the insect vector in the case of epimastigotes, or in the cytosol of the host cell in the case of the intracellular amastigotes. In this regard, transformation of epimastigotes into metacyclic trypomastigotes is accompanied by an increase in expression of antioxidant enzymes, such as ascorbate peroxidase, tryparedoxin peroxidase, tryparedoxin, trypanothione synthase, and iron superoxide dismutase,[2] a phenomenon that was proposed to indicate a preadaptation of metacyclic forms to withstand the potential respiratory burst of phagocytic cells in the mammalian host.[2] This deficiency in the metabolism of $H_2O_2$ also explains in part the susceptibility of *T. cruzi* to $H_2O_2$-generating drugs, such as napthoquinones,[89,90,101−108] and nifurtimox,[109−111] one of the drugs used against Chagas disease.

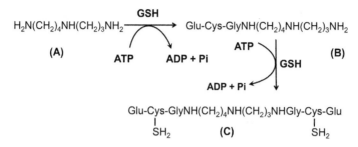

**Figure 17.4** Trypanothione synthesis occurs by condensation of spermidine (A) with GSH to give glutathionyl spermidine (B). Addition of a second GSH leads to the formation of dihydrotrypanothione (T(SH)$_2$) (C). Both reactions consume ATP and are catalyzed by trypanothione synthase.

## The trypanothione system

In contrast to its mammalian hosts, which maintain their intracellular thiol homeostasis using glutathione/glutathione reductases, as well as thioredoxin/thioredoxin reductases, *T. cruzi* redox metabolism depends on the trypanothione/trypanothione reductase couple.[92]

Trypanothione ($N^1,N^8$-bis(glutathionyl)spermidine) is synthesized from glutathione and spermidine (Fig. 17.4). The biosynthesis of glutathione has not been studied in detail in *T. cruzi* although it has been reported that 1-buthionine (S,R) sulfoximine (BSO), an inhibitor of gamma glutamylcysteine synthetase, which is the first enzyme in the synthesis of glutathione (GSH), decreases GSH levels and increases the toxicity of nifurtimox and benznidazole in epimastigotes.[112] *T. cruzi* is auxotrophic for polyamines and unable to carry out de novo biosynthesis of putrescine.[113] Spermidine can be taken up by a transporter[114,115] or derived from putrescine through the reaction catalyzed by spermidine synthase. However, this enzyme has not been characterized in *T. cruzi*. An ATP-dependent enzyme then attaches GSH and spermidine covalently into a glutathionylspermidine conjugate, or monoglutathionylspermidine (GSH-SPD). Subsequently a second molecule of GSH is added to yield dihydrotrypanothione (T(SH)$_2$). Both steps are catalyzed in *T. cruzi* by a trypanothione synthetase with the consumption of two ATPs[116] (Fig. 17.4). Oxidation of dihydrotrypanothione leads to the formation of trypanothione disulfide (TS$_2$), and thypanothione reductase[117] catalyzes its reduction back to T(SH)$_2$ (Fig. 17.5).

Apart from its synthetase activity, trypanothione synthetase has an opposite hydrolytic activity (T(SH)$_2$ amidase) located in its N-terminal region. These two activities were proposed to be relevant for the regulation of polyamine levels in response to their availability and growth phase.[116] Although *T. cruzi* has a gene homologous to the glutathionylspermidine synthase present in *Crihidia fasciculata*,[118] the function of this enzyme in the parasite has not been investigated. The trypanothione synthetase is a potential target for drugs and high throughput screenings of compounds against this enzyme are underway.[119]

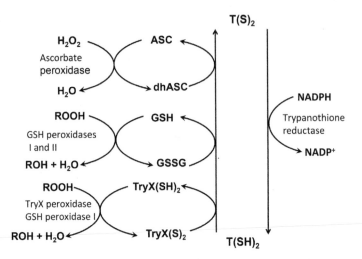

**Figure 17.5** Redox metabolism in *T. cruzi*. Reduction of trypanothione (T(S)$_2$) to dihydrotrypanothione (T(SH)$_2$) is catalyzed by trypanothione reductase with conversion of NADPH into NADP$^+$. Oxidation of dihydrotrypanothione to trypanothione is coupled to the reduction of tryparedoxin (TryX(S)$_2$), GSSG, and dehydroascorbate (dhASC), and these compounds are generated by the action of peroxidases catalyzing the decomposition of H$_2$O$_2$ (ascorbate peroxidase and tryparedoxin peroxidases) or hydroperoxides (ROOH; GSH peroxidases I and II, and tryparedoxin peroxidases).

    The intracellular concentration of dihydrotrypanothione has been reported to be $0.12 \pm 0.06$ and $6.4$ nmol/$10^8$ cells in epimastigotes grown in polyamine-deficient medium and in the presence of $100\,\mu$M extracellular putrescine, respectively, and $0.95 \pm 0.34$ nmol/$10^8$ cells in tissue culture derived trypomastigotes.[120] In another report the concentration of T(SH)$_2$ was indicated as $0.18 \pm 0.04$, $0.25 \pm 0.10$, and $0.12 \pm 0.04$ nmol/$10^8$ cells in epimastigotes, trypomastigotes, and amastigotes, respectively.[121] Interestingly, the intracellular concentration of GSH in epimastigotes ($2.10 \pm 0.53$ nmol/$10^8$ cells) and of cysteine ($0.40 \pm 0.27$ and $0.61 \pm 0.12$ nmol/$10^8$ cells for trypomastigotes and amastigotes, respectively), and GSH ($0.29 \pm 0.13$ and $0.42 \pm 0.04$ nmol/$10^8$ cells in trypomastigotes and amastigotes, respectively) in the mammalian stages, are higher than those of T(SH)$_2$. Taking into account the cell volumes of different stages of *T. cruzi* calculated by the inulin method ($34.8 \pm 3.3$, $11.1 \pm 1.9$ and $14.6 \pm 1.1\,\mu$L/$10^9$ cells for epimastigotes, trypomastigotes, and amastigotes, respectively[122]), the intracellular concentration of T(SH)$_2$ in epimastigotes (unsupplemented with exogenous polyamines), trypomastigotes, and amastigotes would be: $35-52$, $225-855$, and $82\,\mu$M, respectively, and could reach $1.88$ mM in epimastigotes supplemented with $100\,\mu$M putrescine. These values are important when considering the noncatalyzed reactions of T(SH)$_2$ with other molecules and reactions for which the $K_m$ for T(SH)$_2$ is in the micromolar level.

    Trypanothione reductase was purified to homogeneity from *T. cruzi*[123] and the gene cloned and expressed to characterize the enzymatic properties of the recombinant enzyme,[124] which were similar to those of the native enzyme.[123] This enzyme catalyzes the NADPH-dependent reduction of trypanothione disulfide, but not gluta-thione. The enzyme is highly specific for trypanothione and has striking homology to glutathione reductase. Its crystal structure was solved alone or in complex with its substrate or inhibitors.[125−130] A number of compounds, such as nitrofurans and naphthoquinones,[117,131] phenothiazines and related tricyclics,[132−135] crystal vio-let,[136] diphenylsulfide derivatives,[137] polyamine derivatives,[138−141] dibenzaze-pines,[142] bisbenzylisoquinoline alkaloids,[143] ajoene,[144] acridines,[145] terpyridine platinum complexes,[146] Mannich bases,[147] as well as some natural products[148] have been shown to inhibit *T. cruzi* trypanothione reductase and affect parasite growth in vitro or in vivo. However, most inhibitors have $K_i$s in the micromolar range, and none has been curative against *T. cruzi* infection in mice. Because recombinant try-panothione reductase from *T. cruzi* was the first to be obtained, it has been used regularly in high throughput screening campaigns to identify inhibitors.[149,150] The enzyme is predominantly cytosolic although it cannot be ruled out that it could also be present in the mitochondria and glycosomes.[92]

Oxidation of dihydrotrypanothione leads to the reduction of intermediates (oxidized glutathione (GSSG), dehydroascorbate, or the dithiol protein tryparedox-in), which are then used as a source of electrons for peroxidases: ascorbate peroxi-dase, cysteine-dependent glutathione peroxidases, and tryparedoxin peroxidases (Fig. 17.5). Ascorbate peroxidase is reduced by ascorbate, which is regenerated by dihydrotrypoanothione, and decomposes $H_2O_2$ but not organic hydroperoxides.[93,94] The enzyme localizes in the endoplasmic reticulum,[94] although early work found it in the glycosomes,[93] which is the site where ascorbate synthesis occurs.[151] There are two cysteine-dependent glutathione peroxidases, which are characterized by the presence of cysteine instead of selenocysteine in their active site, in contrast to the mammalian homologues. Glutathione peroxidase I can be reduced by trypare-doxin or GSH and is localized in the glycosomes and cytosol.[152,153] Its crystal structure has been solved.[154] Glutathione peroxidase II can be reduced only by GSH and is present in the endoplasmic reticulum.[155] These peroxidases can decom-pose organic hydroperoxides but not $H_2O_2$.[152,155] Tryparedoxin peroxidases (or per-oxiredoxins) belong to the family of 2-cysteine peroxiredoxins and can decompose $H_2O_2$ and are reduced by tryparedoxin.[99,156,157] There are two isoforms, one is cyto-solic and the other mitochondrial.[99] They can also decompose peroxinitrite.[158−161] Their expression is enhanced in *T. cruzi* strains resistant to benznidazole.[162] The crystal structure of the cytosolic tryparedoxin peroxidase has been solved.[163] The roles of these peroxiredoxins in defense against macrophages-generated oxida-tive and nitrosative stresses have been reported.[164] In all cases the activities of these peroxidases depend on the presence of trypanothione, which has therefore a central role in redox metabolism in *T. cruzi*, and have been considered as virulence factors as their levels increase in the infective stages.[96]

## *Other thiols*

Several novel trypanothione analogues derived from spermine or other physiological polyamines have also been found in *T. cruzi* when supplemented with polyamines in the culture medium, among them homotrypanothione, $N^1$, $N^{12}$-bis(glutathionyl)spermine, $N^1$-glutathionyl-$N^8$-acetylspermidine, and $N^1$-glutathionyl-$N^{12}$-acetylspermine.[116,121] These compounds result from the condensation of GSH with polyamines other than spermidine such as cadaverin, spermine, N-acetylspermine, and $N^1$- and $N^8$-acetylspermine in reactions catalyzed by the trypanothione synthetase.[121] The physiological relevance of these thiols as well as ovothiol ($N^1$-methyl-4-mercaptohistidine),[120] which is also present in all three life cycle stages of this parasite is not known.

## Superoxide dismutases

Superoxide dismutases (SODs) catalyze the dismutation of superoxide anion ($O_2^{-}$) to $H_2O_2$ and $O_2$. T. cruzi has four genes encoding for iron-dependent SODs, two of which have been cloned and the recombinant proteins characterized.[165,166] One of these enzymes is cytosolic (TcSODA) while the other (TcSODB) is mitochondrially-localized. The recombinant enzymes are inactivated by peroxynitrite and the crystal structure of TcSODA has been reported.[167] Inhibitors of the iron-containing superoxide dismutases of trypanosomatids have been found and proposed as possible trypanocidal agents.[168] However, it is not self-evident that in an organism deficient in hydrogen peroxide detoxification, superoxide dismutase inhibition will be toxic. This assumption takes for granted that superoxide is the ultimate toxic species. However, it is conceivable that the hydrogen peroxide formed by the action of superoxide dismutase, and the hydroxyl radical eventually derived from it, are more cytotoxic than superoxide itself. If this is so, superoxide dismutase produces the toxic agent and superoxide dismutase inhibition may be protective as long as hydrogen peroxide cannot adequately be detoxified. Interestingly, a superoxide dismutase inhibitor was shown to decrease the parasitemia levels of T. cruzi in infected mice.[169] Overexpression of cytosolic/glycosomal SOD (SODB1) in T. cruzi increases their susceptibility to benznidazole and crystal violet but has no effect on the action of nifurtimox.[166] The reason for these effects is unknown.

## Chemotherapeutic agents used against Chagas disease and redox metabolism

The enzymatic deficiencies of T. cruzi against oxygen toxicity were correlated with their sensitivity to both intracellularly generated and phagocyte-derived by-products of $O_2$ reduction.[15,17] The chemotherapeutic potential of these enzyme deficiencies was first recognized during work on the mode of action of the trypanocidal o-naphthoquinone β-lapachone and derivatives.[15,17] These studies showed that the metabolism of these compounds by T. cruzi involved, at least in part, the generation of superoxide anion and hydrogen peroxide. $H_2O_2$ accumulated in the cells to cytotoxic levels and was also excreted.[15,17]

The chemotherapeutic implications of these deficiencies were also apparent in the case of nifurtimox (Fig. 17.1). One-electron reduction of nifurtimox to a nitro anion radical followed by autoxidation of this radical with generation of superoxide anion and other oxygen reduction by-products, such as $H_2O_2$, and hydroxyl radical were implicated in the trypanocidal and mammalian toxic effects of this drug.[17] More recent work in this area revealed the presence in *T. cruzi* of alternative activation mechanisms of nifurtimox by two enzymes that apparently catalyze its two-electron reduction. One is the Old Yellow Enzyme, also known as prostaglandin F2α synthase[170] and the other is a type I nitroreductase (TcNTR)[171] that generates nitrile metabolites as final products.[172] Interestingly, Kubata et al.[170] could detect the one-electron reduction of naphthoquinones to semiquinones but not of nifurtimox to nitro anion radicals using the recombinant Old Yellow Enzyme. These negative results, which were not shown, contradict the well-known ability of flavoproteins to catalyze reduction of naphthoquinones and nitrofurans equally well.[173] Furthermore, no evidence was presented for the postulated two-electron reduction of nifurtimox.[170] Detection of nitro anion radicals requires more strict anaerobic conditions than detection of semiquinones, which evidently were not obtained by the authors. However, these negative results were used by other authors[172,174] to propose that two-electron reduction could be more relevant for *T. cruzi* toxicity, although not for mammalian toxicity, than the one-electron reduction catalyzed by type II nitroreductases, with generation of reactive oxygen species (ROS). It is important to also mention that these works[172,174] were done with either the recombinant enzymes or with the epimastigote (culture) form of *T. cruzi*, while a nitro anion radical derivative of nifurtimox as well as redox cycling with generation of superoxide anion and $H_2O_2$ are easily detected using *T. cruzi* amastigote and trypomastigote homogenates.[111] In addition, evidence of oxidative stress by nifurtimox, as revealed by increased steady state concentration of $H_2O_2$ and lipid peroxidation in intact epimastigotes[175] or depletion of low molecular weight thiols in different strains and life cycle stages of *T. cruzi*[174,176] was presented by several authors. In the case of the studies with the recombinant TcNTR the authors[172] found that 100 μM nifurtimox in the presence of NADH generated an increase in $O_2$ consumption (compatible with redox cycling) although they did not test other concentrations, or the generation of ROS, or studied if it was possible to detect a nitro anion radical under anaerobic conditions.

In conclusion, there is evidence of one-electron reduction of nifurtimox with generation of ROS in live epimastigotes[109,175] and by enzymes present in amastigotes and trypomastigotes.[111] It is possible that two-electron reduction could also occur (in epimastigotes) but one-electron reduction of nifurtimox and subsequent redox cycling with generation of ROS in *T. cruzi* cannot be ruled out as a mechanism of toxicity against *T. cruzi* if nifurtimox accumulates to high levels in the parasite.

In contrast to nifurtimox, the direct involvement of oxygen reduction products in the trypanocidal action of benznidazole, which is a 2-nitroimidazole (Fig. 17.1), could be ruled out.[17] As the rate of reduction of benznidazole is very low because of its lower reduction potential, redox cycling is considered a detoxification reaction that occurs by inhibition of the net reduction of the drug. The resultant low steady state concentration of superoxide anion might be easily detoxified by the superoxide dismutases present in *T. cruzi*.[17,177] Reduction of benznidazole by recombinant TcNTR was reported to result in the generation of the cytotoxic metabolite glyoxal.[178] However, recent studies indicated that benznidazole treatment of epimastigotes resulted in significant decrease in redox active thiols, apparently by covalent adduct formation with reduced benznidazole, but no formation of glyoxal was detected.[179]

Reactive oxygen species are also involved in the photodynamic action of crystal violet that has been described in *T. cruzi*.[180] Visible light causes photoreduction of crystal violet to a carbon-centered radical. Under aerobic conditions this free radical autooxidizes generating superoxide anion whose dismutation yields $H_2O_2$.[180] Reducing agents known to enhance free radical formation from crystal violet in the presence of light enhance redox cycling of this dye.[181] In contrast to other photosensitizers, irradiation of crystal violet with visible light does not generate detectable amount of singlet oxygen.[181] The trypanocidal effect of crystal violet on *T. cruzi* epimastigotes and trypomastigotes is also enhanced by light.[180] The chemoprophylactic potential of the photodynamic action of crystal violet for the prevention of blood transmission of Chagas disease was also explored.[182] It was demonstrated that photoreduction with visible light in the presence of ascorbate reduces the effective dose and time of contact of the dye with *T. cruzi*-infected blood.[182] The scheme shown in Fig. 17.6 has been proposed to explain the enhancement of the cytotoxicity of crystal violet against *T. cruzi* by ascorbate.[182] In reaction A, ascorbate anion reduces crystal violet under illumination. Under aerobic conditions, the crystal violet carbon-centered free radical then reduces $O_2$ to superoxide anion (reaction B); dismutation of superoxide anion produces $H_2O_2$ (reaction C). Superoxide dismutase increases the rate of $H_2O_2$ formation by catalyzing reaction C. The oxidation of ascorbate by superoxide anion contributes to the formation of $H_2O_2$ and is responsible for the generation of the ascorbyl radical that is detected in incubations of *T. cruzi*-infected blood upon illumination.[182] When catalase is present (as occurs in red and white blood cells but not in *T. cruzi*) $H_2O_2$ is detoxified. Formation of $H_2O_2$ may explain the photodynamic action of crystal violet/ascorbate on *T. cruzi*[182] since the sensitivity of different *T. cruzi* stages to reagent $H_2O_2$, enzymatically generated $H_2O_2$, $H_2O_2$-generating drugs, and $H_2O_2$-generating phagocytic cells has been well documented.[17]

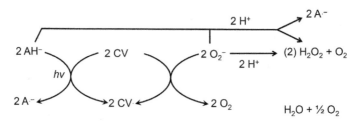

**Figure 17.6** Mechanism of ascorbate enhancement of crystal violet toxicity. Light (*hv*) catalyzes the conversion of crystal violet into a carbon-centered radical (CV) in the presence of ascorbate (AH⁻), which generates ascorbyl radical (A⁻) (reaction A). Autoxidation of the carbon-centered radical generates superoxide anion ($O_2^-$) (reaction B) that dismutates to $H_2O_2$ (reaction C) in the presence of SOD or reacts with ascorbate to generate more ascorbyl radical. $H_2O_2$ can be decomposed by catalase (CAT).

# Acidocalcisome biochemistry and osmoregulation

## The role of acidocalcisomes in T. cruzi metabolism

The acidocalcisome is an acidic organelle rich in phosphorus, calcium, and other cations.[183–186] Phosphorus is present as pyrophosphate and polyphosphate (polyP) and is complexed with calcium, and other cations. PolyP is linear polymer of phosphate linked by high-energy phosphoanhydride bonds that could have from a few to several hundreds phosphate units. The acidocalcisome membrane in *T. cruzi* contains a number of pumps ($Ca^{2+}$-ATPase, V-$H^+$-ATPase, and $H^+$-PPase), and at least a channel (aquaporin), while its matrix contains enzymes related to pyrophosphate and polyP metabolism[183–186] (Fig. 17.7). Acidocalcisomes in *T. cruzi* are also rich in basic amino acids such as arginine, ornithine, and lysine, probably also complexed with polyP.[122] Some of the functions of acidocalcisomes in *T. cruzi* are the storage of cations, phosphorus, and amino acids, pyrophosphate and polyphosphate metabolism, and osmoregulation. The finding of novel enzymes in this organelle that are absent from mammalian cells has led to the discovery of novel targets for drug action.[183–186]

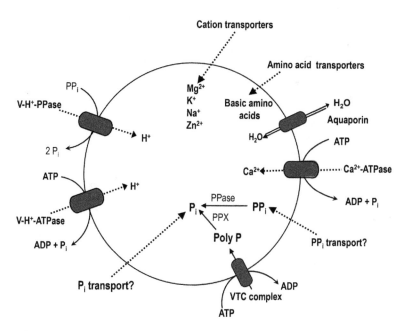

**Figure 17.7** Scheme of a *T. cruzi* acidocalcisome. The matrix contains $P_i$, $PP_i$, and polyP combined with a variety of cations ($Ca^{2+}$, $Mg^{2+}$, $K^+$, $Na^+$, and $Zn^{2+}$) and basic amino acids, and also a pyrophosphatase (PPase) and exopolyphosphatase (PPX) activities. The membrane possesses proton pumps (V-$H^+$-ATPase and V-$H^+$-PPase), a calcium pump ($Ca^{2+}$-ATPase), a water channel (aquaporin), and a polyP kinase complex (VTC complex). Other transporters for cations, $P_i$, $PP_i$, and basic amino acids are also probably present (dashed lines).

## Acidocalcisomes and osmoregulation in T. cruzi

*T. cruzi* encounters severe environmental stressors to which it must adapt as it progresses through its life cycle. One example is the parasite ability to cope with fluctuations in osmolarity that occur within the gut of the vector[187,188] and also as the parasite moves from the insect gut through the acidic phagolysosome to the cytosol of the host cell. The infective form of the parasite passes out of the vector in the highly concentrated excreta (600–700 mOsm)[187] and rapidly encounters the interstitial fluid of the mammalian host with a much lower osmolarity (330 mOsm). Evidently, the parasite has mechanisms that allow it to adapt to both hyperosmotic and hyposmotic stresses. Both the responses of the parasite to hyposmotic,[122,189–191] and hyperosmotic[192] stresses have been studied and the mechanisms involved have been reviewed elsewhere.[193] Two organelles that have fundamental roles in these adaptations are the acidocalcisomes and the contractile vacuole complex. The contractile vacuole complex was described long ago in *T. cruzi* although its function was unknown for a long time.[191] In addition to its role in osmoregulation the contractile vacuole is also a trafficking hub involved in the transport of proteins to the cell surface[48,194] and to the acidocalcisomes.[48]

Upon exposure to a reduction in external osmolarity, cells initially swell but soon regain nearly normal cell volume by a process that has been known as the Regulatory Volume Decrease (RVD; reviewed in Refs. [195,196]), which is accomplished by the efflux of various inorganic ions (such as $Na^+$ and $K^+$) and organic osmolytes to the extracellular environment. An RVD mechanism is present in amastigotes, epimastigotes, and trypomastigotes of *T. cruzi*[122] and is due to the release of amino acids, $K^+$ and water.[191] This process is rapid and essentially complete in all *T. cruzi* stages by 5 min. Uncharged or acidic amino acids are mobilized during hyposmotic stress in all three stages and are probably released through an anion channel with properties similar to those previously described in other cells.[195,196]

Cell swelling causes a spike in intracellular cyclic AMP through activation of an adenyl cyclase, and results in a microtubule-dependent fusion of acidocalcisomes with the CV.[190] A simultaneous rise in ammonia, and its sequestration in acidocalcisomes as $NH_4^+$,[197] increases their pH and probably activates an acidocalcisomal exopolyphosphatase, which cleaves polyP, releasing inorganic phosphate residues and also the various polyP-chelated osmolytes, such as basic amino acids and calcium.[191] The resulting osmotic gradient sequesters water through the aid of an aquaporin, which is subsequently ejected into the flagellar pocket.[191] This pathway would terminate by hydrolysis of cyclic AMP by a phosphodiesterase C,[198] and this phosphodiesterase C[199] could be a potential target against *T. cruzi*.

## Acidocalcisomes as drug targets

A vacuolar proton translocating pyrophosphatase (V-H$^+$-PPase) is involved in the acidification of the organelle in *T. cruzi*.[200] The enzyme uses pyrophosphate instead of ATP as an energy source, is $K^+$-stimulated (type I), and can be used as a marker for acidocalcisome purification.[200] The gene encoding this pump has been functionally expressed in yeast.[201] This enzyme is also found in the Golgi complex and in the plasma membrane of *T. cruzi*,[202] but is absent in mammalian cells.

Pyrophosphate analogues, bisphosphonates (containing a nonhydrolyzable P-C-P, rather than a P-O-P, backbone) as well as imidodiphosphate (containing a nonhydrolyzable P-N-P group), are inhibitors of the plant (mung bean, *Vigna radiata*) V-$H^+$-PPase.[203] Imidodiphosphate and aminomethylenediphosphonate (AMDP), one of the best known inhibitors of the V-$H^+$-PPase, inhibits the *T. cruzi* enzyme.[200]

Acidocalcisomes possess another enzyme that is absent in mammalian cells: a polyP kinase, also known as vacuolar transporter chaperone (VTC) complex.[204,205] This complex is formed in yeast by four subunits: Vtc1−4, with Vtc4 the catalytic subunit.[206] *T. cruzi* has genes homologous to those encoding Vtc1 and Vtc4 (204) and TcVtc4 is its catalytic subunit.[207]

Acidocalcisomes are also known to accumulate drugs. Ormerod observed that these organelles, known at that time as volutin granules, become more visible under light microscopy when cells are treated with drugs.[208] Further work showed that drugs like stilbamidine, quinapyramine, suramin, hydroxystilbamidine, and acriflavine accumulated in these organelles.[209,210] For this reason they were also named as "chemotherapy granules."[211] Interestingly, some of these drugs are first concentrated in the kinetoplast and nucleus, then diffuse to the cytosol, and finally concentrate in acidocalcisomes. Such is also the case of diamidines like DB75 (furamidine) and DB820, which have been in phase III clinical trials against human African trypanosomiasis.[212,213] However, the impact that acidocalcisome accumulation has on the mechanism of action of these compounds is not known.

# Conclusion

Studies on metabolic pathways in *T. cruzi* have in some cases revealed the reason for their susceptibility to drugs effective in vivo against this parasite. That is for example the case for nifurtimox and benznidazole (Fig. 17.1), the drugs currently used in the treatment of Chagas disease. These studies have also helped to understand the effect of antifungal azoles, which have been tested in clinical trials against Chagas disease. In other cases, studies on the metabolism of *T. cruzi* have shed light on potential targets for drug action (such as the acidocalcisomes) or have helped in the identification of compounds (such as bisphosphonates and prenyl transferase inhibitors) that could be of potential use against this disease. We should expect that the use of some of these compounds could result in an adequate treatment for the acute and chronic forms of Chagas disease. The advantage of some of these compounds is that many of them are under development for other uses by pharmaceutical companies and some are already FDA-approved.

The usefulness of specific anti-*T. cruzi* treatment of acute and chronic Chagasic patients suggests that treatment is always beneficial. Even if the situation exists that cardiopathy or megas are not prevented in all those treated, eradication of parasitemia will prevent transmission by blood transfusion and, in female children, congenital transmission years later.

## Acknowledgments

Work in our laboratory was supported by a grant from the U.S. National Institutes of Health (AI-107663).

## References

1. El-Sayed NM, Myler PJ, Bartholomeu DC, Nilsson D, Aggarwal G, Tran AN, et al. The genome sequence of *Trypanosoma cruzi*, etiologic agent of Chagas disease. *Science* 2005;**309**:409−15.
2. Atwood III JA, Weatherly DB, Minning TA, Bundy B, Cavola C, Opperdoes FR, et al. The *Trypanosoma cruzi* proteome. *Science* 2005;**309**:473−6.
3. Cordero EM, Nakayasu ES, Gentil LG, Yoshida N, Almeida IC, da Silveira JF. Proteomic analysis of detergent-solubilized membrane proteins from insect-developmental forms of *Trypanosoma cruzi*. *J Proteome Res* 2009;**8**:3642−52.
4. Nakayasu ES, Gaynor MR, Sobreira TJ, Ross JA, Almeida IC. Phosphoproteomic analysis of the human pathogen *Trypanosoma cruzi* at the epimastigote stage. *Proteomics* 2009;**9**:3489−506.
5. Sant'Anna C, Nakayasu ES, Pereira MG, Lourenco D, de Souza W, Almeida IC, et al. Subcellular proteomics of *Trypanosoma cruzi* reservosomes. *Proteomics* 2009;**9**: 1782−94.
6. Nakayasu ES, Yashunsky DV, Nohara LL, Torrecilhas AC, Nikolaev AV, Almeida IC. GPIomics: global analysis of glycosylphosphatidylinositol-anchored molecules of *Trypanosoma cruzi*. *Mol Syst Biol* 2009;**5**:261.
7. Ferella M, Nilsson D, Darban H, Rodrigues C, Bontempi EJ, Docampo R, et al. Proteomics in *Trypanosoma cruzi*—localization of novel proteins to various organelles. *Proteomics* 2008;**8**:2735−49.
8. Brunoro GV, Caminha MA, Ferreira AT, Leprevost Fda V, Carvalho PC, Perales J, et al. Reevaluating the *Trypanosoma cruzi* proteomic map: the shotgun description of bloodstream trypomastigotes. *J Proteomics* 2015;**115**:58−65.
9. Queiroz RM, Charneau S, Mandacaru SC, Schwammle V, Lima BD, Roepstorff P, et al. Quantitative proteomic and phosphoproteomic analysis of *Trypanosoma cruzi* amastigogenesis. *Mol Cell Proteomics* 2014;**13**:3457−72.
10. de Godoy LM, Marchini FK, Pavoni DP, Rampazzo Rde C, Probst CM, Goldenberg S, et al. Quantitative proteomics of *Trypanosoma cruzi* during metacyclogenesis. *Proteomics* 2012;**12**:2694−703.
11. Nakayasu ES, Sobreira TJ, Torres Jr. R, Ganiko L, Oliveira PS, Marques AF, et al. Improved proteomic approach for the discovery of potential vaccine targets in *Trypanosoma cruzi*. *J Proteome Res* 2012;**11**:237−46.

12. Ulrich PN, Jimenez V, Park M, Martins VP, Atwood 3rd J, Moles K, et al. Identification of contractile vacuole proteins in *Trypanosoma cruzi*. *PLoS ONE* 2011;**6**:e18013.

13. Bayer-Santos E, Aguilar-Bonavides C, Rodrigues SP, Cordero EM, Marques AF, Varela-Ramirez A, et al. Proteomic analysis of *Trypanosoma cruzi* secretome: characterization of two populations of extracellular vesicles and soluble proteins. *J Proteome Res* 2013;**12**:883−97.

14. Brener Z. Present status of chemotherapy and chemoprophylaxis of human trypanosomiasis in the Western Hemisphere. *Pharmacol Ther* 1979;**7**:71−90.

15. Docampo R, Moreno SN. Free radical metabolites in the mode of action of chemotherapeutic agents and phagocytic cells on *Trypanosoma cruzi*. *Rev Infect Dis* 1984;**6**: 223−38.

16. Marr JJ, Docampo R. Chemotherapy for Chagas' disease: a perspective of current therapy and considerations for future research. *Rev Infect Dis* 1986;**8**:884−903.

17. Docampo R. Sensitivity of parasites to free radical damage by antiparasitic drugs. *Chem Biol Interact* 1990;**73**:1−27.

18. Docampo R, Schmunis GA. Sterol biosynthesis inhibitors: potential chemotherapeutics against Chagas disease. *Parasitol Today* 1997;**13**:129−30.

19. Urbina JA, Docampo R. Specific chemotherapy of Chagas disease: controversies and advances. *Trends Parasitol* 2003;**19**:495−501.

20. Urbina JA. Ergosterol biosynthesis and drug development for Chagas disease. *Mem Inst Oswaldo Cruz RJ* 2009;**104**:311−18.

21. Urbina JA. Recent clinical trials for the etiological treatment of chronic chagas disease: advances, challenges and perspectives. *J Eukaryot Microbiol* 2015;**62**:149−56.

22. Cerisola JA. Serologic findings in patients with acute Chagas' disease treated with Bay 2502. *Bol Chil Parasitol* 1969;**24**:54−9.

23. Cerisola JA, Alvarez M, Lugones H, Rebosolan JB. Sensitivity of serological tests in the diagnosis of Chagas' disease. *Bol Chil Parasitol* 1969;**24**:2−8.

24. Schmunis GA, Szarfman A, Coarasa L, Guilleron C, Peralta JM. Anti-*Trypanosoma cruzi* agglutinins in acute human Chagas' disease. *Am J Trop Med Hyg* 1980;**29**: 170−8.

25. Cançado JR, Brener Z. Treatment of Chagas disease. In: Brener Z, Andrade Z, editors. *Trypanosoma cruzi e Doença de Chagas*. Rio de Janeiro: Guanabara Koogan; 1979. p. 362−424.

26. Viotti R, Vigliano C, Armenti H, Segura E. Treatment of chronic Chagas' disease with benznidazole: clinical and serologic evolution of patients with long-term follow-up. *Am Heart J* 1994;**127**:151−62.

27. Viotti R, Vigliano C, Alvarez MG, Lococo B, Petti M, Bertocchi G, et al. Impact of aetiological treatment on conventional and multiplex serology in chronic Chagas disease. *PLoS NTD* 2011;**5**:e1314.

28. de Andrade AL, Zicker F, de Oliveira RM, Almeida Silva S, Luquetti A, Travassos LR, et al. Randomised trial of efficacy of benznidazole in treatment of early *Trypanosoma cruzi* infection. *Lancet* 1996;**348**:1407−13.

29. Viotti R, Vigliano C, Lococo B, Bertocchi G, Petti M, Alvarez MG, et al. Long-term cardiac outcomes of treating chronic Chagas disease with benznidazole versus no treatment: a nonrandomized trial. *Ann Intern Med* 2006;**144**:724−34.

30. Andrade SG, Freitas LA, Peyrol S, Pimentel AR, Sadigursky M. Experimental chemotherapy of *Trypanosoma cruzi* infection: persistence of parasite antigens and positive serology in parasitologically cured mice. *Bull World Health Org* 1991;**69**: 191−7.

31. Tarleton RL, Zhang L, Downs MO. "Autoimmune rejection" of neonatal heart transplants in experimental Chagas disease is a parasite-specific response to infected host tissue. *Proc Natl Acad Sci USA* 1997;**94**:3932−7.

32. Tarleton RL, Zhang L. Chagas disease etiology: autoimmunity or parasite persistence? *Parasitol Today* 1999;**15**:94−9.

33. Docampo R, Moreno SN. Biochemical toxicology of antiparasitic drugs used in the chemotherapy and chemoprophylaxis of American trypanosomiasis (Chagas' disease). *Rev Biochem Toxicol* 1985;**7**:159−204.

34. Docampo R, Moreno SN. Bisphosphonates as chemotherapeutic agents against trypanosomatid and apicomplexan parasites. *Curr Drug Targets Infect Disord* 2001;**1**: 51−61.

35. Gelb MH, Van Voorhis WC, Buckner FS, Yokoyama K, Eastman R, Carpenter EP, et al. Protein farnesyl and *N*-myristoyl transferases: piggy-back medicinal chemistry targets for the development of antitrypanosomatid and antimalarial therapeutics. *Mol Biochem Parasitol* 2003;**126**:155−63.

36. Eberl M, Hintz M, Reichenberg A, Kollas AK, Wiesner J, Jomaa H. Microbial isoprenoid biosynthesis and human gammadelta T cell activation. *FEBS Lett* 2003;**544**:4−10.

37. Banthorpe DV, Charlwood BV, Francis MJ. The biosynthesis of monoterpenes. *Sogo Kango* 1972;**72**:115−55.

38. Montalvetti A, Bailey BN, Martin MB, Severin GW, Oldfield E, Docampo R. Bisphosphonates are potent inhibitors of *Trypanosoma cruzi* farnesyl pyrophosphate synthase. *J Biol Chem* 2001;**276**:33930−7.

39. Ferella M, Montalvetti A, Rohloff P, Miranda K, Fang J, Reina S, et al. A solanesyl-diphosphate synthase localizes in glycosomes of *Trypanosoma cruzi*. *J Biol Chem* 2006;**281**:39339−48.

40. Ferella M, Li ZH, Andersson B, Docampo R. Farnesyl diphosphate synthase localizes to the cytoplasm of *Trypanosoma cruzi* and *T. brucei*. *Exp Parasitol* 2008;**119**:308−12.

41. Parsons M. Glycosomes: parasites and the divergence of peroxisomal purpose. *Mol Microbiol* 2004;**53**:717−24.

42. Docampo R, Moreno SN, Turrens JF, Katzin AM, Gonzalez-Cappa SM, Stoppani AO. Biochemical and ultrastructural alterations produced by miconazole and econazole in *Trypanosoma cruzi*. *Mol Biochem Parasitol* 1981;**3**:169−80.

43. Parodi AJ, Quesada-Allue LA. Protein glycosylation in *Trypanosoma cruzi*. I. Characterization of dolichol-bound monosaccharides and oligosaccharides synthesized "in vivo." *J Biol Chem* 1982;**257**:7637−40.

44. Docampo R, de Boiso JF, Stoppani AO. Tricarboxylic acid cycle operation at the kinetoplast-mitochondrion complex of *Trypanosoma cruzi*. *Biochim Biophys Acta* 1978; **502**:466−76.

45. Cuevas IC, Rohloff P, Sanchez DO, Docampo R. Characterization of farnesylated protein tyrosine phosphatase TcPRL-1 from *Trypanosoma cruzi*. *Eukaryot Cell* 2005;**4**: 1550−61.

46. Nepomuceno-Silva JL, Yokoyama K, de Mello LD, Mendonca SM, Paixao JC, Baron R, et al. TcRho1, a farnesylated Rho family homologue from *Trypanosoma cruzi:* cloning, trans-splicing, and prenylation studies. *J Biol Chem* 2001;**276**:29711−18.

47. Yokoyama K, Trobridge P, Buckner FS, Scholten J, Stuart KD, Van Voorhis WC, et al. The effects of protein farnesyltransferase inhibitors on trypanosomatids: inhibition of protein farnesylation and cell growth. *Mol Biochem Parasitol* 1998;**94**:87−97.

48. Niyogi S, Docampo R. A novel role of Rab11 in trafficking GPI-anchored trans-sialidase to the plasma membrane of *Trypanosoma cruzi*. *Small GTPases* 2015;**6**:8−10.

49. Blanchard L, Karst F. Characterization of a lysine-to-glutamic acid mutation in a conservative sequence of farnesyl diphosphate synthase from *Saccharomyces cerevisiae*. *Gene* 1993;**125**:185−9.

50. Song L, Poulter CD. Yeast farnesyl-diphosphate synthase: site-directed mutagenesis of residues in highly conserved prenyltransferase domains I and II. *Proc Natl Acad Sci USA* 1994;**91**(8):3044−8.

51. Gabelli SB, McLellan JS, Montalvetti A, Oldfield E, Docampo R, Amzel LM. Structure and mechanism of the farnesyl diphosphate synthase from *Trypanosoma cruzi*: implications for drug design. *Proteins* 2006;**62**:80−8.

52. Huang CH, Gabelli SB, Oldfield E, Amzel LM. Binding of nitrogen-containing bisphosphonates (N-BPs) to the *Trypanosoma cruzi* farnesyl diphosphate synthase homodimer. *Proteins* 2010;**78**:888−99.

53. Aripirala S, Szajnman SH, Jakoncic J, Rodriguez JB, Docampo R, Gabelli SB, et al. Design, synthesis, calorimetry, and crystallographic analysis of 2-alkylaminoethyl-1,1-bisphosphonates as inhibitors of *Trypanosoma cruzi* farnesyl diphosphate synthase. *J Med Chem* 2012;**55**(14):6445−54.

54. Rodan GA. Mechanisms of action of bisphosphonates. *Annu Rev Pharmacol Toxicol* 1998;**38**:375−88.

55. Martin MB, Grimley JS, Lewis JC, Heath 3rd HT, Bailey BN, Kendrick H, et al. Bisphosphonates inhibit the growth of *Trypanosoma brucei*, *Trypanosoma cruzi*, *Leishmania donovani*, *Toxoplasma gondii*, and *Plasmodium falciparum*: a potential route to chemotherapy. *J Med Chem* 2001;**44**:909−16.

56. Urbina JA, Moreno B, Vierkotter S, Oldfield E, Payares G, Sanoja C, et al. *Trypanosoma cruzi* contains major pyrophosphate stores, and its growth in vitro and in vivo is blocked by pyrophosphate analogs. *J Biol Chem* 1999;**274**:33609−15.

57. Garzoni LR, Caldera A, Meirelles Mde N, de Castro SL, Docampo R, Meints GA, et al. Selective in vitro effects of the farnesyl pyrophosphate synthase inhibitor risedronate on *Trypanosoma cruzi*. *Int J Antimicrob Agents* 2004;**23**:273−85.

58. Garzoni LR, Waghabi MC, Baptista MM, de Castro SL, Meirelles Mde N, Britto CC, et al. Antiparasitic activity of risedronate in a murine model of acute Chagas' disease. *Int J Antimicrob Agents* 2004;**23**:286−90.

59. Bouzahzah B, Jelicks LA, Morris SA, Weiss LM, Tanowitz HB. Risedronate in the treatment of Murine Chagas' disease. *Parasitol Res* 2005;**96**:184−7.

60. Turunen M, Olsson J, Dallner G. Metabolism and function of coenzyme Q. *Biochim Biophys Acta* 2004;**1660**:171−99.

61. Ohnuma S, Koyama T, Ogura K. Purification of solanesyl-diphosphate synthase from *Micrococcus luteus*. A new class of prenyltransferase. *J Biol Chem* 1991;**266**:23706−13.

62. Kawamukai M. Biosynthesis, bioproduction and novel roles of ubiquinone. *J Biosci Bioeng* 2002;**94**:511−17.

63. Ashby MN, Kutsunai SY, Ackerman S, Tzagoloff A, Edwards PA. COQ2 is a candidate for the structural gene encoding para-hydroxybenzoate:polyprenyltransferase. *J Biol Chem* 1992;**267**:4128−36.

64. Forsgren M, Attersand A, Lake S, Grunler J, Swiezewska E, Dallner G, et al. Isolation and functional expression of human COQ2, a gene encoding a polyprenyl transferase involved in the synthesis of CoQ. *Biochem J* 2004;**382**:519−26.

65. Szajnman SH, Garcia Linares GE, Li ZH, Jiang C, Galizzi M, Bontempi EJ, et al. Synthesis and biological evaluation of 2-alkylaminoethyl-1,1-bisphosphonic acids against *Trypanosoma cruzi* and *Toxoplasma gondii* targeting farnesyl diphosphate synthase. *Bioorg Med Chem* 2008;**16**:3283−90.

66. Glomset JA, Gelb MH, Farnsworth CC. Prenyl proteins in eukaryotic cells: a new type of membrane anchor. *Trends Biochem Sci* 1990;**15**:139—42.
67. Glomset JA, Farnsworth CC. Role of protein modification reactions in programming interactions between ras-related GTPases and cell membranes. *Annu Rev Cell Biol* 1994; **10**:181—205.
68. Yokoyama K, Goodwin GW, Ghomashchi F, Glomset J, Gelb MH. Protein prenyltransferases. *Biochem Soc Trans* 1992;**20**:489—94.
69. Casey PJ, Seabra MC. Protein prenyltransferases. *J Biol Chem* 1996;**271**:5289—92.
70. Leonard DM. Ras farnesyltransferase: a new therapeutic target. *J Med Chem* 1997;**40**: 2971—90.
71. Sealey-Cardona M, Cammerer S, Jones S, Ruiz-Perez LM, Brun R, Gilbert IH, et al. Kinetic characterization of squalene synthase from *Trypanosoma cruzi*: selective inhibition by quinuclidine derivatives. *Antimicrob Agents Chemother* 2007;**51**:2123—9.
72. Veiga-Santos P, Li K, Lameira L, de Carvalho TM, Huang G, Galizzi M, et al. SQ109, a new drug lead for Chagas disease. *Antimicrob Agents Chemother* 2015;**59**:1950—61.
73. Chao MN, Matiuzzi CE, Storey M, Li C, Szajnman SH, Docampo R, et al. Aryloxyethyl thiocyanates are potent growth inhibitors of *Trypanosoma cruzi* and *Toxoplasma gondii*. *ChemMedChem* 2015;**10**:1094—108.
74. Shang N, Li Q, Ko TP, Chan HC, Li J, Zheng Y, et al. Squalene synthase as a target for Chagas disease therapeutics. *PLoS Pathog* 2014;**10**:e1004114.
75. Buckner FS, Griffin JH, Wilson AJ, Van Voorhis WC. Potent anti-*Trypanosoma cruzi* activities of oxidosqualene cyclase inhibitors. *Antimicrob Agents Chemother* 2001;**45**:1210—15.
76. Benaim G, Sanders JM, Garcia-Marchan Y, Colina C, Lira R, Caldera AR, et al. Amiodarone has intrinsic anti-*Trypanosoma cruzi* activity and acts synergistically with posaconazole. *J Med Chem* 2006;**49**:892—9.
77. Lepesheva GI, Zaitseva NG, Nes WD, Zhou W, Arase M, Liu J, et al. CYP51 from *Trypanosoma cruzi*: a phyla-specific residue in the B' helix defines substrate preferences of sterol 14alpha-demethylase. *J Biol Chem* 2006;**281**:3577—85.
78. Chen CK, Leung SS, Guilbert C, Jacobson MP, McKerrow JH, Podust LM. Structural characterization of CYP51 from *Trypanosoma cruzi* and *Trypanosoma brucei* bound to the antifungal drugs posaconazole and fluconazole. *PLoS NTD* 2010;**4**:e651.
79. Lepesheva GI, Hargrove TY, Anderson S, Kleshchenko Y, Furtak V, Wawrzak Z, et al. Structural insights into inhibition of sterol 14alpha-demethylase in the human pathogen *Trypanosoma cruzi*. *J Biol Chem* 2010;**285**:25582—90.
80. Hargrove TY, Wawrzak Z, Alexander PW, Chaplin JH, Keenan M, Charman SA, et al. Complexes of *Trypanosoma cruzi* sterol 14alpha-demethylase (CYP51) with two pyridine-based drug candidates for Chagas disease: structural basis for pathogen selectivity. *J Biol Chem* 2013;**288**:31602—15.
81. McCabe RE, Remington JS, Araujo FG. Ketoconazole inhibition of intracellular multiplication of *Trypanosoma cruzi* and protection of mice against lethal infection with the organism. *J Infect Dis* 1984;**150**:594—601.
82. Raether W, Seidenath H. Ketoconazole and other potent antimycotic azoles exhibit pronounced activity against *Trypanosoma cruzi, Plasmodium berghei* and *Entamoeba histolytica* in vivo. *Z Parasitenkd* 1984;**70**:135—8.
83. Goad LJ, Berens RL, Marr JJ, Beach DH, Holz Jr. GG. The activity of ketoconazole and other azoles against *Trypanosoma cruzi*: biochemistry and chemotherapeutic action in vitro. *Mol Biochem Parasitol* 1989;**32**:179—89.
84. Beach DH, Goad LJ, Holz Jr. GG. Effects of ketoconazole on sterol biosynthesis by *Trypanosoma cruzi* epimastigotes. *Biochem Biophys Res Commun* 1986;**136**:851—6.

85. McCabe RE, Remington JS, Araujo FG. In vitro and in vivo effects of itraconazole against *Trypanosoma cruzi. Am J Trop Med Hyg* 1986;**35**:280—4.

86. Urbina JA, Vivas J, Lazardi K, Molina J, Payares G, Piras MM, et al. Antiproliferative effects of delta 24(25) sterol methyl transferase inhibitors on *Trypanosoma (Schizotrypanum) cruzi*: in vitro and in vivo studies. *Chemotherapy* 1996;**42**:294—307.

87. Docampo R, Moreno SN. Free radical metabolism of antiparasitic agents. *Fed Proc* 1986;**45**:2471—6.

88. Boveris A, Sies H, Martino EE, Docampo R, Turrens JF, Stoppani AO. Deficient metabolic utilization of hydrogen peroxide in *Trypanosoma cruzi. Biochem J* 1980;**188**: 643—8.

89. Docampo R, De Souza W, Cruz FS, Roitman I, Cover B, Gutteridge WE. Ultrastructural alterations and peroxide formation induced by naphthoquinones in different stages of *Trypanosoma cruzi. Z Parasitenkd* 1978;**57**:189—98.

90. Docampo R, Cruz FS, Boveris A, Muniz RP, Esquivel DM. Lipid peroxidation and the generation of free radicals, superoxide anion, and hydrogen peroxide in beta-lapachone-treated *Trypanosoma cruzi* epimastigotes. *Arch Biochem Biophys* 1978;**186**: 292—7.

91. Krauth-Siegel RL, Comini MA. Redox control in trypanosomatids, parasitic protozoa with trypanothione-based thiol metabolism. *Biochim Biophys Acta* 2008;**1780**: 1236—48.

92. Irigoin F, Cibils L, Comini MA, Wilkinson SR, Flohe L, Radi R. Insights into the redox biology of *Trypanosoma cruzi*: trypanothione metabolism and oxidant detoxification. *Free Radic Biol Med* 2008;**45**:733—42.

93. Docampo R, de Boiso JF, Boveris A, Stoppani AO. Localization of peroxidase activity in *Trypanosoma cruzi* microbodies. *Experientia* 1976;**32**:972—5.

94. Wilkinson SR, Obado SO, Mauricio IL, Kelly JM. *Trypanosoma cruzi* expresses a plant-like ascorbate-dependent hemoperoxidase localized to the endoplasmic reticulum. *Proc Natl Acad Sci USA* 2002;**99**:13453—8.

95. Boveris A, Stoppani AO. Hydrogen peroxide metabolism in *Trypanosoma cruzi. Medicina (B Aires)* 1978;**38**:259—65.

96. Piacenza L, Zago MP, Peluffo G, Alvarez MN, Basombrio MA, Radi R. Enzymes of the antioxidant network as novel determiners of *Trypanosoma cruzi* virulence. *Int J Parasitol* 2009;**39**:1455—64.

97. Taylor MC, Lewis MD, Fortes Francisco A, Wilkinson SR, Kelly JM. The *Trypanosoma cruzi* vitamin C dependent peroxidase confers protection against oxidative stress but is not a determinant of virulence. *PLoS NTD* 2015;**9**:e0003707.

98. Nogueira FB, Rodrigues JF, Correa MM, Ruiz JC, Romanha AJ, Murta SM. The level of ascorbate peroxidase is enhanced in benznidazole-resistant populations of *Trypanosoma cruzi* and its expression is modulated by stress generated by hydrogen peroxide. *Mem Inst Oswaldo Cruz* 2012;**107**:494—502.

99. Wilkinson SR, Temperton NJ, Mondragon A, Kelly JM. Distinct mitochondrial and cytosolic enzymes mediate trypanothione-dependent peroxide metabolism in *Trypanosoma cruzi. J Biol Chem* 2000;**275**:8220—5.

100. Turrens JF. Possible role of the NADH-fumarate reductase in superoxide anion and hydrogen peroxide production in *Trypanosoma brucei. Mol Biochem Parasitol* 1987; **25**:55—60.

101. Docampo R, Lopes JN, Cruz FS, Souza W. *Trypanosoma cruzi*: ultrastructural and metabolic alterations of epimastigotes by beta-lapachone. *Exp Parasitol* 1977;**42**:142—9.

102. Boveris A, Docampo R, Turrens JF, Stoppani AO. Effect of beta and alpha-lapachone on the production of $H_2O_2$ and on the growth of *Trypanosoma cruzi*. *Rev Asoc Argent Microbiol* 1977;**9**:54—61.

103. Lopes JN, Cruz FS, Docampo R, Vasconcellos ME, Sampaio MC, Pinto AV, et al. In vitro and in vivo evaluation of the toxicity of 1,4-naphthoquinone and 1,2-naphthoquinone derivatives against *Trypanosoma cruzi*. *Ann Trop Med Parasitol* 1978;**72**:523—31.

104. Boveris A, Docampo R, Turrens JF, Stoppani AO. Effect of beta-lapachone on superoxide anion and hydrogen peroxide production in *Trypanosoma cruzi*. *Biochem J* 1978;**175**:431—9.

105. Cruz FS, Docampo R, Boveris A. Generation of superoxide anions and hydrogen peroxide from beta-lapachone in bacteria. *Antimicrob Agents Chemother* 1978;**14**:630—3.

106. Cruz FS, Docampo R, de Souza W. Effect of beta-lapachone on hydrogen peroxide production in *Trypanosoma cruzi*. *Acta Trop* 1978;**35**:35—40.

107. Boveris A, Stoppani AO, Docampo R, Cruz FS. Superoxide anion production and trypanocidal action of naphthoquinones on *Trypanosoma cruzi*. *Comp Biochem Physiol C* 1978;**61C**:327—9.

108. Goncalves AM, Vasconcellos ME, Docampo R, Cruz FS, de Souza W, Leon W. Evaluation of the toxicity of 3-allyl-beta-lapachone against *Trypanosoma cruzi* bloodstream forms. *Mol Biochem Parasitol* 1980;**1**:167—76.

109. Docampo R, Stoppani AO. Generation of superoxide anion and hydrogen peroxide induced by nifurtimox in *Trypanosoma cruzi*. *Arch Biochem Biophys* 1979;**197**:317—21.

110. Docampo R, Stoppani AO. Mechanism of the trypanocidal action of nifurtimox and other nitro-derivatives on *Trypanosoma cruzi*. *Medicina (B Aires)* 1980;**40**:10—16.

111. Docampo R, Moreno SN, Stoppani AO, Leon W, Cruz FS, Villalta F, et al. Mechanism of nifurtimox toxicity in different forms of *Trypanosoma cruzi*. *Biochem Pharmacol* 1981;**30**:1947—51.

112. Faundez M, Pino L, Letelier P, Ortiz C, Lopez R, Seguel C, et al. Buthionine sulfoximine increases the toxicity of nifurtimox and benznidazole to *Trypanosoma cruzi*. *Antimicrob Agents Chemother* 2005;**49**:126—30.

113. Algranati ID. Polyamine metabolism in *Trypanosoma cruzi*: studies on the expression and regulation of heterologous genes involved in polyamine biosynthesis. *Amino Acids* 2010;**38**:645—51.

114. Le Quesne SA, Fairlamb AH. Regulation of a high-affinity diamine transport system in *Trypanosoma cruzi* epimastigotes. *Biochem J* 1996;**316**:481—6.

115. Carrillo C, Canepa GE, Algranati ID, Pereira CA. Molecular and functional characterization of a spermidine transporter (TcPAT12) from *Trypanosoma cruzi*. *Biochem Biophys Res Commun* 2006;**344**:936—40.

116. Oza SL, Tetaud E, Ariyanayagam MR, Warnon SS, Fairlamb AH. A single enzyme catalyses formation of trypanothione from glutathione and spermidine in *Trypanosoma cruzi*. *J Biol Chem* 2002;**277**(39):35853—61.

117. Jockers-Scherubl MC, Schirmer RH, Krauth-Siegel RL. Trypanothione reductase from *Trypanosoma cruzi*. Catalytic properties of the enzyme and inhibition studies with trypanocidal compounds. *Eur J Biochem* 1989;**180**:267—72.

118. Oza SL, Ariyanayagam MR, Fairlamb AH. Characterization of recombinant glutathionylspermidine synthetase/amidase from *Crithidia fasciculata*. *Biochem J* 2002;**364**:679—86.

119. Torrie LS, Wyllie S, Spinks D, Oza SL, Thompson S, Harrison JR, et al. Chemical validation of trypanothione synthetase: a potential drug target for human trypanosomiasis. *J Biol Chem* 2009;**284**:36137−45.

120. Ariyanayagam MR, Fairlamb AH. Ovothiol and trypanothione as antioxidants in trypanosomatids. *Mol Biochem Parasitol* 2001;**115**:189−98.

121. Ariyanayagam MR, Oza SL, Mehlert A, Fairlamb AH. Bis(glutathionyl)spermine and other novel trypanothione analogues in *Trypanosoma cruzi*. *J Biol Chem* 2003;**278**:27612−19.

122. Rohloff P, Rodrigues CO, Docampo R. Regulatory volume decrease in *Trypanosoma cruzi* involves amino acid efflux and changes in intracellular calcium. *Mol Biochem Parasitol* 2003;**126**:219−30.

123. Krauth-Siegel RL, Enders B, Henderson GB, Fairlamb AH, Schirmer RH. Trypanothione reductase from *Trypanosoma cruzi*. Purification and characterization of the crystalline enzyme. *Eur J Biochem* 1987;**164**:123−8.

124. Borges A, Cunningham ML, Tovar J, Fairlamb AH. Site-directed mutagenesis of the redox-active cysteines of *Trypanosoma cruzi* trypanothione reductase. *Eur J Biochem* 1995;**228**:745−52.

125. Zhang Y, Bond CS, Bailey S, Cunningham ML, Fairlamb AH, Hunter WN. The crystal structure of trypanothione reductase from the human pathogen *Trypanosoma cruzi* at 2. 3 A resolution. *Protein Sci* 1996;**5**:52−61.

126. Bond CS, Zhang Y, Berriman M, Cunningham ML, Fairlamb AH, Hunter WN. Crystal structure of *Trypanosoma cruzi* trypanothione reductase in complex with trypanothione, and the structure-based discovery of new natural product inhibitors. *Structure* 1999;**7**:81−9.

127. Krauth-Siegel RL, Sticherling C, Jost I, Walsh CT, Pai EF, Kabsch W, et al. Crystallization and preliminary crystallographic analysis of trypanothione reductase from *Trypanosoma cruzi*, the causative agent of Chagas' disease. *FEBS Lett* 1993;**317**: 105−8.

128. Lantwin CB, Schlichting I, Kabsch W, Pai EF, Krauth-Siegel RL. The structure of *Trypanosoma cruzi* trypanothione reductase in the oxidized and NADPH reduced state. *Proteins* 1994;**18**:161−73.

129. Jacoby EM, Schlichting I, Lantwin CB, Kabsch W, Krauth-Siegel RL. Crystal structure of the *Trypanosoma cruzi* trypanothione reductase.mepacrine complex. *Proteins* 1996; **24**:73−80.

130. Saravanamuthu A, Vickers TJ, Bond CS, Peterson MR, Hunter WN, Fairlamb AH. Two interacting binding sites for quinacrine derivatives in the active site of trypanothione reductase: a template for drug design. *J Biol Chem* 2004;**279**:29493−500.

131. Aguirre G, Cabrera E, Cerecetto H, Di Maio R, Gonzalez M, Seoane G, et al. Design, synthesis and biological evaluation of new potent 5-nitrofuryl derivatives as anti-*Trypanosoma cruzi* agents. Studies of trypanothione binding site of trypanothione reductase as target for rational design. *Eur J Med Chem* 2004;**39**:421−31.

132. Benson TJ, McKie JH, Garforth J, Borges A, Fairlamb AH, Douglas KT. Rationally designed selective inhibitors of trypanothione reductase. Phenothiazines and related tricyclics as lead structures. *Biochem J* 1992;**286**:9−11.

133. Chan C, Yin H, Garforth J, McKie JH, Jaouhari R, Speers P, et al. Phenothiazine inhibitors of trypanothione reductase as potential antitrypanosomal and antileishmanial drugs. *J Med Chem* 1998;**41**:148−56.

134. Khan MO, Austin SE, Chan C, Yin H, Marks D, Vaghjiani SN, et al. Use of an additional hydrophobic binding site, the Z site, in the rational drug design of a new class of stronger trypanothione reductase inhibitor, quaternary alkylammonium phenothiazines. *J Med Chem* 2000;**43**:3148−56.

135. Gutierrez-Correa J, Fairlamb AH, Stoppani AO. *Trypanosoma cruzi* trypanothione reductase is inactivated by peroxidase-generated phenothiazine cationic radicals. *Free Radic Res* 2001;**34**:363−78.

136. Moreno SN, Carnieri EG, Docampo R. Inhibition of *Trypanosoma cruzi* trypanothione reductase by crystal violet. *Mol Biochem Parasitol* 1994;**67**:313−20.

137. Baillet S, Buisine E, Horvath D, Maes L, Bonnet B, Sergheraert C. 2-Amino diphenylsulfides as inhibitors of trypanothione reductase: modification of the side chain. *Bioorg Med Chem* 1996;**4**:891−9.

138. O'Sullivan MC, Dalrymple DM, Zhou Q. Inhibiting effects of spermidine derivatives on *Trypanosoma cruzi* trypanothione reductase. *J Enzyme Inhib* 1996;**11**:97−114.

139. Bonnet B, Soullez D, Davioud-Charvet E, Landry V, Horvath D, Sergheraert C. New spermine and spermidine derivatives as potent inhibitors of *Trypanosoma cruzi* trypanothione reductase. *Bioorg Med Chem* 1997;**5**:1249−56.

140. O'Sullivan MC, Zhou Q, Li Z, Durham TB, Rattendi D, Lane S, et al. Polyamine derivatives as inhibitors of trypanothione reductase and assessment of their trypanocidal activities. *Bioorg Med Chem* 1997;**5**:2145−55.

141. Li Z, Fennie MW, Ganem B, Hancock MT, Kobaslija M, Rattendi D, et al. Polyamines with *N*-(3-phenylpropyl) substituents are effective competitive inhibitors of trypanothione reductase and trypanocidal agents. *Bioorg Med Chem Lett* 2001;**11**:251−4.

142. Garforth J, Yin H, McKie JH, Douglas KT, Fairlamb AH. Rational design of selective ligands for trypanothione reductase from *Trypanosoma cruzi*. Structural effects on the inhibition by dibenzazepines based on imipramine. *J Enzyme Inhib* 1997;**12**:161−73.

143. Fournet A, Inchausti A, Yaluff G, Rojas De Arias A, Guinaudeau H, Bruneton J, et al. Trypanocidal bisbenzylisoquinoline alkaloids are inhibitors of trypanothione reductase. *J Enzyme Inhib* 1998;**13**:1−9.

144. Gallwitz H, Bonse S, Martinez-Cruz A, Schlichting I, Schumacher K, Krauth-Siegel RL. Ajoene is an inhibitor and subversive substrate of human glutathione reductase and *Trypanosoma cruzi* trypanothione reductase: crystallographic, kinetic, and spectroscopic studies. *J Med Chem* 1999;**42**:364−72.

145. Bonse S, Santelli-Rouvier C, Barbe J, Krauth-Siegel RL. Inhibition of *Trypanosoma cruzi* trypanothione reductase by acridines: kinetic studies and structure−activity relationships. *J Med Chem* 1999;**42**:5448−54.

146. Bonse S, Richards JM, Ross SA, Lowe G, Krauth-Siegel RL. (2,2':6',2''-Terpyridine) platinum(II) complexes are irreversible inhibitors of *Trypanosoma cruzi* trypanothione reductase but not of human glutathione reductase. *J Med Chem* 2000;**43**:4812−21.

147. Lee B, Bauer H, Melchers J, Ruppert T, Rattray L, Yardley V, et al. Irreversible inactivation of trypanothione reductase by unsaturated Mannich bases: a divinyl ketone as key intermediate. *J Med Chem* 2005;**48**:7400−10.

148. Cota BB, Rosa LH, Fagundes EM, Martins-Filho OA, Correa-Oliveira R, Romanha AJ, et al. A potent trypanocidal component from the fungus *Lentinus strigosus* inhibits trypanothione reductase and modulates PBMC proliferation. *Mem Inst Oswaldo Cruz* 2008;**103**:263−70.

149. Holloway GA, Baell JB, Fairlamb AH, Novello PM, Parisot JP, Richardson J, et al. Discovery of 2-iminobenzimidazoles as a new class of trypanothione reductase inhibitor by high-throughput screening. *Bioorg Med Chem Lett* 2007;**17**:1422−7.

150. Holloway GA, Charman WN, Fairlamb AH, Brun R, Kaiser M, Kostewicz E, et al. Trypanothione reductase high-throughput screening campaign identifies novel classes of inhibitors with antiparasitic activity. *Antimicrob Agents Chemother* 2009;**53**:2824−33.

151. Logan FJ, Taylor MC, Wilkinson SR, Kaur H, Kelly JM. The terminal step in vitamin C biosynthesis in *Trypanosoma cruzi* is mediated by a FMN-dependent galactonolactone oxidase. *Biochem J* 2007;**407**:419−26.

152. Wilkinson SR, Meyer DJ, Taylor MC, Bromley EV, Miles MA, Kelly JM. The *Trypanosoma cruzi* enzyme TcGPXI is a glycosomal peroxidase and can be linked to trypanothione reduction by glutathione or tryparedoxin. *J Biol Chem* 2002;**277**: 17062−71.

153. Wilkinson SR, Meyer DJ, Kelly JM. Biochemical characterization of a trypanosome enzyme with glutathione-dependent peroxidase activity. *Biochem J* 2000;**352**:755−61.

154. Patel S, Hussain S, Harris R, Sardiwal S, Kelly JM, Wilkinson SR, et al. Structural insights into the catalytic mechanism of *Trypanosoma cruzi* GPXI (glutathione peroxidase-like enzyme I). *Biochem J* 2010;**425**:513−22.

155. Wilkinson SR, Taylor MC, Touitha S, Mauricio IL, Meyer DJ, Kelly JM. TcGPXII, a glutathione-dependent *Trypanosoma cruzi* peroxidase with substrate specificity restricted to fatty acid and phospholipid hydroperoxides, is localized to the endoplasmic reticulum. *Biochem J* 2002;**364**:787−94.

156. Guerrero SA, Lopez JA, Steinert P, Montemartini M, Kalisz HM, Colli W, et al. His-tagged tryparedoxin peroxidase of *Trypanosoma cruzi* as a tool for drug screening. *Appl Microbiol Biotechnol* 2000;**53**:410−14.

157. Lopez JA, Carvalho TU, de Souza W, Flohe L, Guerrero SA, Montemartini M, et al. Evidence for a trypanothione-dependent peroxidase system in *Trypanosoma cruzi*. *Free Radic Biol Med* 2000;**28**:767−72.

158. Thomson L, Denicola A, Radi R. The trypanothione-thiol system in *Trypanosoma cruzi* as a key antioxidant mechanism against peroxynitrite-mediated cytotoxicity. *Arch Biochem Biophys* 2003;**412**:55−64.

159. Trujillo M, Budde H, Pineyro MD, Stehr M, Robello C, Flohe L, et al. *Trypanosoma brucei* and *Trypanosoma cruzi* tryparedoxin peroxidases catalytically detoxify peroxynitrite via oxidation of fast reacting thiols. *J Biol Chem* 2004;**279**:34175−82.

160. Piacenza L, Peluffo G, Alvarez MN, Kelly JM, Wilkinson SR, Radi R. Peroxiredoxins play a major role in protecting *Trypanosoma cruzi* against macrophage- and endogenously-derived peroxynitrite. *Biochem J* 2008;**410**:59−68.

161. Pineyro MD, Arcari T, Robello C, Radi R, Trujillo M. Tryparedoxin peroxidases from *Trypanosoma cruzi*: high efficiency in the catalytic elimination of hydrogen peroxide and peroxynitrite. *Arch Biochem Biophys* 2011;**507**:287−95.

162. Nogueira FB, Ruiz JC, Robello C, Romanha AJ, Murta SM. Molecular characterization of cytosolic and mitochondrial tryparedoxin peroxidase in *Trypanosoma cruzi* populations susceptible and resistant to benznidazole. *Parasitol Res* 2009;**104**: 835−44.

163. Pineyro MD, Pizarro JC, Lema F, Pritsch O, Cayota A, Bentley GA, et al. Crystal structure of the tryparedoxin peroxidase from the human parasite *Trypanosoma cruzi*. *J Struct Biol* 2005;**150**:11−22.

164. Alvarez MN, Peluffo G, Piacenza L, Radi R. Intraphagosomal peroxynitrite as a macrophage-derived cytotoxin against internalized *Trypanosoma cruzi*: consequences for oxidative killing and role of microbial peroxiredoxins in infectivity. *J Biol Chem* 2011;**286**:6627−40.

165. Ismail SO, Paramchuk W, Skeiky YA, Reed SG, Bhatia A, Gedamu L. Molecular cloning and characterization of two iron superoxide dismutase cDNAs from *Trypanosoma cruzi*. *Mol Biochem Parasitol* 1997;**86**:187−97.

166. Temperton NJ, Wilkinson SR, Meyer DJ, Kelly JM. Overexpression of superoxide dismutase in *Trypanosoma cruzi* results in increased sensitivity to the trypanocidal agents gentian violet and benznidazole. *Mol Biochem Parasitol* 1998;**96**:167−76.
167. Martinez A, Peluffo G, Petruk AA, Hugo M, Pineyro D, Demicheli V, et al. Structural and molecular basis of the peroxynitrite-mediated nitration and inactivation of *Trypanosoma cruzi* iron-superoxide dismutases (Fe-SODs) A and B: disparate susceptibilities due to the repair of Tyr35 radical by Cys83 in Fe-SODB through intramolecular electron transfer. *J Biol Chem* 2014;**289**:12760−78.
168. Meshnick SR, Kitchener KR, Trang NL. Trypanosomatid iron-superoxide dismutase inhibitors. Selectivity and mechanism of N1, N6-bis(2,3-dihydroxybenzoyl)-1,6-diaminohexane. *Biochem Pharmacol* 1985;**34**:3147−52.
169. Olmo F, Urbanova K, Rosales MJ, Martin-Escolano R, Sanchez-Moreno M, Marin C. An in vitro iron superoxide dismutase inhibitor decreases the parasitemia levels of *Trypanosoma cruzi* in BALB/c mouse model during acute phase. *Int J Parasitol Drugs Drug Resist* 2015;**5**:110−16.
170. Kubata BK, Kabututu Z, Nozaki T, Munday CJ, Fukuzumi S, Ohkubo K, et al. A key role for old yellow enzyme in the metabolism of drugs by *Trypanosoma cruzi*. *J Exp Med* 2002;**196**:1241−51.
171. Wilkinson SR, Taylor MC, Horn D, Kelly JM, Cheeseman I. A mechanism for crossresistance to nifurtimox and benznidazole in trypanosomes. *Proc Natl Acad Sci USA* 2008;**105**:5022−7.
172. Hall BS, Bot C, Wilkinson SR. Nifurtimox activation by trypanosomal type I nitroreductases generates cytotoxic nitrile metabolites. *J Biol Chem* 2011;**286**:13088−95.
173. Mason RP, Holtzman JL. The mechanism of microsomal and mitochondrial nitroreductase. Electron spin resonance evidence for nitroaromatic free radical intermediates. *Biochemistry* 1975;**14**:1626−32.
174. Boiani M, Piacenza L, Hernandez P, Boiani L, Cerecetto H, Gonzalez M, et al. Mode of action of nifurtimox and N-oxide-containing heterocycles against *Trypanosoma cruzi*: is oxidative stress involved? *Biochem Pharmacol* 2010;**79**:1736−45.
175. Giulivi C, Turrens JF, Boveris A. Chemiluminescence enhancement by trypanocidal drugs and by inhibitors of antioxidant enzymes in *Trypanosoma cruzi*. *Mol Biochem Parasitol* 1988;**30**:243−51.
176. Maya JD, Repetto Y, Agosin M, Ojeda JM, Tellez R, Gaule C, et al. Effects of nifurtimox and benznidazole upon glutathione and trypanothione content in epimastigote, trypomastigote and amastigote forms of *Trypanosoma cruzi*. *Mol Biochem Parasitol* 1997;**86**:101−6.
177. Moreno SN, Docampo R, Mason RP, Leon W, Stoppani AO. Different behaviors of benznidazole as free radical generator with mammalian and *Trypanosoma cruzi* microsomal preparations. *Arch Biochem Biophys* 1982;**218**:585−91.
178. Hall BS, Wilkinson SR. Activation of benznidazole by trypanosomal type I nitroreductases results in glyoxal formation. *Antimicrob Agents Chemother* 2012;**56**:115−23.
179. Trochine A, Creek DJ, Faral-Tello P, Barrett MP, Robello C. Benznidazole biotransformation and multiple targets in *Trypanosoma cruzi* revealed by metabolomics. *PLoS NTD* 2014;**8**:e2844.
180. Docampo R, Moreno SN, Muniz RP, Cruz FS, Mason RP. Light-enhanced free radical formation and trypanocidal action of gentian violet (crystal violet). *Science* 1983;**220**:1292−5.
181. Reszka K, Cruz FS, Docampo R. Photosensitization by the trypanocidal agent crystal violet. Type I versus type II reactions. *Chem Biol Interact* 1986;**58**:161−72.

182. Docampo R, Moreno SN, Cruz FS. Enhancement of the cytotoxicity of crystal violet against *Trypanosoma cruzi* in the blood by ascorbate. *Mol Biochem Parasitol* 1988;**27**:241−7.

183. Docampo R, de Souza W, Miranda K, Rohloff P, Moreno SN. Acidocalcisomes-conserved from bacteria to man. *Nat Rev Microbiol* 2005;**3**:251−61.

184. Docampo R, Moreno SN. The acidocalcisome as a target for chemotherapeutic agents in protozoan parasites. *Curr Pharm Des* 2008;**14**:882−8.

185. Moreno SN, Docampo R. The role of acidocalcisomes in parasitic protists. *J Eukaryot Microbiol* 2009;**56**:208−13.

186. Docampo R, Moreno SN. Acidocalcisomes. *Cell Calcium* 2011;**50**:113−19.

187. Kollien AH, Grospietsch T, Kleffmann T, Zerbst-Boroffka I, Schaub GA. Ionic composition of the rectal contents and excreta of the reduviid bug *Triatoma infestans*. *J Insect Physiol* 2001;**47**:739−47.

188. Kollien AH, Schaub GA. The development of *Trypanosoma cruzi* in triatominae. *Parasitol Today* 2000;**16**:381−7.

189. Montalvetti A, Rohloff P, Docampo R. A functional aquaporin co-localizes with the vacuolar proton pyrophosphatase to acidocalcisomes and the contractile vacuole complex of *Trypanosoma cruzi*. *J Biol Chem* 2004;**279**:38673−82.

190. Rohloff P, Montalvetti A, Docampo R. Acidocalcisomes and the contractile vacuole complex are involved in osmoregulation in *Trypanosoma cruzi*. *J Biol Chem* 2004;**279**:52270−81.

191. Rohloff P, Docampo R. A contractile vacuole complex is involved in osmoregulation in *Trypanosoma cruzi*. *Exp Parasitol* 2008;**118**:17−24.

192. Li ZH, Alvarez VE, De Gaudenzi JG, Sant'Anna C, Frasch AC, Cazzulo JJ, et al. Hyperosmotic stress induces aquaporin-dependent cell shrinkage, polyphosphate synthesis, amino acid accumulation, and global gene expression changes in *Trypanosoma cruzi*. *J Biol Chem* 2011;**286**:43959−71.

193. Docampo R, Jimenez V, Lander N, Li ZH, Niyogi S. New insights into roles of acidocalcisomes and contractile vacuole complex in osmoregulation in protists. *Int Rev Cell Mol Biol* 2013;**305**:69−113.

194. Niyogi S, Mucci J, Campetella O, Docampo R. Rab11 regulates trafficking of trans-sialidase to the plasma membrane through the contractile vacuole complex of *Trypanosoma cruzi*. *PLoS Pathog* 2014;**10**:e1004224.

195. Lang F, Busch GL, Ritter M, Volkl H, Waldegger S, Gulbins E, et al. Functional significance of cell volume regulatory mechanisms. *Physiol Rev* 1998;**78**:247−306.

196. Lang F, Busch GL, Volkl H. The diversity of volume regulatory mechanisms. *Cell Physiol Biochem* 1998;**8**:1−45.

197. Rohloff P, Docampo R. Ammonium production during hypo-osmotic stress leads to alkalinization of acidocalcisomes and cytosolic acidification in *Trypanosoma cruzi*. *Mol Biochem Parasitol* 2006;**150**:249−55.

198. Schoijet AC, Miranda K, Medeiros LC, de Souza W, Flawia MM, Torres HN, et al. Defining the role of a FYVE domain in the localization and activity of a cAMP phosphodiesterase implicated in osmoregulation in *Trypanosoma cruzi*. *Mol Microbiol* 2011;**79**:50−62.

199. King-Keller S, Li M, Smith A, Zheng S, Kaur G, Yang X, et al. Chemical validation of phosphodiesterase C as a chemotherapeutic target in *Trypanosoma cruzi*, the etiological agent of Chagas' disease. *Antimicrob Agents Chemother* 2010;**54**: 3738−45.

200. Scott DA, de Souza W, Benchimol M, Zhong L, Lu HG, Moreno SN, et al. Presence of a plant-like proton-pumping pyrophosphatase in acidocalcisomes of *Trypanosoma cruzi*. *J Biol Chem* 1998;**273**:22151−8.

201. Hill JE, Scott DA, Luo S, Docampo R. Cloning and functional expression of a gene encoding a vacuolar-type proton-translocating pyrophosphatase from *Trypanosoma cruzi*. *Biochem J* 2000;**351**:281−8.

202. Martinez R, Wang Y, Benaim G, Benchimol M, de Souza W, Scott DA, et al. A proton pumping pyrophosphatase in the Golgi apparatus and plasma membrane vesicles of *Trypanosoma cruzi*. *Mol Biochem Parasitol* 2002;**120**:205−13.

203. Kim EJ, Zhen RG, Rea PA. Heterologous expression of plant vacuolar pyrophosphatase in yeast demonstrates sufficiency of the substrate-binding subunit for proton transport. *Proc Natl Acad Sci USA* 1994;**91**:6128−32.

204. Fang J, Rohloff P, Miranda K, Docampo R. Ablation of a small transmembrane protein of *Trypanosoma brucei* (TbVTC1) involved in the synthesis of polyphosphate alters acidocalcisome biogenesis and function, and leads to a cytokinesis defect. *Biochem J* 2007;**407**:161−70.

205. Lander N, Ulrich PN, Docampo R. *Trypanosoma brucei* vacuolar transporter chaperone 4 (TbVtc4) is an acidocalcisome polyphosphate kinase required for in vivo infection. *J Biol Chem* 2013;**288**:34205−16.

206. Hothorn M, Neumann H, Lenherr ED, Wehner M, Rybin V, Hassa PO, et al. Catalytic core of a membrane-associated eukaryotic polyphosphate polymerase. *Science* 2009;**324**:513−16.

207. Ulrich PN, Lander N, Kurup SP, Reiss L, Brewer J, Soares Medeiros LC, et al. The acidocalcisome vacuolar transporter chaperone 4 catalyzes the synthesis of polyphosphate in insect-stages of *Trypanosoma brucei* and *T. cruzi*. *J Eukaryot Microbiol* 2014;**61**:155−65.

208. Ormerod WE. The study of volutin granules in trypanosomes. *Trans R Soc Trop Med Hyg* 1961;**55**:313−32.

209. Macadam RF, Williamson J. Drug effects on the fine structure of *Trypanosoma rhodesiense*: suramin, tryparsamide and mapharside. *Ann Trop Med Parasitol* 1974;**68**: 301−6.

210. Ormerod WE, Shaw JJ. A study of granules and other changes in phase-contrast appearance produced by chemotherapeutic agents in trypanosomes. *Br J Pharmacol Chemother* 1963;**21**:259−72.

211. Ormerod WE. A study of basophilic inclusion bodies produced by chemotherapeutic agents in trypanosomes. *Br J Pharmacol Chemother* 1951;**6**:334−41.

212. Mathis AM, Holman JL, Sturk LM, Ismail MA, Boykin DW, Tidwell RR, et al. Accumulation and intracellular distribution of antitrypanosomal diamidine compounds DB75 and DB820 in African trypanosomes. *Antimicrob Agents Chemother* 2006;**50**: 2185−91.

213. Mathis AM, Bridges AS, Ismail MA, Kumar A, Francesconi I, Anbazhagan M, et al. Diphenyl furans and aza analogs: effects of structural modification on in vitro activity, DNA binding, and accumulation and distribution in trypanosomes. *Antimicrob Agents Chemother* 2007;**51**:2801−10.

# Ultrastructure of *Trypanosoma cruzi* and its interaction with host cells

*W. de Souza[1,2], T.U. de Carvalho[1] and E.S. Barrias[3]*
[1]Universidade Federal do Rio de Janeiro, Rio de Janeiro, Brazil, [2]Instituto Nacional de Ciência e Tecnologia em Biologia Estrutural e Bioimagens, Rio de Janeiro, Brazil, [3]Instituto nacional de Metrologia, Normalização e Qualidade - Inmetro, Rio de Janeiro, Brazil; Avenida Nossa Senhora das Graças, Rio de Janeiro, Brazil

## Chapter Outline

## Structural organization of *Trypanosoma cruzi*

Structural features of Protozoa of the Trypanosomatidae family include structures/organelles such as the kinetoplast, the glycosome, the paraflagellar rod, a highly specialized flagellar pocket, and a layer of subpellicular microtubules (Fig. 18.1).

American Trypanosomiasis Chagas Disease. DOI: http://dx.doi.org/10.1016/B978-0-12-801029-7.00018-6

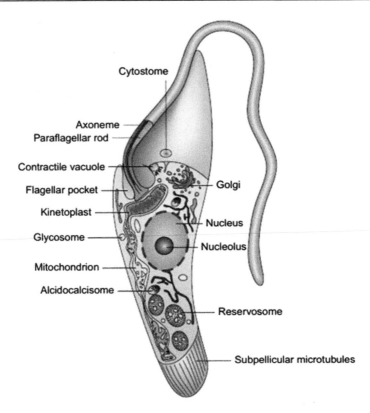

**Figure 18.1** Schematic representation of longitudinal section of an epimastigote showing the main structures and organelles found in *T. cruzi*. The scheme is modified from a drawing by Flavia Moreira-Leite, University of Oxford.
*Source*: After Docampo R, De Souza W, Miranda K, Roheloff P, Moreno S. Acidocalcisomes—conserved from bacteria to man. *Nat Rev Microbiol* 2005;**3**:251−61.

They have the ability to change shape during their life cycle, a process described as protozoan differentiation or transformation.[1,2] Among the trypanosomatids, *Trypanosoma cruzi* proceeds through several developmental stages in the vertebrate and invertebrate hosts, living both in the bloodstream and inside the cells of the vertebrate host (Fig. 18.2).

The infection of mammals usually occurs following an insect bite (member of Reduvidae family), when the metacyclic trypomastigote penetrates directly through the ocular mucosa or skin lesion. Another route of infection is via the ingestion of food that is contaminated with *T. cruzi*, especially juices from fruits, such as açaí and guava, in the Amazon region and sugar cane in other regions.[3,4] Once in the vertebrate host, the metacyclic trypomastigotes invade the nucleate forming a vacuole known as the parasitophorous vacuole (PV). A few hours after infection, trypomastigotes are gradually turned into amastigote (a stage that is rounded and with a

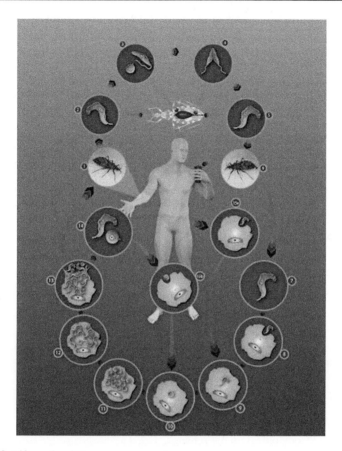

**Figure 18.2** Life cycle of *Trypanosoma cruzi*.

short flagellum) and the PV structure are digested, allowing the amastigotes to come into direct contact with host cell organelles. In the cytoplasm, the amastigotes divide almost synchronously, with a generation time that varies according to the *T. cruzi* strain.[5]

# The nucleus

Initial observations showed a nucleus enveloped by typical membranes with pores, condensed chromatin dispersed throughout the nucleoplasm, and a typical nucleolus found in epimastigotes, but not in amastigote or trypomastigote.[6,7] The nucleolar material persists throughout the closed mitosis process. It was also shown that the nuclear membrane remains intact throughout mitosis, which is characterized by the appearance of intranuclear microtubules, dispersion of the chromatin, and the appearance of dense plates whose number varies according to the trypanosomatid

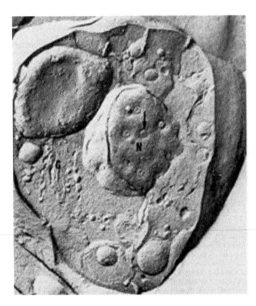

**Figure 18.3** Freeze-fracture images showing the distribution of the nuclear pores as well as the intramembranous particles seen on the nuclear membrane.
*Source*: After Esponda P, Souto-Padrón T, De Souza W. Fine structure and cytochemistry of the nucleus and the kinetoplast of epimastigotes of Trypanosoma cruzi. *J Protozool* 1983;**30** (1):105−10.

species. The nuclear membrane presents a high density of pores thus indicating a high rate of nucleocytoplasmic interchange (Fig. 18.3).[8]

# The kinetoplast—mitochondrion complex

The kinetoplast is situated close to the nucleus, and its shape and structural organization vary according to the developmental stage of the protozoan. The trypanosomatids possess a unique and highly ramified mitochondrion. The kinetoplast appears as a dense structure and is made of kinetoplast DNA (kDNA), found in a specialized portion of the mitochondrion (Fig. 18.4) within the mitochondrial matrix, perpendicular to the axis of the flagellum.

Two types of circular DNA are present in the kinetoplast: minicircles and maxicircles. There are several thousand minicircles, which range in size from about 0.5 to 2.5 kb (depending on the species), and a few dozen maxicircles, which range from 20 to 40 kb.[9] Together, maxicircles and minicircles represent approximately 30% of the total cellular genome.[10] The minicircles present high heterogeneity but also have a conserved region where replication origin sites are localized. Minicircles also encode guide RNAs that modify the maxicircle transcripts by

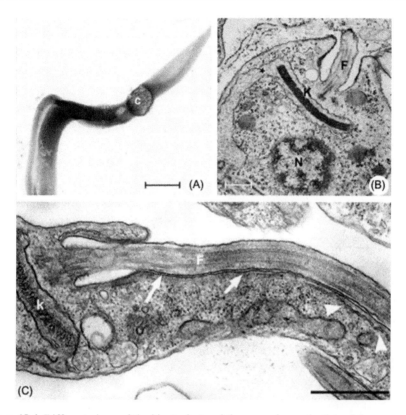

**Figure 18.4** Different views of the kinetoplast and the general organization of the trypomastigote (A), amastigote (B), and epimastigote (C) forms of *Trypanosoma cruzi*. F: flagellum; K: kinetoplast; N: nucleus. The white arrows point to the area of adhesion of the flagellum to the cell body. White arrowheads point to profiles of the endoplasmic reticulum. Bar, 1 μm.
*Source*: After (A and B) De Souza, W. Growth and transformation of Trypanosoma cruzi. In: Briggs AP, Coburn, JA, editors, *Handbook of cell proliferation*. Nova Science Publishers; 2009; (C) Rocha GM, Brandao BA, Mortara RA, Attias M, De Souza W, Carvalho TM. The flagellar attachment zone of Trypanosoma cruzi epimastigote forms. *J Struct Biol* 2006;**154**:89−99.

extensive uridylate insertion or deletion, a process known as RNA editing. The maxicircles are structurally and functionally analogous to the mitochondrial DNA. In situ analysis of the kinetoplast DNA structure showed that the network is formed not by circles, but by irregular polygonal structures (Fig. 18.5). The association of kDNA and mitochondrion membrane are made by filaments known as unilateral filaments. The connection between outer portion of the mitochondrial membrane to the basal body are made by another filaments. Together, the probasal body and the two cytoskeletal structures have been designated as the Tripartite Attachment Complex (TAC) of the kinetoplast.[11−13]

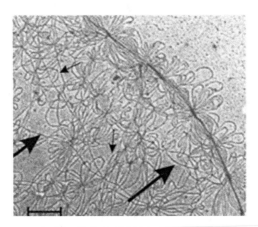

**Figure 18.5** Organization of the kinetoplast DNA fibers in maxicircles and minicircles. The kinetoplast DNA network was dispersed in water, collected in a grid and shadowed at low angle with platinum. Bar, 0.3 μm.
*Source*: Courtesy of David Pérez-Morga.

## The glycosome

All trypanosomatids contain spherical structures with a homogeneous matrix that are surrounded by a unit membrane and distributed throughout the cell. They are a special type of peroxisome, designated as the glycosome due to the concentration of glycolytic pathway enzymes in this organelle.[14–16] Since catalase is found in the glycosomes of monogenetic but not digenetic trypanosomatids, this organelle is now considered to be a special type of peroxisome. In addition to catalase, the peroxisomes of mammalian cells have more than 50 different enzymes involved in metabolic pathways, such as peroxide metabolism, ß-oxidation of fatty acids, and ether phospholipid synthesis. Studies have found that, in addition to the pathways described above, other metabolic pathways that occur in the cytosol of other cells also take place in the glycosomes of trypanosomatids, including carbon dioxide fixation,[17] purine salvage and de novo pyrimidine biosynthesis, fatty acid elongation, isoprenoid biosynthesis, and sterol biosynthesis.[14] The glycosome does not possess a genome. Therefore, all of the proteins found in it are encoded by nuclear genes, translated on free ribosomes and then posttranslationally imported into the organelle.

The biogenesis of the glycosome seems to be similar to that of peroxisome.[18]

## The acidocalcisome

Since the first morphological observations of *T. cruzi*, there have been descriptions of spherical structures distributed throughout the cell body. Only in 1994 was it shown that this organelle, which contains electron dense deposits (Fig. 18.6), is

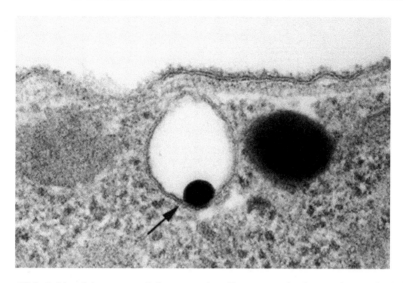

**Figure 18.6** Acidocalcisome morphology seen in cells processed using routine methods for electron microscopy. Bar, 200 nm.
*Source*: After De Souza, W. Growth and transformation of *Trypanosoma cruzi*. In: Briggs AP, Coburn, JA, editors, *Handbook of cell proliferation*. Nova Science Publishers; 2009.

capable of transporting protons and calcium, thus prompting its designation as the "acidocalcisome."[19]

The organelles can also be visualized in whole cells dried on a grid using an electron microscope, especially if the microscope is equipped with an energy filter, as shown in Fig. 18.7. Nowadays, it is known that the acidocalcisome contains calcium, phosphorous, sodium, potassium, and zinc. In some trypanosomatids, iron has also been found.[20]

The acidocalcisomes have many functions as: (1) the storage of calcium, magnesium, sodium, potassium, zinc, iron, and phosphorous compounds, especially inorganic pyrophosphate and polyphosphate, as determined by biochemical analysis and X-ray microanalysis; (2) pH homeostasis; and (3) osmoregulation, a function that involves interaction of the acidocalcisome with the contractile vacuole.[19] This involvement is associated with the rapid hydrolysis or synthesis of acidocalcisome poly-P during hypo- or hyperosmotic stress, respectively, in *T. cruzi*.[21]

One key function of the acidocalcisomes is the accumulation of phosphate, pyrophosphate, and polyphosphate. The latter molecule is formed via the polymerization of a few to thousands of phosphate residues. These molecules are involved in the process of osmoregulation and are vital for *T. cruzi* survival during its life cycle, during which it comes in contact with diverse environmental conditions. Polyphosphate hydrolysis has been shown to occur during hypoosmotic stress in *T. cruzi*, leading to an increase in the acidocalcisome osmotic pressure, which facilitates the movement of water.[22,23]

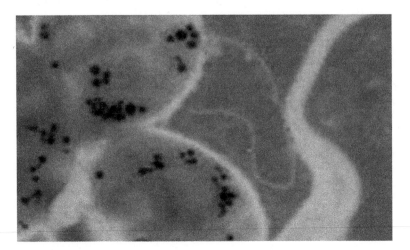

**Figure 18.7** Acidocalcisome morphology seen in whole cells examined using electron spectroscopic imaging. Bar, 2 μm.
*Source*: After De Souza, W. Growth and transformation of *Trypanosoma cruzi*. In: Briggs AP, Coburn, JA, editors, *Handbook of cell proliferation*. Nova Science Publishers; 2009.

## The contractile vacuole

Studies carried out with several protozoa, especially free-living ones, have shown that the contractile vacuole plays a fundamental role in the regulation of osmotic processes. There have been few reports on the presence of such a structure in trypanosomes. The structure was reported to consist of several tubules connected to a central vacuole located close to the flagellar pocket.[24] Aquaporin, a protein involved in water transport, was identified in *T. cruzi* epimastigotes and localized to both the acidocalcisomes and contractile vacuole.[25] It was shown that the fusion of acidocalcisomes to the contractile vacuole takes place in a process mediated by cyclic AMP.[26] Recently, the contractile vacuole has been shown to be important for the regulatory volume decrease that occurs after hypoosmotic stress[27] and for cell shrinking after hyperosmotic stress.[21] In addition, the contractile vacuole is also involved in the trafficking of glycosylphosphatidylinositol (GPI)-anchored proteins to the plasma membrane.[28] Proteomic, bioinformatic, and ultrastructural analyses demonstrated that a number of proteins are involved in trafficking, such as SNARE 2.1 and SNARE 2.2, VAMP1 (an orthologue of mammalian VAMP7), AP180, and the small GTPases Rab11 and Rab32.[29] It has been suggested that the contractile vacuole could be an evolutionary precursor to the recycling endosomal system in other eukaryotes.[30,31] Recently, the participation of Rab32 (present in the contractile vacuole) in the biogenesis of the acidocalcisome was suggested.[23] Evidence of acidocalcisome-contractile vacuole fusion was also observed[25] and advances in ultrastructural techniques have allowed the observation of intimate contact between structures, such as the contractile vacuole, the acidocalcisome, and the spongiome (Fig. 18.8).[23,32]

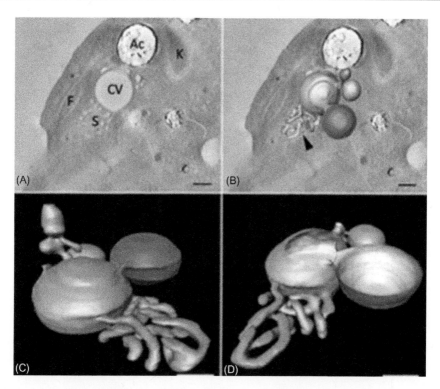

**Figure 18.8** 3D model of the contractile vacuole and flagellar pocket showing the interconnected spongiome connected to the contractile vacuole (arrows) and concentrated in the anterior region of the contractile vacuole. Some vesicles were also connected to the spongiome (arrowheads).
*Source*: After Girard-Dias W, Alcântara CL, Cunha-e-Silva N, de Souza W, Miranda K. On the ultrastructural organization of Trypanosoma cruzi using cryopreparation methods and electron tomography. *Histochem Cell Biol* 2012;**138(6)**:821−31.

# The cytoskeleton

Transmission electron microscopy of thin sections of trypanosomatids showed the presence of subpellicular microtubules distributed throughout the cell body, except in the flagellar pocket region. Profiles of the endoplasmic reticulum can be seen in between and below the subpellicular microtubules (Fig. 18.9).[33]

In addition to the subpellicular microtubules, other sets of a few microtubules have been visualized in trypanosomatids. First, a triplet of microtubules is associated with the cytostome−cytopharynx complex. These microtubules start underneath the cytostome membrane and follow part of the cytopharynx, sometimes disappearing when the cytopharynx lumen becomes thinner. Second, a set of four microtubules appears to originate (or to end) underneath the opening of the flagellar pocket, follow the path of the preoral ridge, and associate with the cytopharynx. These two sets of microtubules appear to be a characteristic feature of *T. cruzi* (and

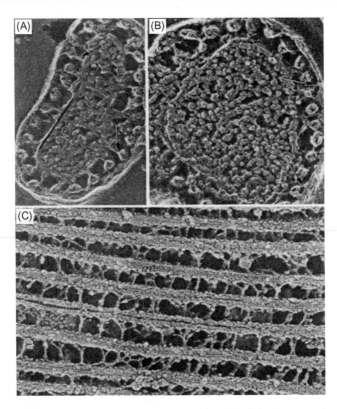

**Figure 18.9** Deep-etching view reveals that subpelicular microtubules connecting with endoplasmic reticulum (A), with plasma membrane (B) and between them (arrows—C). Bar, 100 nm.
*Source*: After Souto-Padron T, De Souza W, Heuser JE. Quick-freeze, deep-etch rotary replication of *Trypanosoma cruzi* and *Herpetomonas megaseliae*. *J Cell Sci* 1984;**69**:167−8.

possibly other members of the Trypanosomatidae family that contain a cytostome). Third, another set of four microtubules is also observed in *T. brucei*[33]; these microtubules originate close to the basal bodies and underlie a portion of the flagellar pocket, forming a channel through which extracellular components may have access to the lumen of the flagellar pocket. This microtubule complex has been designated as MtQ (microtubule quartet) in *T. brucei*.[33] In *T. cruzi*, this complex also surrounds a domain of the flagellar pocket, following a helicoidal pattern and approaching the subpellicular microtubules near the opening of the flagellar pocket.[34] Fourth, single microtubules were observed running through the cytoplasm. One of these microtubules passed through a tunnel-like structure of the mitochondrion (Fig. 18.10).

Microfilaments have never been observed in the cytoplasm of *T. cruzi*. However, it has been shown[35,36] that cytochalasin B treatment leads to morphological alterations in the cytoskeletal elements associated with the cytostome−cytopharynx complex, which is responsible for transferrin uptake. Actin and actin-binding proteins were characterized in *T. cruzi*.[37] Cevallos and colleagues[38] demonstrated that

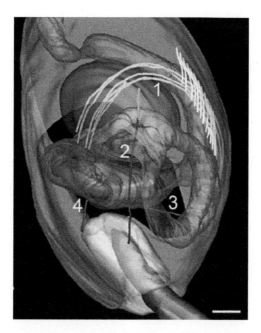

**Figure 18.10** 3D model of *T. cruzi* amastigotes demonstrating a tunnel-like mitochondrion structure in green. Nucleus and *kinetoplast* are represented in blue, microtubules are represented in yellow, *flagelum* is represented in orange, and cell body in gray.
*Source*: After Girard-Dias W, Alcântara CL, Cunha-e-Silva N, de Souza W, Miranda K. On the ultrastructural organization of *Trypanosoma cruzi* using cryopreparation methods and electron tomography. *Histochem Cell Biol* 2012;**138(6)**:821−31.

*T. cruzi* genome encodes for a diverse group of actins, actin-like and actin-related proteins that are conserved among trypanosomatids.

## The flagellum

The flagellum is enveloped by a typical flagellar membrane, which exhibits some interesting features. Freeze-fracture and biochemical studies have shown that there are relatively few proteins in the flagellar membrane and that the content of sterol is relatively high. The main proteins found in the flagellar membrane are (1) the $Ca^{2+}$-binding protein FCaBP, which was initially described in *T. cruzi*; (2) the calflagins, which are found in *T. brucei*; (3) SMP-1, which was found in *Leishmania* and appears to be localized in the inner leaflet of the flagellar membrane; (4) ESAG-4, which is found in *T. brucei* and has a functional adenylate cyclase domain that is also localized in the cytoplasmic portion of the membrane; and (5) a glucose transporter, which was found in Leishmania.[39] All trypanosomatids have one flagellar complex, with a canonical basal body at the base of the flagellum. Even in the so-called intracellular amastigote form, a short flagellum is observed.

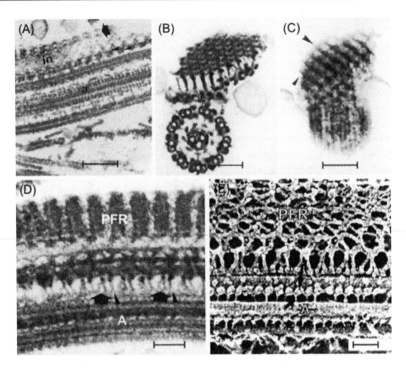

**Figure 18.11** Different views of the flagellum of trypanosomatids as seen in longitudinal
(A, D) and transversal (B, C) views of thin sections and in a replica of quick-frozen, freeze-
fractured, deep-etched, and rotary replicated samples (E). The axonemal (A) microtubules, as
well as filaments which make the paraflagellar rod structure (PFR), can be seen. Bridges
connecting the axoneme to the paraflagellar rod (arrows) and the plates which form the PFR
are seen. Bar, 50 (A—C) and 100 nm (D, E).
*Source*: After Farina M, Attias M, Souto-Padron T, De Souza W. Further studies on the
organization of the paraxial rod of trypanosomatids. *J Protozool* 1986;**33**:552—7.

The flagellum consists of the typical array of nine pairs of peripheral microtubule
doublets and one central pair (Fig. 18.11A).

In addition, it contains an intriguing structure made up of a complex array of
filaments that, due to its location, is called the paraxial or paraflagellar rod (PFR).
The PFR is made of a complex array of filaments linked to the axoneme. Two
regions, designated as proximal (consisting of two plates) and distal (consisting of
several plates), were identified in the PFR (Fig. 18.11B—E). The plates are formed
by an association of 25-nm and 7-nm thick filaments that are oriented at an angle
of 50 degrees in relation to the major axis of the axoneme.[40] Biochemical analyses
have shown that the PFR is composed of a large number of proteins, most of which
have not been yet characterized. However, two major proteins have been characterized in some detail. These proteins, known as PFR 1 and 2, have molecular weights
of 73 and 79 kDa, respectively. The available evidence indicates that the PFR is an
essential structure for parasite survival.[41] Recently, using a CRISPR (clustered

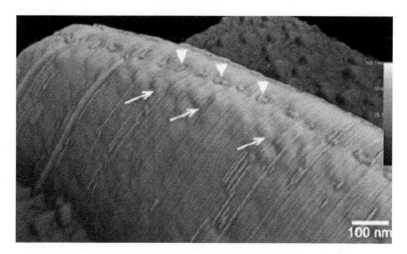

**Figure 18.12** AFM image of the flagellum of a slightly detergent-extracted epimastigote from *T. cruzi*. A furrow along the major axis of the flagellum is clearly seen. Periodically organized protrusions can be seen in the furrow (arrowheads).
*Source*: After Rocha GM, Brandao BA, Mortara RA, Attias M, De Souza W, Carvalho TM. The flagellar attachment zone of *Trypanosoma cruzi* epimastigote forms. *J Struct Biol* 2006;**154**:89−99.

regularly interspaced short palindromic repeats)/Cas9 (CRISPR-associated gene 9) system for disrupting genes in the parasite supported the suggestion that PFR1, PFR2, and GP72 are all important to flagellar attachment to the cell body and motility of the parasites.[42]

Atomic Force Microscopy (AFM) views of the flagellum revealed the presence of a furrow that separates the axoneme-containing portion of the flagellum the PFR-containing portion.[43] Periodic structures associated with the furrow were also observed (Fig. 18.12).

## The flagellar pocket

In all trypanosomatids, the flagellum emerges from a deep sac-like invagination of the plasma membrane close to the region where the basal body-kinetoplast complex is localized. At the deeper portion of the invagination, the membrane continues as the flagellar membrane. At the emergence site, the flagellar membrane comes into contact with the membrane that lines the cell body. Recent studies have shown that some cytoskeletal components concentrate in this region, forming what has been described as the flagellar pocket collar (FPC) that surrounds the whole flagellum and establishes contact with the subpellicular microtubules. A structure known as the bilobe, which is considered to be a Golgi complex-associated structure and contains centrin 2 and several other proteins, is also associated with the FPC. One protein complex that is designated as BILBO1 is involved in the formation of the FPC in *T. brucei*. The knockout of this complex using RNAi disrupts the formation of the FPC. This molecular complex can form polymers in vitro.[44] The complex organization of this system that establishes the membrane invagination forms a nearly complete and dynamic compartment that is the flagellar pocket.[45]

## The secretory pathway

The secretory pathway in *T. cruzi* involves the endoplasmic reticulum (ER), the Golgi complex, and a system of vesicles that bud from the Golgi cisternae and migrate toward the flagellar pocket, where they fuse and discharge their contents into the flagellar pocket. ER cisternae are seen around the nucleus, and these radiate toward all regions of the cell, especially the peripheral microtubule-containing region. Both rough and smooth ER cisternae are present. The Golgi complex is always located close to the flagellar pocket and is essentially similar to that found in other cells. Rab7, a small GTPase involved in membrane trafficking, was also detected in the Golgi complex of trypanosomes.[46] These vesicles present a rich collection of proteins involved in metabolism, signaling, nucleic acid binding, and parasite survival and virulence.[47] The vesicles released by *T. cruzi* also contain a homogeneous population of tRNA- and rRNA-derived small RNAs. Extracellular vesicle cargo could be delivered to other parasites and to susceptible mammalian cells, promoting metacyclogenesis and conferring susceptibility to infection, respectively.[48] Fernandez-Calero[49] compared the small RNA cargo of extracellular vesicles from *T. cruzi* epimastigotes with the respective intracellular compartment using deep sequencing. Compared with the intracellular compartment, the shed extracellular vesicles showed a specific extracellular signature that included distinctive patterns of small RNAs derived from rRNA, tRNA, sno/snRNAs, and protein coding sequences, which evidenced specific secretory small RNA processing pathways. The shed extracellular vesicles are also enriched with glycoproteins of the gp85/ trans-sialidase superfamily and other α-galactosyl-containing glycoconjugates, such as mucins. Depending on the origin (strain) of the extracellular microvesicles, different immune responses are triggered.[50] These shedding vesicles can also increase the inflammatory response in cardiac tissues.[6]

## The endocytic pathway

Trypanosomatids are highly polarized cells, and their endocytic activity is restricted to the flagellar pocket and cytostome regions.[2] Studies of *T. cruzi* have shown that this protozoan exhibits certain peculiarities in its endocytic pathway that distinguish it from other cells. First, endocytosis only occurs at high levels in the epimastigote. Second, epimastigotes have two sites in which macromolecule uptake takes place: the flagellar pocket, and a highly specialized structure known as the cytostome. Third, the cargo of the endocytic vesicles is delivered to unusual structures called reservosomes, which are located at the posterior end of the cell. The cytostome is a plasma membrane invagination coupled to a few special microtubules that penetrate the cell almost to the nucleus. The opening of this complex has a diameter of up to 0.3 μm. There is a specialized region of the membrane lining the parasite that starts in the opening of the cytostome and projects toward the flagellar pocket. The cystostome is the most responsible for ingestion of macromolecules[51] and has an acidic nature.[52] In relation to the ultrastructure of the cytostome and the cytopharynx, it was observed that cytostome presents a cytoskeleton composed of two microtubule sets (a triplet that starts underneath the cytostome membrane and a quartet that originates underneath the flagellar-pocket membrane and follows the preoral ridge before reaching the cytopharynx).[34] Following binding to the cytostome and flagellar pocket, macromolecules are rapidly internalized and appear in small endocytic vesicles, which bud from regions of these structures.[35,36]

The fusion of endocytic vesicles with the tubule-vesicular network can be observed from the perinuclear region to the posterior tip of the cell.

Macromolecules from the extracellular medium or from the ER-Golgi system are concentrated in structures known as reservosomes.[53] The main function of reservosomes in *T. cruzi* epimastigotes is to store macromolecules, although they also contain high concentrations of lysosomal hydrolases. In fact, reservosomes are also considered the main site of protein degradation and regulation. Each epimastigote has several reservosomes, primarily in the posterior region of the cell (Fig. 18.13).

Reservosomes have been described as a structure unique to epimastigotes and several studies demonstrates thar typical reservosomes disappear during the transformation of epimastigotes into metacyclic trypomastigotes in vitro. While lipid and protein uptake has never been demonstrated in either trypomastigotes or amastigotes, intracellular organelles that share many reservosomal features were recently described in the *T. cruzi* mammalian stages.[54] Like reservosomes, these organelles

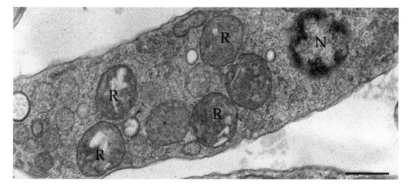

**Figure 18.13** Transmission electron microscopy of *T. cruzi* reservosomes. (A) Ultrathin section of an epimastigote showing reservosomes (R) in situ, with their typical morphology and position, between nucleus (N) and posterior end of the cell. Bar, 1 μm.
*Source*: After Sant'Anna et al. (2009).

are concentrated in the parasite's posterior region. Additionally, they accumulate cruzipain, as well as its natural inhibitor chagasin and serine carboxypetidase. The organelles are acidic and have a P-type $H^+$-ATPase.

# Other cytoplasmic structures

A close view of the cytoplasm of trypanosomatids reveals the presence of many ribosomes. Some ribosomes are scattered randomly throughout the cytoplasm and some are associated with the endoplasmic reticulum and others form granules composed of mRNAs released from polysomes and RNA binding proteins involved in translational regulation.[55]

## The cell surface

The observation of T. cruzi epimastigotes cell surface by freeze fracture makes it evident that the plasma membrane is not homogeneous in terms of density and distribution of intramembranous particles.[56] Indeed, this technique made it possible to identify at least three macrodomains of the membrane[1,56,57]: the cell body, the flagellum, and the flagellar pocket. Each of these macrodomains possesses specific microdomains, such as (1) the flagellar necklace, localized at the basal portion of the flagellum; (2) the zone of attachment of the flagellum to the cell body, where a linear array of intramembranous particles exists on both fracture faces of the flagellar membrane lining the adhesion region; and (3) the cytostome region, observed in epimastigote and amastigote forms of T. cruzi.

The FAZ region of the epimastigote shows a row of IMP clusters and a linear array of IMPs on both the PF and EF faces that could be involved with the FAZ region. The IMPs were longitudinally oriented in relation to the main axis of the flagellum.[58]

## Fine structure of the interaction of T. cruzi with host cells

The first steps of the T. cruzi—mammalian host cell interaction process can be divided into three stages: (1) adhesion and recognition; (2) signaling; and (3) invasion. The adhesion step involves the recognition of molecules present on the surface of both the parasite and the host cell. Initially, the interaction process with the host cell was described as split into two mechanisms: active penetration and phagocytosis. The term active penetration was first used by Romana and Meyer[12] as a process in which mechanical activity of the protozoan is prevalent, and the parasites penetrate into the cell through the plasma membrane. In this classic paper, it was stated that "in general, the active penetration was more visible with metacyclic forms that, with their great motility, easily crossed the cell surface, penetrating into the protoplasm of fibroblasts and myocytes." Posteriorly, Meyer and Xavier de Oliveira[59] demonstrated that the parasite "can touch the surface of the host cells without penetration. Occasionally, they adhere to the cell surface and suddenly penetrate into the cell." The same idea was presented in 1973 by Dvorak and Hyde.[60,61] In the 1970s, electron microscopy data demonstrated the parasite is always present in an intracellular vacuole surrounded by a membrane originated from the host cell plasma membrane, without direct contact with the host cell cytoplasm. The early step to internalization known as adhesion is a process that depends on receptors restricted to membrane domains.

Different strains of *T. cruzi* as well as different forms of the parasite (tissue culture-derived trypomastigotes, metacyclic trypomastigotes, and amastigotes) express different molecules on their surface. In the case of trypomastigotes, several surface-exposed glycoproteins have been described that play roles in the interaction process, including the following: (1) gp90, which seems to have glycosidase activity, downregulates host cell invasion probably due to its lack of $Ca^{2+}$ signal-inducing activity.[62,63] (2) Mucins, which are the major *T. cruzi* surface glycoproteins, have sugar residues that interact with mammalian cells.[64,65] Many mucins have been implicated in the host cell infection process.[65−67] (3) The Tc85 molecule, which is abundant in trypomastigotes, is part of the gp85/trans-sialidase family, which includes other proteins such as gp85, gp82, TSA-1, and trans-sialidases. Tc85 forms a population of heterogeneous GPI-glycoproteins with similar molecular masses but different electric charges.[68−71] Because the Tc85 family is composed of multiadhesive glycoproteins, its members are capable of binding to different receptor molecules either located on the cell surface, like host cell cytokeratin 18,[72] or belonging to components of the extracellular matrix, like fibronectin[73] and laminin.[72] (4) Two groups of glycoproteins, gp82 and gp35/50, are also involved in parasite invasion. Both proteins are expressed on the surface of metacyclic trypomastigotes.[74] In 1998, Favoretto and colleagues[75] demonstrated that gp82 is the signaling receptor that mediates protein tyrosine phosphorylation, which is necessary for host cell invasion. Phospholipase C and IP3 are also involved in this signaling cascade, which is initiated at the parasite cell surface by gp82 and leads to the $Ca^{2+}$ mobilization required to target cell invasion.[75,76] Besides these glycoproteins, a new class of surface proteins of *T. cruzi* was described: the TcSMP[77] expressed in all developmental stages of *T. cruzi* and also present in other members of the *Trypanosoma* genus. (5) Present in all strains of *T. cruzi*, Gp83 is a ligand employed by the parasite to attach and enter both professional and nonprofessional phagocytic cells.[78,79] It is expressed only in infective trypomastigotes.[80] (6) Some *T. cruzi* proteases, including cruzipain, oligopeptidase B and Tc80, have been implicated in the process of host-cell infection. Oligopeptidase B, a serine endopeptidase, is secreted by *T. cruzi* trypomastigotes.[81,82] This soluble factor is generated by the action of a 120-kDa alkaline peptidase on precursors present only in infective trypomastigotes. This 80-kDa cytosolic serine peptidase indirectly induces $[Ca^{2+}]_i$-transients during *T. cruzi* invasion.[82,83] Tc80 is a prolyl oligopeptidase and a member of the serine protease family that hydrolyzes human collagens type I and IV at neutral pH. Fibronectin is important for the parasite's transit through the extracellular matrix[84,85] showed that the parasite's entry into the host cell was blocked by treatment with selective inhibitors of Tc80.

Several surface-exposed molecules on the host cell have been shown to be involved in the process of *T. cruzi*—host cell interaction. These include proteins/glycoproteins released by trypsin and/or neuraminidase, lectin-binding sites, and lectin-like molecules.[86,87] Galectin-3,[88] a β-galactosyl-binding lectin, is a type of lectin involved in *T. cruzi* attachment, and its binding has been suggested to mediate parasite attachment and entry into both dendritic cells and smooth muscle cells.[89] This molecule is recruited during parasite invasion of host cells and influences the intracellular trafficking of amastigotes.[84] Besides, Reignault and coworkers[90] demonstrated that galectin 3 is recruited to parasitophorous vacuole of *T. cruzi* and the in presence of galectin 3 this vacuole remains for 3 h, and may be involved in the lysis process. Another galectin that is involved in *T. cruzi* infection is galectin-1.[91] Galectin-1 not only reduced infection by *T. cruzi* but also diminished parasite phosphatidylserine exposure. Tc85, which is present in the *T. cruzi* membrane and has been associated with parasite invasion, contains fibronectin-like binding sequences[92] and a laminin-binding domain.[72] Besides functioning as a cellular link to laminin or fibronectin, integrins also function as receptors that can activate PI-3 kinase signaling pathways. Another host cell receptor utilized by trypomastigotes that trigger PI3K is LDL receptor.[93] Tc85 can bind to cytokeratin 18, a cytoskeletal protein that was suggested to function as a *T. cruzi* receptor.[86] However, when cytokeratin 18 expression was silenced by RNAi, the binding of trypomastigotes to host cells was not affected.[92] Another molecule present on the host cell surface and involved in trypomastigote entry is the TGFβ receptor. Signal transduction through TGF-β receptors facilitates *T. cruzi* entry into epithelial cells.[84,94] The trypomastigote molecule that is capable of binding to the TGFβ receptor has not yet been identified. Ming and colleagues[95] proposed that infective stages of *T. cruzi* secrete a TGFβ-like molecule or a factor capable of activating latent host TGFβ. The exposure of phosphatidylserine on the surface of *T. cruzi* trypomastigotes[96] and its deactivating effect on macrophages by the induction of TGFβ suggests that phosphatidylserine is a possible activator of host-cell TGFβ receptor.

## *Triggering of endocytosis*

Following binding to and recognition of the parasite by the host cell surface, a series of cell signaling processes takes place, which culminate in the invasion of the host cell. The available evidence indicates that the *T. cruzi* trypomastigotes use several mechanisms of invasion, including the following: (1) phagocytosis/macropinocytosis, an actin-mediated process in which the cells emit pseudopods. In professional phagocytes such as macrophages, the activation of tyrosine kinase proteins occurs, followed by the recruitment of PI-3 kinase and actin filaments (a process that has been associated with the mechanism of phagocytosis) at the trypomastigote entry site[97] (Fig. 18.14); (2) endocytosis, without the emission of pseudopods but with the participation of actin filaments; and (3) invagination of the membrane, without the participation of actin filaments. This latter process has been regarded as an active mechanism for parasite entry that wastes energy.[98]

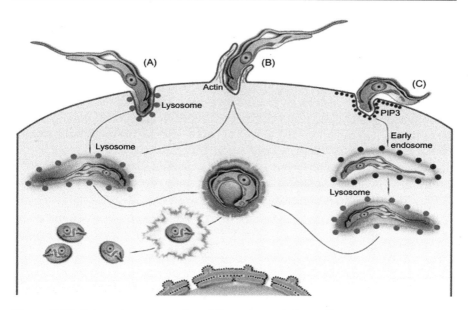

**Figure 18.14** Schematic representation of *T. cruzi* entry in host cells.

In the initial moments of the recognition between *T. cruzi* and the host cell, a transient increase of cytoplasmic levels of calcium occurs in both the parasite and the host cell.[3,99,100] If this transient increase in cytoplasmic calcium is blocked (by treatment with thapsigargin, for example), there is a reduction in parasite invasion.[101] Additionally, in nonprofessional phagocytic cells, there is a recruitment of lysosomes to the place of parasite invasion, although this phenomenon occurs in only about 20% of parasites that enter. Recently, Cortez and Yoshida[102] observed that the participation of lysosomes in the site of entry into host cells may be related to the origin of the trypomastigote used. When nonphagocytic host cells are deprived of nutrients, metacyclic trypomastigotes (released by the insect vector) recruit lysosomes to penetrate. Cultured trypomastigotes use a lysosome-independent pathway. This difference occurs primarily because metacyclic trypomastigotes stimulate the biogenesis/dispersion of lysosomes after gp82-mediated parasite adhesion to the host. The lysosome-dependent pathway is initiated by targeted $Ca^{2+}$-regulated exocytosis of lysosomes at the plasma membrane. Another pathway used for parasite internalization in nonphagocytic cells is the lysosome-independent pathway. In this model, parasites enter cells through plasma membrane invaginations that accumulate PIP3, the major product of class I PI3K activation. As a result of this mode of entry, around 50% of total internalized parasites are contained in vacuoles enriched in plasma membrane markers, and about 20% are in early endosomes (EEA1 labeled) at 10 min postinfection. In this case, the immature vacuole becomes filled with lysosomes within 60 min.[103] Several studies using host cells treated with cytochalasins D or B (agents that depolymerize actin filaments) before the process of interaction with trypomastigotes produced controversial data.

Some authors say that the treatment inhibits the entry of trypomastigote forms,[104–106] while others describe a sharp increase in entry,[107] and still others report almost no effect. Participation of actin cytoskeleton has been discussed in the retention of trypomastigotes in the cytoplasm of the host cell.[106,108,109] Woolsey and Burleigh described that cytochalasin-treated host cells showed a reduction in the number of parasites inside them, confirming earlier data[101] that showed a decrease in infection of cytochalasin pretreated host cells after 40 min of interaction with trypomastigotes.[14,105] More recently, Teixeira et al.[109] also demonstrated using amastigotes that actin participates in *T. cruzi* entry. This participation is followed by the accumulation of Arf6 and Anexin 2 around the parasitophorous vacuole. Actin is also involved in a process known as macropinocytosis. Recently, Barrias and coworkers[109] demonstrated that macropinocytosis is involved in *T. cruzi* entry, as rabankirin, PAK1, actin, and PI3K are recruited to the entry site of the parasite. In addition, host cell treatment with classic inhibitors of the macropinocytosis pathway impairs parasite entry. The entry of the trypomastigote activates signaling processes in the host cell and parasite that lead to parasite invasion. In professional phagocytes, tyrosine kinase activation and recruitment of PI-3 kinase and actin to the site of parasite entry also occur.[99,105]

Host cell plasma membrane microdomains were also shown to be involved in *T. cruzi* entry both in nonphagocytic and phagocytic cells.[111,112] Both groups demonstrated that cholesterol, major membrane raft components, and microdomain molecular markers like flotillin1 colocalize with *T. cruzi* entry site suggesting the microdomains' participation in internalization (Fig. 18.15).

Another mechanism involved in trypomastigote internalization into host cells is trogocytosis. Trogocytosis is a phenomenon involved in the bidirectional transfer of molecules between interacting cells or to cells to which the cell is conjugated via the exchange of plasma membrane fragments. The transferred membrane and associated molecules become part of the recipient cell.[113]

## *Lysis of the parasitophorous vacuole (PV) membrane*

A few hours after internalization, the trypomastigote gradually transforms into an amastigote via an epimastigote-like intermediate stage. In the PV, trypomastigotes release trans-sialidase/neuraminidase, which removes sialic acid residues from the PV membrane, making it sensitive to the action of Tc-Tox (a peptide that shares homology with human complement factor 9).[114] At the acidic pH of the PV, this molecule begins to destroy the PV membrane, possibly by pore formation[114,115] (Fig. 18.15).

Some authors refer to this process as "escape" of the parasite from the PV. Following this disruption, the amastigote then enters into direct contact with the host cell cytoplasm and starts a process of binary division.

After several cycles of intracellular division, the amastigotes start the process of transforming into trypomastigotes, which are subsequently released into the intercellular space. These trypomastigotes eventually reach the bloodstream and infect other cells.

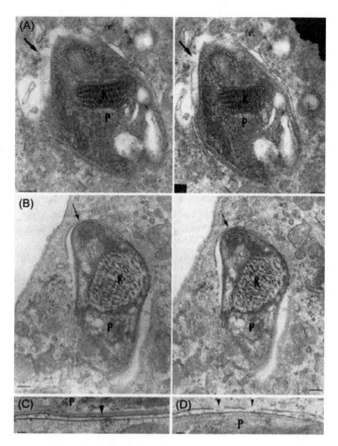

**Figure 18.15** Transmission electron microscopy (TEM) of thin sections of macrophages infected with trypomastigote forms of *T. cruzi*. Focal disruption of the membrane lining the vacuole is observed (arrows in A and B) and especially in C and D; K, kinetoplast; P, parasite. Bar, 1 μm. *Source*: After Carvalho and De Souza (1983).

# Acknowledgments

The author thanks several colleagues who have worked in his laboratory over the last 30 years and contributed with their work and enthusiasm to the progress of studies related to the cell biology of *T. cruzi* and its interaction with host cells. Their contributions are indicated in the legends of the figures used in this review.

# References

1. De Souza W. An introduction to the structural organization of parasitic protozoa. *Curr Pharm Des*. 2008;**14**:822−38.
2. De Souza W. Growth and transformation of *Trypanosoma cruzi*. In: Briggs AP, Coburn JA, editors. *Handbook of cell proliferation*. Nova Science Publishers; 2009.

3. Yoshida N. Molecular mechanisms of *Trypanosoma cruzi* infection by oral route. *Mem Inst Oswaldo Cruz* 2009;**104**:101−7.

4. Coura JR. Special issue on Chagas disease. *Mem Inst Oswaldo Cruz* 2009;**110** (3):275−6. Available from: http://dx.doi.org/10.1590/0074-0276150001.

5. Crane MS, Dvorak JA. *Trypanosoma cruzi*: interaction with vertebrate cells. DNA synthesis and growth of intracellular amastigotes and their relationship to host cell DNA synthesis and growth. *J Protozool* 1979;**26**(4):599−604.

6. De Souza W, Meyer H. An electron microscopic and cytochemical study of the cell coat of *Trypanosoma cruzi* in tissue cultures. *Z Parasitenkd* 1975;**46**(3):179−87.

7. Elias MC, Marques-Porto R, Freymuller E, Schenckman S. Transcription rate modulation through the *Trypanosoma cruzi* life cycle occurs in parallel with changes in nuclear organization. *Mol Biochem Parasitol* 2001;**112**:79−90.

8. Esponda P, Souto-Padrón T, De Souza W. Fine structure and cytochemistry of the nucleus and the kinetoplast of epimastigotes of *Trypanosoma cruzi*. *J Protozool* 1983;**30**(1):105−10.

9. Shapiro TA, Englund PT. The structure and replication of kinetoplast DNA. *Ann Rev Microbiol* 1995;**49**:117−43.

10. Fidalgo LM, Gille L. Mitochondria and trypanosomatids: targets and drugs. *Pharm Res* 2011;**28**(11):2758−70.

11. Povelones ML. Beyond replication: division and segregation of mitochondrial DNA in kinetoplastids. *Mol Biochem Parasitol* 2014;**196**:53−60.

12. Souto-Padron T, De Souza W, Heuser JE. Quick-freeze, deep-etch rotary replication of *Trypanosoma cruzi* and *Herpetomonas megaseliae*. *J Cell Sci* 1984;**69**:167−8.

13. Ogbadoiyi EO, Robinson DR, Gull K. A high-order trans-membrane structural linkage is responsible for mitochondrial genome positioning and segregation by flagellar basal bodies in trypanosomes. *Mol Biol Cell* 2003;**14**:1769−79.

14. Opperdoes FR. Compartmentalization of carbohydrate metabolism in trypanosomes. *Ann Rev Microbiol* 1987;**41**:127−51.

15. Opperdoes FR, Borst P. Localization of nine glycolytic enzymes in a microbody-like organelle in *Trypanosoma brucei*. *FEBS Lett* 1977;**80**:360−4.

16. Haanstra JR, Bakker BM, Michels PA. In or out? On the tightness of glycosomal compartmentalization of metabolites and enzymes in *Trypanosoma brucei*. *Mol Biochem Parasitol* 2014;**198**(1):18−28.

17. Opperdoes FR, Cotton D. Involvement of the glycosome of *Trypanosoma brucei* in carbon dioxide fixation. *FEBS Lett* 1982;**143**:60−4.

18. Haanstra JR, González-Marcano EB, Gualdrón-López M, Michels PA. Biogenesis, maintenance and dynamics of glycosomes in trypanosomatid parasites. *Biochim Biophys Acta* 2016;**1863**(5):1038−48.

19. Docampo R, De Souza W, Miranda K, Roheloff P, Moreno S. Acidocalcisomes - conserved from bacteria to man. *Nat Rev Microbiol* 2005;**3**:251−61.

20. Miranda K, Benchimol M, Docampo R, De Souza W. The fine structure of acidocalcisomes in *Trypanosoma cruzi*. *Parasitol Res* 2000;**86**:373−84.

21. Li FJ, He CY. Acidocalcisome is required for autophagy in *Trypanosoma brucei*. *Autophagy* 2014;**10**(11):1978−88.

22. Furuya T, Okura M, Ruiz FA, Scott DA, Docampo R. TcSCA complements yeast mutants defective in $Ca^{2+}$ pumps and encodes a $Ca^{2+}$-ATPase that localizes to the endoplasmic reticulum of *Trypanosoma cruzi*. *J Biol Chem* 2001;**276**(35):32437−45.

23. Niyogi S, Jimenez V, Girard-Dias W, de Souza W, Miranda K, Docampo R. Rab32 is essential for maintaining functional acidocalcisomes, and for growth and infectivity of *Trypanosoma cruzi*. *J Cell Sci* 2015;**128**:2363−73.

24. Linder JC, Staehelin LA. Plasma membrane specialization in a trypanosomatid flagellate. *J Ultrastruct Res* 1977;**60**:246−62.
25. Montalvetti A, Rohloff P, Docampo R. A functional aquaporin co-localizes with the vacuolar proton pyrophosphatase to acidocalcisomes and the contractile vacuole complex of *Trypanosoma cruzi*. *J Biol Chem* 2004;**279**:3867−82.
26. Rohloff P, Docampo R. A contractile vacuole complex is involved in osmoregulation in *Trypanosoma cruzi*. *Exp Parasitol* 2008;**118**:17−24.
27. Rohloff P, Montalvetti A, Docampo R. Acidocalcisomes and the contractile vacuole complex are involved in osmoregulation in *Trypanosoma cruzi*. *J Biol Chem.* 2004;**279**(50):52270−81.
28. Schoijet AC, Miranda K, Medeiros LC, de Souza W, Flawiá MM, Torres HN, et al. Defining the role of a FYVE domain in the localization and activity of a cAMP phosphodiesterase implicated in osmoregulation in *Trypanosoma cruzi*. *Mol Microbiol* 2011;**79**(1):50−62.
29. Ulrich PN, Jimenez V, Park M, Martins VP, Atwood III J, Moles K, et al. Identification of contractile vacuole proteins in *Trypanosoma cruzi*. *PLoS ONE* 2011;**6**(3):e18013.
30. Docampo R, Jimenez V, Lander N, Li ZH, Niyogi S. New insights into roles of acidocalcisomes and contractile vacuole complex in osmoregulation in protists. *Int Rev Cell Mol Biol* 2013;**305**:69−113.
31. Harris E, Yoshida K, Cardelli J, Bush J. Rab11-like GTPase associates with and regulates the structure and function of the contractilevacuole system in dictyostelium. *J Cell Sci* 2001;**114**(Pt 16):3035−45.
32. Girard-Dias W, Alcântara CL, Cunha-e-Silva N, de Souza W, Miranda K. On the ultrastructural organization of *Trypanosoma cruzi* using cryopreparation methods and electron tomography. *Histochem Cell Biol* 2012;**138**(6):821−31.
33. Pimenta PF, De Souza W. Fine structure and cytochemistry of the endoplasmic reticulum and its association with the plasma membrane of *Leishmania mexicana amazonensis*. *J Submicroscop Cytol* 1985;**17**:413−19.
34. Alcantara CL, Vidal JC, de Souza W, Cunha e Silva NL. The three-dimensional structure of the cytostome−cytopharinx complex of *Trypanosoma cruzi* epimastigotes. *J. Cell Sci* 2014;**127**:2227−37.
35. Corrêa JR, Atella GC, Menna-Barreto RS, Soares MJ. Clathrin in *Trypanosoma cruzi*: in silico gene identification, isolation, and localization of protein expression sites. *J Euk Microbiol* 2007;**54**:297−302.
36. Correa Corrêa JR, Atella GC, Batista MM, Soares M. Transferrin uptake in *Trypanosoma cruzi* is impaired by interference on cytostome-associated cytoskeleton elements and stability of membrane cholesterol, but not by obstruction of clathrin-dependent endocytosis. *Exp Parasitol* 2008;**119**:58−66.
37. De Melo LD, Sant'Anna C, Reis SA, Lourenço D, De Souza W, Lopes UG, et al. Evolutionary conservation of actin-binding proteins in *Trypanosoma cruzi* and unusual subcellular localization of the actin homologue. *Parasitology* 2008;**135**:955−65.
38. Cevallos AM, Segura-Kato YX, Merchant-Larios H, Manning-Cela R, Alberto Hernández-Osorio L, Márquez-Dueñas C, et al. *Trypanosoma cruzi*: multiple actin isovariants are observed along different developmental stages. *Exp Parasitol.* 2010;**127**(1):249−59.
39. Landfear SM, Tran KD, Sanchez MA. Flagellar membrane proteins in kinetoplastid parasites. *IUBMB Life* 2015;**67**:668−76.
40. Farina M, Attias M, Souto-Padron T, De Souza W. Further studies on the organization of the paraxial rod of trypanosomatids. *J Protozool* 1986;**33**:552−7.
41. Bastin P, Gull K. Assembly and function of complex flagellar structures illustrated by the paraflagellar rod of trypanosomes. *Protist* 1999;**150**:113−23.

42. Lander N, Li ZH, Niyogi S, Docampo R. CRISPR/Cas9-induced disruption of parafla-gellar rod protein 1 and 2 genes in *Trypanosoma cruzi* reveals their role in flagellar attachment. *MBio* 2015;**6**(4):e01012 21.

43. Rocha GM, Miranda K, Weissmuller G, Bisch PM, De Souza W. Ultrastructure of *Trypanosoma cruzi* revisited by atomic force microscopy. *Mic Res Tech* 2007;**71**:133−9.

44. Florimond C, Sahin A, Vidiiaseris K, Dong G, Landrein N, Dacheux D, et al. BILBO1 is a scaffold protein of the flagellar pocket collar in the pathogen *Trypanosoma brucei*. *PLoS Pathol* 2015. Available from: http://dx.doi.org/10.1371/journal.ppat.1004654.

45. Field MC, Carrington M. The trypanosome flagellar pocket. *Nat Rev Microbiol* 2009;**7**:775−86.

46. Araripe JR, Ramos FP, Cunha e Silva NL, Urmenyi TP, Silva R, Leite Fontes CF, et al. Characterization of a RAB5 homologue in *Trypanosoma cruzi*. *Biochem Biophys Res Commun* 2005;**329**:638−45.

47. Bayer-Santos E, Cunha-e-Silva NL, Yoshida N, Franco da Silveira J. Expression and cellular trafficking of GP82 and GP90 glycoproteins during *Trypanosoma cruzi* metacy-clogenesis. *Parasit Vectors* 2013;**6**:127.

48. Neves RF, Fernandes AC, Meyer-Fernandes JR, Souto-Padrón T. *Trypanosoma cruzi*-secreted vesicles have acid and alkaline phosphatase activities capable of increasing par-asite adhesion and infection. *Parasitol Res* 2014;**113**(8):2961−72.

49. Pereira MG, Visbal G, Salgado LT, Vidal JC, Godinho JLP, De Cicco NNT, et al. *Trypanosoma cruzi* epimastigotes are able to manage internal cholesterol levels under nutritional lipid stress conditions. *PLoS ONE* 2015;**10**(6).e0128949. Available from: http://dx.doi.org/10.1371/journal.pone.0128949.

50. Nogueira PM, Ribeiro K, Silveira AC, Campos JH, Martins-Filho OA, Bela SR, et al. Vesicles from different *Trypanosoma cruzi* strains trigger differential innate and chronic immune responses. *J Extracell Vesicles* 2015;**4**:28734.

51. Vickerman K. On the surface coat and flagellar adhesion in trypanosomes. *J Cell Sci* 1969;**5**:163−93.

52. Vieira M, Rohloff P, Luo S, Cunha-e-Silva NL, de Souza W, Docampo R. Role for a P-type H + -ATPase in the acidification of the endocytic pathway of *Trypanosoma cruzi*. *Biochem J* 2005;**392**:467−74.

53. Soares MJ, Souto-Padron T, De Souza W. Identification of a large pre-lysosomal com-partment in the pathogenic protozoon *Trypanosoma cruzi*. *J Cell Sci* 1992;**102**:157−67.

54. Sant'Anna C, Parussini F, Lourenço D, de Souza W, Cazzulo JJ, Cunha-E-Silva NL. All *Trypanosoma cruzi* developmental forms present lysosome-related organelles. *Histochem Cell Biol* 2008;**130**:1187−98.

55. Seto E, Onizuka Y, Nakajima-Shimada J. Host cytoplasmic processing bodies assembled by *Trypanosoma cruzi* during infection exert anti-parasitic activity. *Parasitol Int* 2015;**64**(6):540−6.

56. Martinez-Palomo A, De Souza W, Gonzales-Robles A. Topographical differences in the distribution of surface coat components and intramembranous particles. A cytochemical and freeze-fracture study in culture forms of *Trypanosoma cruzi*. *J Cell Biol* 1976;**69**:507−13.

57. De Souza W, Martinez-Palomo A, Gonzáles-Robles A. The cell surface of *Trypanosoma cruzi*: cytochemistry and freeze-fracture. *J Cell Sci* 1978;**33**:285−99.

58. Rocha GM, Brandao BA, Mortara RA, Attias M, De Souza W, Carvalho TM. The fla-gellar attachment zone of *Trypanosoma cruzi* epimastigote forms. *J Struct Biol* 2006;**154**:89−99.

59. Souto-Padrón T, De Souza W. Cytochemical analysis at the fine-structural level of try-panosomatids stained with phosphotungstic acid. *J Protozool* 1979;**26**:551−7.

60. Weatherly DB, Boehlke C, Tarleton RL. Chromosome level assembly of the hybrid Trypanosoma cruzi genome. *BMC Genomics* 2009;**10**:255.
61. Souto-Padron T, Campetella OE, Cazzulo JJ, de Souza W. Cysteine proteinase in *Trypanosoma cruzi*: immunocytochemical localization and involvement in parasite-host cell interaction. *J Cell Sci* 1990;**96**:485–90.
62. Dorta ML, Ferreira AT, Oshiro ME, Yoshida N. $Ca^{2+}$ signal induced by *Trypanosoma cruzi* metacyclic trypomastigote surface molecules implicated in mammalian cell invasion. *Mol Biochem Parasitol* 1995;**73**(1–2):285–9.
63. Yoshida N. Molecular basis of mammalian cell invasion by *Trypanosoma cruzi*. *Ann Acad Bras Cienc* 2006;**78**:87–111.
64. Villalta F, Kierszenbaum F. Host cell invasion by *Trypanosoma cruzi*: role of cell surface galactose residues. *Biochem Biophys Res Commun* 1984;**119**:228–35.
65. Yoshida N, Mortara RA, Araguth MF, Gonzalez JC, Russo M. Metacyclic neutralizing effect of monoclonal antibody 10D8 directed to the 35- and 50-kilodalton surface glycoconjugates of *Trypanosoma cruzi*. *Infect Immun* 1989;**57**:1663–7.
66. Di Noia JM, Sánchez DO, Frasch AC. The protozoan *Trypanosoma cruzi* has a family of genes resembling the mucin genes of mammalian cells. *J Biol Chem* 1995;**270**(41):24146–9.
67. Buscaglia CA, Campo VA, Frasch AC, Di Noia JM. *Trypanosoma cruzi* surface mucins: host-dependent coat diversity. *Nat Rev Microbiol* 2006;**4**:229–36.
68. Abuin G, Colli W, de Souza W, Alves MJ. A surface antigen of *Trypanosoma cruzi* involved in cell invasion (Tc-85) is heterogeneous in expression and molecular constitution. *Mol Biochem Parasitol* 1989;**35**:229–37.
69. Katzin AM, Colli W. Lectin receptors in *Trypanosoma cruzi*. An *N*-acetyl-D-glucosamine-containing surface glycoprotein specific for the trypomastigote stage. *Biochim Biophys Acta* 1983;**727**:403–11.
70. Giordano R, Chammas R, Veiga SS, Colli W, Alves MJ. *Trypanosoma cruzi* binds to laminin in a carbohydrate-independent way. *Braz J Med Biol Res* 1994;**27**:2315–18.
71. Andrews NW, Katzin AM, Colli W. Mapping of surface glycoproteins of *Trypanosoma cruzi* by two-dimensional electrophoresis. A correlation with the cell invasion capacity. *Eur J Biochem* 1984;**140**:599–604.
72. Giordano R, Fouts DL, Tewari D, Colli W, Manning JE, Alves MJ. Cloning of a surface membrane glycoprotein specific for the infective form of *Trypanosoma cruzi* having adhesive properties to laminin. *J Biol Chem* 1999;**274**:3461–8.
73. Ouaissi MA, Cornette J, Afchain D, Capron A, Gras-Masse H, Tartar A. *Trypanosoma cruzi* infection inhibited by peptides modeled from a fibronectin cell attachment domain. *Science* 1986;**234**:603–7.
74. Teixeira MM, Yoshida N. Stage-specific surface antigens of metacyclic trypomastigotes of *Trypanosoma cruzi* identified by monoclonal antibodies. *Mol Biochem Parasitol* 1986;**18**:271–82.
75. Favoreto S, Dorta ML, Yoshida N. *Trypanosoma cruzi* 175-kDa protein tyrosine phosphorylation is associated with host cell invasion; 1998.
76. Yoshida N, Cortez M. *Trypanosoma cruzi*: parasite and host cell signaling during the invasion process. *Subcell Biochem* 2008;**47**:82–91.
77. Cazzulo JJ, Franke MC, Martinez J, Franke de Cazullo BM. Some kinetic properties of a cysteine proteinase (cruzipain) from *Trypanosoma cruzi*. *Biochim Biophys Acta* 1990;**1037**:186–91.
78. Lima MF, Villalta F. Host-cell attachment by *Trypanosoma cruzi*: identification of an adhesion molecule. *Biochem Biophys Res Commun* 1988;**155**:256–62.

79. Villalta F, Madison MN, Kleshchenko YY, Nde PN, Lima MF. Molecular analysis of early host cell infection by *Trypanosoma cruzi*. *Front Biosci* 2008;**13**:3714—34.

80. Villalta F, Lima MF, Ruiz-Ruano A, Zhou L. Attachment of *Trypanosoma cruzi* to host cells: a monoclonal antibody recognizes a trypomastigote stage-specific epitope on the gp 83 required for parasite attachment. *Biochem Biophys Res Commun* 1992;**182**:6—13.

81. Burleigh BA, Andrews NW. A 120-kDa alkaline peptidase from *Trypanosoma cruzi* is involved in the generation of a novel Ca$^{2+}$-signaling factor for mammalian cells. *J Biol Chem* 1995;**270**:5172—80.

82. Burleigh BA, Caler EV, Webster P, Andrews NW. A cytosolic serine endopeptidase from *Trypanosoma cruzi* is required for the generation of Ca$^{2+}$ signaling in mammalian cells. *J Cell Biol* 1997;**136**:609—20.

83. Burleigh BA, Woolsey AM. Cell signalling and *Trypanosoma cruzi* invasion. *Cell Microbiol* 2002;**4**:701—11.

84. Santana JM, Grellier P, Schrével J, Teixeira ARA. *Trypanosoma cruzi*-secreted 80 kDa proteinase with specificity for human collagen types I and IV. *Biochem J.* 1997;**325**:129—37.

85. Grellier P, Vendeville S, Joyeau R, Bastos IM, Drobecq H, Frappier F, et al. *Trypanosoma cruzi* prolyl oligopeptidase Tc80 is involved in nonphagocytic mammalian cell invasion by trypomastigotes. *J Biol Chem* 2001;**276**:47078—86.

86. Magdesian MH, Giordano R, Ulrich H, Juliano MA, Juliano L, Schumacher RI, et al. Infection by *Trypanosoma cruzi*. Identification of a parasite ligand and its host cell receptor. *J Biol Chem* 2001;**276**:19382—9.

87. Scharfstein J, Morrot A. A role for extracellular amastigotes in the immunopathology of Chagas disease. *Mem Inst Oswaldo Cruz* 1999;**94**:51—63.

88. Vray B, Camby I, Vercruysse V, Mijatovic T, Bovin NV, Ricciardi-Castagnoli P, et al. Up-regulation of galectin-3 and its ligands by *Trypanosoma cruzi* infection with modulation of adhesion and migration of murine dendritic cells. *Glycobiology* 2004;**14**:647—57.

89. Kleshchenko YY, Moody TN, Furtak VA, Ochieng J, Lima MF, Villalta F. Human galectin-3 promotes *Trypanosoma cruzi* adhesion to human coronary artery smooth muscle cells. *Infect Immun* 2004;**72**:6717—21.

90. Ochatt CM, Ulloa RM, Torres HN, Téllez-Iñón MT. Characterization of the catalytic subunit of *Trypanosoma cruzi* cyclic AMP-dependent protein kinase. *Mol Biochem Parasitol* 1993;**57**:73—81.

91. Nogueira N, Cohn Z. *Trypanosoma cruzi*: mechanism of entry and intracellular fate in mammalian cells. *J Exp Med* 1976;**143**:1402—20.

92. Claser C, Curcio M, de Mello SM, Silveira EV, Monteiro HP, Rodrigues MM. Silencing cytokeratin 18 gene inhibits intracellular replication of *Trypanosoma cruzi* in HeLa cells but not binding and invasion of trypanosomes. *BMC Cell Biol* 2008;**17**:68.

93. Weinkauf C, Pereira-Perrin M. *Trypanosoma cruzi* promotes neuronal and glial cell survival through the neurotrophic receptor TrkC. *Infect Immun* 2009;**77**:1368—75.

94. Hall BS, Pereira MA. Dual role for transforming growth factor beta-dependent signaling in *Trypanosoma cruzi* infection of mammalian cells. *Infect Immun* 2000;**68**:2077—81.

95. Ming M, Ewen ME, Pereira ME. Trypanosome invasion of mammalian cells requires activation of the TGF beta signaling pathway. *Cell* 1995;**82**:287—96.

96. Kipnis TL, Calich VL, da Silva WD. Active entry of bloodstream forms of *Trypanosoma cruzi* into macrophages. *Parasitology* 1979;**8**:89—98.

97. Vieira M, Dutra JM, Carvalho TM, Cunha-e-Silva NL, Souto-Padrón T, Souza W. Cellular signaling during the macrophage invasion by *Trypanosoma cruzi*. *Histochem Cell Biol* 2002;**118**:491—500.

98. Schenkman S, Mortara RA. HeLa cells extend and internalize pseudopodia during active invasion by *Trypanosoma cruzi* trypomastigotes. *J Cell Sci* 1992;**101**:895—905.

99. Wilkowsky SE, Wainszelbaum MJ, Isola EL. *Trypanosoma cruzi*: participation of intra-cellular $Ca^{2+}$ during metacyclic trypomastigote−macrophage interaction. *Biochem Biophys Res Commun* 1996;**222**:386−9.

100. Garzoni LR, Masuda MO, Capella MM, Lopes AG, de Meirelles Mde N. Characterization of $[Ca^{2+}]_i$ responses in primary cultures of mouse cardiomyocytes induced by *Trypanosoma cruzi* trypomastigotes. *Mem Inst Oswaldo Cruz* 2003;**98**:487−93.

101. Rodríguez A, Rioult MG, Ora A, Andrews NW. A trypanosome-soluble factor induces IP3 formation, intracellular Ca2 + mobilization and microfilament rearrangement in host cells. *J Cell Biol* 1995;**129**(5):1263−73.

102. Cortez MR, Pinho AP, Cuervo P, Alfaro F, Solano M, Xavier SC, et al. *Trypanosoma cruzi* (Kinetoplastida Trypanosomatidae): ecology of the transmission cycle in the wild environment of the Andean valley of Cochabamba, Bolivia. *Exp Parasitol* 2006;**114**:305−13.

103. Burleigh B. Host cell signaling and *Trypanosoma cruzi* invasion: do all roads leads to lysosome? *Sci STKE* 2005;**293**:36.

104. de Meirelles MN, de Araújo Jorge TC, de Souza W. Interaction of *Trypanosoma cruzi* with macrophages *in vitro*: dissociation of the attachment and internalization phases by low temperature and cytochalasin B. *Z Parasitenkd* 1982;**68**:7−14.

105. Barbosa HS, Meirelles MN. Evidence of participation of cytoskeleton of heart muscle cells during the invasion of *Trypanosoma cruzi*. *Cell Struct Funct* 1995;**20**:275−84.

106. Rosestolato CT, Dutra Jda M, De Souza W, de Carvalho TM. Participation of host cell actin filaments during interaction of trypomastigote forms of *Trypanosoma cruzi* with host cells. *Cell Struct Funct* 2002;**27**:91−8.

107. Tardieux I, Nathanson MH, Andrews NW. Role in host cell invasion of *Trypanosoma cruzi*-induced cytosolic-free $Ca^{2+}$ transients. *J Exp Med* 1994;**179**:1017−22.

108. Woolsey AM, Burleigh BA. Host cell actin polymerization is required for cellular retention of *Trypanosoma cruzi* and early association with endosomal/lysosomal compartments. *Cell Microbiol* 2004;**6**:829−38.

109. Barrias ES, Reignault LC, De Souza W, Carvalho TM. *Trypanosoma cruzi* uses macropinocytosis as an additional entry pathway into mammalian host cell. *Microbes Infect* 2012;**14**(14):1340−51.

110. Ley V, Robbins ES, Nussenzweig V, Andrews NW. The exit of *Trypanosoma cruzi* from the phagosome is inhibited by raising the pH of acidic compartments. *J Exp Med* 1990;**171**:401−13.

111. Barrias ES, Dutra JM, De Souza W, Carvalho TM. Participation of macrophage membrane rafts in *Trypanosoma cruzi* invasion process. *Biochem Biophys Res Commun* 2007;**363**:828−34.

112. Fernandes MC, Cortez M, Geraldo Yoneyama KA, Straus AH, Yoshida N, Mortara RA. Novel strategy in *Trypanosoma cruzi* cell invasion: implication of cholesterol and host cell microdomains. *Int J Parasitol* 2007;**37**:1431−41.

113. Hall BF, Furtado GC, Joiner KA. Characterization of host cell-derived membrane proteins of the vacuole surrounding different intracellular forms of *Trypanosoma cruzi* in J774 cells. Evidence for phagocyte receptor sorting during the early stages of parasite entry. *J Immunol* 1991;**147**:4313−21.

114. Andrews NW, Abrams CK, Slatin SL, Griffiths G. A *T. cruzi*-secreted protein immunologically related to the complement component C9: evidence for membrane pore-forming activity at low pH. *Cell* 1990;**61**:1277−87.

115. Carvalho TMU, De Souza W. Early events related with the behavior of *Trypanosoma cruzi* within an endocytic vacuole in mouse peritoneal macrophages. *Cell Struct Funct* 1989;**14**:383−92.

# Genetics of *Trypanosoma cruzi*

# 19

D.C. Bartholomeu[1], S.M.R. Teixeira[2] and N.M.A. El-Sayed[3]

[1]University of Minas Gerais, Belo Horizonte, MG, Brazil, [2]Federal University
of Minas Gerais, Belo Horizonte, MG, Brazil, [3]University of Maryland, College Park,
MD, United States

## Chapter Outline

# Nuclear genome

## Sequencing of the CL Brener reference strain—a historical perspective

In April 1994, an international group of parasitologists along with representatives
of the World Health Organization met in Rio de Janeiro, Brazil, to discuss the initiation of efforts towards the sequencing of the genome of several human parasites,
among them *Trypanosoma cruzi*. The clone CL Brener was selected as the reference
strain for sequencing since it is well characterized biologically. This clone, isolated
by Professors Brener and Pereira (Centro de Pesquisa René Rachou, Fiocruz, Belo
Horizonte, Brazil) presents important *T. cruzi* characteristics: (1) it was isolated

American Trypanosomiasis Chagas Disease. DOI: http://dx.doi.org/10.1016/B978-0-12-801029-7.00019-8

from the domiciliary vector *Triatoma infestans*; (2) its pattern of infectivity in mice is very well known; (3) it has preferential tropism for heart and muscle cells; (4) it shows a clear acute phase in accidentally infected humans; and (5) it is susceptible to drugs used clinically in Chagas disease.[1] Because funds were limited at the time, initial priorities were set to generate karyotype data, physical maps and EST sequences.[2–6] These activities were distributed among approximately 20 laboratories in 15 countries. In 1999, additional funds were obtained from the National Institutes of Allergy and Infectious Diseases/National Institutes of Health (NIAID/NIH) by a consortium formed by three genome centers, The Institute for Genomic Research (Rockville, USA), the Seattle Biomedical Research Institute (Seattle, USA), and Karolinska Institute (Stockholm, Sweden), which allowed deciphering the nuclear genome of the parasite. Approximately 80 researchers from 14 countries contributed to the data analysis that was published[7] in 2005 along with the *Trypanosoma brucei*[8] and *Leishmania major*[9] genomes and a comparative analysis of the genome architecture of the three parasites.[10] The genome information is central for a better understanding of the biology of these parasites and will hopefully aid in the translation of basic research into clinical therapies.

## Sequencing strategy, genome organization, and content

The CL Brener strain is a representative of the *T. cruzi* hybrid lineage VI.[11] The parasite genome is diploid, but displays a high degree of polymorphism between homologous chromosomes. Also, heterologous chromosomes may have similar sizes and triploidy has been reported.[4,12,13] In addition to its hybrid nature,[14–16] CL Brener remains one of the most repetitive parasite genomes sequenced to date, with a repeat content close to 50%. The genome consortium's choice of sequencing strategy was constrained. The high complexity of the *T. cruzi* molecular karyotype precluded the use of a whole chromosome shotgun (WCS) approach and the high repeat content complicated the bacterial artificial chromosome (BAC) "map-as-you-go" clone-by-clone strategy in the early stages of the project. A whole genome shotgun (WGS) strategy was finally adopted. As expected, the high level of allelic variation between the CL Brener haplotypes and the overall repeat content made the genome assembly quite challenging. Long repeats are problematic because genome assemblers cannot differentiate true reads overlaps from those caused by repeats. In addition, typical assemblers are not able to handle highly polymorphic genomes. Ambiguities derived from allelic variations need to be discriminated from sequencing errors. This is possible because base-calling errors are frequently associated with low quality values and are not confirmed by other reads. Highly polymorphic genomes, however, require much higher level of sequence coverage to ensure these inferences are reliable. In the case of *T. cruzi*, 14× coverage was achieved. The assembly of this polymorphic genome generated a redundant dataset. This is because homologous regions displaying high level of polymorphism were assembled separately, hence generating sets of contigs corresponding to each haplotype.

Based on sequence coverage in CL Brener genomic regions represented by the two haplotypes, it was estimated that the diploid genome is around 106–110 Mb.[7]

The genome assembly resulted in 67 Mb, represented by 5489 scaffolds containing 8740 contigs. Of these, 60.4 Mb were used as substrate for gene finding and the downstream analysis such as annotation; this is because contigs in scaffolds smaller than 5 kb or contigs not incorporated into scaffolds and smaller than 5 kb were excluded. The rationale behind excluding this dataset was that its fragmented nature would hamper the gene prediction. Nevertheless, a large proportion of nonannotated sequences correspond to long, near identical segmental duplications, including non-coding sequences and members of nonpolymorphic multigene families organized in tandem which were collapsed and/or misassembled.[7,17] For instance, the *T. cruzi* 195-bp satellite DNA is the most abundant repetitive DNA sequence of the parasite.[18] Copies of this repetitive element can be duplicated as tandem arrays of ~30 kb.[19] By analyzing CL Brener individual reads, it was estimated that this repeat corresponds to approximately 5% of the CL Brener genome, but it represents only 0.09% of the annotated dataset, indicating that a large number of satellite copies were not incorporated into the assembled data.[20] It is important to emphasize that the nonannotated dataset and the individual reads are also available in Genbank and should always be analyzed before strong statements regarding gene content are made.

To be able to distinguish the two haplotypes, postassembly sequence comparisons with sequences from a representative of the parental subgroup IIb (Esmeraldo strain) were performed.[7] Approximately 120 Mb of Esmeraldo sequences (2.5× genome coverage) were generated and compared with CL Brener annotated contigs, which were then classified into the following categories: (1) similar to the Esmeraldo haplotype (lineage IIb); (2) dissimilar to Esmeraldo haplotype; (3) homozygous or haploid regions; (4) repetitive regions; and (5) merged regions. When an Esmeraldo read matched exactly two contigs, the contig region that displayed higher identity match with the Esmeraldo read was classified as Esmeraldo-like haplotype and the corresponding region of the other contig was classified as non-Esmeraldo haplotype. Regions where the Esmeraldo reads matched only a single contig were considered to represent haploid regions corresponding to the IIb parent, if the coverage and/or single nucleotide polymorphism (SNP) density was low. On the other hand, if the coverage and/or SNP density was high, these regions were classified as homozygous or heterozygous regions with very similar sequence that had merged during assembly. Conversely, contigs showing no match to Esmeraldo reads (or matches covering less than 90% of the Esmeraldo read) were presumed to represent haploid regions from the non-Esmeraldo-like haplotype, although they may represent unsampled regions of the Esmeraldo because of low sequence coverage. When the Esmeraldo reads matched three or more contigs, the corresponding regions were classified as repetitive. Around 50.5% of the annotated dataset corresponds to heterozygous regions (Esmeraldo-like or non-Esmeraldo-like haplotype), 37.2% to repeats not merged, 9% to merged sequences (repeats and homozygous regions), and 3.3% to haploid regions.

The two haplotypes display high levels of gene synteny, with most differences due to insertion/deletions in intergenic and subtelomeric regions and/or amplification of repetitive sequences. The average sequence divergence between the two CL

Brener haplotypes is 5.4%. As expected, this value is smaller when comparing the Esmeraldo-like haplotype and Esmeraldo reads (2.5%) and larger when comparing the non-Esmeraldo-like haplotype and Esmeraldo reads (6.5%). Pairs of alleles were identified for approximately half of the CL Brener genes. The average divergence between the coding regions of CL Brener genes is 2.2% (vs 5.4% overall difference), indicating that the large difference between the two haplotypes is due to polymorphism in the intercoding regions. The haplotype classification for each single CL Brener gene based on the type of match with Esmeraldo reads is available through Genbank and Tritryp database (www.tritryp.org).

The initial annotated genome dataset corresponded to 838 scaffolds, built from 4008 contigs and totaling 60.4 Mbases. The diploid genome contains ~23,000 genes, with more than 50% of the genome consisting of repeated sequences. Those include retrotransposons and members of large multigene families encoding surface proteins such as the trans-sialidases (TS) superfamily, mucins, the surface glycoprotein 63 proteases (gp63), and a novel family of about 1400 mucin-associated surface protein (MASP) genes.[7,21] These gene families are mostly *T. cruzi*-specific, account for one fifth of the total protein-coding genes and occur in dispersed clusters of tandem and interspersed repeats. Putative functions were assigned to approximately 50.8% of the annotated protein-coding genes, based on significant sequence similarities with previously characterized proteins and/or the presence of functional domains. All datasets and genome annotations continue to be available through GeneDB (www.genedb.org) and TriTryp database (www.tritryp.org).

# Comparative genome sequencing and analyses

## Comparative genome analysis with other trypanosomatids

The simultaneous availability of the complete genome sequences of two other trypanosomatids, *T. brucei*[8] and *L. major*,[9] allowed comparisons of the gene content and genome architecture of the three parasites and a better understanding of the genetic and evolutionary bases of the shared and distinct parasitic modes and lifestyles of these pathogens. These analyses revealed that the three genomes display striking synteny (Fig. 19.1) and share a conserved core of ~6200 genes, 94% of which are arranged in syntenic directional gene clusters.[10] An amino acid alignment of a large subset of the three-way clusters of orthologous genes (COGs) revealed an average 57% identity between *T. cruzi* and *T. brucei*, and 44% identity between *T. cruzi* and *L. major*, reflecting the expected phylogenetic relationships.[22-25] Most species-specific genes—of which *T. cruzi* (32%) and *T. brucei* (26%) have a much greater proportion than *L. major* (12%)—were found to occur at nonsyntenic chromosome (internal and subtelomeric) regions and consisted of members of large surface antigen families. Retroelements, structural RNAs, and gene family expansion are often associated with breaks in conservation of gene synteny, which, along with gene divergence, acquisition and loss, and rearrangements within syntenic regions, have shaped the genomes of each parasite.[10]

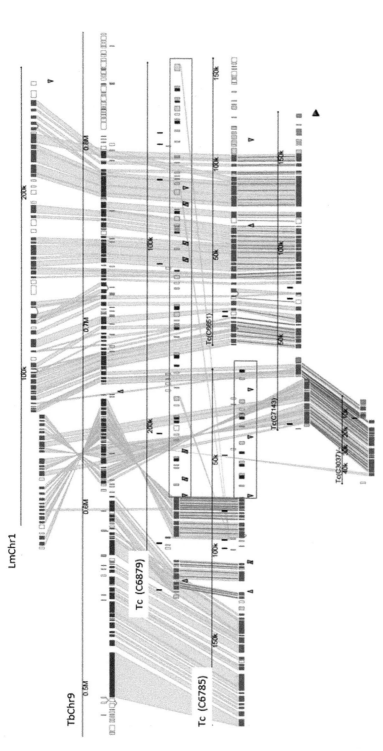

**Figure 19.1** Comparative architecture of *T. cruzi* CL Brener haplotypes (Tc), *T. brucei* (Tb) and *L. major* (Lm) genomes. Lm chromosome 1 was selected as reference to illustrate the organization of the three genomes and their striking degree of synteny. Lm, Tb, and Tc genes are colored in red, purple, and blue, respectively. Gray lines link genes that belong to the same cluster of orthologous genes (COGs). Genes colored in white represent singletons, while those in gray belong to COGs that are not shown. Yellow and black rectangles represent retrotransposons and telomeric repeats, respectively. Blue lines link pair of alleles of each CL Brener haplotype. Tc colored genes represent surface protein-coding genes. Tc arrays of surface protein genes are boxed in red. Tc scaffolds are labeled with the last digits of a unique identifier (10470535 1xxxx).

Compared with the other two trypanosomatids, a remarkable feature of the *T. cruzi* genome is the extensive expansion of species-specific genes, the large majority encoding surface proteins, such as trans-sialidase superfamily, mucin-associated surface proteins, mucins TcMUC, GP63, among others, all of them involved in important host—parasite interactions.[10] The *T. cruzi* surface protein-encoding genes are often clustered into large arrays that can be as large as 600 kb, preferentially associated with large chromosomes.[21,26-28] The available data clearly demonstrates that the clusters of surface proteins are internal in the chromosomes at regions of synteny breaks with *T. brucei* and *L. major* (Fig. 19.1). The synteny breaks of the hybrid CL Brener at the arrays of surface protein genes (Fig. 19.1), suggests that these regions are or were subject to intense rearrangements during the parasite's evolution.[7,21] It is likely therefore that much of the striking polymorphism among the *T. cruzi* isolates that is reflected in several epidemiological and pathological aspects of Chagas disease maybe in part due to variability within these regions (Fig. 19.2).

More recently, the genome of Sylvio X10/1, a nonhybrid strain belonging to *T. cruzi* I DTU and highly divergent from TcVI, was sequenced. TcI is the

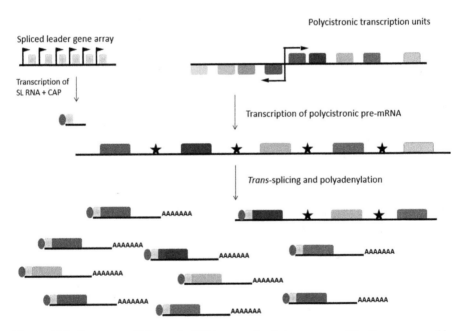

**Figure 19.2** Gene transcription and mRNA processing in trypanosomatids. Genes arranged in the genome as polycistronic transcription units are transcribed into polycistronic pre-mRNAs that are processed by *trans*-splicing and polyadenylation reactions. Capped, spliced leader RNAs are transcribed from the SL gene cluster. Polypyrimidine tracts present in intergenic regions (represented by stars) guide the insertion of a capped-SL sequence at 5′ end and the polyA tail at the 3′ end of transcripts, generating monocistronic mature mRNAs that accumulate at different levels in the cytoplasm.

predominant agent of Chagas disease in the North Amazon region, although generally less pathogenic to humans, and is found in a larger number of reservoirs compared to TcVI.[29] In agreement with the comparative analysis of the two CL Brener haplotypes,[7] the core genomes of Sylvio X10/1 and CL Brener are highly similar and the differences in terms of gene content are almost exclusively restricted to the cluster of genes encoding surface proteins. In the Sylvio genome, several multigene families, such as DGF, mucins, MASP, and GP63, contain fewer copy numbers compared to CL Brener genome.[29] The larger repertoire of genes encoding surface proteins in CL Brener genome may at least in part be related to its hybrid nature. Because surface protein-encoding genes are often clustered into large haploid polymorphic arrays in the hybrid CL Brener genome, the reduction of these regions to a diploid condition after the hybridization event may not have happened and/or may be driven by distinct mechanisms from those acting on the core conserved genomic regions. Improved assembly resolution of hybrid and nonhybrid *T. cruzi* genomes using third-generation single molecule sequencing will allow investigating the implications of hybridization events on genomic organization and architecture of the parasite.

Comparative genomic analysis of TcVI (CL Brener) and TcI (Sylvio X10/1) reinforces the notion that surface protein-encoding genes are a major source of genomic variability among *T. cruzi* isolates. Sequencing a larger number of *T. cruzi* strains belonging to distinct lineages will allow a better assessment of the role and pattern of diversification of these gene families and may disclose other parasite related factors associated to the wide range of virulence patterns and pathologies found within the *T. cruzi* lineages (see chapter: Experimental and Natural Recombination in *Trypanosoma cruzi*).

The recent genome sequencing of other Trypanosomatid species, including the mammalian nonpathogenic *Trypanosoma rangeli*,[30] the bat parasite *Trypanosoma cruzi marinkellei*,[31] and the monoxenic insect parasites *Angomonas deanei* and *Strigomonas culicis*,[32] has contributed to the identification of parasite factors that may be related to the distinct lifestyle adopted by each parasite. Although these studies further confirmed the conservation of the core proteome among Trypanosomatids, some genomic features shared by parasites unable to establish a productive infection in mammals and several species-specific factors were identified. For instance, the genetic basis of the nonpathogenic nature of *T. rangeli* in mammals may be related to the reduced expansion of multigene families encoding key players in host—parasite interaction mechanisms such as MASPs, trans-sialidases and mucins. Also, *T. rangeli* has a smaller number of antioxidant defense enzymes, in agreement with its high susceptibility to oxidative stress.[30] *Trypanosoma cruzi marinkellei* is a subspecies of *T. cruzi*, which infects bats, but no other mammalian host. Comparative genomic analysis of *T. c. marinkellei* and *T. c. cruzi* Sylvio X10 also revealed a reduction in the copy number of the majority of surface protein-encoding genes. Furthermore, retroelements such as VIPER and L1Tc, which are believed to be involved in genome plasticity and therefore may favor the generation of sequence variability, are also reduced in the *T. c. marinkellei* genome.[31] Sequence analysis of *Angomonas deanei* and *Strigomonas culicis*, both monoxenic parasites unable to infect mammals, revealed the absence of mucin-like glycoprotein and trans-sialidase genes.[32] A common pattern clearly emerging from these distinct comparative genomic studies is the absence/reduction of the repertoire of genes encoding surface proteins in the genomes of parasites that are avirulent to mammals, highlighting the importance of these proteins in the parasite interactions with their hosts.

Comparative genomics among Trypanosomatids that have distinct modes of life may also shed light into other aspects of the biology of these parasites, such as intracellular parasitism. An analysis was performed on all predicted protein-coding sequences from 15 Trypanosomatid genomes divided in two groups of parasites based on their ability to invade and survive inside host cells.[33] The analysis of genes present exclusively in intracellular parasites showed that, from a total of 3340 clusters of orthology identified by OrthoMCL, only 37 (~1%) are shared by all parasites able to establish an intracellular infection (the two *T. cruzi* strains CL Brener and Sylvio X10, *T. cruzi marinkellei*, and six species of *Leishmania*). Although some virulence factors known to be involved in host cell invasion and intracellular survival were identified, the majority of these 37 clusters (60%) contain genes annotated as hypothetical proteins, reflecting our limited understanding of the mechanisms associated to the intracellular parasitism.

As additional Trypanosomatid genomes become available, more refined comparative genomics will allow a better understanding of the evolutionary processes underlying parasite survival strategies and will continue providing a powerful framework for selecting genes for functional characterization.

# Transcription mechanisms and genetic expression in *T. cruzi*

## Unique mechanisms of control of gene expression and gene expression profiling

There are marked differences in the way prokaryotes and eukaryotes regulate their gene expression. Being part of a group of early branching eukaryotes, trypanosomatids have attracted the attention of parasitologists not only for their medical relevance but also because they present distinctive features in their mechanisms for controlling gene expression. The absence of defined RNA polymerase II promoter sequences controlling the expression of individual protein-coding genes, the RNA polymerase I-mediated transcription of a select group of genes, and the requirement of pre-mRNA *cis*-splicing as a RNA processing event are major characteristics of eukaryotic gene transcription.[34] In trypanosomatids, transcription is polycistronic, i.e., several genes are transcribed in one large pre-mRNA, and because of the lack of introns, with only four exceptions,[9] *cis*-splicing does not occur in these organisms. However, since primary transcripts are polycistronic, cleavage of the pre-mRNA has to occur in the nucleus in order to produce monocistronic mRNAs that are capped and polyadenylated. In trypanosomes, cleavage of the pre-mRNA is linked to the addition of the 39 nucleotide miniexon (or spliced leader, SL) containing a methylated cap at the 5' end and the poly (A) tail at the 3' end of each mRNA.[35] mRNA biosynthesis in these organisms is also notable because of the fact that most mitochondrial mRNAs have to undergo extensive RNA editing before mitochondrial proteins can be produced.[36]

Adaptation of trypanosomes to distinct environments in the vertebrate and invertebrates hosts as well as differentiation in distinct parasite forms, calls for major changes in morphology, surface composition, biochemical pathways, and thus, complex mechanisms to control gene expression. In most eukaryotes, transcriptional regulation is a major step of gene expression control. In trypanosomes, there is a total lack of evidence for differential regulation of RNA polymerase II transcription and no identifiable RNA polymerase II promoter consensus sequence in the genomes. Thus, the lack of transcription initiation control implies that the knowledge of elements involved in posttranscriptional processes, such as *trans*-splicing, mRNA stabilization, and translation is crucial for the understanding of gene expression in these organisms. As previously indicated, gene organization in trypanosome chromosomes is also very peculiar. Large polycistronic transcription units encoding 20 or more proteins in one strand separated by strand switch regions (i.e., changes of the coding strand) were found initially in the *L. major* genome[37] and later in the Tritryp genomes.[10] Before transcription is completed, the long pre-mRNA is processed in the nucleus by cleavage reactions that are coupled to two cotranscriptional RNA-processing events: *trans*-splicing of a small capped RNA of 39−41 nucleotides, the spliced leader RNA (SL-RNA) which is added to the 5'-terminus of all known protein-encoding RNAs, and 3'-end polyadenylation. Both events are dependent on polypyrimidine motifs (polyPY) located within the intergenic regions.[35] Again, in contrast to most eukaryotes, no canonical polyA addition signal has been identified, and only AG dinucleotides situated downstream from a polyPY motif are used as SL acceptor site.[10,38] Since mRNAs derived from the same polycistronic mRNA precursor can present vast differences in their steady state levels, gene expression modulation must depend heavily on regulatory pathways acting at the control of mRNA half-life. It is believed that by employing this type of regulation, trypanosomes can ensure that rapid changes associated with transmission between insect vector and mammalian host are followed by an instant reprogramming of genetic expression.

Most of the early studies on gene expression in trypanosomatids were focused on the process of antigenic variation, the powerful survival strategy devised by African trypanosomes and allowing *T. brucei* bloodstream forms to escape the immune defenses from the mammalian host. Variant Surface Glycoproteins (VSGs)[39] are the main surface molecules present at the surface of *T. brucei* bloodstream forms. While the genome of this parasite contains about 1000 VSG genes, only one VSG, present in telomeric locations called VSG bloodstream expression site (BES), is active at a time.[40] Understanding the mechanisms controlling VSG expression, particularly the in situ switch (i.e., the mechanism responsible for the activation of one telomeric BES concomitantly with the inactivation of all other

~15 VSG BES), has been a difficult task, but has allowed the discovery of a large body of information about gene expression in this group of organisms (for a recent review, see Stockdale et al.[41]). Notably, transcription of the VSG located in a BES is mediated by an RNA polymerase I that is present in an extranucleolar location identified as expression site body.[42] Compared to *T. brucei*, studies on gene expression in *T. cruzi* had a late start. Whereas the first *T. cruzi* gene was cloned in 1986,[43] characterization of some of the key players involved in gene expression control in this parasite has only recently begun.

Initial studies on stage-specific gene expression in *T. cruzi* indicated that, similar to what had already been described for *T. brucei* and *Leishmania*, the majority of *T. cruzi* genes are constitutively transcribed in epimastigotes, trypomastigotes, and amastigotes.[44−46] Further studies on a number of gene models showed that change in mRNA stability is a main mechanism employed by *T. cruzi* to control stage-specific gene expression of protein-coding genes.[44−48] From these studies, the 3′ UTR has emerged as a main regulatory site involved in controlling mRNA stability. Using transient transfections with CAT or luciferase reporter genes, various groups have demonstrated the presence of elements in the 3′ UTR of several mRNAs that confer developmental regulation of the reporter genes.[46,49,50] The two examples below illustrate some of these studies. In the *T. cruzi* genome a tandem array of alternating genes encoding amastin, a surface glycoprotein, and tuzin, a G-like protein, is polycistronically transcribed in all three forms of the parasites' life cycle. In spite of the constitutive transcription, steady state levels of amastin genes are 60-fold higher in amastigotes compared to epimastigote forms, whereas tuzin mRNA levels do not change significantly. It has been shown that the half-life of amastin mRNAs is sevenfold longer in amastigotes than in epimastigotes and that a 180-nt sequence present in the 3′ UTR is responsible for amastin upregulation.[51] This positive effect is likely mediated by a sequence that binds to a RNA stabilizing factor present in amastigotes.[46,51] Mucin genes are part of an even larger family of cell surface proteins of *T. cruzi* with hypervariable regions and with members of distinct subfamilies expressed in various stages of the parasite life cycle[52,53] have shown that mRNAs for one group of mucins, SMUG mucin mRNAs, are more abundant in the insect stage and that the mRNA turnover is controlled by an AU-rich element (ARE) located in their 3′-UTR. These authors have also demonstrated that an RNA-binding protein named TcUBP-1 is involved in mRNA destabilization in vivo through binding to the ARE of SMUG mucin mRNAs.[54] They have gone further in characterizing this trans-acting factor, showing that TcUBP-1 is part of a ~450 kDa ribonucleoprotein complex with a poly(A)-binding protein and a novel 18 kDa RNA-binding protein, named TcUBP-2.[55] The two examples above show that both positive and negative regulatory elements controlling mRNA stability are found in the genome of *T. cruzi* and that these sequences are recognized by trans-acting factors. Trypanosomatid genomes encode for numerous proteins containing an RNA recognition motif (RRM).[56] It is thus likely that a large number of these proteins are key players in processes controlling pre-mRNA *trans*-splicing, transport and mRNA decay, but so far, only a few of them have been characterized in *T. cruzi*.[57−59] More recently, the identification of the glucosylated thymine DNA base (β-D-glucosyl-hydroxymethyluracil) (or base J) in the *T. cruzi* genome revealed the existence of epigenetic mechanisms controlling transcription in this parasite.[60] Base J is also present in silent telomeric repeats in the *T. brucei* genome as well as in *Leishmania* where it was found to be essential for proper transcription termination of the polycistronic transcription units.[61,62]

Transitions in gene expression that occur during differentiation of *T. cruzi* have also been analyzed using high throughput strategies that recently became available. Reports on microarray analyses confirm that it is a valuable screening tool for identifying stage-regulated genes in *T. cruzi*.[63−65] From these studies, we can infer that a total of almost 5000 transcripts (approx. 50% of *T. cruzi* genes) are regulated during the parasite life cycle, supporting the conclusion that transcript abundance is one of the main levels of gene expression regulation in *T. cruzi*. Together with more recent studies using next generation cDNA sequencing technologies, these analyses allow researchers to identify groups of genes that are part what has been called "posttranscriptional regulons," consisting of mRNAs that show almost identical patterns of regulation.[66] Using RNA-seq and ribosome profiling, Smircich et al. were able to assess the extent of regulation of the transcriptome and the translatome during differentiation from epimastigotes to the infective metacyclic trypomastigote stage.[67] This study showed that translational regulation, in addition to regulation of steady state level of mRNA, is a significant mechanism controlling gene expression in the parasite. Also using RNA-seq, a recent study investigated global transcriptome dynamics simultaneously captured in *T. cruzi* parasite and host cells in an infection time course of human fibroblasts.[68] Extensive remodeling of the *T. cruzi* transcriptome was observed during the early establishment of intracellular infection, coincident with a major developmental transition in the parasite. The findings suggested that transcriptome remodeling is required to establish a modified template to guide developmental transitions in the parasite, whereas homeostatic functions are regulated independently of transcriptomic changes, similar to that reported in related trypanosomatids. Thus, in addition to the biological inferences gained from gene ontology and functional enrichment analysis of differentially expressed genes in parasite and host, this comprehensive, high resolution transcriptomic dataset provided a substantially more detailed interpretation of *T. cruzi* infection biology and offered a basis for future drug and vaccine discovery efforts.[68]

## Genetic manipulation of T. cruzi

Most of our current knowledge of the mechanisms controlling gene expression in trypanosomatids resulted from the development of transfection protocols, which allowed the manipulation of genes, the generation of knockout mutants and the introduction of reporter genes and genetic markers in parasite genomes. In contrast to *T. brucei*, in which homologous recombination of the foreign sequences with the parasite genome is the main strategy that allows the generation of stable transfection lineages, two types of transfection vectors are used in *T. cruzi* and in various *Leishmania* species. Vectors containing the foreign gene flanked by *T. cruzi* sequences allow the integration of the foreign DNA, by homologous recombination in the parasite genome. Episomal vectors have also been used to obtain high levels of expression of foreign genes, if they contain SL/polyadenylation addition sites present both upstream (for *trans*-splicing) and downstream (for polyadenylation) from the exogenous gene (for a review, see Teixeira and daRocha[69]). Work from our lab has identified sequences derived from various genes that can be used to provide efficient *trans*-splicing and polyadenylation.[70,71] With regards to the choice of promoters that can be used in *T. cruzi* expression vectors, we are quite limited. While VSG and procyclin promoters (both of them recognized by RNA polymerase I) work well in *T. brucei* expression vectors, the only option currently available in *T. cruzi* is the rRNA promoter. However, similar to what has been observed in various species of *Leishmania*, it is also possible to obtain relatively high levels of expression of foreign genes using episomal vectors that do not contain promoter sequences at all.[46,72]

An important breakthrough allowing a better control of genetic manipulation in trypanosomatids was achieved with the development of inducible expression of gene products under the control of tetracycline repressor. In this system, which has been initially developed for *T. brucei*, transgenic parasites expressing the tetracycline repressor of *E. coli* exhibit inducer (tetracycline)-dependent expression of a reporter gene cloned downstream from a trypanosome promoter bearing one or more copies of the Tet operator.[73] Although such an inducible expression system has been developed in *T. cruzi*,[71,74] its efficiency in controlling transcription in response to tetracycline does not seem to be as high as in *T. brucei*. More efforts are still needed to create better vectors to allow tight regulated, inducible expression of foreign genes in *T. cruzi* since the availability of such repressor/operator system is an excellent tool for dissecting function of essential genes and for expression of toxic gene products in the parasite.

A second major advance that provided a powerful tool for genetic manipulation in trypanosomes was described by Ngô et al.[75] who were able to generate "knockdown" mutants by targeting mRNA degradation through the mechanisms of RNA interference (RNAi). RNAi is a very specific gene silencing mechanism guided by double strand RNA (dsRNA) bearing sequences derived from a target gene. Briefly, exogenously synthesized or internally expressed dsRNAs homologous to the coding sequence of a target gene are processed into 20−24−nt-long RNAs which work as active guides for mRNA degradation.[76] RNAi is particularly convenient as a methodology to study trypanosomatid genes where conventional gene knockout is hindered by the fact that several genes are present in multiple copies.[77] In addition to *T. brucei*, reports of successful RNAi knock-downs have been described for *Trypanosoma congolense*[78] and in *Leishmania braziliensis*.[79,80] Unfortunately, although RNAi has revolutionized genetic manipulation in *T. brucei*, the lack of an RNA silencing pathway in *T. cruzi* [71] and in old world *Leishmania* species[79] has resulted in a much slower progress in similar studies in *T. cruzi* and in *Leishmania*.

Gene targeting by homologous recombination (HR) remains one of the most powerful techniques to investigate gene function since it allows the generation of parasites with defined mutations in their genome. If the target is not an essential gene, gene deletion by HR is initiated with the replacement of the first allele by a drug resistance marker and, in a second step, by transfecting the heterozygous mutant with a second resistance marker flanked by sequences corresponding to the second allele of the targeted gene. Although the first report of a *T. cruzi* gene knockout by HR was 20 years ago, this approach is time-consuming (3 months on average) and consequently, a limited number of studies involving generation of *T. cruzi* null mutants have been described.

More recently, new technologies developed to improve genetic manipulation in different organisms have been adapted for *T. cruzi*. Among the highly effective new tools that are now available to facilitate genome editing in *T. cruzi* are Cre-recombinases and the CRISPR-Cas9 system. Kangussu-Marcolino et al.[81] showed that it is possible to create *T. cruzi* mutants using the conditional deletion DiCRE system by expressing the split CRE recombinase in epimastigotes. Following insertion of an expression cassette containing the gene encoding for puromycin-N-acetyl-transferase (purR) flanked by loxP sites in the *T. cruzi* genome, the report shows that induction of DiCRE recombinase by addition of rapamycin to the culture medium, resulted in the removal of the selectable marker with high efficiency. Soon thereafter, Peng et al.[82] generated epimastigote cell lines stably expressing GFP and Cas9 nuclease and, after transfection with in vitro transcribed sgRNAs that target eGFP, these authors showed deletion of gfp sequences in 50–60% of parasites as early as day 2 after sgRNA transfection. Importantly, these authors also demonstrated that CRISPR-Cas9 system can be an effective in disrupting genes present in the parasite genome as multigene families such as α-tubulin and β-galactofuranosyl glycosyl-transferase (β-GalGT) genes. Subsequently, Lander et al.[83] also reported the disruption of *T. cruzi* genes using CRISPR-Cas9 technology. These authors described two different transfection strategies, a single transfection vector carrying both the Cas9 nuclease and sgRNA sequences transcribed from the rRNA promoter and a strategy involving transfection of parasites with two separate plasmids, one containing Cas9 gene and the other carrying the sgRNA sequence, that allow generating knockout cell lines for genes encoding GP72 and paraflagellar rod proteins, which are protein required for flagellar attachment or components of the parasite flagellum. Certainly, entirely new avenues have been opened towards a more comprehensive functional analysis of this parasite's genome.

# References

1. Zingales B, Pereira MES, Oliveira RP, Almeida KA, Umezawa ES, Souto RP, et al. *Trypanosoma cruzi* genome project: biological characteristics and molecular typing of clone CL Brener. *Acta Trop* 1997;**68**:159–73.
2. Brandão A, Urmenyi T, Rondinelli E, Gonzalez A, de Miranda AB, Degrave W. Identification of transcribed sequences (ESTs) in the *Trypanosoma cruzi* genome project. *Mem Inst Oswaldo Cruz* 1997;**92**:863–6.
3. Cano MI, Gruber A, Vazquez M, Cortés A, Levin MJ, González A, et al. Molecular karyotype of clone CL Brener chosen for the *Trypanosoma cruzi* Genome Project. *Mol Biochem Parasitol* 1995;**71**:273–8.

4. Henriksson J, Porcel B, Rydåker M, Ruiz A, Sabaj V, Galanti N, et al. Chromosome specific markers reveal conserved linkage groups in spite of extensive chromosomal size variation in *Trypanosoma cruzi. Mol Biochem Parasitol* 1995;**73**:63−74.

5. Porcel BM, Tran AN, Tammi M, Nyarady Z, Rydker M, Urmenyi TP, et al. Gene survey of the pathogenic protozoan *Trypanosoma cruzi. Genome Res* 2000;**10**:1103−7.

6. Verdun RE, Di Paolo N, Urmenyi TP, Rondinelli E, Frasch AC, Sanchez DO. Gene discovery through expressed sequence Tag sequencing in *Trypanosoma cruzi. Infect Immun* 1998;**66**:5393−8.

7. El-Sayed NM, Myler PJ, Bartholomeu DC, Nilsson D, Aggarwal G, Tran A-N, et al. The genome sequence of *Trypanosoma cruzi*, etiologic agent of Chagas disease. *Science* 2005; **309**:409−15.

8. Berriman M, Ghedin E, Hertz-Fowler C, Blandin G, Renauld H, Bartholomeu DC, et al. The genome of the African trypanosome *Trypanosoma brucei. Science* 2005;**309**:416−22.

9. Ivens AC, Peacock CS, Worthey EA, Murphy L, Aggarwal G, Berriman M, et al. The genome of the kinetoplastid parasite, *Leishmania major. Science* 2005;**309**:436−42.

10. El-Sayed NM, Myler PJ, Blandin G, Berriman M, Crabtree J, Aggarwal G, et al. Comparative genomics of trypanosomatid parasitic protozoa. *Science* 2005;**309**:404−9.

11. Zingales B, Andrade SG, Briones MRS, Campbell DA, Chiari E, Fernandes O, et al. A new consensus for *Trypanosoma cruzi* intraspecific nomenclature: second revision meeting recommends TcI to TcVI. *Mem Inst Oswaldo Cruz* 2009;**104**:1051−4.

12. Branche C, Ochaya S, Aslund L, Andersson B. Comparative karyotyping as a tool for genome structure analysis of *Trypanosoma cruzi. Mol Biochem Parasitol* 2006; **147**:30−8.

13. Obado SO, Taylor MC, Wilkinson SR, Bromley EV, Kelly JM. Functional mapping of a trypanosome centromere by chromosome fragmentation identifies a 16-kb GC-rich transcriptional "strand-switch" domain as a major feature. *Genome Res* 2005;**15**:36−43.

14. Brisse S, Barnabé C, Bañuls AL, Sidibé I, Noël S, Tibayrenc M. A phylogenetic analysis of the *Trypanosoma cruzi* genome project CL Brener reference strain by multilocus enzyme electrophoresis and multiprimer random amplified polymorphic DNA fingerprinting. *Mol Biochem Parasitol* 1998;**92**:253−63.

15. Machado C a, Ayala FJ. Nucleotide sequences provide evidence of genetic exchange among distantly related lineages of Trypanosoma cruzi. *Proc Natl Acad Sci USA* 2001;**98**:7396−401.

16. Westenberger SJ, Barnabé C, Campbell DA, Sturm NR. Two hybridization events define the population structure of *Trypanosoma cruzi. Genetics* 2005;**171**:527−43.

17. Arner E, Kindlund E, Nilsson D, Farzana F, Ferella M, Tammi MT, et al. Database of *Trypanosoma cruzi* repeated genes: 20,000 additional gene variants. *BMC Genomics* 2007;**8**:391.

18. Gonzalez A, Prediger E, Huecas ME, Nogueira N, Lizardi PM. Minichromosomal repetitive DNA in *Trypanosoma cruzi*: its use in a high-sensitivity parasite detection assay. *Proc Natl Acad Sci USA* 1984;**81**:3356−60.

19. Elias MCQB, Vargas NS, Zingales B, Schenkman S. Organization of satellite DNA in the genome of *Trypanosoma cruzi. Mol Biochem Parasitol* 2003;**129**:1−9.

20. Martins C, Baptista CS, Ienne S, Cerqueira GC, Bartholomeu DC, Zingales B. Genomic organization and transcription analysis of the 195-bp satellite DNA in *Trypanosoma cruzi. Mol Biochem Parasitol* 2008;**160**:60−4.

21. Bartholomeu DC, Cerqueira GC, Leão ACA, DaRocha WD, Pais FS, Macedo C, et al. Genomic organization and expression profile of the mucin-associated surface protein

(masp) family of the human pathogen *Trypanosoma cruzi*. *Nucleic Acids Res* 2009;**37**:3407−17.

22. Haag J, O'hUigin C, Overath P. The molecular phylogeny of trypanosomes: evidence for an early divergence of the Salivaria. *Mol Biochem Parasitol* 1998;91. Available from: http://dx.doi.org/10.1016/S0166-6851(97)00185-0

23. Lukeš J, Jirků M, Doležel D, Kral'ová I, Hollar L, Maslov DA. Analysis of ribosomal RNA genes suggests that trypanosomes are monophyletic. *J Mol Evol* 1997;**44**:521−7.

24. Stevens JR, Noyes H a, Dover G a, Gibson WC. The ancient and divergent origins of the human pathogenic trypanosomes, *Trypanosoma brucei* and *T. cruzi*. *Parasitology* 1999;**118(Pt 1)**:107−16.

25. Wright ADG, Li S, Feng S, Martin DS, Lynn DH. Phylogenetic position of the kineto-plastids, *Cryptobia bullocki*, *Cryptobia catostomi*, and *Cryptobia salmositica* and mono-phyly of the genus Trypanosoma inferred from small subunit ribosomal RNA sequences. *Mol Biochem Parasitol* 1999;**99**:69−76.

26. Baida RCP, Santos MRM, Carmo MS, Yoshida N, Ferreira D, Ferreira AT, et al. Molecular characterization of serine-, alanine-, and proline-rich proteins of *Trypanosoma cruzi* and their possible role in host cell infection. *Infect Immun* 2006;**74**:1537−46.

27. Di Noia JM, Sánchez DO, Frasch AC. The protozoan *Trypanosoma cruzi* has a family of genes resembling the mucin genes of mammalian cells. *J Biol Chem* 1995;**270**:24146−9.

28. Vargas N, Pedroso A, Zingales B. Chromosomal polymorphism, gene synteny and genome size in *T. cruzi* I and *T. cruzi* II groups. *Mol Biochem Parasitol* 2004;**138**:131−41.

29. Franzén O, Ochaya S, Sherwood E, Lewis MD, Llewellyn MS, Miles MA, et al. Shotgun sequencing analysis of *Trypanosoma cruzi* I Sylvio X10/1 and comparison with *T. cruzi* VI CL Brener. *PLoS NTD* 2011;**5**:e984.

30. Stoco PH, Wagner G, Talavera-Lopez C, Gerber A, Zaha A, Thompson CE, et al. Genome of the avirulent human-infective trypanosome—*Trypanosoma rangeli*. *PLoS NTD* 2014;**8**:e3176.

31. Franzén O, Talavera-López C, Ochaya S, Butler CE, Messenger L a, Lewis MD, et al. Comparative genomic analysis of human infective *Trypanosoma cruzi* lineages with the bat-restricted subspecies *T. cruzi marinkellei*. *BMC Genomics* 2012;**13**:531.

32. Motta MCM, Martins AC, de A, de Souza SS, Catta-Preta CMC, Silva R, et al. Predicting the proteins of *Angomonas deanei*, *Strigomonas culicis* and their respective endosymbionts reveals new aspects of the trypanosomatidae family. *PLoS ONE* 2013;**8**: e60209.

33. Bartholomeu DC, de Paiva RMC, Mendes TAO, DaRocha WD, Teixeira SMR. Unveiling the intracellular survival gene kit of trypanosomatid parasites. *PLoS Pathogens* 2014;**10**:e1004399.

34. Licatalosi DD, Darnell RB. RNA processing and its regulation: global insights into biological networks. *Nat Rev Genet* 2010;**11**:75−87.

35. Matthews KR, Tschadi C, Ullu E. A common pyrimidine-rich motif governs trans-splicing and polyadenylation of tubulin polycistronic pre-mRNA in trypanosomes. *Genes Dev* 1994;**8**:491−501.

36. Stuart K, Panigrahi AK. RNA editing: complexity and complications. *Mol Microbiol* 2002;**45**:591−6. Available from: http://dx.doi.org/10.1046/j.1365-2958.2002.03028.x.

37. Myler PJ, Audleman L, DeVos T, Hixson G, Kiser P, Lemley C, et al. Leishmania major Friedlin chromosome 1 has an unusual distribution of protein-coding genes. *Proc Natl Acad Sci USA* 1999;**96**:2902−6.

38. Campos PC, Bartholomeu DC, DaRocha WD, Cerqueira GC, Teixeira SMR. Sequences involved in mRNA processing in *Trypanosoma cruzi*. *Int J Parasitol* 2008;**38**:1383−9.

39. Boothroyd JC, Cross GA, Hoeijmakers JH, Borst P. A variant surface glycoprotein of *Trypanosoma brucei* synthesized with a C-terminal hydrophobic "tail" absent from purified glycoprotein. *Nature* 1980;**288**:624−6.

40. Donelson JE. Antigenic variation and the African trypanosome genome. *Acta Trop* 2003;**85**:391−404.

41. Stockdale C, Swiderski MR, Barry JD, McCulloch R. Antigenic variation in *Trypanosoma brucei*: joining the DOTs. *PLoS Biol* 2008;**6**:1386−91.

42. Navarro M, Gull K. A pol I transcriptional body associated with VSG mono-allelic expression in *Trypanosoma brucei*. *Nature* 2001;**414**:759−63.

43. Peterson DS, Wrightsman RA, Manning JE. Cloning of a major surface-antigen gene of *Trypanosoma cruzi* and identification of a nonapeptide repeat. *Nature* 1986;**322**:566−8.

44. Bartholomeu DC, Silva RA, Galvão LMC, El-Sayed NMA, Donelson JE, Teixeira SMR. *Trypanosoma cruzi*: RNA structure and post-transcriptional control of tubulin gene expression. *Exp Parasitol* 2002;**102**:123−33.

45. Gentil LG, Cordero EM, do Carmo MS, dos Santos MRM, da Silveira JF. Posttranscriptional mechanisms involved in the control of expression of the stage-specific GP82 surface glycoprotein in *Trypanosoma cruzi*. *Acta Trop* 2009;**109**:152−8.

46. Teixeira SMR, Kirchhoff LV, Donelson JE. Post-transcriptional elements regulating expression of mRNAs from the amastin/tuzin gene cluster of *Trypanosoma cruzi*. *J Biol Chem* 1995;**270**:22586−94.

47. Abuin G, Freitas-Junior LH, Colli W, Alves MJ, Schenkman S. Expression of trans-sialidase and 85-kDa glycoprotein genes in *Trypanosoma cruzi* is differentially regulated at the post-transcriptional level by labile protein factors. *J Biol Chem* 1999; **274**:13041−7.

48. D'Orso I, Frasch AC. Functionally different AU- and G-rich cis-elements confer developmentally regulated mRNA stability in *Trypanosoma cruzi* by interaction with specific RNA-binding proteins. *J Biol Chem* 2001;**276**:15783−93.

49. Lu HY, Buck GA. Expression of an exogenous gene in *Trypanosoma cruzi* epimastigotes. *Mol Biochem Parasitol* 1991;**44**:109−14.

50. Nozaki T, Cross GA. Effects of 3' untranslated and intergenic regions on gene expression in *Trypanosoma cruzi*. *Mol Biochem Parasitol* 1995;**75**:55−67.

51. Coughlin BC, Teixeira SMR, Kirchhoff LV, Donelson JE. Amastin mRNA abundance in *Trypanosoma cruzi* is controlled by a 3'-untranslated region position-dependent cis-element and an untranslated region-binding protein. *J Biol Chem* 2000;**275**:12051−60.

52. Buscaglia CA, Campo VA, Frasch ACC, Di Noia JM. *Trypanosoma cruzi* surface mucins: host-dependent coat diversity. *Nat Rev Microbiol* 2006;**4**:229−36.

53. Di Noia JM, D'Orso I, Sánchez DO, Frasch AC. AU-rich elements in the 3'-untranslated region of a new mucin-type gene family of *Trypanosoma cruzi* confers mRNA instability and modulates translation efficiency. *J Biol Chem* 2000;**275**:10218−27.

54. D'Orso I, Frasch ACC. TcUBP-1, an mRNA destabilizing factor from trypanosomes, homodimerizes and interacts with novel AU-rich element- and Poly(A)-binding proteins forming a ribonucleoprotein complex. *J Biol Chem* 2002;**277**:50520−8.

55. De Gaudenzi JG, D'Orso I, Frasch ACC. RNA recognition motif-type RNA-binding proteins in *Trypanosoma cruzi* form a family involved in the interaction with specific transcripts in vivo. *J Biol Chem* 2003;**278**:18884−94.

56. De Gaudenzi J, Frasch AC, Clayton C. RNA-binding domain proteins in Kinetoplastids: a comparative analysis. *Eukaryot Cell* 2005;**4**:2106—14.

57. Alves LR, Avila AR, Correa A, Holetz FB, Mansur FCB, Manque PA, et al. Proteomic analysis reveals the dynamic association of proteins with translated mRNAs in *Trypanosoma cruzi*. *Gene* 2010;**452**:72—8.

58. Noé G, De Gaudenzi JG, Frasch AC. Functionally related transcripts have common RNA motifs for specific RNA-binding proteins in trypanosomes. *BMC Mol Biol* 2008;**9**:107.

59. Pérez-Díaz L, Duhagon MA, Smircich P, Sotelo-Silveira J, Robello C, Krieger MA, et al. *Trypanosoma cruzi*: molecular characterization of an RNA binding protein differentially expressed in the parasite life cycle. *Exp Parasitol* 2007; **117**:99—105.

60. Ekanayake DK, Minning T, Weatherly B, Gunasekera K, Nilsson D, Tarleton R, et al. Epigenetic regulation of transcription and virulence in *Trypanosoma cruzi* by O-linked thymine glucosylation of DNA. *Mol Cell Biol* 2011;**31**:1690—700.

61. Genest P-A, Baugh L, Taipale A, Zhao W, Jan S, van Luenen HGAM, et al. Defining the sequence requirements for the positioning of base J in DNA using SMRT sequencing. *Nucleic Acids Res* 2015;**43**:2102—15.

62. Borst P, Sabatini R, Base J. discovery, biosynthesis, and possible functions. *Annu Rev Microbiol* 2008;**62**:235—51.

63. Baptista CS, Vêncio RZN, Abdala S, Valadares MP, Martins C, De Bragança Pereira CA, et al. DNA microarrays for comparative genomics and analysis of gene expression in *Trypanosoma cruzi*. *Mol Biochem Parasitol* 2004;**138**:183—94.

64. Minning TA, Bua J, Garcia GA, McGraw RA, Tarleton RL. Microarray profiling of gene expression during trypomastigote to amastigote transition in *Trypanosoma cruzi*. *Mol Biochem Parasitol* 2003;**131**:55—64.

65. Minning TA, Weatherly DB, Atwood J, Orlando R, Tarleton RL. The steady-state transcriptome of the four major life-cycle stages of *Trypanosoma cruzi*. *BMC Genomics* 2009;**10**:370.

66. Queiroz R, Benz C, Fellenberg K, Hoheisel JD, Clayton C. Transcriptome analysis of differentiating trypanosomes reveals the existence of multiple post-transcriptional regulons. *BMC Genomics* 2009;**10**:495.

67. Smircich P, Eastman G, Bispo S, Duhagon MA, Guerra-Slompo EP, Garat B, et al. Ribosome profiling reveals translation control as a key mechanism generating differential gene expression in *Trypanosoma cruzi*. *BMC Genomics* 2015;**16**:443.

68. Li Y, Shah-Simpson S, Okrah K, Belew AT, Choi J, Caradonna KL, et al. Transcriptome remodeling in *Trypanosoma cruzi* and human cells during intracellular infection. *PLoS Pathogens* 2016.

69. Teixeira SMR, daRocha WD. Control of gene expression and genetic manipulation in the Trypanosomatidae. *Genet Mol Res* 2003;**2**:148—58.

70. DaRocha WD, Silva RA, Bartholomeu DC, Pires SF, Freitas JM, Macedo AM, et al. Expression of exogenous genes in *Trypanosoma cruzi*: improving vectors and electroporation protocols. *Parasitol Res* 2004;**92**:113—20.

71. Darocha WD, Otsu K, Teixeira SMR, Donelson JE. Tests of cytoplasmic RNA interference (RNAi) and construction of a tetracycline-inducible T7 promoter system in *Trypanosoma cruzi*. *Mol Biochem Parasitol* 2004;**133**:175—86.

72. Laban A, Wirth DF. Transfection of *Leishmania enriettii* and expression of chloramphenicol acetyltransferase gene. *Proc Natl Acad Sci USA* 1989;**86**:9119—23.

73. Wirtz E, Clayton C. Inducible gene expression in trypanosomes mediated by a prokaryotic repressor. *Science* 1995;**268**:1179—83.

74. Wen LM, Xu P, Benegal G, Carvaho MR, Butler DR, Buck GA. *Trypanosoma cruzi*: exogenously regulated gene expression. *Exp Parasitol* 2001;**97**:196−204.

75. Ngô H, Tschudi C, Gull K, Ullu E. Double-stranded RNA induces mRNA degradation in *Trypanosoma brucei*. *Proc Natl Acad Sci USA* 1998;**95**:14687−92.

76. Filipowicz W. RNAi: the nuts and bolts of the RISC machine. *Cell* 2005;**122**:17−20.

77. Ullu E, Tschudi C, Chakraborty T. RNA interference in protozoan parasites. *Cell Microbiol* 2004;**6**:509−19. Available from: http://dx.doi.org/10.1111/j.1462-5822.2004.00399.x

78. Inoue N, Otsu K, Ferraro DM, Donelson JE. Tetracycline-regulated RNA interference in *Trypanosoma congolense*. *Mol Biochem Parasitol* 2002;**120**:309−13.

79. Lye LF, Owens K, Shi H, Murta SMF, Vieira AC, Turco SJ, et al. Retention and loss of RNA interference pathways in trypanosomatid protozoans. *PLoS Pathogens* 2010;**6**.

80. de Paiva RMC, Grazielle-Silva V, Cardoso MS, Nakagaki BN, Mendonça-Neto RP, Canavaci AMC, et al. Amastin knockdown in *Leishmania braziliensis* affects parasite−macrophage interaction and results in impaired viability of intracellular amastigotes. *PLoS Pathogens* 2015;**11**:e1005296.

81. Kangussu-Marcolino MM, Cunha AP, Avila AR, Herman J-P, DaRocha WD. Conditional removal of selectable markers in *Trypanosoma cruzi* using a site-specific recombination tool: proof of concept. *Mol Biochem Parasitol* 2014;**198**:71−4.

82. Peng D, Kurup SP, Yao PY, Minning TA, Tarleton RL. CRISPR-Cas9-mediated single-gene and gene family disruption in *Trypanosoma cruzi*. *MBio* 2015;**6**.

83. Lander N, Li ZH, Niyogi S, Docampo R. CRISPR/Cas9-induced disruption of paraflagellar rod protein 1 and 2 genes in *Trypanosoma cruzi* reveals their role in flagellar attachment. *MBio* 2015;**6**.

# Kinetoplast genome

*J. Telleria[1] and M. Svoboda[2]*
[1]Unité Mixte de Recherche: Institut de recherche pour le développement (IRD)/CIRAD, Montpellier, France, [2]Université Libre de Bruxelles, Brussels, Belgium

## Introduction

The protozoan parasite *Trypanasoma cruzi* belongs to the kinetoplastida order.

Like other kinetoplastid flagellates, *T. cruzi* possesses a unique mitochondrion containing an unusually complex assembly of mitochondrial DNA known as kinetoplastid DNA (kDNA).

## kDNA organization

The morphology of the kinetoplast varies, dependent on the species. Either it has the structure of a disk (poly kDNA), or its form is less well defined and known as pankinetoplastid. The kinetoplast in *Trypanosoma cruzi* has the poly kDNA structure and contains $4.9 \times 10^7$ nucleotide pairs $(5.4 \times 10^{-14} \text{ g})$.[1] It represents a nonnegligible part of the total DNA, approximately 15% of the total DNA cells.[2]

The DNA of the kinetoplast presents a particular structure, its size and shape is variable in the different developmental stages of the protozoan. In trypomastigotes, the kinetoplast appears like a basket due to a particular arrangement of the DNA loops in several layers, whereas in epimastigotes and amastigotes the kDNA presents a rod-like aspect.

The kinetoplast appears as a dense structure. It forms a giant network composed of interlocked DNA rings: maxicircles and minicircles concatenated between them.

The maxicircles are present in a few dozen copies and represent the equivalent of classical mitochondrial DNA; apparently, they are identical copies varying between 20 and 38 kb, which have slipped into the concatenated single layer of minicircles.

Each *T. cruzi* kinetoplast contains approximately 20,000–30,000 DNA minicircles. The size of *T. cruzi* minicircles is relatively constant, approximately 1.4 kb, but in heterogeneous sequences.

Despite the high heterogeneity of minicircle sequences, similar sequence features are present in all *T. cruzi* minicircles. Each minicircle contains four regions of approximately 100 bp with a nucleotide sequence which is almost identical for all minicircles, of all *T. cruzi* lineages. These constant domains are equidistant, located on 3, 6, 9, and 12 o'clock of the minicircle. Segments separating conserved domains contain 280–320 pb and are called hypervariable region (HVR).[3,4]

# Replication model of kDNA

The structure of the kDNA network has an unusual replication mechanism.

Replication of kDNA minicircles has been first characterized in *Crithidia fasciculata* (for review see Shapiro and Englund[5]). Nevertheless, the replication mechanism is similar to that of *T. cruzi*.[6] The minicircles are not linked to the network when they replicate themselves.

Their replication is initiated at dodecamer 5′-GGGGTTGGTGTA-3′ called the universal minicircle sequence (UMS). During the early stages of replication, this dodecamer binds specifically to a zing finger protein called UMS-binding protein. This UMS sequence is identical for trypanosomid minicircles and the UMS-binding protein sequence presents a high similarity between various *Trypanosoma* species.[7]

The minicircles may be freed by the enzyme topoisomerase II, enabling them to replicate freely. They are in a natural state closed covalently in their replication. The first step is replication in θ like structures, then, in the second step, Okazaki fragments are synthesized and their descendants, which contain gaps, are subsequently reconnected to the periphery of the network.[6] This mechanism is fundamentally different from that of all others cells. In either prokaryotes or eukaryotes, Okazaki fragments are ligated immediately after their synthesis.[8]

When the network is being replicated, the central region which is not involved diminishes in size, and the peripheral region containing the new replicates of the minicircles with gaps, grows bigger. Once the minicircles have replicated (minicircles containing the gaps), the number has doubled.

Whereas the connection sites are opposed, the new minicircles containing gaps are rapidly uniformly distributed around the periphery of the network in a sequential manner. This uniform distribution is considered to be a movement relative to the kinetoplast disk as well as to the protein complexes. It has been suggested that the kinetoplast disk rotates between the two protein complexes. Due to the distribution of recently replicated minicircles in the network, it has been called the "annular" replication mechanism.[6] This kind of movement during replication of *T. cruzi* kDNA is similar in *Crithidia fasciculata*, and *Leishmania* species but is distinct in *T. brucei* where minicircles are during replication removed from the central region and reattached at the poles adjacent to theantipodal sites.[9]

In order for this mechanism to function, it is necessary for the gaps between the Okazaki fragments to be repaired, and then the network divides into two. The latter process is possibly mediated by the enzymes contained in the antipodal site such as endonuclease I (SSE-1), responsible for primer removing and which colocalizes with the kinetoplast topoisomerase II and DNA polymerase β during replication.[10] These enzymes then untie neighboring minicircles along the cleavage line of the network.[6]

Following primer removal, the gaps between fragments are repaired by DNA polymerase β and DNA ligase kβ as well as mitochondrial DNA helicase.[4] The new replicates of the minicircles are connected, in two opposite positions, to the periphery of the network. Several authors have suggested that these positions are adjacent to two protein complexes, known to contain topoisomerase II and a DNA polymerase β.[11] As the structure trypanosomids topoisomerases is specific, this class of enzyme represents a potential therapeutic drug target.[12] They use berenil, which inhibits the minicircle decatenation of the network and thus produces significant changes in kDNA arrangement affecting *T. cruzi* proliferation, has been described.[13]

## Maxicircles and minicircles: kDNA coding

Maxicircles contain mitochondrial rRNA genes and genes which encode hydrophobic mitochondrial proteins. These proteins are predominantly involved in the process of oxidative phosphorylation. *T. cruzi* uses this pathway in its transformation to the epimastigote stage in the vector. Other proteins take part in the glycolytic pathway, used by the parasite in its mammal host.

For *T. cruzi*, the genome of maxicircles has been mounted and annotated for the CL Brener and Esmeraldo strains by the TIGR-SBRI-KI *T. cruzi* Sequencing Consortium (TSK-TSC). This maxicircle genome is schematized in Fig. 19.3 (reprinted from the original paper of Westenberger et al.[14]).

The order of the rRNAs and protein genes on the *T. cruzi* maxicircle is identical with both the *T. brucei* and *L. tarentolae* maxicircles.

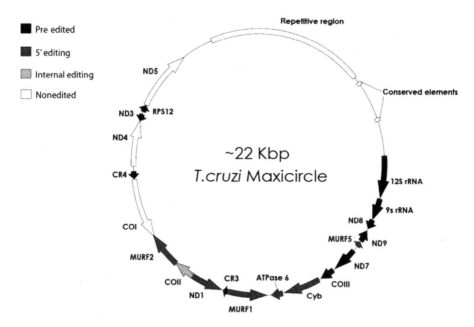

**Figure 19.3** Maxicircle of the *Trypanosoma cruzi* CL Brener and Esmeraldo reference strains (from Westenberger et al.[14]). All annotated genes are shown as arrows indicating coding direction. The noncoding regions of both genomes are distinct from one another, with the exception of a duplicated conserved element lying between the repetitive region and the *12S rRNA*.

The selective pressure requirement for active gene production is noticeable in the sequence comparison of the maxicircle coding domain. Comparison of maxicircle encoded genes of *T. cruzi* with *T. brucei*, *T. lewisi*, and *T. tarantolae* demonstrated that whereas nonedited genes (*ND5, ND4, COI, COII, ND1, MURF1, MURF2, Cyb*) have a similarity of more than 75%, extensively-edited genes (*COIII, ATPase6, ND7, ND8, ND9, CR4, CR5, RPS12*) have a similarity of less than 50% only at the DNA level. The similarity of translated edited genes rose however to 75% for the majority of comparisons.[15]

The absence of selective pressure is obvious in the noncoding domain of maxicircles: no similarity was found between *T. cruzi* with *T. brucei* and *T. tarantolae*. Furthermore, almost no homology was evidenced between two sequenced maxicircles of two different lineages of *T. cruzi*. Variable sequences of maxicircles could also be potentially used for the determination of *T. cruzi* lineages. However, the variable sequences of maxicircles of each lineage have not yet been published and it has been considered that the number of maxicircles is 100 times lower than the number of minicircles. Nevertheless, sequences of amplicons of maxicircles fragment contributed to determine *T. cruzi* strains such Cyb as in Chile isolates (Arenas 2011) or more recently COII-NDI fragment for the parasites isolated from the vector *Triatoma protracta* in California.[16]

In 1986, Bonne et al. described the presence of four nonencoded uridylate (U) residues in the mRNA of the maxicircle gene encoding subunit 2 of cytochrome c oxidase (cox) of two kinetoplastids, *Trypanosoma brucei* and *Crithidia fasciculate* (for review see Benne[17]).

Now, we know that the DNA of maxicircles encodes 20 genes, corresponding to edited and nonedited genes. However, the majority of primary transcriptions of the maxicircles cannot be directly translated because they often contain many errors relating to the ORF (open reading frame) and should be "published" before the translation. That is why, at first sight, the genome seems to be lacking several genes characteristic of mitochondrial genomes, whereas other genes lack key elements for the translation, such as initiation codons or contiguous ORFs.

Whereas the information contained in a genomic sequence is, in most cases, accurately reproduced in the RNA, in the case of *T. cruzi*, the transcription undergoes a genuine correction which modifies its sequence, thanks to the process referred to as "RNA edition." It regroups addition mechanisms, the suppression, and more rarely, the conversion of nucleotides in precise positions of the coding region of maxicircle primary transcriptions (for review see Stuart et al.[18] This process may be defined as a programmed alteration of RNA primary structure enabling the production of a functional sequence. Thus, initiation codons are created, or the correction of internal reading is realized, if not, the transcriptions are unrecognizable for the creation of the ORF.[14]

Since the discovery of mitochondrial RNA editing, we know that this process is the result of a perfect collaboration between genes contained in the maxicircles and the minicircles. The maxicircles provide preedited RNA and the minicircles contribute RNA guides (gRNA). The existence of these gRNA in *T. cruzi* and their role in the edition of the transcribed RNA maxicircle has been demonstrated by Avila and Simpson[19] and Thomas et al.[20] This RNA edition must be extremely accurate in order to avoid the insertion or the suppression of a wrong number of uridines, which would falsify the DNA edition.

The consequence of such errors could lead to the synthesis of an untranslatable reading frame, or modify a senseless sequence giving rise to a full reading frame. The key to this precision lies with the RNA guides.[21] They possess a complementary sequence of the edited region which determines the precise number of uridines to add, suppress, or convert.

Nevertheless, the level of the variability in the gRNA sequence, without loss of functional information, is impressive, due to the fact that any link with G or residues of U in the RNAm is not affected by the transition mutations in the gRNA.[14] But the genes in the maxicircle must maintain a certain degree of fidelity to the gRNA genes in order that the correction be made.[2]

The gRNA, in their 5′ region, present a sequence called "inking sequence," which pairs with preedited transcriptions, and their 3′ region, particular to RNAg, is a poly tail (U) which could be involved in the stabilization of the mRNA−gRNA complex.

The formation of the first mRNA−gRNA complex is crucial to the activation of the edition process. The gRNA associated with the transcription serves as a matrix for the insertion or suppression of uridines. In some cases, the edition creates a new inking site for a second gRNA. The consecutive action of the gRNA means that the edition is a $3''-5'$ oriented process which repeats itself until the mRNA is completely edited.

A series of enzymatic reactions triggered by the pairing of the gRNA enables the endonuclease to cleave the RNA messenger at the level of the first wrongly paired base. The 5' fragment thus formed, is maintained close to the 3' fragment via RNA−RNA interactions bringing into play the poly tail (U) of the gRNA[22] and proteins. This group is called "editosome."

Secondly, in the 3' of 5' fragment, takes place the addition, suppression or the conversion of uridines, thanks to 3' terminal uridylyl transferases (TUTases). The newly added uridines pair with the gRNA. The two RNA fragments (5' and 3'), which remain together due to complementarity with gRNA, are finally linked by an RNA ligase giving rise to the mature transcription.[21] This multisubunit enzymatic RNA editing complex and its function in *T. brucei* was recently reviewed by Aphasizheva and Aphasizhev.[23]

The edition process of maxicircle transcriptions contributes to the evolution of the stages of cellular life and the unusual energetic metabolism of *T. cruzi* in certain stages of life, passing through rich glucose sanguine trypomastigotes to intracellular amastigotes, and to the poorest epimastigotes living in the energy environment of insects' intestines.

# Determination of *T. cruzi* lineages analyzing minicircles DNA sequences

*T. cruzi* undergoes essentially clonal evolution with only very rare sexual recombination as described by Tibayrenc et al.[24]. The occurrence of hybridization in natural populations of *T. cruzi* has been unequivocally demonstrated.[14,25,26] Nevertheless, the rarity of such sexual recombination allows propagation of clonal genotypes over long periods of time.[26] Consequently, lineages of this parasite are identifiable on the basis of their genotype and phenotype. Recently, the nomenclature of *T. cruzi* intraspecific variability has been revised, taking into account the six principal genotypes.[27]

The identification of the lineage could be based either on genomic DNA sequences, on the polymorphism of isoenzymes (i.e., products of genomic DNA) or, on the presence of specific sequences in hypervariable kDNA region. It is largely accepted that at least two hybridization events occurred in *T. cruzi* natural populations in which a fusion between ancestral TC I−II (former DTU I and DTU IIb, respectively) genotypes gave rise to a heterozygous hybrid that homogenized its genome to become the homozygous progenitor of TC III−TC IV (former DTU IIa and DTU IIc, respectively). The second hybridization was between TC II and TC III (former DTU IIb and DTU IIc, respectively) strains that generated TC V and TC VI (former DTUs IId and DTU IIe, respectively). It is noteworthy that the reference strain CL Brener, whose genome was first sequenced, pertains to a hybrid TC VI (former DTU IIe) lineage.

For various reasons developed later, the genetic pressure to maintain the constant gRNA encoding domain of minicircles appears to be low. It is therefore not surprising that the long and separate evolution of parasites led to the evolution of the sequence diversity of hypervariable domain minicircles. The relationships between nuclear genotypes specific to given lineages and sets of minicircles sequences is, however, maintained. Consequently, each lineage may be characterized by a set of minicircle sequences roughly specific to this lineage. The sequence diversity of minicircles is the foundation of various typing methods determining parasite lineage.

A first approach to *T. cruzi* kDNA characterization, described by Mattei et al.[28] was based on the variability of restriction fragment length polymorphism (RFLP) of the minicircles. The kDNA should be purified, which requires extraction of kDNA from a large number of cultured parasites. Later, Morel et al.,[29] used this method for genotyping *T. cruzi* strains and proposed the term "schizodeme" to refer to groups of parasites presenting the same pattern of kDNA.

Schizodeme typing is based on the separation of fragments of the digested kDNA by electrophoresis. Most of the digestions for schizodeme analysis were performed in polyacrylamide gels. When agarose gels were used, the resolution was not sufficient, and hybridization (southern blot) was necessary. These methods are time-consuming.

PCR amplification of hypervariable domain of minicircles was already described in 1989 by Sturm et al.[30] Hypervariable domains are amplified using primers based on the constant region. An amplicon of approximately 320 bp was obtained. This amplicon contains the hypervariable domain but also about 100 bp of the constant domain (primers plus 60 bp of relatively constant sequence).

This PCR approach yielded good results with relatively pure parasites isolated from bugs, but did not allow direct identification of parasites in blood samples. In order to increase sensitivity and specificity, hybridization of amplicons was proposed.[32] This approach was developed by Veas et al.,[31] who amplified the kDNA hypervariable domain using modified primer containing restriction sites, allowing subsequent elimination of constant domains from amplicons (HVRm).

Probes prepared by Veas et al.[31] were used for strain typing. Brenière et al. demonstrated that probes obtained by amplification of kDNA from clonet 39, hybridized only with DNA from clonet 39, probes obtained from clonet 43, hybridized only with DNA of clonet 43, and probes from clonet 20, hybridized with clonet 19 and 20, respectively[32,33] Subsequently, the method was validated for epidemiological purposes, using total kDNA as probes.[34] More recently it was used for typification of the Chile *T. cruzi* isolates.[35]

Systematic sequencing of large numbers of hypervariable sequences originating from different lineages confirmed sequence specificity of each group and demonstrated that if some hypervariable sequences are rare or unique, other sequences are frequently repeated in one lineage but, in proportion, varying from one strain to another. This was observed mainly in lineage TC V (former DTU IId).[36]

# References

1. Lanar DE, Levy LS, Manning JE. *Mol Biochem Parasitol* 1981;**3**:327−41.
2. Baptista CS, Vencio RZ, Abdala S, Carranza JC, Westenberger SJ, Silva MN, et al. *Mol Biochem Parasitol* 2006;**150**:236−48.
3. Degrave W, Fragoso SP, Britto C, van Heuverswyn H, Kidane GZ, Cardoso MA, et al. *Mol Biochem Parasitol* 1988;**27**:63−70.
4. Liu B, Liu Y, Motyka SA, Agbo EE, Englund PT. *Trends Parasitol* 2005;**21**:363−9.
5. Shapiro TA, Englund PT. *Annu Rev Microbiol* 1995;**49**:117−43.
6. Guilbride DL, Englund PT. *J Cell Sci* 1998;**111(Pt 6)**:675−9.
7. Coelho ER, Urmenyi TP, Franco dS, Rondinelli E, Silva R. *Int J Parasitol* 2003;**33**:853−8.
8. Kunkel TA, Burgers PM. *Trends Cell Biol* 2008;**18**:521−7.
9. Povelones ML. *Mol Biochem Parasitol* 2014;**196**:53−60.
10. Engel ML, Ray DS. *Proc Natl Acad Sci USA* 1999;**96**:8455−60.
11. Abu-Elneel K, Robinson DR, Drew ME, Englund PT, Shlomai J. *J. Cell Biol* 2001;**153**:725−34.
12. Balana-Fouce R, Alvarez-Velilla R, Fernandez-Prada C, Garcia-Estrada C, Reguera RM. *Int J Parasitol Drugs Drug Resist* 2014;**4**:326−37.
13. Zuma AA, Cavalcanti DP, Zogovich M, Machado AC, Mendes IC, Thiry M, et al. *Parasitol Res* 2015;**114**:419−30.
14. Westenberger SJ, Barnabe C, Campbell DA, Sturm NR. *Genetics* 2005;**171**:527−43.
15. Lin RH, Lai DH, Zheng LL, Wu J, Lukes J, Hide G, et al. *Parasit Vectors* 2015;**8**:665.
16. Shender LA, Lewis MD, Rejmanek D, Mazet JA. *PLoS NTD* 2016;**10**:e0004291.
17. Benne R. *Eur J Biochem* 1994;**221**:9−23.
18. Stuart KD, Schnaufer A, Ernst NL, Panigrahi AK. *Trends Biochem Sci* 2005;**30**:97−105.
19. Avila HA, Simpson L. *RNA* 1995;**1**:939−47.
20. Thomas S, Martinez LL, Westenberger SJ, Sturm NR. *BMC Genomics* 2007;**8**:133.
21. Blanc V, Davidson NO. *J Biol Chem* 2003;**278**:1395−8.
22. Blum B, Simpson L. *Cell* 1990;**62**:391−7.
23. Aphasizheva I, Aphasizhev R. *Trends Parasitol* 2016;**32**:144−56.
24. Tibayrenc M, Ward P, Moya A, Ayala FJ. *Proc Natl Acad Sci USA* 1986;**83**:115−19.
25. Machado CA, Ayala FJ. *Proc Natl Acad Sci USA* 2001;**98**:7396−401.
26. De Freitas JM, Augusto-Pinto L, Pimenta JR, Bastos-Rodrigues L, Goncalves VF, Teixeira SM, et al. *PLoS Pathogens* 2006;**2**:e24.
27. Zingales B, Andrade SG, Briones MR, Campbell DA, Chiari E, Fernandes O, et al. *Mem Inst Oswaldo Cruz* 2009;**104**:1051−4.
28. Mattei DM, Goldenberg S, Morel C. *FEBS Lett* 1977;**74**:264−8.
29. Morel C, Chiari E, Camargo EP, Mattei DM, Romanha AJ, Simpson L. *Proc Natl Acad Sci USA* 1980;**77**:6810−14.
30. Sturm NR, Degrave W, Morel C, Simpson L. *Mol Biochem Parasitol* 1989;**33**:205−14.
31. Veas F, Cuny G, Breniere SF, Tibayrenc M. *Acta Trop* 1990;**48**:79−82.
32. Breniere SF, Bosseno MF, Revollo S, Rivera MT, Carlier Y, Tibayrenc M. *Am J Trop Med Hyg* 1992;**46**:335−41.
33. Breniere SF, Bosseno MF, Telleria J, Bastrenta B, Yacsik N, Noireau F, et al. *Exp Parasitol* 1998;**89**:285−95.
34. Breniere SF, Bosseno MF, Noireau F, Yacsik N, Liegeard P, Aznar C, et al. *Mem Inst Oswaldo Cruz* 2002;**97**:289−95.

35. Arenas M, Campos R, Coronado X, Ortiz S, Solari A. *Vector Borne Zoonotic Dis* 2012;**12**:196−205.
36. Telleria J, Lafay B, Virreira M, Barnabe C, Tibayrenc M, Svoboda M. *Exp Parasitol* 2006;**114**:279−88.

# Experimental and natural recombination in *Trypanosoma cruzi*

*M.D. Lewis[1], M.S. Llewellyn[2], M. Yeo[1], L.A. Messenger[1] and M.A. Miles[1]*
[1]London School of Hygiene and Tropical Medicine, London, United Kingdom,
[2]University of Glasgow, Glasgow, United Kingdom

## Chapter Outline

## Introduction

The disease manifestations of *Trypanosoma cruzi* infection in individual patients and in different geographical regions are diverse, as is the response to chemotherapy. This is thought to be partially dependent on the very high degree of intraspecific genetic diversity in *T. cruzi*. Genetic diversity is shaped by several evolutionary forces, including mutations, migration of individuals, genetic drift, and natural selection. Genetic exchange can also have a dramatic impact because it generates new combinations of alleles. Recombination classically occurs during meiosis as part of the process of sexual reproduction in most eukaryotes. Meiosis is a specialized form of cell division involving a halving of the number of chromosomes to generate gametes (gametogenesis). Gametes subsequently fuse to form progeny (fertilization) with a full complement of chromosomes restored.

While sexual reproduction involving canonical meiosis is obligatory in almost all multicellular eukaryotes, this is not necessarily true of protozoa. The life cycles of these unicellular eukaryotes typically involve repeated rounds of binary

*American Trypanosomiasis Chagas Disease. DOI: http://dx.doi.org/10.1016/B978-0-12-801029-7.00020-4*

fission (mitosis). In some cases, e.g., the apicomplexan protozoa (*Toxoplasma*, *Plasmodium*), clonal stages are interspersed with obligatory episodes of sexual reproduction. For many other protozoa (e.g., *Giardia*, *Trichomonas*, *Kinetoplastidae*) sex may occur but is not an essential part of the life cycle. The key advantage of sex is that it can rapidly generate diverse, new genotype combinations, however, its occurrence in many protozoa was considered rare and of little consequence to their evolution.[1,2] It is important to note that populations of genetically identical individuals can also be generated via sexual selfing, a process that may frequently occur in the case of parasitic protozoa such as *T. cruzi*. Moreover, recombination between genetically similar, but not identical, individuals will tend to generate progeny with very low genetic diversity. Without careful, high-resolution analysis, this situation may be indistinguishable from a reproductively clonal population. More recent data from diverse protozoa are leading to a less rigid framework for understanding their population structures in order to account for the range of possibilities between panmixia and long-term asexuality.[3]

The population structure of disease-causing microorganisms, such as *T. cruzi*, is determined by the relative rates of recombination and clonality. They may differ between geographical locations and vary over time. Understanding these processes is important because they influence the spread of epidemiologically relevant traits such as virulence, transmission potential, or resistance to therapeutic drugs. Accurate knowledge of such factors can thus be important in designing disease control strategies. In this chapter we will examine our understanding of recombination in *T. cruzi*. Research in this area is not only important for the reasons laid out above with respect to Chagas disease epidemiology; it is also of intrinsic biological interest due to its potential evolutionary novelty.

# Genetic diversity of *T. cruzi*

*T. cruzi* is still considered to be a single species. Early comparisons between strains suggested a diverse range of phenotypic characteristics. The application of biochemical methods, especially multilocus enzyme electrophoresis (MLEE) to study intraspecific diversity led to the description of distinct genetic lineages (or discrete typing units, DTUs). Initially three main groups were described called principal zymodemes. Further application of MLEE revealed six discrete genetic lineages. A plethora of molecular biological methods was subsequently applied, largely confirming the existence of six major genetic lineages. These corresponded with those originally defined by MLEE but also uncovered appreciable diversity within some of the lineages, dependent on the degree of resolution of the molecular method used. From a recent consensus review of the subspecific nomenclature of *T. cruzi* these six lineages or DTUs were designated as TcI to TcVI.[4] It is anticipated that as sampling coverage of endemic areas improves, novel *T. cruzi* lineages might be described. For example, a somewhat diverse group, provisionally named TcBat, presenting distinctive genotypic characteristics has been described.[5] This group appears most closely related to TcI and there is not yet consensus that it should be treated as a seventh DTU. In addition a subspecies of *T. cruzi* that is restricted to bats is named *T. cruzi marinkellei*.

TcI to TcVI have distinctive, yet partially overlapping geographical distributions and ecological associations.[6,7] TcI is the most diverse and widespread DTU; it has a primarily arboreal cycle between *Didelphis* species and the triatomine tribe *Rhodniini* with secondary transmission among terrestrial rodents and sylvatic *Triatoma* species; in humans it is the main agent of Chagas disease in endemic regions north of the Amazon, e.g., in Venezuela.[8] Although a high level of genetic diversity is present within TcI, perhaps two thirds of human TcI infections are associated with a subset of closely related "domestic" strains.[9] TcII, TcV, and TcVI are less genetically diverse than TcI and are almost exclusively described from domestic transmission cycles in the Southern Cone region of South America and parts of Brazil. All four of these lineages are agents of Chagas disease in this region, though TcV and TcII predominate in human infections.[10,11] TcII is presumed to have sylvatic cycles but these appear scarce,, and remain poorly understood. TcIII is geographically widespread and has a dispersed terrestrial sylvatic cycle that principally involves the armadillo, *Dasypus novemcinctus*,[12] but also occurs in (peri)domestic cycles and occasionally infects humans.[13,14] TcIV is little studied but has divergent genotypes in South and North America, is a secondary disease agent in Venezuela, and has been implicated in recent outbreaks of orally transmitted acute Chagas disease in the Brazilian Amazon.[8,15] Thus, both TcIII and TcIV are generally associated with sylvatic hosts and vectors and although both can cause human infection, they as yet only sporadically invade domestic transmission cycles. This present understanding of the genetic diversity of *T. cruzi* is a valid framework but needs to remain dynamic as more extensive sampling and research continue.

## Experimental recombination

Experimental attempts to produce recombinants between TcI and TcII, then referred to as Z1 and Z2, were first undertaken in the 1970s (M. Miles, unpublished data). The experimental approach was either simply to passage together mixed populations of the two lineages in blood agar cultures or sequentially from mouse to triatomine to mouse and back into culture, then re-characterizing the population mixtures. No recombinants were detected and either a mixture of TcI and TcII or TcII alone were recovered from these experiments. In retrospect it was ambitious to attempt an experimental cross between these genetically divergent lineages. Furthermore, there were no genetic markers available for the selection of recombinants, which would have been undetectable if they had been present as minor populations in the output of such experiments.

Experimental genetics for *T. cruzi* became feasible with the development of recombinant DNA technology that allowed genetic transformation of parasite populations to confer resistance to different drugs. Trypanosomes could now be marked to carry a wide range of reporter genes including fluorescent markers of various colors: it is possible to direct such markers to intracellular organelles of special interest or to tag genes of interest that are expressed during different life cycle stages.

In 1996, putative parental homozygous and recombinant heterozygous genotypes of TcI were described on the basis of phosphoglucomutase (PGM) isoenzyme phenotypes in isolates from a single locality in the Amazon basin of Brazil, potentially compatible with active intra-lineage recombination.[16] Accordingly, two putative parental strains from this locality were transformed with episomal recombinant DNA plasmids bearing genes conferring resistance to specific antibiotics, either hygromycin B or G418. Experimental crosses were attempted *in vitro* in mammalian cell cultures, and *in vivo* in mice and triatomine bugs by coinfection with both transgenic parental strains.[17] Parasite populations subsequently derived from the co-infections were subjected to selection with both drugs simultaneously. Six double drug-resistant *T. cruzi* recombinant hybrid clones were obtained from mixed infections in the mammalian cell cultures and were shown to contain both drug resistance marker genes indicating that they were the products of genetic exchange between the co-infecting strains. The six clones were characterized by MLEE, karyotypes, microsatellites, and sequencing of some housekeeping genes. This analysis demonstrated that parental genetic markers had not been inherited in typical Mendelian ratios. Rather than inheriting one allele per locus from each of the parent strains, as expected in typical meiotic $F_1$ heterozygous progeny, the hybrid clones contained all alleles from both parents at most loci. However, at a small minority of loci, some parental alleles were not present. Each of the six hybrid clones had one of the parental kDNA maxicircle genotypes but not both. It was concluded that fusion of the diploid parental strains had occurred to produce a tetraploid hybrid, with limited subsequent genome erosion and an unclear level of concomitant genetic recombination between parental sequences.

In terms of virulence, pathogenesis, and epidemiological relevance it was of considerable interest to see how these hybrid *T. cruzi* clones behaved in experimental infections. The hybrid clones proved to be at least as a virulent as the parental strains in immunocompromised mice.[18] They produced abundant pseudocysts in heart and skeletal muscle, with some detectable infection of smooth muscle of the alimentary tract. This showed that these *in vitro* generated hybrids were capable of all the morphogenic transitions required to complete a full life cycle, and were able to survive in a mammalian host. Whether the hybrid clones display increased virulence or "hybrid vigor" in comparison with their parents, or would compete with the parents in co-infections, is a topic that requires further study.

Flow cytometric analysis of DNA content provided further insight into the genomic composition and ploidy of the experimental hybrid clones and the process of genome erosion. This approach was originally applied to *T. cruzi* by James Dvorak in the 1980s and revealed substantial variation in the DNA content of natural isolates.[19] The DNA content analysis demonstrated that all six hybrids had, on average, 69% more DNA that the parental strains. This was compatible with an aneuploid chromosome complement intermediate between 3n and 4n, and so the hybrids were considered to be subtetraploid.[18] There was no dramatic decline in DNA content when the clones were recovered from infected mice or in response to stressful growth conditions, such as heat shock, indicating that their genomes were relatively stable. The DNA content analysis thus further supported the hypothesis that the hybrids underwent limited genome erosion from a tetraploid fusion product.

The ploidy level, however, is not absolutely stable. Following prolonged passage in axenic cultures a gradual, progressive decline in DNA content has been observed (M. Lewis, unpublished data), with a pattern that is not compatible with any true meiotic reductive division that would result in rapid, ordered reduction of ploidy. Further comparisons are ongoing of the parental and experimental hybrid karyotypes and genotypes, particularly using heterozygous parental allelic markers, to understand the mechanism of genome erosion in *T. cruzi*. Meanwhile, it is clear these *in vitro*-generated *intra-lineage* TcI hybrids are not the result of the typical eukaryotic programme of genetic exchange, because neither the parents nor the hybrids underwent a meiotic reductive division. The process of fusion of diploids followed by genome erosion is reminiscent of the parasexual reproductive cycle of the pathogenic yeast *Candida albicans*, which is characterized by cellular and nuclear fusion of diploid cells producing tetraploid intermediates, followed by random, concerted chromosome losses, giving rise to recombinant progeny with an approximately diploid chromosome complement.[20] Whether the diploid fusion—genome erosion model of genetic exchange applies to wild populations of *T. cruzi* or whether sexual reproduction involving normal meiosis could occur under different conditions or between different strains remains an open question.

Performing experimental crosses in *T. brucei* using transgenic strains expressing different fluorescent proteins cytoplasmically or tagged to specific proteins has proven to be a powerful tool for studying recombination under laboratory conditions since hybrid organisms co-expressing multiple markers due to inheritance can be identified microscopically. This has helped to pinpoint the developmental stage of the parasite that is involved in genetic exchange.[21,22] The same approach may prove fruitful for experimental crosses in *T. cruzi*. Red and green fluorescent strains of *T. cruzi* as well as the closely related species *T. rangeli* have been described, and the potential for exploiting these reporters to track co-infections *in vitro* and in mice and triatomine bugs *in vivo* has now been demonstrated.[23,24] As yet no hybrid parasites have been recovered from such experiments, although relatively few conditions or strains appear to have been tested.

In *T. cruzi* the experimental hybrid clones described above were derived from mammalian cell cultures but it was not proven that hybridization was an intracellular event. In *T. brucei* and *Leishmania* sp. recombination occurs in their invertebrate vectors—the tsetse fly and sand fly, respectively.[25,26] In the *T. cruzi* cross the mammalian cells were infected with a mixture of metacyclic trypomastigotes and epimastigotes from stationary phase cultures. It is therefore possible that hybridization occurred between epimastigotes prior to invasion and establishment of intracellular forms. Alternatively hybridization may have taken place between trypomastigotes emerging from the mammalian cells during the prolonged infection, which could have encompassed up to four rounds of invasion and intracellular multiplication. This implies that hybridization between extracellular forms that would be found in natural infections of triatomine bug vectors should not be ruled out. This possibility requires further investigation, ideally with transgenic *T. cruzi* strains carrying both drug resistance and fluorescent markers to allow visualization of interactions between coinfecting strains. This will require careful experimental design because there are around 140 known species of triatomines, and the 6 known lineages of *T. cruzi* each encompassing considerable genetic diversity. Triatomine species appear to differ in their susceptibilities to infection with different *T. cruzi* lineages and so the behavior of *T. cruzi* strains in one combination of triatomine species and *T. cruzi* lineage will not necessarily be typical.

The experimental demonstration of hybridization was a milestone in research on *T. cruzi*. It proved that *T. cruzi* has an extant capacity for genetic exchange. It also revealed an unusual, nonmeiotic mechanism involving fusion of diploids followed by genome erosion, for which the precise details remain to be understood. This mechanism may be operating among natural populations of *T. cruzi*, but the occurrence of other genetic mechanisms among natural populations cannot be excluded.

# Recombination in natural populations

## Inter-lineage (inter DTU) recombination: TcV and TcVI

The clonal theory of parasitic protozoa implied that genetic exchange was either absent or a rare event in *T. cruzi* and of little or no epidemiological significance.[1,2] This hypothesis was supported by several features of the genetic diversity of *T. cruzi*, including strong linkage disequilibrium, identical genotypes spread over vast geographical distances, and phylogenetic correlation between independent sets of genetic markers. Nevertheless, early MLEE studies of isolates from Bolivia and Paraguay, now incorporated within lineage TcV and TcVI, respectively, revealed highly distinctive, heterozygous MLEE profiles, with at least one corresponding homozygous profile seen among other isolates from the same locality.[13,27] For example, the dimeric enzyme glucose phosphate isomerase (GPI) had the profile of three equidistantly separated bands, with a central band that was more intense as would be expected for recombinant strains. Furthermore, this profile was sustained in clones so could not be due to a mixture of populations. The TcV and TcVI profiles were similar in that both showed a high level of heterozygosity but they also had some distinguishing isoenzyme bands.

TcV and TcVI have an unusual geographical distribution: they were found to be particularly common in the foothills of the Andes and the greater Gran Chaco regions of Bolivia, Chile, Paraguay, northern Argentina, and in the extreme south of Brazil, where there were wider fluctuations in environmental temperature than in the Amazon and Atlantic forests. This suggested that the heterozygous MLEE profiles might be adaptive, giving enhanced fitness in triatomine bugs through metabolic flexibility over a range of environmental temperatures. Such an adaptive advantage was proven to occur in other systems, e.g., in fish moving between warm and cold climatic conditions. Hybridization is also known to be associated with the generation of new phenotypes in *Leishmania* sp.[28] The metabolic significance of the predominantly heterozygous profiles of TcV and TcVI was explored by purifying the GPI isoenzymes and testing their catalytic rates at different temperatures. Although the isoenzymes certainly differed in temperature stability, as was readily seen directly by their differing persistence on incubated MLEE gels, there was no proof of differences in catalytic efficiency at diverse temperatures for the purified isoenzymes.[29] Nevertheless, the maintenance of high levels of heterozygosity in TcV and TcVI suggests that such experiments to test for associations with fitness remain worthwhile.

The hybrid nature of TcV and TcVI was confirmed by other molecular methods, notably by sequencing of housekeeping genes.[30–32] Comparison of nucleotide sequences showed that TcV and TcVI must have arisen through hybridization between genetically distinct parents because they were found to possess fully intact alleles from two other DTUs (TcII and TcIII) that are so distinct that they could not possibly have arisen independently. As in the experimental hybrids described in the previous section, sequencing of kDNA maxicircle genes showed they were inherited uniparentally by TcV and TcVI, with the TcIII parent being the donor in each case.

Lewis et al.[32] conducted a comprehensive analysis of TcV and TcVI based on nuclear and mitochondrial gene sequences as well as a panel of 28 microsatellite loci. These markers evolve at very different rates, which allowed the relationships between hybrid and nonhybrid DTUs to be studied with high resolution at multiple timescales. Overall, TcV and TcVI each closely resembled the sterile $F_1$ meiotic progeny of a relatively recent cross between TcII and TcIII. The hybrid genotypes were found to be highly heterozygous, with low intra-DTU diversity. Very few unique polymorphisms were identified, consistent with limited clonal diversification after hybrid formation. Consistent with this, multilocus sequence analysis of coding genes showed that intra-TcV and intra-TcVI differences were essentially restricted to loss of heterozygosity (LOH) events, such that some strains had become homozygous for TcII or TcIII parental alleles.[33]

The close genetic similarity between TcV and TcVI has made it difficult to determine whether they are the products of a single hybridization event followed by limited clonal diversification or of two independent events involving genetically similar TcII and TcIII parental strains. Analyses of housekeeping gene sequences supported the hypothesis of a single hybridization event followed by divergence to form TcV and TcVI.[34,35] In contrast, microsatellite data based on five loci[36] and other coding gene phylogenies[37] have indicated that two independent events are the most likely explanation. However, these studies used relatively few strains and/or low resolution data such that they were probably underpowered to address the question. The multilocus microsatellite analysis conducted by Lewis et al.[32] showed that the two hybrid groups had highly distinct profiles composed of different combinations of alleles that were shared with TcII and TcIII strains. This, combined with the many known coding sequence differences, strongly suggested that TcV and TcVI had not evolved by diversification from a common ancestor. Two scenarios for the origins of TcV and TcVI were proposed to fit these data: two independent hybridization events between distinct TcII and TcIII strains or two independent progeny from a single TcII × TcIII cross.

Comparison of hybrid and parental genotypes has been used as a way to identify extant TcII and TcIII strains that most closely resemble the ancestral parents that hybridized to form TcV and TcVI. For example, analysis of 5S rDNA sequences has shown that the TcII-like allele for these sequences found in the hybrid strains is more similar to TcII isolates from Bolivia and Chile than to others from Brazil.[38] Similarly, TcII-like GPI sequences and microsatellite alleles in the hybrids were phylogenetically closer to those in modern strains from Chile, Paraguay, and Bolivia than those from Brazil.[32] The TcIII alleles present in the hybrids supported a closer genetic relationship with modern TcIII from Bolivia, Paraguay, or Peru than strains from Brazil, Colombia, or Venezuela. Mitochondrial kDNA maxicircle sequences, inherited by the hybrids uniparentally from TcIII, point more specifically to a smaller subset of TcIII strains, most commonly found in Paraguay.[31,32] Although the current distribution of TcII and TcIII strains may not coincide with the situation when TcV/VI were formed, their genotypes are most consistent with an origin in the Gran Chaco or adjoining Andean valleys in southwestern South America. Emerging data show that the rare occurrence of TcV and TcVI genotypes in Colombia is almost certainly a result of dispersal rather than more ancient (or additional) hybridization events (L. Messenger, unpublished data). This does, however, demonstrate that the discovery of new TcV or TcVI strains, particularly from sylvatic sources, will necessitate reevaluation of their evolutionary origins.

Intuitively, the more recent the natural hybridization event(s) that gave rise to TcV and TcVI, the more likely it is that new natural hybrid lineages could be expected to emerge. Moreover, given the abundance of hybrids, particularly TcV, in human infections across large endemic areas, there may be a significant risk associated with newly emergent recombinant strains. In an effort to estimate the evolutionary timeframe for the origin of TcV and TcVI, Lewis et al.[32] conducted a phylogenetic molecular clock analysis on a large set of nuclear and mitochondrial sequences from hybrid and non-hybrid strains. These authors concluded that the extant TcV and TcVI strains last shared a common ancestor within approximately the last 60,000 years. Such a recent timescale is close to the limits of resolution for the sequences that were used, however, so the actual origin may well be more recent, especially considering the lack of diversity at microsatellite loci, which typically have very fast mutation rates. Furthermore, the calibration point for the molecular clock used may have been overly conservative.[39] Such a recent origin for natural TcII−III hybrids, together with evidence for genetic exchange within TcI in the laboratory[17] and the field[40,41] indicate that sexual recombination continues to be available as a reproductive mode to a broad range of *T. cruzi* strains.

The ecological circumstances of the origin of TcV and TcVI are not known and can only be inferred based on the balance of probabilities. These hybrids are strongly associated with domestic vectors, humans, and domestic animals. Records of nondomestic TcV/VI are extremely rare and wild populations of their principal vector, *T. infestans*, appear to be overwhelmingly associated with TcI.[42] The formative hybridization events must have occurred in either a mammalian host or a triatomine bug coinfected with TcII and TcIII. However, wild populations of these DTUs have apparently little overlap.[6] Lewis et al.[32] suggested that the most likely circumstances for TcII−TcIII coinfections to occur were in domestic transmission cycles because they provide an environment where they can and do overlap. Even though molecular clock analysis indicated the hybrids arose prior to the arrival of humans in South America there is enough leeway in the dating estimates (see above) to accommodate a more recent, anthropogenic origin. The apparent lack of modern day genetic diversity within both hybrid DTUs from isolates covering a vast geographic area is most plausibly a result of a recent spread of TcV and TcVI as two clonal lineages in association with the spread of domiciliated *T. infestans*, which evidence indicates is itself due to human activities and population movements.[43]

If TcV and TcVI were, like the experimental hybrids, products of genome fusion of diploids to yield aneuploid progeny, the redundant extra copies of genes might confer versatility and evolutionary advantage, in that those genes would potentially be free to evolve rapidly and independently and to acquire alternative independent functions. Accordingly, flow cytometric analysis of DNA content and multilocus genotyping has been applied to natural isolates of *T. cruzi* representing the known *T. cruzi* lineages.[18] Unlike experimental TcI hybrids, the natural TcV and TcVI hybrids were found to have DNA contents consistent with diploidy and equivalent to the average DNA contents of isolates representative of their TcII and TcIII parents. All the available evidence indicates that TcV and TcVI are typical (sterile) $F_1$ meiotic progeny — they possess one TcII allele and one TcIII allele for most loci and the limited cases of homozygosity are best explained by LOH through gene conversion.[12,32] There are, therefore, fundamental differences between the naturally occurring hybrid strains and the experimental hybrids both in terms of allelic inheritance patterns and overall DNA content. It is not clear whether these differences reflect the operation of distinct mechanisms of genetic exchange. It is possible that developmental cues that would cause the experimental hybrids to return to diploidy were absent under laboratory conditions. Alternatively, if TcV and TcVI are indeed derived from fusion of diploids, genome reduction may have progressed sufficiently to result in reversion to a heterozygous diploid state.[32] The mechanism of genetic exchange in natural populations is thus yet to be fully understood and potentially differs from that documented so far from experimental observations.

While the precise biological circumstances that governed the origin and spread of TcV and TcVI remain to be fully understood, the epidemiological impact of these hybrids is striking. They are highly abundant in domestic transmission cycles and TcV predominates among human infections in Bolivia and northern Argentina. More limited data indicate these hybrids are also common causes of human infection in Chile, Paraguay, and southern Brazil. Chagas disease manifestations are often severe in these regions and chagasic cardiomyopathy, megaoesophagus, megacolon, and congenital transmission are all common. In this context, the epidemiological importance of genetic exchange in *T. cruzi* is clear: it has been and may still be profoundly important.

## Interlineage (inter DTU) recombination: other lineages

It has been proposed that TcIII and TcIV are themselves the products of a more ancient interlineage hybridization event between TcI and TcII.[35,44] The evolutionary relationships between TcIII and TcIV had been unclear for some time. In phylogenetic analyses of various nuclear loci TcI and TcII were consistently found to be the most genetically distant lineages. The position of TcIII and TcIV, however, could not be satisfactorily resolved since some markers indicated close relationships with TcI while others indicated a stronger affinity with TcII. A multilocus sequence typing (MLST) analysis of nine nuclear genes,[35] showed that the copies of each gene carried by TcIII and TcIV strains contained single nucleotide polymorphisms (SNPs) that were otherwise only found in TcI or TcII strains. The TcIII and TcIV sequences contained both TcI-like and TcII-like SNPs in mosaic patterns, with the ratio of TcI-like to TcII-like SNPs varying between genes. This potentially explained the incongruent phylogenetic trees that were observed for different genes. The authors concluded that the number of SNPs contributing to these mosaic patterns was too high to be a result of the same mutations arising in each lineage independently (homoplasy) and so must have been a result of genetic exchange between TcI and TcII ancestral populations. TcIII and TcIV also had their own unique SNPs interspersed between the TcI- and TcII-like SNPs, reflecting independent evolution since their divergence. This interpretation has since been brought into question by Tomasini and Diosque[37] on the basis that no appropriate outgroup had been included. By comparing TcI−IV sequences for four genes with orthologous sequences from *T. cruzi marinkellei*, these authors showed that many of the polymorphisms present in TcIII/IV that appeared to have been inherited from TcII were in fact ancestral states shared with the outgroup as well as TcII. This substantially reduced the number of polymorphisms that would need to be explained by homoplasy instead of hybridization. This led to the conclusion that TcII diverged basally with respect to TcI−III−IV and that TcIV and TcIII diverged sequentially without any recombination events. However, two of the four genes reanalyzed by Tomasini and Diosque[37] were not sufficiently diverse to make well-supported phylogenetic inferences and other authors found that TcIII/IV *GPI* gene sequences resembled TcII−III mosaics even when appropriate outgroup sequences were included.[32]

Two alternative evolutionary scenarios for TcI−IV have been proposed that differ according to whether or not TcIII and TcIV are considered to have a hybrid origin. Westenberger et al.[35] concluded that two homozygous lineages (TcI and TcII) diverged from a universal *T. cruzi* common ancestor and subsequently representatives of these lineages underwent hybridization. The mosaic-like sequences in the modern day TcIII and TcIV genomes were suggested to be the product of homologous recombination between the TcI and TcII-like alleles. Extensive genome homogenization fixed these mosaic alleles in a homozygous state and novel mutations accumulated over time during clonal diversification. In contrast Tomasini and Diosque[37] proposed TcI−III−IV as a monophyletic group, from within which TcIV diverged first, making TcI and TcIII sister clades. Thus, the evolution of the TcIII and TcIV DTUs was explicable without inter-DTU hybridization events or any genetic contribution from TcII. The true evolutionary relationships of these *T. cruzi* lineages is likely to become clearer when a sufficient number of whole genome sequences become available for analysis.

Analysis of the current diversity within TcIII and TcIV shows that although ancient recombination events may have contributed to their origin, their multilocus genotypes are consistent with long-term evolution in isolation from the other major lineages and they should be treated as distinct in applied studies. TcIII also has a characteristic DNA content that is significantly greater than the other DTUs.[18] Furthermore, as mentioned above, TcIII has distinct ecological associations, being commonly isolated from *Dasypus* spp. over a wide geographical range.[12] TcIV is not a well-sampled *T. cruzi* lineage but analysis of the limited isolates available has pointed toward abundant intralineage genetic diversity with highly distinct subgroups present in North and South America.[30,32,45]

## *Mitochondrial introgression as a signature of genetic exchange*

There are four distinct monophyletic *T. cruzi* clades based on nuclear haplotypes (TcI−TcIV), with TcV and TcVI containing one haplotype derived from TcII and one from TcIII. In contrast, there are only three corresponding mitochondrial maxicircle sequence clades.[31,36] The hybrids TcV and TcVI only have the TcIII parental maxicircle genotype.[32] The TcI and TcII DTUs carry highly distinct maxicircles, but the TcIII and TcIV maxicircle sequences are surprisingly similar given their nuclear gene sequence divergence. This is unexpected because mitochondrial genes typically evolve more rapidly, not slower, than nuclear ones. This was originally suggested to be the result of relatively recent mitochondrial introgression between TcIII and TcIV.[31]

Incongruence in the phylogenetic relationships inferred by nuclear and mitochondrial sequences also identified putative inter-lineage genetic exchange via mitochondrial introgression between TcIV and TcI populations in North America—in this case one strain possessing TcI-like nuclear genes was found to have virtually identical maxicircle sequences to specific TcIV strains.[31] Some North American TcI and TcIV strains have been shown to have unexpectedly high DNA contents, potentially linking mitochondrial introgression in this region to hybridization events.[18] There is now mounting evidence that TcIV may frequently be involved in this type of recombination event.[32,45−47] The genetic composition of TcIV is heterogeneous and requires much further study to understand its evolution, e.g., TcIV strains can have at least three alternative miniexon genotypes, including the TcI type, three alternative 24Sα rDNA genotypes, including the TcII type, and they contain multiple microsatellite alleles that are otherwise specific to other DTUs.[18,48]

Improved sampling and the use of higher resolution genotyping methods have shown that mitochondrial introgression is also frequent at the intralineage level, particularly among TcI populations, which have been studied most extensively.[49−52] It is unclear whether the apparent prevalence of introgression in TcI is due to the examination of representatives from intensely sampled populations that are minimally subdivided spatially and temporally, and therefore more likely to undergo hybridization, or if it truly reflects the analysis of strains that are more permissive to recombination.[3,53] It has been suggested that incongruence between nuclear and mitochondrial phylogenies might be an artefact of differences in evolutionary rates between noncoding microsatellites and coding maxicircle genes.[54] However, it is highly improbable that mutation rate variation could account for the observation of nearly identical nuclear genotypes with radically divergent mitochondrial genomes, particularly when putative donors and recipients are identified within the same population[47,49] and when multilocus microsatellite genotypes are stable enough to infer all six DTUs.[32] Microsatellite data are concatenated from many chromosomes making it difficult to know whether the incongruence with mitochondrial sequences holds across the nuclear genome.

A recent study from Colombia, indirectly identified biparental mitochondrial inheritance as a putative consequence of genetic exchange events.[49] Specifically, a mosaic maxicircle sequence was detected in a human TcI isolate and the presence of a recombination breakpoint confirmed by allele-specific PCR. Such a sequence can be explained by intermolecular maxicircle recombination, which requires the inheritance of mixed mitochondrial complements, or uniparental inheritance of highly heteroplasmic maxicircles. However, mitochondrial heteroplasmy (the presence of multiple different mitochondrial haplotypes in an individual organism) in *T. cruzi* appears rare.[47] This favors the former interpretation, although homoplasy cannot be completely ruled out. Parallel observations from some experimental crosses of *T. brucei*,[21] suggest that biparental mitochondrial inheritance might be a general feature of trypanosomatid hybridization.

Overall there is good evidence that both inter- and intra-DTU exchange of kDNA maxicircles occurs between *T. cruzi* strains. It remains unclear whether these transfers are coupled to the exchange of chromosomal DNA, i.e., that they occur during hybridization events that involve nuclear fusion. Comparative genomic analysis of strains associated with introgression events will be required to address this question. Such studies would therefore be an important source of new insight into recombination mechanisms in natural populations of *T. cruzi*.

## *Intralineage (intra DTU) recombination*

The existence of natural hybrid lineages shows that while inter-lineage genetic exchange may well be rare in *T. cruzi*, it has had a major impact on its evolution and current diversity. The current genetic lineages, including hybrids, appear to be stable and independently propagating with little gene flow between them, with the exception of the small number of mitochondrial introgression events. The frequency of recombination within lineages and, more importantly, at the population level, remains relatively unexplored. Molecular epidemiological studies on *T. cruzi* have not generally permitted meaningful analysis of recombination rates at this scale because of a lack of sufficiently diverse markers or insufficient sampling. The availability of *T. cruzi* genome sequences[55,56] allowed the development of genetic markers covering a wide range of evolutionary rates and hence levels of resolution for comparisons between strains. Consequently, comparative genomics, MLST, and multilocus microsatellite typing (MLMT) have led to dramatically improved understanding of *T. cruzi* evolution, population genetics, and disease epidemiology.

MLST of nuclear or mitochondrial genes is more broadly applicable than MLMT for formal genetic, phylogenetic, and taxonomic studies. It has the advantage that the functional roles of many genes are known, lower mutation rates means they are less prone to homoplasy, selective pressures can be inferred, and the mutational mechanism is well characterized. This means that selection of appropriate targets can permit both recent and potentially ancient recombination events to be deduced. A basic MLST approach for *T. cruzi*, comparing incongruence between individual phylogenetic trees, was employed by Machado and Ayala in their 2001 study[31] of genetic recombination in natural populations that confirmed TcV and TcVI were interlineage hybrids. A standardized panel of suitable MLST loci for *T. cruzi* has more recently been developed, which has demonstrated accurate lineage assignment, incongruent phylogenetic topologies, potential gene mosaics within DTUs, and putative intra-lineage hybrid and parental isolates based on patterns of SNPs.[33,57,58]

Microsatellites display a far higher degree of intra-lineage polymorphism than protein-coding nucleotide sequences. MLMT thus has the advantage of being a high resolution approach to investigating recent evolutionary history, population structure, multiclonality, and evidence of recombination among closely related isolates, and is particularly applicable to intra-lineage recombination. More than 50 microsatellite loci have been validated,[9,59] providing a powerful means of unraveling the microdynamics of *T. cruzi* in different epidemiological situations.

Analysis by MLMT involves genotyping isolates at a large number of microsatellite loci distributed on many different chromosomes. Microsatellites are composed of short tandem repeats of di-, tri-, or tetranucleotide motifs (e.g., TCTCTCTC, GATGATGAT, and TTTATTTATTTA). Because of the repetitive nature of these sequences they are prone to replication errors that result in frequent expansion or contraction of the tandem repeat, e.g., from 10 repeat units to 12. Over time these mutations accumulate at a far higher rate than nucleotide substitutions and so microsatellite loci are typically highly polymorphic, enabling resolution at an intra-lineage level. At each locus the number of repeats present in any strain can be determined using PCR and used to build up multilocus genotypes that can then be compared between different strains. Improved population sampling combined with the use of these high resolution markers, is now beginning to provide a better understanding of intralineage population structures.

In recent years MLMT has been applied to analyze the population substructures of most *T. cruzi* DTUs, including some in multiple endemic areas, revealing extensive intra-lineage diversity that had previously been hidden.[9,49–52,60] Patterns of diversity among isolates that form genetic subpopulations can be analyzed to detect signatures of recombination at a local scale. Population genetic theory provides us with numerous tools to do this, useful so long as we are careful to interpret their output in the light of the assumptions on which they are based. Fundamental among these tools are statistics that measure the statistical likelihood for co-occurrence of alleles (linkage) at different loci among samples,[61] although allele frequencies at individual loci and the frequency of repeated genotypes can also be informative. In general, recombination should disrupt such associations between alleles whereas clonal reproduction will maintain them. MLMT analysis has shown that, at the intralineage level, the co-occurrence of alleles at different loci among samples is commonplace in those *T. cruzi* populations so far examined, suggesting that widespread clonality prevails at this level, without sufficient amounts of recombination to break up associations between microsatellite alleles.[9,60] However, not all observations of *T. cruzi* intra-lineage population structures are consistent with a total lack of recombination. Strictly asexual (diploid) populations are expected to be characterized by fixed heterozygosity due to alleles at the same locus independently acquiring different mutations over time, a process often referred to as the "Meselson effect."[62] However, this phenomenon is not observed for TcI or TcIII; natural sylvatic populations actually show unexpectedly low levels of heterozygosity. This also appears to also be true of TcII and TcIV although sampling of these lineages has been far less comprehensive.[31,35] Explanations for the high levels of homozygosity in TcI−IV may include frequent LOH due to high rates of gene conversion or mitotic recombination. Alternatively, sexual recombination, even at relatively low frequencies could prevent allelic divergence; this could occur between individuals that are genetically identical (selfing), closely related (inbreeding), or genetically distinct (outcrossing).[31]

Perhaps the most important issue with intra-DTU population genetic analyses is that they do not represent the situation occurring at the population scale. Grouping of divergent non-recombining subgroups (in the case of *T. cruzi*, major DTUs) can inflate genetic linkage statistics and mask recombination events occurring between more closely related individuals.[61] Appropriately sampled populations, with samples minimally subdivided in space and time are difficult to obtain for protozoa like *T. cruzi* but they are, nevertheless, required to draw accurate conclusions regarding the frequency of recombination from population genetic data.[53] The high possibility of mixed infections also means that multiple parasite clones should ideally be isolated from individual hosts and vectors for analysis.[63] Efforts to conduct studies of this type have begun to bear fruit. For example, sexually recombining populations of TcI have been identified in Ecuador and Bolivia.[40,41] Importantly, in both cases these populations were in relatively close geographical proximity to others that appeared to be predominantly clonal. This highlights the fact that different population structures may be present in different ecological and epidemiological contexts.

# Conclusions and future research

In conclusion, the concept that genetic exchange is of little importance to *T. cruzi* is no longer tenable. Experimental work has demonstrated that *T. cruzi* has an extant capacity for genetic exchange, albeit by a somewhat unusual mechanism of fusion of diploids and genome erosion. Inter-lineage genetic exchange, though infrequent, has clearly shaped the evolution of the species, giving rise to at least two of the principal DTUs, TcV and TcVI. Furthermore, this has had a profound epidemiological impact: TcV and TcVI are widespread and probably recently dispersed agents of Chagas disease. Mechanisms of genetic exchange in natural populations may be more varied and distinct from fusion of diploids and genome erosion discovered in the laboratory. Mitochondrial introgression is emerging as a common feature of both inter- and Inter-lineage recombination events. Analyses of spatiotemporally appropriate, multiclonal samples have identified cases of frequently recombining TcI populations. Further experimental crosses, combined with genome-scale sequence analysis of parents and hybrids, as well as higher resolution analysis of natural hybrids and their putative parents, should soon yield insights into the mechanisms of genetic exchange in *T. cruzi*.

In terms of control of Chagas disease, it is important to re-examine the association of *T. cruzi* genotypes with drug susceptibility, virulence, and pathogenesis, all of which are traits that may be rapidly spread by genetic exchange within and between lineages. Given the high level of genetic diversity within *T. cruzi* and the complexity of its population structure(s), new drugs should be tested against representatives of all the lineages, including hybrid strains.

## Acknowledgments

We thank the Wellcome Trust, the European Union Seventh Framework Program, and the BBSRC (UK) for financial support of our research. We especially thank all current and previous research collaborators working on *T. cruzi* and Chagas disease, particularly those in Latin America.

## References

1. Tibayrenc M, Ayala FJ. The clonal theory of parasitic protozoa: 12 years on. *Trends Parasitol* 2002;**18**:405—10.
2. Tibayrenc M, Kjellberg F, Ayala FJ. A clonal theory of parasitic protozoa: the population structures of *Entamoeba, Giardia, Leishmania, Naegleria, Plasmodium, Trichomonas* and *Trypanosoma* and their medical and taxonomical consequences. *Proc Natl Acad Sci USA* 1990;**87**:2414—18.
3. Ramírez JD, Llewellyn MS. Reproductive clonality in protozoan pathogens—truth or artefact? *Mol Ecol* 2014;**23**:4195—202.
4. Zingales B, Andrade SG, Briones MRS, et al. A new consensus for *Trypanosoma cruzi* intraspecific nomenclature: second revision meeting recommends TcI to TcVI. *Mem Inst Oswaldo Cruz* 2009;**104**:1051—4.
5. Marcili A, Lima L, Cavazzana M, et al. A new genotype of *Trypanosoma cruzi* associated with bats evidenced by phylogenetic analyses using SSU rDNA, cytochrome b and Histone H2B genes and genotyping based on ITS1 rDNA. *Parasitology* 2009;**136**:641—55.
6. Miles MA, Llewellyn MS, Lewis MD, et al. The molecular epidemiology and phylogeography of *Trypanosoma cruzi* and parallel research on *Leishmania*: looking back and to the future. *Parasitology* 2009;**136**:1509—28.

7. Messenger LA, Miles MA, Bern C. Between a bug and a hard place: *Trypanosoma cruzi* genetic diversity and the clinical outcomes of Chagas disease. *Exp Rev Antiinfect Therapy* 2015;**13**:995−1029.

8. Carrasco HJ, Segovia M, Llewellyn MS, et al. Geographical distribution of *Trypanosoma cruzi* genotypes in Venezuela. *PLoS NTD* 2012;**6**:e1707.

9. Llewellyn MS, Miles MA, Carrasco HJ, et al. Genome-scale multilocus microsatellite typing of *Trypanosoma cruzi* discrete typing unit I reveals phylogeographic structure and specific genotypes linked to human infection. *PLoS Pathogens* 2009;**5**:e1000410.

10. Cura CI, Lucero RH, Bisio M, et al. *Trypanosoma cruzi* discrete typing units in Chagas disease patients from endemic and non-endemic regions of Argentina. *Parasitology* 2012;**139**:516−21.

11. de Oliveira MT, Machado de Assis GF, Oliveira e Silva VJC, et al. *Trypanosoma cruzi* discret typing units (TcII and TcVI) in samples of patients from two municipalities of the Jequitinhonha Valley, MG, Brazil, using two molecular typing strategies. *Parasit Vectors* 2015;**8**:1−11.

12. Yeo M, Acosta N, Llewellyn M, et al. Origins of Chagas disease: *Didelphis* species are natural hosts of *Trypanosoma cruzi* I and armadillos hosts of *Trypanosoma cruzi* II, including hybrids. *Int J Parasitol* 2005;**35**:225−33.

13. Chapman M, Baggaley R, Godfrey-Fausset P, et al. *Trypanosoma cruzi* from the Paraguayan Chaco: isoenzyme profiles of strains isolated at Makthlawaiya. *J Protozool* 1984;**31**:482−6.

14. D'Ávila DA, Macedo AM, Valadares HMS, et al. Probing population dynamics of *Trypanosoma cruzi* during progression of the chronic phase in chagasic patients. *J Clin Microbiol* 2009;**47**:1718−25.

15. Monteiro WM, Magalhães LKC, de Sá ARN, et al. *Trypanosoma cruzi* IV causing outbreaks of acute Chagas disease and infections by different haplotypes in the Western Brazilian Amazonia. *PLoS ONE* 2012;**7**:e41284.

16. Carrasco HJ, Frame IA, Valente SA, Miles MA. Genetic exchange as a possible source of genomic diversity in sylvatic populations of *Trypanosoma cruzi*. *Am J Trop Med Hyg* 1996;**54**:418−24.

17. Gaunt MW, Yeo M, Frame IA, Stothard JR, Carrasco HJ, Taylor MC. Mechanism of genetic exchange in American trypanosomes. *Nature* 2003;421.

18. Lewis MD, Llewellyn MS, Gaunt MW, Yeo M, Carrasco HJ, Miles MA. Flow cytometric analysis and microsatellite genotyping reveal extensive DNA content variation in *Trypanosoma cruzi* populations and expose contrasts between natural and experimental hybrids. *Int J Parasitol* 2009;**39**:1305−17.

19. Dvorak J, Hall T, Crane M, Engel J, McDaniel J, Uriegas R. *Trypanosoma cruzi*: flow cytometric analysis. I. Analysis of total DNA/organism by means of mithramycin-induced fluorescence. *J Protozool* 1982;**29**:430−7.

20. Bennett RJ, Johnson AD. Completion of a parasexual cycle in *Candida albicans* by induced chromosome loss in tetraploid strains. *EMBO J* 2003;**22**:2505−15.

21. Gibson W, Peacock L, Ferris V, Williams K, Bailey M. The use of yellow fluorescent hybrids to indicate mating in *Trypanosoma brucei*. *Parasit Vector* 2008;**1**:4.

22. Peacock L, Ferris V, Sharma R, et al. Identification of the meiotic life cycle stage of *Trypanosoma brucei* in the tsetse fly. *Proc Natl Acad Sci* 2011;**108**:3671−6.

23. Guevara P, Dias M, Rojas A, et al. Expression of fluorescent genes in *Trypanosoma cruzi* and *Trypanosoma rangeli* (Kinetoplastida: Trypanosomatidae): its application to parasite-vector biology. *J Med Entomol* 2005;48−56.

24. Pires SF, DaRocha WD, Freitas JM, et al. Cell culture and animal infection with distinct *Trypanosoma cruzi* strains expressing red and green fluorescent proteins. *Int J Parasitol* 2008;**38**:289−97.

25. Akopyants NS, Kimblin N, Secundino N, et al. Demonstration of genetic exchange during cyclical development of *Leishmania* in the Sand Fly Vector. *Science* 2009; **324**:265−8.

26. Jenni L, Marti S, Schweizer J, et al. Hybrid formation between African trypanosomes during cyclical transmission. *Nature* 1986;**322**:173−5.

27. Tibayrenc M, Miles MA. A genetic comparison between Brazilian and Bolivian zymodemes of *Trypanosoma cruzi*. *Trans R Soc Trop Med Hyg* 1983;**77**:76−83.

28. Volf P, Benkova I, Myskova J, Sadlova J, Campino L, Ravel C. Increased transmission potential of *Leishmania major/Leishmania infantum* hybrids. *Int J Parasitol* 2007; **37**:589−93.

29. Widmer G, Dvorak J, Miles M. Temperature modulation of growth rates and glucosephosphate isomerase isozyme activity in *Trypanosoma cruzi*. *Mol Biochem Parasitol* 1987;**23**:55−62.

30. Brisse S, Henriksson J, Barnabé C, et al. Evidence for genetic exchange and hybridization in *Trypanosoma cruzi* based on nucleotide sequences and molecular karyotype. *Infect Genet Evol* 2003;**2**:173−83.

31. Machado CA, Ayala FJ. Nucleotide sequences provide evidence of genetic exchange among distantly related lineages of *Trypanosoma cruzi*. *Proc Natl Acad Sci USA* 2001;**98**:7396−401.

32. Lewis MD, Llewellyn MS, Yeo M, Acosta N, Gaunt MW, Miles MA. Recent, independent and anthropogenic origins of *Trypanosoma cruzi* hybrids. *PLoS NTD* 2011;**5**:e1363.

33. Yeo M, Mauricio IL, Messenger LA, et al. Multilocus sequence typing (MLST) for lineage assignment and high resolution diversity studies in *Trypanosoma cruzi*. *PLoS NTD* 2011;**5**:e1049.

34. Flores-López CA, Machado CA. Analyses of 32 loci clarify phylogenetic relationships among *Trypanosoma cruzi* lineages and support a single hybridization prior to human contact. *PLoS NTD* 2011;**5**:e1272.

35. Westenberger SJ, Barnabé C, Campbell DA, Sturm NR. Two hybridization events define the population structure of *Trypanosoma cruzi*. *Genetics* 2005;**171**:527−43.

36. de Freitas JM, Augusto-Pinto L, Pimenta JR, et al. Ancestral genomes, sex, and the population structure of *Trypanosoma cruzi*. *PLoS Pathogens* 2006;**2**:e24.

37. Tomasini N, Diosque P. Evolution of *Trypanosoma cruzi*: clarifying hybridisations, mitochondrial introgressions and phylogenetic relationships between major lineages. *Mem Inst Oswaldo Cruz* 2015;**110**:403−13.

38. Westenberger SJ, Sturm NR, Campbell DA. *Trypanosoma cruzi* 5S rRNA arrays define five groups and indicate the geographic origins of an ancestor of the heterozygous hybrids. *Int J Parasitol* 2006;**36**:337−46.

39. Hamilton PB, Teixeira MMG, Stevens JR. The evolution of *Trypanosoma cruzi*: the "bat seeding" hypothesis. *Trends Parasitol* 2012;**28**:136−41.

40. Ocaña-Mayorga S, Llewellyn MS, Costales JA, Miles MA, Grijalva MJ. Sex, subdivision, and domestic dispersal of *Trypanosoma cruzi* lineage I in Southern Ecuador. *PLoS NTD* 2011;**4**:e915.

41. Barnabe C, Buitrago R, Bremond P, et al. Putative Panmixia in restricted populations of *Trypanosoma cruzi* isolated from wild *Triatoma infestans* in Bolivia. *PLoS ONE* 2013;**8**: e82269.

42. Brenière SF, Aliaga C, Waleckx E, et al. Genetic characterization of *Trypanosoma cruzi* DTUs in wild *Triatoma infestans* from Bolivia: predominance of TcI. *PLoS NTD* 2012; **6**:e1650.

43. Bargues MD, Klisiowicz DR, Panzera F, et al. Origin and phylogeography of the Chagas disease main vector *Triatoma infestans* based on nuclear rDNA sequences and genome size. *Infect Genet Evol* 2006;**6**:46−62.

44. Sturm NR, Vargas NS, Westenberger SJ, Zingales B, Campbell DA. Evidence for multiple hybrid groups in *Trypanosoma cruzi. Int J Parasitol* 2003;**33**:269−79.

45. Roellig DM, Savage MY, Fujita AW, et al. Genetic variation and exchange in *Trypanosoma cruzi* isolates from the United States. *PLoS ONE* 2013;**8**:e56198.

46. Shender LA, Lewis MD, Rejmanek D, Mazet JAK. Molecular diversity of *Trypanosoma cruzi* detected in the vector *Triatoma protracta* from California, USA. *PLoS NTD* 2016;**10**:e0004291.

47. Messenger LA, Llewellyn MS, Bhattacharyya T, et al. Multiple mitochondrial introgression events and heteroplasmy in *Trypanosoma cruzi* revealed by maxicircle MLST and next generation sequencing. *PLoS NTD* 2012;**6**.

48. Lewis MD, Ma J, Yeo M, Carrasco HJ, Llewellyn MS, Miles MA. Genotyping of *Trypanosoma cruzi*: systematic selection of assays allowing rapid and accurate discrimination of all known lineages. *Am J Trop Med Hyg* 2009;**81**:1041−9.

49. Ramírez JD, Guhl F, Messenger LA, et al. Contemporary cryptic sexuality in *Trypanosoma cruzi. Mol Ecol* 2012;**21**:4216−26.

50. Zumaya-Estrada FA, Messenger LA, Lopez-Ordonez T, et al. North American import? Charting the origins of an enigmatic *Trypanosoma cruzi* domestic genotype. *Parasit Vectors* 2012;**5**:1−9.

51. Lima VS, Jansen AM, Messenger LA, Miles MA, Llewellyn MS. Wild *Trypanosoma cruzi* I genetic diversity in Brazil suggests admixture and disturbance in parasite populations from the Atlantic Forest region. *Parasit Vectors* 2014;**7**:1−8.

52. Messenger LA, Garcia L, Vanhove M, et al. Ecological host fitting of *Trypanosoma cruzi* TcI in Bolivia: mosaic population structure, hybridization and a role for humans in Andean parasite dispersal. *Mol Ecol* 2015;**24**:2406−22.

53. Prugnolle F, De Meeûs T. Apparent high recombination rates in clonal parasitic organisms due to inappropriate sampling design. *Heredity* 2010;**104**:135−40.

54. Tibayrenc M, Ayala FJ. How clonal are *Trypanosoma* and *Leishmania*? *Trends Parasitol* 2013;**29**:264−9.

55. El-Sayed NM, Myler PJ, Bartholomeu DC, et al. The genome sequence of *Trypanosoma cruzi*, etiologic agent of Chagas disease. *Science* 2005;**309**:409−15.

56. Franzén O, Ochaya S, Sherwood E, et al. Shotgun sequencing analysis of *Trypanosoma cruzi* I Sylvio X10/1 and comparison with *T. cruzi* VI CL Brener. *PLoS NTD* 2011;**5**: e984.

57. Lauthier JJ, Tomasini N, Barnabe C, et al. Candidate targets for multilocus sequence typing of *Trypanosoma cruzi*: validation using parasite stocks from the Chaco Region and a set of reference strains. *Infect Genet Evol* 2012;**12**.

58. Diosque P, Tomasini N, Lauthier JJ, et al. Optimized multilocus sequence typing (MLST) scheme for *Trypanosoma cruzi. PLoS NTD* 2014;**8**:e3117.

59. Oliveira RP, Broude NE, Macedo AM, Cantor CR, Smith CL, Pena SDJ. Probing the genetic population structure of *Trypanosoma cruzi* with polymorphic microsatellites. *Proc Natl Acad Sci USA* 1998;**95**:3776−80.

60. Llewellyn MS, Lewis MD, Acosta N, et al. *Trypanosoma cruzi* IIc: phylogenetic and phylogeographic insights from sequence and microsatellite analysis and potential impact on emergent Chagas disease. *PLoS NTD* 2009;**3**:e510.
61. Maynard Smith J, Smith NH, O'Rourke M, Spratt BG. How clonal are bacteria? *Proc Natl Acad Sci USA* 1993;**90**:4384–8.
62. Mark Welch DB, Meselson M. Evidence for the evolution of bdelloid rotifers without sexual reproduction or genetic exchange. *Science* 2000;**288**:1211–15.
63. Llewellyn MS, Rivett-Carnac JB, Fitzpatrick S, et al. Extraordinary *Trypanosoma cruzi* diversity within single mammalian reservoir hosts implies a mechanism of diversifying selection. *Int J Parasitol* 2011;**41**:609–14.

# *Trypanosoma cruzi* and the model of predominant clonal evolution

M. Tibayrenc[1] and F.J. Ayala[2]

[1]Maladies Infectieuses et Vecteurs Ecologie, Génétique, Evolution et Contrôle MIVEGEC (Institut de Recherche pour le Développement 224- Centre National de la Recherche Scientifique 5290-Universités de Montpellier 1 and 2), Centre IRD, Montpellier, France, [2]University of California, Irvine, CA, United States

## Chapter Outline

## Introduction

The title of this chapter may sound strange to those who are not familiar with the concepts of evolutionary genetics. It refers to the evolutionary pattern in which discrete genetic lines undergo preponderant separate evolution, partly countered by

American Trypanosomiasis Chagas Disease. DOI: http://dx.doi.org/10.1016/B978-0-12-801029-7.00021-6

occasional bouts of hybridization events and genetic exchange. This situation is reached in many higher plants. It appears to be the best way to summarize the evolutionary strategy of *Trypanosoma cruzi*, as well as that of many other micropathogens, including other parasitic protozoa, fungi, bacteria, and viruses.

# An indispensable recall of evolutionary genetics

## Predominant clonal evolution: what does it mean?

Predominant clonal evolution (PCE) is the basic evolutionary model proposed for *T. cruzi*[1] and other eukaryotic pathogens, with many clarifications and refinements recently proposed.[2−7] Many misleading interpretations have been made, of the model designated by this term. Clarification is hence necessary. It can never be emphasized enough that clonality, according to this model, refers to all cases where offsprings have multilocus genotypes that are identical or extremely similar to parental lines, whatever the cytological mechanism of reproduction may be. PCE, in this genetical meaning, is synonymous with lack or rarity of genetic recombination (reassortment of genotypes occurring at different loci). This situation can originate from: (1) mitotic propagation; (2) several cases of parthenogenesis; (3) gynogenesis, hybridogenesis; (4) self-fertilization in the homozygous state; and (5) extreme cases of homogamy.

Mitotic propagation (1) is the usual case observed in many bacterial species and does occur in *T. cruzi*. However, PCE, again, has a much broader meaning. Cases (2) to (5) are able to generate genetic clones as well. Parthenogenesis (2) is observed in many insects, and even vertebrates.[8] Specific cases of parthenogenesis (gynogenesis, hybridogenesis) are recorded in some fish and salamander species. Interestingly, gynogenetic and hybridogenetic females mate and therefore mimic the behavior of sexuality. Only the genetic analysis of their offspring can evidence that they actually generate clonal lines.[8,9] Cases (4) and (5) have been presented as an alternative hypothesis to clonal evolution in the case of *Leishmania* parasites,[10−13] while according to the PCE model, they obviously constitute only a specific case of it.[2,14,15] Another recurrent source of misunderstanding comes from the fact that the PCE model does not by any means rule out occasional bouts of genetic exchange.[16] It only stipulates that such events are rare and interfere only at an evolutionary scale. The PCE model therefore does not amount to absolute clonality, as sometimes claimed.[17] It does not state either that its evolutionary and epidemiological impact is negligible (as misunderstood by some authors[18−22]), but only that it is not frequent enough to break up the predominance of clonal evolution.

Lack of, or severe restrictions to genetic recombination is the only, necessary, and sufficient criterion to settle the working hypothesis of broad-sense clonality (genetic clonality). This definition is broadly accepted by many scientists working on pathogen population genetics (see many examples cited in Refs. [2−7]). The relevant population genetics statistics is linkage disequilibrium (LD), or nonrandom association of genotypes occurring at different loci. By definition, linkage disequilibrium evaluates the obstacles to recombination and is the only statistical approach able to do this. Unilocus segregation analysis based on *Fis*, *Fst*, Hardy–Weinberg equilibrium analysis,[23] although very useful to explore mating strategies in depth, by its very nature cannot estimate the strength of recombination inhibition. Moreover, segregation tests are based on the hypothesis of diploidy, which has been recently questioned, since not only *Leishmania*,[24–33] but also *Trypanosoma cruzi*[34–37] have been hypothesized to undergo widespread aneuploidy. If this hypothesis is confirmed, tests based on diploidy will be irrelevant, while LD tests remain valid.

LD analysis is based on the very simple principle that the expected frequency of multilocus genotypes is the product of the observed frequencies of the unilocus genotypes they are composed of. For example, if two loci A and B are surveyed, and the observed frequencies of genotypes A1 and B2 are 0.3 and 0.5, respectively, the expected frequency of the bilocus genotype A1 + B2 is $0.3 \times 0.5 = 0.15$. When a large number of loci are surveyed, this analysis becomes very powerful, because the mere fact that a multilocus genotype is recorded more than once could become highly improbable. Calculating this by hand and simple chi-square analysis is possible but rapidly becomes cumbersome. Various indices have been published.[16,38] Biases due to time or geographical separation (Wahlund effect) have been previously discussed.[39]

LD tests evidence severe obstacles to recombination. However, in some cases, they could be positive in situations where the genetic clones in a given species are ephemeral and soon disappear in the common gene pool of the species (epidemic clonality[38]). From an epidemiological and medical point of view, the important parameter to evaluate is the stability of the genetic clones in space and time. For this, LD analysis is usefully completed by two approaches: (1) direct observation and (2) phylogenetic analysis.

1. Direct observation is done at a limited timescale. The *T. cruzi* strains have now been characterized for long enough to score recurrent observations of multilocus genotypes that have been repeatedly sampled for more than 30 years over vast geographical areas. This is in itself a strong indication of stable clonal propagation. Such observations cannot be made in highly recombinant pathogens such as *Helicobacter pylori*.[40]
2. Phylogenetic analysis addresses a much longer timescale than population genetics and aims at reconstructing the evolutionary past of a given species over thousands or millions of years. This chapter is not the place to provide a comprehensive presentation of phylogenetic analysis. Many valuable textbooks have detailed the matter. Instead, I will present a few general principles that are specifically relevant for surveying the subspecific phylogenetic diversity of *T. cruzi*.

## T. cruzi *undergoes some genetic exchange*

In an organism such as *T. cruzi*, in which some recombination is occurring (see Introduction section and further), phylogenetic analysis should be understood in a specific manner. Indeed, by definition, phylogenetic analysis surveys the evolution of discrete lines that are genetically strictly separated from each other (clades). When some genetic exchange occurs between these lines, it clouds the phylogenetic picture of the species under study.[2,15] The observed departures from an ideal phylogenetic reconstruction are in themselves useful information on how and how much occasional recombination is operating. On the other hand, the cleaner the phylogenetic reconstruction is, the stronger the evidence is that recombination is exceptional or absent. Pathogenic microorganisms that are strictly clonal are probably the exception rather than the rule. It would be the case of the African trypanosome *Trypanosoma brucei gambiense* "group I."[41] It is for this reason that we have stated[2] that a strict cladistic approach is not adequate in the case of micropathogens. We have rather recommended a flexible phylogenetic approach based on a congruence criterion inspired by the principle of genealogical concordance between independent genes proposed for the recognition of biological taxa.[9] According to this congruence criterion, adding more relevant data (e.g., more loci, or more molecular markers, or data obtained from different phylogenetic approaches), will reveal a growing phylogenetic signal in the sample under study. We have proposed that such a growing phylogenetic signal is the signature of the "clonality threshold," beyond which the impact of clonal evolution definitely overcomes that of genetic recombination.[7] This clonality threshold concept is neither "pseudoquantitative" nor "vague."[42] Moreover, "predominant" clonal evolution is not open to "wide interpretation."[42] The growing phylogenetic signal, on which the clonality threshold concept is based, is easy to observe with appropriate data (see: *T. cruzi* is a structured species). The clonality threshold concept makes it possible to dismiss vague, subjective terms, such as "gross" incongruences (between phylogenetic trees),[43] "widespread genetic exchange,"[22] and "intense lateral exchange of genetic information,"[42] and to rather rely on a clear-cut parameter that identifies the "clonality border."

## Gene trees and species trees are not the same[44]

The evolutionary history of a given gene often does not reflect the general evolution of the species under study. The gene could undergo strong selective pressures or have a specific evolutionary rapidity (molecular clock). The general, most welcome, tendency is now to base phylogenetic reconstruction of species on a broad range of genes. Although gene sequencing conveys a great deal of information, the use of classical markers such as multilocus enzyme electrophoresis (MLEE) or random amplified polymorphic DNA (RAPD), if it is based on a broad range of loci, could be more reliable than the analysis of the sequence of only one gene or a few genes to reconstruct the evolution of a species. Many studies on *T. cruzi* have relied on the analysis of only one gene or a few genes.[45-47] These studies convey useful information on the precise genes they investigate. However, extrapolation to the entire species should be done with caution. The ideal approach is of course to combine the power of (1) gene sequencing and (2) multilocus analysis. This is done by multilocus sequence typing (MLST[48]), which has been now widely used for *T. cruzi*.[49,50] The last step is accomplished by population genomics, relying on the whole genome analysis of various strains. Such an approach tends to become routine in viruses[51] and bacteria.[52] This has not been done until now in the case of *T. cruzi*.

## Comparing the information of different markers

Different genetic markers explore different regions of the genome that have specific evolutionary patterns. For example, MLEE explores only genes that code for enzyme variants, while RAPD also surveys noncoding sequences and is able to evidence copy-number polymorphism (insertions/deletions/inversions), contrary to both MLEE and MLST. When the phylogenies designed after different markers corroborate each other, this is particularly strong evidence that these phylogenies are valid, according to the congruence criterion above exposed. It is a specific strong case of linkage disequilibrium (correlation between independent sets of genetic markers: criterion g).[16]

## Erroneous concept: microsatellites cannot be used for phylogenetic reconstruction

It has been claimed that microsatellites exhibit too much homoplasy to be useable for phylogenetic reconstruction. Actually the same can be said for the other uses of microsatellites, such as population genetics and strain typing. For example, in population genetics, homoplasy could mimic genetic recombination and lower the observed rate of LD. In strain typing, due to homoplasy, two strains could appear more closely related than they actually are. Microsatellites can be used for phylogenetic reconstruction, but must be used with caution. One has to address micro-evolutionary levels only, in accordance with the fast molecular clock of this marker. Moreover, the risk of homoplasy should be kept in mind.

# The results: how does *T. cruzi* evolve?

Having performed evolutionary analysis based on the principles recalled above, the results presented hereafter have emerged.

## Is T. cruzi a "good" species?

This is the first question to arise from a medical and epidemiological point of view, especially when studying molecular epidemiology (strain typing). Defining what a good species is refers to the very definition of what a species is. Briefly, species are generally defined as: (1) a community of sexual reproduction (the biological species concept); (2) a clade (a monophyletic lineage with only one ancestor; the phylogenetic species concept); or (3) a set of organisms that share specific phenotypic traits (the phenotypic species concept). The biological species concept is not easy to handle and inadequate in those organisms in which sexual reproduction is not a constant and mandatory process, which it is the case for the agent of Chagas disease. On the other hand, there is no doubt that *T. cruzi* meets the criteria for (2) and (3) (phylogenetic and phenotypic species concepts). All phylogenetic studies have brought all *T. cruzi* strains into a single clade that is distinguishable from closely related taxa (*T. cruzi marenkellei*, a close relative of *T. cruzi*, a bat parasite, is the best choice of such an outgroup). Moreover, all *T. cruzi* strains share a set of specific phenotypic characteristics (morphological aspect, vectorial transmission by triatomine bugs, potential host range extended to all mammal species, but restricted to them, geographical distribution limited to the New World, potential pathogenic power all point to Chagas disease). Consequently, according to the phylogenetic and phenotypic concepts, *T. cruzi* is a so-called good species. The fact that *T. cruzi* is a unique clade makes it possible to design various molecular markers that will be specifically shared by all strains of the taxon and only by them (in the cladistic jargon, synapomorphic characteristics).

## T. cruzi *undergoes PCE*

It can actually be said that the agent of Chagas disease is a paradigmatic case of this evolutionary model. Recurrent observations have been made of multilocus genotypes that have persisted unchanged for more than 30 years over vast geographical areas. Moreover, the linkage disequilibrium in *T. cruzi* is considerable and has been verified for a large set of genetic markers, including MLEE,[1,53] restriction-fragment length polymorphism of kinetoplast DNA,[54] RAPD,[55,56] and microsatellites.[57] Linkage disequilibrium is so strong in *T. cruzi* that it also involves the polymorphism of expressed genes surveyed by random amplified differentially expressed sequences (RADES)[58] and genes that undergo strong natural selection.[59]

Again, clonality and clonal evolution are taken here in the genetic sense and the precise cytological mechanism of PCE in *T. cruzi* continues to be debated. Homogamy and self-fertilization[10] could play a role in some cycles, as suggested by results obtained with microsatellite markers.[60] Nevertheless, the important result remains: genetically homogeneous lines isolated from each other (genetic clones by definition) persist over long periods of time and vast geographical areas in natural populations of *T. cruzi*.

Other evidence for PCE in *T. cruzi* comes from the existence of stable genetic subdivisions, within which PCE is also verified (see further).

## *Genetic variants of* T. cruzi *represent clonets, not clones*

Once PCE has been ascertained, it comes to mind that the genotypes identified by MLEE, MLST, RAPD, microsatellites, etc., represent the clones of this parasite. Now let us identify genotypes with 15 MLEE loci. For example, 43 different genotypes can be observed.[1] If we take a broader range of loci, say 22 of them, many of the previously identified presumably homogeneous genotypes split into several additional ones.[53] This is a never-ending story. The only way to exhaust the complete clonal diversity of a given species would be to sequence all the strains of this species, an unfeasible task. Moreover, this would not take into account genomic rearrangements, which also play a role in clonal diversity and could be involved in gene expression.

To overcome this difficulty, the term "clonet" has been coined[14] to refer to those sets of stocks that appear to be identical with a given set of genetic markers in a basically clonal species. *T. cruzi* zymodemes, schizodemes, RAPDdemes, etc., should therefore be considered clonets rather than true clones. From an evolutionary point of view, clonets represent sets of closely related clones.

## Recombination operates at the evolutionary scale: reticulate evolution

The presence of hybrid genotypes in *T. cruzi* natural populations has long been hypothesized.[61−64] The potentiality of genetic recombination in this species has been experimentally demonstrated by Gaunt et al.[65] These experimental hybrids have been obtained from parental genotypes that are genetically only closely related. They seem to be generated by fusion of diploid parents followed by genomic erosion slowly returning to a diploid state. Natural hybrids seem to be of a different nature. They are predominantly diploid and can be the result of hybridization between distantly related parental genotypes.[66] Different scenarios and genealogies have been proposed to explain the generation of the currently observed natural hybrids in *T. cruzi*.[17] This will be detailed further (see: Evolutionary origin of the hybrid near-clades). At this step, a number of important points about recombination in *T. cruzi* should be underlined: (1) these events are exceptional in this parasite's natural populations. By definition, frequent genetic exchange would be incompatible with the strong inhibition of genetic recombination evidenced by linkage disequilibrium. (2) Once generated, the hybrid genotypes are stabilized by clonal propagation and behave like genetic clones. They have been recurrently observed unchanged over long periods of time and large geographical areas. (3) These natural hybrid clones are widespread in domestic chagasic cycles and could represent a specific adaptation to these transmission cycles, in which they behave like successful genotypes.

## T. cruzi *is a structured species*

This means that its natural populations are divided into discrete and stable subdivisions between which the genetic distances convey reliable evolutionary information.[39]

The existence of such clusters was first postulated by the pioneering MLEE studies of Miles et al.[67,68] It is interesting to note that, in spite of a lack of genetic interpretation of these data, the MLEE variants identified at that time (zymodemes I, II, and III) are still there, although the picture has of course been refined by further studies (Table 21.1). Again, the permanency of the multilocus genotypes to which these zymodemes correspond is in itself a strong indication of stable clonal propagation.

## The discrete typing units or "near-clades"

The term "discrete typing units" was coined to overcome the difficulty that occasional hybridization events make it impossible to consider *T. cruzi*'s genetic

**Table 21.1 Correspondence between the most recent nomenclature of *Trypanosoma cruzi* genetic variants and previously published nomenclatures**

| 1 | 2 | 3 | 4 | 5 |
|---|---|---|---|---|
| DTU I | DTU 1 | 1–25 | Z I | X10 cl1, Cuica cl1 |
| DTU II | DTU 2a | 26–29 | Z III | CAN III cl1 |
| DTU III | DTU 2b | 30–34 | Z II | TU 18 cl2 |
| DTU IV | DTU 2c | 35–37 | Z II | M5631, M6241 |
| DTU V | DTU 2d | 38, 39 | Z II | MN cl2, SC43 cl1 |
| DTU VI | DTU 2e | 40, 43 | Z II | CL Brenner, Tulahuen cl2 |

1 = Ref. 69.
2 = Ref. 56.
3 = Ref. 1.
4 = Ref. 67.
5 = Representative stocks.

subdivisions as true clades. Indeed, (1) these subdivisions are not strictly separated from each other, as true clades should be, and (2) hybrid clones have two parental genotypes, while true clades should originate from one ancestral parent only. The concept of discrete typing units (DTUs) has therefore been proposed[70]: sets of stocks that are genetically closer to each other than to any other stock and are identifiable by common molecular, genetic, biochemical, or immunological markers called tags. The genetic subdivisions identified within *T. cruzi* fully match this definition, whereas they very imperfectly fit the definition of clades. More recently, we have proposed the term "near-clades" to design those stable genetic subdivisions within a given microbial species when discreteness is clouded by occasional recombination.[2] Using the convergence criterion above exposed makes it possible to evidence the growing phylogenetic signal that is a typical feature of the near-clades. *T. cruzi* DTUs represent typical near-clades. The near-clade concept is more informative than the DTU concept, since it is based on a precise evolutionary definition. We have proposed that the very existence of near-clades was a typical signature and a main result of PCE in a given species.[2] It has been asserted that the observation of such near-clades within a given species was "self-evident," and therefore would be an artifactual evidence for PCE.[22,42] It is true that, once the near-clades have been clearly evidenced, it is useless and redundant to perform on the whole species population genetic tests such as LD. However, (1) we have read nowhere but in our articles the proposal that near-clades, even considered as "self-evident," were a typical manifestation of PCE; and (2) evidencing near-clades is all the less self-evident (except when arriving long after the battle) because their identification in *T. cruzi* took many years of in-depth population genetic analyses, and because their very numbering still is under dispute[71]. The near-clade concept has a clear evolutionary definition. It makes it possible to replace with a unique term the many, confusing, vague names used in the literature dealing with pathogen population genetics to designate within-species genetic subdivisions (assemblages, clades, clusters, genogroups, lineages, genetic groups, among others).

Detailed analysis by MLEE,[53] RAPD,[56] and gene sequencing[72,73] have congruently evidenced the existence of six DTUs within *T. cruzi* (Fig. 21.1). These DTUs have also been uncovered by RADES,[58] which shows that this structuring persists when surveying coding expressed genes. PCR-RFLP typing[74] and MLST[49] have also corroborated this clustering into six DTUs.

The formerly proposed partition of *T. cruzi* into two major subdivisions,[39,75] DTU 1 and 2,[53,56] named TC I and TC II (TC = *Trypanosoma cruzi*[76]), is presently questioned, although possibly not ruled out. In a recent meeting, Chagas disease experts decided to retain the subdivision of *T. cruzi* into six DTUs as the official reference model for this parasite's genetic variability. However, it was decided to renumber the DTUs into TC I−VI instead of DTUs 1, 2b, 2c, 2a, 2d, and 2e, respectively (Table 21.1), to take into account the present debate on the presence of two major subdivisions.[69,77]

It has proved to be impossible to reliably identify each DTU with unique markers. Instead, a convenient set of three markers has been proposed.[78]

Thus far the six DTUs have been upheld. The studies that have evidenced them have sometimes relied on impressively extensive samples, the most exhaustive of which is the MLEE study by Barnabé et al.[53] which involved no less than 434 different stocks. It is possible that this classification will be slightly modulated by further samplings involving more sylvatic cycles. However, to date these studies have evidenced further variability within the DTUs and have revealed some very interesting new epidemiological features, but have corroborated the classification.[60,79]

A seventh near-clade, referred to as "Tc-Bat" (for it has been isolated only from bats) has been recently evidenced.[47,80−82] Tc-bat has been recorded years apart in Brazil, Colombia, Ecuador, and Panama, in different species of bats, which illustrates the stability in space and time of the near-clades. Lastly, the partitioning into seven near-clades has been recently challenged by Barnabé et al.[71] on a broad sample of strains, but with a limited set of one nuclear gene and two mitochondrial genes. This proposal has obviously to be explored with a broader set of genetic markers. However, it illustrates the fact that even in the extremely well-studied species *T. cruzi*, evidencing near-clades is far from being "self-evident."[42]

## Evolutionary origin of the hybrid near-clades

Some near-clades have a clear hybrid origin. The number of hybrid events and the precise sequence that have generated the present near-clades continues to be debated.[17] It is generally recognized that the evolutionary origin of some near-clades results from the following recombination events: (1) near-clades III and IV probably originated from a hybridization event between ancestral near-clade I and II genotypes[83] and (2) near-clades V and VI probably resulted from the hybridization of genotypes similar to near-clade II with near-clade III.[64,83]

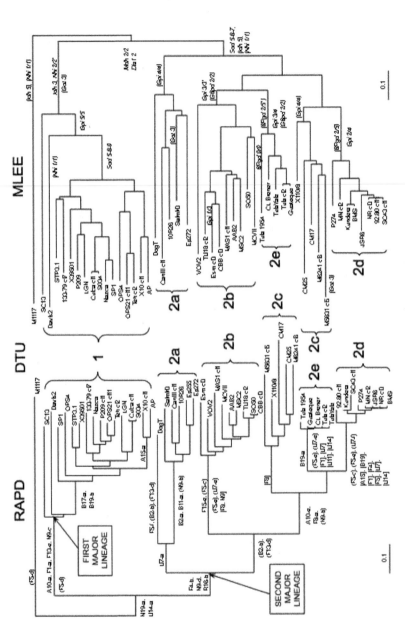

**Figure 21.1** Two phylogenetic trees depicting the evolutionary relationships among *Trypanosoma cruzi* genotypes: isoenzymes (right) and RAPD (left). The strong agreement between the two trees is a clear manifestation of linkage disequilibrium.
*Source:* From Brisse S, Barnabé C, Tibayrenc M. Identification of six *Trypanosoma cruzi* phylogenetic lineages by random amplified polymorphic DNA and multilocus enzyme electrophoresis. *Int J Parasitol* 2000;**30**:35–44.[56]

## Nomenclature considerations

We have already explained why the term "clade" is inappropriate to designate *T. cruzi* genetic subdivisions. "Clusters" and "groups" are also inadequate, because, contrary to near-clades, they have no precise definition.

The recent meeting of experts on *T. cruzi* nomenclature suggested replacing the DTUs with six Linnaean species with binomial Latin names. However, the proposal was not retained until further notice. The group has agreed that new species of pathogenic microorganisms should be based on the congruence of clear phylogenetic and medico-phenotypic characteristics only. The near-clade concept, with its flexible phylogenetic approach, makes it possible to revisit the phylogenetic species concept for microbial pathogens. A newly described species should fulfill two criteria: (1) it should correspond to a clearly-identified near-clade and (2) it should exhibit relevant epidemiological and/or pathogenic features.[5]

## Medical and epidemiological characteristics of T. cruzi *near-clades*

These specificities have often been exaggerated. For example, it is incorrect to consider that near-clade I is specifically linked to sylvatic cycles.[17] It has been recorded many times in classical domestic cycles involving chronic chagasic patients and the vector *Triatoma infestans*. Near-clade IV (zymodeme III), classically considered to be linked to sylvatic Amazonian cycles, has been also recorded in chronic chagasic patients in Ecuador.[84]

Now the null hypothesis that near-clade subdividing is neutral compared to Chagas disease epidemiology and geographical distribution can be reliably rejected.

The geographical distribution of the near-clades is not uniform. Most of them are present in most places of Chagas transmission, including the United States, which shows that *T. cruzi* pertains to the native fauna in the United States.[85] However, the hybrid near-clades V and VI are predominant in the southern part of the area of Chagas transmission and are specifically related to domestic cycles, for example. Near-clade I is largely predominant in Mexico and Venezuela. Still, exhaustive mapping of near-clade geographical distribution remains to be done.

The question of a clinical specificity of *T. cruzi* genetic variants has long been open[86] and has not yet received a final answer. The near-clades show clear pathogenic specificities in animal experiments,[87] but this cannot be extrapolated to human disease.

More generally, *T. cruzi* near-clades often show strong statistical associations between various experimental parameters, such as growth speed in in vitro and in vivo culture, pathogenicity for laboratory animals, transmissibility through insect vectors, and in vitro and in vivo sensitivity to antichagasic drugs.[88] However, these various studies are complex and therefore have investigated a limited number of stocks (approximately 20).

Lastly, there are clear links between near-clade classification and gene expression surveyed by proteomic analysis.[89,90]

## Within-near-clade population genetics: the "Russian doll" model

It has been asserted that recombination could be severely restricted between genetic clusters that subdivide a given species (=near-clades), while it would not be, or would be much less, within each of these near-clades.[22,91] The near-clades would therefore be equivalent to cryptic, biological species. The Russian doll model[3] has been proposed to falsify this hypothesis. It states that within the near-clades, PCE also is verified. Each near-clade exhibits a sort of miniature picture of the whole species, with lesser near-clades and LD (Fig. 21.2).

One has to be careful with the evolutionary scale considered here. Since the within-near-clade evolutionary scale is smaller than the whole-species scale, the level of resolution of the markers used for the latter could not be appropriate for the former. Within near-clade apparent recombination could therefore be due to a statistical type II error (impossibility to reject the null hypothesis of recombination, not because it is verified, but rather, because of a trivial lack of resolution). It is therefore required to rely on markers with resolution power adequate to the microevolutionary scale of within-near-clade genetic diversity.

Typical cases of Russian doll patterns are recorded in *Leishmania*, as well as in *T. cruzi*.[3,7] In *T. cruzi*, the main examples are found within the near-clade I. These lesser subdivisions have been labeled I a to e[92] (Fig. 21.3).

They have been corroborated by various markers.[93,94] These lesser near-clades are distributed over vast geographic areas and are observed in sympatry, which demonstrates their stability in space and time. A typical Russian doll pattern has been

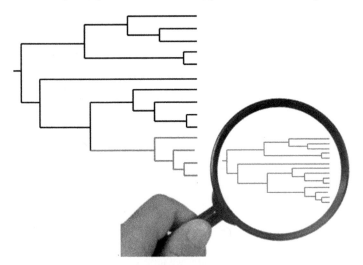

**Figure 21.2** "Russian doll" model. When population genetic tests are performed with adequate markers (of sufficient resolution) within each of the near-clades that subdivide the species under study (large tree, left part of the figure), they reveal a miniature picture of the whole species, with the two main PCE features, namely, linkage disequilibrium and lesser near-clades (small tree, right part of the figure). This is evidence that the near-clades are not cryptic biological species, and that they also undergo predominant clonal evolution.

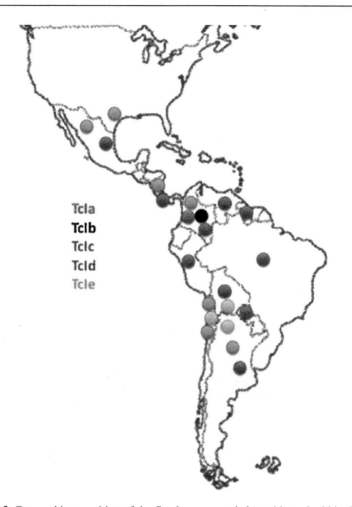

**Figure 21.3** Geographic repartition of the five lesser near-clades evidenced within the *Trypanosoma cruzi* near-clade TCI (see Fig. 21.1). The lesser near-clades are widely distributed and occur in sympatry, which is an evidence of a "Russian doll pattern."[3]
*Source:* After Guhl F, Ramírez JD. *Trypanosoma cruzi* I diversity: towards the need of genetic subdivision? *Acta Tropica* 2011;**119**:14.

recorded also in Argentinean strains pertaining to near-clade I.[50] The few studies that are at odds with the hypothesis of a Russian doll pattern within *T. cruzi* near-clades[43,95–97] definitely need to be confirmed by broader and more reliable samples.

*T. cruzi* Russian doll patterns, if confirmed by further studies, indicate that PCE acts, not only at the level of the whole species, but also, within each of its near-clades.

## Relevance of T. cruzi *genetic variability in applied research*

The concepts of clonet, near-clade, and Russian doll pattern are robust and it is likely that they will not be called into question by further studies.

The clonets and near-clades are convenient units of analysis for molecular epidemiology (epidemiological tracking, strain typing). However, clonet identification should be based on a broad range of markers. A set of three markers has been proposed for reliable, routine characterization of *T. cruzi* near-clades.[78]

Apart from epidemiological tracking, the near-clades should be taken into account for all applied studies investigating *T. cruzi*: clinical studies, drug development, diagnostic testing, and vaccine design.[98] It is crucial, for example, to verify that a new drug is effective in all genetic variants of *T. cruzi*. A set of stocks representative of the near-clade classification should therefore be used for all these types of study.

Lastly, clonets and near-clades, due to their discreteness and stability in space and time, are ideal units of analysis for experimental evolution.[88−90]

# Conclusion: *Trypanosoma cruzi* should be a star in the field of pathogen population genetics

This is unexpected, since the community of scientists working on Chagas disease is very limited by comparison with those working on AIDS, tuberculosis, and malaria. Nevertheless, it can be said that *T. cruzi* is by far the pathogenic microorganism that population genetics knows best and can compete in this domain with the bacterium *Escherichia coli*. In spite of the obstacle that it is a pathogenic agent, it is our hope now to "sell" *Trypanosoma cruzi* as a pet model for basic evolutionary research, together with *Escherichia coli*, *Drosophila melanogaster*, *Mus musculus*, and *Caenorhabditis elegans*.[99]

As far as applied research is concerned, it is our hope that *T. cruzi*'s genetic variability is far from having revealed all its secrets and will continue to make great contributions to the survey, control, and cure of Chagas disease.

# Glossary of specialized terms

**Clade** Evolutionary lineage defined by cladistic analysis. A clade is monophyletic (it has only one ancestor) and is genetically isolated (which means that it evolves independently) from other clades.

**Cladistic analysis** A specific method of phylogenetic analysis based on the polarization of characters, that are divided into ancestral (plesiomorphic) and derived (apomorphic) characteristics.

**Genetic distance** Various statistical measures inferred from genetic data, estimating the genetic dissimilarities among individuals or populations. Genetic distances can be based on the percentage of band mismatches on gels (as for markers such as MLEE or RAPD) or allelic frequency differences or the percentage of sequence divergence.

**Genotype** Genetic constitution of a given organism; cf. phenotype.

**Homoplasy** Possession shared by distinct phylogenetic lines of identical characteristics that do not come from a common ancestry. The origin of homoplasic characteristics can be: (a) convergence (possession of identical characteristics derived from different ancestral characteristics, due to convergent evolutionary pressure; f), (b) parallelism (possession of identical characteristics derived from a single ancestral characteristic, and generated independently in different phylogenetic lines), and (c) reversion (restoration of an ancestral characteristic from a derived characteristic).

**Molecular clock** In its strict, original sense (more appropriately called the DNA clock hypothesis), the concept that the rate of nucleotide substitutions in DNA is constant. In a broader sense, it is simply the evolutionary speed of the part of the genome that encodes the variability of a given marker. This speed is commended by the rate of substitution/mutation. It may be regular or irregular.

**Multilocus genotype** The combined genotype of a given strain or a given individual established with several genetic loci.

**Outgroup** In cladistics or phylogenetics, an outgroup is a (monophyletic) group of organisms that is used as a reference group for determining the phylogenetic relationship in a set of monophyletic groups of organisms. The outgroup is selected to be closely related to the groups under study, but less closely than any single one of the groups under study is to another.

**Phenotype** All observable properties of a given individual or a given population apart from the genotype. The phenotype is not limited to morphological characteristics and can include, e.g., physiological or biochemical parameters. The pathogenicity of a microorganism is a phenotypic property. The phenotype is produced by the interaction between the genotype and the environment.

**Phylogenetics** A branch of genetics that aims at reconstructing the evolutionary past and genetic relationships of taxa, species, strains, or of separate evolutionary lines.

**Phylogeny** Evolutionary relationships between taxa, species, organisms, genes, or molecules.

**Population genetics** Analysis of allele and genotype frequency distribution and modifications under the influence of genetic drift, natural selection, mutation, and gene flow. It also takes into account the factors of population subdivision and population structure.

**Sympatry** Living in the same geographical location.

# Acknowledgment

We thank Jenny Telleria for designing Fig. 21.2.

# References

1. Tibayrenc M, Ward P, Moya A, Ayala FJ. Natural populations of *Trypanosoma cruzi*, the agent of Chagas'disease, have a complex multiclonal structure. *Proc Nat Acad Sci USA* 1986;**83**:115−19.
2. Tibayrenc M, Ayala FJ. Reproductive clonality of pathogens: a perspective on pathogenic viruses, bacteria, fungi, and parasitic protozoa. *Proc Nat Acad Sci USA* 2012;**109**(48): E3305−13.

3. Tibayrenc M, Ayala FJ. How clonal are *Trypanosoma* and *Leishmania*? *Trends Parasitol* 2013;**29**:264−9.
4. Tibayrenc M, Ayala FJ. New insights into Clonality and Panmixia in *Plasmodium* and *Toxoplasma*. *Adv Parasitol* 2014;**84**:253−68.
5. Tibayrenc M, Ayala FJ. *Cryptosporidium, Giardia, Cryptococcus, Pneumocystis* genetic variability: cryptic biological species or clonal near-clades? *PLoS Pathogens* 2014; **10**(4):e1003908 Available from: http://dx.doi.org/10.1371/journal.ppat.1003908.
6. Tibayrenc M, Ayala FJ. Reproductive clonality in protozoan pathogens—truth or artifact? A reply. *Mol Ecol* 2015;**24**:5778−81.
7. Tibayrenc M, Ayala FJ. The population genetics of *Trypanosoma cruzi* revisited in the light of the predominant clonal evolution model. *Acta Tropica* 2015;**151**:156−65.
8. Avise JC. Evolutionary perspectives on clonal reproduction in vertebrate animals. *Proc Nat Acad Sci USA* 2015;**112**:8867−73.
9. Avise JC. *Molecular markers, natural history and evolution*. 2nd ed. New York. London: Chapman & Hall; 2004.
10. Rougeron V, De Meeûs T, Hide M, Waleckx E, Bermudez H, Arevalo J, et al. Extreme inbreeding in *Leishmania braziliensis*. *Proc Nat Acad Sci USA* 2009; **25**:10224−9.
11. Rougeron V, De Meeûs T, Kako Ouraga S, Hide M, Bañuls AL. "Everything You Always Wanted to Know About Sex (but Were Afraid to Ask)" in *Leishmania* after two decades of laboratory and field analyses. *PLoS Pathogens* 2010;**6**(8):e1001004. Available from: http://dx.doi.org/10.1371/journal.ppat.1001004.
12. Rougeron V, De Meeûs T, Bañuls AL. A primer for *Leishmania* population genetic studies. *Trends Parasitol* 2014;**31**:52−9.
13. Rougeron V, De Meeûs T, Bañuls AL. Response to Tibayrenc et al.: can recombination in *Leishmania* parasites be so rare? *Trends Parasitol* 2015;**31**:280−1.
14. Tibayrenc M, Ayala FJ. Towards a population genetics of microorganisms: the clonal theory of parasitic protozoa. *Parasitol Today* 1991;**7**:228−32.
15. Tibayrenc M, Ayala FJ. The clonal theory of parasitic protozoa: 12 years on. *Trends Parasitol* 2002;**18**:405−10.
16. Tibayrenc M, Kjellberg F, Ayala FJ. A clonal theory of parasitic protozoa: the population structure of *Entamoeba, Giardia, Leishmania, Naegleria, Plasmodium, Trichomonas* and *Trypanosoma*, and its medical and taxonomical consequences. *Proc Nat Acad Sci USA* 1990;**87**:2414−18.
17. Sturm N, Campbell DA. Alternative lifestyles: the population structure of *Trypanosoma cruzi*. *Acta Tropica* 2010;**115**:35−43.
18. Calo S, Billmyre BB, Heitman J. Generators of phenotypic diversity in the evolution of pathogenic microorganisms. *PLoS Pathogens* 2013;**9**(3):e1003181. Available from: http://dx.doi.org/10.1371/journal.ppat.1003181.
19. Messenger LA, Miles MA. Evidence and importance of genetic exchange among field populations of *Trypanosoma cruzi*. *Acta Tropica* 2015;**151**:150−5.
20. Miles MA, Llewellyn MS, Lewis MD, Yeo M, Baleela R, Fitzpatrick S, et al. The molecular epidemiology and phylogeography of *Trypanosoma cruzi* and parallel research on *Leishmania*: looking back and to the future. *Parasitology* 2009;**136**: 1509−28.
21. Ramírez JD, Guhl F, Messager LA, Lewis MD, Montilla M, Cucunubá Z, et al. Contemporary cryptic sexuality in *Trypanosoma cruzi*. *Mol Ecol* 2012;**17**:4216−26.
22. Ramírez JD, Llewellyn JD. Reproductive clonality in protozoan pathogens—truth or artefact? *Mol Ecol* 2014;**23**:4195−202.

23. de Meeûs T, McCoy KD, Prugnolle F, Chevillon C, Durand P, Hurtrez-Boussès S, et al. Population genetics and molecular epidemiology or how to "débusquer la bête." *Infect Genet Evol* 2007;**2007**(7):308−32.

24. Boité MC, Mauricio IL, Miles MA, Cupolillo E. New insights on taxonomy, phylogeny and population genetics of *Leishmania* (*Viannia*) parasites based on multilocus sequence analysis. *PLoS NTD* 2012;**6**(11):e1888. Available from: http://dx.doi.org/10.1371/journal.pntd.0001888.

25. Downing T, Imamura H, Decuypere S, Clark TG, Coombs GH, Cotton JA, et al. Whole genome sequencing of multiple *Leishmania donovani* clinical isolates provides insights into population structure and mechanisms of drug resistance. *Genome Res* 2011;**21**:2143−56.

26. Inbar E, Akopyants NS, Charmoy M, Romano A, Lawyer P, Elnaiem DA, et al. The mating competence of geographically diverse *Leishmania major* strains in their natural and unnatural sand fly vectors. *PLoS Genetics* 2013;**9**(7):e1003672. Available from: http://dx.doi.org/10.1371/journal.pgen.1003672.

27. Lachaud L, Bourgeois N, Kuk N, Morelle C, Crobu L, Merlin G, et al. Constitutive mosaic aneuploidy is a unique genetic feature widespread in the *Leishmania* genus. *Microbes Infect* 2014;**16**:61−6.

28. Mannaert A, Downing T, Imamura H, Dujardin JC. Adaptive mechanisms in pathogens: universal aneuploidy in *Leishmania*. *Trends Parasitol* 2012;**28**:370−6.

29. Rogers MB, Hilley JD, Dickens NJ, Wilkes J, Bates PA, Depledge DP, et al. Chromosome and gene copy number variation allow major structural change between species and strains of *Leishmania*. *Genome Res* 2011;**21**:2129−42.

30. Rogers MB, Downing T, Smith BA, Imamura H, Sanders M, Svobodova M, et al. Genomic confirmation of hybridisation and recent inbreeding in a vector-isolated *Leishmania* population. *PLoS Genet* 2014;**10**(1):e1004092. Available from: http://dx.doi.org/10.1371/journal.pgen.1004092.

31. Sterkers Y, Lachaud L, Crobu L, Bastien P, Pagès M. FISH analysis reveals aneuploidy and continual generation of chromosomal mosaicism in *Leishmania major*. *Cellular Microbiol* 2011;**13**:274−83.

32. Sterkers Y, Lachaud L, Bourgeois N, Crobu L, Bastien P, Pagès M. Novel insights into genome plasticity in Eukaryotes: mosaic aneuploidy in *Leishmania*. *Mol Microbiol* 2012; **86**:15−23.

33. Sterkers Y, Crobu L, Lachaud L, Pagès M, Bastien P. Parasexuality and mosaic aneuploidy in *Leishmania*: alternative genetics. *Trends Parasitol* 2014;**30**:429−35.

34. Buscaglia CA, Kissinger JC, Agüero F. Neglected tropical diseases in the post-genomic era. *Trends Genet* 2015;**31**:539−55.

35. Minning TA, Weatherly DB, Flibotte S, Tarleton R. Widespread, focal copy number variations (CNV) and whole chromosome aneuploidies in *Trypanosoma cruzi* strains revealed by array comparative genomic hybridization. *BMC Genomics* 2011; **12**:139.

36. Reis-Cunha JL, Rodrigues-Luiz GF, Valdivia HO, Baptista RP, Mendes TAO, de Morais GL, et al. Chromosomal copy number variation reveals differential levels of genomic plasticity in distinct *Trypanosoma cruzi* strains. *BMC Genomics* 2015;**16**:499.

37. Souza RT, Lima FM, Moraes Barros R, Cortez DR, Santos MF, Cordero EM, et al. Genome size, karyotype polymorphism and chromosomal evolution in *Trypanosoma cruzi*. *PLoS ONE* 2011;**6**(8):e23042. Available from: http://dx.doi.org/10.1371/journal.pone.0023042.

38. Maynard Smith J, Smith NH, O'Rourke M, Spratt BG. How clonal are bacteria? *Proc Natl Acad Sci USA* 1993;**90**:4384−8.

39. Tibayrenc M. Population genetics of parasitic protozoa and other microorganisms. *Adv Parasitol* 1995;**36**:47−115.

40. Go MF, Kapur V, Graham D, Musser JM. Population genetic analysis of *Helicobacter pylori* by multilocus enzyme electrophoresis: extensive allelic diversity and recombinational population structure. *J Bacteriol* 1997;**178**:3934−8.

41. Weir W, Capewell P, Foth B, Clucas C, Pountain A, Steketee P, et al. Population genomics reveals the origin and asexual evolution of human infective trypanosomes. *eLIFE* 2016;**5**:e11473.

42. Ramírez JD, Llewellyn MS. Response to Tibayrenc and Ayala: reproductive clonality in protozoan pathogens—truth or artefact? *Mol Ecol* 2015;**24**:5782−4.

43. Messenger LA, Llewellyn MS, Bhattacharyya T, Franzén O, Lewis MD, Ramírez JD, et al. Multiple mitochondrial introgression events and heteroplasmy in *Trypanosoma cruzi* revealed by maxicircle MLST and next generation sequencing. *PLoS NTD* 2012;**6**: e1584. Available from: http://dx.doi.org/10.1371/journal.pntd.0001584.

44. Nichols R. Gene trees and species trees are not the same. *Trends Ecol Evol* 2001;**16**: 358−64.

45. O'Connor O, Bosseno MF, Barnabé C, Douzery EJP, Brenière SF. Genetic clustering of *Trypanosoma cruzi* I lineage evidenced by intergenic miniexon gene sequencing. *Infect Genet Evol* 2007;**7**:587−93.

46. Spotorno AE, Córdova L, Solari A. Differentiation of *Trypanosoma cruzi* I subgroups through characterization of cytochrome b gene sequences. *Infect Genet Evol* 2008;**8**: 898−900.

47. Marcili A, Lima L, Cavazzsana M, Junqueira ACV, Veludo HH, Maia Da Silva F, et al. A new genotype of *Trypanosoma cruzi* associated with bats evidenced by phylogenetic analyses using SSU rDNA, cytochrome b and Histone H2B genes and genotyping based on ITS1 rDNA. *Parasitology* 2009;**136**:641−55.

48. Maiden MCJ, Bygraves JA, Feil E, Morelli G, Russell JE, Urwin R, et al. Multilocus sequence typing: a portable approach to the identification of clones within populations of pathogenic microorganisms. *Proc Natl Acad Sci USA* 1998;**95**:3140−5.

49. Lauthier JJ, Tomasini N, Barnabé C, Monje Rumi MM, Alberti D'Amato AM, Ragone PG, et al. Candidate targets for multilocus sequence typing of *Trypanosoma cruzi*: validation using parasite stocks from the Chaco region and a set of reference strains. *Infect Genet Evol* 2012;**12**:350−8.

50. Tomasini N, Lauthier JJ, Monje Rumi MM, Ragone PG, Alberti D'Amato AM, et al. Preponderant clonal evolution of *Trypanosoma cruzi* I from Argentinean Chaco revealed by Multilocus Sequence Typing (MLST). *Infect Genet Evol* 2014;**27**:348−54.

51. Holmes EC. The evolutionary genetics of emerging viruses. *Ann Rev Ecol Evol Syst* 2009; **40**:353−72.

52. Wong VK, Baker S, Pickard DJ, Parkhill J, Page AJ, Feasey NA, et al. Phylogeographical analysis of the dominant multidrug-resistant H58 clade of *Salmonella typhi* identifies inter- and intracontinental transmission events. *Nat Genet* 2015;**47**: 632−9.

53. Barnabé C, Brisse S, Tibayrenc M. Population structure and genetic typing of *Trypanosoma cruzi*, the agent of Chagas' disease: a multilocus enzyme electrophoresis approach. *Parasitology* 2000;**150**:513−26.

54. Tibayrenc M, Ayala FJ. Forte corrélation entre classification isoenzymatique et variabilité de l'ADN kinétoplastique chez *Trypanosoma cruzi*. *C R Acad Sci Paris* 1987; **304**:89−93.

55. Tibayrenc M, Neubauer K, Barnabé C, Guerrini F, Sarkeski D, Ayala FJ. Genetic characterization of six parasitic protozoa: parity of random-primer DNA typing and multilocus isoenzyme electrophoresis. *Proc Natl Acad Sci USA* 1993;**90**:1335–9.

56. Brisse S, Barnabé C, Tibayrenc M. Identification of six *Trypanosoma cruzi* phylogenetic lineages by random amplified polymorphic DNA and multilocus enzyme electrophoresis. *Int J Parasitol* 2000;**30**:35–44.

57. Oliveira RP, Broude NE, Macedo AM, Cantor CR, Smith CL, Pena SDJ. Probing the genetic population structure of *Trypanosoma cruzi* with polymorphic microsatellites. *Proc Natl Acad Sci USA* 1998;**95**:3776–80.

58. Telleria J, Barnabé C, Hide M, Bañuls AL, Tibayrenc M. Predominant clonal evolution leads to a close parity between gene expression profiles and subspecific phylogeny in *Trypanosoma cruzi*. *Mol Biochem Parasitol* 2004;**137**:133–41.

59. Lima L, Ortiz PA, da Silva FM, Alves JMP, Serrano MG, Cortez AP, et al. Repertoire, genealogy and genomic organization of cruzipain and homologous genes in *Trypanosoma cruzi*, *T. cruzi*-like and other trypanosome species. *PLoS ONE* 2012;**7**(6): e38385. Available from: http://dx.doi.org/10.1371/journal.pone.0038385.

60. Llewellyn MS, Miles MA, Carrasco HJ, Lewis MD, Yeo M, Vargas J, et al. Genome-scale multilocus microsatellite typing of *Trypanosoma cruzi* discrete typing unit I reveals phylogeographic structure and specific genotypes linked to human infection. *PLoS Pathogens* 2009;**5**(5):e1000410. Available from: http://dx.doi.org/10.1371/journal.ppat.1000410.

61. Bogliolo AR, Lauriapires L, Gibson WC. Polymorphisms in *Trypanosoma cruzi*: evidence of genetic recombination. *Acta Tropica* 1996;**61**:31–40.

62. Carrasco HJ, Frame IA, Valente SA, Miles MA. Genetic exchange as a possible source of genomic diversity in sylvatic populations of *Trypanosoma cruzi*. *Am J Trop Med Hyg* 1996;**54**:418–24.

63. Machado CA, Ayala FJ. Nucleotide sequences provide evidence of genetic exchange among distantly related lineages of *Trypanosoma cruzi*. *Proc Natl Acad Sci USA* 2001; **98**:7396–401.

64. Brisse S, Henriksson J, Barnabé C, Douzery EJP, Berkvens D, Serrano M, et al. Evidence for genetic exchange and hybridization in *Trypanosoma cruzi* based on nucleotide sequences and molecular karyotype. *Infect Genet Evol* 2003;**2**:173–83.

65. Gaunt MW, Yeo M, Frame IA, Tothard JR, Carrasco HJ, Taylor MC, et al. Mechanism of genetic exchange in American trypanosomes. *Nature* 2003;**421**:936–9.

66. Lewis MD, Llewellyn MS, Gaunt MW, Yeo M, Carrasco HJ, Miles MA. Flow cytometric analysis and microsatellite genotyping reveal extensive DNA content variation in *Trypanosoma cruzi* populations and expose contrasts between natural and experimental hybrids. *Int J Parasitol* 2009;**39**:1305–17.

67. Miles MA, Toyé PJ, Oswald SC, Godfrey DG. The identification by isoenzyme patterns of two distinct strain-groups of *Trypanosoma cruzi*, circulating independently in a rural area of Brazil. *Trans R Soc Trop Med Hyg* 1977;**71**:217–25.

68. Miles MA, Souza A, Povoa M, Shaw JJ, Lainson R, Toyé PJ. Isozymic heterogeneity of *Trypanosoma cruzi* in the first autochtonous patients with Chagas' disease in Amazonian Brazil. *Nature* 1978;**272**:819–21.

69. Zingales B, Andrade SG, Briones MRS, Campbell DA, Chiari E, Fernandes O, et al. A new consensus for *Trypanosoma cruzi* intraspecific nomenclature: second revision meeting recommends TcI to TcVI. *Mem Inst Oswaldo Cruz RJ* 2009;**104**:1051–4.

70. Tibayrenc M. Genetic epidemiology of parasitic protozoa and other infectious agents: the need for an integrated approach. *Int J Parasitol* 1998;**28**:85–104.

71. Barnabé C, Mobarec HI, Jurado MR, Cortez JA, Brenière SF. Reconsideration of the seven discrete typing units within the species *Trypanosoma cruzi*, a new proposal of three reliable mitochondrial clades. *Infect Genet Evol* 2016;**39**:176−86.

72. Brisse S, Dujardin JC, Tibayrenc M. Identification of six *Trypanosoma cruzi* lineages by sequence-characterised amplified region markers. *Mol Biochem Parasitol* 2000;**111**: 95−105.

73. Brisse S, Verhoef J, Tibayrenc M. Characterisation of large and small subunit rRNA and mini-exon genes further supports the distinction of six *Trypanosoma cruzi* lineages. *Int J Parasitol* 2001;**31**:1218−26.

74. Rozas M, De Doncker S, Adaui V, Coronado W, Barnabé C, Tibayrenc M, et al. Multilocus polymerase chain reaction restriction fragment−length polymorphism genotyping of *Trypanosoma cruzi* (Chagas disease): taxonomic and clinical applications. *J Infect Dis* 2007;**195**:1381−8.

75. Souto RP, Fernandes O, Macedo AM, Campbell DA, Zingales B. DNA markers define two major phylogenetic lineages of *Trypanosoma cruzi*. *Mol Biochem Parasitol* 1996; **83**:141−52.

76. Anonymous. Taxonomy of *Trypanosoma cruzi*: a commentary on characterization and nomenclature. *Mem Inst Oswaldo Cruz* 1999;**94**:181−4.

77. Zingales B, Miles MA, Campbell D, Tibayrenc M, Macedo AM, Teixeira MM, et al. The revised *Trypanosoma cruzi* subspecific nomenclature: rationale, epidemiological relevance and research applications. *Infect Genet Evol* 2012;**12**:240−53.

78. Lewis MD, Ma J, Yeo M, Carrasco HJ, Llewellyn MS, Miles MA. Genotyping of *Trypanosoma cruzi*: systematic selection of assays allowing rapid and accurate discrimination of all known lineages. *Am J Trop Med Hyg* 2009;**81**:1041−9.

79. Llewellyn MS, Lewis MD, Acosta N, Yeo M, Carrasco HJ, Segovia M, et al. *Trypanosoma cruzi* IIc: phylogenetic and phylogeographic insights from sequence and microsatellite analysis and potential impact on emergent Chagas disease. *PLoS NTD* 2009;**3**(9):e510. Available from: http://dx.doi.org/10.1371/journal.pntd.0000510.

80. Lima L, Espinosa-Álvarez O, Ortiz PA, Trejo-Varón JA, Carranza JC, Pinto CM, et al. Genetic diversity of *Trypanosoma cruzi* in bats, and multilocus phylogenetic and phylogeographical analyses supporting Tcbat as an independent DTU (discrete typing unit). *Acta Tropica* 2015;**151**:166−77.

81. Pinto CM, Kalko EKV, Cottontail I, Wellinghausen N, Cottontail VM. TcBat a bat-exclusive lineage of *Trypanosoma cruzi* in the Panama Canal Zone, with comments on its classification and the use of the 18S rRNA gene for lineage identification. *Infect Genet Evol* 2012;**12**:1328−32.

82. Pinto CM, Ocaña-Mayorga S, Tapia EE, Lobos SE, Zurita AP, Aguirre-Villacís F, et al. Bats, Trypanosomes, and Triatomines in Ecuador: new insights into the diversity, transmission, and origins of *Trypanosoma cruzi* and Chagas disease. *PLoS ONE* 2016;**10**(10): e0139999. Available from: http://dx.doi.org/10.1371/journal.pone.0139999.

83. Westenberger SJ, Barnabé C, Campbell DA, Sturm NR. Two hybridization events define the population structure of *Trypanosoma cruzi*. *Genetics* 2005;**171**:527−43.

84. Garzón EA, Barnabé C, Córdova X, Bowen C, Paredes W, Gómez E, et al. *Trypanosoma cruzi* isoenzyme variability in Ecuador: first observation of zymodeme III genotypes in chronic chagasic patients. *Trans R Soc Trop Med Hyg* 2002;**96**:378−82.

85. Barnabé C, Yaeger R, Pung O, Tibayrenc M. Considerable phylogenetic diversity indicates that *Trypanosoma cruzi*, the agent of Chagas disease, is indigenous to the native fauna of the USA. *Exp Parasitol* 2001;**99**:73−9.

86. Miles MA, Povoa M, Prata A, Cedillos RA, De Souza AA, Macedo V. Do radically dissimilar *Trypanosoma cruzi* strains (zymodemes) cause Venezuelan and Brazilian forms of Chagas'disease? *Lancet* 1981;**8234**:1336—40.

87. De Lana M, Pinto A, Bastrenta B, Barnabé C, Noël S, Tibayrenc M. *Trypanosoma cruzi*: infectivity of clonal genotypes infections in acute and chronic phases in mice. *Exp Parasitol* 2000;**96**:61—6.

88. Revollo S, Oury B, Laurent JP, Barnabé C, Quesney V, Carrière V, et al. *Trypanosoma cruzi*: impact of clonal evolution of the parasite on its biological and medical properties. *Exp Parasitol* 1998;**89**:30—9.

89. Telleria J, Biron DG, Brizard JP, Demettre E, Seveno M, Barnabé C, et al. Phylogenetic character mapping of proteomic diversity shows high correlation with subspecific phylogenetic diversity in *Trypanosoma cruzi*, the agent of Chagas disease. *Proc Natl Acad Sci USA* 2010;**107**:20411—16.

90. Machin A, Telleria J, Brizard JP, Demettre E, Séveno M, Ayala FJ, et al. *Trypanosoma cruzi*: gene expression surveyed by proteomic analysis reveals interaction between different genotypes in mixed in vitro cultures. *PLoS ONE* 2014;**9**(4):e95442. ISSN 1932-6203.

91. Campbell LT, Currie BJ, Krockenberger M, Malik R, Meyer W, Heitman J, et al. Clonality and recombination in genetically differentiated subgroups of *Cryptococcus gattii*. *Eukaryotic Cell* 2005;**4**:1403—9.

92. Guhl F, Ramírez JD. *Trypanosoma cruzi* I diversity: towards the need of genetic subdivision? *Acta Tropica* 2011;**119**:1—4.

93. Cura CI, Mejía-Jaramillo AM, Duffy T, Burgos JM, Rodriguero M, Cardinal MV, et al. *Trypanosoma cruzi* I genotypes in different geographical regions and transmission cycles based on a microsatellite motif of the intergenic spacer of spliced-leader genes. *Int J Parasitol* 2010;**40**:1599—607.

94. Ramírez JD, Duque MC, Guhl F. Phylogenetic reconstruction based on Cytochrome b (Cytb) gene sequences reveals distinct genotypes within Colombian *Trypanosoma cruzi* I populations. *Acta Tropica* 2011;**119**:61—5.

95. Barnabé C, Buitrago R, Brémond P, Aliaga C, Salas R, Vidaurre P, et al. Putative Panmixia in restricted populations of *Trypanosoma cruzi* isolated from wild *Triatoma infestans* in Bolivia. *PLoS ONE* 2013;**8**(11):e82269. Available from: http://dx.doi.org/10.1371/journal.pone.0082269.

96. de Paula Baptista R, Alchaar D'Ávila D, Segatto M, Faria do Valle I, Regina Franco G, Silva Valadares HM, et al. Evidence of substantial recombination among *Trypanosoma cruzi* II strains from Minas Gerais. *Infect Genet Evol* 2014;**22**:183—91.

97. Ocaña-Mayorga S, Llewellyn MS, Costales JA, Miles MA, Grijalva MJ. Sex, subdivision, and domestic dispersal of *Trypanosoma cruzi* lineage I in Southern Ecuador. *PLoS NTD* 2010;**4**(12):e915. Available from: http://dx.doi.org/10.1371/journal.pntd.0000915.

98. Zingales B, Miles MA, Moraes CB, Luquetti A, Guhl F, Schijman AG, et al. Drug discovery for Chagas disease should consider *Trypanosoma cruzi* strain diversity. *Mem Inst Oswaldo Cruz RJ* 2014;**109**:828—33.

99. Tibayrenc M. Modeling the transmission of *Trypanosoma cruzi*: the need for an integrated genetic epidemiological and population genomics approach. In: Michael E, editor. *Infectious disease transmission modeling and management of parasite control*. Eurekah: Landes Bioscience; 2009.

# Vector transmission: how it works, what transmits, where it occurs

*S.F. Brenière[1], A. Villacis[2] and C. Aznar[3]*
[1]Institut de Recherche pour le Développement (IRD), Montpellier, France,
[2]Center for Infectious and Chronic Disease Research, School of Biological Sciences,
Pontifical Catholic University of Ecuador, Quito, Ecuador, [3]Université des Antilles
et de la Guyane, Cayenne, French Guyana

## Chapter Outline

## How does transmission work?

Chagas disease is commonly transmitted by bloodsucking triatomine vectors living in residential dwellings (domestic vectors) in close contact with humans. Indeed, the main interventions implemented to decrease transmission focus on eliminating vectors that live in dwellings. Generally, transmission occurs during the night when the insects are most active, at which time they take their blood meal on sleeping humans. The parasite is transmitted during this contact, but the free-infection form (flagellated) is in the feces of the insect rather than the salivary glands, as in most other arthropod vectors. The parasites are concentrated in the rectal bulb in the terminal part of the digestive tube of the insect, and during the blood meal or soon after, the bugs defecate and deposit the infected feces on the skin or near mucosa. The bite causes a skin abrasion that allows the parasite to enter underneath the skin. This transmission is complex, and all the steps are not well understood. Its load

*American Trypanosomiasis Chagas Disease.* DOI: http://dx.doi.org/10.1016/B978-0-12-801029-7.00023-X

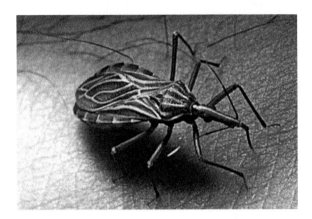

**Figure 22.1** *Rhodnius prolixus* taking a meal on human skin.
*Source*: Electronic publication from "Centro de Análisis de Imágenes Biomédicas Computarizadas," CAIBCO, Instituto de Medicina, Tropical, Facultad de Medicina, Universidad Central de Venezuela.

depends on many factors including those that promote human−vector contact and those that allow the parasite to enter its host (Fig. 22.1).

The first step is the contact between the vector and the mammal. What attracts the bugs to their prey? Heat, carbon dioxide, and odors could be cues and lures that direct the bugs. *Triatoma dimidiata* and *Rhodnius prolixus* are major vectors of Chagas disease in Central and South America: in experimental tests, these vectors were more attracted by heat or $CO_2$ alone than by selected chemicals.[1] In experiments where the breathing of a host was mimicked by pulses of $CO_2$ and where a continuous flow of $CO_2$ was provided, *Triatoma infestans*, the main vector in the Southern Cone, was attracted.[2] However, $CO_2$ may not be an essential component to attract triatomines.[3] In 2002, it was speculated that *T. infestans* possess thermoreceptors as do other animals and insects, which aids in hunting and feeding.[4] Additional studies have shown that heat has a significant attractive effect, such as the heat emitted by the face, which can attract a triatomine bug from a distance of 2 m.[5] Furthermore, moisture could increase the attraction of a hot spot, but this effect may be limited to short distances.[6] A double-choice olfactometer was used to test volatile substances and showed that *R. prolixus* is also attracted by the odors of human skin and even microflora compounds present mainly on the face, which would explain why the bites frequently occur on the human face.[7] Among the factors that influence the movement of the bugs toward their prey, infrared radiation could be a cue, as recently suggested when analyzing the infrared emission in landscapes from sunset to the early hours of the night.[8]

The duration of the blood meal of triatomines is long because the insect must obtain a large quantity of blood. It is important that the host does not react in a hostile manner because of the pain caused by the bite. A number of biological properties of triatomine saliva are similar to that of other arthropods and help the vector obtain its meal while also facilitating the transmission of the pathogenic agents. Among others, the saliva proteomic analyses have identified a large number of these factors.[9] Thus, saliva contains anesthetic factors, anticoagulants, and vasodilators that facilitate the intake of blood.[10,11] Although the anesthetic effect has been little studied, parasitological xenodiagnosis was used with different species of triatomine. The patient was exposed to the bite of 30—40 nymphs, and the bites were rather painless.[12] Interestingly, the use of triatomines to obtain blood from small animals with cryptic veins was proposed as an alternative to conventional blood sampling[13]; the authors reported that the animals may be less stressed and possibly did not notice the bloodsucking insect. However, it should be noted that the inhabitants of hyperendemic areas frequently testified that the bug density was so high in their house (*T. infestans*) that they would be awakened at night by the attack of bugs, and they were forced to sleep elsewhere ("nos sacaban de la casa").

The parasites contained in feces can penetrate skin cells through the abrasion made by the bite. In fact, intact skin is an effective barrier against *Trypanosoma cruzi*, but very small abrasions of the skin (e.g., triggered by scraping) could allow the parasite to penetrate the skin. In experimental trials on mice of the natural route of infection via skin, cells were invaded very quickly.[14] The results showed that the parasite spread rapidly (<15 min) from the site of inoculation. At least a few parasitic forms can be immediately transported, possibly through the lymphatic or blood system, and then disseminated to other tissues of the host. Of course, if the parasites are transmitted via the mucosa, cells are easier to infect. In the invasion process, triatomine saliva still plays a role. It has an inhibitory effect on the activation of the classical complement pathway that acts in the lysis of foreign agents.[15] The role of the complex salivary secretion of triatomines is not well known, but immunomodulating proteins exist in the saliva of several hematophagous arthropods, and it has been widely observed that saliva can enhance the infectivity of pathogens.[16] Saliva particularly affects the activation of T- and B-lymphocytes, macrophages, and dendritic cells. Interestingly, lysophosphatidylcholine, a component present in the saliva of *R. prolixus*, acts as a powerful chemoattractant for inflammatory cells at the site of the bug bite, leading to a concentration of available cells for infection.[17] Thus, saliva is able to create a local environment conducive to cell invasion by the parasite.

Human infection requires the multiplication of the parasite, which occurs only in the host cells in the amastigote form. In fact, *T. cruzi* invades a wide variety of vertebrate cells by endocytosis, including phagocytic cells, using a mechanism distinct from phagocytosis.[18] There are many mechanisms of recognition between the parasite and host cells, and *T. cruzi* has adapted to invade a wide variety of specialized cells.[19–21]

## Who transmits the parasite?

At present, 140 species of the subfamily Triatominae have been described.[22] These are grouped into 15 genera, which include species that are important vectors of Chagas disease or live in the human environment and therefore constitute a potential danger: *Dipetalogaster* (Usinger, 1939), *Eratyrus* (Stål, 1859), *Meccus*

(Stål, 1859), *Panstrongylus* (Berg, 1879), *Rhodnius* (Stål, 1859), and *Triatoma* (Laporte, 1832). The vector capacity of each species is difficult to determine. However, several indicators are usually used for laboratory colonies, and most often, several species are compared under the same experimental conditions.[23] However, the vector capacity appears to be shaped by environmental conditions mainly related to food availability.

## Vector capacity

The vector capacity of a species depends on the ability of *T. cruzi* to complete its life cycle along the gut of the insect and to produce infective forms at the rectal gland (metacyclogenesis process) that are then deposited near skin abrasions or on mucous membranes. Metacyclogenesis is the transformation of epimastigote forms (noninfective) to trypomastigotes, which are metacyclic forms that are capable of infecting mammalian cells when released into the feces. The transitions to metacyclic forms seem to occur primarily in situ in the rectal gland, where both epimastigotes and trypomastigotes are attached by the flagellum.[24,25] In the small intestine, transitional forms occur but are scarce. Several molecules play a role in the redox status of the triatomine gut microenvironment that influence metacyclogenesis,[26] which appears to be vector-dependent.[27–29] For example, during experimental comparisons of several species (*R. prolixus*, *Rhodnius neglectus*, *Panstrongylus megistus*, *Triatoma sordida*, *T. infestans*, *Triatoma brasiliensis*, *Triatoma rubrovaria*, *Triatoma pseudomaculata*, and *T. dimidiata*) reared in the laboratory, the authors observed a significant difference in the rate of metacyclic forms between species at the 120th day of infection, where metacyclic forms comprised 50% of the individuals in *R. neglectus* and 37% in its congener *R. prolixus* but were dramatically lower in the majority of *Triatoma* species (5% in *T. sordida*, 3% in *T. brasiliensis*, and 0% in *T. pseudomaculata*).[27] Several studies have also shown that the rate of metacyclogenesis varies from one strain of *T. cruzi* to another. In *T. infestans*, a strain belonging to the *T. cruzi* discrete typing unit (DTU) TcI nearly always reached higher trypomastigote density in the rectum than another strain belonging to TcII DTUs.[30] Another experimental work, comparing the percentage of infected insects, and the number of flagellates and metacyclic forms per insect, confirmed that parasites belonging to TcI are more efficiently transmitted in *T. infestans* than TcII and TcV.[31] Several studies have examined the metacyclogenesis process in vitro. The incubation of epimastigote forms in an appropriate medium induced metacyclogenesis, and different strains exhibited highly heterogeneous differentiation rates, and in particular TcI strains exhibited the highest level of differentiation.[32,33] Another factor that influences metacyclogenesis is the meal of the triatomine. Starvation reduces the total number of parasites and the number and percentage of trypomastigotes. Moreover, feeding the vector after 40 days of starvation induces the appearance of pure populations of trypomastigotes.[34] These observations indicate that vector capacity depends on the availability of food sources.

Another important factor determining the vector capacity of triatomine species is their feeding behavior and defecation reflex resulting in the feces being deposited near the bite. Several indices were measured in laboratory colonies using the main vector species (*T. infestans* and *R. prolixus*) as references. Voracity (i.e., the delay before initiating a meal), the meal period, and especially the time to postfeed defecation were analyzed. It is impossible to formulate a comprehensive description of the feeding behavior of triatomines, but it is important to note that the main vector species are not the only species that exhibit eating and defecation behaviors that favor transmission of the parasite. Some species that are not currently recognized as vectors may be adapting to the human environment (e.g., *Triatoma patagonica*). For example, 69% and 58% of the nymphs of *T. patagonica* and *T. infestans*, respectively, produced their first defecation within 5 min after being fed, and the nymphs of *T. patagonica* were capable of defecating during or immediately after feeding.[35] Similarly, several Mexican species exhibit a short time to defecation (<10 min for *Triatoma lecticularia*, *Triatoma protracta*, and the youngest nymphs of *Triatoma gerstaeckeri*), which suggests that these three species may be important potential vectors of *T. cruzi* for human populations in areas of Mexico where these species are currently present.[36] In general, the experimental studies on laboratory-reared triatomine species tend to evaluate a set of parameters to conclude whether the vector studied has good transmission competencies. The species *T. protracta* and *Triatoma rubida* are common triatomines in southwestern North America and were considered poor vectors.[37] However, other studies have shown that of the three sympatric Mexican species, *Triatoma recurva*, *T. protracta*, and *T. rubida*, only the last one should be considered as an important potential vector.[38,39] *Triatoma williami*, a species belonging to the *T. oliveira* complex that occurs in the Pantanal ecosystem (Mato Grosso, Brazil), also shows a short time to defecation, so this species found in intradomicile and peridomicile locations in rural and urban areas should be considered as a competent vector.[40] This is also the case of *Triatoma boliviana*, a new species recently described in some valleys in the Department of La Paz in Bolivia.[41] In the Gran Chaco region, *Triatoma guasayana* is a species commonly found in peridomiciles and exhibits a vectorial capacity very similar to that of *T. infestans*, the principal vector in the region.[29]

## Eclectic species

Some species of triatomines are adapted to specialist niches, but many others are generalists, more eclectic, and may be a danger to humans by transmitting Chagas disease. These species, classified as secondary, are a concern because the strictly domesticated species of vectors have been targeted for extermination through various regional initiatives fighting Chagas disease in most endemic countries. In more general terms, in many areas the problem is made worse by wild species of triatomines now playing a role in transmission. This transmission relates to sylvatic zoonotic foci and generally results in sporadic occurrences of human cases. However, these regions must be under entomological supervision because an increased risk of contact between humans and infected vectors might emerge from uncontrolled environmental factors. *T. brasiliensis* is now considered the most important Chagas disease vector in the semiarid zones of northeastern Brazil. In a study on domiciliary infestation from 1993 to 1999, 21 triatomine species were captured within the geographic range of *T. brasiliensis* in Brazil, but the highest domiciliary infestation rate was for *T. brasiliensis*.[42] In the Brazilian Caatinga region, reinfestation by *T. brasiliensis* occurred after treatments of habitats. Based on genetic markers and population genetics, there appeared to be a triatomine flow (*T. brasiliensis*) between the neighboring sylvatic and artificial environments, such that the peridomestic area was a main interface function[43] and the elimination of *T. brasiliensis* was more complex. Lastly, for the first time, a study reported the capture of *T. brasiliensis* in a sylvatic environment, using light traps, indicating that *T. brasiliensis* is attracted by light and that the colonization of houses might also be due to artificial light sources.[44] In Mexico, *Meccus longipennis*, a species first identified in domiciles and peridomiciles, mostly in Jalisco State, is a truly wild species that colonizes artificial structures such as rock pile boundary walls separating crop fields[45] and natural structures such as the common cliff and rock formations in the region.[46,47] Surprisingly, two different vector dynamic models of this species could operate in the villages. In the first village studied, there was a high peridomestic colonization with one-third of the visited structures infested by *M. longipennis*[48,49]; in this case the triatomine entering the home could originate from peridomicile colonies. In the second village, the peridomicile colonization by *M. longipennis* was much lower and the triatomines entering the home probably originated from the wild[50]; most remarkable was the high proportion of *M. longipennis* males collected by the inhabitants in this village. This could explain the very low colonization load of the peridomicile, whereas peridomestic structures offered to colonization were highly abundant, such as in the first village.

Among the unexpected species, *Triatoma tibiamaculata*, which is often associated with *P. megistus* and *T. sordida*, was found inside houses in Saõ Paulo State, Brazil. The triatomines captured within the domiciles were mostly adults, but about half of them had fed upon humans.[51,52] Further south on the west coast of Brazil in the state of Santa Catalina (municipality of Navegantes), an outbreak of acute human cases occurred in 2005 because humans had ingested sugar cane juice contaminated by the feces of triatomines. This was the first report involving *T. tibiamaculata* in peridomestic areas.[53] In an area 1630 km further north, in the state of San Salvador, the main habitat of *T. tibiamaculata* is marsupial and rodent nests in bromeliads; in this area, it was suspected that *T. tibiamaculata* was transmitting Chagas disease.[54] Similarly, in a periurban zone in Santiago, Chile, a study on the prevalence of blood sources in *Mepraia spinolai* (regarded as a sylvatic species) identified several human feeding sources. This suggests that the wild insect might become a vector of greater epidemiological importance.[55] Various entomological studies highlight complex situations where several triatomine species coexist in environments neighboring developed areas, and many of these species are capable of entering dwellings. In communities in the northeastern province of Corrientes, Argentina, several species were identified in domestic ecotopes. *T. infestans* was the most dominant species. The second most dominant species was *T. sordida*, which is widely distributed in South America and most frequently found in extradomiciliary ecotopes. Although it is rarely domiciliated, it could be considered capable of colonizing human dwellings.[56] In the same province, a study showed a remarkable rate of infestation by *T. sordida* of palm trees on a farm (96−100% of *Butia yatay* and *Acrocomia aculeate*, respectively). The use of fronds in walls and roofs can favor the passive transport of wild triatomines to the domestic environment, as has been reported for *Rhodnius* spp. in tropical forests.[57] Although *T. sordida* has not been considered dangerous, in 1995 in the Velasco province, Bolivia, it was the only species that colonized houses, and some autochthonous cases of infection were detected.[58] The case of palm trees (*Livistona australis*) infested with *R. neglectus* in a square opposite the church in the city of Monte Alto in Brazil, where public notifications of domiciliary invasions were made, should also be noted.[59] In the United States, a country considered to be nonendemic, the transmission of Chagas disease may occur at a very low level, given that six autochthonous human cases have been detected.[60] Interestingly, a study used geographical information system and survey analyses of Chagas infection patterns to predict the impact of an increase in temperature in the year 2030 on the geographical distribution of three triatomine species (*Triatoma sanguisuga*, *T. lecticularia*, and *T. protracta*) in the southern United States; the results indicated that there is a risk of Chagas disease emerging in this country[61] (Fig. 22.2).

## Chagas disease in the Amazonian region

Particular attention should be paid to the Amazonian region. Indeed, this region has become a focus of scientific investigation, and Chagas disease is now a public health priority in the region. In 2004, the countries concerned launched "The Initiative for the Prevention and Control of Chagas Disease" (Pan American Health Organization; AMCHA: Initiative of the Amazon Countries for Surveillance and Control of Chagas Disease; http://www.paho.org/english/ad/dpc/cd/dch-amcha.htm). Since the 1970s, the number of autochthonous cases has increased, with 205 cases identified as of 2000.[62] This region covers nine countries and 44% of the area of South America. At least 24 species of triatomines have been found infected, and 14 of these were recently recorded exclusively in French Guiana.[63] Regarding the *Rhodnius* genus, which is widely involved in vector transmission in the Amazon, it is associated with palm trees, which are also present in urban areas.[64] An extremely broad range of mammals (e.g., marsupials, bats, rodents, and toothless and carnivorous primates) have been infected, indicating the complexity of this enzootic disease. Environmental and social changes in the last 30 years have led to the transmission of *T. cruzi* to humans. This transformation in the disease's epidemiological pattern in the Amazon can be explained by new human settlements near forested areas (especially with palm trees), seasonal and permanent rural−urban migrations, deforestation, cattle raising, mining, sedentary living, and an increase in the presence of domestic animals.[65−67] Among the reported acute cases, oral infections comprise a large portion, but vector transmission is also involved. Therefore, continuous entomological surveillance is necessary.

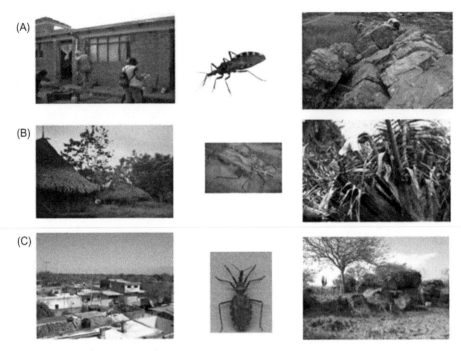

**Figure 22.2** New patterns of vector transmission linked to wild populations of triatomines. (A) A typical suburban house in Quillacollo city (Department of Cochabamba, Bolivia) at risk of invasion by a population of *Triatoma infestans* living in rocky outcrops near the home. (B) A typical house in the Sierra Nevada, Colombia, at risk of invasion by wild populations of *Rhodnius* sp. and *Triatoma dimidiata* that are living in the forest where palm trees provide habitat. (C) A typical village in the Ameca Valley (Jalisco State, Mexico). Wild populations of *Meccus longipennis* are widely distributed in the surrounding countryside and are concentrated especially in the dry stone walls separating fields; the dwellings are at risk of invasion.
*Source*: Photographs by (A) S.F. Brenière; (B) J. Dib and (C) S.F. Brenière and E. Magallón.

# Where does the transmission occur?

## *In dwellings*

Unlike other vector-borne diseases, the vector transmission of Chagas disease occurs almost exclusively in the home, because it involves vectors that live in or occasionally enter the home. Historically, areas in which Chagas disease was found were rapidly associated with the presence of domiciliated triatomines. Several studies have demonstrated this association. For example, in the Northern Goias State of Brazil, the presence of triatomines in dwellings or evidence of triatomine colonization has been found to be statistically correlated with seropositivity in children.[68] Similarly, in an area in Argentina where *T. infestans* was endemic, there was a high correlation between an indicator of entomological risk (the number of risky bites per human) and the seroprevalence in children.[69] Some primarily wild species became domestic in specific areas; this is the case in Caracas city in Venezuela[70] and in the province of Loja in Ecuador[71]; in these studies, a correlation was found between triatomine infestation of dwellings and the presence of close sylvatic habitats.

## In rural, urban, and periurban areas

Furthermore, the traditional idea of vector transmission is that transmission takes place in rural areas where the habitat is more favorable to infestation by bugs, but in fact, urban areas are not spared. The demographic transition of human populations from rural areas to large urban centers often results in the development of slums as well as disordered occupation of forest remnants, parks, and protected areas, and consequently favorable situations for *T. cruzi* transmission.[72] Chagas disease can also be considered an urban health problem. In Cochabamba, Bolivia, vector transmission persists in periurban areas.[73] In the city of Arequipa, Peru, 10 years ago, scientists started to be concerned about the possible emergence of transmission in periurban areas due to the infestation of houses by *T. infestans*. Today, this problem remains current.[74–76] Additionally, *T. dimidiata* has been found in several cities and towns in Costa Rica[77] as well as in Mérida, Mexico, where infestation was more related to environmental factors (e.g., location of houses on the outskirts of the city, near abandoned land) than to the quality of the dwelling.[78] More surprising, a huge colony of *T. infestans* was discovered in a hen building for egg production in an urban neighborhood of Greater Buenos Aires.[79] *T. infestans* was found in apartments in an urban neighborhood of the capital city of the province of San Juan, Argentina. Its occurrence was related to the proximity of poor housing areas, and dispersal by flight from this area was assumed to be a main mechanism of infestation.[80] Also, a study on triatomines from the Nearctic Region of Mexico reports the domestication of vector species such as *T. rubida* and *T. protracta* in urban areas, which was almost unheard of two decades before.[81] Indeed, several triatomine species have survived the modification of the landscape and have taken advantage of alternative sources of shelters and food to keep their populations in the new anthropized environments.

## Risk factors of domiciliary infestation by triatomines

Because the disease is transmitted within human dwellings, many studies have examined the types of building that facilitate the development of triatomine colonies. However, an approach based on identifying risk factors for intradomiciliary infestation revealed the human activities that play a role in the disease's epidemiological cycle. The results of these studies clearly showed that infestation is multifactorial and differs by region. Increasingly, it appears that the manner in which society and individuals position themselves and act against the disease and the vectors is crucial.[82] Several studies found a strong association of disease prevalence with the type of construction, the materials used for walls and roofs, and the conditions of the materials. These factors facilitate triatomine colonizations inside a house, but other factors play a large role, including limited knowledge about the disease, socioeconomic status, crowded rooms, cleanliness (household hygiene), conviviality, and household pets.[69,83−88] For example, intervention by the inhabitants themselves through better household hygiene and housing construction would have the advantage of reducing the risk of infestation by triatomines for a longer duration than the standard intervention using insecticides.[89] In the same way, the construction of an antitriatomine house model was developed in the province of Loja, involving the local population in the construction of houses.[90]

In addition, the peridomestic space is often a source of domestic infestation. The vectors may colonize several structures primarily related to domestic animals, but different vector species may colonize different structures. In rural localities in the state of Ceara, Brazil, *T. brasiliensis* primarily colonized brick piles and roofing tiles, *T. pseudomaculata* preferred wood poles and woodpiles, and *R. nasutus* was mainly found in roofing straw.[91] Also, studies based on multivariate logistic regression analysis can rationally identify, among different structural and management factors, those that are associated with the infestation with triatomines.[92−94] In a rural community in western Mexico, peridomestic infestation risks by *T. longipennis* and *T. barberi* (evaluated with multivariate logistic regression analysis) were related to the density of permanent and temporal structures but not with domestic animals because the main food source of triatomines was *Rattus rattus*.[49,95] In Guatemala, the persistence of *T. dimidiata* was associated with the conservation of habitats for dogs, chickens, and rodents.[96] In the home, residents must rely on management changes to limit the infestation of triatomines in peridomestic areas. In other cases, attention must be paid to the immediate vegetation. For example, *T. guasayana* is a semisylvatic species that invades peridomestic sites in rural northwestern Argentina, and its spatial distribution is related to the local abundance of goats, but also with the density of vegetation habitats near houses including bromeliads, dry cacti, and firewood.[97] The importance of the immediate environment in neotropical regions is even more striking because most species of *Rhodnius* are primarily associated with palm trees.[98,99] Interestingly, in Panama an association was found between dog infections and the presence of palm trees in the peridomicile where the dog live and in the two nearest peridomiciles.[100] Recently, a review of the relationships between palm trees and triatomines showed that the infestation of palm trees is not limited to rural areas but also occurs in urban areas; the palm trees that maintain the populations of triatomines, mostly species of the *Rhodnius* genus, favor the low continuous transmission of Chagas disease.[101] Given that many triatomine species are attracted to light, or rather light guides their movements,[102] house lights and street lighting undoubtedly play a role in the dispersal of triatomine bugs. A study in a village in Yucatan favors this hypothesis, showing a higher house infestation rate depending on their proximity to a public electric pole.[103] Another study based on field collection and modeling explored the effect of different levels of illumination in a village: the model showed that increments in light could very significantly increase vector−human contacts.[104]

## Does vector transmission occur outside human dwellings?

The existence of vector-borne transmission outside dwellings is virtually undocumented; however, it may exist. Only one report suggests this kind of transmission. In the northern part of the state of Amazonas, three cases of chronic chagasic cardiopathy have been reported in patients who were bitten several times by triatomine bugs in their camping huts while gathering pia ava fibers.[105] Moreover, some species are aggressive, and one of the authors has personally experienced severe attacks by *T. guasayana* and *T. sordida* outdoors at dusk in the Gran Chaco region, Bolivia. For the Indians of the Sierra Nevada in Colombia, the economy is based on agriculture located in different climatic zones. They travel into the mountains to reach their crops and commonly stay in camps. In addition to the classic transmission related to colonization of dwellings by *R. prolixus* and *T. dimidiata*, the practice of camping results in people being exposed to triatomine bites independent of human dwellings (Dib, personal communication). Moreover, a Yucatan farmer reported to us that he had collected wild *T. dimidiata* specimens during a 1-month camping trip in the forest where he hunted; every day at dusk he was attacked by about five triatomines when he was resting in his hammock. Another interesting case occurred during light trap collection of triatomines in Southern Ecuador[106]: a male *Rhodnius ecuadoriensis*, attracted by the light, remained a long moment on the leg of a person sitting approximately 6 m from the light trap.

Indirectly, the identification of blood meals taken on humans by specimens of *T. infestans*, including nymphs, caught in a wild environment in Bolivia shows that the risk exists.[107–109] Lastly, human blood meals in *T. sanguisuga* captured in a wild environment were also reported in Louisiana.[110] These experiences show that travelers in the Americas should be informed that camping in the forest or in other uninhabited environments where natural populations of triatomines exist is dangerous; self-protection is indispensable during the night.

# The perception of vectors and a need for education

Unfortunately, even now, humans in the affected regions do not associate the presence of triatomines in their home with the transmission of any illnesses. The ignorance surrounding Chagas disease works against efforts to control it. Indeed to fight against Chagas disease, people should become aware that living with triatomines could be dangerous to their health. It is urgent that people exposed to vector transmission be made aware of this danger so that they can become involved in combating Chagas disease. In recent years, several initiatives have been developed to involve residents in the fight against vectors. This has been done in Mexico (Yucatan), Guatemala, and Bolivia in two regions (Andean valleys and lowlands), as well as in other countries. Consultations and discussions were carried out during meetings implemented between the group of researchers and the inhabitants to evaluate different strategies and then have a better exchange within the population for the actions that they decided to implement.[89,111,112] Also, the experience in the

United States on information dissemination and collection of triatomines through different media is very interesting: printed pamphlets, radio, phone, website, and a dedicated email address were all used.[113]

Knowledge about Chagas disease should be disseminated throughout the at-risk population so that testimonies such as José's are not repeated. "Montero is a town 100 km from Santa Cruz de la Sierra in Bolivia. A large family of ten children live in a house near the sawmill on the outskirts of the city. The nuisance is so great that the mother regularly struggles against the triatomines and cockroaches invading the house. She periodically removes the mattresses and places them in the sun. José remembers: 'Frequently at night, we'd catch *Triatoma infestans*, and then Mom would send us to sleep with our uncle as she treated the house with insecticide overnight. But it is impossible to get rid of these disgusting insects. When did I know that the *Triatoma infestans* transmitted disease? When my sister, Juana, began her nursing studies, she discovered that she was chagasic and began treatment but soon discontinued her treatment because she had adverse reactions. No one in the family realized that Chagas disease could be a problem for the other members of the family, and everyone needed a checkup. A few years later in 2000, my brother suffered a heart attack during a football game and died. He was 46 years old. The autopsy showed infection by *T. cruzi*. Then we were all concerned about our health, and my brothers and sisters are all chagasic. Juana is in Italy and I am in France, the countries to which we immigrated a few years ago. During recent years, two other siblings died, both suddenly. We did not know about the bugs, the insects that transmit Chagas disease. And then later, we heard only that Chagas disease could not be treated, and that we should live with it without worrying about it.' I talked with José, and I explained several things. I told him that parasites are in the feces and that the parasite is not in the salivary glands; he did not know. He remembered that when he was a young boy, he and his siblings frequently found *Triatoma infestans* in the bedroom, usually engorged with blood, and they would remove the head, but they had not taken any precautions, and they would get blood and feces on their hands."

The lack of satisfactory treatments and a vaccine for Chagas disease is a huge problem at the clinical, educational social, and psychological levels. For this reason, prevention is the best alternative to fight against this disease, and education is key of sustained prevention.

# References

1. Milne MA, Ross EJ, Sonenshine DE, Kirsch P. Attraction of *Triatoma dimidiata* and *Rhodnius prolixus* (Hemiptera: Reduviidae) to combinations of host cues tested at two distances. *J Med Entomol* 2009;**46**:1062−73.
2. Barrozo RB, Lazzari CR. Orientation response of haematophagous bugs to $CO_2$: the effect of the temporal structure of the stimulus. *J Comp Physiol A Neuroethol Sens Neural Behav Physiol* 2006;**192**:827−31.
3. Lazzari CR, Pereira MH, Lorenzo MG. Behavioural biology of Chagas disease vectors. *Mem Inst Oswaldo Cruz* 2013;**108**(Suppl 1):34−47.

4. Campbell AL, Naik RR, Sowards L, Stone MO. Biological infrared imaging and sensing. *Micron* 2002;**33**:211−25.

5. Lorenzo MG, Manrique G, Pires HH, de Brito Sanchez MG, Diotaiuti L, Lazzari CR. Yeast culture volatiles as attractants for *Rhodnius prolixus*: electroantennogram responses and captures in yeast-baited traps. *Acta Trop* 1999;**72**:119−24.

6. Barrozo RB, Manrique G, Lazzari CR. The role of water vapour in the orientation behaviour of the blood-sucking bug *Triatoma infestans* (Hemiptera, Reduviidae). *J Insect Physiol* 2003;**49**:315−21.

7. Ortiz MI, Molina J. Preliminary evidence of (Hemiptera: Triatominae) attraction to human skin odour extracts. *Acta Trop* 2010;**113**:174−9.

8. Catala SS. The infra-red (IR) landscape of *Triatoma infestans*. An hypothesis about the role of IR radiation as a cue for Triatominae dispersal. *Infect Genet Evol* 2011;**11**: 1891−8.

9. de Araujo CN, Bussacos AC, Sousa AO, Hecht MM, Teixeira AR. Interactome: smart hematophagous triatomine salivary gland molecules counteract human hemostasis during meal acquisition. *J Proteomics* 2012;**75**:3829−41.

10. Santos A, Ribeiro JM, Lehane MJ, Gontijo NF, Veloso AB, Sant'Anna MR, et al. The sialotranscriptome of the blood-sucking bug *Triatoma brasiliensis* (Hemiptera, Triatominae). *Insect Biochem Mol Biol* 2007;**37**:702−12.

11. Assumpcao TC, Francischetti IM, Andersen JF, Schwarz A, Santana JM, Ribeiro JM. An insight into the sialome of the blood-sucking bug *Triatoma infestans*, a vector of Chagas' disease. *Insect Biochem Mol Biol* 2008;**38**:213−32.

12. WHO. Reducing risks, promoting healthy life. *World Health Rep* 2002;192−7.

13. Voigt CC, Peschel U, Wibbelt G, Frolich K. An alternative, less invasive blood sample collection technique for serologic studies utilizing triatomine bugs (Heteroptera; Insecta). *J Wildl Dis* 2006;**42**:466−9.

14. Schuster JPS, Schaub GA. *Trypanosoma cruzi*: skin-penetration kinetics of vector-derived metacyclic trypomastigotes. *Int J Parasitol* 2000;**30**:1475−9.

15. Cavalcante RR, Pereira MH, Gontijo NF. Anti-complement activity in the saliva of phlebotomine sand flies and other haematophagous insects. *Parasitology* 2003;**127**:87−93.

16. Titus RG, Bishop JV, Mejia JS. The immunomodulatory factors of arthropod saliva and the potential for these factors to serve as vaccine targets to prevent pathogen transmission. *Parasite Immunol* 2006;**28**:131−41.

17. Silva-Neto MA, Carneiro AB, Silva-Cardoso L, Atella GC. Lysophosphatidylcholine: a novel modulator of *Trypanosoma cruzi* transmission. *J Parasitol Res* 2012;**2012**:625838.

18. De Araujo-Jorge TC, Barbosa HS, Meirelles MN. *Trypanosoma cruzi* recognition by macrophages and muscle cells: perspectives after a 15-year study. *Mem Inst Oswaldo Cruz* 1992;**87**(Suppl 5):43−56.

19. Snary D. Receptors and recognition mechanisms of *Trypanosoma cruzi*. *Trans R Soc Trop Med Hyg* 1985;**79**:587−90.

20. Andrews NW. Living dangerously: how *Trypanosoma cruzi* uses lysosomes to get inside host cells, and then escapes into the cytoplasm. *Biol Res* 1993;**26**:65−7.

21. Stafford JL, Neumann NF, Belosevic M. Macrophage-mediated innate host defense against protozoan parasites. *Crit Rev Microbiol* 2002;**28**:187−248.

22. Schofield CJ, Galvao C. Classification, evolution, and species groups within the Triatominae. *Acta Trop* 2009;**110**:88−100.

23. WHO. Control of Chagas' disease. *Technical report series*, Geneva; 1991, No. 811.

24. Schaub GA. Direct transmission of *Trypanosoma cruzi* between vectors of Chagas' disease. *Acta Trop (Basel)* 1988;**45**:11−19.

25. Zeledon R, Bolanos R, Rojas M. Scanning electron microscopy of the final phase of the life cycle of *Trypanosoma cruzi* in the insect vector. *Acta Trop* 1984;**41**:39−43.

26. Nogueira NP, Saraiva FM, Sultano PE, Cunha PR, Laranja GA, Justo GA, et al. Proliferation and differentiation of *Trypanosoma cruzi* inside its vector have a new trigger: redox status. *PLoS One* 2015;**10**:e0116712.

27. Perlowagora-Szumlewicz A, Moreira CJ. In vivo differentiation of *Trypanosoma cruzi*. Experimental evidence of the influence of vector species on metacyclogenesis. *Mem Inst Oswaldo Cruz* 1994;**89**:603−18.

28. Carvalho-Moreira CJ, Spata MC, Coura JR, Garcia ES, Azambuja P, Gonzalez MS, et al. In vivo and in vitro metacyclogenesis tests of two strains of *Trypanosoma cruzi* in the triatomine vectors *Triatoma pseudomaculata* and *Rhodnius neglectus*: short/long-term and comparative study. *Exp Parasitol* 2003;**103**:102−11.

29. Loza-Murguia M, Noireau F. Vectorial capacity of *Triatoma guasayana* (Wygodzinsky & Abalos) (Hemiptera: Reduviidae) compared with two other species of epidemic importance. *Neotrop Entomol* 2010;**39**:799−809.

30. Schaub GA. *Trypanosoma cruzi*: quantitative studies of development of two strains in small intestine and rectum of the vector *Triatoma infestans*. *Exp Parasitol* 1989;**68**: 260−73.

31. de Lana M, da Silveira Pinto A, Barnabé C, Quesney V, Noël S, Tibayrenc M. *Trypanosoma cruzi*: compared vectorial transmissibility of three major clonal genotypes by *Triatoma infestans*. *Exp Parasitol* 1998;**90**:20−5.

32. Sanchez G, Wallace A, Olivares M, Diaz N, Aguilera X, Apt W, et al. Biological characterization of *Trypanosoma cruzi* zymodemes: in vitro differentiation of epimastigotes and infectivity of culture metacyclic trypomastigotes in mice. *Exp Parasitol* 1990;**71**:125−33.

33. Laurent JP, Barnabé C, Quesney V, Noël S, Tibayrenc M. Impact of clonal evolution on the biological diversity of *Trypanosoma cruzi*. *Parasitology* 1997;**114**:213−18.

34. Kollien AH, Schaub GA. Development of *Trypanosoma cruzi* after starvation and feeding of the vector—a review. *Tokai J Exp Clin Med* 1998;**23**:335−40.

35. Rodriguez CS, Carrizo SA, Crocco LB. Comparison of feeding and defecation patterns between fifth-instar nymphs of *Triatoma patagonica* (Del Ponte, 1929) and *Triatoma infestans* (Klug, 1934) under laboratory conditions. *Rev Soc Bras Med Trop* 2008;**41**: 330−3.

36. Martinez-Ibarra JA, Alejandre-Aguilar R, Paredes-Gonzalez E, Martinez-Silva MA, Solorio-Cibrian M, Nogueda-Torres B, et al. Biology of three species of North American Triatominae (Hemiptera: Reduviidae: Triatominae) fed on rabbits. *Mem Inst Oswaldo Cruz* 2007;**102**:925−30.

37. Klotz SA, Dorn PL, Klotz JH, Pinnas JL, Weirauch C, Kurtz JR, et al. Feeding behavior of triatomines from the Southwestern United States: an update on potential risk for transmission of Chagas disease. *Acta Trop* 2009;**111**:114−18.

38. Martinez-Ibarra JA, Paredes-Gonzalez E, Licon-Trillo A, Montanez-Valdez OD, Rocha-Chavez G, Nogueda-Torres B. The biology of three Mexican-American species of Triatominae (Hemiptera: Reduviidae): *Triatoma recurva*, *Triatoma protracta* and *Triatoma rubida*. *Mem Inst Oswaldo Cruz* 2012;**107**:659−63.

39. Reisenman CE, Gregory T, Guerenstein PG, Hildebrand JG. Feeding and defecation behavior of *Triatoma rubida* (Uhler, 1894) (Hemiptera: Reduviidae) under laboratory conditions, and its potential role as a vector of Chagas disease in Arizona, USA. *Am J Trop Med Hyg* 2011;**85**:648−56.

40. Lunardi RR, Gomes LP, Peres Camara T, Arrais-Silva WW. Life cycle and vectorial competence of *Triatoma williami* (Galvao, Souza e Lima, 1965) under the influence of different blood meal sources. *Acta Trop* 2015;**149**:220−6.

41. Duran P, Sinani E, Depickère S. Biological cycle and preliminary data on vectorial competence of *Triatoma boliviana* in laboratory conditions. *Acta Trop* 2014;**140**:124−9.

42. Costa J, Almeida CE, Dotson EM, Lins A, Vinhaes M, Silveira AC, et al. The epidemiologic importance of *Triatoma brasiliensis* as a Chagas disease vector in Brazil: a revision of domiciliary captures during 1993-1999. *Mem Inst Oswaldo Cruz* 2003;**98**: 443−9.

43. Borges EC, Dujardin JP, Schofield CJ, Romanha AJ, Diotaiuti L. Dynamics between sylvatic, peridomestic and domestic populations of *Triatoma brasiliensis* (Hemiptera: Reduviidae) in Ceara State, Northeastern Brazil. *Acta Trop* 2005;**93**:119−26.

44. Carbajal de la Fuente AL, Minoli SA, Lopes CM, Noireau F, Lazzari CR, Lorenzo MG. Flight dispersal of the Chagas disease vectors *Triatoma brasiliensis* and *Triatoma pseudomaculata* in Northeastern Brazil. *Acta Trop* 2007;**101**:115−19.

45. Magallón-Gastelúm E, Lozano-Kasten F, Bosseno MF, Cardenas-Contreras R, Ouaissi A, Brenière SF. Colonization of rock pile boundary walls in fields by sylvatic triatomines (Hemiptera: Reduviidae) in Jalisco State, Mexico. *J Med Entomol* 2004;**41**:484−8.

46. Bosseno MF, Barnabé C, Sierra MJ, Kengne P, Guerrero S, Lozano F, et al. Wild ecotopes and food habits of *Triatoma longipennis* infected by *Trypanosoma cruzi* lineages I and II in Mexico. *Am J Trop Med Hyg* 2009;**80**:988−91.

47. Magallón-Gastelúm E, Lozano-Kasten F, Flores-Perez A, Bosseno MF, Brenière SF. Sylvatic triatominae of the phyllosoma complex (Hemiptera: Reduviidae) around the community of Carrillo Puerto, Nayarit, Mexico. *J Med Entomol* 2001;**38**:638−40.

48. Brenière SF, Bosseno MF, Magallón-Gastelúm E, Castillo Ruvalcaba EG, Gutierrez MS, Montano Luna EC, et al. Peridomestic colonization of *Triatoma longipennis* (Hemiptera, Reduviidae) and *Triatoma barberi* (Hemiptera, Reduviidae) in a rural community with active transmission of *Trypanosoma cruzi* in Jalisco State, Mexico. *Acta Trop* 2007;**101**:249−57.

49. Walter A, Lozano-Kasten F, Bosseno MF, Ruvalcaba EG, Gutierrez MS, Luna CE, et al. Peridomicilary habitat and risk factors for triatoma infestation in a rural community of the Mexican occident. *Am J Trop Med Hyg* 2007;**76**:508−15.

50. Brenière SF, Bosseno MF, Gastelúm EM, Soto Gutierrez MM, de Jesus Kasten Monges M, Barraza Salas JH, et al. Community participation and domiciliary occurrence of infected *Meccus longipennis* in two Mexican villages in Jalisco State. *Am J Trop Med Hyg* 2010;**83**:382−7.

51. Carvalho ME, da Silva RA, Barata JM, Domingos Mde F, Ciaravolo RM, Zacharias F. Chagas' disease in the southern coastal region of Brazil. *Rev Saude Publica* 2003;**37**: 49−58.

52. de Carvalho ME, da Silva RA, Rodrigues VL, de Oliveira CD. The Chagas disease control program of the Sao Paulo State: the contribution of serology to the epidemiological investigation of triatomine-infested domiciliary units during the 1990s. *Cad Saude Publica* 2002;**18**:1695−703.

53. Steindel M, Kramer Pacheco L, Scholl D, Soares M, de Moraes MH, Eger I, et al. Characterization of *Trypanosoma cruzi* isolated from humans, vectors, and animal reservoirs following an outbreak of acute human Chagas disease in Santa Catarina State, Brazil. *Diagn Microbiol Infect Dis* 2008;**60**:25−32.

54. Dias-Lima AG, Sherlock IA. Sylvatic vectors invading houses and the risk of emergence of cases of Chagas disease in Salvador, State of Bahia, Northeast Brazil. *Mem Inst Oswaldo Cruz* 2000;**95**:611−13.
55. Canals M, Cruzat L, Molina MC, Ferreira A, Cattan PE. Blood host sources of *Mepraia spinolai* (Heteroptera: Reduviidae), wild vector of Chagas disease in Chile. *J Med Entomol* 2001;**38**:303−7.
56. Damborsky MP, Bar ME, Oscherov EB. Detection of triatomines (Hemiptera: Reduviidae) in domiciliary and extra-domiciliary ecotopes. Corrientes, Argentina. *Cad Saude Publica* 2001;**17**:843−9.
57. Bar ME, Wisnivesky-Colli C. *Triatoma sordida* stal 1859 (Hemiptera, Reduviidae: Triatominae) in palms of Northeastern Argentina. *Mem Inst Oswaldo Cruz* 2001;**96**: 895−9.
58. Noireau F, Brenière F, Ordonez J, Cardozo L, Morochi W, Gutierrez T, et al. Low probability of transmission of *Trypanosoma cruzi* to humans by domiciliary *Triatoma sordida* in Bolivia. *Trans R Soc Trop Med Hyg* 1997;**91**:653−6.
59. Carvalho DB, Almeida CE, Rocha CS, Gardim S, Mendonca VJ, Ribeiro AR, et al. A novel association between *Rhodnius neglectus* and the *Livistona australis* palm tree in an urban center foreshadowing the risk of Chagas disease transmission by vectorial invasions in Monte Alto city, Sao Paulo, Brazil. *Acta Trop* 2014;**130**:35−8.
60. Garcia MN, Woc-Colburn L, Aguilar D, Hotez PJ, Murray KO. Historical perspectives on the epidemiology of human Chagas disease in Texas and recommendations for enhanced understanding of clinical Chagas disease in the southern United States. *PLoS Negl Trop Dis* 2015;**9**:e0003981.
61. Lambert R, Kolivras KN, Resler LM, Brewster CC, Paulson SL. The potential for emergence of Chagas disease in the United States. *Geospat Health* 2008;**2**:227−39.
62. Coura JR, Junqueira AC, Boia MN, Fernandes O, Bonfante C, Campos JE, et al. Chagas disease in the Brazilian Amazon: IV. A new cross-sectional study. *Rev Inst Med Trop Sao Paulo* 2002;**44**:159−65.
63. Bérenger JM, Pluot-Sigwalt D, Pagès F, Blanchet D, Aznar C. The triatominae species of French Guiana (Heteroptera: Reduviidae). *Mem Inst Oswaldo Cruz* 2009;**104**:1111−16.
64. Ricardo-Silva AH, Lopes CM, Ramos LB, Marques WA, Mello CB, Duarte R, et al. Correlation between populations of *Rhodnius* and presence of palm trees as risk factors for the emergence of Chagas disease in Amazon region, Brazil. *Acta Trop* 2012;**123**: 217−23.
65. Aguilar HM, Abad-Franch F, Dias JC, Junqueira AC, Coura JR. Chagas disease in the Amazon region. *Mem Inst Oswaldo Cruz* 2007;**102**:47−56.
66. Briceno-Leon R. Chagas disease in the Americas: an ecohealth perspective. *Cad Saude Publica* 2009;**25**(Suppl 1):S71−82.
67. Coura JR, Junqueira AC. Risks of endemicity, morbidity and perspectives regarding the control of Chagas disease in the Amazon region. *Mem Inst Oswaldo Cruz* 2012;**107**: 145−54.
68. de Andrade AL, Zicker F, Silva IG, Souza JM, Martelli CM. Risk factors for *Trypanosoma cruzi* infection among children in Central Brazil: a case-control study in vector control settings. *Am J Trop Med Hyg* 1995;**52**:183−7.
69. Catala SS, Crocco LB, Munoz A, Morales G, Paulone I, Giraldez E, et al. Entomological aspects of Chagas' disease transmission in the domestic habitat, Argentina. *Rev Saude Publica* 2004;**38**:216−22.

70. Reyes-Lugo M, Rodriguez-Acosta A. Domiciliation of the sylvatic Chagas disease vector *Panstrongylus geniculatus* latreille, 1811 (triatominae: Reduviidae) in Venezuela. *Trans R Soc Trop Med Hyg* 2000;**94**:508.

71. Grijalva MJ, Suarez-Davalos V, Villacis AG, Ocana-Mayorga S, Dangles O. Ecological factors related to the widespread distribution of sylvatic *Rhodnius ecuadoriensis* populations in Southern Ecuador. *Parasit Vectors* 2012;**5**:17.

72. Ribeiro Jr. G, Gurgel-Goncalves R, Reis RB, Santos CG, Amorim A, Andrade SG, et al. Frequent house invasion of *Trypanosoma cruzi*-infected triatomines in a suburban area of Brazil. *PLoS Negl Trop Dis* 2015;**9**:e0003678.

73. Medrano-Mercado N, Ugarte-Fernandez R, Butron V, Uber-Busek S, Guerra HL, Araujo-Jorge TC, et al. Urban transmission of Chagas disease in Cochabamba, Bolivia. *Mem Inst Oswaldo Cruz* 2008;**103**:423−30.

74. Delgado S, Ernst KC, Pumahuanca ML, Yool SR, Comrie AC, Sterling CR, et al. A country bug in the city: urban infestation by the Chagas disease vector *Triatoma infestans* in Arequipa, Peru. *Int J Health Geogr* 2013;**12**:48.

75. Levy MZ, Bowman NM, Kawai V, Plotkin JB, Waller LA, Cabrera L, et al. Spatial patterns in discordant diagnostic test results for Chagas disease: links to transmission hotspots. *Clin Infect Dis* 2009;**48**:1104−6.

76. Levy MZ, Bowman NM, Kawai V, Waller LA, Cornejo del Carpio JG, Cordova Benzaquen E, et al. Periurban *Trypanosoma cruzi*-infected *Triatoma infestans*, Arequipa, Peru. *Emerg Infect Dis* 2006;**12**:1345−52.

77. Zeledon R, Calvo N, Montenegro VM, Lorosa ES, Arevalo C. A survey on *Triatoma dimidiata* in an urban area of the province of Heredia, Costa Rica. *Mem Inst Oswaldo Cruz* 2005;**100**:507−12.

78. Guzman-Tapia Y, Ramirez-Sierra MJ, Dumonteil E. Urban infestation by *Triatoma dimidiata* in the city of Merida, Yucatan, Mexico. *Vector Borne Zoonotic Dis* 2007;**7**:597−606.

79. Gajate P, Pietrokovsky S, Abramo Orrego L, Perez O, Monte A, Belmonte J, et al. *Triatoma infestans* in greater Buenos Aires, Argentina. *Mem Inst Oswaldo Cruz* 2001; **96**:473−7.

80. Vallve SL, Rojo H, Wisnivesky-Colli C. Urban ecology of *Triatoma infestans* in San Juan, Argentina. *Mem Inst Oswaldo Cruz* 1996;**91**:405−8.

81. Pfeiler E, Bitler BG, Ramsey JM, Palacios-Cardiel C, Markow TA. Genetic variation, population structure, and phylogenetic relationships of *Triatoma rubida* and *T. recurva* (Hemiptera: Reduviidae: Triatominae) from the Sonoran Desert, insect vectors of the Chagas' disease parasite *Trypanosoma cruzi*. *Mol Phylogenet Evol* 2006;**41**:209−21.

82. Walter A. Human activities and American trypanosomiasis. Review of the literature. *Parasite* 2003;**10**:191−204.

83. Gurtler RE, Chuit R, Cecere MC, Castanera MB, Cohen JE, Segura EL. Household prevalence of seropositivity for *Trypanosoma cruzi* in three rural villages in Northwest Argentina: environmental, demographic, and entomologic associations. *Am J Trop Med Hyg* 1998;**59**:741−9.

84. Sanmartino M, Crocco L. Knowledge about Chagas' disease and risk factors in Argentina communities with different epidemiological trends. *Rev Panam Salud Publica* 2000;**7**:173−8.

85. Campbell-Lendrum DH, Angulo VM, Esteban L, Tarazona Z, Parra GJ, Restrepo M, et al. House-level risk factors for triatomine infestation in Colombia. *Int J Epidemiol* 2007;**36**:866−72.

86. Feliciangeli MD, Sanchez-Martin MJ, Suarez B, Marrero R, Torrellas A, Bravo A, et al. Risk factors for *Trypanosoma cruzi* human infection in Barinas State, Venezuela. *Am J Trop Med Hyg* 2007;**76**:915–21.

87. Rojas ME, Varquez P, Villarreal MF, Velandia C, Vergara L, Moran-Borges YH, et al. An entomological and seroepidemiological study of Chagas' disease in an area in Central-Western Venezuela infested with *Triatoma maculata* (Erichson 1848). *Cad Saude Publica* 2008;**24**:2323–33.

88. Bustamante DM, Monroy C, Pineda S, Rodas A, Castro X, Ayala V, et al. Risk factors for intradomiciliary infestation by the Chagas disease vector *Triatoma dimidiata* in Jutiapa, Guatemala. *Cad Saude Publica* 2009;**25**(Suppl 1):S83–92.

89. Monroy C, Bustamante DM, Pineda S, Rodas A, Castro X, Ayala V, et al. House improvements and community participation in the control of *Triatoma dimidiata* re-infestation in Jutiapa, Guatemala. *Cad Saude Publica* 2009;**25**(Suppl 1):S168–78.

90. Nieto-Sanchez C, Baus EG, Guerrero D, Grijalva MJ. Positive deviance study to inform a Chagas disease control program in Southern Ecuador. *Mem Inst Oswaldo Cruz* 2015; **110**:299–309.

91. Sarquis O, Sposina R, de Oliveira TG, Mac Cord JR, Cabello PH, Borges-Pereira J, et al. Aspects of peridomiciliary ecotopes in rural areas of Northeastern Brazil associated to triatomine (Hemiptera, Reduviidae) infestation, vectors of Chagas disease. *Mem Inst Oswaldo Cruz* 2006;**101**:143–7.

92. Rossi JC, Duarte EC, Gurgel-Goncalves R. Factors associated with the occurrence of *Triatoma sordida* (Hemiptera: Reduviidae) in rural localities of Central-West Brazil. *Mem Inst Oswaldo Cruz* 2015;**110**:192–200.

93. Grijalva MJ, Villacis AG, Ocana-Mayorga S, Yumiseva CA, Moncayo AL, Baus EG. Comprehensive survey of domiciliary triatomine species capable of transmitting Chagas disease in Southern Ecuador. *PLoS Negl Trop Dis* 2015;**9**:e0004142.

94. Villacis AG, Ocana-Mayorga S, Lascano MS, Yumiseva CA, Baus EG, Grijalva MJ. Abundance, natural infection with trypanosomes, and food source of an endemic species of triatomine, *Panstrongylus howardi* (neiva 1911), on the Ecuadorian central coast. *Am J Trop Med Hyg* 2015;**92**:187–92.

95. Bosseno MF, Garcia LS, Baunaure F, Gastelúm EM, Gutierrez MS, Kasten FL, et al. Identification in triatomine vectors of feeding sources and *Trypanosoma cruzi* variants by heteroduplex assay and a multiplex miniexon polymerase chain reaction. *Am J Trop Med Hyg* 2006;**74**:303–5.

96. Bustamante DM, De Urioste-Stone SM, Juarez JG, Pennington PM. Ecological, social and biological risk factors for continued *Trypanosoma cruzi* transmission by *Triatoma dimidiata* in Guatemala. *PLoS One* 2014;**9**:e104599.

97. Vazquez-Prokopec GM, Cecere MC, Kitron U, Gurtler RE. Environmental and demographic factors determining the spatial distribution of *Triatoma guasayana* in peridomestic and semi-sylvatic habitats of rural Northwestern Argentina. *Med Vet Entomol* 2008; **22**:273–82.

98. Abad-Franch F, Palomeque FS, Aguilar HMt, Miles MA. Field ecology of sylvatic *Rhodnius* populations (Heteroptera, Triatominae): risk factors for palm tree infestation in Western Ecuador. *Trop Med Int Health* 2005;**10**:1258–66.

99. Villacis AG, Grijalva MJ, Catala SS. Phenotypic variability of *Rhodnius ecuadoriensis* populations at the Ecuadorian Central and Southern Andean region. *J Med Entomol* 2010;**47**:1034–43.

100. Saldana A, Calzada JE, Pineda V, Perea M, Rigg C, Gonzalez K, et al. Risk factors associated with *Trypanosoma cruzi* exposure in domestic dogs from a rural community in Panama. *Mem Inst Oswaldo Cruz* 2015;**110**:936−44.

101. Abad-Franch F, Lima MM, Sarquis O, Gurgel-Goncalves R, Sanchez-Martin M, Calzada J, et al. On palms, bugs, and Chagas disease in the Americas. *Acta Trop* 2015; **151**:126−41.

102. Minoli SA, Lazzari CR. Take-off activity and orientation of triatomines (Heteroptera: Reduviidae) in relation to the presence of artificial lights. *Acta Trop* 2006;**97**:324−30.

103. Pacheco-Tucuch FS, Ramirez-Sierra MJ, Gourbière S, Dumonteil E. Public street lights increase house infestation by the Chagas disease vector *Triatoma dimidiata*. *PLoS One* 2012;**7**:e36207.

104. Erazo D, Cordovez J. The role of light in Chagas disease infection risk in Colombia. *Parasit Vectors* 2016;**9**:9.

105. Vinas Albajar P, Laredo SV, Terrazas MB, Coura JR. Dilated cardiomyopathy in patients with chronic chagasic infection: report of two fatal autochthonous cases from Rio Negro, State of Amazonas, Brazil. *Rev Soc Bras Med Trop* 2003;**36**:401−7.

106. Grijalva MJ, Villacis AG. Presence of *Rhodnius ecuadoriensis* in sylvatic habitats in the Southern highlands (Loja province) of Ecuador. *J Med Entomol* 2009;**46**:708−11.

107. Buitrago R, Waleckx E, Bosseno MF, Zoveda F, Vidaurre P, Salas R, et al. First report of widespread wild populations of *Triatoma infestans* (reduviidae, triatominae) in the valleys of La Paz, Bolivia. *Am J Trop Med Hyg* 2010;**82**:574−9.

108. Buitrago R, Bosseno MF, Depickère S, Waleckx E, Salas R, Aliaga C, et al. Blood meal sources of wild and domestic Triatoma infestans (Hemiptera: Reduviidae) in Bolivia: connectivity between cycles of transmission of Trypanosoma cruzi. *Parasit Vectors* 2016;**9**:214.

109. Buitrago NL, Bosseno MF, Waleckx E, Brémond P, Vidaurre P, Zoveda F, et al. Risk of transmission of *Trypanosoma cruzi* by wild *Triatoma infestans* (Hemiptera: Reduviidae) in Bolivia supported by the detection of human blood meals. *Infect Genet Evol* 2013;**19**:141−4.

110. Waleckx E, Suarez J, Richards B, Dorn PL. *Triatoma sanguisuga* blood meals and potential for Chagas disease, Louisiana, USA. *Emerg Infect Dis* 2014;**20**:2141−3.

111. Lardeux F, Depickère S, Aliaga C, Chavez T, Zambrana L. Experimental control of *Triatoma infestans* in poor rural villages of Bolivia through community participation. *Trans R Soc Trop Med Hyg* 2015;**109**:150−8.

112. Waleckx E, Camara-Mejia J, Ramirez-Sierra MJ, Cruz-Chan V, Rosado-Vallado M, Vazquez-Narvaez S, et al. An innovative ecohealth intervention for Chagas disease vector control in Yucatan, Mexico. *Trans R Soc Trop Med Hyg* 2015;**109**:143−9.

113. Curtis-Robles R, Wozniak EJ, Auckland LD, Hamer GL, Hamer SA. Combining public health education and disease ecology research: using citizen science to assess Chagas disease entomological risk in Texas. *PLoS Negl Trop Dis* 2015;**9**:e0004235.

# Maternal–fetal transmission of *Trypanosoma cruzi*

*Y. Carlier[1,2] and C. Truyens[1]*
[1]Université Libre de Bruxelles (ULB), Brussels, Belgium,
[2]Tulane University, New Orleans, LA, United States

## Chapter Outline

American Trypanosomiasis Chagas Disease. DOI: http://dx.doi.org/10.1016/B978-0-12-801029-7.00024-1

# From maternal–fetal transmission of *Trypanosoma cruzi* to congenital Chagas disease: definitions and limits

Maternal–fetal *transmission* of *Trypanosoma cruzi* induces congenital infection (from its Latin etymology "cum" (with), and "genitus" (engendered)) when transmitted live parasites persist and multiply in fetuses and/or after birth (*development of infection*). Maternal–fetal transmission can be "prenatal" (in utero) or "perinatal" (at the time of delivery). It excludes the "postnatal" transmission of parasites (mainly through maternal milk by breast feeding) and the transmission of dead parasites, parasitic DNA, or other molecules released from parasites in the mother and likely to be found in fetal blood.

The terms "mother-to-child transmission" or "vertical transmission" have a broader connotation corresponding to transmission from one generation to the next, including prenatal, perinatal, as well as postnatal transmission of live parasites. The term "congenital infection with *T. cruzi*" refers to asymptomatic as well as symptomatic cases of infection, whereas the term "congenital Chagas disease" should be used only for symptomatic cases, though, often, both terms are confounded. In order to facilitate the reading of this chapter, the terms "mother" or "maternal" will be also used for pregnant women (before delivery), albeit such terms normally refer to the status of women having delivered.

The present chapter updates the previously one published in the first edition of the book in 2010.[1] The critical review of interactions between *T. cruzi* parasites, pregnant women, placenta, and fetuses recently published by the authors[2] can usefully complete the reading of the present chapter.

# Epidemiological aspects of congenital infection with *Trypanosoma cruzi*

## Situation in Latin American endemic countries

Historically, Carlos Chagas himself, in 1911, referred to the possibility of congenital transmission of *T. cruzi* infection when he found trypomastigotes in the blood smear of a 2-month-old child whose mother was infected.[3] Dao, in 1949, was the first in reporting cases of congenital Chagas disease from Venezuela.[4]

According a recent WHO estimation,[5] 1,125,000 women in fertile age are infected with *T. cruzi* in the 21 Latin American countries where Chagas disease is currently endemic. The incidence of congenital infection is estimated to be 8668 cases per year, with nearly 50% of such cases grouped in Mexico, Argentina, and Colombia. Congenital transmission would be responsible for 90 to 100% of new annual cases of infection in countries declared free of transmission by the vector *Triatoma infestans* (such as Brazil, Chile, Uruguay) and for 6 to 90% in other countries depending on the achievement of their vector control programs (e.g., Colombia: 16.5%; Mexico: 22.6%; Argentina: 57.5%) (Table 23.1).

The maternal—fetal transmission rate, classically defined as the number of congenital cases/number of *T. cruzi*-infected mothers, can gain in precision by including multiple births if expressed as the number of congenitally infected infants divided by the number of infants born to infected mothers. Well defined, it occurs in an average of 4.7% of chronically infected mothers in endemic areas,[6] though differences can be observed between countries.[7,8]

## Globalization of congenital infection with Trypanosoma cruzi

Migration of Latin American people particularly during these last decades has promoted Chagas disease as a global disease, now observed in areas deprived from vector transmission (Europe, Canada, Japan, Australia) or with exceptional vector transmission to humans, such as the United States. The current trend toward the feminization of such migration[9] is relevant for an increased risk of congenital transmission into nonendemic areas. Cases of congenital Chagas disease have been reported mainly in Spain,[10,11] but also in Sweden,[12] Switzerland,[13] and more recently in the United States,[14] Canada,[15] and Japan.[16] The congenital route is the main transmission mode of *T. cruzi* in nonendemic areas, over blood transfusions and organ transplantations (occurring in an average of 2.7% of chronically infected mothers[6]).

## Epidemiological features specific to congenital infection with Trypanosoma cruzi

Congenital transmission of *T. cruzi*, in contrast with toxoplasmosis, can arise in both acute and chronic phases of maternal infection and be repeated at each pregnancy, i.e., throughout the fertile period of woman life (most cases of congenital infection derive from chronically infected mothers, having been infected by insect

Table 23.1 **WHO estimations of women in fertile age infected with *T. cruzi* and congenital cases in Latin American countries for the year 2010[5]**

| Country | Population | Prevalence of infection (%) | Nb of infected women aged 15–44 years | Congenital cases | | |
|---|---|---|---|---|---|---|
| | | | | Annual nb | Incidence (%) | Annual new infection cases[b] (%) |
| **South America** | | | | | | |
| Argentina | 41,343,000 | 3.640 | 211,102 | 1 457 | 0.210 | 57.5 |
| Bolivia | 9,947,000 | 6.104 | 199,351 | 616 | 0.235 | 7.1 |
| Brazil | 190,755,799 | 0.030 | 119,298 | 571 | 0.020 | 92.5 |
| Chile | 17,095,000 | 0.699 | 11,771 | 115 | 0.046 | 100.0 |
| Colombia | 48,805,000 | 0.956 | 116,221 | 1046 | 0.114 | 16.5 |
| Ecuador | 14,483,499 | 1.379 | 62,898 | 696 | 0.317 | 25.4 |
| Guyanas[a] | 1,501,962 | 0.838 | 3818 | 18 | 0.075 | 6.0 |
| Paraguay | 8,668,000 | 2.130 | 63,385 | 525 | 0.340 | 63.9 |
| Peru | 28,948,000 | 0.439 | 28,132 | 232 | 0.038 | 10.1 |
| Uruguay | 3,301,000 | 0.237 | 1858 | 20 | 0.040 | 100.0 |
| Venezuela | 27,223,000 | 0.710 | 40,223 | 665 | 0.110 | 43.2 |
| **Central America** | | | | | | |
| Belize | 315,000 | 0.330 | 272 | 25 | 0.333 | 71.4 |
| Costa Rica | 4,516,000 | 0.169 | 1728 | 61 | 0.080 | 85.9 |
| El Salvador | 6,952,000 | 1.297 | 18,211 | 234 | 0.187 | 19.4 |
| Guatemala | 13,550,000 | 1.230 | 32,759 | 164 | 0.035 | 11.4 |
| Honduras | 7,989,000 | 0.917 | 16,149 | 257 | 0.126 | 21.8 |
| Nicaragua | 5,604,000 | 0.522 | 5822 | 138 | 0.124 | 26.5 |
| Panama | 3,557,687 | 0.515 | 6332 | 40 | 0.056 | 18.6 |
| **North America** | | | | | | |
| Mexico | 112,468,855 | 0.779 | 185,600 | 1788 | 0.089 | 22.6 |
| Total | 543,877,115 | 1.055 | 1,124,930 | 8 668 | 0.089 | 22.5 |

Nb/nb=number
[a]including French Guyana, Guyana and Surinam.
[b]calculated from WHO data[5] as: estimated annual number of congenital infection cases/estimated annual infection cases due to congenital + vector transmissions.

vectors since childhood by residing in endemic areas of Latin America).[1,17] Moreover, transgenerational (vertical) transmission of parasites can occur from an infected mother to her daughter who in turn transmits parasites to her own infants, etc. All these elements can contribute to the familial clustering of congenital cases.[18,19] Such epidemiological features specific to *T. cruzi* infection suggest a particularly long-term risk of mother-to-offspring transmission through the pool of currently infected pregnant women in endemic, as well as in nonendemic areas.

This pinpoints congenital infection with *T. cruzi* as an important public health problem which can easily extend in space (through migrations of infected fertile women) and time (for the reasons mentioned above).[1,20]

# Routes of maternal−fetal transmission of *Trypanosoma cruzi*

## Possible transmission routes of Trypanosoma cruzi *parasites*

A possible mode of maternal−fetal transmission might be through parasites released into amniotic fluid (AF) (Fig. 23.1; see section: Histopathologic studies of placentas from infected or uninfected neonates).[21,22] The latter might contaminate the fetuses by oral or pulmonary routes, or eventually by skin penetration (fetuses are bathing in AF and continuously absorbing it). Lung and skin infections with *T. cruzi* have been reported in macerated fetuses and stillborns.[23,24] However, AF contains potent antimicrobial peptides[25] and *T. cruzi* parasites are not found by microscopic observation and parasitic DNA is hardly detected in AF or aspirated gastric fluid content of infected asymptomatic newborns.[26,27]

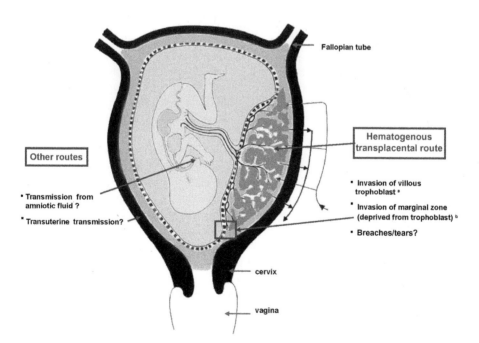

**Figure 23.1 Possible routes of maternal−fetal transmission of *T. cruzi*.** [a]In case of huge parasite amounts in the placental intervillous space; [b]in case of moderate parasite amounts in the placental intervillous space.
*Source*: According to Carlier Y, Truyens C. Maternal-fetal transmission of Trypanosoma cruzi. In: Telleria J, Tibayrenc M, editors. *American trypanosomiasis-Chagas disease. One hundred years of research*. London, Burlington: Elsevier; 2010. p. 539−81.

The possibility of placental/fetal invasion directly from the uterine wall (transuterine route) remains to be determined, since *T. cruzi* amastigote nests are observed in placental deciduas of mothers having delivered infected neonates[28] (Fig. 23.1).

Although outside of the scope of this chapter, it is interesting to mention the possible postnatal transmission of parasites through maternal milk by breast feeding. Only one report mentions a possible infant contamination during lactation.[29] Another one indicates the presence of parasites in milk during maternal infection,[30] but their detection might have been related to a contamination of collected milk with maternal blood.[31] Others studies do not observe parasites in milk of infected women.[32−34] Moreover, blood trypomastigotes, by contrast with metacyclic trypomastigotes expressing Tcgp82, can hardly adhere and migrate through the gastric mucin layer and survive into the gastric milieu.[35,36]

Whether fetal contamination with parasites coming from AF or uterine wall, and/or eventually by breast feeding remains a possibility in acute or reactivated infection,[37] these routes are unlikely in chronic infection.

Placenta is therefore the key fetal organ facing the parasites present into the intervillous blood space and from which transmission depends. Such a route requires parasites to cross or skirt the trophoblastic barrier (first placental line of defense) (Fig. 23.1).

## The hematogenous transplacental route: strengths and weaknesses of the trophoblastic barrier

Villi of the human placenta are covered by two layers of trophoblast: an outer layer called syncytiotrophoblast and an inner layer termed cytotrophoblast ("Langhans" cells). Extravillous cytotrophoblast cells also cover nonvillous structures (e.g., the chorionic plate) and migrate from the placenta into the uterine wall. To a great degree, only the syncytiotrophoblast is interposed between maternal blood and fetal tissues, since the cytotrophoblast cell number decreases during the gestation period.[38]

Besides the physical barrier formed by the syncytiotrophoblast that forgoes intercellular junctions, the placenta is an active immunological organ also able to initiate an innate immune response. It can release pro-inflammatory cytokines, chemokines, reactive oxygen- and nitrogen-intermediates (NO), and antimicrobial peptides,[39] through Toll-like receptors (TLRs) recognizing pathogen-associated molecular patterns (PAMPs).[40]

However, the placental barrier displays some weaknesses since some areas are not covered by trophoblast, such as the marginal zone joining the membranes to the chorionic and basal plates. The latter is constituted with smooth muscle cells embedded in an extracellular fibrinoid matrix (fibronectin, collagen, laminin), only covered by a nontrophoblastic epithelium.[41]

## Ex vivo/in vitro interactions between Trypanosoma cruzi and placenta

Ex vivo studies show the inhibiting role of placental subfractions on trypomastigote infectivity,[42] the slow multiplication of parasites in villous explants and their killing by NO produced by placental cells,[43] arguing for an activation of placental innate defenses in the presence of parasites. Other studies show that low concentrations of parasites induce proliferation, differentiation, and finally a turnover of the syncytio-trophoblast of such explants, considered as another mechanism to clear parasites out of the placental environment.[44] However, high concentrations of parasites induce massive destruction of the trophoblastic cells of villi by infecting them. *T. cruzi* attaches to trophoblastic cells through interactions with calreticulin and C1q and induces a disassembly of actin in cytosqueletton, the placental alkaline phosphatase contributing to such invasion.[45–47]

## Histopathologic studies of placentas from infected or uninfected neonates

In placentas of severe and mortal cases of congenital Chagas disease (abortions, still-births, or premature newborns dead in the neonatal period; rarely observed today), a severe placentitis/villitis occurs with large areas of trophoblast destruction and necrosis. Amastigote parasites are found in villous trophoblast and stromal cells.[48,49] Immunohistochemical studies show important inflammatory responses in such placentas, with infiltrates mainly composed of CD68[+] macrophages, CD8[+] T lymphocytes, and few natural killer (NK) cells, and an intense production of TNF-α.[50]

In placentas of live neonates suffering mild congenital *T. cruzi* infection (frequent today), villitis is much less marked or not observed (despite some degree of reorganization of extracellular matrix). Parasites are not, or hardly, identified in villous and extravillous trophoblast. Necrosis and lysis associated with infiltration of neutrophils and lymphocytes are more frequently detected in chorionic plate and membranes surrounding the fetus (chorioamnionitis) and umbilical cord (funisitis).[28,50,51] In serial biopsies performed in 19 placentas from infected live Bolivian newborns, we observed an unexpected high density of parasites at the level of marginal zone, joining the membranes to the chorionic and basal plates, with gradually decreasing densities in the chorionic plate and distant membranes.[1,22]

Histopathology of placentas of uninfected neonates born to infected mothers is similar to that of control newborns of uninfected mothers (or display slight inflammation without lymphocyte infiltration).[17,28]

## Interpretation attempt of Trypanosoma cruzi–placenta interactions

Based on the observations mentioned above, we can depict four scenarios of interactions between the parasite and the placenta, considering the importance of placental lesions and the occurrence of transmission (Fig. 23.1).

1. The huge parasite load in the intervillous space overflows the placental defenses, leading to infection and rupture of the trophoblastic barrier. This results in the transmission of large quantities of free trypomastigotes as well as of amastigote-infected cells, and to severe and mortal congenital Chagas disease. In such a situation, the placental inflammation (placentitis) is strongly marked and has pathological instead of protective effects,

with the substantial release of TNF-α contributing to the trophoblast rupture, as well as to fetal and neonatal mortality.[52] The high local production of other inflammatory mediators, such as reactive oxygen species, NO and peroxynitrite, has deleterious effects on placental vascularization.[53] This is probably what occurs in acute or reactivated infection during pregnancy displaying the highest parasitemias (see section: Parasitic load during pregnancy and transmission of congenital infection).

2. In the presence of moderate parasite amounts in the intervillous space, the placental innate defenses are only slightly activated. Indeed, *T. cruzi*, being partially deficient in strong PAMPs,[54] can hardly stimulate the TLRs expressed on the trophoblast.[40] This does not induce the rupture of the trophoblastic barrier and transmission can occur by the marginal zone deprived of trophoblast (see section: Histopathologic studies of placentas from infected or uninfected neonates[41]). Parasites invade cells of this zone, and those surviving the mesenchymal defense (second placental line of defense) can easily spread by successive infections of fibroblasts, myofibroblasts, and macrophages (Hofbauer cells) within the chorion. They finally infect myocytes and endothelial cells lining fetal vessels embedded in chorionic plate or umbilical cord, and gain access to the fetal circulation.[1,22] This situation likely corresponds to the common mild congenital *T. cruzi* infections observed in roughly 5% of live newborns of chronically infected women (see section: Situation in Latin American endemic countries). Additionally, the infection spreads in membranes surrounding the fetus, inducing their embrittlement. This leads to their premature rupture and contribute to the premature birth, frequently observed in these cases.[55]

3. Parasite transmission (of trypomastigotes as well as amastigote-infected cells) occurs at delivery, when placental breaches/tears appear naturally with labor contractions. This route, which can be avoided by cesarean delivery (see section: Timing of maternal—fetal transmission of *Trypanosoma cruzi*) is used for transmission of HIV-infected leukocytes.[56] It is independent of the activation of placental innate defenses.

4. There is neither parasite transmission, nor disruption of the trophoblastic barrier, nor inflammation; placental innate defenses are not activated by the too low blood parasite amount; this might concern the 95% of chronically infected pregnant women displaying weak parasitemias (see section: Parasitic load during pregnancy and transmission of congenital infection) and delivering uninfected newborns.

A placental microbiome has been recently discovered.[57] Its role in the transmission of congenital infection deserves further investigations.

Mutations in the placental genes for the disintegrin and metalloproteinases ADAM12 and MMP2 are associated to the susceptibility to congenital infection with *T. cruzi*.[58] Whether such mutations in placental genes are sufficiently frequent to contribute to transmission remains to be determined.

# Timing of maternal—fetal transmission of *Trypanosoma cruzi*

There is likely little or no transmission of blood trypomastigotes during the first trimester of pregnancy, since the placental intervillous space is not open. Maternal blood supply becomes continuous and diffuse in the entire placenta only after the 12th week of gestation.[59] The absence of developmental malformations in live newborns congenitally infected with *T. cruzi* (see section: Clinical manifestations of congenital Chagas disease) also suggests there is no transmission at the early stages of organogenesis in the embryo.

Abortions, stillbirths, and premature births in *T. cruzi*-infected women are more frequent for gestational ages between 19 and 37 weeks of pregnancy, but the proof of congenital infection as responsible for such pejorative outcomes has not been systematically investigated.[51,60] The rare reported cases of acute *T. cruzi* infection during pregnancy indicate possible transmission around the 20th week of pregnancy.[61] However, in most pregnant women who are in the chronic phase of infection (see section: Epidemiological features specific to congenital infection with *Trypanosoma cruzi*), it is impossible to pinpoint the timing of maternal—fetal transmission of *T. cruzi*. Transmission rates in vaginal and cesarean deliveries of infected women are similar (see Ref. [62], unpublished own data), indicating that most transmissions are prenatal, though possible later additional perinatal transmission during labor cannot be excluded (see section: Interpretation attempt of *Trypanosoma cruzi*—placenta interactions).

# Parasitic factors involved in transplacental transmission and development of *Trypanosoma cruzi* infection in fetuses/newborns

Based on different molecular approaches, *T. cruzi* has been classified into six phylogenetic lineages, so-called "discrete typing units" (DTUs) named TcI to TcVI,[63] though recent studies propose to reconsider such classification into only three reliable mitochondrial clades.[64]

Five *T. cruzi* DTUs (TcI, TcII, TcIII, TcV, and TcVI) and associations of them (coinfections) have been identified in human cases of congenital infection. The DTU TcV has been reported in 80—100% of congenital cases in Argentina, Bolivia, Southern Brazil, Chile, and Paraguay.[65—74] DTUs TcII and TcVI have been reported in neonates from Argentina, Bolivia, Brazil (Bahia state), and Chile,[65,67,71,73,75] whereas TcIII has been identified in Paraguay[76] and TcI in some neonates from Argentina, Chile, and Colombia.[71,72,77]

The distribution of DTUs identified in congenital cases is similar to that found in the local population.[65,67,68] The same DTUs are generally detected in mothers and their infected newborns, as well as in congenitally infected twins or siblings born in consecutive gestations.[66,67] However, when multiclonal infections occur with different DTUs or DTU variants,[65,67,68,70,71,73,74] slight differences can be observed between clones infecting mothers and those found in congenitally infected infants, suggesting that a natural selection of transmitted parasite populations might occur,[67,71,74] perhaps through interactions with placental cells and/or the host immune system (see sections: Interpretation attempt of *Trypanosoma cruzi*—placenta interactions and Immunity in pregnant women and transmission of congenital infection). So, at this time, there is no clear evidence of a relationship between *T. cruzi* DTUs (defined by the currently used molecular markers) and congenital infection in humans.

# Maternal factors involved in transmission and development of *Trypanosoma cruzi* infection

## Parasitic load during pregnancy and transmission of congenital infection

A lot of data has now well established that blood parasite amount during pregnancy is a key factor for congenital transmission. Although parasitemia slightly increases during pregnancy (on second and third trimesters),[78,79] congenital transmission during chronic infection increases with parasitemias and occurs mainly in women displaying around 10−20 p/mL (i.e., 10−20 times higher than in non-transmitting women.[62,66,80−84] Transmission rates are much higher in acute infection (in 6/11−54% of reported cases in acutely infected mothers[17,61]) and reactivated Chagas disease (100%, in case of coinfection with HIV[85,86]), displaying extremely high and huge parasitemias, respectively (Fig. 23.2).

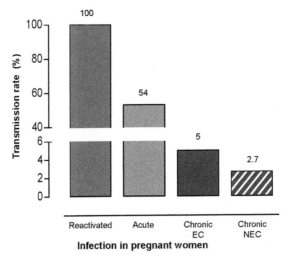

**Figure 23.2 Maternal−fetal transmission rates of *T. cruzi* infection, according to the clinical phase/form of infection in pregnant women.**
*Source*: Reactivated Chagas disease: data according to Freilij H, Altcheh J, Muchinik G. Perinatal human immunodeficiency virus infection and congenital Chagas' disease. Pediatr *Infect Dis* 1995;**14**:161−162 and Scapellato PG, Bottaro EG, Rodriguez-Brieschke MT. Mother-child transmission of Chagas disease: could coinfection with human immunodeficiency virus increase the risk? *Rev Soc Bras Med Trop* 2009;**42**:107−109; acute Chagas disease: data according to Bittencourt AL. Possible risk factors for vertical transmission of Chagas' disease. *Rev Inst Med Trop Sao Paulo* 1992;**34**:403−408 and Moretti E, Basso B, Castro I, Carrizo P, Chaul M, Barbieri G, et al. Chagas' disease: study of congenital transmission in cases of acute maternal infection. *Rev Soc Bras Med Trop* 2005;**38**:53−55; chronic Chagas disease: average transmission rates in endemic and nonendemic countries (EC and NEC, respectively) according to Howard EJ, Xiong X, Carlier Y, Sosa-Estani S, Buekens P. Frequency of the congenital transmission of Trypanosoma cruzi: a systematic review and meta-analysis. *Brit J Obst Gyn* 2014;**121**:22−33.

## Immunity in pregnant women and transmission of congenital infection

Maternal immunity is likely a factor limiting transmission of infections in fetus/ neonate. *T. cruzi*-specific IgG antibodies play a protective role by favoring the clearance of circulating parasites through activated phagocytes expressing FcR, likewise contributing to limiting parasitemia (reviewed in Chapter 25, Protective host response to *Trypanosoma cruzi* and its limitations).

Analyses of innate immune defences in pregnant women by us and others show that monocytes from transmitting women display a less activated phenotype and release less TNF-α as compared to non-transmitting subjects.[80,87,88] Conversely, we also showed that blood cells from non-transmitting women produce higher levels of TNF-α, IL-1β, and IL-6 in response to *T. cruzi* or LPS/PHA than uninfected controls.[89]

As expected, infected pregnant women display an adaptive response to parasites with higher blood cell production and circulating levels of IFN-γ than in non-infected ones.[80,89,90] However, T cells from those transmitting *T. cruzi* to their fetuses produce three times less IFN-γ than cells from non-transmitting women (Fig. 23.3), which probably contributes to increase their parasitemia[80] (see section: Parasitic load during pregnancy and transmission of congenital infection).

Altogether, and as schematically shown in Fig. 23.4, such results indicate that (1) a strong innate immune response is associated with the absence of congenital transmission (in non-transmitting women); (2) women transmitting congenital infection present

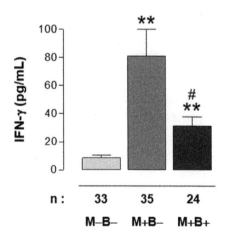

**Figure 23.3 IFN-γ production by whole blood cells of mothers either noninfected (M−) or infected (M+) having delivered infected neonates (B+) or uninfected newborns (B−).** Cells were stimulated with *T. cruzi* lysate for 24 h; IFN-γ levels were determined in supernatants of whole blood cells by ELISA; results are expressed as arithmetic means ± SEM; **$p < 0.01$ versus M−B−; #$p < 0.05$ M+B+ versus M + B−. *Source*: Data from Hermann E, Truyens C, Alonso-Vega C, Rodriguez P, Berthe A, Torrico F, et al. Congenital transmission of *Trypanosoma cruzi* is associated with maternal enhanced parasitemia and decreased production of interferon-gamma in response to parasite antigens. *J Infect Dis* 2004;**189**:1274−81.

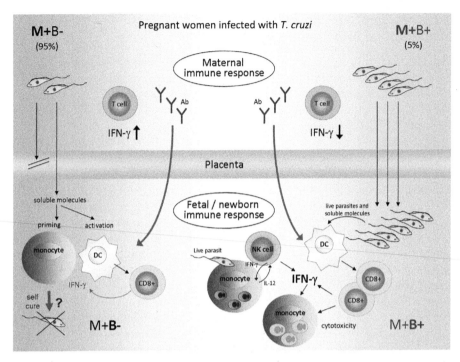

**Figure 23.4 Schematical view of immune responses in infected pregnant women transmitting (M+B+) or not (M+B−) parasites and their fetuses according to the occurrence (M+B+) or not of congenital infection (M+B−).**

some defect of their innate and adaptive immune responses, and (3) such defect mainly relies on a lower capacity to produce IFN-γ in response to *T. cruzi*.

## *Other maternal factors involved in transmission of congenital infection*

The fact that around 95% of chronically infected pregnant women do not transmit parasites to their fetuses (see section: Situation in Latin American endemic countries) suggests that the physiological immune environment of pregnancy is likely not contributing to the immune defect of transmitting women. The pro-inflammatory environment occurring at different stages of gestation[91] might rather reboost the innate responses during chronic infection to keep infected women away from congenital transmission. However, as observed by our team,[55] but not by others,[62] primiparity (and young age) might be an additional factor contributing to parasite transmission.

Malnutrition and poverty also favor the congenital transmission of *T. cruzi*,[17,55,92,93] probably by worsening the deficiency of immune responses during pregnancy.[94] These factors might play a role in the difference observed between transmission rates in endemic and nonendemic countries (5% vs 2.7%, respectively[6]).

Maternal coinfection with *T. cruzi* and HIV results in increasing frequency and severity of congenital Chagas disease (see section: Pregnancy outcomes, clinical manifestations, and long-term consequences of congenital Chagas disease),[85,86] highlighting the important role of maternal immunity and high parasitemia in favoring parasite transmission to the fetus (see sections: Parasitic load during pregnancy and transmission of congenital infection; Immunity in pregnant women and transmission of congenital infection). Interestingly, in vitro infection of human placenta with *T. cruzi* reduces HIV replication.[95]

The role of maternal genetic factors in favoring parasite transmission remains to be explored. Indeed, the familial clustering of congenital cases (see section: Epidemiological features specific to congenital infection with *Trypanosoma cruzi*),[18,19] as well as the persistence after delivery of the defective capacity of IFN-γ response to parasites in transmitting mothers (see section: Immunity in pregnant women and transmission of congenital infection),[80] suggest that some mothers might display a "transmitter" phenotype.

The diversity of intestinal microbiota and its impact on maternal immune responses has not been studied yet, nor has the role of the mode of delivery in transmitting it to the neonate. A cesarean section instead of a vaginal delivery prevents the transmission of the maternal vaginal and gut microbiota (recognized as essential immune-modulating factors in neonates and infants).[96] Particularly, the gut microbiota induces the production of anti-Gal antibodies which are lytic for *T. cruzi*[97] (reviewed in Chapter 25, Protective host response to *Trypanosoma cruzi* and its limitations).

# Interactions between the maternal and fetal immune systems

## Main biorelevant transferred molecules

Besides transmission of parasites resulting in congenital infection, other biologically relevant elements can be transferred to congenitally infected as well as uninfected fetuses from infected pregnant women.

The transplacental transfer of maternal IgG through the FcRn expressed on trophoblast[98] occurs in Chagas disease as in other infections.[99—102] The levels of *T. cruzi*-specific-antibodies in neonates and their repertoire are similar to those of their mothers,[100] indicating that the mild and focused placentitis often observed in chronically infected pregnant women (see sections: Histopathologic studies of placentas from infected or uninfected neonates; Interpretation attempt of *Trypanosoma cruzi*—placenta interactions) does not affect their transfer. Such transferred antibodies can persist up to 8—9 months after birth.[103—105]

Parasitic-circulating antigens (excreted and secreted), parasitic-breakdown molecules with pro-inflammatory activity and/or antigen surrogates (such as antibody idiotypes) are likely transferred through the placenta, as suggested in human and experimental infections with *T. cruzi*.[101,106—108]

This is probably also the case for parasitic-breakdown DNA (from dead or live parasites)[109,110] and the recently discovered small RNAs which are secreted by parasites as extracellular vesicles.[111] Indeed, transmission of maternal cells (microchimerism) and circulating cell-free DNA (ccfDNA) to fetuses is known to occur in normal pregnancy and to persist into adulthood.[112—114]

Except for IL-6, contradictory results have been reported on maternal—fetal transfer of cytokines.[115]

## Maternal immunological imprinting/priming of infant immune responses

Besides the direct effects of transferred antibodies, the elements mentioned above (see section: Main biorelevant transferred molecules) can imprint/prime the fetal/neonatal immune system with long-term unexpected consequences (epigenetic effects). They can promote specific immunological memory or, conversely, immune tolerance, increasing resistance or susceptibility to further *T. cruzi* (re)infection, respectively (see section: Fetal/neonatal factors involved in the development of congenital Chagas disease), leading to more or less severe clinical forms of Chagas disease. Moreover, this imprinting in early life can also have consequences for responses toward other infections or vaccinations (reviewed in Refs. [116,117]). Our team showed that uninfected infants from infected mothers displayed stronger type 1 response to BCG (producing IFN-γ) and that congenitally infected infants developed this stronger response to hepatitis B, diphtheria, and tetanus vaccines, as well as enhanced antibody production to hepatitis B vaccine, compared to controls from uninfected mothers.[118] This might be related to an activation of fetal/neonatal dendritic cells (DCs) (induced by soluble parasite-derived molecules transferred from their mother).[119,120]

# Fetal/neonatal factors involved in the development of congenital Chagas disease

## Parasite amounts in newborns and severity of congenital Chagas disease

Parasitemias in congenitally infected newborns depend on: (1) the amount of parasites transmitted from the mothers (see section: Parasitic load during pregnancy and transmission of congenital infection); (2) the capacity of the infecting parasite strain(s) to invade and multiply into cells/tissues (virulence) and/or limit the efficiency of immune responses in fetuses/neonates; (3) the time allowed for parasite multiplication from the transmission time point during pregnancy (see section: Timing of maternal—fetal transmission of *Trypanosoma cruzi*);[72] and, finally (4) the amplitude of the own individual fetal/neonatal innate and/or adaptive immune responses against parasites, modulated according to the maternal imprinting/priming (see section: Maternal immunological imprinting/priming of infant immune responses). Parasitemias in newborns are generally higher than in their mothers and can reach more than 60,000 p/mL at birth (umbilical cord), though, in some cases, parasites are more easily detectable weeks or months after birth[66,72,82,103,121,122] (Fig. 23.5). Indeed, neonatal parasitic loads increase up to 1—3 months after birth, before decreasing as infection enters in the chronic phase.[103] As shown in Fig. 23.6, morbidity and mortality of congenital disease are associated with the highest parasitemias.[122]

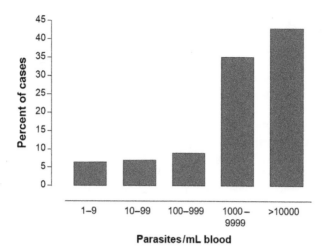

**Figure 23.5 Distribution of parasitemias in Bolivian newborns congenitally infected with *T. cruzi*.** Parasitemias were determined by qPCR.
*Source*: Data from Virreira M, Truyens C, Alonso-Vega C, Brutus L, Jijena J, Torrico F, et al. Comparison of *Trypanosoma cruzi* lineages and levels of parasitic DNA in infected mothers and their newborns. *Am J Trop Med Hyg* 2007;**77**:102−6.

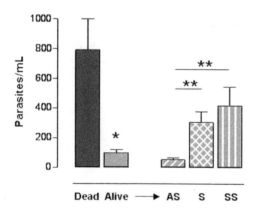

**Figure 23.6 Mean parasitemias, morbidity and mortality at birth in Bolivian newborns congenitally infected with *T. cruzi*.** *AS*, asymptomatic; *S*, symptomatic; *SS*, severe symptoms. Parasitemias were determined by microscopic examination of blood collected in microhematocrit tubes; results are expressed as geometric means; $^*p < 0.05$; $^{**}p < 0.01$.
*Source*: Data from Torrico F, Alonso-Vega C, Suarez E, Rodriguez P, Torrico MC, Dramaix M, et al. Maternal *Trypanosoma cruzi* infection, pregnancy outcome, morbidity, and mortality of congenitally infected and non-infected newborns in Bolivia. *Am J Trop Med Hyg* 2004;**70**:201−9; Torrico MC, Solano M, Guzman JM, Parrado R, Suarez E, Alonzo-Vega C, et al. Estimation of the parasitemia in *Trypanosoma cruzi* human infection: high parasitemias are associated with severe and fatal congenital Chagas disease. *Rev Soc Bras Med Trop* 2005;**38**(Suppl 2):58−61.

## Immune responses in newborns of Trypanosoma cruzi-*infected mothers*

*T. cruzi*-congenitally infected newborns display lower circulating levels of TNF-α, IFN-γ, and IL-18 compared to uninfected neonates of infected mothers,[88,123,124] as well as a decreased proportion of CD56[bright] NK cells (innate immune response).[125] By contrast, we have also shown that such neonates can mount a strong *T. cruzi*-specific T cell response (adaptive immune response) with activated CD8 T cells having cytotoxic activities and producing IFN-γ, but not IL-4.[126] They stimulate also a B cell response producing IgG, IgM, and IgA antibodies.[127−129] However, as shown in Fig. 23.7, the capacity of blood cells (mainly T cells) of congenitally infected neonates to produce IFN-γ in response to *T. cruzi*, is variable from one neonate to another, and inversely related to their parasitemias and the severity of infection (see section: Parasite amounts in newborns and severity of congenital Chagas disease),[2] confirming the key role of IFN-γ in controlling the severity of *T. cruzi* infection (see section: Immunity in pregnant women and transmission of congenital infection), as previously reported in adult subjects.[130]

By contrast, uninfected neonates from infected mothers display an unexpected strong inflammatory status. We and others showed that their blood cells are activated and produce higher levels of IL-1β, IL-6, and TNF-α, in response to *T. cruzi* or LPS/PHA than control uninfected neonates born to uninfected

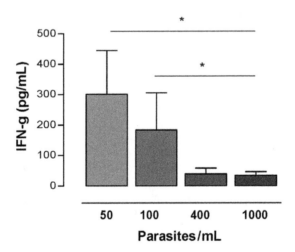

**Figure 23.7 IFN-γ production by whole blood cells of congenitally infected neonates according to their parasitemias at birth.** Cells were stimulated with *T. cruzi* lysate for 24 h; IFN-γ levels were determined in supernatants of whole blood cells by ELISA; results are expressed as arithmetic means ± SEM; *$p < 0.05$; parasitemias were determined by microscopic examination of the buffy coat from blood collected in microhematocrit heparinized tubes. *Source*: According to Carlier Y, Truyens C. Congenital Chagas disease as an ecological model of interactions between *Trypanosoma cruzi* parasites, pregnant women, placenta and fetuses. *Acta Trop* 2015;**151**:103−15.

mothers,[88–90,101] whereas they display no or low degrees of specific T cell activation and responses to *T. cruzi* antigens or surrogates.[101,106,131] However, their B cell responses seem more stimulated with the production of IgA and overall IgM antibodies.[1,101,129] Since live parasites have, apparently, not entered in contact with these fetuses/neonates, such cell activation and responses result from transmission of maternally derived molecules (see section: Interactions between the maternal and fetal immune systems).

Altogether, and as schematically shown in Fig. 23.4, such results indicate that (1) more inflammation (innate immune response) than specific T cell response is observed in uninfected newborns from infected mothers, such status deriving from maternal priming; (2) congenitally infected neonates display weak innate immune responses, but stronger T cell responses, mainly based on CD8[+] T cells with cytotoxic activities and producing IFN-γ (type 1 immune response); (3) such adaptive response seems partially able to control parasitic load, but insufficient, to completely cure the congenital infection; and (4) the cell capacity of congenitally infected neonates to produce IFN-γ determines their parasitic load and the subsequent severity of congenital Chagas disease.

## Interpretation attempt of fetal/neonatal immune responses to Trypanosoma cruzi

Neonatal immunity is usually polarized toward a type 2 environment which appears essential for the survival of the fetus. This, in combination with the hypermethylation of the IFN-γ gene in CD4[+] T cells, limits the development of type 1 immunity in early life.[132] Thwarting such limitation, as in newborns of *T. cruzi*-infected mothers, requires an activation of fetal/neonatal monocytes and DCs. Monocytes produce IL-12 that synergizes with IL-15 to activate in turn NK cell subpopulations releasing IFN-γ.[133,134] DCs trigger T cell proliferation (preferentially CD8[+] T cells) and more IFN-γ release.[119,120] Activation of neonatal DCs can be obtained in the presence of live *T. cruzi* trypomastigotes (as in congenital cases) or, like for monocytes, with soluble molecules released from parasites (e.g., cruzipain, Tc52, HSP70; as in uninfected infants of infected mothers), and antibodies (present in both infant groups; see section: Main biorelevant transferred molecules). The expression of FcR on DC and monocyte membrane can explain the role of antibodies in such activation.

From these observations, it can be postulated that some newborns from *T. cruzi*-infected mothers might naturally auto-cure their congenital infection, either before or at a short time after birth ("unsuccessful" congenital infection in parasitological terms). This could have important consequences both in interpreting neonatal results of laboratory diagnosis, as well as in management of public health control programs related to congenital *T. cruzi* infection (see sections: Laboratory diagnosis of congenital infection with *Trypanosoma cruzi*; Prevention and control of congenital *Trypanosoma cruzi* infection).

## Other fetal/neonatal factors susceptible to interfere with the development of congenital Chagas disease

As discussed for mothers, the familial clustering of congenital *T. cruzi* infections (see section: Epidemiological features specific to congenital infection with *Trypanosoma cruzi*) suggests that some neonates might be predisposed to a lower capacity of immune responses, raising the question of a possible role of fetal/neonatal genetic background (different from the maternal one, since it also derives from the father) and/or environmental factors (e.g., malnutrition, poverty, bacterial gut colonization—see section: Other maternal factors involved in transmission of congenital infection) in the susceptibility and outcome of congenital Chagas disease.

Fetal sex is probably not a risk factor for congenital infection, since most studies report similar frequency in both sexes.[19,55,62,135]

It has been shown that living in areas of high vector density during pregnancy (resulting in multiple re-infections with metacyclic trypomasigotes in a previously established chronic infection) is associated with a serious risk of more severe and mortal congenital Chagas disease.[93,136]

# Vertical transmission of *Trypanosoma cruzi* in other mammals

## Vertical transmission in the natural mammal reservoir of Trypanosoma cruzi

The vertical transmission in mammals involved in the sylvatic cycle of *T. cruzi* (see Chapter 11, Ecological aspects of *Trypanosoma cruzi*: wild hosts and reservoirs) has to be considered as a possible complementary mode, beside vector transmission, of maintaining the parasite reservoir. It does not seem involved in the natural infection of the opossum *Didelphis marsupialis* in endemic areas.[137] Vertical transmission has been observed in some eutherian mammals naturally infected, as dogs, bats,[138–140] and nonhuman primates living in wild conditions or primate centers.[141,142] There is no evidence that chronic maternal *T. cruzi* infection causes fetal loss in nonhuman primates.[143] However, the importance of this vertical mode in the transmission of *T. cruzi* has not been evaluated on a large scale.

## Vertical transmission in experimental infection with Trypanosoma cruzi

Guinea pigs were historically the first mammals to be studied for such transmission,[144,145] and one study documents vertical transmission of *T. cruzi* in dogs.[146]

Experiments in mice show acute infection inducing high rates of fetal resorptions and/or pup mortality, in relation to high blood parasite- and TNF-$\alpha$-levels.[147–150] Indeed, no or rare maternal–fetal transmissions are observed regardless of the time the parasites were inoculated, before or during gestation of mice and rats.[109,147,149,151–160] However, transmission can occur when a blockade of placental phagocytic activity or placental lesions are induced.[161,162] Two works (by the same team) found transmission being associated with the virulent RA (TcVI)- and not with the CA1 or K98 (TcI)-*T. cruzi* strains.[149,159] Other studies reported high percentages of positive PCR (see section: Detection of neonatal infection (0–4 weeks after birth)) in offspring of mice chronically infected with TcI, TcIV, or TcV, but congenital infection (with live parasites) was not demonstrated in such pups.[163,164] A recent work of our team[110] studied congenital transmission from mouse dams acutely or chronically infected with the *T. cruzi* strains X10 (TcI), Y (TcII), and Tulahuen (TcVI). It showed that congenital infection (detected by blood microscopic examination in offspring submitted to cyclophosphamide-induced immunosuppression in order to activate possible cryptic infection) occurred in approximately 4% of living pups born to dams acutely infected with Y or Tulahuen strains, but not with X10 strain and not in those born to chronically infected animals. Interestingly, this study also shows that (1) parasitemias in transmitting dams are higher than in nontransmitting animals (see section: Parasitic load during pregnancy and transmission of congenital infection); (2) re-inoculation of parasites during gestation in chronically infected mice, strongly increases pup mortality (see section: Other fetal/neonatal factors susceptible to interfere with the development of congenital Chagas disease); and (3) PCR detection of parasitic DNA is unrelated to congenital infection (see section: Detection of neonatal infection (0–4 weeks after birth)). Parasites were not found in rat AF[160] and postnatal transmission by murine milk was not observed[37,160,165] (see section: Possible transmission routes of *Trypanosoma cruzi* parasites). Interestingly, a study showed that the administration of the trypanocidal drug benznidazole to pregnant rats is able to cross the placenta and reach the fetus.[166]

So, despite experimental data confirming some bioclinical observations, mice and rats display lower yield of maternal–fetal parasite transmission than humans and do not bring relevant information on the *T. cruzi*-DTU-congenital infection relationship. Although they have hemochorial placentas like humans, their layer architecture (labyrinthine interdigitation into the murine decidua vs. the villous structure of human placenta; see section: The hematogenous transplacental route: strengths and weaknesses of the trophoblastic barrier) and/or their maternal–fetal blood flow interrelations are different, in addition to their shorter duration of gestation.[38] This makes it difficult to extrapolate data obtained from these animals to the maternal–fetal transmission occurring in human and should encourage further studies in nonhuman higher primates.

# Pregnancy outcomes, clinical manifestations, and long-term consequences of congenital Chagas disease

## Trypanosoma cruzi *infection and pregnancy outcomes*

The proportions of abortions and stillbirths in women chronically infected with *T. cruzi* were reported to be either similar[167,168] or slightly higher than in uninfected women.[51,60,169–171] Whether they are due to congenital infection and/or placental dysfunction remains unknown in most cases. However, such records are difficult, and recent and reliable data on abortions or stillbirths in Chagas disease are lacking, which perhaps underestimates rates of maternal—fetal transmission.

Neonatal mortality can occur in untreated severe congenital Chagas disease. We reported mortality rates up to 13% in a Bolivian cohort of congenitally infected newborns studied between 1992 and 1994, while the rate dropped to 2% in another study in 1999—2001, when Bolivia benefited from improved socioeconomic conditions, better maternal care, and extended its vector control programs.[55,93] This latter factor is in line with the role of re-infections in the morbidity and mortality of congenital Chagas disease mentioned in Section, Other fetal/neonatal factors susceptible to interfere with the development of congenital Chagas disease. Neonatal pejorative outcomes are also much higher when acute or reactivated infection (coinfection with HIV) occurs during pregnancy (see sections: Parasitic load during pregnancy and transmission of congenital infection; Other maternal factors involved in transmission of congenital infection).[61,85,86]

## *Clinical manifestations of congenital Chagas disease*

Congenital *T. cruzi* infection, though an acute infection, is frequently asymptomatic at birth, as observed in 40—100% of cases.[55,135,172−177]

Clinical manifestations of congenital Chagas disease can appear within days or weeks after birth, depending on the transplacental transmission time (see section: Timing of maternal—fetal transmission of *Trypanosoma cruzi*). Signs and symptoms that can be observed are non-specific. They are generally similar to those reported in other common congenital infections, due, e.g., to cytomegalovirus and Herpes simplex virus (commonly identified in the acronym TORCH).[178] This and the high frequency of asymptomatic cases highlight the mandatory need for sensitive diagnostic tools to detect such infection close to birth (see section: Laboratory diagnosis of congenital infection with *Trypanosoma cruzi*). *T. cruzi*-infected newborns can exhibit fever, low birth weight (<2500 g), prematurity (gestational age <37 weeks), hepato-splenomegaly, and pneumonitis and more rarely jaundice.[24,49,51,55,62,135,173,175,179−181] The premature rupture of membranes frequently observed in congenital Chagas disease (see section: The hematogenous transplacental route: strengths and weaknesses of the trophoblastic barrier) can result in the birth of premature newborns with immature pulmonary function. Pneumonitis in such cases can be more severe and evolve into respiratory distress syndromes.[55] Growth retardation can be associated with a multisystemic diffusion of parasites in fetus, in addition to being a consequence of placentitis (see section: The hematogenous transplacental route: strengths and weaknesses of the trophoblastic barrier).

More severe clinical manifestations can be also observed in congenital Chagas disease, such as meningoencephalitis (inducing a large range of signs from slight tremors of face or limbs to generalized convulsions) and/or acute myocarditis (resulting in alterations of cardiac rhythm and cardiomegaly),[55,135,179,182−184] particularly in case of maternal coinfection with HIV (see section: Other maternal factors involved in transmission of congenital infection[85,180]).

Purpura and edema (anasarca/fetal hydrops in severe forms) can be also observed.[49,55,185] Anemia and thrombocytopeny have been reported as the main hematological alterations of congenital Chagas disease.[19,49,62,173–175,179,183,185] Megaesophagus or megacolon have been rarely reported in congenital cases.[186–190] Ocular involvement has been also exceptionally mentioned though the possibility of coinfection with *Toxoplasma* has not been eliminated.[179,191] No malformations are detected in such infected newborns.

It is interestingly to note that the oldest clinical reports on congenital Chagas disease from Argentina, Brazil, and Chile indicate the highest morbidity rates, whereas, by contrast, the recent studies in endemic as well as nonendemic countries, more frequently report congenital cases, either asymptomatic or suffering from mild symptoms.

Except in women presenting severe cardiac or digestive forms of Chagas disease before pregnancy,[192,193] gestation generally does not enhance the development of disease in chronically infected women. This allows considering congenital infection and placentitis as being the main short-term consequences of *T. cruzi* infection during pregnancy.

## Long-term consequences of congenital infection with Trypanosoma cruzi

Untreated congenital *T. cruzi* infection, whatever the neonatal morbidity, can develop into chronic chagasic myocardiopathy or digestive megaviscera 25–35 years after birth[194] (see Chapter 28, Clinical phases and forms of Chagas disease). However evolution toward severe cardiopathy seems less frequent than in subjects residing in endemic areas and infected by the vector route.[195] This might be related to the maternal imprinting of the fetal/neonatal immune system (mentioned in section: Maternal immunological imprinting/priming of infant immune responses) which can stimulate the immune responses to *T. cruzi*. Untreated cases with meningoencephalitis can suffer severe neurologic sequelae.[196] The transgenerational transmission of parasites (see section: Epidemiological features specific to congenital infection with *Trypanosoma cruzi*) is also a potential long-term consequence of congenital infection.

## Laboratory diagnosis of congenital infection with Trypanosoma cruzi

The laboratory diagnosis of congenital infection with *T. cruzi* involves, first, the detection of infection in pregnant women, and, second, the confirmation of infection in newborns of positive mothers. Detailed aspects of the laboratory diagnosis of Chagas disease are covered in Chapter 29, Diagnosis of *Trypanosoma cruzi* infection. The present paragraph will focus on the specific aspects of the biological diagnosis of congenital *T. cruzi* infection.

## Detection of infection in pregnant women

Positive results to two standard serological tests detecting *T. cruzi*-specific antibodies (indirect hemaglutination, indirect immunofluorescence, or enzyme-linked immunosorbent assay (ELISA)) are necessary for confirming a latent chronic infection in pregnant women as in other patients.[197] Such tests are commercially available at low cost at primary health care level. They have to be performed as soon as pregnancy has been diagnosed, or, if not possible, at any time during pregnancy, including at the time of delivery, or in umbilical cord blood (detecting transferred maternal antibodies).[102] In case of doubtful or discordant results, the tests can be repeated and a third confirmatory test can also be used, such as the radioimmunoprecipitation assays, immunoblot assays using recombinant antigens, and western blot assays using trypomastigote excreted-secreted antigens (TESA-blot).

Sometimes more rapid and simple tests (such as inmunochromatographic, immunodot, immunofiltration tests) are necessary (e.g., when a pregnant woman enter into the maternity just before delivery without previous serodiagnosis, or at primary health care level in rural endemic areas). Positive results obtained with these screening tests need further confirmation with standard serological tests.[102]

However, sensitivity and specificity of serological assays for the diagnosis of Chagas disease appear to be less than previously thought and discordant results can be observed,[198-201] justifying even more the need of using at least two different tests to ensure an accurate diagnosis in pregnant women. If the test results are negative, there is no possible congenital transmission.

## In utero detection of fetal infection

As mentioned in Section, Possible transmission routes of *Trypanosoma cruzi* parasites, *T. cruzi* DNA is rarely detected in AF and amniocentesis is currently not recommended for the prenatal diagnosis of *T. cruzi* congenital infection.[27]

Fetal blood sampling (cordocentesis to be performed by experienced clinical practitioners) for standard parasitological or molecular testing has been rarely used for the prenatal diagnosis of congenital *T. cruzi* infections.[202]

## Detection of neonatal infection (0–4 weeks after birth)

Blood samples can be collected either at birth, from the umbilical cord (easy to collect without trauma for newborns and mothers) or later in neonates by peripheral venipuncture (from heel, arm, or finger). In case of symptoms suggesting meningoencephalitis, cerebrospinal fluid can also be collected in neonates.

*Parasitological tests*: Live *T. cruzi* trypomastigotes can be detected in blood samples by microscopic examination of buffy coat from centrifuged heparinized microhematocrit tubes. The latter method is rapid, cheap, affordable, one of both currently recommended gold standards, since detecting around 40 p/mL using four to six tubes (more sensitive than the other parasitological methods, such as microscopic examination of fresh blood samples, fixed blood smears, or thick smear) and, overall, because detection of parasites in blood definitively confirms congenital infection.[105] The sample has to be examined within 24 h to avoid a decrease of sensitivity due to parasite lysis. Examination of parasites can be done after cutting the tube.[203,204] However, to avoid possible contamination of the examiner, buffy coat can be also examined in the tube without previous rupture using immersion oil[205,206] or by rotating it.[55,122]

The alternative Strout concentration method (so-called microstrout using Eppendorf tubes),[207,208] as well as indirect parasitological methods, such as hemo-culture (more expensive and needing weeks before obtaining results), can also be used for detecting blood parasites in congenital *T. cruzi* infection.[55,204] All these parasitological methods, which indisputably confirm infection by showing live parasites, need well-skilled personnel and regular quality controls.

*PCR assays*: Molecular tests are able to detect low amounts of *T. cruzi* DNA in blood samples of neonates born to infected mothers.[121,204,209–211] *T. cruzi* PCR proto-cols have been recently compared and efforts have been done to standardize them.[212] Despite of its high sensitivity, PCR does not detect 100% of congenital cases and a negative PCR does not completely exclude a possible congenital infection.

The main question about molecular tests concerns the association between the detection of parasitic DNA and the real presence of live parasites in biological fluids (see section: From maternal–fetal transmission of *Trypanosoma cruzi* to congenital Chagas disease: definitions and limits). As mentioned in section, Main biorelevant transferred molecules, ccfDNA released by *T. cruzi* (dead or live) transferred from mother to uninfected fetuses might be detected by PCR, complicating the interpretation of results, particularly in the case of low inten-sity amplicons susceptible to correspond to trace amounts of parasitic DNA instead of live parasites. So, an early positive PCR is not absolutely indicative of a congenital infection and even less for its treatment (see section: Treatment of congenital infection with *T. cruzi*). It might be considered that blood sampling later after birth might provide more reliable PCR positive results. However, critical information is still lacking on the stability and duration of parasitic DNA in maternal and umbilical cord blood, and ccfTcDNA might be also produced in some fetuses that have naturally auto-cured their congenital infection (see section: Interpretation attempt of fetal/neonatal immune responses to *Trypanosoma cruzi*).

This probably explains the apparent high maternal–fetal transmission rates reported from human studies considering only results of PCR tests close to birth,[204,209,213,214] as well as in experimental infections,[163,164] whereas reports con-firming congenital infection by parasitological or late serological tests display lower rates.[6,110]

Quantitative (real time) PCR that estimates parasite DNA levels, might be useful in completing the results of PCR if protocols are more standardized and a discrimi-nant cut-off value to predict parasite infection is determined.[66,72,82,215,216] New molecular tests targeting exclusively live parasites (e.g., detecting mRNA by reverse transcriptase PCR) or other markers are urgently needed to improve such diagnosis.

*Detection of T. cruzi-specific total IgM and IgA antibodies*: Antibody isotypes not transferred by mothers are not present in all infected newborns and are also detected in uninfected newborns of infected mothers (see section: Immune responses in newborns of *Trypanosoma cruzi*-infected mothers).[1,101,128,129,217,218] Such detection is presently not recommended for the diagnosis of congenital *T. cruzi* infection.

*Detection of IgG/IgM antibodies recognizing Shed Acute Phase Antigen (SAPA)*: A dot-blot assay detecting IgG antibodies recognizing SAPA has been developed in order to diagnose congenital cases, considering such antibodies as being synthesized by acutely infected fetus/neonates and not transferred from mother.[127] However, further studies indicated that the SAPA-specific antibodies are also detected in chronic patients (including around 50% of infected mothers) and could also be transferred.[219]

A TESA blot (see section: Detection of infection in pregnant women) allows detecting IgM antibodies recognizing a band at 130−200 kDa corresponding to SAPA in blood of congenital cases.[220] The specificity of this TESA (SAPA) blot-IgM is close to 100%, but its sensitivity varies according to the studies.[103,220]

*Detection of parasite soluble antigens*: Detection of *T. cruzi* soluble antigens in urine and serum by capture ELISA has been proposed for diagnosis of congenital cases. However, these tests did not detect all infected cases.[221,222] Recently, a new test has been developed using nanoparticles to capture, concentrate (by 100-fold), and preserve such antigens in urine (so-called "Chunap"). The antigens are eluted and detected by Western Blot using a monoclonal antibody against *T. cruzi* lipophosphoglycan.[223] This method remains to be validated at a larger scale for the diagnosis of congenital infection.

*Placental histopathology*: Standard histopathological or immunoenzymatic studies, PCR analyses or in vitro cultures of placental biopsies have been also considered for the diagnosis of congenital *T. cruzi* infection. However, placental parasitism can be either not detected in congenitally infected neonates, or, conversely, observed in uninfected newborns.[22,49,51,70,176,224] So, placental analysis is presently not recommended for the diagnosis of congenital *T. cruzi* infection.

## Infant detection of Trypanosoma cruzi *congenital infection* *(1−12 months after birth)*

If newborns of mothers infected with *T. cruzi* display negative results with the above mentioned tests (mainly parasitological and/or PCR), or if it was not possible to perform such tests, detection of specific antibodies using standard serological assays (as for diagnosis in mothers; see section: Detection of infection in pregnant women) can be carried out in infants when IgG antibodies transferred from the mother have been eliminated. Different studies agree to consider there are no more maternal antibodies 8−9 months after birth.[104,176,225] Such delayed IgG antibody detection is the second currently recommended gold standard method for the diagnosis of congenital infection: a negative serological result indicates the absence of congenital infection, whereas a positive result indicates that the infant is currently infected. The congenital origin of the *T. cruzi* contamination 8 or more months after birth can be established in areas where possibilities of vector or other transmission routes have been ruled out (i.e., in nonendemic areas or in areas previously endemic but having developed vector and blood bank control programs).[176]

Congenital cases might be also detected at 1—3 months of age with an IgG ELISA using recombinant SAPA, since such maternally transmitted antibodies disappear earlier in babies than conventional antibodies.[218,226] By subtracting the maternal ELISA absorbance values of this test from those in the infant samples, it is possible to detect 90% of congenital cases.[227,228] The beneficial advantage of this simple serological method remains to be validated at a larger scale.

## Recommendations

A reliable biological diagnosis of congenital infection is essential to take the decision to initiate a treatment (see section: Treatment of congenital infection with *Trypanosoma cruzi*). So, the criteria defining a "successful" *T. cruzi* congenital infection (to be treated) have to be carefully and clearly specified for public health programs aiming to control such infection (see section: Prevention and control of congenital *Trypanosoma cruzi* infection).[7]

The 2011 conclusions of the WHO technical group on congenital Chagas disease were based on a consensus considering the detection of blood parasites at any time after birth, and/or a positive serology after 8 months of age, as both gold standards for the diagnosis of such infection.[105] An early diagnosis allows a rapid initiation of the treatment and an easier follow-up of the newborns, avoiding their escape from the health system.[229] However, different recent studies have clearly shown a detrimental lack of sensitivity of the parasitological detection.[72,103] Examination of other biological samples of the same neonate week(s) after birth should increase the sensitivity of parasitological detection since neonatal parasitic loads can increase up to 1—3 months after delivery.[72,103,229]

In such a context, what might be the place of PCR for such a diagnosis? Practically, if a PCR is positive in neonates of infected mothers close to birth, it can be considered as alerting the health system to search congenital infection on subsequent samples of these neonates, by using parasitological and/or serological later tests while repeating PCR. This might allow maintaining a more straight contact with the family in order to limit patient escape (see above), and generate a greater efficiency in the management of congenital cases.[230]

# Treatment of congenital infection with *Trypanosoma cruzi*

The treatment of *T. cruzi* infection/Chagas disease is reviewed in detail in Chapter 31, Treatment of Chagas disease. The present paragraph will focus on the pediatric application of such treatment. In order to limit the morbidity and mortality of acute infection and prevent the development of further chronic disease at adult age (see section: Pregnancy outcomes, clinical manifestations, and long-term consequences of congenital Chagas disease), there is a consensus to treat with standard trypanocidal drugs all congenital *T. cruzi* infection detected in newborns or infants, as soon as the diagnosis has been confirmed.[105] Both drugs, benznidazole[55,105,121,175,209,231,232] and nifurtimox,[121,135,175,233,234] can be used to treat congenital cases. Although no comparative and randomized trials have been achieved for congenital infection, it seems that that they have similar curative effects.[121]

The recommended standard doses to be used for both drugs are 10 mg/kg/day (in two to three divided oral subdoses) in neonates and infants till 1 year of age, and 7 mg/kg/day for infants above 1 year, with a 60 day duration of treatment.[105] However, a recent trial using benznidazole at 5 mg/kg in two daily doses for 60 days or at 7.5 mg/kg in a single daily dose for 30 days showed similar efficacy and good tolerance in both regimens, indicating that short treatment should be preferred as it allows reducing its cost.[235]

Such a treatment regimen with doses adapted to increasing body weight is not easy to carry out since pediatric formulations (e.g., liquid formulation) of these drugs remain unavailable. Precautions have to be taken to obtain appropriate dosage since tablets have to be fractionated, crushed, and used as suspension. Full adherence of mothers to scheduled treatment requires a firm relationship between the pediatrician and affected families.[236]

Side effects currently seen in adults (see Chapter 31, Treatment of Chagas disease) are rare, generally mild, and similar in neonates and children treated with benznidazole or nifurtimox.[237,238] The cytogenetic damage and chromosomal aberrations initially reported in chagasic children treated with benznidazole and nifurtimox, respectively,[239] have never been further confirmed. Such low proportion of side effects in neonates efficiently treated with benznidazole is likely related to their lower plasma concentrations of drug (and higher weight-corrected clearance rate) compared to adults.[232]

A negative standard serology is required to confirm cure and this result is generally obtained 3−16 months after the initiation of treatment.[104] The use of PCR/qPCR can help to assess cure (see section: Detection of neonatal infection (0−4 weeks after birth)).[121,209,240] Therapeutic efficacy is around 90−100% in most studies if treatment is applied before 1 year of age.[55,105,121,135,175,176,209]

# Prevention and control of congenital *Trypanosoma cruzi* infection

*Primary prevention* (prophylaxis) of fetal infection with *T. cruzi* aims to prevent infection of pregnant women. This can be obtained by limiting the risk of contamination through vector contacts (see Chapter 10, Control strategies against Triatominae and Chapter 22, Vector transmission: how it works, what transmits, where it occurs) or blood transfusion (see Chapter 24, Other forms of transmission: blood transfusion, organ transplantation, laboratory accidents, oral and sexual transmission). Another strategy which has now clearly shown its efficacy consists of treating infected girls before they enter into their child bearing years[241,242] (see Chapter 31, Treatment of Chagas disease).

*Secondary prophylaxis* would aim to avoid maternal–fetal parasite transmission from a previously infected pregnant woman using trypanocidal safe drugs. However, the potential teratogenic effects of both currently used trypanocidal drugs, benznidazole and nifurtimox, are not known in humans. Moreover, the side effects of both drugs in adults are hardly acceptable during pregnancy and their curative efficacy is limited in the chronic phase of infection presented by most infected pregnant women (see Chapter 31, Treatment of Chagas disease). For all these reasons, the treatment of *T. cruzi* infection during pregnancy is currently not recommended.[105] Moreover, a recent ex vivo study shows benznidazole and nifurtimox unable to impair parasite invasion of human placental chorionic villi explants and nifurtimox displaying toxic effects on such tissue.[243] However, two other recent reports indicate the use of benznidazole during pregnancy to fight acute or reactivated infections, either because pregnancy was not known[244] or the maternal life was threated.[245] Such treatment prevented congenital transmission with no evidence of side effects either in the mother or the baby. Of course, more studies are necessary to validate these in vivo findings.

So, there is presently an international consensus to consider the best control strategy as associating the detection of congenital infection based on laboratory diagnosis (see section: Laboratory diagnosis of congenital infection with *Trypanosoma cruzi*) with the systematic treatment of positive neonates (see section: Treatment of congenital infection with *Trypanosoma cruzi*).[105] The cost/benefit of this control strategy has been evaluated and shown to be much cheaper than the cumulative costs of managing chagasic patients over years.[246,247] Obviously, its benefit remains fully effective if infants are reintegrated in areas where vector transmission has been controlled. Mathematical models have been proposed to estimate the time period it will take to eliminate congenital transmission in regions where vector transmission was reduced to close to zero.[20] Such a control strategy has been applied successfully in different endemic countries.[175,218,231,248,249] This strategy is presently also recommended in some nonendemic countries, but currently only applied in Spain (Catalonia).[250]

Interestingly, the observation of an association between dwelling in areas of high vector density during pregnancy and the severity of congenital Chagas disease (see section: *Trypanosoma cruzi* infection and pregnancy outcomes)[93] suggests that vector control programs in endemic Latin American areas might unexpectedly contribute to limit the mortality and morbidity of a nonvector-borne infection.

Restriction of breast-feeding in infected mothers has no rational base (see section: Possible transmission routes of *Trypanosoma cruzi* parasites). A recent case report and prospective study of lactating women with Chagas disease treated with benznidazole or nifurtimox showed the limited transference of such drugs into breast milk and the normal clinical evolution of the breastfed babies (with no adverse reactions), suggesting that maternal treatment for Chagas disease during breast feeding is unlikely to present a risk for the breastfed infant.[251–253]

Although out of the scope of this chapter, it is important to mention that cord blood from neonates born to infected mothers should not be used for bone marrow transplantation, due to the risk of inducing an acute CD in an immunosuppressed recipient.[254]

# Conclusions

Maternal—fetal transmission of *T. cruzi* can have severe outcomes by compromising survival and/or growth of fetus/neonate, and/or lead to severe clinical forms of chronic infection later in adult life, if infant remains untreated. Congenital *T. cruzi* infection can be found worldwide since such transmission can occur in endemic, as well as nonendemic areas receiving immigrants from endemic regions. Though often asymptomatic at birth and neglected, this congenital infection must be considered as an important public health problem requiring the development of reasonable prevention or control strategies, based on a deep understanding of mechanisms and multiple involved factors. Targeting the group of infected pregnant women at risk of transmission and a reliable diagnosis of neonates displaying a "successful" congenital infection (particularly molecular tests identifying live parasites) are two particularly important points to be improved for a better efficacy of health systems in charge of controlling congenital Chagas disease.

# References

1. Carlier Y, Truyens C. Maternal-fetal transmission of *Trypanosoma cruzi*. In: Telleria J, Tibayrenc M, editors. *American trypanosomiasis-Chagas disease. One hundred years of research*. London, Burlington: Elsevier; 2010. p. 539—81.
2. Carlier Y, Truyens C. Congenital Chagas disease as an ecological model of interactions between *Trypanosoma cruzi* parasites, pregnant women, placenta and fetuses. *Acta Trop* 2015;**151**:103—15.
3. Chagas C. Nova entidade morbida do homen. Resumo geral de estudos etiologicos e clinicos. *Mem Inst Oswaldo Cruz* 1911;**3**:219—75.
4. Dao L. Otros casos de la enfermedad de Chagas en el Estado de Guarico (Venezuela): Formas agudas y crónicas; observación sobre la enfermedad de Chagas congénita. *Rev Policlin (Caracas)* 1949;**17**:17—32.
5. World Health Organization. Chagas disease in Latin America: an epidemiological update based on 2010 estimates. *Wkly Epidemiol Rec* 2015;**90**:33—44.
6. Howard EJ, Xiong X, Carlier Y, Sosa-Estani S, Buekens P. Frequency of the congenital transmission of *Trypanosoma cruzi*: a systematic review and meta-analysis. *Brit J Obst Gyn* 2014;**121**:22—33.
7. Carlier Y, Sosa-Estani S, Luquetti AO, Buekens P. Congenital Chagas disease: an update. *Mem Inst Oswaldo Cruz* 2015;**110**:363—8.
8. Luquetti AO, Tavares SB, Siriano Lda R, Oliveira RA, Campos DE, de Morais CA, et al. Congenital transmission of *Trypanosoma cruzi* in central Brazil. A study of 1,211 individuals born to infected mothers. *Mem Inst Oswaldo Cruz* 2015;**110**:369—76.
9. Pellegrino. Migration from Latin America to Europe: trends and policy challenges. *IOM Migration Res* 2004;**16**.
10. Barona-Vilar C, Giménez-Martí MJ, Fraile T, González-Steinbauer C, Parada C, Gil-Brusola A, et al. Prevalence of *Trypanosoma cruzi* infection in pregnant Latin American women and congenital transmission rate in a non-endemic area: the experience of the Valencian Health Programme (Spain). *Epidemiol Infect* 2012;**140**: 1896—903.

11. Otero S, Sulleiro E, Molina I, Espiau M, Suy A, Martín-Nalda A, et al. Congenital transmission of *Trypanosoma cruzi* in non-endemic areas: evaluation of a screening program in a tertiary care hospital in Barcelona, Spain. *Am J Trop Med Hyg* 2012;**87**:832—6.

12. Pehrson PO, Wahlgren M, Bengtsson E. Intracranial calcifications probably due to congenital Chagas' disease. *Am J Trop Med Hyg* 1982;**31**:449—51.

13. Jackson Y, Myers C, Diana A, Marti HP, Wolff H, Chappuis F, et al. Congenital transmission of Chagas disease in Latin American immigrants in Switzerland. *Emerg Infect Dis* 2009;**15**:601—3.

14. Lazarte RA, Litman-Mazo F, Crewalk AJ, Keim DE, Baram M, Klassen-Fischer MK, et al. Congenital transmission of Chagas disease—Virginia, 2010. *MMWR Morb Mortal Wkly Rep* 2012;**61**:26.

15. Fearon MA, Scalia V, Huang M, Dines I, Ndao M, Lagacé-Wiens P. A case of vertical transmission of Chagas disease contracted via blood transfusion in Canada. *Can J Infect Dis Med Microbiol* 2013;**24**:32—4.

16. Imai K, Maeda T, Sayama Y, Mikita K, Fujikura Y, Misawa K, et al. Mother-to-child transmission of congenital Chagas disease, Japan. *Emerg Infect Dis* 2014;**20**:146—8.

17. Bittencourt AL. Possible risk factors for vertical transmission of Chagas' disease. *Rev Inst Med Trop Sao Paulo* 1992;**34**:403—8.

18. Schenone H, Gaggero M, Sapunar J, Contreras MC, Rojas A. Congenital Chagas disease of second generation in Santiago, Chile. Report of two cases. *Rev Inst Med Trop Sao Paulo* 2001;**43**:231—2.

19. Sanchez NO, Mora MC, Basombrio MA. High prevalence of congenital *Trypanosoma cruzi* infection and family clustering in Salta, Argentina. *Pediatrics* 2005;**115**:e668—72.

20. Raimundo SM, Massad E, Yang HM. Modelling congenital transmission of Chagas' disease. *Biosystems* 2010;**99**:215—22.

21. Carlier Y. Factors and mechanisms involved in the transmission and development of congenital infection with *Trypanosoma cruzi*. *Rev Soc Bras Med Trop* 2005;**38**(Suppl 2):105—7.

22. Fernandez-Aguilar S, Lambot MA, Torrico F, Alonso-Vega C, Cordoba M, Suarez E, et al. Placental lesions in human *Trypanosoma cruzi* infection. *Rev Soc Bras Med Trop* 2005;**38**(Suppl 2):84—6.

23. Bittencourt AL. Anatomo-pathological aspects of the skin in congenital Chagas' disease. *Rev Inst Med Trop Sao Paulo* 1975;**17**:135—9.

24. Bittencourt AL, Rodrigues de Freitas LA, Galvao de Araujo MO, Jacomo K. Pneumonitis in congenital Chagas' disease. A study of ten cases. *Am J Trop Med Hyg* 1981;**30**:38—42.

25. Soto E, Espinoza J, Nien JK, Kusanovic JP, Erez O, Richani K, et al. Human beta-defensin-2: a natural antimicrobial peptide present in amniotic fluid participates in the host response to microbial invasion of the amniotic cavity. *J Matern Fetal Neonatal Med* 2007;**20**:15—22.

26. Nilo M, Alvarado J, Ramirez M, Espejo E. Hallazgo de tripomastigoto en estudio citoquimico de liqido amniotico. *Parasitologia al dia* 2000;**24**:49—51.

27. Virreira M, Martinez S, Alonso-Vega C, Torrico F, Solano M, Torrico MC, et al. Amniotic fluid is not useful for diagnosis of congenital *Trypanosoma cruzi* infection. *Am J Trop Med Hyg* 2006;**75**:1082—4.

28. Moya PR, Villagra L, Risco J. Congenital Chagas disease: anatomopathological findings in the placenta and umbilical cord. *Rev Fac Cienc Med Cordoba* 1979;**37**:21—7.

29. Medina-Lopes MD. Transmission of *Trypanosoma cruzi* in a case, during lactation, in a non-endemic area. *Rev Soc Bras Med Trop* 1988;**21**:151—3.

30. Mazza S, Montana A, Benitez C, Janzi E. Transmision del *Schizotrypanum cruzi* al nino por leche de la madre con enfermedad de Chagas. Pubicaciones Mision de Estudios de Patologia Regional Argentina (MEPRA). *Universidad de Buenos-Aires* 1936;**28**:41–6.

31. Jörg ME. The transmission of *Trypanosoma cruzi* via human milk. *Rev Soc Bras Med Trop* 1992;**25**:83.

32. Bittencourt AL, Sadigursky M, Da Silva AA, Menezes CA, Marianetti MM, Guerra SC, et al. Evaluation of Chagas' disease transmission through breast-feeding. *Mem Inst Oswaldo Cruz* 1988;**83**:37–9.

33. Amato NV, Matsubara L, Campos R, Moreira AA, Pinto PL, Facciol R, et al. *Trypanosoma cruzi* in the milk of women with chronic Chagas disease. *Rev Hosp Clin Fac Med Sao Paulo* 1992;**47**:10–11.

34. Norman FF, López-Vélez R. Chagas disease and breast-feeding. *Emerg Inf Dis* 2013;**19**:1561–6.

35. Hoft DF. Differential mucosal infectivity of different life stages of *Trypanosoma cruzi*. *Am J Trop Med Hyg* 1996;**55**:360–4.

36. Cortez C, Yoshida N, Bahia D, Sobreira TJ. Structural basis of the interaction of a *Trypanosoma cruzi* surface molecule implicated in oral infection with host cells and gastric mucin. *PLoS One* 2012;**7**:e42153.

37. Martins LP, Castanho RE, Nogueira AB, Silva OT, Gusmão AS. Incidence of *Trypanosoma cruzi* transmission through breastfeeding during acute experimental Chagas disease. *Braz J Infect Dis* 2011;**15**:116–18.

38. Benirschke K, Kaufmann P, Baergen R. *Pathology of the human placenta*. New York: Springer Science + Business Media; 2006.

39. Zeldovich VB, Clausen CH, Bradford E, Fletcher DA, Maltepe E, Robbins JR, et al. Placental syncytium forms a biophysical barrier against pathogen invasion. *PLoS Pathog* 2013;**9**:e1003821.

40. Koga K, Izumi G, Mor G, Fujii T, Osuga Y. Toll-like receptors at the maternal-fetal interface in normal pregnancy and pregnancy complications. *Am J Reprod Immunol* 2014;**72**:192–205.

41. Nanaev AK, Kosanke G, Kemp B, Frank HG, Huppertz B, Kaufmann P. The human placenta is encircled by a ring of smooth muscle cells. *Placenta* 2000;**21**:122–5.

42. Frank F, Sartori MJ, Asteggiano C, Lin S, de Fabro SP, Fretes RE. The effect of placental subfractions on *Trypanosoma cruzi*. *Exp Mol Pathol* 2000;**69**:144–51.

43. Díaz-Luján C, Triquell MF, Schijman A, Paglini P, Fretes RE. Differential susceptibility of isolated human trophoblasts to infection by *Trypanosoma cruzi*. *Placenta* 2012;**33**:264–70.

44. Liempi A, Castillo C, Duaso J, Droguett D, Sandoval A, Barahona K, et al. *Trypanosoma cruzi* induces trophoblast differentiation: a potential local antiparasitic mechanism of the human placenta? *Placenta* 2014;**35**:1035–42.

45. Sartori MJ, Lin S, Frank FM, Malchiodi EL, de Fabro SP. Role of placental alkaline phosphatase in the interaction between human placental trophoblast and *Trypanosoma cruzi*. *Exp Mol Pathol* 2002;**72**:84–90.

46. Duaso J, Rojo G, Cabrera G, Galanti N, Bosco C, Maya JD, et al. *Trypanosoma cruzi* induces tissue disorganization and destruction of chorionic villi in an ex vivo infection model of human placenta. *Placenta* 2010;**31**:705–11.

47. Castillo C, Ramírez G, Valck C, Aguilar L, Maldonado I, Rosas C, et al. The interaction of classical complement component C1 with parasite and host calreticulin mediates *Trypanosoma cruzi* infection of human placenta. *PLoS Negl Trop Dis* 2013;**7**:e2376.

48. Bittencourt AL. Chagasic placentitis and congenital transmission of Chagas' disease. *Rev Inst Med Trop Sao Paulo* 1963;**5**:62−7.

49. Bittencourt AL. Congenital Chagas disease. *Am J Dis Child* 1976;**130**:97−103.

50. Altemani AM, Bittencourt AL, Lana AM. Immunohistochemical characterization of the inflammatory infiltrate in placental Chagas disease: a qualitative and quantitative analysis. *Am J Trop Med Hyg* 2000;**62**:319−24.

51. Azogue E, La Fuente C, Darras C. Congenital Chagas' disease in Bolivia: epidemiological aspects and pathological findings. *Trans R Soc Trop Med Hyg* 1985;**79**:176−80.

52. Haider S, Knofler M. Human tumour necrosis factor: physiological and pathological roles in placenta and endometrium. *Placenta* 2009;**30**:111−23.

53. Myatt L, Cui X. Oxidative stress in the placenta. *Histochem Cell Biol* 2004;**122**: 369−82.

54. Kurup SP, Tarleton RL. Perpetual expression of PAMPs necessary for optimal immune control and clearance of a persistent pathogen. *Nat Commun* 2013;**4**:2616.

55. Torrico F, Alonso-Vega C, Suarez E, Rodriguez P, Torrico MC, Dramaix M, et al. Maternal *Trypanosoma cruzi* infection, pregnancy outcome, morbidity, and mortality of congenitally infected and non-infected newborns in Bolivia. *Am J Trop Med Hyg* 2004;**70**:201−9.

56. Biggar RJ, Lee TH, Wen L, Broadhead R, Kumwenda N, Taha TE, et al. The role of transplacental microtransfusions of maternal lymphocytes in HIV transmission to newborns. *AIDS* 2008;**22**:2251−6.

57. Aagaard K, Ma J, Antony KM, Ganu R, Petrosino J, Versalovic J. The placenta harbors a unique microbiome. *Sci Transl Med* 2014;**6**:237ra65.

58. Juiz NA, Cayo NM, Burgos M, Salvo ME, Nasser JR, Búa J, et al. Human polymorphisms in placentally expressed genes and their association with susceptibility to congenital *Trypanosoma cruzi* infection. *J Infect Dis* 2016;**213**:1299−306.

59. Jauniaux E, Gulbis B, Burton GJ. Physiological implications of the materno-fetal oxygen gradient in human early pregnancy. *Reprod Biomed Online* 2003;**7**:250−3.

60. Bittencourt AL, Barbosa HS. Incidence of congenital transmission of Chagas' disease in abortion. *Rev Inst Med Trop Sao Paulo* 1972;**14**:257−9.

61. Moretti E, Basso B, Castro I, Carrizo P, Chaul M, Barbieri G, et al. Chagas' disease: study of congenital transmission in cases of acute maternal infection. *Rev Soc Bras Med Trop* 2005;**38**:53−5.

62. Salas NA, Cot M, Schneider D, Mendoza B, Santalla JA, Postigo J, et al. Risk factors and consequences of congenital Chagas disease in Yacuiba, south Bolivia. *Trop Med Int Health* 2007;**12**:1498−505.

63. Zingales B, Miles MA, Campbell DA, Tibayrenc M, Macedo AM, Teixeira MM, et al. The revised *Trypanosoma cruzi* subspecific nomenclature: rationale, epidemiological relevance and research applications. *Infect Genet Evol* 2012;**12**:240−53.

64. Barnabé C, Mobarec HI, Jurado MR, Cortez JA, Brenière SF. Reconsideration of the seven discrete typing units within the species *Trypanosoma cruzi*, a new proposal of three reliable mitochondrial clades. *Infect Genet Evol* 2016;**39**:176−86.

65. Virreira M, Alonso-Vega C, Solano M, Jijena J, Brutus L, Bustamante Z, et al. Congenital Chagas disease in Bolivia is not associated with DNA polymorphism of *Trypanosoma cruzi*. *Am J Trop Med Hyg* 2006;**75**:871−9.

66. Virreira M, Truyens C, Alonso-Vega C, Brutus L, Jijena J, Torrico F, et al. Comparison of *Trypanosoma cruzi* lineages and levels of parasitic DNA in infected mothers and their newborns. *Am J Trop Med Hyg* 2007;**77**:102−6.

67. Burgos JM, Altcheh J, Bisio M, Duffy T, Valadares HM, Seidenstein ME, et al. Direct molecular profiling of minicircle signatures and lineages of *Trypanosoma cruzi* bloodstream populations causing congenital Chagas disease. *Int J Parasitol* 2007;**37**: 1319−27.

68. Corrales RM, Mora MC, Negrette OS, Diosque P, Lacunza D, Virreira M, et al. Congenital Chagas disease involves *Trypanosoma cruzi* sub-lineage IId in the northwestern province of Salta, Argentina. *Infect Genet Evol* 2009;**9**:278−82.

69. Diez C, Lorenz V, Ortiz S, Gonzalez V, Racca A, Bontempi I, et al. Genotyping of *Trypanosoma cruzi* sublineage in human samples from a North-East Argentina area by hybridization with DNA probes and specific polymerase chain reaction (PCR). *Am J Trop Med Hyg* 2010;**82**:67−73.

70. Bisio M, Seidenstein ME, Burgos JM, Ballering G, Risso M, Pontoriero R, et al. Urbanization of congenital transmission of *Trypanosoma cruzi*: prospective polymerase chain reaction study in pregnancy. *Trans R Soc Trop Med Hyg* 2011;**105**:543−9.

71. Ortiz S, Zulantay I, Solari A, Bisio M, Schijman A, Carlier Y, et al. Presence of *Trypanosoma cruzi* in pregnant women and typing of lineages in congenital cases. *Acta Trop* 2012;**124**:243−6.

72. Bua J, Volta BJ, Perrone AE, Scollo K, Velazquez EB, Ruiz AM, et al. How to improve the early diagnosis of *Trypanosoma cruzi* infection: relationship between validated conventional diagnosis and quantitative DNA amplification in congenitally infected children. *PLoS Negl Trop Dis* 2013;**10**:e2476.

73. Garcia A, Ortiz S, Iribarren C, Bahamonde MI, Solari A. Congenital co-infection with different *Trypanosoma cruzi* lineages. *Parasitol Int* 2014;**63**:138−9.

74. Llewellyn MS, Messenger LA, Luquetti AO, Garcia L, Torrico F, Tavares SB, et al. Deep sequencing of the *Trypanosoma cruzi* GP63 surface proteases reveals diversity and diversifying selection among chronic and congenital Chagas disease patients. *PLoS Negl Trop Dis* 2015;**9**:e0003458.

75. Bittencourt AL, Mota E, Povoa M. Isoenzyme characterization of *Trypanosoma cruzi* from congenital cases of Chagas' disease. *Ann Trop Med Parasitol* 1985;**79**:393−6.

76. del Puerto F, Sanchez Z, Nara E, Meza G, Paredes B, Ferreira E, et al. *Trypanosoma cruzi* lineages detected in congenitally infected infants and *Triatoma infestans* from the same disease-endemic region under entomologic surveillance in Paraguay. *Am J Trop Med Hyg* 2010;**82**:386−90.

77. Pavia PX, Montilla M, Florez C, Herrera G, Ospina JM, Manrique F, et al. The first case of congenital Chagas' disease analyzed by AP-PCR in Colombia. *Biomedica* 2009;**29**:513−22.

78. Brutus L, Ernould JC, Postigo J, Romero M, Schneider D, Santalla JA. Influence of pregnancy on *Trypanosoma cruzi* parasitemia in chronically infected women in a rural Bolivian community. *Am J Trop Med Hyg* 2011;**84**:808−12.

79. Siriano L, da R, Luquetti AO, Boaventura Avelar J, Marra NL, de Castro AM. Chagas disease: increased parasitemia during pregnancy detected by hemoculture. *Am J Trop Med Hyg* 2011;**84**:569−74.

80. Hermann E, Truyens C, Alonso-Vega C, Rodriguez P, Berthe A, Torrico F, et al. Congenital transmission of *Trypanosoma cruzi* is associated with maternal enhanced parasitemia and decreased production of interferon-gamma in response to parasite antigens. *J Infect Dis* 2004;**189**:1274−81.

81. Brutus L, Castillo H, Bernal C, Salas NA, Schneider D, Santalla JA, et al. Detectable *Trypanosoma cruzi* parasitemia during pregnancy and delivery as a risk factor for congenital Chagas disease. *Am J Trop Med Hyg* 2010;**83**:1044−7.

82. Bua J, Volta BJ, Velazquez EB, Ruiz AM, Rissio AM, Cardoni RL. Vertical transmission of *Trypanosoma cruzi* infection: quantification of parasite burden in mothers and their children by parasite DNA amplification. *Trans R Soc Trop Med Hyg* 2012;**106**:623–8.
83. Kaplinski M, Jois M, Galdos-Cardenas G, Rendell VR, Shah V, Do RQ, et al. Sustained domestic vector exposure is associated with increased Chagas cardiomyopathy risk but decreased parasitemia and congenital transmission risk among young women in Bolivia. *Clin Infect Dis* 2015;61918–26.
84. Rendell VR, Gilman RH, Valencia E, Galdos-Cardenas G, Verastegui M, Sanchez L, et al. *Trypanosoma cruzi*-infected pregnant women without vector exposure have higher parasitemia levels: implications for congenital transmission risk. *PLoS One* 2015;**10**: e0119527.
85. Freilij H, Altcheh J, Muchinik G. Perinatal human immunodeficiency virus infection and congenital Chagas' disease. *Pediatr Infect Dis* 1995;**14**:161–2.
86. Scapellato PG, Bottaro EG, Rodriguez-Brieschke MT. Mother-child transmission of Chagas disease: could coinfection with human immunodeficiency virus increase the risk? *Rev Soc Bras Med Trop* 2009;**42**:107–9.
87. Cardoni RL, Garcia MM, De Rissio AM. pro-inflammatory and anti-inflammatory cytokines in pregnant women chronically infected with *Trypanosoma cruzi*. *Acta Trop* 2004;**90**:65–72.
88. Garcia MM, de Rissio AM, Villalonga X, Mengoni E, Cardoni RL. Soluble tumor necrosis factor (TNF) receptors (sTNF-R1 and -R2) in pregnant women chronically infected with *Trypanosoma cruzi* and their children. *Am J Trop Med Hyg* 2008;**78**:499–503.
89. Vekemans J, Truyens C, Torrico F, Solano M, Torrico MC, Rodrigue P, et al. Maternal *Trypanosoma cruzi* infection upregulates capacity of uninfected neonate cells to produce pro- and anti-inflammatory cytokines. *Infect Immun* 2000; **68**:5430–4.
90. Cuna WR, Choque AG, Passera R, Rodriguez C. Pro-inflammatory cytokine production in chagasic mothers and their uninfected newborns. *J Parasitol* 2009;**95**:891–4.
91. Racicot K, Kwon JY, Aldo P, Silasi M, Mor G. Understanding the complexity of the immune system during pregnancy. *Am J Reprod Immunol* 2014;**72**:107–16.
92. Azogue E. Women and congenital Chagas' disease in Santa Cruz, Bolivia: epidemiological and sociocultural aspects. *Soc Sci Med* 1993;**37**:503–11.
93. Torrico F, Alonso-Vega C, Suarez E, Tellez T, Brutus L, Rodriguez P, et al. Are maternal re-infections with *Trypanosoma cruzi* associated with higher morbidity and mortality of congenital Chagas disease?. *Trop Med Int Health* 2006;**11**:628–35.
94. Rytter MJ, Kolte L, Briend A, Friis H, Christensen VB. The immune system in children with malnutrition—a systematic review. *PLoS One* 2014;**9**:e105017.
95. Dolcini GL, Solana ME, Andreani G, Celentano AM, Parodi LM, Donato AM, et al. *Trypanosoma cruzi* (Chagas' disease agent) reduces HIV-1 replication in human placenta. *Retrovirology* 2008;**5**:53.
96. Romano-Keeler J, Weitkamp JH. Maternal influences on fetal microbial colonization and immune development. *Pediatr Res* 2015;**77**:189–95.
97. Galili U. Anti-Gal: an abundant human natural antibody of multiple pathogeneses and clinical benefits. *Immunology* 2013;**140**:1–11.
98. Simister NE. Placental transport of immunoglobulin G. *Vaccine* 2003;**21**:3365–9.
99. Miles MA, Castro C, Macedo V, Draper CC. Letter: *Trypanosoma cruzi*—prenatal transfer of maternal antibody in man. *Trans R Soc Trop Med Hyg* 1975;**69**:286.

100. Breniere SF, Bailly M, Carrasco R, Carlier Y. Transmission transplacentaire des anticorps anti-*Trypanosoma cruzi*. *Cah ORSTOM Ser Ent Med et Parasitol* 1983;**21**: 139−40.

101. Truyens C, Hermann E, Alonso-Vega C, Rodriguez P, Vekemans J, Torrico F, et al. Immune responses of non-infected neonates of mothers infected with *Trypanosoma cruzi*. *Rev Soc Bras Med Trop* 2005;**38**(Suppl 2):96−100.

102. Sosa-Estani S, Gamboa-Leon MR, Cid-Lemus J, Althabe F, Alger J, Almendares O, et al. Use of a rapid test on umbilical cord blood to screen for *Trypanosoma cruzi* infection in pregnant women in Argentina, Bolivia, Honduras, and Mexico. *Am J Trop Med Hyg* 2008;**79**:755−9.

103. Bern C, Verastegui M, Gilman RH, Lafuente C, Galdos-Cardenas G, Calderon M, et al. Congenital *Trypanosoma cruzi* transmission in Santa Cruz, Bolivia. *Clin Infect Dis* 2009;**49**:1667−74.

104. Chippaux JP, Clavijo AN, Santalla JA, Postigo JR, Schneider D, Brutus L. Antibody drop in newborns congenitally infected by *Trypanosoma cruzi* treated with benznidazole. *Trop Med Int Health* 2010;**15**:87−93.

105. Carlier Y, Torrico F, Sosa-Estani S, Russomando G, Luquetti L, Freilij H, et al. Congenital Chagas disease: recommendations for diagnosis, treatment and control of newborns, siblings and pregnant women. *PLoS Negl Trop Dis* 2011;**5**:e1250.

106. Neves SF, Eloi-Santos S, Ramos R, Rigueirinho S, Gazzinelli G, Correa-Oliveira R. In utero sensitization in Chagas' disease leads to altered lymphocyte phenotypic patterns in the newborn cord blood mononuclear cells. *Parasite Immunol* 1999;**21**:631−9.

107. Rivera MT, Marques de Araujo S, Lucas R, Deman J, Truyens C, Defresne MP, et al. High tumor necrosis factor alpha (TNF-alpha) production in *Trypanosoma cruzi*-infected pregnant mice and increased TNF-alpha gene transcription in their offspring. *Infect Immun* 1995;**63**:591−5.

108. Didoli GL, Davila HO, Feldman S, di Masso R, Revelli SS, Bottasso OA. Protected *Trypanosoma cruzi* infection in rats born to mothers receiving interferon-gamma during gestation is associated with a decreased intramacrophage parasite growth and preferential synthesis of specific IgG2b antibodies. *Int J Immunopharmacol* 2000;**22**:45−55.

109. Alarcón M, Pérez MC, Villarreal J, Araujo S, Goncalves L, González A, et al. Detection of *Trypanosoma cruzi* DNA in the placenta and fetuses of mice with Chagasic acute infection. *Invest Clin* 2009;**50**:335−45.

110. Cencig S, Coltel N, Truyens C, Carlier Y. Fertility, gestation outcome and parasite congenital transmissibility in mice infected with TcI, TcII and TcVI genotypes of *Trypanosoma cruzi*. *PLoS Negl Trop Dis* 2013;**7**:e2271.

111. Garcia-Silva MR, Cabrera-Cabrera F, das Neves RF, Souto-Padrón T, de Souza W, Cayota A. Gene expression changes induced by *Trypanosoma cruzi* shed microvesicles in mammalian host cells: relevance of tRNA-derived halves. *Biomed Res Int* 2014;**2014**:305239.

112. Maloney S, Smith A, Furst DE, Myerson D, Rupert K, Evans PC, et al. Microchimerism of maternal origin persists into adult life. *J Clin Invest* 1999;**104**:41−7.

113. Jonsson AM, Uzunel M, Götherström C, Papadogiannakis N, Westgren M. Maternal microchimerism in human fetal tissues. *Am J Obstet Gynecol* 2008;**198**:325.e1−6.

114. AbdelHalim RM, Ramadan DI, Zeyada R, Nasr AS, Mandour IA. Circulating maternal total cell-free DNA, cell-free fetal DNA and soluble endoglin levels in preeclampsia: predictors of adverse fetal outcome? A cohort study. *Mol Diagn Ther* 2016;**2**:135−49.

115. Jonakait GM. The effects of maternal inflammation on neuronal development: possible mechanisms. *Int J Dev Neurosci* 2007;**25**:415—25.

116. Carlier Y, Truyens C. Influence of maternal infection on offspring resistance towards parasites. *Parasitol Today* 1995;**11**:94—9.

117. Dauby N, Goetghebuer T, Kollmann TR, Levy J, Marchant A. Uninfected but not unaffected: chronic maternal infections during pregnancy, fetal immunity, and susceptibility to postnatal infections. *Lancet Infect Dis* 2012;**12**:330—40.

118. Dauby N, Alonso-Vega C, Suarez E, Flores A, Hermann E, Cordova M, et al. Maternal infection with *Trypanosoma cruzi* and congenital Chagas disease induce a trend to a type 1 polarization of infant immune responses to vaccines. *PLoS Neg Trop Dis* 2009;**3**:e571.

119. Rodriguez P, Carlier Y, Truyens C. Activation of cord blood myeloid dendritic cells by *Trypanosoma cruzi* and parasite-specific antibodies, proliferation of CD8+ T cells, and production of IFN-γ. *Med Microbiol Immunol* 2012;**201**:157—69.

120. Rodriguez P, Carlier Y, Truyens C. *Trypanosoma cruzi* activates cord blood myeloid dendritic cells independently of cell infection. *Med Microbiol Immunol* 2012;**201**:287—96.

121. Schijman AG, Altcheh J, Burgos JM, Biancardi M, Bisio M, Levin MJ, et al. Aetiological treatment of congenital Chagas' disease diagnosed and monitored by the polymerase chain reaction. *J Antimicrob Chemother* 2003;**52**:441—9.

122. Torrico MC, Solano M, Guzman JM, Parrado R, Suarez E, Alonzo-Vega C, et al. Estimation of the parasitemia in *Trypanosoma cruzi* human infection: high parasitemias are associated with severe and fatal congenital Chagas disease. *Rev Soc Bras Med Trop* 2005;**38**(Suppl 2):58—61.

123. Mayer JP, Biancardi M, Altcheh J, Freilij H, Weinke T, Liesenfeld O. Congenital infections with *Trypanosoma cruzi* or *Toxoplasma gondii* are associated with decreased serum concentrations of interferon-gamma and interleukin-18 but increased concentrations of interleukin-10. *Ann Trop Med Parasitol* 2010;**104**:485—92.

124. Fernández-Villegas A, Thomas MC, Carrilero B, Téllez C, Marañón C, Murcia L, et al. The innate immune response status correlates with a divergent clinical course in congenital Chagas disease of twins born in a non-endemic country. *Acta Trop* 2014;**140**:84—90.

125. Hermann E, Alonso-Vega C, Berthe A, Truyens C, Flores A, Cordova M, et al. Human congenital infection with *Trypanosoma cruzi* induces phenotypic and functional modifications of cord blood NK cells. *Pediatr Res* 2006;**60**:38—43.

126. Hermann E, Truyens C, Alonso-Vega C, Even J, Rodriguez P, Berthe A, et al. Human fetuses are able to mount an adultlike CD8T-cell response. *Blood* 2002;**100**:2153—8.

127. Reyes MB, Lorca M, Munoz P, Frasch AC. Fetal IgG specificities against *Trypanosoma cruzi* antigens in infected newborns. *Proc Natl Acad Sci USA* 1990;**87**:2846—50.

128. Di Pentima MC, Edwards M. Enzyme-linked immunosorbent assay for IgA antibodies to *Trypanosoma cruzi* in congenital infection. *Am J Trop Med Hyg* 1999;**60**:211—14.

129. Rodriguez P, Truyens C, Alonso-Vega C, Flores A, Cordova M, Suarez E, et al. Serum levels of IgM and IgA antibodies to anti-*Trypanosoma cruzi* in samples of blood from newborns from mothers with positive serology for Chagas disease. *Rev Soc Bras Med Trop* 2005;**38**(Suppl 2):62—4.

130. Laucella SA, Postan M, Martin D, Hubby Fralish B, Albareda MC, Alvarez MG, et al. Frequency of interferon-gamma-producing T cells specific for *Trypanosoma cruzi*

inversely correlates with disease severity in chronic human Chagas disease. *J Infect Dis* 2004;**189**:909−18.

131. Eloi-Santos SM, Novato-Silva E, Maselli VM, Gazzinelli G, Colley DG, Correa-Oliveira R. Idiotypic sensitization in utero of children born to mothers with schistosomiasis or Chagas' disease. *J Clin Invest* 1989;**84**:1028−31.

132. Prabhudas M, Adkins B, Gans H, King C, Levy O, Ramilo O, et al. Challenges in infant immunity: implications for responses to infection and vaccines. *Nat Immunol* 2011;**12**:189−94.

133. Guilmot A, Bosse J, Carlier Y, Truyens C. Monocytes play an IL-12-dependent crucial role in driving cord blood NK cells to produce IFN-g in response to *Trypanosoma cruzi*. *PLoS Negl Trop Dis* 2013;**7**:e2291.

134. Guilmot A, Carlier Y, Truyens C. Differential IFN-γ production by adult and neonatal blood CD56+ natural killer (NK) and NK-like-T cells in response to *Trypanosoma cruzi* and IL-15. *Parasite Immunol* 2014;**36**:43−52.

135. Freilij H, Altcheh J. Congenital Chagas' disease: diagnostic and clinical aspects. *Clin Infect Dis* 1995;**21**:551−5.

136. Brutus L, Schneider D, Postigo J, Romero M, Santalla J, Chippaux JP. Congenital Chagas disease: diagnostic and clinical aspects in an area without vectorial transmission, Bermejo, Bolivia. *Acta Trop* 2008;**106**:195−9.

137. Jansen AM, Madeira FB, Deane MP. *Trypanosoma cruzi* infection in the opossum *Didelphis marsupialis*: absence of neonatal transmission and protection by maternal antibodies in experimental infections. *Mem Inst Oswaldo Cruz* 1994;**89**:41−5.

138. Villela EA. A transmissao intra-uterina da moléstia de Chagas. Encefalite congênita pelo *Trypanosoma cruzi* (Nota prévia). *Folia Méd* 1923;**4**:41−3.

139. Barr SC, Van Beek O, Carlisle-Nowak MS, Lopez JW, Kirchhoff LV, Allison N, et al. *Trypanosoma cruzi* infection in Walker hounds from Virginia. *Am J Vet Res* 1995;**56**:1037−44.

140. Añez N, Crisante G, Soriano PJ. *Trypanosoma cruzi* congenital transmission in wild bats. *Acta Trop* 2009;**109**:78−80.

141. Dorn PL, Daigle ME, Combe CL, Tate AH, Stevens L, Phillippi-Falkenstein KM. Low prevalence of Chagas parasite infection in a nonhuman primate colony in Louisiana. *J Am Assoc Lab Anim Sci* 2012;**51**:443−7.

142. Minuzzi-Souza TT, Nitz N, Knox MB, Reis F, Hagström L, Cuba CA, et al. Vector-borne transmission of Trypanosoma cruzi among captive Neotropical primates in a Brazilian zoo. *Parasit Vectors* 2016;**9**:39.

143. Grieves JL, Hubbard GB, Williams JT, Vandeberg JL, Dick Jr EJ, Lopez-Alvarenga JC, et al. *Trypanosoma cruzi* in non-human primates with a history of stillbirths: a retrospective study (*Papio hamadryas* spp.) and case report (*Macaca fascicularis*). *J Med Primatol* 2008;**37**:318−28.

144. Mayer M, Rocha-Lima H. Zum verhalten von *Schizotrypanum cruzi* in warm blutern und arthropoden. *Arch FU Schiffs-u Tropenhyg* 1914;**18**:257−92.

145. Nattan-Larrier L. Hérédité des infections expérimentales à *Schizotrypanum cruzi*. *Bull Soc Pathol Exot* 1921;**14**:232−8.

146. Rodríguez-Morales O, Ballinas-Verdugo MA, Alejandre-Aguilar R, Reyes PA, Arce-Fonseca M. *Trypanosoma cruzi* connatal transmission in dogs with Chagas disease: experimental case report. *Vector Borne Zoonotic Dis* 2011;**11**:1365−70.

147. Mjihdi A, Lambot MA, Stewart IJ, Detournay O, Noel JC, Carlier Y, et al. Acute *Trypanosoma cruzi* infection in mouse induces infertility or placental parasite invasion

and ischemic necrosis associated with massive fetal loss. *Am J Pathol* 2002;**161**: 673–80.

148. Mjihdi A, Truyens C, Detournay O, Carlier Y. Systemic and placental productions of tumor necrosis factor contribute to induce fetal mortality in mice acutely infected with *Trypanosoma cruzi*. *Exp Parasitol* 2004;**107**:58–64.

149. Solana ME, Celentano AM, Tekiel V, Jones M, Gonzalez Cappa SM. *Trypanosoma cruzi*: effect of parasite subpopulation on murine pregnancy outcome. *J Parasitol* 2002; **88**:102–6.

150. Solana ME, Alba Soto CD, Fernandez MC, Poncini CV, Postan M, Gonzalez Cappa SM. Reduction of parasite levels in blood improves pregnancy outcome during experimental *Trypanosoma cruzi* infection. *Parasitology* 2009;**136**:627–39.

151. Apt W, Naquira C, Strozzi L. Congenital transmission of trypanosomiasis cruzi. III. In mice with acute and chronic infection. *Bol Chil Parasitol* 1968;**23**:15–19.

152. Apt W, Naquira C, Tejada A, Strozzi L. Congenital transmission of *Trypanosoma cruzi*. II. In rats with acute and chronic infections. *Bol Chil Parasitol* 1968;**23**:9–15.

153. Werner H, Egger I. Congenital chagas—influence of *Trypanosoma cruzi* infection on embryonic development in pregnant mice. *Z Tropenmed Parasitol* 1971;**22**:224–34.

154. Cabeza MP, Chambo GJ, Laguens RP. Congenital disease secondary to the chronic infection of mice with *Trypanosoma cruzi*. Experimental model of congenital Chagas disease. *Medicina (B Aires)* 1980;**40**(Suppl 1):40–4.

155. de Cunio RW, Olmos JA, de Mercau TN, Blanca RL, de Marteau DF, Ontivero MI, et al. Experimental congenital Chagas-Mazza disease. *Medicina (B Aires)* 1980;**40** (Suppl 1):50–5.

156. Andrade S. The influence of the strain of Trypanosoma cruzi in placental infections in mice. *Trans R Soc Trop Med Hyg* 1982;**76**:123–8.

157. Carlier Y, Rivera MT, Truyens C, Puissant F, Milaire J. Interactions between chronic murine Trypanosoma cruzi infection and pregnancy: fetal growth retardation. *Am J Trop Med Hyg* 1987;**37**:534–40.

158. Davila HO, Revelli SS, Moreno HS, Valenti JL, Musso OC, Poli HO, et al. Infection with *Trypanosoma cruzi* during pregnancy in rats and a decrease in chronic myocardial lesions in their infected offspring. *Am J Trop Med Hyg* 1994;**50**:506–11.

159. Gonzalez Cappa SM, Mirkin GA, Solana ME, Tekiel VS. *Trypanosoma cruzi* pathology. Strain dependent? *Medicina (B Aires)* 1999;**59**(Suppl 2):69–74.

160. Moreno EA, Rivera IM, Moreno SC, Alarcon ME, Lugo-Yarbuh A. Vertical transmission of *Trypanosoma cruzi* in Wistar rats during the acute phase of infection. *Invest Clin* 2003;**44**:241–54.

161. Werner H, Kunert H. Causes of congenital Protozoa infection. *Z Tropenmed Parasitol* 1958;**9**:17–27.

162. Delgado MA, Santos-Buch CA. Transplacental transmission and fetal parasitosis of *Trypanosoma cruzi* in outbred white Swiss mice. *Am J Trop Med Hyg* 1978;**27**: 1108–15.

163. Hall CA, Pierce EM, Wimsatt AN, Hobby-Dolbeer T, Meers JB. Virulence and vertical transmission of two genotypically and geographically diverse isolates of *Trypanosoma cruzi* in mice. *J Parasitol* 2010;**96**:371–6.

164. Alkmim-Oliveira SM, Costa-Martins AG, Kappel HB, Correia D, Ramirez LE, Lages-Silva E. *Trypanosoma cruzi* experimental congenital transmission associated with TcV and TcI subpatent maternal parasitemia. *Parasitol Res* 2013;**112**:671–8.

165. Davila HO, Revelli S, Moreno HS, Valenti JL, Musso OC, Poli HO, et al. Attenuated Trypanosoma cruzi infection in young rats nursed on infected mothers undergoing interferon-gamma treatment during pregnancy. *Immunopharmacology* 1997;**37**:1−6.

166. de Toranzo EG, Masana M, Castro JA. Administration of benznidazole, a chemotherapeutic agent against Chagas disease, to pregnant rats. Covalent binding of reactive metabolites to fetal and maternal proteins. *Arch Int Pharmacodyn Ther* 1984;**272**: 17−23.

167. Oliveira FC, Chapadeiro E, Alonso MT, Lopes ER, Pereira FE. Chagas disease and pregnancy. I. Incidence of trypanosomiasis and spontaneous abortion in pregnant women with chronic Chagas disease. *Rev Inst Med Trop Sao Paulo* 1966;**8**:184−5.

168. Teruel JR, Nogueira JL. Fetal losses in a high prevalence area of chronic Chagas' disease. *Rev Inst Med Trop Sao Paulo* 1970;**12**:239−44.

169. Castilho EA, Silva GR. Infecçao chagásica materna e prematuridade. *Rev Inst Med Trop Sao Paulo* 1976;**18**:258−60.

170. Hernandez-Matheson IM, Frankowski RF, Held B. Foeto-maternal morbidity in the presence of antibodies to *Trypanosoma cruzi*. *Trans R Soc Trop Med Hyg* 1983;**77**:405−11.

171. Schenone H, Contreras MC, Borgono JM, Rojas A, Villarroel F. Congenital Chagas' disease in Chile. Longitudinal study of the reproductivity of women with or without Chagas' disease and of some parasitological and clinical parameters of them and their corresponding children. *Bol Chil Parasitol* 1985;**40**:24−9.

172. Streiger M, Fabbro D, del Barco M, Beltramino R, Bovero N. Congenital Chagas disease in the city of Santa Fe. Diagnosis and treatment. *Medicina (B Aires)* 1995; **55**:125−32.

173. Zaidenberg M. Congenital Chagas' disease in the province of Salta, Argentina, from 1980 to 1997. *Rev Soc Bras Med Trop* 1999;**32**:689−95.

174. Contreras S, Fernandez MR, Aguero F, Desse DJ, Orduna T, Martino O. Congenital Chagas-Mazza disease in Salta, Argentina. *Rev Soc Bras Med Trop* 1999;**32**:633−6.

175. Blanco SB, Segura EL, Cura EN, Chuit R, Tulian L, Flores I, et al. Congenital transmission of *Trypanosoma cruzi*: an operational outline for detecting and treating infected infants in north-western Argentina. *Trop Med Int Health* 2000;**5**:293−301.

176. Carlier Y, Torrico F. Congenital infection with *Trypanosoma cruzi*: from mechanisms of transmission to strategies for diagnosis and control. *Rev Soc Bras Med Trop* 2003; **6**:767−71.

177. Munoz J, Portus M, Corachan M, Fumado V, Gascon J. Congenital *Trypanosoma cruzi* infection in a non-endemic area. *Trans R Soc Trop Med Hyg* 2007;**101**:1161−2.

178. Klein JO, Baker C, Remington JS, Wilson C. Current concepts of infections of the fetus and newborn infant. In: Remington JS, Klein JO, Wilson C, Baker C, editors. *Infectious diseases of the fetus and newborn infant*. Philadelphia, PA: Elsevier Saunders; 2006. p. 13−25.

179. Munoz M, Thiermann E, Atias A, Acevedo C. Enfermedad de Chagas congenita sintomatica en recien nacidos y lactantes. *Rev Chil Pediatr* 1992;**63**:196−202.

180. Nisida IV, Amato Neto V, Braz LM, Duarte MI, Umezawa ES. A survey of congenital Chagas' disease, carried out at three health institutions in Sao Paulo City, Brazil. *Rev Inst Med Trop Sao Paulo* 1999;**41**:305−11.

181. Oliveira I, Torrico F, Muñoz J, Gascon J. Congenital transmission of Chagas disease: a clinical approach. *Expert Rev Anti Infect Ther* 2010;**8**:945−56.

182. Rubio M, Allende N, Roman C, Ebensperger I, Moreno L. Involvement of the central nervous system in a case of congenital Chagas' disease. *Bol Chil Parasitol* 1967;**22**: 119−22.

183. Saleme AE, Yanicelli GL, Inigo LA, Valperga SM, Alonso E, Paz d E, et al. Congenital Chagas-Mazza disease in Tucuman. Concerning 8 doubtful and 2 probable cases diagnosed in the Dept. of Pediatrics of the S. M. Institute of Maternity during the period October 1967—September 1968. *Arch Argent Pediatr* 1971;**69**:162—9.

184. Vieira GO, Maguire J, Bittencourt AL, Fontes JA. Congenital Chagas' disease. Report of a case with cerebral palsy. *Rev Inst Med Trop Sao Paulo* 1983;**25**:305—9.

185. Howard J, Rubio M. Congenital Chagas' disease. I. Clinical and epidemiological study of 30 cases. *Bol Chil Parasitol* 1968;**23**:107—12.

186. Rubio M. Esophageal involvement in 2 cases of congenital Chagas' disease. *Bol Chil Parasitol* 1968;**23**:157—63.

187. Bittencourt AL, Vieira GO, Tavares HC, Mota E, Maguire J. Esophageal involvement in congenital Chagas' disease. Report of a case with megaesophagus. *Am J Trop Med Hyg* 1984;**33**:30—3.

188. de Almeida MA, Barbosa HS. Congenital Chagas megacolon. Report of a case. *Rev Soc Bras Med Trop* 1986;**19**:167—9.

189. Atias A. A case of congenital chagasic megaesophagus: evolution until death caused by esophageal neoplasm, at 27 years of age. *Rev Med Chil* 1994;**122**:319—22.

190. Costa-Pinto EA, Almeida EA, Figueiredo D, Bucaretchi F, Hessel G. Chagasic megaesophagus and megacolon diagnosed in childhood and probably caused by vertical transmission. *Rev Inst Med Trop Sao Paulo* 2001;**43**:227—30.

191. Atias A, Morales M, Munoz P, Barria M. Ocular involvement in congenital Chagas' disease. *Rev Chil Pediatr* 1985;**56**:137—41.

192. Sologuren Acha R, Oliveira Rezende M, Guzman Heredia R, Coehlo da Silva A, Santos Rezende E, Oliveira Souza C. Prevalence of cardiac arrhythmias during and after pregnancy in women with Chagas disease without apparent heart disease. *Arq Bras Cardiol* 2002;**79**:5—9.

193. Avila WS, Rossi EG, Ramires JA, Grinberg M, Bortolotto MR, Zugaib M, et al. Pregnancy in patients with heart disease: experience with 1,000 cases. *Clin Cardiol* 2003;**26**:135—42.

194. Carlier Y, Pinto Dias JC, Ostermayer Luquetti A, Hontebeyrie M, Torrico F, Truyens C. Trypanosomiase américaine ou maladie de Chagas. In: *Editions Scientifiques et Médicale. Encycl Med Chir, Maladies infectieuses*, Paris: Elsevier SAS; 2002. p. 21.8-505-A-20.

195. Storino R, Auger S, Caravello O, Urrutia MI, Sanmartino M, Jorg M. Chagasic cardiopathy in endemic area versus sporadically infected patients. *Rev Saude Publica* 2002; **36**:755—8.

196. Howard J. Clinical aspects of congenital Chagas disease. In: Pan American Health Organization Scientific Publications. American trypanosomiasis research. 1975. p. 212—15.

197. World Health Organization. Control of Chagas disease. *World Health Organ Tech Rep* 2002;**905**:1—109.

198. Verani JR, Seitz A, Gilman RH, LaFuente C, Galdos-Cardenas G, Kawai V, et al. Geographic variation in the sensitivity of recombinant antigen-based rapid tests for chronic *Trypanosoma cruzi* infection. *Am J Trop Med Hyg* 2009;**80**:410—15.

199. Gamboa-León R, Gonzalez-Ramirez C, Padilla-Raygoza N, Sosa-Estani S, Caamal-Kantun A, Buekens P, et al. Do commercial serologic tests for *Trypanosoma cruzi* infection detect Mexican strains in women and newborns? *J Parasitol* 2011;**97**: 338—43.

200. Afonso AM, Ebell MH, Tarleton RL. A systematic review of high quality diagnostic tests for Chagas disease. *PLoS Negl Trop Dis* 2012;**6**:e1881.

201. Guzmán-Gómez D, López-Monteon A, de la Soledad Lagunes-Castro M, Álvarez-Martínez C, Hernández-Lutzon MJ, Dumonteil E, et al. Highly discordant serology against *Trypanosoma cruzi* in central Veracruz, Mexico: role of the antigen used for diagnostic. *Parasit Vectors* 2015;**8**:466.

202. Okumura M, Aparecida dos Santos V, Camargo ME, Schultz R, Zugaib M. Prenatal diagnosis of congenital Chagas' disease (American trypanosomiasis). *Prenat Diagn* 2004;**24**:179–81.

203. Freilij H, Muller L, Gonzalez Cappa SM. Direct micromethod for diagnosis of acute and congenital Chagas' disease. *J Clin Microbiol* 1983;**18**:327–30.

204. Mora M, Sanchez NO, Marco D, Barrio A, Ciaccio M, Segura MA, et al. Early diagnosis of congenital *Trypanosoma cruzi* infection using PCR, hemoculture, and capillary concentration, as compared with delayed serology. *J Parasitol* 2005;**91**:1468–73.

205. Woo PT. The haematocrit centrifuge for the detection of trypanosomes in blood. *Can J Zool* 1969;**47**:921–3.

206. La Fuente C, Saucedo E, Urjel R. The use of microhaematocrit tubes for the rapid diagnosis of Chagas disease and malaria. *Trans R Soc Trop Med Hyg* 1984;**78**:278–9.

207. Moya P, Basso B, Moretti E. Congenital Chagas disease in Cordoba, Argentina: epidemiological, clinical, diagnostic, and therapeutic aspects. Experience of 30 years of follow up. *Rev Soc Bras Med Trop* 2005;**38**(Suppl 2):33–40.

208. de Rissio AM, Scollo K, Cardoni RL. Maternal-fetal transmission of *Trypanosoma cruzi* in Argentina. *Medicina (B Aires)* 2009;**69**:529–35.

209. Russomando G, de Tomassone MM, de Guillen I, Acosta N, Vera N, Almiron M, et al. Treatment of congenital Chagas' disease diagnosed and followed up by the polymerase chain reaction. *Am J Trop Med Hyg* 1998;**59**:487–91.

210. Virreira M, Torrico F, Truyens C, Alonso-Vega C, Solano M, Carlier Y, et al. Comparison of polymerase chain reaction methods for reliable and easy detection of congenital *Trypanosoma cruzi* infection. *Am J Trop Med Hyg* 2003;**68**:574–82.

211. Diez CN, Manattini S, Zanuttini JC, Bottasso O, Marcipar I. The value of molecular studies for the diagnosis of congenital Chagas disease in northeastern Argentina. *Am J Trop Med Hyg* 2008;**78**:624–7.

212. Schijman AG, Bisio M, Orellana L, Sued M, Duffy T, Mejia Jaramillo AM, et al. International study to evaluate PCR methods for detection of *Trypanosoma cruzi* DNA in blood samples from Chagas disease patients. *PLoS Negl Trop Dis* 2011;**5**:e931.

213. Diez C, Manattini S, Imaz MS, Zanuttini JC, Marcipart A. PCR (polymerase chain reaction) in neonatal Chagas disease. An alternative for its early diagnosis? *Medicina (B Aires)* 1998;**58**:436–7.

214. Garcia A, Bahamonde M, Verdugo S, Correa J, Pastene C, Solari A, et al. Infeccion transplacentaria por *Trypanosoma cruzi:* situacion en Chile. *Rev Med Chile* 2001;**129**:330–2.

215. Piron M, Fisa R, Casamitjana N, López-Chejade P, Puig L, Vergés M, et al. Development of a real-time PCR assay for *Trypanosoma cruzi* detection in blood samples. *Acta Trop* 2007;**103**:195–200.

216. Duffy T, Cura CI, Ramirez JC, Abate T, Cayo NM, Parrado R, et al. Analytical performance of a multiplex real-time PCR assay using TaqMan probes for quantification of *Trypanosoma cruzi* satellite DNA in blood samples. *PLoS Negl Trop Dis* 2013;**7**:e2000.

217. Lorca M, Veloso C, Munoz P, Bahamonde MI, Garcia A. Diagnostic value of detecting specific IgA and IgM with recombinant *Trypanosoma cruzi* antigens in congenital Chagas' disease. *Am J Trop Med Hyg* 1995;**52**:512–15.

218. Russomando G, Almiron M, Candia N, Franco L, Sanchez Z, de Guillen I, et al. Implementation and evaluation of a locally sustainable system of prenatal diagnosis to detect cases of congenital Chagas disease in endemic areas of Paraguay. *Rev Soc Bras Med Trop* 2005;**38**(Suppl 2):49–54.

219. Breniere SF, Yaksic N, Telleria J, Bosseno MF, Noireau F, Wincker P, et al. Immune response to *Trypanosoma cruzi* shed acute phase antigen in children from an endemic area for Chagas' disease in Bolivia. *Mem Inst Oswaldo Cruz* 1997;**92**:503–7.

220. Umezawa ES, Nascimento MS, Kesper Jr N, Coura JR, Borges-Pereira J, Junqueira AC, et al. Immunoblot assay using excreted-secreted antigens of *Trypanosoma cruzi* in serodiagnosis of congenital, acute, and chronic Chagas' disease. *J Clin Microbiol* 1996;**34**:2143–7.

221. Freilij HL, Corral RS, Katzin AM, Grinstein S. Antigenuria in infants with acute and congenital Chagas' disease. *J Clin Microbiol* 1987;**25**:133–7.

222. Corral RS, Altcheh J, Alexandre SR, Grinstein S, Freilij, Katzin AM. Detection and characterization of antigens in urine of patients with acute, congenital, and chronic Chagas' disease. *J Clin Microbiol* 1996;**34**:1957–62.

223. Castro-Sesquen YE, Gilman RH, Galdos-Cardenas G, Ferrufino L, Sanchez G, Valencia Ayala E, et al. Use of a novel chagas urine nanoparticle test (chunap) for diagnosis of congenital chagas disease. *PLoS Negl Trop Dis* 2014;**8**:e3211.

224. Azogue E, Darras C. Congenital Chagas in Bolivia: comparative study of the effectiveness and cost of diagnostic methods. *Rev Soc Bras Med Trop* 1995;**28**:3943.

225. Moya P, Moretti E, Paolasso R, Basso B, Blanco S, Sanmartino C, et al. Neonatal Chagas disease: laboratory diagnosis during the first year of life. *Medicina (B Aires)* 1989;**49**:595–9.

226. Russomando G, Sánchez Z, Meza G, de Guillen Y. Shed acute-phase antigen protein in an ELISA system for unequivocal diagnosis of congenital Chagas disease. *Expert Rev Mol Diagn* 2010;**10**:705–7.

227. Mallimaci MC, Sosa-Estani S, Russomando G, Sanchez Z, Sijvarger C, Alvarez IM, et al. Early diagnosis of congenital *Trypanosoma cruzi* infection, using shed acute phase antigen, in Ushuaia, Tierra del Fuego, Argentina. *Am J Trop Med Hyg* 2010;**82**: 55–9.

228. Volta BJ, Russomando G, Bustos PL, Scollo K, De Rissio AM, Sánchez Z, et al. Diagnosis of congenital *Trypanosoma cruzi* infection: a serologic test using shed acute phase antigen (SAPA) in mother-child binomial samples. *Acta Trop* 2015;**147**:31–7.

229. de Rissio AM, Riarte AR, García MM, Esteva MI, Quaglino M, Ruiz AM. Congenital *Trypanosoma cruzi* infection. Efficacy of its monitoring in an urban reference health center in a non-endemic area of Argentina. *Am J Trop Med Hyg* 2010;**82**:838–45.

230. Velázquez EB, Rivero R, De Rissio AM, Malagrino N, Esteva MI, Riarte AR, et al. Predictive role of polymerase chain reaction in the early diagnosis of congenital *Trypanosoma cruzi* infection. *Acta Trop* 2014;**137**:195–200.

231. Luquetti AO, Dias J, Prata A. Diagnosis and treatment of congenital infection caused by *Trypanosoma cruzi* in Brazil. *Rev Soc Bras Med Trop* 2005;**38**(Suppl 2):27–8.

232. Altcheh J, Moscatelli G, Mastrantonio G, Moroni S, Giglio N, Marson ME, et al. Population pharmacokinetic study of benznidazole in pediatric Chagas disease suggests efficacy despite lower plasma concentrations than in adults. *PLoS Negl Trop Dis* 2014;**8**:e2907.

233. Moya PR, Paolasso RD, Blanco S, Lapasset M, Sanmartino C, Basso B, et al. Treatment of Chagas' disease with nifurtimox during the first months of life. *Medicina (B Aires)* 1985;**45**:553—8.

234. Altcheh J, Biancardi M, Lapena A, Ballering G, Freilij H. Congenital Chagas disease: experience in the Hospital de Ninos, Ricardo Gutierrez, Buenos Aires, Argentina. *Rev Soc Bras Med Trop* 2005;**38**(Suppl 2):41—5.

235. Chippaux JP, Salas-Clavijo AN, Postigo JR, Schneider D, Santalla JA, Brutus L. Evaluation of compliance to congenital Chagas disease treatment: results of a randomised trial in Bolivia. *Trans R Soc Trop Med Hyg* 2013;**107**:1—7.

236. Suarez E, Alonso-Vega, Torrico F, Cordova M. Integral treatment of congenital Chagas disease: the Bolivian experience. *Rev Soc Bras Med Trop* 2005;**38**(Suppl 2): 21—3.

237. Altcheh J, Moscatelli G, Moroni S, Garcia-Bournissen F, Freilij H. Adverse events after the use of benznidazole in infants and children with Chagas disease. *Pediatrics* 2011;**127**:e212—18.

238. Bianchi F, Cucunubá Z, Guhl F, González NL, Freilij H, Nicholls RS, et al. Follow-up of an asymptomatic Chagas disease population of children after treatment with nifurtimox (Lampit) in a sylvatic endemic transmission area of Colombia. *PLoS Negl Trop Dis* 2015;**9**:e0003465.

239. Castro JA, de Mecca MM, Bartel LC. Toxic side effects of drugs used to treat Chagas' disease (American trypanosomiasis). *Hum Exp Toxicol* 2006;**25**:471—9.

240. Solari A, Ortíz S, Soto A, Arancibia C, Campillay R, Contreras M, et al. Treatment of *Trypanosoma cruzi*-infected children with nifurtimox: a 3 year follow-up by PCR. *J Antimicrob Chemother* 2001;**48**:515—19.

241. Fabbro DL, Danesi E, Olivera V, Codebó MO, Denner S, Heredia C, et al. Trypanocide treatment of women infected with *Trypanosoma cruzi* and its effect on preventing congenital Chagas. *PLoS Negl Trop Dis* 2014;**8**:e3312.

242. Moscatelli G, Moroni S, García-Bournissen F, Ballering G, Bisio M, Freilij H, et al. Prevention of congenital Chagas through treatment of girls and women of childbearing age. *Mem Inst Oswaldo Cruz* 2015;**110**:507—9.

243. Rojo G, Castillo C, Duaso J, Liempi A, Droguett D, Galanti N, et al. Toxic and therapeutic effects of Nifurtimox and Benznidazol on *Trypanosoma cruzi* ex vivo infection of human placental chorionic villi explants. *Acta Trop* 2014;**132**:112—18.

244. Corrêa VR, Barbosa FG, Melo Junior CA, D'Albuquerque e Castro LF, Andrade Junior HF, Nascimento N. Uneventful benznidazole treatment of acute Chagas disease during pregnancy: a case report. *Rev Soc Bras Med Trop* 2014;**47**:397—400.

245. Bisio M, Altcheh J, Lattner J, Moscatelli G, Fink V, Burgos JM, et al. Benznidazole treatment of chagasic encephalitis in pregnant woman with AIDS. *Emerg Infect Dis* 2013;**19**:1490—2.

246. Billot C, Torrico F, Carlier Y. Cost effectiveness study of a control program of congenital Chagas disease in Bolivia. *Rev Soc Bras Med Trop* 2005;**38**(Suppl 2):108—13.

247. Sicuri E, Muñoz J, Pinazo MJ, Posada E, Sanchez J, Alonso PL, et al. Economic evaluation of Chagas disease screening of pregnant Latin American women and of their infants in a non endemic area. *Acta Trop* 2011;**118**:110—17.

248. Torrico F, Alonso Vega C, Billot C, Truyens C, Carlier Y. Relaciones materno-fetales en la infeccion con *T. cruzi* y la implementacion de un programa nacional de deteccion y tratamiento de Chagas congenito en Bolivia. *Enf Emerg* 2007;**9**:9—16.

249. Alonso-Vega C, Billot C, Torrico F. Achievements and challenges upon the implementation of a program for national control of congenital Chagas in Bolivia: results 2004–2009. *PLoS Negl Trop Dis* 2013;**7**:e2304.
250. Soriano-Arandes A, Angheben A, Serre-Delcor N, Treviño-Maruri B, Prat JG, Jackson Y. Control and management of congenital Chagas disease in Europe and other non-endemic countries: current policies and practices. *Trop Med Int Health* 2016;**21**:590–6.
251. Garcia-Bournissen F, Altcheh J, Panchaud A, Ito S. Is use of nifurtimox for the treatment of Chagas disease compatible with breast feeding? A population pharmacokinetics analysis. *Arch Dis Child* 2010;**95**:224–8.
252. García-Bournissen F, Moroni S, Marson ME, Moscatelli G, Mastrantonio G, Bisio M, et al. Limited infant exposure to benznidazole through breast milk during maternal treatment for Chagas disease. *Arch Dis Child* 2015;**100**:90–4.
253. Vela-Bahena LE, Vergara R, Vite L, Ramos C. Postpartum treatment without interrupting breastfeeding in a patient with Chagas disease. *Ginecol Obstet Mex* 2015;**83**:487–93.
254. Forés R, Sanjuán I, Portero F, Ruiz E, Regidor C, López-Vélez R, et al. Chagas disease in a recipient of cord blood transplantation. *Bone Marrow Transplant* 2007;**39**:127–8.

# Other forms of transmission: blood transfusion, organ transplantation, laboratory accidents, oral and sexual transmission

S.F. Brenière[1], E. Waleckx[2] and C. Aznar[3]
[1]Institut de Recherche pour le Développement (IRD), Montpellier, France, [2]Universidad Autónoma de Yucatán, Mérida, Mexico, [3]Université des Antilles et de la Guyane, Cayenne, French Guiana

## Chapter Outline

## Introduction

In addition to vector-borne transmission (see chapter: Vector Transmission: How It Works, What Transmits, Where It Occurs) and maternal—fetal transmission (see chapter: Maternal—Fetal Transmission of *Trypanosoma cruzi*), *Trypanosoma cruzi* may be transmitted by transfusion of infected blood, through organ transplantation from infected donors, during a laboratory accident, or via the oral route. These four

American Trypanosomiasis Chagas Disease. DOI: http://dx.doi.org/10.1016/B978-0-12-801029-7.00025-3

modes of transmission are discussed in this chapter. Other secondary mechanisms of transmission, such as breastfeeding transmission (see chapter: Maternal—Fetal Transmission of *Trypanosoma cruzi*) and sexual transmission are sometimes mentioned, and we have added a short review of the latter.

# Blood transfusion

Due to the persistence of the parasite in the organism, infected individuals may be responsible for parasite transmission by blood donation throughout their life, even when they are asymptomatic carriers and unaware of their infection. Fever is the most common and sometimes the only manifestation of acute Chagas disease following transfusion of infected blood, but in the most severe cases (lymphadenopathy, hepatospleno-megaly, and cardiac arrhythmia), central nervous system involvement may be present.[1]

## *Current situation in endemic countries*

In the past, the risk of transmission of *T. cruzi* during blood transfusion was high in endemic areas because of the lack of controls in blood banks. The first cases of people who acquired the infection by blood transfusion were described in 1952 in Brazil.[2] It was only with the spread of HIV in the 1980s that effective blood control programs were implemented in most Latin American countries.[3] This opened the way to preventing other widespread infectious diseases and in many of the endemic countries, blood transmission of *T. cruzi* dramatically decreased in the 1990s after the implementation of mandatory blood bank controls.[4–12] The blood banks of Brazil and Uruguay are now totally controlled for Chagas disease and Chile is finishing this control.[13]

However, despite these successes, blood bank control remains a great challenge, because some endemic countries have not yet introduced complete controls of their blood donors or have done so only recently, and there is no consensus on the methods to apply.[7] For example, in Mexico, one of the countries with the lowest level of screening coverage in Latin America, cases of *T. cruzi* transmission by blood transfusion have been described in the last decade and great efforts have been necessary to increase the donor *T. cruzi* screening coverage of 36.5% in 2005 to 92% in 2012.[12,14]

## *Current situation in nonendemic countries*

Transmission of *T. cruzi* through blood transfusion is not only a concern in endemic countries. Indeed, many nonendemic countries are currently receiving a continuous flow of migrants from endemic areas who carry the parasite. Among these are the United States (this country is considered as "nonendemic," even if autochthonous cases of vector transmission to humans have been increasingly described the last few years),[15–17] Canada,[18] Spain, France, the United Kingdom, and other countries in Europe (see below), Asia,[19–21] and Oceania.[22,23]

The United States and Europe are currently receiving most of the seropositive Latin American migrants.[12] In Spain, where the number of residents from endemic areas is the highest in Europe, the prevalence of *T. cruzi* infection may reach 5% in the Latin American population.[24] In Berlin, Germany, a prevalence of 2% in the Latin American population has been reported.[25] Additional reports show that these populations participate in blood donations. For instance, in Paris, France, a study reported 0.31% *T. cruzi* infection prevalence in blood donors born in Latin America.[26] In Italy, 3.9% of 128 blood donors originating from Latin America were reported seropositive.[27] Similar situations are reported in Switzerland,[28] Sweden,[29] and England.[30] In the United States there is a particularly large donor population at risk in California.[31−33]

A recently published comprehensive estimation of affected people in Europe, based on the number of legal immigrants and the *T. cruzi* prevalence in their country of origin, indicates that 14,000−180,000 persons are *T. cruzi* carriers.[34] However, only a small proportion of these individuals have been diagnosed. Until 2009, less than 4300 cases had been reported, of which 89% were in Spain,[35,36] while in the United States, an estimated 300,000 of the approximately 13 million people from endemic areas now living there carry the parasite.[37]

Importantly, most Latin American immigrants are asymptomatic for Chagas disease and do not know that they are carrying the parasite.[36] Actually, 70% of *T. cruzi*-infected people are believed to be in an asymptomatic chronic phase, and the acute phase of the infection is not often detected due to a lack of specific clinical symptoms.

Cases of *T. cruzi* transmission through blood donations were first detected in the United States.[38,39] Up to date, a dozen cases have been detected in this country,[40−42] including the case of a 3.5-year-old girl published in 2007[43] and two other cases that received a leukoreduced apheresis platelet unit from the same Argentinean donor.[44] Likewise, some cases have been reported in Europe: one in Belgium, completely unexpected, in a 7-year-old child whose parents were from Burundi,[45] and five in Spain including one fatal case.[46,47] According to the above-mentioned reports, greater attention must be paid to the risk of *T. cruzi* transmission with transfused platelet products than with other blood components.[48]

## Strategies to combat T. cruzi *transmission risk through blood transfusion*

Two main strategies to prevent *T. cruzi* transmission through blood transfusion can be mentioned. The first one consists in eliminating *T. cruzi* in blood units by adding a chemical product with trypanocidal activity. The second one, adopted nearly universally, is based on the selection of donors based on questionnaires and/or serological screening.

Gentian violet, already added to sterilize blood before transfusion in early attempts[49] is still being used to eliminate *T. cruzi* in the chemoprophylaxis of Chagas disease infection via blood transfusion when prior laboratory control is not possible or under emergency circumstances in endemic areas. The addition of gentian violet blackens blood samples, scaring patients and sometimes leading to their refusal of blood transfusion.[50] Also, some degree of genotoxicity has been described for this product.[51] Given these defects, some studies are currently looking for antiparasitic drugs to sterilize blood samples infected by *T. cruzi*.[51–53]

In most endemic countries, blood screening for anti-*T. cruzi* antibodies was adopted in blood banks to identify the potential blood samples that were carriers of the parasite. At the beginning, there was uncertainty regarding which *T. cruzi* serological tests were the most effective (i.e., the most sensitive). Different antigens were tested in different multicentric assays as well as in research laboratories.[54–59] Today, only commercial kits are used, but there is no gold standard. Most blood banks use one serologic test for screening and then they add other tests for confirmatory serodiagnosis (e.g., in Mexico).[60] The current recommendation to use two simultaneous serological tests for serodiagnosis is still in effect to confirm any suspected case of infection at the blood bank. A recent review of available commercial ELISA tests revealed substantial heterogeneity in sensitivity, specificity, or both among the tests, and the overestimation of these indices.[61] Consequently, unresolved serologies due to discrepancies between tests sometimes force blood banks to discard blood from possibly uninfected people. Moreover, some cases of negative serology, as previously described in Bolivia, can exist,[62] but their frequency remains unknown.

Since the late 1980s, many studies have attempted to detect parasite DNA in the blood of infected patients using molecular methods.[63–67] However, their usefulness remains to be clarified and there is not consensus on their routine use.[61,68] It is worth noting that their sensitivity is limited to the presence of the parasite in the processed sample, and that some strains of *T. cruzi* give very low parasitemia, which may be under these methods' threshold of detection.[67,69]

In nonendemic countries, it is assumed that prevention efficacy depends on the selection of donors and the use of questionnaires.[70–74] The serologic screening is then applied to the donors at risk. Spain (2005) and the United States (2007) were the first countries to implement blood screening for at-risk donors (i.e., people originating from an endemic area, donors with mothers originating from these areas and individuals who had lived in or traveled to endemic areas). In the United States, blood bank regulation is organized by the CDC (Centers for Disease Control).[75] Most European countries have also adopted similar safety policies to avoid *T. cruzi* transmission by transfusion, but the situation varies from one country to another[12] (e.g., questionnaire established by the Etablissement français du sang [EFS] in France, https://www.dondusang.net/rewrite/article/4276/ou-donner/conseils-pratiques/infos-pre-don/infos-pre-don.htm?idRubrique = 1402).

It is important to note that the serological kits used to diagnose *T. cruzi* infection in Latin America cannot systematically be used in nonendemic countries because of a possibly different cut-off between the pool of normal uninfected sera from endemic and nonendemic countries.[76,77] As mentioned above, unresolved cases stemming from discrepancies between tests sometimes force blood banks to discard blood from possibly uninfected people. Research is therefore oriented toward the development of 100% reliable tests and alternative detection of the parasite through biomarkers.[78,79]

Blood donor counseling is now well developed in most countries because it is considered a key in the blood transfusion system. Historically, guidelines were first developed in response to HIV's specific challenges, but now guidelines have been extended to the different health problems that can be acquired by transfusion, including Chagas disease.[80]

# Organ transplantation

## *Organ transplantation from* T. cruzi-*infected donors*

There is little experience and information related to transmission of *T. cruzi* during organ transplantations from infected donors, but, as in the case of blood transfusion, persons receiving an organ from an infected donor may be infected with the parasite and develop acute Chagas disease.[81-91] Due to immunosuppressive treatment in the organ receiver, a small number of parasites present in the graft are able to develop very quickly.

Among the recently reviewed cases of solid organ transplantations from *T. cruzi*-infected donors to naive recipients in Argentina and Brazil, and in the United States (for the 2001−11 period), most of them are related to kidney, liver, and heart transplantations, but transmission through lung transplantation has also been reported.[89,90] Also, these reviews show that transmission of *T. cruzi* from an infected donor is not a general rule, and the proportion of recipients infected during organ transplantation appears to depend on the organ type (heart transplantation from a *T. cruzi*-infected donor seems to have the most serious implications). Moreover, while some of the recipients infected during transplantation died from Chagas disease, in most of the cases reviewed, prompt treatment of infected recipients with trypanocidal drugs was effective. The use of organs from infected donors continues to be debated, but it is distorted by the disparity between the number of organ transplantation candidates on the waiting list, the available organs, and the intense pressure that exists to safely expand the donor pool. In this context, several guidelines and recommendations related to organ transplants from *T. cruzi*-infected donors have been published in Argentina,[89] the United States,[92] and Spain.[93] Generally speaking, the different working groups state that the transplantation of an organ from an infected donor is acceptable and feasible when intensive monitoring for *T. cruzi* infection in the recipient is followed and prompt therapy with trypanocidal drugs can be administered. All working groups recommend avoiding transplanting hearts from *T. cruzi*-infected donors; in Argentina, hearts from infected donors are currently discarded.[89] For other organs from *T. cruzi*-infected donors, the informed consent of the recipient is needed. In Argentina, all organ donors are tested for *T. cruzi* infection at the time of organ procurement, while in the United States and Spain, screening of potential donors born in Latin America is recommended. Moreover, infected living donors should receive trypanocidal treatment for 30 days prior to donation to allow clearance of parasitemia, and donation should take place as soon as possible after completion of treatment. More research is needed to improve experience and information related to the transmission of *T. cruzi* during organ transplantations from infected donors, and it should be a top priority of the governments of endemic and nonendemic countries to adapt safety policies aiming to prevent potential transmission occurring under these circumstances.

### Organ transplantation in T. cruzi-*infected recipients*

Although these cases are not related to acquired infection of *T. cruzi* by organ transplantation, it seems appropriate to recall here that *T. cruzi*-infected patients need specific medical care in the context of organ transplantation. Due to reactivation of the parasite, an infected patient who is receiving an organ transplant may develop high parasitemia and clinical signs of Chagas disease when immunosuppressive treatment is implemented before transplantation.

However, heart transplantation is recommended for patients with chronic Chagas heart disease in its terminal phase because it is the only treatment able to modify the progression of the disease.[94,95] In this case, parasitemia in recipients should be monitored throughout the transplantation process, but also after because of possible reactivation.[96] A survey of parasitemia and PCR control in the myocardium has been recommended.[97–99] Early diagnosis and rapid trypanocidal treatment has a good prognosis.[100,101]

# Laboratory-acquired contamination

Individuals working in research or clinical laboratories are at risk of being infected with *T. cruzi*, particularly through the handling of materials containing viable parasites (e.g., infective trypomastigotes, infective amastigotes, or meta-cyclic trypomastigotes). Since they may occur in many circumstances and often may be unnoticed or undiagnosed, laboratory-acquired cases of *T. cruzi* infection are likely underreported.[102–106] Moreover, there is generally no interest in their disclosure (they may even be hidden or denied), since it may mean inappropriate safety rules or lack of technical expertise on the part of the laboratory or researcher involved.[107]

In 2001, 65 documented laboratory-acquired cases of infection with *T. cruzi* were reviewed, showing that the most frequent contamination source results from accidental self-inoculation of parasites with contaminated needlesticks during the development of experiments involving infection of laboratory animals or from skin or mucosal contact with aerosol or droplets of infected materials (*T. cruzi* tissue culture supernatants, triatomine feces, and infected blood).[106] Additionally, special tubes for cryogenic preservation of *T. cruzi* strains can suddenly break when they are thawed, causing a significant risk situation (S.F. Brenière, personal communication). Infections may result from a very low quantity of parasites and these may also be present in very small droplets of infective culture or contaminated blood present on a laboratory bench, for instance. Moreover, even if epimastigote cultures are considered to be noninfective, old cultures are enriched in metacyclic trypomastigotes and are infectious.

Laboratory-acquired infections can be prevented by wearing appropriate personal protective equipment (gloves, face mask, lab coat, closed shoes, etc.), cultivating the parasite in a Biosafe laboratory, and by using appropriate facilities for animals.[108] Moreover, rigorous training of the personnel working with *T. cruzi* is essential, and every professional handling *T. cruzi* should undergo serological diagnosis upon recruitment, and when negative, every year.[107,109] Also, for further comparisons, it is important to keep aliquots of the different control sera to avoid repeated freezing and thawing. Finally, trypanocidal drugs should be available in every laboratory that works with infectious *T. cruzi* to allow for a prompt response in case of an accident. However, many countries are not authorized to trade these drugs, and in this case, the laboratory needs a governmental agreement to import them, mainly from Brazil or Argentina.

*T. cruzi* multiply in the human host from a very few parasites. If one suspects that some parasites have been in contact with a mucosa or if one's skin has been scratched by a contaminated needle, it is necessary to immediately disinfect the inoculation site and initiate preventive treatment with trypanocidal drugs under medical control. Then infection can be confirmed by direct examination of the blood, specific serology, or by using trial molecular methods such as PCR, which allows a very early and sensitive parasitic diagnosis.[110]

# Oral transmission

While oral transmission was already described in 1913 by Brumpt,[111] it did not receive much attention until the last decade. At that time, it was also suggested as a natural infection route for wild and domestic animals eating infected triatomines.[112,113]

## Experimental and natural infections of mammals via the oral route

The first experimental demonstration of this route of transmission was made by successfully infecting rats after feeding them with blood containing trypomastigote forms of *T. cruzi*.[114] Then many other experiments conducted with mammals confirmed the transmission of *T. cruzi* via the oral route through eating infected triatomines, contaminated triatomine feces, or food directly contaminated with the parasite or with contaminated triatomine feces.[115–121]

Successful infection of mice after eating food contaminated with parasites present in the anal glands of *Didelphis marsupialis* highlighted the risk of being infected through eating food contaminated with opossum dejections.[122] Finally, effective oral transmission of *T. cruzi* was also demonstrated by feeding *Didelphis albiventris* with *T. cruzi*-infected rodents.[123]

These data on the natural or experimental infections of wild and domestic animals show the possible oral transmission of *T. cruzi* by eating (1) infected triatomines; (2) infected animals; (3) food contaminated with contaminated feces of triatomines or anal gland secretions of opossums; and (4) directly contaminated feces of triatomines or anal gland secretions of opossums.

## Human outbreaks of acute Chagas disease acquired by oral transmission

In humans, the possibility of oral transmission of *T. cruzi* has recently been considered a serious issue because microepidemic or epidemic episodes of acute Chagas disease have been increasingly reported in areas without domiciliated triatomines or with a low level of domestic infestation by triatomines. When various serious acute cases appear at the same time in a family or a community, or during a common meal (meetings, celebrations), systematic inquiry generally raises suspicion of an oral route of contamination and its origin. Several cases are reported below.

The first outbreak of acute Chagas disease due to oral transmission was reported in 1968[124]: 17 simultaneous cases with acute myocarditis occurred in March 1965, in a rural school from Teutônia, situated in Estrêla, the Rio Grande do Sul state in Brazil. The inquiry showed that the first clinical signs appeared 13−19 days after the infection, and during this epidemic period, five people died before 40 days. The points suggesting oral transmission were (1) the occurrence of 17 serious cases at the same time; (2) the lack of cutaneous or mucosal injury in the patients; (3) the lack of triatomines in the school; and (4) the presence of a *Didelphis* spp. infected with *T. cruzi* in the school. Accordingly, the authors favored the hypothesis that food contaminated by the anal gland secretions of the opossum were ingested.

In the Amazon region, reports of acute cases due to oral transmission are more common. In October 1986, 7−22 days after a meeting at a farm in Catolé do Rocha, in the Paraíba state in Brazil, 26 acute cases of Chagas disease were identified.[125] The patients had a febrile illness associated with bilateral eyelid and lower limb edema, mild hepatosplenomegaly, lymphadenopathy, and occasionally a skin rash. One 74-year-old patient died. In this outbreak, it seemed that an infected opossum could have deposited infective anal gland secretions over the sugar cane crusher. Between 1988 and 2005, 233 cases including 183 (78.5%) during outbreaks (mean, four individuals), probably due to oral transmission, were reported in Pará, Amapá, and Maranhão, Brazil.[126] In these cases, the most frequent clinical signs were fever, headache, myalgia, pallor, dyspnea, swelling of the legs, facial edema, abdominal pain, myocarditis, and exanthema. These grouped cases appeared mostly in July (19 cases) and August (25 cases), with the highest numbers in October (40 cases) and November (43 cases). This seasonality raised the suspicion of the consumption of contaminated beverages as the source of oral transmission because at that time there was a very high production and consumption of different juices from palm tree fruits, sugar cane, and other sources. In 2005 in Santa Catarina, Brazil, sugar cane juice was implicated as the source of infection (24 cases and several deaths),[127] while the consumption of açaí, the fruit of a palm of the Aracaceae family, was reported to be the source of infection in several outbreaks in the Brazilian Amazon.[128,129]

Outside Brazil, where it is estimated that over 1500 patients in 6 states of the Amazon region have been infected through oral transmission,[130] several outbreaks have been reported in Columbia and Venezuela,[131–133] where the largest outbreak described occurred with 103 cases in the same school in Caracas city, 1 in French Guyana,[134] and 1 in Bolivia.[135] Through all these reports, the main sources of oral transmission were clearly the homemade fruit juices contaminated by infected triatomine feces or infected Didelphidae secretions.[136] Note that the consumption of crude or undercooked meat of a *T. cruzi*-infected animal—even if very unusual and never evidenced—might also be a source of oral transmission.

The recent increase of oral transmission in the Amazon is related to the new scenarios of Chagas disease, which are related to the human impact on fauna and triatomines.[7,131] Due to the deforestation associated with new human settlements, the forest balance of zoonotic cycles of *T. cruzi* is disturbed. The triatomines move in search of new hosts and new habitats to urban areas, most often attracted by lights. Accordingly, oral transmission should be considered in areas of humid tropical forest other than the Amazon, particularly those suffering from deforestation, because in this context, forest triatomine species may adapt to the anthropized medium. The approximation of the vectors to humans creates a situation of transmission risk, especially via the oral route.

## Prevention of oral transmission

Over the last few years, research centers have emerged in the Amazonian region and elsewhere, which has led to an increase in the knowledge of vectors, reservoirs and the symptomatology of acute cases found in the areas where few sporadic cases or chronic cases have been reported. The transmission of *T. cruzi* through contaminated food and beverages was evaluated in a technical consultation of PAHO/WHO.[137] It was concluded that oral transmission of *T. cruzi* was an important consideration that warranted inclusion in the National Programs of Prevention and Control of Chagas disease.

Risk factors involved in oral transmission are directly bound to the consumption of food or beverages contaminated by the parasite. These food and beverages are either naturally contaminated or contaminated during their preparation.

In 2007, Brazil's Ministry of Health, with the departments of surveillance and prevention, in conjunction with the Evandro Chagas Institute, FUNASA, ANVISA, the Ministry of Agriculture and Fishing, and other institutions, proposed several measures to prevent and survey the preparation and production of food and beverages likely to be contaminated with *T. cruzi*, including açaí juice, which is very important to the economy of northern Brazil. At the industrial level, it was recommended that açaí juice should be pasteurized. For small producers (on the family scale), recommendations were proposed to improve hygiene and minimize the risk of juice contamination during fruit collection, transportation, and handling. While kissing bugs are primarily responsible for the contamination of food and beverages, it is obvious that to prevent oral transmission, vector control with insecticides and/ or improvements to homes do not apply. The only alternative is education for the communities exposed to the risk of oral transmission and improving hygiene when preparing homemade food and beverages.[132]

## Sexual transmission

While the possibility of sexual transmission of *T. cruzi* has been discussed since the discovery of Chagas disease, very few studies have been published on the subject. The first conclusive evidence of such transmission in a model has only been published very recently.[138]

Previous observations of *T. cruzi* colonization in several tissues of the urogenital system in infected mice as well as the presence of parasites mixed with spermatozoa suggested that *T. cruzi* could potentially be transmitted via the sexual route.[139,140] Moreover, successful infections of healthy mice were obtained by intravaginal instillation of blood trypomastigote forms of *T. cruzi* and also by similar instillation in the penis.[141] In a recent study, a low probability of sexual transmission by crossbreeding of immunosuppressive females with acutely infected males was evidenced in a murine model.[142] Finally, *T. cruzi* sexual transmission in mice was successfully obtained (100% mating) through mating between chronically infected males and naive females or infected females and naive males[138]; the transmission was corroborated by both serological and molecular techniques in all cases. Moreover, almost all offspring of sexually infected females were then congenitally infected.

Few data exist in humans, but the presence of *T. cruzi* was reported in seminiferous tubes and ovarian cells of children who succumbed to Chagas disease, or in menstrual blood of infected patients.[143,144] Also, *T. cruzi* amastigote forms were observed in epithelial cells of cervical tissues in a reactivation case of *T. cruzi* infection in a young immunocompromised patient.[145]

If this route of transmission is also possible in humans, e.g., in the particular immunological state of the partners, then the paradigm of Chagas disease could considerably change. Indeed, this route of transmission could represent a frightening potential for spreading Chagas disease worldwide. Moreover, if confirmed, this could suggest that a much larger number of people than estimated may be at risk of acquiring *T. cruzi*.

## References

1. Wendel S. Transfusion transmitted Chagas disease: is it really under control? *Acta Trop* 2010;**115**:28−34.
2. Pedreira De Freitas JL, Amato Neto V, Nussenzweig V, Sonntag R, Barreto JG. Primeiras verificações de transmissão acidental da moléstia de Chagas ao homem por transfusão de sangue. *Rev Paul Med* 1952;**40**:36−40.

3. Pinto-Dias JC, Brener Z. Chagas' disease and blood transfusion. *Mem Inst Oswaldo Cruz* 1984;**79**:139−47.

4. Moncayo A, Silveira AC. Current epidemiological trends for Chagas disease in Latin America and future challenges in epidemiology, surveillance and health policy. *Mem Inst Oswaldo Cruz* 2009;**104**(Suppl. 1):17−30.

5. Moncayo A. Chagas disease: current epidemiological trends after the interruption of vectorial and transfusional transmission in the Southern Cone countries. *Mem Inst Oswaldo Cruz* 2003;**98**:577−91.

6. Schmunis GA. Epidemiology of Chagas disease in non-endemic countries: the role of international migration. *Mem Inst Oswaldo Cruz* 2007;**102**(Suppl. 1):75−85.

7. Coura JR. The main sceneries of Chagas disease transmission. The vectors, blood and oral transmissions—a comprehensive review. *Mem Inst Oswaldo Cruz* 2015;**110**:277−82.

8. Schmunis GA, Zicker F, Cruz JR, Cuchi P. Safety of blood supply for infectious diseases in Latin American countries, 1994−1997. *Am J Trop Med Hyg* 2001;**65**: 924−30.

9. Schmunis GA, Cruz JR. Safety of the blood supply in Latin America. *Clin Microbiol Rev* 2005;**18**:12−29.

10. Schmunis GA. Risk of Chagas disease through transfusions in the Americas. *Medicina (B Aires)* 1999;**59**(Suppl. 2):125−34.

11. Schmunis GA. *Trypanosoma cruzi*, the etiologic agent of Chagas' disease: status in the blood supply in endemic and nonendemic countries. *Transfusion* 1991;**31**:547−57.

12. Angheben A, Boix L, Buonfrate D, Gobbi F, Bisoffi Z, Pupella S, et al. Chagas disease and transmission medicine: a perspective from non-endemic countries. *Blood Transfusion* 2015;**13**:540−50.

13. Coura JR. Chagas disease: control, elimination and eradication. Is it possible? *Mem Inst Oswaldo Cruz* 2013;**108**:962−7.

14. Medina JR. Blood safety in the XXI century. Transfusion transmitted infectious diseases. International and Mexican view. *Gaceta Medica De Mexico* 2014;**150**:78−83.

15. Cantey PT, Stramer SL, Townsend RL, Kamel H, Ofafa K, Todd CW, et al. The United States *Trypanosoma cruzi* infection study: evidence for vector-borne transmission of the parasite that causes Chagas disease among United States blood donors. *Transfusion* 2012;**52**:1922−30.

16. Garcia MN, Aguilar D, Gorchakov R, Rossmann SN, Montgomery SP, Rivera H, et al. Evidence of autochthonous Chagas disease in Southeastern Texas. *Am J Trop Med Hyg* 2015;**92**:325−30.

17. Navin TR, Roberto RR, Juranek DD, Limpakarnjanarat K, Mortenson EW, Clover JR, et al. Human and sylvatic *Trypanosoma cruzi* infection in California. *Am J Public Health* 1985;**75**:366−9.

18. Steele LS, MacPherson DW, Kim J, Keystone JS, Gushulak BD. The sero-prevalence of antibodies to *Trypanosoma cruzi* in Latin American refugees and immigrants to Canada. *J Immigr Minor Health* 2007;**9**:43−7.

19. Ueno Y, Nakamura Y, Takahashi M, Inoue T, Endo S, Kinoshita M, et al. A highly suspected case of chronic Chagas' heart disease diagnosed in Japan. *Jpn Circ J* 1995;**59**:219−23.

20. Imai K, Maeda T, Sayama Y, Osa M, Mikita K, Kurane I, et al. Chronic Chagas disease with advanced cardiac complications in Japan: case report and literature review. *Parasitol Int* 2015;**64**:240−2.

21. Imai K, Maeda T, Sayama Y, Mikita K, Fujikura Y, Misawa K, et al. Mother-to-child transmission of congenital Chagas disease, Japan. *Emerg Infect Dis* 2014;**20**:146−8.

22. Pinto A, Pett S, Jackson Y. Identifying Chagas disease in Australia: an emerging challenge for general practitioners. *Aust Fam Physician* 2014;**43**:440−2.
23. Jackson Y, Pinto A, Pett S. Chagas disease in Australia and New Zealand: risks and needs for public health interventions. *Trop Med Int Health* 2014;**19**:212−18.
24. Schmunis GA, Yadon ZE. Chagas disease: a Latin American health problem becoming a world health problem. *Acta Trop* 2010;**115**:14−21.
25. Frank M, Hegenscheid B, Janitschke K, Weinke T. Prevalence and epidemiological significance of *Trypanosoma cruzi* infection among Latin American immigrants in Berlin, Germany. *Infection* 1997;**25**:355−8.
26. El Ghouzzi MH, Boiret E, Wind F, Brochard C, Fittere S, Paris L, et al. Testing blood donors for Chagas disease in the Paris area, France: first results after 18 months of screening. *Transfusion* 2010;**50**:575−83.
27. Gabrielli S, Girelli G, Vaia F, Santonicola M, Fakeri A, Cancrini G. Surveillance of Chagas disease among at-risk blood donors in Italy: preliminary results from Umberto I Polyclinic in Rome. *Blood Transfusion* 2013;**11**:558−62.
28. Jackson Y, Getaz L, Wolff H, Holst M, Mauris A, Tardin A, et al. Prevalence, clinical staging and risk for blood-borne transmission of Chagas disease among Latin American migrants in Geneva, Switzerland. *PLoS NTD* 2010;**4**:e592.
29. Sandahl K, Botero-Kleiven S, Hellgren U. Chagas' disease in Sweden—great need of guidelines for testing. Probably hundreds of seropositive cases, only a few known. *Lakartidningen* 2011;**108**:2368−71.
30. Kitchen AD, Hewitt PE, Chiodini PL. The early implementation of *Trypanosoma cruzi* antibody screening of donors and donations within England: preempting a problem. *Transfusion* 2012;**52**:1931−9.
31. Galel SA, Kirchhoff LV. Risk factors for *Trypanosoma cruzi* infection in California blood donors. *Transfusion* 1996;**36**:227−31.
32. Leiby DA, Herron Jr. RM, Read EJ, Lenes BA, Stumpf RJ. *Trypanosoma cruzi* in Los Angeles and Miami blood donors: impact of evolving donor demographics on seroprevalence and implications for transfusion transmission. *Transfusion* 2002;**42**:549−55.
33. Kerndt PR, Waskin HA, Kirchhoff LV, Steurer F, Waterman SH, Nelson JM, et al. Prevalence of antibody to *Trypanosoma cruzi* among blood donors in Los Angeles, California. *Transfusion* 1991;**31**:814−18.
34. Strasen J, Williams T, Ertl G, Zoller T, Stich A, Ritter O. Epidemiology of Chagas disease in Europe: many calculations, little knowledge. *Clin Res Cardiol* 2014;**103**:1−10.
35. Basile L, Jansa JM, Carlier Y, Salamanca DD, Angheben A, Bartoloni A, et al. Chagas disease in European countries: the challenge of a surveillance system. *Euro Surveill* 2011;16.
36. Gascon J, Bern C, Pinazo MJ. Chagas disease in Spain, the United States and other non-endemic countries. *Acta Trop* 2010;**115**:22−7.
37. Bern C, Montgomery SP. An estimate of the burden of Chagas disease in the United States. *Clin Infect Dis* 2009;**49**:E52−4.
38. Grant IH, Gold JW, Wittner M, Tanowitz HB, Nathan C, Mayer K, et al. Transfusion-associated acute Chagas disease acquired in the United States. *Ann Intern Med* 1989;**111**:849−51.
39. Nickerson P, Orr P, Schroeder ML, Sekla L, Johnston JB. Transfusion-associated *Trypanosoma cruzi* infection in a non-endemic area. *Ann Intern Med* 1989;**111**:851−3.
40. Cimo PL, Luper WE, Scouros MA. Transfusion-associated Chagas' disease in Texas: report of a case. *Tex Med* 1993;**89**:48−50.

41. Leiguarda R, Roncoroni A, Taratuto AL, Jost L, Berthier M, Nogues M, et al. Acute CNS infection by *Trypanosoma cruzi* (Chagas' disease) in immunosuppressed patients. *Neurology* 1990;**40**:850−1.
42. Leiby DA, Lenes BA, Tibbals MA, Tames-Olmedo MT. Prospective evaluation of a patient with *Trypanosoma cruzi* infection transmitted by transfusion. *N Engl J Med* 1999;**341**:1237−9.
43. Young C, Losikoff P, Chawla A, Glasser L, Forman E. Transfusion-acquired *Trypanosoma cruzi* infection. *Transfusion* 2007;**47**:540−4.
44. Kessler DA, Shi PA, Avecilla ST, Shaz BH. Results of lookback for Chagas disease since the inception of donor screening at New York blood center. *Transfusion* 2013; **53**:1083−7.
45. Blumental S, Lambermont M, Heijmans C, Rodenbach MP, El Kenz H, Sondag D, et al. First documented transmission of *Trypanosoma cruzi* infection through blood transfusion in a child with sickle-cell disease in Belgium. *PLoS NTD* 2015;**9**:e0003986.
46. Flores-Chavez M, Fernandez B, Puente S, Torres P, Rodriguez M, Monedero C, et al. Transfusional Chagas disease: parasitological and serological monitoring of an infected recipient and blood donor. *Clin Infect Dis* 2008;**46**:e44−7.
47. Benjamin RJ, Stramer SL, Leiby DA, Dodd RY, Fearon M, Castro E. *Trypanosoma cruzi* infection in North America and Spain: evidence in support of transfusion transmission. *Transfusion* 2012;**52**:1913−21, quiz 2.
48. Cancino-Faure B, Fisa R, Riera C, Bula I, Girona-Llobera E, Jimenez-Marco T. Evidence of meaningful levels of *Trypanosoma cruzi* in platelet concentrates from seropositive blood donors. *Transfusion* 2015;**55**:1249−55.
49. Nussenzweig V, Sonntag R, Biancalana A, De Freitas JL, Amato Neto V, Kloetzel J. Effect of triphenylmethane dyes on *Trypanosoma cruzi in vitro*; use of gentian violet in prevention of transmission of Chagas disease by blood transfusion. *Hospital (Rio J)* 1953;**44**:731−44.
50. Nussenzweig V, Biancalana A, Amato Neto V, Sonntag R, De Freitas JP, Kloetzel J. Effect of gentian violet on *Trypanosoma cruzi in vitro*; importance in the sterilization of blood for transfusion. *Rev Paul Med* 1953;**42**:57−8.
51. Díaz Gómez MI, Castro JA. Genotoxicidad en leucocitos por la quimioprofilaxis de sangre con violeta de genciana y su prevención con antioxidantes. *Acta Bioq Clín Latinoamer* 2013;**47**:719−26.
52. Moraes-Souza H, Bordin JO. Strategies for prevention of transfusion-associated Chagas' disease. *Transfus Med Rev* 1996;**10**:161−70.
53. Moraes-Souza H, Bordin JO, Bardossy L, Blajchman MA. Treatment of *T. cruzi* infected human platelet concentrates with aminomethyltrimethyl psoralen (AMT) and ultraviolet a (UV-A) light: preliminary results. *Rev Soc Bras Med Trop* 1996;**29**:47−9.
54. Levin MJ. Molecular mimicry and Chagas' heart disease: High anti-R-13 autoantibody levels are markers of severe Chagas heart complaint. *Res Immunol* 1991;**142**:157−9.
55. Carvalho MR, Krieger MA, Almeida E, Oelemann W, Shikanai-Yassuda MA, Ferreira AW, et al. Chagas' disease diagnosis: evaluation of several tests in blood bank screening. *Transfusion* 1993;**33**:830−4.
56. Vergara U, Veloso C, Gonzalez A, Lorca M. Evaluation of an enzyme-linked immunosorbent assay for the diagnosis of Chagas' disease using synthetic peptides. *Am J Trop Med Hyg* 1992;**46**:39−43.
57. Gomes ML, Galvao LM, Macedo AM, Pena SD, Chiari E. Chagas' disease diagnosis: comparative analysis of parasitologic, molecular, and serologic methods. *Am J Trop Med Hyg* 1999;**60**:205−10.

58. Umezawa ES, Luquetti AO, Levitus G, Ponce C, Ponce E, Henriquez D, et al. Serodiagnosis of chronic and acute Chagas' disease with *Trypanosoma cruzi* recombinant proteins: results of a collaborative study in six latin American countries. *J Clin Microbiol* 2004;**42**:449−52.

59. Pirard M, Iihoshi N, Boelaert M, Basanta P, Lopez F, Van der Stuyft P. The validity of serologic tests for *Trypanosoma cruzi* and the effectiveness of transfusional screening strategies in a hyperendemic region. *Transfusion* 2005;**45**:554−61.

60. Escamilla-Guerrero G, Martinez-Gordillo MN, Riveron-Negrete L, Aguilar-Escobar DV, Bravo-Lindoro A, Cob-Sosa C, et al. *Trypanosoma cruzi*: seroprevalence detected in the blood bank of the Instituto Nacional de Pediatria, Mexico city, in the period 2004 through 2009. *Transfusion* 2012;**52**:595−600.

61. Brasil PE, Castro R, Castro L. Commercial enzyme-linked immunosorbent assay versus polymerase chain reaction for the diagnosis of chronic Chagas disease: a systematic review and meta-analysis. *Mem Inst Oswaldo Cruz* 2016;**111**:1−19.

62. Brenière SF, Poch O, Selaes H, Tibayrenc M, Lemesre JL, Antezana G, et al. Specific humoral depression in chronic patients infected by *Trypanosoma cruzi*. *Rev Inst Med Trop Sao Paulo* 1984;**26**:254−8.

63. Degrave W, Fragoso SP, Britto C, van Heuverswyn H, Kidane GZ, Cardoso MA, et al. Peculiar sequence organization of kinetoplast DNA minicircles from *Trypanosoma cruzi*. *Mol Biochem Parasitol* 1988;**27**:63−70.

64. Avila HA, Pereira JB, Thiemann O, De Paiva E, DeGrave W, Morel CM, et al. Detection of *Trypanosoma cruzi* in blood specimens of chronic Chagasic patients by polymerase chain reaction amplification of kinetoplast minicircle DNA: comparison with serology and xenodiagnosis. *J Clin Microbiol* 1993;**31**:2421−6.

65. Wincker P, Bosseno MF, Britto C, Yaksic N, Cardoso MA, Morel CM, et al. High correlation between Chagas' disease serology and PCR-based detection of *Trypanosoma cruzi* kinetoplast DNA in Bolivian children living in an endemic area. *FEMS Microbiol Lett* 1994;**124**:419−23.

66. Wincker P, Telleria J, Bosseno MF, Cardoso MA, Marques P, Yaksic N, et al. PCR-based diagnosis for Chagas' disease in Bolivian children living in an active transmission area: comparison with conventional serological and parasitological diagnosis. *Parasitology* 1997;**114**(Pt 4):367−73.

67. Brenière SF, Bosseno MF, Noireau F, Yacsik N, Liegeard P, Aznar C, et al. Integrate study of a Bolivian population infected by *Trypanosoma cruzi*, the agent of Chagas disease. *Mem Inst Oswaldo Cruz* 2002;**97**:289−95.

68. Schijman AG, Bisio M, Orellana L, Sued M, Duffy T, Mejia Jaramillo AM, et al. International study to evaluate PCR methods for detection of *Trypanosoma cruzi* DNA in blood samples from Chagas disease patients. *PLoS NTD* 2011;**5**:e931.

69. Anez N, Carrasco H, Parada H, Crisante G, Rojas A, Gonzalez N, et al. Acute Chagas' disease in Western Venezuela: a clinical, seroparasitologic, and epidemiologic study. *Am J Trop Med Hyg* 1999;**60**:215−22.

70. Reesink HW. European strategies against the parasite transfusion risk. *Transfus Clin Biol* 2005;**12**:1−4.

71. Appleman MD, Shulman IA, Saxena S, Kirchhoff LV. Use of a questionnaire to identify potential blood donors at risk for infection with *Trypanosoma cruzi*. *Transfusion* 1993;**33**:61−4.

72. O'Brien SF, Ram SS, Vamvakas EC, Goldman M. The Canadian blood donor health assessment questionnaire: lessons from history, application of cognitive science principles, and recommendations for change. *Transfus Med Rev* 2007;**21**:205−22.

73. O'Brien SF, Scalia V, Goldman M, Fan W, Yi QL, Dines IR, et al. Selective testing for *Trypanosoma cruzi*: the first year after implementation at Canadian blood services. *Transfusion* 2013;**53**:1706−13.

74. O'Brien SF, Chiavetta JA, Fan W, Xi G, Yi QL, Goldman M, et al. Assessment of a travel question to identify donors with risk of *Trypanosoma cruzi*: operational validity and field testing. *Transfusion* 2008;**48**:755−61.

75. Galel SA, Lifson JD, Engleman EG. Prevention of AIDS transmission through screening of the blood supply. *Annu Rev Immunol* 1995;**13**:201−27.

76. Aznar C, Liegeard P, Mariette C, Lafon S, Levin MJ, Hontebeyrie M. A simple *Trypanosoma cruzi* enzyme-linked immunoassay for control of human infection in nonendemic areas. *FEMS Immunol Med Microbiol* 1997;**18**:31−7.

77. Verani JR, Seitz A, Gilman RH, LaFuente C, Galdos-Cardenas G, Kawai V, et al. Geographic variation in the sensitivity of recombinant antigen-based rapid tests for chronic *Trypanosoma cruzi* infection. *Am J Trop Med Hyg* 2009;**80**:410−15.

78. Nagarkatti R, de Araujo FF, Gupta C, Debrabant A. Aptamer based, non-PCR, non-serological detection of Chagas disease biomarkers in *Trypanosoma cruzi* infected mice. *PLoS NTD* 2014;**8**:e2650.

79. Pinazo MJ, Thomas MC, Bustamante J, Almeida IC, Lopez MC, Gascon J. Biomarkers of therapeutic responses in chronic Chagas disease: state of the art and future perspectives. *Mem Inst Oswaldo Cruz* 2015;**110**:422−32.

80. WHO. *Blood donor counselling: implementation guidelines*, Geneva: World Health Organization; 2014.

81. Vazquez MC, Riarte A, Pattin M, Lauricella M. Chagas-disease can be transmitted through kidney-transplantation. *Transpl Proc* 1993;**25**:3259−60.

82. CDC. From the Centers for Disease Control and Prevention. Chagas disease after organ transplantation—United States, 2001. *JAMA* 2002;**287**:1795−6.

83. (CDC) CfDCaP. Chagas disease after organ transplantation—Los Angeles, California, 2006. *MMWR* 2006;**55**:798−800.

84. Defaria JBL, Alves G. Transmission of Chagas-disease through cadaveric renal-transplantation. *Transplantation* 1993;**56**:1583−4.

85. Ferraz AS, Figueiredo JFC. Transmission of Chagas' disease through transplanted kidney: occurrence of the acute form of the disease in two recipients from the same donor. *Rev Inst Med Trop Sao Paulo* 1993;**35**:461−3.

86. Riarte A, Luna C, Sabatiello R, Sinagra A, Schiavelli R, De Rissio A, et al. Chagas' disease in patients with kidney transplants: 7 years of experience 1989−1996. *Clin Infect Dis* 1999;**29**:561−7.

87. D'Albuquerque LA, Gonzalez AM, Filho HL, Copstein JL, Larrea FI, Mansero JM, et al. Liver transplantation from deceased donors serologically positive for Chagas disease. *Am J Transplant* 2007;**7**:680−4.

88. Kun H, Moore A, Mascola L, Steurer F, Lawrence G, Kubak B, et al. Transmission of *Trypanosoma cruzi* by heart transplantation. *Clin Infect Dis* 2009;**48**:1534−40.

89. Lattes R, Altclas J, Arselan S, Barcan L, Diez M, Gadano A, et al. Chagas' disease and solid organ transplantation. *Transplant Proc* 2010;**42**:3354−9.

90. Huprikar S, Bosserman E, Patel G, Moore A, Pinney S, Anyanwu A, et al. Donor-derived *Trypanosoma cruzi* infection in solid organ recipients in the United States, 2001−2011. *Am J Transplant* 2013;**13**:2418−25.

91. Souza FF, Castro ESO, Marin Neto JA, Sankarankutty AK, Teixeira AC, Martinelli AL, et al. Acute Chagasic myocardiopathy after orthotopic liver transplantation with donor and recipient serologically negative for *Trypanosoma cruzi*: a case report. *Transplant Proc* 2008;**40**:875−8.

92. Chin-Hong PV, Schwartz BS, Bern C, Montgomery SP, Kontak S, Kubak B, et al. Screening and treatment of Chagas disease in organ transplant recipients in the United States: recommendations from the Chagas in transplant working group. *Am J Transplant* 2011;**11**:672−80.

93. Pinazo MJ, Miranda B, Rodriguez-Villar C, Altclas J, Brunet Serra M, Garcia-Otero EC, et al. Recommendations for management of Chagas disease in organ and hematopoietic tissue transplantation programs in nonendemic areas. *Transplant Rev (Orlando)* 2011;**25**:91−101.

94. Bertolino ND, Villafanha DF, Cardinalli-Neto A, Cordeiro JA, Arcanjo MJ, Theodoropoulos TA, et al. Prognostic impact of Chagas' disease in patients awaiting heart transplantation. *J Heart Lung Transplant* 2010;**29**:449−53.

95. Kransdorf EP, Czer LS, Luthringer DJ, Patel JK, Montgomery SP, Velleca A, et al. Heart transplantation for Chagas cardiomyopathy in the United States. *Am J Transplant* 2013;**13**:3262−8.

96. Sadala ML, Stolf NA, Bicudo MA. Heart transplantation: the experience of patients with Chagas disease. *Rev Esc Enferm USP* 2009;**43**:588−95.

97. Diez M, Favaloro L, Bertolotti A, Burgos JM, Vigliano C, Lastra MP, et al. Usefulness of PCR strategies for early diagnosis of Chagas' disease reactivation and treatment follow-up in heart transplantation. *Am J Transplant* 2007;**7**:1633−40.

98. Benvenuti LA, Roggerio A, Sambiase NV, Fiorelli A, Higuchi Mde L. Polymerase chain reaction in endomyocardial biopsies for monitoring reactivation of Chagas' disease in heart transplantation: a case report and review of the literature. *Cardiovasc Pathol* 2005;**14**:265−8.

99. Freitas HF, Chizzola PR, Paes AT, Lima AC, Mansur AJ. Risk stratification in a Brazilian hospital-based cohort of 1220 outpatients with heart failure: role of Chagas' heart disease. *Int J Cardiol* 2005;**102**:239−47.

100. Fiorelli AI, Santos RH, Oliveira Jr. JL, Lourenco-Filho DD, Dias RR, Oliveira AS, et al. Heart transplantation in 107 cases of Chagas' disease. *Transplant Proc* 2011;**43**:220−4.

101. Bestetti RB, Theodoropoulos TA. A systematic review of studies on heart transplantation for patients with end-stage Chagas' heart disease. *J Card Fail* 2009;**15**:249−55.

102. Coudert J, Despeignes J, Battesti MR, Michel-Brun J. A case of Chagas' disease caused by accidental laboratory contamination by *T. cruzi*. *Bull Soc Pathol Exot Filiales* 1964; **57**:208−13.

103. Pizzi T, Niedmann G, Jarpa A. Report of 3 cases of acute Chagas' disease produced by accidental laboratory infections. *Bol Chil Parasitol* 1963;**18**:32−6.

104. Brener Z. Laboratory-acquired Chagas' disease: an endemic disease among parasitologists. In: Morel CME, editor. *Genes and antigens of parasites: a laboratory manual*. Rio de Janeiro, Brazil: Fundaçao Oswaldo Cruz; 1984. p. 39.

105. Hofflin JM, Sadler RH, Araujo FG, Page WE, Remington JS. Laboratory-acquired Chagas disease. *Trans R Soc Trop Med Hyg* 1987;**81**:437−40.

106. Herwaldt BL. Laboratory-acquired parasitic infections from accidental exposures. *Clin Microbiol Rev* 2001;**14**:659−88, table of contents.

107. Dias JCP, Amato Neto V. Prevenção referente às modalidades alternativas de transmissão do *Trypanosoma cruzi* no Brasil. *Rev Soc Brasil Med Trop* 2011;**44**:68−72.

108. Brener Z, Alquezar AS, Luquetti AS. Normas de segurança para infecções acidentais com o *Trypanosoma cruzi*, agente causador da doença de Chagas. *Rev Patol Trop* 1997;**26**:129−30.

109. Andrade JP, Marin Neto JA, Paola AA, Vilas-Boas F, Oliveira GM, Bacal F, et al. I Latin American guidelines for the diagnosis and treatment of Chagas' heart disease: Executive summary. *Arq Bras Cardiol* 2011;**96**:434−42.

110. Kinoshita-Yanaga AT, Toledo MJ, Araújo SM, Vier BP, Gomes ML. Accidental infection by *Trypanosoma cruzi* follow-up by the polymerase chain reaction: Case report. *Rev Inst Med Trop São Paulo* 2009;**51**:295−8.

111. Brumpt E. *Précis de parasitologie*. Paris: Masson et Cie; 1927.

112. Dias E. Xenodiagnostico e algumas verificaçoes epidemiologicas na moléstia de Chagas. In: Regional RdSdP, editor. Buenos Aires, vol. 1; 1935, p. 89−119.

113. Dias E. *Estudos sobre o Schizotrypanum cruzi*. Rio de Janeiro: Universidade de Rio de Janeiro; 1933.

114. Nattan-Larrier L. Infections à Trypanosomes et voies de pénétrations des virus. *Bull Soc Path Exot* 1921;**26**:2579.

115. Torrico RA. Conocimientos actuales sobre la enfermedad de Chagas en Bolivia. *Bol Of Sanit Panam* 1950;**29**:827−41.

116. Diaz-Ungria C. Transmision del *Trypanosoma cruzi* en los vertebrados. *Rev Ibér Parasitol Today* 1965;**25**:1−44.

117. Mayer HF. Infeccion experimental con *Trypanosoma cruzi* por via digestive. *Anales Inst Med Regional* 1961;**5**:43−8.

118. Baretto MP, Ribeiro RD, Belda Neto FM. Estudos sobre reservatorios e vectores silvestres do *Trypanosoma cruzi*. Lxviii: Infeccao de mamiferos pela via oral. *Rev Bras Biol* 1978;**38**:45569.

119. Schenone H, Gonzalez H, Schenone H, Rojas A. Infeccion experimental de ratas con *Trypanosoma cruzi* por via oral. *Bol Chile Parasit* 1982;**37**:29.

120. Calvo MML, Nogueda B, Aguilar RA. Oral route: a probable way of transmission of *Trypanosoma cruzi*. *Rev Lat-amer Microbiol* 1992;**34**:39−42.

121. Marsden PD. *Trypanosoma cruzi* infections in CFI mice. II. Infections induced by different routes. *Ann Trop Med Parasitol* 1967;**61**:62−7.

122. Jansen AM, Moriearty PL, Castro BG, Deane MP. *Trypanosoma cruzi* in the opossum *Didelphis marsupialis*: an indirect fluorescent antibody test for the diagnosis and follow-up of natural and experimental infections. *Trans R Soc Trop Med Hyg* 1985;**79**: 474−7.

123. Ribeiro DR, Rissato e Garcia TA, Bonomo WC. Contribuiçao para o estudo dos mecanismos de transmissao do agente etiologico da doença de Chagas. *Rev Saude Publ Sao Paulo* 1987;**21**:51−4.

124. da Silva NN, Clausell DT, Nolibos H, de Mello AL, Ossanai J, Rapone T, et al. Epidemic outbreak of Chagas disease probably due to oral contamination. *Rev Inst Med Trop Sao Paulo* 1968;**10**:265−76.

125. Shikanai-Yasuda MA, Marcondes CB, Guedes LA, Siqueira GS, Barone AA, Dias JC, et al. Possible oral transmission of acute Chagas' disease in Brazil. *Rev Inst Med Trop Sao Paulo* 1991;**33**:351−7.

126. Neves Pinto AY, Valente SA, Valente VC, Ferreira AG, Coura JR. Fase aguda da doença de Chagas na Amazonia Brasileira. Estudo de 233 casos de para, amapae maranhao observados entre 1988 e 2005. *Rev Soc Bras Med Trop* 2008;**41**:602−14.

127. Steindel M, Kramer Pacheco L, Scholl D, Soares M, de Moraes MH, Eger I, et al. Characterization of *Trypanosoma cruzi* isolated from humans, vectors, and animal reservoirs following an outbreak of acute human Chagas disease in Santa Catarina State, Brazil. *Diagn Microbiol Infect Dis* 2008;**60**:25−32.

128. Valente S.A.S., Valente V.C., Pin A.Y. Epidemiologia e transmissao oral da doença de Chagas na Amazonia Brasiliera. In: Organizacion Panamericana de la Salud/ Organizacion Mundial de la Salud W, editor. *Informe de la consulta técnica em epidemiologia, prevencion y manejo de la transmission de la enfermedad de Chagas como enfermedad transmitida por alimentos (ETA)*; 2006. p. 21—6.

129. Nobrega AA, Garcia MH, Tatto E, Obara MT, Costa E, Sobel J, et al. Oral transmission of Chagas disease by consumption of acai palm fruit, Brazil. *Emerg Infect Dis* 2009;**15**:653—5.

130. Coura JR, Junqueira AC. Surveillance, health promotion and control of Chagas disease in the Amazon region-medical attention in the Brazilian Amazon region: a proposal. *Mem Inst Oswaldo Cruz* 2015;**110**:825—30.

131. de Noya BA, Gonzalez ON. An ecological overview on the factors that drives to *Trypanosoma cruzi* oral transmission. *Acta Trop* 2015;**151**:94—102.

132. Coura JR. Special issue on Chagas disease. *Mem Inst Oswaldo Cruz* 2015;**110**:275—6.

133. Alarcon de Noya B, Diaz-Bello Z, Colmenares C, Ruiz-Guevara R, Mauriello L, Zavala-Jaspe R, et al. Large urban outbreak of orally acquired acute Chagas disease at a school in Caracas, Venezuela. *J Infect Dis* 2010;**201**:1308—15.

134. Blanchet D, Brenière SF, Schijman AG, Bisio M, Simon S, Veron V, et al. First report of a family outbreak of Chagas disease in French Guiana and posttreatment follow-up. *Infect Genet Evol* 2014;**28**:245—50.

135. Santalla-Vargas J, Oporto P, Espinoza E, Ríos T, Brutus L. Primer brote reportado de la enfermedad de Chagas en la Amazonía Boliviana: reporte de 14 casos agudos por transmisión oral de *Trypanosoma cruzi* en Guayaramerín, Beni-bolivia. *BIOFARBO* 2011;**19**:52—8.

136. Coura JR, Junqueira AC, Fernandes O, Valente SA, Miles MA. Emerging Chagas disease in Amazonian Brazil. *Trends Parasitol* 2002;**18**:171—6.

137. PAHO/WHO, Organizacion Panamericana de la Salud/Organizacion Mundial de la Salud W, editor. Informe de la consulta técnica em epidemiologia, prevencion y manejo de la transmission de la enfermedad de Chagas como enfermedad transmitida por alimentos (ETA) 2006.

138. Ribeiro M, Nitz N, Santana C, Moraes A, Hagstrom L, Andrade R, et al. Sexual transmission of *Trypanosoma cruzi* in murine model. *Exp Parasitol* 2016;**162**:1—6.

139. Carvalho LO, Abreu-Silva AL, Hardoim Dde J, Tedesco RC, Mendes VG, da Costa SC, et al. *Trypanosoma cruzi* and myoid cells from seminiferous tubules: interaction and relation with fibrous components of extracellular matrix in experimental Chagas' disease. *Int J Exp Pathol* 2009;**90**:52—7.

140. Carvalho TL, Ribeiro RD, Lopes RA. The male reproductive organs in experimental Chagas' disease. I. Morphometric study of the vas deferens in the acute phase of the disease. *Exp Pathol* 1991;**41**:203—14.

141. Herrera L, Urdaneta-Morales S. Experimental transmission of *Trypanosoma cruzi* through the genitalia of albino mice. *Mem Inst Oswaldo Cruz* 2001;**96**:713—17.

142. Martin DL, Lowe KR, McNeill T, Thiele EA, Roellig DM, Zajdowicz J, et al. Potential sexual transmission of *Trypanosoma cruzi* in mice. *Acta Trop* 2015;**149**:15—18.

143. Teixeira AR, Roters F, Mott KE. Acute Chagas disease. *Gaz Med Bahia* 1970;**70**:176e—86e.

144. Jorg ME, Oliva R. Presencia de tripomastigotes en sangue menstrual de mujeres con *Trypanosoma cruzi*. *Rev Arg Parasitol* 1980;**1**.

145. Concetti H, Retegui M, Perez G, Perez H. Chagas' disease of the cervix uteri in a patient with acquired immunodeficiency syndrome. *Hum Pathol* 2000;**31**:120—2.

# Protective host response to *Trypanosoma cruzi* and its limitations

C. Truyens[1] and Y. Carlier[1,2]

[1]Université Libre de Bruxelles (ULB), Brussels, Belgium, [2]Tulane University, New Orleans, LA, United States

## Chapter Outline

*T. cruzi* induces a complex immune response owing to the simultaneous presence in the vertebrate host of extracellular trypomastigotes disseminating in biological fluids and intracellular amastigotes multiplying in the cytoplasm of a wide variety of cell types, requiring different effector mechanisms to be controlled.

American Trypanosomiasis Chagas Disease. DOI: http://dx.doi.org/10.1016/B978-0-12-801029-7.00026-5

Knowledge mainly comes from the experimental mouse model of infection, widely used as the infection progresses similarly in mouse and humans, resulting after the acute parasitemic phase, in chronic parasite persistence. However, experimental data cannot be systematically extrapolated to human infection since mouse and human immune systems display subtle differences.[1] In addition, most mouse models uses specific pathogen-free animals, therefore, they are not comparable to humans as they have not experienced other infections responsible for trained immunity.[2]

This chapter deals with current knowledge on innate and adaptive immune responses involved in the control of acute *T. cruzi* infection, from initiation to effector mechanisms, as well as immunoregulation and escape mechanisms allowing the parasite to persist lifelong at low levels in tissues. It is an update of the previous edition, in which much more detail and precision can been found.[3]

# Innate immune response in *T. cruzi* infection

## Soluble components of the innate system

When invading its vertebrate host, the parasite is facing soluble microbicidal factors such as the complement system, natural antibodies, and antimicrobial peptides rapidly produced by epithelial cells and infiltrating leucocytes. *T. cruzi* trypomastigotes and amastigotes activate the lectin and/or the alternative pathways of the complement.[4] They however express various molecules rendering them resistant to complement lysis, allowing them to invade cells. Natural antibodies produced by B-1 B cells are also involved in early protection against *T. cruzi*.[5] In humans, part of natural Abs, called anti-Gal Ab, can lyse trypomastigotes by binding to surface α-galactosyl residues.[6] Infected epithelial cells rapidly produce the antimicrobial peptide defensin α-1 able to induce irreversible damages to trypomastigotes and amastigotes.[7]

## Innate recognition of *T. cruzi* infection

Pattern recognition receptors (PRRs) recognize molecular motifs shared by different types of microbes and activate the transcription of genes involved in inflammation and antimicrobial responses.[8] TLR2, TLR4 (surface receptors), TLR7, and TLR9 (endosomal receptors) have to date been implicated in the recognition of *T. cruzi*. TLR2 (in association with TLR6) recognizes the glycosylphosphatidylinositol (GPI) anchors of surface mucins of blood trypomastigotes (tGPI).[9] How their lipid moiety buried in the plasma membrane are accessible for TLR recognition is not clear. Structural requirements are incompatible with the site of cleavage by the parasite GPI-PLC, which in addition is not expressed by trypomastigotes.[10] tGPI anchors might be released with vesicles shed by trypomastigotes.[11] TLR2 also recognizes Tc52 shed by trypomastigotes and amastigotes.[12] TLR4 recognizes surface ceramide-containing GPI-anchors known as glycoinositolphospholipids (GIPLs),[13] and may also be activated by the parasite trans-sialidase (TS) independently of GIPL recognition.[14] TLR7 is involved in *T. cruzi* recognition, though no more information is available.[15] TLR9 recognizes unmethylated CpG sequences of *T. cruzi* DNA.[16]

*T. cruzi* also engages other PRRs such as the surface mannose receptor, the lectin-like receptor mMGL,[17] and the cytosolic NLRs NOD-1 and NOD-2.[18] The parasites have recently been shown to also activate the inflammasome NLRP3.[19]

TLRs and NOD-1 significantly contribute to control the acute infection. TLR9 plays a dominant role, TLR2 exerts an activating or immunoregulatory role depending on cell type, while TLR4 seems to play a minor role,[13,20–22] whereas the TRIF pathway synergizes with the Myd88 one.[23] Importantly, when the parasite invades its vertebrate host, several days are needed before parasite TLR-ligands become available for TLR recognition, delaying potent innate immune recognition.[24]

## Cells of the innate immune system

### Natural killer (NK) and other innate cells

Both cytotoxic and IFN-γ producing NK cells are quickly induced upon *T. cruzi* infection.[25] NK cell depletion reveals their crucial role in the control of acute infection.[26] The protective role of NK cells likely preferentially relies on IFN-γ production than on cytotoxicity. Indeed, NK cells expressing granulysin, a cytotoxic protein expressed by humans (absent in mouse) and able to kill intracellular amastigotes,[27] do not significantly contribute to the control of infection.[28] However, cytotoxic NK cells can directly kill trypomastigotes in vitro.[29] IFN-γ production by NK cells requires the indirect action of parasites on accessory cells producing IL-12[30,31]. The protective effect of IFN-γ released by NK cells mainly relies on activation of macrophages and other cells to limit *T. cruzi* replication during the early acute phase of the infection.[25]

Innate lymphoid cells[32] other than NK cells have to date not been investigated in *T. cruzi* infection, at odds of "innate-like" lymphocytes such as B1-B cells, invariant natural killer T (iNKT) cells and γδ-T cell subsets.[33] Plasma B cells, recently identified has important rapid producers of cytokines,[34] are discussed later in this chapter.

*T. cruzi* associated with IL-12 triggers rapid production of IFN-γ by iNKT cells. Depending on the cytokine environment, they might exert beneficial or harmful effects,[3,35] as γδ-T lymphocytes, probably in relation to subsets presenting different properties in different tissues.[36,37] Liver γδ T could contribute to the particularly efficient control of parasite multiplication in this organ.[38]

### Neutrophils

Neutrophils are rapidly recruited at the site of infection[39] and infiltrate infected organs. They contribute to eliminate parasites by uptaking and killing trypomastigotes (overall if they are opsonizd by Abs)[40] as well as amastigotes released from infected tissues.[41] A nice study showed recently that neutrophils generate extracellular traps (NETs) in the presence of *T. cruzi* in a TLR2 and TLR4-dependent manner,[42] that help limit the infection by affecting the infectivity/pathogenicity of parasites.[42] Neutrophils also produce cytokines/chemokines involved in shaping the immune response.[43]

## Monocytes/macrophages

Macrophages have received much attention as crucial players in host defense against *T. cruzi* as they simultaneously act as host cells and antigen-presenting cells.

### Macrophage activation

Macrophage activation is a complex process involving coordinate/synergistic action of signals from cytokines, chemokines, and PAMPs.[44] IFN-γ is the most potent macrophage-activating factor, inducing "inflammatory" macrophages, called "M1."[45] Full macrophage activation requires previous priming that may be provided by low levels of IFNs. Some tissular macrophages are likely physiologically primed under homeostatic conditions.[44] To avoid toxicity associated with excessive activation, IFNs concurrently induce the expression of the inhibitory proteins SOCS whereas TLR engagement induces the production of the macrophage deactivator IL-10.[46]

Priming of macrophages in *T. cruzi* infection may relate to type 1 IFNs produced at the site of parasite entry[47] and IFN-γ produced by iNKT cells. NK cell-derived IFN-γ would play a role in a second step.[39] Macrophage activation is strengthened later on when higher amounts of IFN-γ are produced by T lymphocytes.[48]

*T. cruzi* activates mouse macrophages to produce IL-1, IL-12, TNF-α, IL-10, nitric oxide (NO), and ROS,[49–51] and likely also IL-18 and IL-27.[52,53] tGPI, Tc52, Ssp4, AgC10, and galactose moieties are all *T. cruzi* molecules able to directly activate macrophages.[17,54–56] Inflammasomes play also a significant role in the IL-1β response.[51,57] The parasite also activates human monocytes.[58,59]

### Trypanocidal action of macrophages

IFN-γ[60,61] and macrophages[62] play a crucial role in the control of *T. cruzi* infection. ROS mediate intraphagosomal killing of *T. cruzi* before they escape in the cytoplasm,[63,64] though they would have a limited role in controlling parasite multiplication[65] owing to several antioxidant enzymes.[66] However, ROS may also favor parasite entry and multiplication.[67] NO is the principal effector molecule involved in macrophage-mediated killing of *T. cruzi*,[68] at least in mouse.[62] Production of NO is much slower in human monocytes than mouse macrophages. More parasites might therefore escape in the cytoplasm before being killed in the phagosome,[64] resulting in less efficient NO-dependent control in humans.

NO production is triggered by IFN-γ, upregulated by TNF-α and type 1 IFNs,[65,69] and downregulated by IL-10 and TGF-β in "alternatively" activated macrophages (see Section, Modulation of immune responses by macrophages). Moreover, TGF-β induces polyamine synthesis that favors parasite replication and persistence.[63,70]

Other mechanisms also contribute to limit parasite multiplication, involving indoleamine 2,3-dioxygenase (IDO),[71] the immunity-related GTPases IRG47 and LRG47.[23,72,73]

### Modulation of immune responses by macrophages

"Classically" IFN-γ-activated "M1" macrophages produce IL-12 which drives type 1 immune responses. In the presence of IL-10, glucocorticoïds or apoptotic cells, macrophages are "alternatively" activated ("M2"),[74] producing mainly IL-10 and TGF-β which antagonize the protective action of IFN-γ.

IL-12 plays a crucial role in resistance to *T. cruzi* infection[75] due to its ability to promote IFN-γ and TNF-α-dependent NO production.[76] IL-18 may contribute to trigger IFN-γ.[77] Its early production, combined with IL-12, improves resistance to infection.[52]

IL-27 is involved in protection[78] by favoring Th1-dependent control of parasite multiplication and limiting Th2 responses and alternative macrophage activation. It has also a beneficial effect for the host by controlling excessive production of pro-inflammatory cytokines, like IL-6 and TNF-α, known to be involved in mortality when released at high levels during acute infection.[79]

IL-10 limits the potential harmful effects of excessive inflammatory cytokines.[46] When produced in higher quantities by M2 macrophages, it prevents the activating action of IFN-γ. IL-10 also regulates the interplay between macrophages and NK cells.[25] The balance between IFN-γ and IL-10 expression is crucial in modulating the resistance or susceptibility to *T. cruzi* infection and depends on the host genetic background: cruzipain favors M2 macrophage activation in Balb/c mice,[80] while in C57BL/6 mice it generates a predominant Th1 response.[81]

Other immunosuppressive or anti-inflammatory mediators like TGF-β and PGE2 are produced during the acute phase of infection.[82,83] Interestingly, the parasite activates this cytokine to invade cells bearing TGF-β receptors while TGF-β limits IFN-γ-activation of macrophages.[84,85] On the other hand, PGE2 limits the production of IFN-γ and TNF-α[83] known to have harmful effects when present at too high levels,[86,79] while preserving the NO-dependent trypanocidal action. Yet it exerts a detrimental effect by inhibiting lymphocyte proliferation and IL-2 production.[87]

## Macrophages as antigen-presenting cells

*T. cruzi* macrophage infection impairs Ag presentation to CD4[+] T cells, leading to a reduced proliferation.[88] This is related to impeded ability to take up and catabolize exogenous antigen, decreased expression of MHC class II molecules, and/or defective adhesion to T cells (see Section 4.1), but likely not to deficient delivery of co-stimulatory signals.[88,89]

On the contrary, *T. cruzi* does not inhibit MHC class I Ag presentation to CD8[+] T cells.[90] However, MHC I-dependent Ag presentation may take time to become efficient, through a delay in immunoproteasome synthesis, as well as in MHC class I mRNA synthesis and cell surface expression.[91] Such delay results from transient inhibition by the parasite of protein tyrosine phosphatase in macrophage. Thus, in the first hours after invasion, the parasite could delay early CTL-mediated immunity long enough to facilitate parasite establishment inside the host.[91]

# Dendritic cells (DCs) and the initiation of the adaptive immune response

*T. cruzi* increases expression of MHC-I, -II, and costimulatory molecules on myeloid DCs.[92,93] Activated DCs are critical for inducing protective immune response by producing IL-12 to induce IFN-$\gamma$ release by CD4$^+$ and CD8$^+$ T cells.[94-96] Cruzipain (see hereunder), HSP70,[92,97] and Tc52[12] have been shown to activate DCs, while sialylated structures of *T. cruzi* limit their IL-12 response by engaging the inhibitory receptor Siglec-E.[98] TLRs engagement on DCs is not absolutely required to develop a Th1 response to *T. cruzi*.[94] Intracellular Ca$^{2+}$ mobilization is rather the activating signal of DCs.[94,95] Ca$^{2+}$ mobilization is triggered by parasite entry into the cell as well as by bradykinin produced upon the action of the parasite protease cruzipain on kininogen.[95] TLR-2 indirectly potentiates the bradykinin-dependent activation of DC.[99] Macrophage migration inhibitory factor (MIF) and C5a (produced upon complement activation) also contributes to DC activation.[100,101]

# Adaptive immune response: induction, characterization, and role of the T cell response

## T cell epitopes

Epitopes presented by MHC class II molecules to mouse or human CD4$^+$ T cells have been identified in the catalytic domain of *T. cruzi* TS,[102] in the variant SA85-1.1 of TS,[103] in cruzipain,[80] in KMP1,[104] and in the amastigote surface protein 2 (ASP-2).[105] A particular epitope of SA85-1.1 seems to be a major Th1 inducer,[103] while cruzipain preferentially induces Th2 cells.[80]

CD8$^+$ T cell responses develop against an array of parasite antigens.[106,107] Target antigens of mouse and human CD8$^+$ T cells have been described in the TS family of *T. cruzi* molecules like TSA-1 (trypomastigote surface antigen−1), ASP-1 and -2 (amastigote surface proteins), FL-160 (flagellar-associated antigen family specific of trypomastigotes).[108−111,112] In mouse, the paraflagellar rod proteins 2, 3 (PFR2 and PFR3), and 4 (PAR4), and MASP family members have more recently been identified as targets of CD8$^+$ T cells.[113−115] Other human MHC class I-binding peptides have been found in the parasite cruzipain, the calcium-binding protein (CaBP), LYT1 protein,[111,116,117] the ribosomal protein TcP2beta,[118] KMP1,[119] and HSP70.[120] Interestingly, despite the fact that parasites concomitantly express a large number of polymorphic proteins of the TS family, the CD8$^+$ T cell response is highly focused on a restricted repertoire of TS epitopes.[121−123]

## T lymphocytes in the control of the infection

The T cell response to *T. cruzi* exhibits a mixed Th1/Th2/Th17 profile. NK-derived IFN-$\gamma$ and IL-12 produced by DCs and/or macrophages contribute in establishing a type 1 environment, while IL-18 would rather exert an immunomodulatory effect.[3,124,125] The CD8$^+$ T cell response may develop independently of TLR engagement, IFNs, and CD4$^+$ T cell help,[126−128] though CD4$^+$ T cells allowed to reach CD8$^+$ T cell frequency are able to control the infection.[122] A role for signals associated with NADPH oxidase activation in macrophages has recently been reported.[129]

The critical dependence on both CD8$^+$ and CD4$^+$ T cell-mediated responses for control of acute *T. cruzi* infection in mouse is unequivocal.[123,130] The protective effect of CD4$^+$ Th1 cells relates to IFN-γ activation of trypanocidal action of macrophages and to their help for inducing CD8$^+$ T cells and B cell switch to produce protective Ab isotypes.[131] Even if IFN-γ released by CD8$^+$ T cells also contribute to the control of the infection,[132] the main protective function of CD8$^+$ T cells is likely related to their cytotoxic properties.[127] Of note, human but not mouse CD8$^+$ T cells express granulysin, able to kill intracellular amastigotes, at odds with perforin and granzyme.[28] Studies of the group of Tarleton have provided a lot of information on CD8$^+$ T cells in *T. cruzi* infection.[123,133] The mechanisms underlying the inability to totally eliminate *T. cruzi*-infected cells are to date not precisely known. Data suggest that TGF-β, regulatory CD4$^+$ T cells, or exhaustion do not play a major role in this,[134–137] though exhausted CD8$^+$ T cells may.[138] In humans, a weakening of CD8$^+$ T cell response can be observed,[123,139] likely associated with the expression of inhibitory receptors such as PD-1, CTLA-4, 2B4, CD160, and TIM-3[140] and perturbed IL-7/IL-7R T cell signaling in chronically infected patients.[141]

## Regulatory T cells

Few data are available about regulatory T cells (Treg) during *T. cruzi* acute infection (most studies address the role of Treg in the pathology of chronic cardiopathy, which is not the topic of this chapter). CD4$^+$CD25$^+$ Tregs expressing PD-1 or CTLA-4 have been detected during acute *T. cruzi* infection.[142,143] The amastigote protein SSP4 is involved in the induction of TGF-β-producing Treg,[144] as well as a galectine-1-dependent mechanism.[145] Tregs favor parasite growth by limiting IFN-γ production. However, their immunosuppressive activity may be rather beneficial by restraining inflammation, thereby prolonging survival.[143]

## The recently disclosed role of IL-17 in T. cruzi infection

Since its discovery in 1993, IL-17 represented the hallmark of the Th17 cell subset, having an important role in protecting the host against extracellular pathogens (particularly fungi) by activating neutrophils. It has more recently been documented that other T cell subsets such as γδT and natural killer T (NKT) cells, as well a subset of ILCs, can also produce IL-17 in response to innate stimuli.[32,146]

Interest in IL-17 in *T. cruzi* infection has followed the demonstration, in 2010, of the crucial beneficial involvement of IL-17 in the control of acute infection.[147,148] It was shown that IL-17 was mainly produced by CD4$^+$ T cells during the acute infection, though CD8$^+$ T cells[58] and NKT and γδT cells[149] also contribute. Of note, the ability to induce IL-17 production may vary according to the parasite strain/DTU.[58]

A still more fascinating discovery is that B cells have been recently disclosed as a major early source of IL-17 in *T. cruzi* infection through an unprecedented way, independent of Ag recognition by BCR or of TLR engagement.[150] The authors showed that parasite TS modifies the glycosylation pattern of surface CD45 molecule of B cells, leading to IL-17 release by a noncanonical signaling mechanism. This constitutes one of the rare examples described to date that B cells bring more than antibodies to the fight against pathogens.[151]

Maximal IL-17 levels are reached during the acute phase of *T. cruzi* infection. IL-17 is thought to reduce inflammation and mortality by recruiting suppressive IL-10-producing neutrophils.[152] The mechanism by which IL-17 limits parasite multiplication is less clear. It might rely to restriction of IFN-$\gamma$-related control mechanisms (Th17 cells may inhibit Th1 response[148]). It has however recently been shown that IL-17 is able to limit parasite multiplication in macrophages through a particular mechanism: though favoring the entry of parasites into macrophages, IL-17 facilitates their killing by prolonging their residency in endosomal/lysosomal compartments, which enhances exposure to antimicrobial effectors.[153] This mechanism may be strongly strain-dependent.

# Adaptive immune response: the B cell response and production of antibodies

*T. cruzi* infection is characterized by the production of both parasite-specific and unspecific Ab arising from polyclonal B cell stimulation.[154,155] Polyclonal activation is discussed later in this chapter.

## Targets of T. cruzi-specific Ab

Molecules of the TS family (expressed by trypomastigotes but not or poorly by amastigotes) are major targets of Ab. The major B epitope is a repetitive sequence called SAPA (shed acute phase antigen). SAPA-repeats induce an early Ab response[156] and promotes the production of Ab directed to the catalytic domain that inhibit TS enzyme activity.[157] Cruzipain is also strongly immunogenic and elicits Ab.[158] Other *T. cruzi*-specific Ab neutralize parasite molecules involved in parasite−host interaction, like CRP (complement-regulatory proteins),[159] T-DAF,[160] "TIF" (trypanosomal immunosuppressive factor),[161] HSP70,[162] the flagellar calcium-binding protein (FCaBP 24 kDa),[163] and the adhesion sequence RGD.[164] In humans only, Ab directed against $\alpha$-galactosyl residues abundantly expressed on surface mucins of trypomastigotes strongly increases during infection.[165]

## Isotypes of specific Ab

In human infection, IgA Abs appear first, followed by IgM and IgG. Ab levels peak during the acute phase. IgA and IgM are generally no more detectable in the chronic phase, while IgG persist lifelong in untreated patients. IgG1 subclass predominates among IgG, followed by IgG3. Such isotypes are known to be associated with type 1-responses.[166] A similar kinetics is observed in mouse *T. cruzi* infection, though IgM Ab persist in the chronic phase of the infection (probably related to the short time span as compared to years-long chronic phase in humans).[154] In mouse, the IgG specific response is also dominated by an isotype known to be driven by Th1 immune responses, i.e., IgG2a,[167] over IgG1 Ab associated with Th2 responses.[154]

## Effector mechanisms of Ab

The production of specific Ab in *T. cruzi* infection starts rather late. High levels of Ab are reached when parasitemia starts to decrease and there have an important protective role in the transition from acute to chronic phase of infection.[168] Mechanisms of clearance of extracellular trypomastigotes by Ab mainly relate to direct lysis of parasites and to phagocytosis of opsonized parasites. These are reviewed elsewhere.[3,169] Briefly, some Abs induce complement-dependent lysis of parasites by neutralizing the molecules that protect the parasite against complement lysis,[170] while anti-Gal Abs induce lysis of trypomastigotes.[6] Anti-$\alpha$-Gal Ab would however be lytic only before the parasite covers itself very quickly with sialic acid residues that mask $\alpha$-Gal epitopes, preventing this lysis mechanism.

Ab-opsonized parasites are also eliminated after phagocytosis by activated cells expressing the Fc$\gamma$R. The Ab isotypes able to bind to these Fc$\gamma$R, i.e., IgG2a, IgG2b, and IgG1 (in mouse), have a preferential role in parasite clearance.[171] Ab-opsonization also leads to deposition of complement components on their membrane, allowing their uptake by phagocytic cells expressing complement receptors.[172] Macrophages and neutrophils can mediate parasite immune clearance,[169] mainly occurring in liver and spleen.[173]

# Deregulations of T and B lymphocyte responses

## Defective lymphocyte responses

Immunosuppression has been broadly documented in *T. cruzi*-infected humans. It results from both direct and indirect action of parasites on lymphocytes. Mechanisms are detailed by Truyens and Carlier.[3] Briefly, suboptimal B and T lymphoproliferative responses result from insufficient activation of Ag presenting cells and perturbations of the IL-2/IL-2R pathway. Myeloid-derived suppressor cells (MDSC)[174,175] and PGE2[83] also contribute to immunosuppression. MDSC may however also exert a beneficial role by preventing excessive inflammation.[176] The recently disclosed interaction of the parasite cruzipain with the inhibitory receptor Siglec-E[177] might also contribute to dampen the immune response.[178]

Besides, apoptosis of B and T lymphocytes, particularly pronounced during the acute phase of infection,[179] likely contributes to delay the Ab response.[180] B and T cell depletion depends on Fas/FasL, TNF-$\alpha$, and NO pathways, as well as the action of the parasite trans-sialidase.[3,181] Apoptosis of CD4$^+$ T cells, but not of CD8$^+$ T cells, in chronic infection is rather related to the physiological process of activation-induced programmed cell death.[182]

Finally, suboptimal specific response also relates to the abundant expression by *T. cruzi* of polymorphic molecules of the TS superfamily. Some T cell epitopes of these molecules are major CD4$^+$ T cell antigens (the variant SA85-1.1, for instance) and have a low affinity for T cell TCRs. They therefore induce incomplete or anergic T cell rather than optimal responses.[183] Such "altered peptide presentation" may have a substantial impact in biasing the global response to suboptimal (though Th1) levels.[103]

## Polyclonal activation

*T. cruzi* induces in mouse an abundant and long-lasting polyclonal plasma cell response producing mostly nonparasite specific antibodies,[154,184] in which B1-B cells would play an important role.[185] Several parasite molecules are involved in polyclonal B cell activation (reviewed by Truyens and Carlier[3]). Polyclonal activation is thought to constitute an immune evasion mechanism by masking/deviating the specific responses, thereby limiting the control of infection. Moreover, it might participate to enlarge the B repertoire to self-antigens, favoring the production of autoreactive Ab participating in the pathology of the chronic infection.

# Escape mechanisms of *T. cruzi* to the immune responses

Lymphocyte immunosuppression and polyclonal B cell activation indubitably facilitate the parasite to establish in its host. However, as said by Tarleton, "failure to completely eliminate the parasites during acute infection might rather reflects the success of *T. cruzi* in evading host immune responses than results from a suppressed or dysregulated immune response."[133] Indeed, the parasite also makes use of other remarkable evasion strategies to slow down the initiation of the immune response and limit its effector action. Points discussed hereunder do not constitute an exhaustive list of escape mechanisms, summarized in excellent recent reviews.[186−188]

## Resistance to complement lysis

Trypomastigotes must evade this powerful mechanism of killing before entry into host cells and again after they emerge. They possess membrane-bound proteins that impair complement activation, such as complement regulatory proteins (160-CRP),[189] decay-accelerating factor (T-DAF),[190] gp58/68,[191] and calreticulin[192] expressed by trypomastigotes, and a 27−32 kDa protein expressed by metacyclic trypomastigotes.[193] Amastigotes resist complement lysis through a mechanism totally different from trypomastigotes.[194]

## Intracellular survival

*T. cruzi* possesses a large arsenal of antioxidant enzymes allowing it to resist to the trypanocidal action of phagocytes.[66] The parasite also takes advantage when low amounts of NO are produced in resident macrophages, as it favors parasite proliferation instead of impeding it.[63] Next, GIPLs and GPI-anchors rapidly induce apoptosis of resident macrophages, an effect reinforced by IFN-γ. This leads to the release of amastigotes before they are killed intracellularly, which may then infect other cells.[195] Moreover, amastigotes preferentially invade nonactivated macrophages, i.e., not armed to kill the parasite. This may be related to their use of the mannose receptor (MR) for entry, the expression of which is decreased on IFN-γ-activated macrophages.[196] Trypomastigotes do not bind to MR, conferring to amastigotes an advantage to achieve the persistence of the infection.

Besides, cruzipain limits macrophage activation by inducing proteolysis or the transcription factor NF-kB, leading to unresponsiveness of the macrophage during early infection. This immune evasion mechanism may be critical for *T. cruzi* survival during early infection with a low number of trypmastigotes,[197] while abundant lymphocyte apoptosis associated with the acute phase of infection triggers alternatively activated macrophages less able to control parasite replication.[198]

The question still remains as to how *T. cruzi* is able to persist, albeit at very low levels, in muscle cells, some neurons, and adipose tissue. Muscle cells produce less NO and more polyamines than phagocytes, which favor parasite multiplication.[63] Additionally, myoglobin and neuroglobin are known to scavenge toxic reactive oxygen and nitrogen species,[199] while parasite cruzipain and TS induce in cardiomyocytes the production of antiapoptotic molecules. This will protect the host cell from apoptosis induced by oxidative stress, TNF-α, and Fas-FasL pathway and is expected to help the completion of the multiplicative cycle by increasing the life span of the host cell.[200,201] Survival of *T. cruzi* in muscle cells is associated with its ability to limit the expression of NF-κB-dependent genes in these cells, contrary to what happens in epithelial and endothelial cells and fibroblasts.[202] It is also proposed that particular metabolic features of muscle and adipose tissue provide a survival advantage for *T. cruzi* in these cells.[24]

## *Escape from the action of Ab*

*T. cruzi* can limit the Fc-dependent effector functions of specific Ab bound to its surface by two mechanisms. First, cruzipain can digest the Fc part of IgG, impairing their binding to FcR.[203] Second, it expresses on its surface a factor that binds mammalian Igs through their Fc fragment,[204] inhibiting Ig-mediated attachment and penetration of *T. cruzi* into macrophages.

*T. cruzi* TS also contributes to parasite survival. During the acute phase, TS molecules bearing SAPA repeats are abundantly released by the parasite. The immunodominance of SAPA prevents the early formation of neutralizing Ab directed against the catalytic site, situated away on the molecule. As long as TS enzyme is active, it profits the parasite by favoring host cell invasion[205] and conferring resistance to lytic anti-α-GAL Ab.[6] Later on, when SAPA sequences are masked by Abs, TS-neutralizing Ab are produced. Neutralization of TS activity favors survival of the host by limiting massive cell invasion by the parasite.[205]

## Being a stealth parasite, dampening and disturbing T cell responses

Tarleton has nicely pointed out various mechanisms allowing the parasite to delay the initiation of the immune response and its efficacy to favor its persistence.[133] It results from the ability of the parasite to delay its recognition by TLRs, to modify surface sialylation of CD8[+] T cells (which dampens the CD8[+] T cell response) and to simultaneously express many variant TS epitopes. Another report studying the CD8[+] T cell response against the amastigote protein ASP2 supports that immunodominance, by avoiding broad immune response, constitutes an advantage for the parasite.[206]

The dominant response of CD8[+] T cells against TS might also override a more efficient response directed against other targets. Tarleton reported that the T cell epitope PAR4 was presented earlier than molecules of the trans-sialidase family.[114] PAR4-specific CD8[+] T cells provide significant protection by killing infected cells. This beneficial response might be thereafter thwarted by the dominant CD8[+] T cell response against TS epitopes which on the contrary seem to be dispensable to control infection.[207]

# Conclusion

Control of *T. cruzi* infection requires the activation of multiple immune effector mechanisms in relation to the presence of both extracellular trypomastigotes and intracellular amastigotes. Host protection is mainly governed by IFNs and IL-17. IFN-γ is required for controlling parasite multiplication, while IL-17 rather prevents damage due to excessive inflammation. The role of this latter cytokine has been more recently disclosed and surprisingly, shown to be produced early during the infection by B cells through an unprecedented mechanism. It is also worth noting that neutrophils and iNKT cells seem to have an important role in the very initial steps of the infection, without forgetting the essential contribution of NK cells and macrophages later on, as well as CD8[+] T cells. The parasite disposes of various mechanisms allowing it to establish slowly as well as to escape the diversified immune response. Its ability to temporarily limit Ag presentation through MHC class I molecules (delaying the recognition of infected host cells by cytotoxic lymphocytes) and to favor the release of amastigotes (through host cell apoptosis) that invade preferentially unactivated macrophages, is particular. Late chronic infection in humans is associated with the progressive disappearance of early activated T cells and waning of T cell responses, at least in the absence of reinfections.

Trans-sialidases, mucins, and cruzipain are the main parasite molecules regulating the host response in conjunction with several parasite PRR-ligands, not all identified to date. Variations in the expression of these polymorphic molecules between parasite genotypes/DTUs are more and more recognized as determining the virulence of *T. cruzi*. The host genetic background also accounts for susceptibility or resistance to infection in relation to its ability to produce better and more rapidly protective or immunoregulatory cytokines.

Among microbicidal molecules produced by host cells, nitric oxide has for long been identified as pivotal in infected mice, since the parasite is well equipped to resist reactive oxygen species. However, it has to be kept in mind that NO also exerts dramatically adverse effects for the host by inducing immunosuppression and lymphocyte apoptosis. This dampens the immune response and induces alternatively activated macrophages unable to control the infection. IRG proteins might be more important than thought for controlling parasite multiplication in humans.

Comprehension of the inability to eliminate the parasite is progressing and should, hopefully, come up with immunotherapeutic strategies helping to cure lifelong chronically infected people, keeping in mind that it remains to be known if the host would actually benefit from a better efficient immune response in the long term, since it might have pathological consequences in some chronically infected individuals.

# References

1. Mestas J, Hughes CC. Of mice and not men: differences between mouse and human immunology. *J Immunol* 2004;**172**:2731−8.
2. Boysen P, Eide DM, Storset AK. Natural killer cells in free-living *Mus musculus* have a primed phenotype. *Mol Ecol* 2011;**20**:5103−10.
3. Truyens C, Carlier Y. *Protective host response to parasite and its limitations. American Trypanosomiasis Chagas disease—One hundred years of research.* Burlington: Jenny Telleria and Michel Tibayrenc; 2010. p. 601−68.
4. Cestari I, Evans-Osses I, Schlapbach LJ, de Messias-Reason I, Ramirez MI. Mechanisms of complement lectin pathway activation and resistance by trypanosomatid parasites. *Mol Immunol* 2013;**53**:328−34.
5. Santos-Lima EC, Vasconcellos R, Reina-San-Martin B, Fesel C, Cordeiro-Da-Silva A, Berneman A, et al. Significant association between the skewed natural antibody repertoire of Xid mice and resistance to *Trypanosoma cruzi* infection. *Eur J Immunol* 2001;**31**:634−45.
6. Pereira-Chioccola VL, Acosta-Serrano A, Correia de AI, Ferguson MA, Souto-Padron T, Rodrigues MM, et al. Mucin-like molecules form a negatively charged coat that protects *Trypanosoma cruzi* trypomastigotes from killing by human anti-alpha-galactosyl antibodies. *J Cell Sci* 2000;**113**(Pt 7):1299−307.
7. Johnson CA, Rachakonda G, Kleshchenko YY, Nde PN, Madison MN, Pratap S, et al. Cellular response to *Trypanosoma cruzi* infection induces secretion of defensin α-1, which damages the flagellum, neutralizes trypanosome motility, and inhibits infection. *Infect Immun* 2013;**81**:4139−48.
8. Mogensen TH. Pathogen recognition and inflammatory signaling in innate immune defenses. *Clin Microbiol Rev* 2009;**22**:240−73. Table of Contents.
9. Campos MA, Almeida IC, Takeuchi O, Akira S, Valente EP, Procopio DO, et al. Activation of Toll-like receptor-2 by glycosylphosphatidylinositol anchors from a protozoan parasite. *J Immunol* 2001;**167**:416−23.
10. Salto ML, Furuya T, Moreno SN, Docampo R, de Lederkremer RM. The phosphatidylinositol-phospholipase C from *Trypanosoma cruzi* is active on inositolphosphoceramide. *Mol Biochem Parasitol* 2002;**119**:131−3.

11. Nogueira PM, Ribeiro K, Silveira ACO, Campos JH, Martins-Filho OA, Bela SR, et al. Vesicles from different *Trypanosoma cruzi* strains trigger differential innate and chronic immune responses. *J Extracell Vesicles* 2015;**4**:28734.

12. Ouaissi A, Guilvard E, Delneste Y, Caron G, Magistrelli G, Herbault N, et al. The *Trypanosoma cruzi* Tc52-released protein induces human dendritic cell maturation, signals via Toll-like receptor 2, and confers protection against lethal infection. *J Immunol* 2002;**168**:6366−74.

13. Oliveira AC, Peixoto JR, de Arruda LB, Campos MA, Gazzinelli RT, Golenbock DT, et al. Expression of functional TLR4 confers proinflammatory responsiveness to *Trypanosoma cruzi* glycoinositolphospholipids and higher resistance to infection with *T. cruzi*. *J Immunol* 2004;**173**:5688−96.

14. Amith SR, Jayanth P, Franchuk S, Finlay T, Seyrantepe V, Beyaert R, et al. Neu1 desialylation of sialyl alpha-2,3-linked beta-galactosyl residues of TOLL-like receptor 4 is essential for receptor activation and cellular signaling. *Cell Signal* 2010;**22**:314−24.

15. Caetano BC, Carmo BB, Melo MB, Cerny A, dos Santos SL, Bartholomeu DC, et al. Requirement of UNC93B1 reveals a critical role for TLR7 in host resistance to primary infection with *Trypanosoma cruzi*. *J Immunol Baltim Md 1950* 2011;**187**:1903−11.

16. Bartholomeu DC, Ropert C, Melo MB, Parroche P, Junqueira CF, Teixeira SM, et al. Recruitment and endo-lysosomal activation of TLR9 in dendritic cells infected with *Trypanosoma cruzi*. *J Immunol* 2008;**181**:1333−44.

17. Vázquez A, Ruiz-Rosado J, de D, Terrazas LI, Juárez I, Gomez-Garcia L, et al. Mouse macrophage galactose-type lectin (mMGL) is critical for host resistance against *Trypanosoma cruzi* infection. *Int J Biol Sci* 2014;**10**:909−20.

18. Gurung P, Kanneganti T-D. Immune responses against protozoan parasites: a focus on the emerging role of Nod-like receptors. *Cell Mol Life Sci CMLS* 2016. Available from: http://dx.doi.org/10.1007/s00018-016-2212-3.

19. Gonçalves VM, Matteucci KC, Buzzo CL, Miollo BH, Ferrante D, Torrecilhas AC, et al. NLRP3 controls *Trypanosoma cruzi* infection through a caspase-1-dependent IL-1R-independent NO production. *PLoS NTD* 2013;**7**:e2469.

20. Silva GK, Gutierrez FR, Guedes PM, Horta CV, Cunha LD, Mineo TW, et al. Cutting edge: nucleotide-binding oligomerization domain 1-dependent responses account for murine resistance against *Trypanosoma cruzi* infection. *J Immunol* 2010;**184**:1148−52.

21. Gravina HD, Antonelli L, Gazzinelli RT, Ropert C. Differential use of TLR2 and TLR9 in the regulation of immune responses during the infection with *Trypanosoma cruzi*. *PLoS ONE* 2013;**8**:e63100.

22. Bafica A, Santiago HC, Goldszmid R, Ropert C, Gazzinelli RT, Sher A. Cutting edge: TLR9 and TLR2 signaling together account for MyD88-dependent control of parasitemia in *Trypanosoma cruzi* infection. *J Immunol* 2006;**177**:3515−19.

23. Koga R, Hamano S, Kuwata H, Atarashi K, Ogawa M, Hisaeda H, et al. TLR-dependent induction of IFN-beta mediates host defense against *Trypanosoma cruzi*. *J Immunol* 2006;**177**:7059−66.

24. Padilla AM, Simpson LJ, Tarleton RL. Insufficient TLR activation contributes to the slow development of CD8+ T cell responses in *Trypanosoma cruzi* infection. *J Immunol* 2009;**183**:1245−52.

25. Cardillo F, Voltarelli JC, Reed SG, Silva JS. Regulation of *Trypanosoma cruzi* infection in mice by gamma interferon and interleukin 10: role of NK cells. *Infect Immun* 1996;**64**:128−34.

26. Duthie MS, Kahn SJ. NK cell activation and protection occur independently of natural killer T cells during *Trypanosoma cruzi* infection. *Int Immunol* 2005;**17**:607−13.

27. Jacobs T, Bruhn H, Gaworski I, Fleischer B, Leippe M. NK-lysin and its shortened analog NK-2 exhibit potent activities against *Trypanosoma cruzi*. *Antimicrob Agents Chemother* 2003;**47**:607–13.

28. Dotiwala F, Mulik S, Polidoro RB, Ansara JA, Burleigh BA, Walch M, et al. Killer lymphocytes use granulysin, perforin and granzymes to kill intracellular parasites. *Nat Med* 2016;**22**:210–16.

29. Lieke T, Graefe SE, Klauenberg U, Fleischer B, Jacobs T. NK cells contribute to the control of *Trypanosoma cruzi* infection by killing free parasites by perforin-independent mechanisms. *Infect Immun* 2004;**72**:6817–25.

30. Antunez MI, Cardoni RL. IL-12 and IFN-gamma production, and NK cell activity, in acute and chronic experimental *Trypanosoma cruzi* infections. *Immunol Lett* 2000;**71**:103–9.

31. Guilmot A, Bosse J, Carlier Y, Truyens C. Monocytes play an IL-12-dependent crucial role in driving cord blood NK cells to produce IFN-g in response to *Trypanosoma cruzi*. *PLoS NTD* 2013;**7**:e2291.

32. Sonnenberg GF, Artis D. Innate lymphoid cells in the initiation, regulation and resolution of inflammation. *Nat Med* 2015;**21**:698–708.

33. Bendelac A. Innate-like lymphocytes. *Curr Opin Immunol* 2006;**18**:517–18.

34. Dang VD, Hilgenberg E, Ries S, Shen P, Fillatreau S. From the regulatory functions of B cells to the identification of cytokine-producing plasma cell subsets. *Curr Opin Immunol* 2014;**28**:77–83.

35. Duthie MS, Kahn M, White M, Kapur RP, Kahn SJ. Both CD1d antigen presentation and interleukin-12 are required to activate natural killer T cells during *Trypanosoma cruzi* infection. *Infect Immun* 2005;**73**:1890–4.

36. Santos Lima EC, Minoprio P. Chagas' disease is attenuated in mice lacking gamma delta T cells. *Infect Immun* 1996;**64**:215–21.

37. Nomizo A, Cardillo F, Postol E, de Carvalho LP, Mengel J. V gamma 1 gammadelta T cells regulate type-1/type-2 immune responses and participate in the resistance to infection and development of heart inflammation in *Trypanosoma cruzi*-infected BALB/c mice. *Microbes Infect* 2006;**8**:880–8.

38. Sardinha LR, Elias RM, Mosca T, Bastos KR, Marinho CR, D'Imperio Lima MR, et al. Contribution of NK, NK T, gamma delta T, and alpha beta T cells to the gamma interferon response required for liver protection against *Trypanosoma cruzi*. *Infect Immun* 2006;**74**:2031–42.

39. Chessler AD, Unnikrishnan M, Bei AK, Daily JP, Burleigh BA. *Trypanosoma cruzi* triggers an early type I IFN response in vivo at the site of intradermal infection. *J Immunol* 2009;**182**:2288–96.

40. Docampo R, Casellas AM, Madeira ED, Cardoni RL, Moreno SN, Mason RP. Oxygen-derived radicals from *Trypanosoma cruzi*-stimulated human neutrophils. *FEBS Lett* 1983;**155**:25–30.

41. Villalta F, Kierszenbaum F. Role of polymorphonuclear cells in Chagas' disease. I. Uptake and mechanisms of destruction of intracellular (amastigote) forms of *Trypanosoma cruzi* by human neutrophils. *J Immunol* 1983;**131**:1504–10.

42. Sousa-Rocha D, Thomaz-Tobias M, Diniz LFA, Souza PSS, Pinge-Filho P, Toledo KA. *Trypanosoma cruzi* and its soluble antigens induce NET release by stimulating toll-like receptors. *PLoS ONE* 2015;**10**:e0139569.

43. Luna-Gomes T, Filardy AA, Rocha JDB, Decote-Ricardo D, LaRocque-de-Freitas IF, Morrot A, et al. Neutrophils increase or reduce parasite burden in *Trypanosoma cruzi*-infected macrophages, depending on host strain: role of neutrophil elastase. *PLoS ONE* 2014;**9**:e90582.

44. Schultze JL, Schmidt SV. Molecular features of macrophage activation. *Semin Immunol* 2016. Available from: http://dx.doi.org/10.1016/j.smim.2016.03.009.

45. Wang N, Liang H, Zen K. Molecular mechanisms that influence the macrophage m1−m2 polarization balance. *Front Immunol* 2014;**5**:614.

46. Hu X, Chakravarty SD, Ivashkiv LB. Regulation of interferon and Toll-like receptor signaling during macrophage activation by opposing feedforward and feedback inhibition mechanisms. *Immunol Rev* 2008;**226**:41−56.

47. Vaena de Avalos S, Blader IJ, Fisher M, Boothroyd JC, Burleigh BA. Immediate/early response to *Trypanosoma cruzi* infection involves minimal modulation of host cell transcription. *J Biol Chem* 2002;**277**:639−44.

48. Rodrigues MM, Ribeirao M, Boscardin SB. CD4 Th1 but not Th2 clones efficiently activate macrophages to eliminate *Trypanosoma cruzi* through a nitric oxide dependent mechanism. *Immunol Lett* 2000;**73**:43−50.

49. Camargo MM, Almeida IC, Pereira ME, Ferguson MA, Travassos LR, Gazzinelli RT. Glycosylphosphatidylinositol-anchored mucin-like glycoproteins isolated from *Trypanosoma cruzi* trypomastigotes initiate the synthesis of proinflammatory cytokines by macrophages. *J Immunol* 1997;**158**:5890−901.

50. Camargo MM, Andrade AC, Almeida IC, Travassos LR, Gazzinelli RT. Glycoconjugates isolated from *Trypanosoma cruzi* but not from *Leishmania* species membranes trigger nitric oxide synthesis as well as microbicidal activity in IFN-gamma-primed macrophages. *J Immunol* 1997;**159**:6131−9.

51. Dey N, Sinha M, Gupta S, Gonzalez MN, Fang R, Endsley JJ, et al. Caspase-1/ASC inflammasome-mediated activation of IL-1β-ROS-NF-κB pathway for control of *Trypanosoma cruzi* replication and survival is dispensable in NLRP3−/− macrophages. *PLoS ONE* 2014;**9**:e111539.

52. Antunez MI, Cardoni RL. Early IFN-gamma production is related to the presence of interleukin (IL)-18 and the absence of IL-13 in experimental *Trypanosoma cruzi* infections. *Immunol Lett* 2001;**79**:189−96.

53. Hamano S, Himeno K, Miyazaki Y, Ishii K, Yamanaka A, Takeda A, et al. WSX-1 is required for resistance to *Trypanosoma cruzi* infection by regulation of proinflammatory cytokine production. *Immunity* 2003;**19**:657−67.

54. Almeida IC, Gazzinelli RT. Proinflammatory activity of glycosylphosphatidylinositol anchors derived from *Trypanosoma cruzi*: structural and functional analyses. *J Leukoc Biol* 2001;**70**:467−77.

55. Fernandez-Gomez R, Esteban S, Gomez-Corvera R, Zoulika K, Ouaissi A. *Trypanosoma cruzi*: Tc52 released protein-induced increased expression of nitric oxide synthase and nitric oxide production by macrophages. *J Immunol* 1998;**160**:3471−9.

56. Ramos-Ligonio A, Lopez-Monteon A, Talamas-Rohana P, Rosales-Encina JL. Recombinant SSP4 protein from *Trypanosoma cruzi* amastigotes regulates nitric oxide production by macrophages. *Parasit Immunol* 2004;**26**:409−18.

57. Silva GK, Costa RS, Silveira TN, Caetano BC, Horta CV, Gutierrez FRS, et al. Apoptosis-associated speck-like protein containing a caspase recruitment domain inflammasomes mediate IL-1β response and host resistance to *Trypanosoma cruzi* infection. *J Immunol Baltim Md 1950* 2013;**191**:3373−83.

58. Magalhães LMD, Viana A, Chiari E, Galvão LMC, Gollob KJ, Dutra WO. Differential activation of human monocytes and lymphocytes by distinct strains of *Trypanosoma cruzi*. *PLoS NTD* 2015;**9**:e0003816.

59. Abel LCJ, Ferreira LRP, Cunha Navarro I, Baron MA, Kalil J, Gazzinelli RT, et al. Induction of IL-12 production in human peripheral monocytes by *Trypanosoma cruzi* is mediated by glycosylphosphatidylinositol-anchored mucin-like glycoproteins and potentiated by IFN- γ and CD40−CD40L interactions. *Mediators Inflamm* 2014;**2014**: 345659.

60. Torrico F, Heremans H, Rivera MT, Van Marck E, Billiau A, Carlier Y. Endogenous IFN-gamma is required for resistance to acute *Trypanosoma cruzi* infection in mice. *J Immunol* 1991;**146**:3626−32.

61. Cummings KL, Tarleton RL. Inducible nitric oxide synthase is not essential for control of *Trypanosoma cruzi* infection in mice. *Infect Immun* 2004;**72**:4081−9.

62. Lykens JE, Terrell CE, Zoller EE, Divanovic S, Trompette A, Karp CL, et al. Mice with a selective impairment of IFN-gamma signaling in macrophage lineage cells demonstrate the critical role of IFN-gamma-activated macrophages for the control of protozoan parasitic infections in vivo. *J Immunol Baltim Md 1950* 2010;**184**:877−85.

63. Peluffo G, Piacenza L, Irigoin F, Alvarez MN, Radi R. L-arginine metabolism during interaction of *Trypanosoma cruzi* with host cells. *Trends Parasitol* 2004;**20**: 363−9.

64. Piacenza L, Alvarez MN, Peluffo G, Radi R. Fighting the oxidative assault: the *Trypanosoma cruzi* journey to infection. *Curr Opin Microbiol* 2009;**12**:415−21.

65. Metz G, Carlier Y, Vray B. *Trypanosoma cruzi* upregulates nitric oxide release by IFN-gamma-preactivated macrophages, limiting cell infection independently of the respiratory burst. *Parasit Immunol* 1993;**15**:693−9.

66. Piacenza L, Peluffo G, Alvarez MN, Martínez A, Radi R. *Trypanosoma cruzi* antioxidant enzymes as virulence factors in Chagas disease. *Antioxid Redox Signal* 2013;**19**:723−34.

67. Goes GR, Rocha PS, Diniz ARS, Aguiar PHN, Machado CR, Vieira LQ. *Trypanosoma cruzi* needs a signal provided by reactive oxygen species to infect macrophages. *PLoS NTD* 2016;**10**:e0004555.

68. Gutierrez FRS, Mineo TWP, Pavanelli WR, Guedes PMM, Silva JS. The effects of nitric oxide on the immune system during *Trypanosoma cruzi* infection. *Mem Inst Oswaldo Cruz* 2009;**104**(Suppl. 1):236−45.

69. Costa VM, Torres KC, Mendonca RZ, Gresser I, Gollob KJ, Abrahamsohn IA, et al. IFNs stimulate nitric oxide production and resistance to *Trypanosoma cruzi* infection. *J Immunol* 2006;**177**:3193−200.

70. Noel W, Raes G, Hassanzadeh GG, De Baetselier P, Beschin A. Alternatively activated macrophages during parasite infections. *Trends Parasitol* 2004;**20**:126−33.

71. Knubel CP, Martinez FF, Fretes RE, Diaz LC, Theumer MG, Cervi L, et al. Indoleamine 2,3-dioxigenase (IDO) is critical for host resistance against *Trypanosoma cruzi*. *FASEB J* 2010.

72. Santiago HC, Feng CG, Bafica A, Roffe E, Arantes RM, Cheever A, et al. Mice deficient in LRG-47 display enhanced susceptibility to *Trypanosoma cruzi* infection associated with defective hemopoiesis and intracellular control of parasite growth. *J Immunol* 2005;**175**:8165−72.

73. Kim B-H, Shenoy AR, Kumar P, Bradfield CJ, MacMicking JD. IFN-inducible GTPases in host cell defense. *Cell Host Microbe* 2012;**12**:432−44.

74. Porta C, Riboldi E, Ippolito A, Sica A. Molecular and epigenetic basis of macrophage polarized activation. *Semin Immunol* 2015;**27**:237−48.

75. Aliberti JC, Cardoso MA, Martins GA, Gazzinelli RT, Vieira LQ, Silva JS. Interleukin-12 mediates resistance to *Trypanosoma cruzi* in mice and is produced by murine macrophages in response to live trypomastigotes. *Infect Immun* 1996;**64**:1961−7.

76. Munoz-Fernandez MA, Fernandez MA, Fresno M. Synergism between tumor necrosis factor-alpha and interferon-gamma on macrophage activation for the killing of intracellular *Trypanosoma cruzi* through a nitric oxide-dependent mechanism. *Eur J Immunol* 1992;**22**:301−7.

77. Muller U, Kohler G, Mossmann H, Schaub GA, Alber G, Di Santo JP, et al. IL-12-independent IFN-gamma production by T cells in experimental Chagas' disease is mediated by IL-18. *J Immunol* 2001;**167**:3346−53.

78. Böhme J, Roßnagel C, Jacobs T, Behrends J, Hölscher C, Erdmann H. Epstein−Barr virus-induced gene 3 suppresses T helper type 1, type 17 and type 2 immune responses after *Trypanosoma cruzi* infection and inhibits parasite replication by interfering with alternative macrophage activation. *Immunology* 2016;**147**:338−48.

79. Truyens C, Torrico F, Lucas R, De Baetselier P, Buurman WA, Carlier Y. The endogenous balance of soluble tumor necrosis factor receptors and tumor necrosis factor modulates cachexia and mortality in mice acutely infected with *Trypanosoma cruzi*. *Infect Immun* 1999;**67**:5579−86.

80. Giordanengo L, Guinazu N, Stempin C, Fretes R, Cerban F, Gea S. Cruzipain, a major *Trypanosoma cruzi* antigen, conditions the host immune response in favor of parasite. *Eur J Immunol* 2002;**32**:1003−11.

81. Guinazu N, Pellegrini A, Carrera-Silva EA, Aoki MP, Cabanillas AM, Girones N, et al. Immunisation with a major *Trypanosoma cruzi* antigen promotes pro-inflammatory cytokines, nitric oxide production and increases TLR2 expression. *Int J Parasitol* 2007;**37**:1243−54.

82. Lopes MF, Freire-de-Lima CG, DosReis GA. The macrophage haunted by cell ghosts: a pathogen grows. *Immunol Today* 2000;**21**:489−94.

83. Pinge-Filho P, Tadokoro CE, Abrahamsohn IA. Prostaglandins mediate suppression of lymphocyte proliferation and cytokine synthesis in acute *Trypanosoma cruzi* infection. *Cell Immunol* 1999;**193**:90−8.

84. Hall BS, Pereira MA. Dual role for transforming growth factor beta-dependent signaling in *Trypanosoma cruzi* infection of mammalian cells. *Infect Immun* 2000;**68**:2077−81.

85. Ferrão PM, d'Avila-Levy CM, Araujo-Jorge TC, Degrave WM, Gonçalves A, da S, et al. Cruzipain activates latent TGF-β from host cells during *T. cruzi* invasion. *PLoS ONE* 2015;**10**:e0124832.

86. Jacobs F, Dubois C, Carlier Y, Goldman M. Administration of anti-CD3 monoclonal antibody during experimental Chagas' disease induces CD8 + cell-dependent lethal shock. *Clin Exp Immunol* 1996;**103**:233−8.

87. Michelin MA, Silva JS, Cunha FQ. Inducible cyclooxygenase released prostaglandin mediates immunosuppression in acute phase of experimental *Trypanosoma cruzi* infection. *Exp Parasitol* 2005;**111**:71−9.

88. La Flamme AC, Kahn SJ, Rudensky AY, Van Voorhis WC. *Trypanosoma cruzi*-infected macrophages are defective in major histocompatibility complex class II antigen presentation. *Eur J Immunol* 1997;**27**:3085−94.

89. Frosch S, Kuntzlin D, Fleischer B. Infection with *Trypanosoma cruzi* selectively upregulates B7-2 molecules on macrophages and enhances their costimulatory activity. *Infect Immun* 1997;**65**:971−7.

90. Buckner FS, Wipke BT, Van Voorhis WC. *Trypanosoma cruzi* infection does not impair major histocompatibility complex class I presentation of antigen to cytotoxic T lymphocytes. *Eur J Immunol* 1997;**27**:2541−8.

91. Bergeron M, Blanchette J, Rouleau P, Olivier M. Abnormal IFN-gamma-dependent immunoproteasome modulation by *Trypanosoma cruzi*-infected macrophages. *Parasit Immunol* 2008;**30**:280−92.

92. Cuellar A, Santander SP, Thomas MC, Guzman F, Gomez A, Lopez MC, et al. Monocyte-derived dendritic cells from chagasic patients vs healthy donors secrete differential levels of IL-10 and IL-12 when stimulated with a protein fragment of *Trypanosoma cruzi* heat-shock protein-70. *Immunol Cell Biol* 2008;**86**:255−60.

93. Rodriguez P, Carlier Y, Truyens C. Activation of cord blood myeloid dendritic cells by *Trypanosoma cruzi* and parasite-specific antibodies, proliferation of CD8+ T cells, and production of IFN-γ. *Med Microbiol Immunol (Berl)* 2012;**201**:157−9.

94. Kayama H, Koga R, Atarashi K, Okuyama M, Kimura T, Mak TW, et al. NFATc1 mediates Toll-like receptor-independent innate immune responses during *Trypanosoma cruzi* infection. *PLoS Pathogens* 2009;**5**:e1000514.

95. Monteiro AC, Schmitz V, Svensjo E, Gazzinelli RT, Almeida IC, Todorov A, et al. Cooperative activation of TLR2 and bradykinin B2 receptor is required for induction of type 1 immunity in a mouse model of subcutaneous infection by *Trypanosoma cruzi*. *J Immunol* 2006;**177**:6325−35.

96. Miyahira Y, Katae M, Kobayashi S, Takeuchi T, Fukuchi Y, Abe R, et al. Critical contribution of CD28-CD80/CD86 costimulatory pathway to protection from *Trypanosoma cruzi* infection. *Infect Immun* 2003;**71**:3131−7.

97. Planelles L, Thomas M, Pulgar M, Maranon C, Grabbe S, Lopez MC. *Trypanosoma cruzi* heat-shock protein-70 kDa, alone or fused to the parasite KMP11 antigen, induces functional maturation of murine dendritic cells. *Immunol Cell Biol* 2002;**80**:241−7.

98. Erdmann H, Steeg C, Koch-Nolte F, Fleischer B, Jacobs T. Sialylated ligands on pathogenic *Trypanosoma cruzi* interact with Siglec-E (sialic acid-binding Ig-like lectin-E). *Cell Microbiol* 2009;**11**:1600−11.

99. Schmitz V, Svensjo E, Serra RR, Teixeira MM, Scharfstein J. Proteolytic generation of kinins in tissues infected by *Trypanosoma cruzi* depends on CXC chemokine secretion by macrophages activated via Toll-like 2 receptors. *J Leukoc Biol* 2009;**85**:1005−14.

100. Terrazas CA, Huitron E, Vazquez A, Juarez I, Camacho GM, Calleja EA, et al. MIF synergizes with *Trypanosoma cruzi* antigens to promote efficient dendritic cell maturation and IL-12 production via p38 MAPK. *Int J Biol Sci* 2011;**7**:1298−310.

101. Schmitz V, Almeida LN, Svensjö E, Monteiro AC, Köhl J, Scharfstein J. C5a and bradykinin receptor cross-talk regulates innate and adaptive immunity in *Trypanosoma cruzi* infection. *J Immunol Baltim Md 1950* 2014;**193**:3613−23.

102. Fujimura AE, Kinoshita SS, Pereira-Chioccola VL, Rodrigues MM. DNA sequences encoding CD4+ and CD8+ T-cell epitopes are important for efficient protective immunity induced by DNA vaccination with a *Trypanosoma cruzi* gene. *Infect Immun* 2001;**69**:5477−86.

103. Millar AE, Kahn SJ. The SA85-1.1 protein of the *Trypanosoma cruzi* trans-sialidase superfamily is a dominant T-cell antigen. *Infect Immun* 2000;**68**:3574−80.

104. Cuellar A, Rojas F, Bolanos N, Diez H, Del Carmen TM, Rosas F, et al. Natural CD4(+) T-cell responses against *Trypanosoma cruzi* KMP-11 protein in chronic chagasic patients. *Immunol Cell Biol* 2009;**87**:149−53.

105. Rampazo EV, Amorim KNS, Yamamoto MM, Panatieri RH, Rodrigues MM, Boscardin SB. Antigen targeting to dendritic cells allows the identification of a CD4 T-cell epitope within an immunodominant *Trypanosoma cruzi* antigen. *PLoS ONE* 2015;**10**:e0117778.

106. Alvarez MG, Postan M, Weatherly DB, Albareda MC, Sidney J, Sette A, et al. HLA class I-T cell epitopes from trans-sialidase proteins reveal functionally distinct subsets of CD8+ T cells in chronic Chagas disease. *PLoS NTD* 2008;**2**:e288.

107. Teh-Poot C, Tzec-Arjona E, Martínez-Vega P, Ramirez-Sierra MJ, Rosado-Vallado M, Dumonteil E. From genome screening to creation of vaccine against *Trypanosoma cruzi* by use of immunoinformatics. *J Infect Dis* 2015;**211**:258−66.

108. Wizel B, Nunes M, Tarleton RL. Identification of *Trypanosoma cruzi* trans-sialidase family members as targets of protective CD8+ TC1 responses. *J Immunol* 1997;**159**: 6120−30.

109. Wizel B, Palmieri M, Mendoza C, Arana B, Sidney J, Sette A, et al. Human infection with *Trypanosoma cruzi* induces parasite antigen-specific cytotoxic T lymphocyte responses. *J Clin Invest* 1998;**102**:1062−71.

110. Low HP, Santos MA, Wizel B, Tarleton RL. Amastigote surface proteins of *Trypanosoma cruzi* are targets for CD8+ CTL. *J Immunol* 1998;**160**:1817−23.

111. Fonseca SG, Moins-Teisserenc H, Clave E, Ianni B, Nunes VL, Mady C, et al. Identification of multiple HLA-A*0201-restricted cruzipain and FL-160 CD8+ epitopes recognized by T cells from chronically *Trypanosoma cruzi*-infected patients. *Microbes Infect* 2005;**7**:688−97.

112. Nogueira RT, Nogueira AR, Pereira MCS, Rodrigues MM, Galler R, Bonaldo MC. Biological and immunological characterization of recombinant Yellow Fever 17D viruses expressing a *Trypanosoma cruzi* Amastigote Surface Protein-2 CD8+ T cell epitope at two distinct regions of the genome. *Virol J* 2011;**8**:127.

113. Egui A, Thomas MC, Morell M, Marañón C, Carrilero B, Segovia M, et al. *Trypanosoma cruzi* paraflagellar rod proteins 2 and 3 contain immunodominant CD8(+) T-cell epitopes that are recognized by cytotoxic T cells from Chagas disease patients. *Mol Immunol* 2012;**52**:289−98.

114. Kurup SP, Tarleton RL. The *Trypanosoma cruzi* flagellum is discarded via asymmetric cell division following invasion and provides early targets for protective CD8+ T cells. *Cell Host Microbe* 2014;**16**:439−49.

115. Serna C, Lara JA, Rodrigues SP, Marques AF, Almeida IC, Maldonado RA. A synthetic peptide from *Trypanosoma cruzi* mucin-like associated surface protein as candidate for a vaccine against Chagas disease. *Vaccine* 2014;**32**:3525−32.

116. Manning-Cela R, Gonzalez A, Swindle J. Alternative splicing of LYT1 transcripts in *Trypanosoma cruzi*. *Infect Immun* 2002;**70**:4726−8.

117. Laucella SA, Postan M, Martin D, Hubby FB, Albareda MC, Alvarez MG, et al. Frequency of interferon-gamma-producing T cells specific for *Trypanosoma cruzi* inversely correlates with disease severity in chronic human Chagas disease. *J Infect Dis* 2004;**189**:909−18.

118. Garcia F, Sepulveda P, Liegeard P, Gregoire J, Hermann E, Lemonnier F, et al. Identification of HLA-A*0201-restricted cytotoxic T-cell epitopes of *Trypanosoma cruzi* TcP2beta protein in HLA-transgenic mice and patients. *Microbes Infect* 2003;**5**: 351−9.

119. Lasso P, Mesa D, Cuéllar A, Guzmán F, Bolaños N, Rosas F, et al. Frequency of specific CD8+ T cells for a promiscuous epitope derived from *Trypanosoma cruzi* KMP-11 protein in chagasic patients. *Parasit Immunol* 2010;**32**:494−502.

120. Marañón C, Egui A, Carrilero B, Thomas MC, Pinazo MJ, Gascón J, et al. Identification of HLA-A*02:01-restricted CTL epitopes in *Trypanosoma cruzi* heat shock protein-70 recognized by Chagas disease patients. *Microbes Infect Inst Pasteur* 2011;**13**:1025−32.

121. Martin DL, Weatherly DB, Laucella SA, Cabinian MA, Crim MT, Sullivan S, et al. CD8+ T-cell responses to *Trypanosoma cruzi* are highly focused on strain-variant trans-sialidase epitopes. *PLoS Pathogens* 2006;**2**:e77.

122. Padilla A, Xu D, Martin D, Tarleton R. Limited role for CD4 + T-cell help in the initial priming of *Trypanosoma cruzi*-specific CD8+ T cells. *Infect Immun* 2007;**75**: 231−5.

123. Padilla AM, Bustamante JM, Tarleton RL. CD8+ T cells in *Trypanosoma cruzi* infection. *Curr Opin Immunol* 2009;**21**:385−90.

124. Matta Guedes PM, Gutierrez FR, Maia FL, Milanezi CM, Silva GK, Pavanelli WR, et al. IL-17 produced during *Trypanosoma cruzi* infection plays a central role in regulating parasite-induced myocarditis. *PLoS NTD* 2010;**4**:e604.

125. Esper L, Utsch L, Soriani FM, Brant F, Esteves Arantes RM, Campos CF, et al. Regulatory effects of IL-18 on cytokine profiles and development of myocarditis during *Trypanosoma cruzi* infection. *Microbes Infect Inst Pasteur* 2014;**16**:481−90.

126. Cobb D, Guo S, Lara AM, Manque P, Buck G, Smeltz RB. T-bet-dependent regulation of CD8+ T-cell expansion during experimental *Trypanosoma cruzi* infection. *Immunology* 2009;**128**:589−99.

127. Oliveira A-C, de Alencar BC, Tzelepis F, Klezewsky W, da Silva RN, Neves FS, et al. Impaired innate immunity in Tlr4(−/−) mice but preserved CD8+ T cell responses against *Trypanosoma cruzi* in Tlr4-, Tlr2-, Tlr9- or Myd88-deficient mice. *PLoS Pathogens* 2010;**6**:e1000870.

128. Martin DL, Murali-Krishna K, Tarleton RL. Generation of *Trypanosoma cruzi*-specific CD8+ T-cell immunity is unaffected by the absence of type I interferon signaling. *Infect Immun* 2010;**78**:3154−9.

129. Dhiman M, Garg NJ. P47phox−/− mice are compromised in expansion and activation of CD8+ T cells and susceptible to *Trypanosoma cruzi* infection. *PLoS Pathogens* 2014;**10**:e1004516.

130. Tarleton RL, Grusby MJ, Postan M, Glimcher LH. *Trypanosoma cruzi* infection in MHC-deficient mice: further evidence for the role of both class I- and class II-restricted T cells in immune resistance and disease. *Int Immunol* 1996;**8**:13−22.

131. Hoft DF, Schnapp AR, Eickhoff CS, Roodman ST. Involvement of CD4(+) Th1 cells in systemic immunity protective against primary and secondary challenges with *Trypanosoma cruzi*. *Infect Immun* 2000;**68**:197−204.

132. Tarleton RL, Koller BH, Latour A, Postan M. Susceptibility of beta 2-microglobulin-deficient mice to *Trypanosoma cruzi* infection. *Nature* 1992;**356**:338−40.

133. Tarleton RL. CD8+ T cells in *Trypanosoma cruzi* infection. *Semin Immunopathol* 2015;**37**:233−8.

134. Martin DL, Postan M, Lucas P, Gress R, Tarleton RL. TGF-beta regulates pathology but not tissue CD8+ T cell dysfunction during experimental *Trypanosoma cruzi* infection. *Eur J Immunol* 2007;**37**:2764−71.

135. Kotner J, Tarleton R. Endogenous CD4(+) CD25(+) regulatory T cells have a limited role in the control of *Trypanosoma cruzi* infection in mice. *Infect Immun* 2007;**75**: 861−9.

136. Martin DL, Tarleton RL. Antigen-specific T cells maintain an effector memory phenotype during persistent *Trypanosoma cruzi* infection. *J Immunol* 2005;**174**:1594−601.

137. Bustamante JM, Bixby LM, Tarleton RL. Drug-induced cure drives conversion to a stable and protective CD8+ T central memory response in chronic Chagas disease. *Nat Med* 2008;**14**:542–50.

138. Sullivan NL, Eickhoff CS, Sagartz J, Hoft DF. Deficiency of antigen-specific B cells results in decreased *Trypanosoma cruzi* systemic but not mucosal immunity due to CD8 T cell exhaustion. *J Immunol Baltim Md 1950* 2015;**194**:1806–18.

139. Giraldo NA, Bolaños NI, Cuellar A, Roa N, Cucunubá Z, Rosas F, et al. T lymphocytes from chagasic patients are activated but lack proliferative capacity and down-regulate CD28 and CD3ζ. *PLoS NTD* 2013;**7**:e2038.

140. Lasso P, Mateus J, Pavía P, Rosas F, Roa N, Thomas MC, et al. Inhibitory receptor expression on CD8+ T cells is linked to functional responses against *Trypanosoma cruzi* antigens in chronic chagasic patients. *J Immunol Baltim Md 1950* 2015;**195**:3748–58.

141. Albareda MC, Perez-Mazliah D, Natale MA, Castro-Eiro M, Alvarez MG, Viotti R, et al. Perturbed T cell IL-7 receptor signaling in chronic Chagas disease. *J Immunol Baltim Md 1950* 2015;**194**:3883–9.

142. Graefe SE, Jacobs T, Wachter U, Broker BM, Fleischer B. CTLA-4 regulates the murine immune response to *Trypanosoma cruzi* infection. *Parasit Immunol* 2004;**26**:19–28.

143. Borges DC, Araújo NM, Cardoso CR, Lazo Chica JE. Different parasite inocula determine the modulation of the immune response and outcome of experimental *Trypanosoma cruzi* infection. *Immunology* 2013;**138**:145–56.

144. Flores-García Y, Rosales-Encina JL, Rosales-García VH, Satoskar AR, Talamás-Rohana P. CD4+ CD25+ FOXP3+ Treg cells induced by rSSP4 derived from *T. cruzi* amastigotes increase parasitemia in an experimental Chagas disease model. *BioMed Res Int* 2013;**2013**:632436.

145. Poncini CV, Ilarregui JM, Batalla EI, Engels S, Cerliani JP, Cucher MA, et al. *Trypanosoma cruzi* infection imparts a regulatory program in dendritic cells and T cells via Galectin-1-dependent mechanisms. *J Immunol Baltim Md 1950* 2015;**195**:3311–24.

146. Xu S, Cao X. Interleukin-17 and its expanding biological functions. *Cell Mol Immunol* 2010;**7**:164–74.

147. Miyazaki Y, Hamano S, Wang S, Shimanoe Y, Iwakura Y, Yoshida H. IL-17 is necessary for host protection against acute-phase *Trypanosoma cruzi* infection. *J Immunol Baltim Md 1950* 2010;**185**:1150–7.

148. da Matta Guedes PM, Gutierrez FRS, Maia FL, Milanezi CM, Silva GK, Pavanelli WR, et al. IL-17 produced during *Trypanosoma cruzi* infection plays a central role in regulating parasite-induced myocarditis. *PLoS NTD* 2010;**4**:e604.

149. Cobb D, Smeltz RB. Regulation of proinflammatory Th17 responses during *Trypanosoma cruzi* infection by IL-12 family cytokines. *J Immunol Baltim Md 1950* 2012;**188**:3766–73.

150. Bermejo DA, Jackson SW, Gorosito-Serran M, Acosta-Rodriguez EV, Amezcua-Vesely MC, Sather BD, et al. *Trypanosoma cruzi* trans-sialidase initiates a program independent of the transcription factors RORγt and Ahr that leads to IL-17 production by activated B cells. *Nat Immunol* 2013;**14**:514–22.

151. León B, Lund FE. IL-17-producing B cells combat parasites. *Nat Immunol* 2013;**14**:419–21.

152. Tosello Boari J, Amezcua Vesely MC, Bermejo DA, Ramello MC, Montes CL, Cejas H, et al. IL-17RA signaling reduces inflammation and mortality during *Trypanosoma cruzi* infection by recruiting suppressive IL-10-producing neutrophils. *PLoS Pathogens* 2012;**8**:e1002658.

153. Erdmann H, Roßnagel C, Böhme J, Iwakura Y, Jacobs T, Schaible UE, et al. IL-17A promotes macrophage effector mechanisms against *Trypanosoma cruzi* by trapping parasites in the endolysosomal compartment. *Immunobiology* 2013;**218**:910−23.

154. el Bouhdidi A, Truyens C, Rivera MT, Bazin H, Carlier Y. *Trypanosoma cruzi* infection in mice induces a polyisotypic hypergammaglobulinaemia and parasite-specific response involving high IgG2a concentrations and highly avid IgG1 antibodies. *Parasit Immunol* 1994;**16**:69−76.

155. Minoprio P, Burlen O, Pereira P, Guilbert B, Andrade L, Hontebeyrie-Joskowicz M, et al. Most B cells in acute *Trypanosoma cruzi* infection lack parasite specificity. *Scand J Immunol* 1988;**28**:553−61.

156. Affranchino JL, Ibanez CF, Luquetti AO, Rassi A, Reyes MB, Macina RA, et al. Identification of a *Trypanosoma cruzi* antigen that is shed during the acute phase of Chagas' disease. *Mol Biochem Parasitol* 1989;**34**:221−8.

157. Buscaglia CA, Campetella O, Leguizamon MS, Frasch AC. The repetitive domain of *Trypanosoma cruzi* trans-sialidase enhances the immune response against the catalytic domain. *J Infect Dis* 1998;**177**:431−6.

158. Duschak VG, Riarte A, Segura EL, Laucella SA. Humoral immune response to cruzipain and cardiac dysfunction in chronic Chagas disease. *Immunol Lett* 2001;**78**: 135−42.

159. Beucher M, Norris KA. Sequence diversity of the *Trypanosoma cruzi* complement regulatory protein family. *Infect Immun* 2008;**76**:750−8.

160. Tambourgi DV, Cavinato RA, De Abreu CM, Peres BA, Kipnis TL. Detection of *Trypanosoma*-decay accelerating factor antibodies in mice and humans infected with *Trypanosoma cruzi*. *Am J Trop Med Hyg* 1995;**52**:516−20.

161. Kierszenbaum F, Lopez HM, Sztein MB. Inhibition of *Trypanosoma cruzi*-specific immune responses by a protein produced by *T. cruzi* in the course of Chagas' disease. *Immunology* 1994;**81**:462−7.

162. Engman DM, Dragon EA, Donelson JE. Human humoral immunity to hsp70 during *Trypanosoma cruzi* infection. *J Immunol* 1990;**144**:3987−91.

163. Godsel LM, Tibbetts RS, Olson CL, Chaudoir BM, Engman DM. Utility of recombinant flagellar calcium-binding protein for serodiagnosis of *Trypanosoma cruzi* infection. *J Clin Microbiol* 1995;**33**:2082−5.

164. Truyens C, Rivera MT, Ouaissi A, Carlier Y. High circulating levels of fibronectin and antibodies against its RGD adhesion site during mouse *Trypanosoma cruzi* infection: relation to survival. *Exp Parasitol* 1995;**80**:499−506.

165. Schocker NS, Portillo S, Brito CRN, Marques AF, Almeida IC, Michael K. Synthesis of Galα(1,3)Galβ(1,4)GlcNAcα-, Galβ(1,4)GlcNAcα- and GlcNAc-containing neoglycoproteins and their immunological evaluation in the context of Chagas disease. *Glycobiology* 2016;**26**:39−50.

166. Garraud O, Perraut R, Riveau G, Nutman TB. Class and subclass selection in parasite-specific antibody responses. *Trends Parasitol* 2003;**19**:300−4.

167. Snapper CM, Paul WE. Interferon-gamma and B cell stimulatory factor-1 reciprocally regulate Ig isotype production. *Science* 1987;**236**:944−7.

168. Krettli AU, Brener Z. Protective effects of specific antibodies in *Trypanosoma cruzi* infections. *J Immunol* 1976;**116**:755−60.

169. Umekita LF, Mota I. How are antibodies involved in the protective mechanism of susceptible mice infected with *T. cruzi*? *Braz J Med Biol Res* 2000;**33**:253−8.

170. Krautz GM, Kissinger JC, Krettli AU. The targets of the lytic antibody response against *Trypanosoma cruzi*. *Parasitol Today* 2000;**16**:31−4.

171. Brodskyn CI, Silva AM, Takehara HA, Mota I. IgG subclasses responsible for immune clearance in mice infected with *Trypanosoma cruzi*. *Immunol Cell Biol* 1989;**67**(Pt 6): 343−8.

172. Krettli AU, Weisz-Carrington P, Nussenzweig RS. Membrane-bound antibodies to bloodstream *Trypanosoma cruzi* in mice: strain differences in susceptibility to complement-mediated lysis. *Clin Exp Immunol* 1979;**37**:416−23.

173. Sardinha LR, Mosca T, Elias RM, do Nascimento RS, Goncalves LA, Bucci DZ, et al. The liver plays a major role in clearance and destruction of blood trypomastigotes in *Trypanosoma cruzi* chronically infected mice. *PLoS NTD* 2010;**4**:e578.

174. Bronte V, Serafini P, Mazzoni A, Segal DM, Zanovello P. L-arginine metabolism in myeloid cells controls T-lymphocyte functions. *Trends Immunol* 2003;**24**:302−6.

175. Dulgerian LR, Garrido VV, Stempin CC, Cerbán FM. Programmed death ligand 2 regulates arginase induction and modifies *Trypanosoma cruzi* survival in macrophages during murine experimental infection. *Immunology* 2011;**133**:29−40.

176. Arocena AR, Onofrio LI, Pellegrini AV, Carrera Silva AE, Paroli A, Cano RC, et al. Myeloid-derived suppressor cells are key players in the resolution of inflammation during a model of acute infection. *Eur J Immunol* 2014;**44**:184−94.

177. Ferrero MR, Heins AM, Soprano LL, Acosta DM, Esteva MI, Jacobs T, et al. Involvement of sulfates from cruzipain, a major antigen of *Trypanosoma cruzi*, in the interaction with immunomodulatory molecule Siglec-E. *Med Microbiol Immunol (Berl)* 2016;**205**:21−35.

178. Bochner BS, Zimmermann N. Role of siglecs and related glycan-binding proteins in immune responses and immunoregulation. *J Allergy Clin Immunol* 2015;**135**:598−608.

179. Guillermo LV, Silva EM, Ribeiro-Gomes FL, De Meis J, Pereira WF, Yagita H, et al. The Fas death pathway controls coordinated expansions of type 1 CD8 and type 2 CD4 T cells in *Trypanosoma cruzi* infection. *J Leukoc Biol* 2007;**81**:942−51.

180. Acosta Rodriguez EV, Zuniga EI, Montes CL, Merino MC, Bermejo DA, Amezcua Vesely MC, et al. *Trypanosoma cruzi* infection beats the B-cell compartment favouring parasite establishment: can we strike first? *Scand J Immunol* 2007;**66**:137−42.

181. Vasconcelos JR, Bruña-Romero O, Araújo AF, Dominguez MR, Ersching J, de Alencar BCG, et al. Pathogen-induced proapoptotic phenotype and high CD95 (Fas) expression accompany a suboptimal CD8+ T-cell response: reversal by adenoviral vaccine. *PLoS Pathogens* 2012;**8**:e1002699.

182. Nunes MP, Andrade RM, Lopes MF, DosReis GA. Activation-induced T cell death exacerbates *Trypanosoma cruzi* replication in macrophages cocultured with CD4+ T lymphocytes from infected hosts. *J Immunol* 1998;**160**:1313−19.

183. Uhlin M, Masucci M, Levitsky V. Is the activity of partially agonistic MHC: peptide ligands dependent on the quality of immunological help? *Scand J Immunol* 2006;**64**: 581−7.

184. Bermejo DA, Amezcua Vesely MC, Khan M, Acosta Rodríguez EV, Montes CL, Merino MC, et al. *Trypanosoma cruzi* infection induces a massive extrafollicular and follicular splenic B-cell response which is a high source of non-parasite-specific antibodies. *Immunology* 2011;**132**:123−33.

185. Minoprio P, Coutinho A, Spinella S, Hontebeyrie-Joskowicz M. Xid immunodeficiency imparts increased parasite clearance and resistance to pathology in experimental Chagas' disease. *Int Immunol* 1991;**3**:427−33.

186. Nagajyothi F, Machado FS, Burleigh BA, Jelicks LA, Scherer PE, Mukherjee S, et al. Mechanisms of *Trypanosoma cruzi* persistence in Chagas disease. *Cell Microbiol* 2012;**14**:634−43.

187. Flávia Nardy A, Freire-de-Lima CG, Morrot A. Immune evasion strategies of *Trypanosoma cruzi*. *J Immunol Res* 2015;**2015**:178947.

188. Cardoso MS, Reis-Cunha JL, Bartholomeu DC. Evasion of the immune response by *Trypanosoma cruzi* during acute infection. *Front Immunol* 2015;**6**:659.

189. Norris KA, Bradt B, Cooper NR, So M. Characterization of a *Trypanosoma cruzi* C3 binding protein with functional and genetic similarities to the human complement regulatory protein, decay-accelerating factor. *J Immunol* 1991;**147**:2240−7.

190. Tambourgi DV, Kipnis TL, da Silva WD, Joiner KA, Sher A, Heath S, et al. A partial cDNA clone of trypomastigote decay-accelerating factor (T-DAF), a developmentally regulated complement inhibitor of *Trypanosoma cruzi*, has genetic and functional similarities to the human complement inhibitor DAF. *Infect Immun* 1993;**61**:3656−63.

191. Fischer E, Ouaissi MA, Velge P, Cornette J, Kazatchkine MD. gp 58/68, a parasite component that contributes to the escape of the trypomastigote form of *T. cruzi* from damage by the human alternative complement pathway. *Immunology* 1988;**65**: 299−303.

192. Valck C, Ramirez G, Lopez N, Ribeiro CH, Maldonado I, Sanchez G, et al. Molecular mechanisms involved in the inactivation of the first component of human complement by *Trypanosoma cruzi* calreticulin. *Mol Immunol* 2010.

193. Cestari IS, Evans-Osses I, Freitas JC, Inal JM, Ramirez MI. Complement C2 receptor inhibitor trispanning confers an increased ability to resist complement-mediated lysis in *Trypanosoma cruzi*. *J Infect Dis* 2008;**198**:1276−83.

194. Iida K, Whitlow MB, Nussenzweig V. Amastigotes of *Trypanosoma cruzi* escape destruction by the terminal complement components. *J Exp Med* 1989;**169**:881−91.

195. Freire-de-Lima CG, Nunes MP, Corte-Real S, Soares MP, Previato JO, Mendonca-Previato L, et al. Proapoptotic activity of a *Trypanosoma cruzi* ceramide-containing glycolipid turned on in host macrophages by IFN-gamma. *J Immunol* 1998;**161**: 4909−16.

196. Kahn S, Wleklinski M, Aruffo A, Farr A, Coder D, Kahn M. *Trypanosoma cruzi* amastigote adhesion to macrophages is facilitated by the mannose receptor. *J Exp Med* 1995;**182**:1243−58.

197. Doyle PS, Zhou YM, Hsieh I, Greenbaum DC, McKerrow JH, Engel JC. The *Trypanosoma cruzi* protease cruzain mediates immune evasion. *PLoS Pathogens* 2011; **7**:e1002139.

198. de Souza EM, Araujo-Jorge TC, Bailly C, Lansiaux A, Batista MM, Oliveira GM, et al. Host and parasite apoptosis following *Trypanosoma cruzi* infection in in vitro and in vivo models. *Cell Tissue Res* 2003;**314**:223−35.

199. Herold S, Fago A. Reactions of peroxynitrite with globin proteins and their possible physiological role. *Comp Biochem MolIntegr Physiol* 2005;**142**:124−9.

200. Aoki MP, Cano RC, Pellegrini AV, Tanos T, Guinazu NL, Coso OA, et al. Different signaling pathways are involved in cardiomyocyte survival induced by a *Trypanosoma cruzi* glycoprotein. *Microbes Infect* 2006;**8**:1723−31.

201. Chuenkova MV, PereiraPerrin M. *Trypanosoma cruzi* targets Akt in host cells as an intracellular antiapoptotic strategy. *Sci Signal* 2009;**2**:ra74.

202. Hall BS, Tam W, Sen R, Pereira ME. Cell-specific activation of nuclear factor-kappaB by the parasite *Trypanosoma cruzi* promotes resistance to intracellular infection. *Mol Biol Cell* 2000;**11**:153−60.

203. Berasain P, Carmona C, Frangione B, Cazzulo JJ, Goni F. Specific cleavage sites on human IgG subclasses by cruzipain, the major cysteine proteinase from *Trypanosoma cruzi*. *Mol Biochem Parasitol* 2003;**130**:23−9.

204. Campos-Neto A, Suffia I, Cavassani KA, Jen S, Greeson K, Ovendale P, et al. Cloning and characterization of a gene encoding an immunoglobulin-binding receptor on the cell surface of some members of the family Trypanosomatidae. *Infect Immun* 2003;**71**: 5065−76.

205. Frasch AC. Functional diversity in the trans-sialidase and mucin families in *Trypanosoma cruzi*. *Parasitol Today* 2000;**16**:282−6.

206. Dominguez MR, Silveira ELV, de Vasconcelos JRC, de Alencar BCG, Machado AV, Bruna-Romero O, et al. Subdominant/cryptic CD8 T cell epitopes contribute to resistance against experimental infection with a human protozoan parasite. *PLoS ONE* 2011;**6**: e22011.

207. Rosenberg CS, Martin DL, Tarleton RL. CD8+ T cells specific for immunodominant trans-sialidase epitopes contribute to control of *Trypanosoma cruzi* infection but are not required for resistance. *J Immunol Baltim Md 1950* 2010;**185**:560−8.

# Cell invasion by *Trypanosoma cruzi* and the type I interferon response

J.A. Costales

Pontificia Universidad Católica del Ecuador, Quito, Ecuador

## Chapter Outline

## Introduction

The life cycle of *Trypanosoma cruzi* is digenetic, comprising developmental stages in an invertebrate host (vector) as well as a mammalian host. Well over a 100 species of blood feeding triatomines may harbor *T. cruzi*,[1] while a variety of wild and domestic mammals, in addition to humans, can serve as the mammalian hosts.[2] In the triatomine vector, only extracellular developmental forms of the parasite occur. Epimastigotes, which are slender flagellated replicative forms, attach to the lumen

*American Trypanosomiasis Chagas Disease.* DOI: http://dx.doi.org/10.1016/B978-0-12-801029-7.00027-7

of the vector digestive tract, multiply in the anterior midgut,[3] and differentiate into metacyclic trypomastigotes in the hindgut.[4,5] Metacyclic trypomastigotes, which are capable of infecting the mammalian host, are released along with the triatomine feces, from where they are involuntarily placed in the bite wound or the mucous membranes of the eyes by the bitten individual.

Intracellular forms of *T. cruzi*, on the other hand, occur exclusively within mammalian cells. Trypomastigotes are capable of invading a wide variety of nonphagocytic cells in vivo. In addition, the parasite invades virtually every nucleated mammalian cell type in culture. Once trypomastigotes have gained access to the host cell, they transform into amastigotes, which multiply in the host cell cytoplasm for several days.[6] Finally, the parasites transform back into trypomastigotes, which egress the host cell[7] and may infect additional cells or reach the circulation from where they can be taken up by triatomines. Fig. 26.1 summarizes the *T. cruzi* life cycle, indicating the different extracellular and intracellular forms of the parasite.

In terms of experimental models, trypomastigotes equivalent to those found in the circulation of infected mammalian hosts (blood forms) are obtained from infected mammalian cells in tissue culture (tissue culture-derived trypomastigotes), while metacyclic trypomastigotes can be differentiated in vitro from epimastigote cultures.[8]

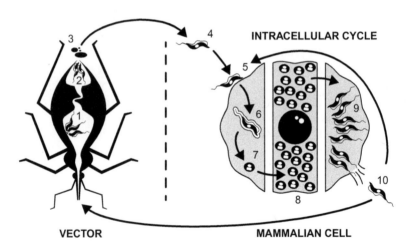

**Figure 26.1** The digenetic life cycle of *T. cruzi*. Infected triatomine bugs harbor *T. cruzi* epimastigotes in the midgut. Epimastigotes attach to the lumen of the midgut and multiply (1). In the triatomine hindgut, the parasite transforms to metacyclic trypomastigotes (2), which are expelled along with triatomine feces (3). The metacyclic trypomastigotes contained in the feces contaminate the mammalian host through either the bite wound or the mucosal membranes (4). The parasite attaches to the surface of nonphagocytic host cells (5) and invades them, entering in a vacuole (6), from which it escapes as it transforms into an amastigote, which resides in the host cell cytoplasm (7). The amastigotes multiply by binary fission for approximately 5 days (8), filling the host cell cytoplasm before transforming back into trypomastigotes (9), which egress from the host cell (10). These free trypomastigotes are then capable of infecting new cells or reaching the circulation, from where they can be taken up and infect a new triatomine bug, reinitiating the cycle.

The invasion of nonphagocytic mammalian cells by *T. cruzi* is a complex and elegant biological process, during which the parasite triggers diverse signaling pathways to subvert cellular processes and facilitate its entry into the host cell. The invasion process by trypomastigotes involves continuous parasite motility and repeated probing by the parasite on the surface of host cells,[9] requiring energy expenditure from the parasite.[10] Initially, *T. cruzi* enters the host cell enveloped in a parasitophorous vacuole, from which it later escapes, gaining access to the host cell cytoplasm.

Infection by *T. cruzi* results in marked changes in host cell gene expression, the most conspicuous of which is the activation of the interferon-beta (IFN-β) gene and interferon-stimulated genes (ISGs). This chapter explores the invasion of nonphagocytic mammalian cells by *T. cruzi* and the IFN-β response initiated by the host cell as response to host cell colonization by the parasite.

## Attachment to the host cell and parasite homing

Prior to entry, *T. cruzi* attaches to the mammalian host cell. A growing number of molecules have been implicated in mediating *T. cruzi* adhesion to the surface of host cells, including members of the gp85/transialidase, mucin-associated surface proteins, and mucin families (reviewed in Romano et al.[11]). These large polymorphic gene families expressed on the parasite surface encompass around one-half of the *T. cruzi* genome,[12,13] and several variants of their members are known to be coexpressed in trypomastigotes.[14] The best characterized among these is the gp85/transialidase family, which is composed of over 1400 members,[12] some of which have been shown to interact with several extracellular matrix components, including laminin and cytokeratins.[15,16] The gp85/transialidase family is specific to tissue culture-derived/bloodstream trypomastigotes and amastigotes,[17] and its members display a conserved amino acid sequence termed the FLY peptide (VTV × NV × LYNR) near the carboxy-terminus.[15,18] Tonelli et al.[19,20] employed phage display methodology and a panel of cultured vascular endothelial cells from different mouse organs to show that the FLY peptide interacts with high avidity with the vascular endothelium of the heart and bladder, and to a lesser extent with the colon. In contrast, only negligible binding was detected to endothelial cells from bone marrow and lung, suggesting that the FLY peptide binds to endothelium in an organ-specific manner. Additionally, when the FLY-displaying phages were intravenously injected into mice, they were showed to home mainly in the heart vasculature (8800-fold over the control phage), followed by the bladder and esophagus. These results suggest that members of the gp85/transialidase family may not only be important for the interaction with the extracellular matrix during infection, but they may influence the tissue tropism of the parasite as well. Furthermore, a similar phage display approach was used to show that TS9, an in silico-identified peptide shared by gp85/transialidase family members, binds to mammalian cell cytokeratins and vimentin, part of the host cell intermediate filaments.[16] Gp82, another member of the gp85/transialidase family which is expressed specifically by metacyclics,[21] has been shown to act as an adhesion molecule, binding specifically to gastric mucin, and is believed to be implicated in *T. cruzi* invasion of the gastric mucosal epithelium during oral transmission of Chagas disease.[22]

# Nonphagocytic cell invasion by *T. cruzi*

Trypomastigotes are capable of invading a wide variety of mammalian cells, through a process that differs from classical phagocytosis in that no pseudopods occur during entry and it is not prevented by actin filament depolymerization.[23,24] Different research groups have characterized at least three processes involved in *T. cruzi* trypomastigote invasion of nonprofessional phagocytic cells, all of which converge in the lysosomal compartment of the infected host cell (reviewed by Caradonna et al.[9]). While initially presented as mechanistically distinct pathways, an invasion model proposing that the three invasion routes are aspects of the same overall process reconciles historical and emerging information. Below, experimental evidence supporting different *T. cruzi* trypomastigote invasion routes/aspects is introduced in separate sections before discussing a unified model of invasion.

## *Lysosome exocytosis invasion route*

Evidence for lysosome involvement in the process cell of invasion by *T. cruzi* originally arose in the early 1990s. Lysosomes on the host cell periphery were shown to be recruited toward the parasite attachment site and fuse with the plasma membrane during invasion of nonphagocytic cells by *T. cruzi*.[25,26] Experimental conditions which facilitate movement of lysosomes toward the host cell surface lead to increased parasite invasion, whereas those which deplete cells from peripheral lysosomes or prevent their fusion with the plasma membrane reduce invasion.[25] For example, parasite entry can be impaired by lysosome agglutination through microinjection of antibodies against lysosomal proteins or by chemical disruption of the microtubules required for lysosome migration.[26]

Trypomastigotes are able to trigger signaling cascades through host cell trimeric guanine nucleotide-binding protein (G-protein) receptors, activating cyclic adenosine monophosphate (cAMP)-dependent pathways and inducing cytosolic $Ca^{2+}$ concentration fluxes in the host cell cytoplasm.[27,28] Liberation of $Ca^{2+}$ from intracellular stores was suggested to activate the phospholipase C/inositol-3-phosphate signaling pathway and results in transient actin fiber reorganization in the host cells,[29] which is known to facilitate parasite entry.[25] Synaptotagmin VII serves as a $Ca^{2+}$ sensor in lysosome−plasma membrane fusion,[30] and blocking its activity causes a significant reduction ($\sim 50\%$) of *T. cruzi* invasion.[31]

*T. cruzi* appears to have evolved redundant mechanisms to elicit $Ca^{2+}$ signaling in host cells. A parasite-derived cytosolic serine endopeptidase, termed oligopeptidase-B, triggers $Ca^{2+}$ transients over a variety of mammalian cells.[32,33] This enzyme has recently been shown to form dimers in solution,[34] and is believed to act by producing a $Ca^{2+}$ agonist through proteolysis in the cytoplasm of the parasite. The agonist, which has not been identified to date, is proposed to act by initiating signaling cascades resulting in $Ca^{2+}$ transients in mammalian cells.[32,33] Parasites carrying oligopeptidase-B gene deletions show defects in cell invasion in vitro and are less infective in the murine model as well.[35] Furthermore, they are defective in the initiation of $Ca^{2+}$ transients in fibroblasts, myoblasts and HeLa cells, an activity which is restored by addition of recombinant oligopeptidase-B, showing that this enzyme plays a key role in invasion of mammalian cells by the parasite.[35]

However, even in parasites carrying a double KO for oligopeptidase-B, a residual capacity to induce $Ca^{2+}$ transients and to infect cells persists; reinforcing the notion that the parasite possesses redundant mechanism involved in the generation of $Ca^{2+}$ transients.[35] In fact, several other *T. cruzi* proteins have been shown to be able to initiate $Ca^{2+}$ signaling in nonphagocytic cells, including cruzipain,[36] members of the gp85/transialidase family (reviewed by Maeda et al.[8]), a novel family of *T. cruzi* surface membrane proteins (TcSMP),[37] the variant of trypomastigote small surface antigen present in *T. cruzi* lineage VI (TSSA VI),[38,39] and *T. cruzi* serine-, alanine-, and proline-rich proteins (SAP).[40] Among these, the mechanisms of action of cruzipain and that of metacyclic trypomastigotes surface glycoproteins are the best characterized, and will be discussed in further detail below.

The major *T. cruzi* protease, cruzipain, initiates signaling through kinin generation. Kinins are short-lived peptidic hormones involved in circulatory homeostasis which signal through the B2 bradykinin receptor (B2R).[41] Scharfstein et al.[36] showed that purified cruzipain triggers robust $Ca^{2+}$ responses in umbilical vein endothelial cells and B2R-expressing Chinese hamster ovary (CHO) cells. HOE, a specific, and E-64, an irreversible inhibitor of cruzipain, were shown to block such $Ca^{2+}$ transients. Furthermore, live tissue culture-derived trypomastigotes induced $Ca^{2+}$ transients in B2R-expressing CHO but not in mock transfected cells, and addition of purified kininogens or physiological concentrations of bradykinin to the culture medium increased parasite entry into B2R-expressing CHO cells.[36,42] These findings imply that cruzipain is capable of initiating $Ca^{2+}$ transients in the host cell by proteolytically cleaving host cell-bound kininogens to generate kinins in umbilical vein endothelial cells and B2R expressing CHO cells.[36] Since protease inhibitors which block cruzipain activity, such as cystatin-C or E-64, do not block parasite entry into the host cells, it has been proposed that the kininogen lysis by cruzipain requires close contact between the cell membranes of the host cell and the parasite,[36,42] although this has not been demonstrated experimentally.

The work by Yoshida and collaborators regarding the signaling of surface glycoproteins in metacyclic trypomastigotes is also compelling. It has been postulated that tissue culture-derived trypomastigotes (equivalent to blood stream forms) and metacyclic trypomastigotes induce $Ca^{2+}$ transients by different mechanisms (reviewed by Maeda et al.[8]). While tissue culture-derived trypomastigotes would induce $Ca^{2+}$ flux through oligopeptidase B and cruzipain, metacyclics of the CL strain are believed to signal through gp82, a gp85/transialidase family member, activating phospholipase C, the mammalian target of rapamycin (mTOR) and phosphoinositide 3-kinase (PI3K), and resulting in $Ca^{2+}$ transients in HeLa cells.[8,43] The less infective G-strain is believed to signal through the gp35/50 surface mucin and to generate $Ca^{2+}$ transients in a cyclic AMP-dependent fashion.[43]

The relative expression of gp82, gp35/50, and gp90 (a nonsignaling member of the gp85/trans-sialidase family) has been proposed to govern the infectivity of *T. cruzi* stocks, where immunoprecipitation, immunoblotting, and FACS analysis with monoclonal antibodies revealed that the poorly infective strains (including G strain) express relatively high levels of gp35/50 and gp90, while highly infective strains (including the CL strain) expressed high levels of gp82 and negligible gp90 on its surface.[44] These three metacyclic trypomastigote-specific surface proteins interact with receptors in the surface of mammalian cells, where gp82 induces a robust $Ca^{2+}$ response, while the response induced by gp35/50 is weaker and that of gp90 is negligible.[44] Experimentally induced reduction of gp90 expression through antisense nucleotides was shown to increase parasite infectivity,[45] and it is believed that gp90 negatively regulate *T. cruzi* infectivity.[46] Furthermore, parasite isolates expressing gp90 variants that are sensitive to gastric peptidases are infective through the oral route in vivo despite showing poor infectivity in vitro. High infectivity in vitro can be induced in such isolates by gp90 degradation though exposure to gastric juice.[47]

## Plasma membrane invasion route

A second cell invasion route employed by *T. cruzi*, which does not depend on lysosome exocytosis, was discovered by Woolsey et al.[48] These authors noted that after infection of mammalian cells in culture with tissue culture-derived trypomastigotes, only 20−30% of the newly formed parasitophorous vacuoles could be stained for the lysosomal marker LAMP-1 (lysosomal-associated membrane protein) in fluorescence microscopy experiments. The remaining vacuoles are formed by invagination of the host cell plasma membrane, without immediate association with lysosomes. The interaction between the invading parasites and the host cell plasma membrane during the early stages of invasion was evidenced by microscopy experiments involving green fluorescent protein (GFP)-tagged plasma membrane markers. Parasites which enter the cells in plasma membrane-derived vacuoles later fuse with early endosomes and lysosomes, as the vacuole matures. This cell invasion route is not cell type-specific, as it was shown to occur in a variety of mammalian cells (including myoblasts, CHO cells, and primary cardiomyocytes).

Additionally, Woolsey et al.[48] showed that cell invasion by *T. cruzi* is a reversible process, i.e., parasites which have entered the cell through plasma membrane invagination may exit from the host cell. The frequency of reversible invasion increased under conditions which prevent lysosome fusion with the parasitophorous vacuole (disruption of actin filaments with cytochalasin D or inhibiting phosphoinositide-3-kinase with wortmannin).[48,49] These results have generated opposing interpretations, since based on microscopy experiments employing wortmannin, Andrade and Andrews[50] concluded that the plasma membrane invasion route results in reversible, nonproductive cell infection. However, wortmannin affects not only lysosome fusion, but also endosome fusion with the parasitophorous vacuole (part of the vacuole maturation according to the plasma membrane invasion model) and autophagosome formation (implicated in a third invasion route discussed in the next section). Therefore, the experiments involving treatment of host cells with wortmannin may not be definitive, and the need for time-lapse experiments to clarify the controversy has been pointed out.[9]

## The autophagosome route

More recently, a third invasion route employed by *T. cruzi* has been described, which involves elements of the autophagy pathway.[11] Autophagy is a conserved catalytic pathway in mammalian cells, involved in the turnover of old or surplus organelles and macromolecules by their engulfment into phagosomes and subsequent delivery to endosomes and/or lysosomes for their degradation and reuse.[51] The products of several autophagy related genes form part of the core molecular autophagy machinery, and are essential for the formation of phagosomes.[51] Among them, microtubule-associated protein 1A/1B-light chain 3 (LC3), a soluble protein distributed ubiquitously in mammalian cells, constitutes one of the best characterized markers used to monitor autophagy and autophagy-related processes.[52]

Using CHO cells overexpressing a GFP-tagged version of the autophagic marker LC3, Romano et al.[11] evidenced colocalization of GFP-LC3 with *T. cruzi* parasitophorous vacuoles by confocal microscopy, indicating interaction of the parasite with the autophagic compartments during host cell invasion. Abundant phagosomes displaying LC3 on their membrane were recruited to the parasite entry site at early time points (1-h postinfection), but no LC3 was detectable in association with the parasite at later time points, when the parasite is free on the cytoplasm and no longer contained in the parasitophorous vacuole (48−72 h).

Induction of autophagy by cell starvation or pharmacological means (rapamycin) increases host cell invasion by the parasite, along with LC3 colocalization with parasitophorous vacuoles.[11] Subsequent studies have shown that the parasitophorous vacuoles for different strains of *T. cruzi* (Brazil, K98, and CL Brenner) associate with LC3 in various other cell types, including rat myoblasts, mouse cardiomyocytes, and epithelial cells, suggesting that the usage of this invasion route is not limited to a particular parasite strain/host cell combination, and that it constitutes a widespread phenomenon.[53] Additionally, Vanrell et al.[54] showed that blocking the synthesis of polyamines (ubiquitous low molecular weight polycations involved in nucleic acid/protein and protein/protein interactions) through the inhibition of the biosynthetic enzyme ornithine decarboxylase with difluoromethylornithine results in suppression of autophagy in mammalian cells, thus preventing cell invasion by *T. cruzi*.[11]

## Toward a unified model for T. cruzi *invasion*

Despite the differences in their surface molecules and signaling pathways they employ for invasion, trypomastigotes, both metacyclic and tissue culture-derived, share the ability to enter a wide variety of mammalian host cells through an actin-independent process which retains in common a similar parasitophorous vacuole formation and maturation, suggesting that shared host cell traits must exist which allow for responsiveness to parasite signals and to support parasite entry.[55]

Injuries compromising the plasma membrane integrity of mammalian cells are repaired by a mechanism dependent on intracellular free $Ca^{2+}$ signaling, in which membrane wound resealing occurs by targeted lysosome exocytosis.[56] Interestingly, the evidence demonstrating that bona fide acidic lysosomes could be mobilized to participate in this wound repair process came from studies of the invasion of nonphagocytic mammalian cells by *T. cruzi*, and it is believed that the parasite triggers this repair pathway and subsequently subverts it, hijacking the lysosomes to form the vacuole in which it gains access to the host cell.[57] More recently, the repair process has been further characterized to demonstrate that pore-forming protein-induced lesions as well as mechanical wounds are removed from the plasma membrane by a coupled endocytosis step[58] promoted by lysosomal acid sphingomyelinase, ASM.[59] Therefore, Fernandes et al.[60] studied whether this enzyme also plays a role during *T. cruzi* invasion, and showed that blocking ASM activity through inhibitors (desipramine) or RNA interference (RNAi) hampers trypomastigote invasion. Additionally, they showed that trypomastigotes cause wounds in the host cells plasma membrane during invasion (presumably through their intense motility and secretion of pore-forming molecules) allowing the flow of extracellular $Ca^{2+}$ into the cell through the lesions. The presence of ceramide in the membranes surrounding >60% of recently invading parasites was shown by immunostaining, and additional lysosomes were shown to progressively fuse with the parasitophorous vacuole.[60] Therefore, the proposed model for invasion of nonphagocytic cells by *T. cruzi* has been recently updated as follows. Lysosome exocytosis toward parasite-induced wounds takes place, and fusion of lysosomes with the host cell plasma membrane occurs as part of the repair process. Upon fusion, lysosome content is released toward the cell surface, liberating ASM, which in turn hydrolyzes sphingomyelin on the external layer of the host cell plasma membrane and generating ceramide microdomains, which invaginate and facilitate the formation of the parasitophorous vacuole and the entrance of the parasite into the cell.[55,60] This invagination of the plasma membrane, which in the lesion repair removes the membrane lesions by endocytosis is likely to represent the "plasma membrane" invasion route described above.[48] Subsequent fusion of lysosomes with the parasitophorous vacuole would ensure parasite retention inside the host cell.[55,60] It has been proposed that the frequency with which striated and cardiac muscle cells undergo plasma membrane injury may be related to the parasite tropism toward these cell types.[55] This unified model thus reconciles the lysosome-dependent and plasma membrane invasion routes as part of the same invasion process. Additionally, in an attempt to include the knowledge about cruzipain-induced kinin signaling within this unified invasion framework, Scharfstein et al.[61] have hypothesized that lipid rafts containing B2R and other G-protein coupled receptors could be internalized during the ASM-mediated invagination of ceramide-rich plasma membrane domains. This hypothesis would predict that during the cell membrane invagination and/or inside the parasitophoruos vacuole the flagellar pocket and the receptors would be in close proximity allowing for the signaling events triggered by the cruzipain-mediated generation of kinins, although experimental support for this is still lacking.

As the unified model of invasion evolves, it is predicted that newer studies will be interpreted within its framework. In some cases, recent findings regarding the *T. cruzi* invasion process have already been presented by the authors within the framework of this unified invasion model. In one such case, Zhao et al.[62] reported that trypomastigotes invade in with parallel orientation to the host cell microtubules. Microtubule cytoplasmic linker associated protein-1 (CLASP1), a plus end-tracking protein involved in microtubule stabilization at the cell periphery, was shown to play a key role in trypomastigote internalization, lysosome fusion with the parasitophorous vacuole and postentry parasite localization near the host cell nucleus.[62] Furthermore, knocking down CLASP1 impaired all of these events without affecting $Ca^{2+}$-mediated lysosome exocytosis. Importantly, besides the findings about *T. cruzi* invasion, this study showed evidence that CLASP1 is involved in the dynamics of intracellular localization of lysosomes in mammalian cells. Fig. 26.2 shows a model for *T. cruzi* invasion where the different invasion routes are unified. Some of the findings in the study by Zhao et al.[62] are also included in Fig. 26.2.

In other cases, even very recent studies are still interpreted within a framework which considers different invasion routes for *T. cruzi* exist. For example, Cortez et al.[63] recently reported that lysosome exocytosis and scattering induced by short-term nutrient deprivation of the host cells, promotes host cell invasion by metacyclic trypomastigotes while reducing invasion by tissue culture-derived trypomastigotes. Rapamycin treatment of the host cells prior to infection produced the opposite effect, where metacyclics infected less. The interpretation of these findings by the authors was that metacyclic trypomastigotes and tissue culture-derived trypomastigotes invasion occur by different mechanisms, where the former invade mainly through a lysosome-dependent route, while the later invade through a lysosome-independent route.[63] These results would argue that even if *T. cruzi* invasion occurs though a unified mechanism, different parasite life cycle forms could favor the usage of different components of it. If this were true, it is likely that different genetic lineages and isolates of *T. cruzi* could display such preferences as well.

## Escape from the lysosome

Once it has invaded the host cell, *T. cruzi* escapes from the phagolysosome to gain access to the cytoplasm, and this process is dependent on phagolysosome acidification.[64] Lysis of the phagolysosome membrane is believed to be mediated by a parasite-derived secreted pore-forming molecule known as Tc-Tox, which works optimally at low pH.[65,66] Tc-Tox cross-reacts with antibodies against complement C9 protein,[66] and this property was used to screen an expression library and identify a *T. cruzi* gene (LYT1) coding for a hemolytic protein acting at low pH, which cross-reacts with anti-C9 antibodies.[67] In addition, *T. cruzi* neuraminidase

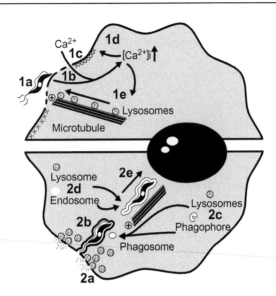

**Figure 26.2** Intracellular invasion by *T. cruzi* trypomastigotes. TOP. Trypomastigotes are highly motile and they attach to the surface of nonphagocytic mammalian cells (1a). The parasite causes increased intracellular $Ca^{2+}$ levels by triggering signaling cascades (1b), and by inducing plasma membrane lesions, through which extracellular $Ca^{2+}$ can flow into the cell (1c). Increased intracellular $Ca^{2+}$ concentrations facilitate parasite entry by inducing transient depolymerization of the cortical actin cytoskeleton (1d) and lysosome anterograde (toward the " + " end) translocation on microtubules to reach the parasite entry site in the cell periphery (1e).
BOTTOM. At the parasite entry site, lysosomes exocytose while sealing membrane wounds, and release acid sphingomyelinase, ASM (2a). ASM generates ceramide domains in the outer leaflet of the plasma membrane and favors its invagination, allowing parasites to enter the cell enveloped in a plasma membrane-derived vacuole, in most cases devoid of lysosomal markers (2b). Phagosomes, formed by the fusion of phagophores with lysosomes, may fuse to the nascent parasitophorous vacuole (2c), which may also fuse with endosomes and additional lysosomes as it matures (2d). The parasitophorous vacuole undergoes retrograde (away from the "plus" end) translocation on microtubules toward the perinuclear region (2e).

(trans-sialidase), which has also been shown to be active at low pH, has also been implicated in the disruption of parasitophorous vacuoles.[68] Interestingly, coinmuno-precipitation experiments suggest that Tc-Tox/LYT1 protein is capable of physically interacting with trans-sialidase.[69] However, direct proof of the proposed functions of these proteins in egress from the parasitophorous vacuole is still lacking.

## Host cellular processes required for *T. cruzi* invasion

An RNAi-based genome-wide functional screen designed to identify mammalian cell genes and processes which support establishment of intracellular infection and intracellular growth by *T. cruzi* was performed by Caradonna et al.[70] The screen employed a multistep process, with an initial library of >25,000 siRNA pools which was assayed on an in vitro culture system using HeLa cells, to determine the effect of silencing individual genes over the *T. cruzi* intracellular infection process. The initial screen was followed by secondary screens with endpoints at 18 h and 72 h postinfection, corresponding to the prereplication phase of infection (i.e., invasion, <24 h after cell infection) and intracellular growth (i.e., amastigote multiplication, >24−90 h after cell infection). Although functional confirmation experiments performed in this study concentrated on host pathways which support the parasites intracellular growth (host metabolic networks and cellular signaling pathways were identified as important for this phase of the parasite life cycle), the screen did identify several dozen candidate host genes involved in the establishment of intracellular residence by *T. cruzi*. Genes that were found to affect parasite invasion included host cell signaling molecules, cytoskeletal proteins (CLASP1, cofilin-1), extracellular matrix proteins (laminin, collagen 1α), and genes involved in protein trafficking and organelle biosynthesis, among others. These findings are in line with what would be expected based on the knowledge regarding mammalian cell invasion described in previous sections of this chapter. The identification of CLASP1 as a protein required for parasite invasion in the RNAi knockdown screen was immediately followed by functional confirmation in subsequent studies,[62] highlighting the validity of the use of unbiased screens to identify functional leads that can be subsequently confirmed and characterized in the pursuit of unveiling the details of the infection process by *T. cruzi*, and intracellular pathogens in general.

## Global transcriptional responses to *T. cruzi* infection: type I IFN response

Interaction with intracellular pathogens produces characteristic transcriptional signatures in host cells.[71] Vaena de Avalos et al.[72] dissected the transcriptional response of human fibroblast to *T. cruzi* infection using microarray technology and showed that the parasite elicits very little transcriptional changes early in the intracellular infection. However, at 24 h postinfection, the transcriptional signature shows very clear upregulation of ISGs due to infected IFN-β production by the infected fibroblasts. Importantly, this transcriptional signature characterized by ISGs was not present in similar studies with other intracellular pathogens, including *T. gondii*[73] and *Salmonella*.[74] Additional studies characterized transcriptional responses to *T. cruzi* infection in three different primary human cell types relevant to the infection in vivo: fibroblasts, smooth muscle cells, and endothelial cells, reporting a shared ISGs induction signature that was driven by soluble/secreted cytokines as demonstrated using transwell plates.[75] When analyzing the gene-ontology functions to which the commonly upregulated genes belonged to, "IFN signaling" and "antigen presentation" emerged as the top signaling pathways induced in all three cell types, consistent with strong increase in IFNβ gene transcription. In conjunction, these studies demonstrate that type I IFN drives the early transcriptional response to *T. cruzi* infection.

## Type I IFNs

The IFNs are classified into type I ( > 20 members), type II (IFN-γ), and type III (three types of IFN-ʎ). IFN-γ is produced by natural killer (NK) and natural killer T (NKT) cells stimulated by IL-12, while type I and III IFNs are generally produced in response to viral infections.[76] Type I IFNs form part of the most diverse family cytokines, and upon binding to the interferon-α/β receptor (IFNAR), induce transcriptional modulation of over 1000 genes with diverse biological properties as part of the innate immune response.[76]

The IFNAR receptor consists of two transmembrane protein chains (IFNAR1 and 2), associated to the cytoplasmic Janus Kinase 1 (JAK1) and tyrosine kinase 2 (TYK2). In the canonical signal transduction pathway, STAT1 (signal transducer and activator of transcription 1) and STAT2 proteins are phosphorylated, bind interferon regulatory factor 9 (IRF9), and this complex translocates to the nucleus to activate ISGs.[77] However, this signal transduction pathway is not isolated, and it is extensively interconnected with signaling pathways from the innate immune system involved in pattern recognition, including the Toll-like receptors (TLRs), RIG-I like receptors (RLGs), NOD-like receptors, and C-type lectin receptors.[78]

There are different mechanisms by which pathogens can activate type I IFN production, namely interaction with TLRs and cytosolic surveillance molecules. TLRs are transmembrane receptors specialized in the recognition of pathogen associated molecular patterns which are expressed in immune and some nonimmune cells. Upon binding of a ligand, TLRs dimerize and signal through the adaptor molecules myeloid differentiation factor 88 (MyD88) and TIR (Toll/interleukin-1 receptor) domain-containing adaptor protein inducing interferon beta (TRIF) (reviewed in Ref. [79]).

The signal transduction networks activated downstream of the innate immunity receptors is vast and complex and a detailed description of it is beyond the scope of this chapter. We refer the reader to the excellent reviews on the subject in Refs. [76,78,79]. However, in the following paragraphs of this section we will mention some of the molecules in the signaling networks downstream of TLRs and other cytoplasmic receptors, which are relevant to the discussion of studies about type I IFN induction during *T. cruzi* infection.

Among the molecules known to act downstream of MyD88 and TRIF are the interferon regulatory transcription factor 3 (IRF3) and TANK-binding kinase 1 (TBK1). IRF3 is sufficient to induce the expression of IFN-β, and upon phosphorylation by TBK1 dimerizes and translocates to the nucleus, binding the IFN-β promoter[80,81] and driving the expression of IFN-β itself (autocrine loop) and of ISGs.[79]

Production of type I IFNs can also occur in a TLR-independent manner. Cytoplasmic pathogens are detected by a different set of receptors, among which the retinoic acid-inducible protein I (RIG-I) and melanoma differentiation-associated gene 5 (MDA5) are cytoplasmic receptors which recognize dsRNA of viral origin, and are required for type I IFN responses against several types of viruses. The signal transduction pathway downstream of RIG-I and MDA5 converges with that of TLRs in the activation of TBK-1, which phosphorylates IRF3.[79] A variety of other DNA cytoplasmic sensors capable of inducing IFN production are known (reviewed by Gurtler and Bowie[82]).

## Signaling pathways involved in type I IFN production in *T. cruzi* infected cells

The signaling pathways responsible for induction of type I IFN production by host cells during *T. cruzi* infection have not been fully characterized. The process has been shown to depend on IRF3/TBK1 (as all known pathways leading to IFN-α and -β production), and to follow the dynamics of an autocrine induction loop.[83] Additionally, type I IFN production by host cells is known to be elicited before *T. cruzi* escapes the parasitophorous vacuole, and can take place in the absence of active infection (since heat-killed trypomastigotes also triggered it).[83]

Despite earlier indications of TLR3 involvement,[84] Chessler et al.[83] found no evidence for TLR-signaling in the process by exploiting mouse fibroblasts (MEFs) and mouse bone marrow-derived macrophages (BMDM) defective for TLR3, TLR4, and their downstream mediators Myd88 and TRIF. Moreover, the cytosolic sensors known at the time (RIG-I and MDA5) were also not required during *T. cruzi*-induced type I IFN production. A possible role for more recently discovered cytoplasmic sensing mechanisms[82,85] remains to be studied. Additionally, it is tempting to speculate that $Ca^{2+}$ signaling associated to perturbations of host cell membrane could activate IRF3, causing type I IFN production during *T. cruzi* cell invasion, as it has been shown to occur during viral infection.[86]

## Type I IFN responses to *T. cruzi* infection in the mouse model

Chagas disease transmission occurs primarily by the vectorial route.[6] Therefore, infection on a dermal or mucosal site would be expected to constitute the first parasite−host contact. Chessler et al.[87] studied the transcriptional responses at the site of intradermal infection with *T. cruzi* in a murine model for dermal infection. As evidenced by transcriptomic analysis of mouse dermal tissue in the inoculation site with Affymetrix microarray chips, strong activation of ISGs occurs at the primary infection site. Similar to what occurs in cultured cells,[72,75] the major pathway activated by *T. cruzi* infection in mouse skin is IFN signaling.[87]

Among the genes activated during dermal infection, several were related to the recruitment or activity of natural killer (NK) cells, macrophages, lymphocytes, neutrophils, and dendritic cells. The presence of these cells in the infection site was confirmed by histologic analysis of dermal tissue, suggesting that neutrophil and NK cells recruited to the infection site could be responsible for IFN-γ production, leading to the strong activation of transcription of ISGs which was observed. Therefore, mice were depleted of NK cells or neutrophils through treatment-specific antibodies. Surprisingly, however, NK cell or neutrophil depletion had little effect over the expression of ISGs, indicating that although they are recruited to the infection site, these cells are not required for the IFN response.[87]

Additionally, microarray analysis showed a robust ISG activation at the *T. cruzi* inoculation site in IFN-γ-deficient mice. On the other hand, when mice lacking the type I IFN receptor were infected with *T. cruzi*, the transcriptional activation of ISGs at the inoculation site is abrogated, clearly showing that type I IFNs are responsible for activation of this transcriptional signature.[87]

Subsequently, the authors measured the IFN-β and ISGs induction by three parasite strains displaying different degrees of virulence. Parasitemia, parasite tissue load, and pathologic manifestations in the infected dermal tissue displayed by the strains correlated directly with the intensity of the IFN-β induction at the dermal inoculation site (Brazil > Y > G). However, the intensity of the overall induction of ISGs did not (Y > Brazil > G).[87]

It has been shown that CD8 T cells play a key role for the control of *T. cruzi* infection, and mice rapidly succumb when infected by the parasite if they are unable to mount CD8 responses.[88,89] Martin et al.[90] studied the impact of IFN-β over the CD8 T cell response in a murine model. Over 30% of the CD8 T cell population of B6 mice infected with the Brazilian strain of *T. cruzi* specifically responded to epitopes of the transialidase peptides TSKB20 (ANYKFTLV) and TSKB18 (ANYDFTL).[90] When mice lacking the type I IFN receptor (IFNAR$^{-/-}$) were infected with *T. cruzi*, the numbers of CD8 T cells, their expansion dynamics, as well as their capacity for IFN-γ production specific for TSKB20 and TSKB18 peptides did not change as compared to wild-type infected mice. This shows that CD8 T cell responses, known to be crucial for *T. cruzi* infection, are independent from type I IFN signaling.[90]

In an additional study, infections with infections in IFNAR$^{-/-}$ mice with Brazil and Y strain were characterized.[91] When sublethal inoculation doses were employed, no differences in parasitemia or mortality between IFNAR$^{-/-}$ and control mice were detected. However, when lethal parasite doses were used, wild-type mice succumbed to the infection while IFNAR$^{-/-}$ mice had significantly better survival rates. No differences were found among the mice in terms of inflammation, parasite burden in tissues, cellular infiltrate, or apoptotic cells in the infected tissues. Additionally, the splenocytes from IFNAR$^{-/-}$ mice produced significantly higher amounts of IFN-γ in response to *T. cruzi* antigen, although both types of mice had a similar number of effector cells present. In summary, according to Chessler et al.,[91] type I IFN appears not to provide protection against *T. cruzi* infection, and to even be harmful for the host when the parasite burden is high (Fig. 26.3).

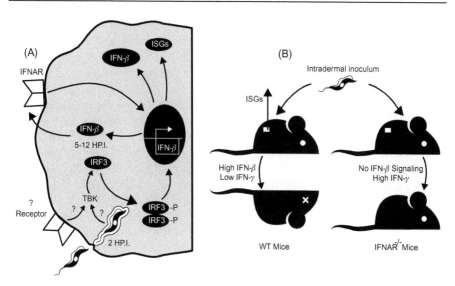

**Figure 26.3** The type I IFN response during *T. cruzi* infection. (A) IFN-β production in a nonphagocytic cell infected by *T. cruzi*. The identity and intracellular/extracellular nature of the receptors and signaling molecules initially triggered by *T. cruzi* remains unknown (indicated by question marks). However, as early as 2-h postinfection, while the parasite is still contained in the parasitophorous vacuole, IRF3 is phosphorylated by TBK. IRF3 dimers activate IFN-β transcription. Through a transcription activation loop involving signaling through the IFNAR receptor, IFN-β intensifies its own production as well as that of ISGs. (B) In vivo intradermal *T. cruzi* infection in a murine model under high parasite burden conditions (lethal dose inoculum). Upon dermal infection with *T. cruzi*, wild-type mice produce high amounts of IFN-β, which in turn activates ISGs. However, low levels of IFN-γ are produced, and the wild-type mice die. On the other hand, mice lacking the type I IFN receptor (IFNAR$^{-/-}$) produce high levels of IFN-γ and survive the infection.

# The balance between type I and type II IFN responses during infection with intracellular pathogens

The fact that type I IFNs do not protect against *T. cruzi* infection, and that they might be harmful to the host under specific circumstances[91] fit a broader trend in the literature regarding the innate responses to intracellular pathogens like *Mycobacterium* spp. and *Leishmania* spp. Studies in human leprosy[92] have demonstrated that polarized clinical manifestations of infection with *M. leprae* correlate with IFN-β and IFN-γ expression profiles. IFN-β and the genes it activates (including IL-10) are preferentially expressed in lepromatous lesions, a disseminated and progressive clinical manifestation of leprosy where abundant bacilli and a Th2 type immune response profile are present. Meanwhile, in tuberculoid leprosy, characterized by self-healing localized lesions, an IFN-γ transcriptional signature, including a vitamin D-dependent antimicrobial peptide response, is present along with a Th1 profile. The responses in tuberculoid leprosy can be inhibited by IFN-β and IL-10, which suggests that the type I versus type II IFN balance in the site of infection might affect protective and pathogenic responses during *M. leprae* infection.[92] Additionally, an IFN-β transcriptional signature was detected in peripheral blood mononuclear cells from symptomatic tuberculosis patients, while an IFN-γ transcriptional profile is present in latent tuberculosis, suggesting that type I versus type II IFN balance can affect the progression of *M. tuberculosis* infection as well.[92]

Several recent reports[93−96] highlight a link between destructive disseminative mucocutaneous leishmaniasis and type I IFN-induced hyperinflammatory Th1 type responses. Interestingly, type I IFN responses have been associated to *Leishmania* isolates carrying the *Leishmania*-specific totivirus LRV1.[93] Infection of macrophages functionally deficient for TLR3, 7, or 9, or for the adaptors MyD88 and TRIF, indicate that the double-stranded genome of LRV1 carried by *L. guayanensis* induces IFN-β production by engaging the TLR3−TRIF-dependent pathway in macrophages. Heavier infection with LRV1 induces more robust IFN-β expression which exacerbates the clinical manifestations of leishmaniasis.[93]

Collectively, these reports support the view that the double-stranded RNA genome of the LRV1 virus within *Leishmania* parasites acts as in innate immunogen which promotes parasite persistence and alters the clinical course of leishmaniasis. This probably occurs when LRV1 particles are liberated from dead *Leishmania* parasites. This knowledge may allow for better prognosis of the risk of developing mucocutaneous leishmaniasis as well as for better treatment options. However, other factors, such as the genetic variability of the host and parasite, may play a role in the clinical outcome as well.

# Concluding remarks

Invasion of nonphagocytic host cells and the concomitant activation of the innate immune response are among the earliest interactions between *T. cruzi* and its mammalian host. An integrated model of nonphagocytic cell invasion by *T. cruzi* is currently favored, which reconciles previously described invasion routes originally considered to be mechanistically independent. Importantly, although it is well established that parasite-triggered signaling cascades initiated by interaction with host cell surface molecules are required for invasion, attaining integrated understanding of the relationship between these signaling events and the different components of the emerging invasion model constitutes a remaining challenge to be tackled in future research efforts.

*T. cruzi* invasion of nonphagocytic host cells results in the activation of the innate immune system, specifically type I IFN production, which in turn drives the global transcriptional profile of infected cells and influences the subsequent adaptive immune response. The signaling mechanisms leading to type I IFN production during *T. cruzi* infection remain poorly understood. Furthermore, the degree to which these early events determine the outcome of the infection with *T. cruzi* is currently unknown, although under conditions of high parasite burden, type I IFN production is detrimental for the host.[83] A negative effect of type I IFN responses is in line with a trend found for infection with other intracellular pathogens, such as mycobacteria and *Leishmania*, and gaining a better understanding of these phenomena may provide clues to new therapeutic options and strategies for prognosis of the clinical manifestations of Chagas disease. Finally, further studies are warranted in order to gain broader understanding of the impact that the full breath of genetic variability of *T. cruzi* might have over individual aspects of infection such as cell invasion and type I IFN responses, and how this might in turn impact the overall immune responses and the clinical outcomes of chagasic patients.

# Acknowledgments

The author wishes to acknowledge Dr. Barbara Burleigh for useful discussions about the contents of this chapter and critical reading of the manuscript.

# Glossary

| | |
|---|---|
| **AMP** | adenosine monophosphate |
| **ASM** | lysosomal acid sphingomyelinase |
| **BMDM** | mouse bone marrow-derived macrophages |
| **B2R** | B2 bradykinin receptor |
| $Ca^{2+}$ | calcium ion |
| **CHO cells** | Chinese hamster ovary cells |
| **CLASP1** | microtubule cytoplasmic linker associated protein-1 |
| **E-64** | an irreversible inhibitor of cysteine proteases. Chemical name (1*S*,2*S*)-2-(((*S*)-1-((4-guanidinobutyl)amino)-4-methyl-1-oxopentan-2-yl)carbamoyl) cyclopropanecarboxylic acid |
| **FACS** | fluorescence-activated cell sorting |
| **G protein** | guanine nucleotide-binding protein |
| **GFP** | green fluorescent protein |
| **Gp82** | *Trypanosoma cruzi* metacyclic trypomastigote-specific surface glycoprotein |
| **Gp85** | *Trypanosoma cruzi* Gp85 glycoproteins, members of the Gp85/Trans-sialidase superfamily |
| **HOE** | a potent antagonist of the bradykynin-2 receptor. Chemical name Arg-(3-hyp-5-thi-7-tic-9-oic)-9-desarg-bradykinin |
| **IFN** | interferon |
| **IFNAR receptor** | interferon-α/β receptor |
| **IFN-β** | interferon β |
| **IFN-γ** | interferon γ |
| **IRF3** | interferon regulatory transcription factor 3 |
| **IRF9** | interferon regulatory factor 9 |
| **ISGs** | interferon-stimulated genes |

| | |
|---|---|
| **JAK1** | Janus Kinase 1 |
| **LAMP-1** | lysosomal-associated membrane protein |
| **LC3** | microtubule-associated protein 1A/1B-light chain 3 |
| **LRV1** | *Leishmania* RNA virus |
| **MDA5** | melanoma differentiation associated gene 5 |
| **mTOR** | mammalian target of rapamycin |
| **MyD88** | myeloid differentiation factor 88 |
| **NK cell** | natural killer cell |
| **NKT cell** | natural killer T cell |
| **NOD receptor** | nucleotide-binding oligomerization domain receptor |
| **PI3K** | phosphoinositide 3-kinase |
| **RIG-I** | retinoic-acid-inducible protein I |
| **RLGs** | RIG-I like receptors |
| **RNAi** | RNA interference |
| **SAP** | *T. cruzi* serine-, alanine-, and proline-rich proteins |
| **STAT1** | signal transducer and activator of transcription 1 |
| **STAT2** | signal transducer and activator of transcription 2 |
| **TBK1** | TANK-binding kinase 1 |
| **TcSMP** | *T. cruzi* surface membrane proteins |
| **TIR** | toll/interleukin-1 receptor |
| **TLR3** | Toll-like receptor 3 |
| **TLR4** | Toll-like receptor 4 |
| **TLRs** | Toll-like receptors |
| **TRIF** | domain-containing adaptor protein inducing interferon beta |
| **TSSA VI** | trypomastigote small surface antigen present in *T. cruzi* lineage VI |
| **TYK2** | tyrosine kinase 2 |

# References

1. Schofield CJ, Galvao C. Classification, evolution, and species groups within the triatominae. *Acta Trop* 2009;**110**:88−100.
2. Noireau F, Diosque P, Jansen AM. *Trypanosoma cruzi*: adaptation to its vectors and its hosts. *Vet Res* 2009;**40**:26.
3. Kollien AH, Schaub GA. The development of *Trypanosoma cruzi* in triatominae. *Parasitol Today* 2000;**16**:381−7.
4. Schmidt J, Kleffmann T, Schaub GA. Hydrophobic attachment of *Trypanosoma cruzi* to a superficial layer of the rectal cuticle in the bug *Triatoma infestans*. *Parasitol Res* 1998;**84**:527−36.
5. Zeledon R, Bolanos R, Espejo Navarro MR, Rojas M. Morphological evidence by scanning electron microscopy of excretion of metacyclic forms of *Trypanosoma cruzi* in vector's urine. *Mem Inst Oswaldo Cruz* 1988;**83**:361−5.
6. Bern C. Chagas' disease. *N Engl J Med* 2015;**373**:1882.
7. Costales J, Rowland EC. A role for protease activity and host-cell permeability during the process of *Trypanosoma cruzi* egress from infected cells. *J Parasitol* 2007;**93**:1350−9.
8. Maeda FY, Cortez C, Yoshida N. Cell signaling during *Trypanosoma cruzi* invasion. *Front Immunol* 2012;**3**:361.

9. Caradonna KL, Burleigh BA. Mechanisms of host cell invasion by *Trypanosoma cruzi*. *Adv Parasitol* 2011;**76**:33–61.

10. Martins RM, Covarrubias C, Rojas RG, Silber AM, Yoshida N. Use of L-proline and ATP production by *Trypanosoma cruzi* metacyclic forms as requirements for host cell invasion. *Infect Immun* 2009;**77**:3023–32.

11. Romano PS, Arboit MA, Vazquez CL, Colombo MI. The autophagic pathway is a key component in the lysosomal dependent entry of *Trypanosoma cruzi* into the host cell. *Autophagy* 2009;**5**:6–18.

12. El-Sayed NM, Myler PJ, Bartholomeu DC, Nilsson D, Aggarwal G, Tran AN, et al. The genome sequence of *Trypanosoma cruzi*, etiologic agent of Chagas disease. *Science* 2005;**309**:409–15.

13. Alves MJ, Colli W. Role of the gp85/trans-sialidase superfamily of glycoproteins in the interaction of *Trypanosoma cruzi* with host structures. *Subcell Biochem* 2008;**47**:58–69.

14. Atwood III JA, Weatherly DB, Minning TA, Bundy B, Cavola C, Opperdoes FR, et al. The *Trypanosoma cruzi* proteome. *Science* 2005;**309**:473–6.

15. Mattos EC, Tonelli RR, Colli W, Alves MJ. The gp85 surface glycoproteins from *Trypanosoma cruzi*. *Subcell Biochem* 2014;**74**:151–80.

16. Teixeira AA, de Vasconcelos Vde C, Colli W, Alves MJ, Giordano RJ. *Trypanosoma cruzi* binds to cytokeratin through conserved peptide motifs found in the laminin-g-like domain of the gp85/trans-sialidase proteins. *PLoS NTD* 2015;**9**:e0004099.

17. Alves MJ, Colli W. *Trypanosoma cruzi*: adhesion to the host cell and intracellular survival. *IUBMB Life* 2007;**59**:274–9.

18. do Carmo MS, dos Santos MR, Cano MI, Araya JE, Yoshida N, da Silveira JF. Expression and genome-wide distribution of the gene family encoding a 90 kDa surface glycoprotein of metacyclic trypomastigotes of *Trypanosoma cruzi*. *Mol Biochem Parasitol* 2002;**125**:201–6.

19. Tonelli RR, Giordano RJ, Barbu EM, Torrecilhas AC, Kobayashi GS, Langley RR, et al. Role of the gp85/trans-sialidases in *Trypanosoma cruzi* tissue tropism: preferential binding of a conserved peptide motif to the vasculature in vivo. *PLoS NTD* 2010;**4**:e864.

20. Tonelli RR, Colli W, Alves MJ. Selection of binding targets in parasites using phage-display and aptamer libraries in vivo and in vitro. *Front Immunol* 2012;**3**:419.

21. Correa PR, Cordero EM, Gentil LG, Bayer-Santos E, da Silveira JF. Genetic structure and expression of the surface glycoprotein gp82, the main adhesin of *Trypanosoma cruzi* metacyclic trypomastigotes. *Sci World J* 2013;**2013**:156734.

22. Staquicini DI, Martins RM, Macedo S, Sasso GR, Atayde VD, Juliano MA, et al. Role of gp82 in the selective binding to gastric mucin during oral infection with *Trypanosoma cruzi*. *PLoS NTD* 2010;**4**:e613.

23. Schenkman S, Andrews NW, Nussenzweig V, Robbins ES. *Trypanosoma cruzi* invade a mammalian epithelial cell in a polarized manner. *Cell* 1988;**55**:157–65.

24. Schenkman S, Robbins ES, Nussenzweig V. Attachment of *Trypanosoma cruzi* to mammalian cells requires parasite energy, and invasion can be independent of the target cell cytoskeleton. *Infect Immun* 1991;**59**:645–54.

25. Tardieux I, Webster P, Ravesloot J, Boron W, Lunn JA, Heuser JE, et al. Lysosome recruitment and fusion are early events required for trypanosome invasion of mammalian cells. *Cell* 1992;**71**:1117–30.

26. Rodriguez A, Samoff E, Rioult MG, Chung A, Andrews NW. Host cell invasion by trypanosomes requires lysosomes and microtubule/kinesin-mediated transport. *J Cell Biol* 1996;**134**:349–62.

27. Tardieux I, Nathanson MH, Andrews NW. Role in host cell invasion of *Trypanosoma cruzi*-induced cytosolic-free $Ca^{2+}$ transients. *J Exp Med* 1994;**179**:1017–22.

28. Rodriguez A, Martinez I, Chung A, Berlot CH, Andrews NW. Camp regulates $Ca^{2+}$-dependent exocytosis of lysosomes and lysosome-mediated cell invasion by trypanosomes. *J Biol Chem* 1999;**274**:16754–9.

29. Rodriguez A, Rioult MG, Ora A, Andrews NW. A trypanosome-soluble factor induces ip3 formation, intracellular $Ca^{2+}$ mobilization and microfilament rearrangement in host cells. *J Cell Biol* 1995;**129**:1263–73.

30. Martinez I, Chakrabarti S, Hellevik T, Morehead J, Fowler K, Andrews NW. Synaptotagmin vii regulates ca(2 + )-dependent exocytosis of lysosomes in fibroblasts. *J Cell Biol* 2000;**148**:1141–9.

31. Caler EV, Chakrabarti S, Fowler KT, Rao S, Andrews NW. The exocytosis-regulatory protein synaptotagmin vii mediates cell invasion by *Trypanosoma cruzi*. *J Exp Med* 2001;**193**:1097–104.

32. Burleigh BA, Andrews NW. A 120-kDa alkaline peptidase from *Trypanosoma cruzi* is involved in the generation of a novel ca(2 + )-signaling factor for mammalian cells. *J Biol Chem* 1995;**270**:5172–80.

33. Burleigh BA, Andrews NW. Signaling and host cell invasion by *Trypanosoma cruzi*. *Curr Opin Microbiol* 1998;**1**:461–5.

34. Motta FN, Bastos IM, Faudry E, Ebel C, Lima MM, Neves D, et al. The *Trypanosoma cruzi* virulence factor oligopeptidase B (OPBTc) assembles into an active and stable dimer. *PLoS ONE* 2012;**7**:e30431.

35. Caler EV, Vaena de Avalos S, Haynes PA, Andrews NW, Burleigh BA. Oligopeptidase B-dependent signaling mediates host cell invasion by *Trypanosoma cruzi*. *EMBO J* 1998;**17**:4975–86.

36. Scharfstein J, Schmitz V, Morandi V, Capella MM, Lima AP, Morrot A, et al. Host cell invasion by *Trypanosoma cruzi* is potentiated by activation of bradykinin B(2) receptors. *J Exp Med* 2000;**192**:1289–300.

37. Martins NO, Souza RT, Cordero EM, Maldonado DC, Cortez C, Marini MM, et al. Molecular characterization of a novel family of *Trypanosoma cruzi* surface membrane proteins (TcSMP) involved in mammalian host cell invasion. *PLoS NTD* 2015;**9**:e0004216.

38. Di Noia JM, Buscaglia CA, De Marchi CR, Almeida IC, Frasch ACA. *Trypanosoma cruzi* small surface molecule provides the first immunological evidence that Chagas' disease is due to a single parasite lineage. *J Exp Med* 2002;**195**:401–13.

39. Canepa GE, Degese MS, Budu A, Garcia CR, Buscaglia CA. Involvement of TSSA (trypomastigote small surface antigen) in *Trypanosoma cruzi* invasion of mammalian cells. *Biochem J* 2012;**444**:211–18.

40. Zanforlin T, Bayer-Santos E, Cortez C, Almeida IC, Yoshida N, da Silveira JF. Molecular characterization of *Trypanosoma cruzi* sap proteins with host-cell lysosome exocytosis-inducing activity required for parasite invasion. *PLoS ONE* 2013;**8**: e83864.

41. Couture R, Blaes N, Girolami JP. Kinin receptors in vascular biology and pathology. *Curr Vasc Pharmacol* 2014;**12**:223–48.

42. Scharfstein J, Lima AP. Roles of naturally occurring protease inhibitors in the modulation of host cell signaling and cellular invasion by *Trypanosoma cruzi*. *Subcell Biochem* 2008;**47**:140–54.

43. Ferreira D, Cortez M, Atayde VD, Yoshida N. Actin cytoskeleton-dependent and -independent host cell invasion by *Trypanosoma cruzi* is mediated by distinct parasite surface molecules. *Infect Immun* 2006;**74**:5522–8.

44. Ruiz RC, Favoreto Jr. S, Dorta ML, Oshiro ME, Ferreira AT, Manque PM, et al. Infectivity of *Trypanosoma cruzi* strains is associated with differential expression of surface glycoproteins with differential Ca$^{2+}$ signalling activity. *Biochem J* 1998;**330**(Pt 1):505–11.

45. Malaga S, Yoshida N. Targeted reduction in expression of *Trypanosoma cruzi* surface glycoprotein gp90 increases parasite infectivity. *Infect Immun* 2001;**69**:353–9.

46. Yoshida N. Molecular mechanisms of *Trypanosoma cruzi* infection by oral route. *Mem Inst Oswaldo Cruz* 2009;**104**(Suppl 1):101–7.

47. Covarrubias C, Cortez M, Ferreira D, Yoshida N. Interaction with host factors exacerbates *Trypanosoma cruzi* cell invasion capacity upon oral infection. *Int J Parasitol* 2007;**37**:1609–16.

48. Woolsey AM, Sunwoo L, Petersen CA, Brachmann SM, Cantley LC, Burleigh BA. Novel pi 3-kinase-dependent mechanisms of trypanosome invasion and vacuole maturation. *J Cell Sci* 2003;**116**:3611–22.

49. Woolsey AM, Burleigh BA. Host cell actin polymerization is required for cellular retention of *Trypanosoma cruzi* and early association with endosomal/lysosomal compartments. *Cell Microbiol* 2004;**6**:829–38.

50. Andrade LO, Andrews NW. Lysosomal fusion is essential for the retention of *Trypanosoma cruzi* inside host cells. *J Exp Med* 2004;**200**:1135–43.

51. Yang Z, Klionsky DJ. Mammalian autophagy: core molecular machinery and signaling regulation. *Curr Opin Cell Biol* 2010;**22**:124–31.

52. Tanida I, Ueno T, Kominami E. Lc3 and autophagy. *Methods Mol Biol* 2008;**445**:77–88.

53. Romano PS, Cueto JA, Casassa AF, Vanrell MC, Gottlieb RA, Colombo MI. Molecular and cellular mechanisms involved in the *Trypanosoma cruzi*/host cell interplay. *IUBMB Life* 2012;**64**:387–96.

54. Vanrell MC, Cueto JA, Barclay JJ, Carrillo C, Colombo MI, Gottlieb RA, et al. Polyamine depletion inhibits the autophagic response modulating *Trypanosoma cruzi* infectivity. *Autophagy* 2013;**9**:1080–93.

55. Fernandes MC, Andrews NW. Host cell invasion by *Trypanosoma cruzi*: a unique strategy that promotes persistence. *FEMS Microbiol Rev* 2012;**36**:734–47.

56. Reddy A, Caler EV, Andrews NW. Plasma membrane repair is mediated by ca(2+)-regulated exocytosis of lysosomes. *Cell* 2001;**106**:157–69.

57. Tan H, Andrews NW. Don't bother to knock—the cell invasion strategy of *Trypanosoma cruzi*. *Trends Parasitol* 2002;**18**:427–8.

58. Idone V, Tam C, Goss JW, Toomre D, Pypaert M, Andrews NW. Repair of injured plasma membrane by rapid Ca$^{2+}$-dependent endocytosis. *J Cell Biol* 2008;**180**:905–14.

59. Tam C, Idone V, Devlin C, Fernandes MC, Flannery A, He X, et al. Exocytosis of acid sphingomyelinase by wounded cells promotes endocytosis and plasma membrane repair. *J Cell Biol* 2010;**189**:1027–38.

60. Fernandes MC, Cortez M, Flannery AR, Tam C, Mortara RA, Andrews NW. *Trypanosoma cruzi* subverts the sphingomyelinase-mediated plasma membrane repair pathway for cell invasion. *J Exp Med* 2011;**208**:909–21.

61. Scharfstein J, Andrade D, Svensjo E, Oliveira AC, Nascimento CR. The kallikrein–kinin system in experimental Chagas disease: a paradigm to investigate the impact of inflammatory edema on GPCR-mediated pathways of host cell invasion by *Trypanosoma cruzi*. *Front Immunol* 2012;**3**:396.

62. Zhao X, Kumar P, Shah-Simpson S, Caradonna KL, Galjart N, Teygong C, et al. Host microtubule plus-end binding protein CLASP1 influences sequential steps in the *Trypanosoma cruzi* infection process. *Cell Microbiol* 2013;**15**:571–84.

63. Cortez C, Real F, Yoshida N. Lysosome biogenesis/scattering increases host cell susceptibility to invasion by *Trypanosoma cruzi* metacyclic forms and resistance to tissue culture trypomastigotes. *Cell Microbiol* 2015.

64. Ley V, Robbins ES, Nussenzweig V, Andrews NW. The exit of *Trypanosoma cruzi* from the phagosome is inhibited by raising the ph of acidic compartments. *J Exp Med* 1990;**171**:401–13.

65. Andrews NW, Whitlow MB. Secretion by *Trypanosoma cruzi* of a hemolysin active at low pH. *Mol Biochem Parasitol* 1989;**33**:249–56.

66. Andrews NW, Abrams CK, Slatin SL, Griffiths G. A *T. cruzi*-secreted protein immunologically related to the complement component C9: evidence for membrane pore-forming activity at low pH. *Cell* 1990;**61**:1277–87.

67. Manning-Cela R, Cortes A, Gonzalez-Rey E, Van Voorhis WC, Swindle J, Gonzalez A. LYT1 protein is required for efficient in vitro infection by *Trypanosoma cruzi*. *Infect Immun* 2001;**69**:3916–23.

68. Hall BF, Webster P, Ma AK, Joiner KA, Andrews NW. Desialylation of lysosomal membrane glycoproteins by *Trypanosoma cruzi*: a role for the surface neuraminidase in facilitating parasite entry into the host cell cytoplasm. *J Exp Med* 1992;**176**:313–25.

69. Lugo-Caballero C, Ballesteros-Rodea G, Martinez-Calvillo S, Manning-Cela R. Identification of protein complex associated with LYT1 of *Trypanosoma cruzi*. *Biomed Res Int* 2013;493525.

70. Caradonna KL, Engel JC, Jacobi D, Lee CH, Burleigh BA. Host metabolism regulates intracellular growth of *Trypanosoma cruzi*. *Cell Host Microbe* 2013;**13**:108–17.

71. Diehn M, Relman DA. Comparing functional genomic datasets: lessons from DNA microarray analyses of host–pathogen interactions. *Curr Opin Microbiol* 2001; **4**:95–101.

72. Vaena de Avalos S, Blader IJ, Fisher M, Boothroyd JC, Burleigh BA. Immediate/early response to *Trypanosoma cruzi* infection involves minimal modulation of host cell transcription. *J Biol Chem* 2002;**277**:639–44.

73. Blader IJ, Manger ID, Boothroyd JC. Microarray analysis reveals previously unknown changes in *Toxoplasma gondii*-infected human cells. *J Biol Chem* 2001; **276**:24223–31.

74. Eckmann L, Smith JR, Housley MP, Dwinell MB, Kagnoff MF. Analysis by high density CDNA arrays of altered gene expression in human intestinal epithelial cells in response to infection with the invasive enteric bacteria salmonella. *J Biol Chem* 2000;**275**:14084–94.

75. Costales JA, Daily JP, Burleigh BA. Cytokine-dependent and -independent gene expression changes and cell cycle block revealed in *Trypanosoma cruzi*-infected host cells by comparative mrna profiling. *BMC Genomics* 2009;**10**:252.

76. Noppert SJ, Fitzgerald KA, Hertzog PJ. The role of type I interferons in TLR responses. *Immunol Cell Biol* 2007;**85**:446–57.

77. Lopez de Padilla CM, Niewold TB. The type I interferons: basic concepts and clinical relevance in immune-mediated inflammatory diseases. *Gene* 2016;**576**:14–21.

78. Takeuchi O, Akira S. Pattern recognition receptors and inflammation. *Cell* 2010;**140**:805–20.

79. Akira S, Uematsu S, Takeuchi O. Pathogen recognition and innate immunity. *Cell* 2006;**124**:783–801.

80. Lin R, Mamane Y, Hiscott J. Structural and functional analysis of interferon regulatory factor 3: localization of the transactivation and autoinhibitory domains. *Mol Cell Biol* 1999;**19**:2465–74.

81. Sharma S, tenOever BR, Grandvaux N, Zhou GP, Lin R, Hiscott J. Triggering the interferon antiviral response through an IKK-related pathway. *Science* 2003; **300**:1148−51.

82. Gurtler C, Bowie AG. Innate immune detection of microbial nucleic acids. *Trends Microbiol* 2013;**21**:413−20.

83. Chessler AD, Ferreira LR, Chang TH, Fitzgerald KA, Burleigh BA. A novel IFN regulatory factor 3-dependent pathway activated by trypanosomes triggers IFN-beta in macrophages and fibroblasts. *J Immunol* 2008;**181**:7917−24.

84. Koga R, Hamano S, Kuwata H, Atarashi K, Ogawa M, Hisaeda H, et al. TLR-dependent induction of IFN-beta mediates host defense against *Trypanosoma cruzi*. *J Immunol* 2006;**177**:7059−66.

85. Bhat N, Fitzgerald KA. Recognition of cytosolic DNA by CGAS and other sting-dependent sensors. *Eur J Immunol* 2014;**44**:634−40.

86. Hare DN, Collins SE, Mukherjee S, Loo YM, Gale Jr. M, Janssen LJ, et al. Membrane perturbation-associated $Ca^{2+}$ signaling and incoming genome sensing are required for the host response to low-level enveloped virus particle entry. *J Virol* 2015;**90**:3018−27.

87. Chessler AD, Unnikrishnan M, Bei AK, Daily JP, Burleigh BA. *Trypanosoma cruzi* triggers an early type I IFN response in vivo at the site of intradermal infection. *J Immunol* 2009;**182**:2288−96.

88. Tarleton RL, Koller BH, Latour A, Postan M. Susceptibility of beta 2-microglobulin-deficient mice to *Trypanosoma cruzi* infection. *Nature* 1992;**356**:338−40.

89. Tarleton RL, Grusby MJ, Postan M, Glimcher LH. *Trypanosoma cruzi* infection in MHC-deficient mice: further evidence for the role of both class I- and class II-restricted T cells in immune resistance and disease. *Int Immunol* 1996;**8**:13−22.

90. Martin DL, Murali-Krishna K, Tarleton RL. Generation of *Trypanosoma cruzi*-specific CD8 + T-cell immunity is unaffected by the absence of type I interferon signaling. *Infect Immun* 2010;**78**:3154−9.

91. Chessler AD, Caradonna KL, Da'dara A, Burleigh BA. Type I interferons increase host susceptibility to *Trypanosoma cruzi* infection. *Infect Immun* 2011;**79**:2112−19.

92. Teles RM, Graeber TG, Krutzik SR, Montoya D, Schenk M, Lee DJ, et al. Type I interferon suppresses type II interferon-triggered human anti-mycobacterial responses. *Science* 2013;**339**:1448−53.

93. Ives A, Ronet C, Prevel F, Ruzzante G, Fuertes-Marraco S, Schutz F, et al. *Leishmania* RNA virus controls the severity of mucocutaneous leishmaniasis. *Science* 2011;**331**:775−8.

94. Ronet C, Beverley SM, Fasel N. Muco-cutaneous leishmaniasis in the New World: the ultimate subversion. *Virulence* 2011;**2**:547−52.

95. Hartley MA, Ronet C, Zangger H, Beverley SM, Fasel N. *Leishmania* RNA virus: when the host pays the toll. *Front Cell Infect Microbiol* 2012;**2**:99.

96. Hartley MA, Drexler S, Ronet C, Beverley SM, Fasel N. The immunological, environmental, and phylogenetic perpetrators of metastatic leishmaniasis. *Trends Parasitol* 2014;**30**:412−22.

# Human genetic susceptibility to Chagas disease

M.-A. Shaw

University of Leeds, St James's University Hospital, Leeds, United Kingdom

## Chapter Outline

Why should we study the genetics of susceptibility to Chagas disease (CD) and associated traits such as cardiomyopathy? At one level, this is to improve our basic knowledge of the biology of disease processes in a range of population groups and settings. In a more practical sense we would hope studies would contribute to development of diagnostic biomarkers and new therapeutics.

## Phenotypes for study

There are a number of phenotypes that have been used in genetic studies of CD. Broadly speaking investigations have been focused on two questions: firstly concerning genetic control of infection per se as the phenotype, and secondly on genetic control of chronic disease phenotypes. One advantage of addressing host genetic susceptibility, as opposed to, e.g., immunological questions, is that it is not necessary to enroll cases showing active disease and under treatment as "susceptible." Nevertheless, for CD, active cases have often been recruited.

With respect to infectious disease, an individual defined as resistant must necessarily have been exposed. Whereas scientists working in highly endemic areas may

American Trypanosomiasis Chagas Disease. DOI: http://dx.doi.org/10.1016/B978-0-12-801029-7.00028-9

be confident that recruits have been exposed, this cannot be taken as a certainty. Many studies employ anti-*Trypanosoma cruzi* antibody levels to classify individuals as seropositive or seronegative. Those who are seropositive will have had the acute phase and entered into the chronic phase of disease. Some studies, less satisfactorily, will use "healthy controls" rather than individuals tested as seronegative, although both groups are relying on individuals being exposed.

Of those individuals for whom disease progresses from a quiescent phase and enters into the chronic phase, the most common phenotype studied is that of cardiomyopathy (CCC). Since 20−30% of infected people may develop CCC, the numbers available for study should not be limiting. In a few instances the information from electrocardiograms (ECGs), used to diagnose CCC, is employed directly as phenotypes.[1] Other phenotypes used for the chronic forms of disease include digestive forms and mixed cardiomyopathic and digestive forms. Since such conditions develop over many years, control groups should be carefully matched for age and sex.

A phenotype receiving little attention, which we might speculate has a genetic component to susceptibility, is congenital CD. Whereas congenital transmission can occur during acute and chronic stages of infection, the majority of cases occur from chronically infected mothers. The transmission rate has been estimated to be 5%, although rates vary across South American countries, which could be due to a number of variables including population diversity.[2,3]

Other phenotypes that have occasionally been used in the context of CD progression include survival analysis and responses to drugs, since the main drugs prescribed, nifurtimox and bedznidazole, have associated adverse side effects.[1] However, the vast majority of the work on susceptibility to CD and disease progression, and the work reviewed here, have been carried out using qualitative, usually dichotomous, traits, such as seropositivity versus seronegativity, or presence or absence of cardiomyopathy. For the future, it is worth considering that use of quantitative traits may more accurately reflect disease states.[4]

In the context of CD, family studies are not common. This limits genetic analyses to case control studies. Family studies are useful for establishing the magnitude of the genetic component of disease. Fortunately, traditional linkage-based approaches for identification of regions of the genome controlling disease susceptibility, requiring family details, are no longer commonly employed in studies of multifactorial disorders, i.e., those controlled by multiple genes plus the environment. Similarly, there is a dearth of longitudinal studies. Longitudinal studies would be especially beneficial for studies of phenotypes relating to disease progression. Many of the studies in the literature for other infectious diseases, have focused on severe consequences of infection. Identifying individuals at high risk of severe consequences or chronic disease, such as CCC, ultimately would enable resources to be targeted to this subset of patients.

## Heritability

How important is genetics for infectious disease susceptibility? Prior to spending time and resources in the search for genes contributing to susceptibility, it is advisable to have an idea of the heritability of relevant phenotypes. Heritability is the proportion of the phenotypic variance due to genetic factors. For infectious diseases it is likely that host genetic diversity will be a major player for some disease outcomes, whereas pathogen or vector diversity will be of paramount importance for others. In general, heritability of susceptibility to infectious disease is not high and findings might be confounded by the difficulties of sorting genetic from shared household effects. Although there are uninfected individuals in areas with a high prevalence of CD, this is not necessarily genetic resistance and household and environmental risk factors need to be understood. Importantly, measures of heritability are time-, place-, and population-dependent. Some of the more robust estimates of heritability in the literature for infectious diseases, other than CD, do not concern genetic control of infection per se, but rather severity or particular manifestations of disease, sometimes many years after the original infection.

For CD, although there are indications of genetic involvement from mouse models, evidence from human studies has been limited. There are a number of indications that may point to a genetic component to any disease, and a number of ways of measuring heritability. Historically, racial differences in susceptibility might have suggested genetic involvement, as is the case for cutaneous leishmaniasis. CD is often prevalent in populations that are racially mixed, but this does not necessarily give clarity and no comments on racial differences in susceptibility appear in the literature. The first measures of heritability for many diseases came from the use of twin studies, where twins are either concordant or discordant for disease. There are few references with any mention of twins in the CD literature. These refer to disease progression in individual twin pairs rather than assessing cohorts of twins.[5] The infrequency of "family studies" in the CD literature is particularly relevant here. There were early estimates of a heritable component to immunoglobulin levels in a CD-infected Brazilian population[6] and an effect of sibling history on Chagas-associated cardiopathy.[7] The involvement in the early 1980s of one of the world's most eminent human geneticists, Newton Morton, is notable.[6] Subsequent substantial work that was carried out in this area for CD is by Williams-Blangero et al.[4,8] In a study of seropositivity for *T. cruzi* in 716 Brazilian adults, 525 of whom were assigned to 146 pedigrees, an estimate of the heritability of infection of 56% was obtained, with a further 23% of the variation due to shared environment/common household.[8] A more recent study by Silva-Grecco et al., also in Brazil, looked at 41 families with 526 individuals and found evidence of familial clustering of seropositivity to *T. cruzi*, with 15 families showing seropositivity in >50% of individuals.[9] A sporadic model of seropositivity was clearly rejected, although the causes of familial aggregation could not be established. They also considered cardiomyopathy in a subset of families, with 6 families showing cardiomyopathy in >50% of individuals.

Whilst most work has focused on qualitative traits, Williams-Blangero et al. have analyzed quantitative traits to determine heritabilities for seropositivity and traits obtained from ECGs, in an ongoing longitudinal study of >1300 individuals.[4] The heritability for seropositivity to *T. cruzi* rose from 56%, obtained using a dichotomous trait, to 64%. ECG-related traits were also highly heritable, though surprisingly less heritable than seropositivity. A subsequent question concerns whether putative genes control more than one of the traits. There was no good evidence that genes controlling seropositivity also controlled cardiovascular traits.[4]

In the context of heritability of susceptibility to infectious disease per se, an estimate of 56% is very high. However such high heritabilities have been calculated sometimes for immunoglobulin/antibody levels. Nevertheless this high estimate gives some cause for optimism that a hunt for genes might be worthwhile.

## Candidate gene studies

Most human genetic studies for CD have employed a candidate gene approach. The choice of candidate genes varies according to the phenotype, whether considering infection per se or development of particular pathologies. Candidates are selected using knowledge of the host–pathogen interaction, of the immune response, from mouse models, or from investigations of other relevant diseases. For example, variation in the ability of mothers to mount an appropriate immune response, or variation in TLR-2 and TLR-9, which recognize pathogen-associated membrane patterns of *T. cruzi*, and are elevated during placental infection, may determine transmission and susceptibility to congenital CD.[2,3] There is considerable knowledge of the host innate and adaptive immune responses in CD,[10,11] and it is clear that variations in inflammatory responses throughout the course of disease will be important. Autoimmune conditions are some of the best studied in the context of genetic predisposition, and genes controlling susceptibility to more than one autoimmune disease have been identified. Hence, the recognition that the cardiac form of CD has an autoimmune component is of interest.[12] For many infectious diseases, candidate genes have been derived from studies of mouse models. The reliability of such extrapolation will in part result from how well murine immune responses and pathologies parallel those seen in humans.[13] Although for CD some questions remain on the appropriateness of models, studies in mice are complementary to those in humans, whether through use of knockouts or mapping of traits.[14,15]

Populations where CD is endemic are often ethnically heterogeneous. That populations are mixed is commented on in some publications, although the majority do not control for ethnic diversity. Since candidate gene studies are likely to use a case control design, appropriate matching of controls is key to preventing spurious associations. As we see more and more studies published, it is clear that knowledge of differences between populations will be extremely important for interpretation.

The majority of early genetic studies for CD have tested one or few single nucleotide polymorphisms (SNPs). This is unlikely to suffice in the future. Study of copy number variation (CNVs) is less common, although here also population differences will be key. The SNPs employed often are those which have shown associations with other diseases, and are perhaps thought to be of functional relevance. A number of the most investigated SNPs are in the promoter regions of immune response genes, rather than coding sequence, potentially controlling levels of expression. However, inferring causality is difficult as in many instances associations are due to a polymorphism being in linkage disequilibrium (LD) with a causative variant. This, nonrandom association of alleles at adjacent loci, together with population differences, may result in the direction of association differing between two studies, i.e., an allele which is associated with resistance in one report may be associated with susceptibility in another. Interpretation will be helped by use of the HapMap project which catalogues human genetic variation in the major population groups and describes LD profiles across the human genome (http://hapmap.ncbi.nlm.nih.gov/).

Sample sizes for CD have lacked power and are sometimes further subdivided according to phenotype. Problems are exacerbated since SNPs are sometimes relatively uninformative with poor information content. A SNP with two alleles each having a frequency of 0.5 provides the maximum information, but many SNPs selected have much lower minor allele frequencies (MAFs). To some extent this can be overcome by the use of multiple polymorphisms and haplotypes, and will improve with changing technologies and better gene coverage.

Where candidate gene studies, particularly for immune response genes, are complemented by expression data, the functional measurements, for practical reasons, are often carried out on a reduced number of patients. It is of course far from simple to marry together simple sequence variation in a gene of interest with levels of expression. Major projects relating regulatory regions to tissue-specific levels of gene expression are currently underway.[16]

In general, findings from the candidate gene studies may or may not tie up with other related literature. Statistical methods vary and correction for multiple testing, particularly for multiallelic systems such as HLA and haplotypic analyses, are not uniformly applied. The last few years has seen publication of meta-analyses of candidate gene association studies for many diseases, including some infectious diseases. Not all published associations are supported reflecting a publication bias for positive findings, and a number of "false positives" from small underpowered studies with a failure to correct for multiple testing. Publication of results on a single SNP when multiple SNPs have been examined is a not unknown approach! Sadly, there have been low estimates of any published association being genuine. For multifactorial disorders, those where both genes and the environment are important, the relative risk for any individual allele is often very small, hence increasing the problems of detection.

Malaria has the longest history in terms of research into human genetic variation determining susceptibility. A relatively recent reappraisal of 27 loci previously associated with severe malaria, with data on 11,890 cases and 17,441 controls from 12 locations, found evidence of association at only 5 of these loci, highlighting the many complexities of case control association studies.[17]

## Genetic associations from candidate gene studies to date

Recent reviews of human genetic susceptibility to CD and CCC have catalogued reported associations, in some cases listing associated alleles and significance levels.[18−21] Since it is early in the investigation of susceptibility to CD, few firm conclusions can be drawn, and because of some of the issues outlined above, this chapter merely attempts to summarize available publications.

The tables list studies to date. They may include studies with elements of replication, where results are not repeated, or studies with patient cohorts in common, but reporting some additional information.[22,23] Phenotypes listed include "seronegatives," where seronegatives are usually presumed to be exposed but not to have had CD, and may also include untested "healthy controls" who would be presumed to be seronegative but from an endemic area, hence exposed. "Asymptomatics" are seropositive and assumed to have had acute infection, and include those categorized as indeterminate. The numbers listed for each of the phenotypes shows the size of the studies and also provides an indication of the questions addressed by the authors, e.g., susceptibility to infection and CD per se through comparison of aysmptomatics with seronegatives, or susceptibility to forms of chronic disease through comparison of these with asymptomatics. It is notable that the most commonly studied chronic form is CCC.

Although more recent investigations often use larger sample sizes, many studies are relatively small and low powered, particularly for considering multiallelic systems or uninformative markers. Associations, whether listed in the tables or described in the text, are as reported by the authors, irrespective of the analytical and statistical methodology employed. The following summaries indicate that investigators have made a good start in the field of human genetic susceptibility to CD.

## HLA

There are a number of studies where HLA class I and class II genotyping has been carried out, in several countries, some with ethnically mixed populations, as summarized in Table 27.1. Because of the high diversity in this region of the genome, the majority of recent studies have genotyped using sequence specific oligonucleotide probes (SSO). Problems of sampling and genotyping have led to some minor inconsistencies in the literature, even in serial publications from the same country.[23] Both susceptibility to CD per se, by comparison of genotypic distributions in seronegatives versus asymptomatic individuals, and susceptibility to severe disease, by comparison of genotypic distributions in asymptomatics versus those with manifestations of chronic disease, have been tested. Due to the presence of LD between potentially "causative" loci, examination of haplotypes is useful, but has only been employed in a handful of studies (Tables 27.1 and 27.2).[29,48] Some have approximated haplotypic analyses, e.g., a very early study by Llop et al. found HLA-B49 conferred protection against CCC in the presence of HLA-Cw3.[26] Similarly, the later study of the class II region by Colorado et al. considered combinations of alleles.[35] Detailed analyses are sometimes precluded by small sample sizes, and hampered by lack of adequately matched controls.[32]

**Table 27.1 The major histocompatibilty complex class I, class II, and related loci**

| Gene | Genotyping | Population | Seronegative | Asymptomatic | CCC (mild/severe) | Digestive | Mixed | Allele | Association | Refs. |
|---|---|---|---|---|---|---|---|---|---|---|
| HLA-G | 3'UTR sequencing | Brazil | 155 | 39 | 52 | 62 | 24 | Allele/genotype/haplotype | Various with infection and clinical variants | 24 |
| HLA-A/HLA-B/HLA-C | Serology | Chile | 32 | | 73 (± CCC) | | | B40 Cw3 | Increase in seropositives without heart disease | 25 |
| HLA-A/HLA-B/HLA-C | Serology | Chile | | 73 | 51 | | | B49 in the presence of Cw3 | Conferred protection against CCC | 26 |
| HLA-A/HLA-B/HLA-C | By SSO | Venezuela | | 35 | 78 (45/33) | | | C*03 in LD with B*40 and B*15 | Conferred susceptibility to CCC | 22 |
| HLA-A/HLA-B/HLA-C/KIR | By SSO | Brazil | 165 | 87 | 44 | | | KIR2DS2 +/2DL2-/C1+ | Increased frequency in patients, particularly CCC | 27 |
| HLA-B/MICA | By SSO | Brazil | 159 | 85 | 44 | | | MICA*007 <br> MICA*008 | Conferred protection against infection <br> Conferred susceptibility to CCC | 28 |
| HLA-A/HLA-B/MICA/MICB/HLA-DRB1/TNF | By sequencing and SSO | Bolivia | | 133 | 60 | 81 | 17 | B*08 and MICA*008-HLA-B*08 <br> DRB1*01 <br> B*1402 | Conferred susceptibility to infection <br> Conferred protection against CCC and digestive forms of disease <br> Conferred protection against CCC and digestive forms of disease | 29 |
| HLA-A/HLA-B/HLA-DR | By SSO and SSP | Mexico | 127 | 34 | 32 | | | DRB1*01-B*14-MICA*011 <br> B39 and DR4 <br> A68 and B39 <br> DR16 | Conferred protection against chronic CD <br> Conferred susceptibility to infection <br> Conferred protection against CCC <br> Conferred susceptibility to CCC | 30 |

(Continued)

**Table 27.1 (Continued)**

| Gene | Genotyping | Population | Seronegative | Asymptomatic | CCC (mild/severe) | Digestive | Mixed | Allele | Association | Refs. |
|---|---|---|---|---|---|---|---|---|---|---|
| HLA-A/HLA-B/HLA-C/ HLA-DR/HLA-DQ | Cytotoxicity and SSO | Brazil | 448 | 33 | 78 (18/60) | 25 | 40 | A30 | Conferred susceptibility to disease | 31 |
| | | | | | | | | DQB1*06 | Conferred protection against development of any form of disease | 32 |
| HLA-DR/HLA-DQA/HLA-DQB | SSP and SSO | Brazil | | 64 | 142 | | | None | With disease progression | 33 |
| HLA-DRB1 | By SSO | Argentina | 81 | | 71 (±CCC) | | | DRB1*0409 | Conferred susceptibility to infection | 33 |
| | | | | | | | | DRB1*1503 | Conferred susceptibility to infection and CCC | |
| | | | | | | | | DRB1*1103 | Conferred protection against infection | |
| HLA-DRB1 | By SSO | Argentina | 41 | 35 | | | | DRB1*0409 | Conferred susceptibility to disease | 34 |
| HLA-DRB1/HLA-DQB1 | By SSO | Venezuela | 156 | | 67 (±CCC) | | | DRB1*14 | Conferred protection against infection | 23 |
| | | | | | | | | DQB1*0303 | Conferred protection against infection | |
| | | | | | | | | DRB1*1501 | Conferred protection against CCC | |
| HLA-DRB1/HLA-DQB1/ HLA-DPB1 | By SSO | Venezuela | | 35 | 76 (43/33) | | | DRB1*01-DQB1*0501 | Conferred susceptibility to CCC | 35 |
| | | | | | | | | DPB1*0401 | Conferred susceptibility to CCC | |
| | | | | | | | | DPB1*0401 | Conferred protection against CCC | |
| HLA-DRB1/HLA-DQB1 | PCR-RFLP and SSO | Peru | 87 | 52 | 33 | | | DRB1*14-DQB1*0301 | Conferred protection against infection | 36 |
| HLA-A/HLA-B/HLA-C/ HLA-DR | By SSO | Spain | 52 | 52 | | | | None B*3505 | With disease progression With moderate to severe cutaneous reaction to benznidazole | 37 |

**Table 27.2 The major histocompatibilty complex continued class III**

| Gene | Genotyping | Population | Seronegative | Asymptomatic | CCC (mild/severe) | Digestive | Mixed | Ref. |
|---|---|---|---|---|---|---|---|---|
| *TNF* | TNF-308 | Brazil | | 62 | 84 | | | 38 |
| *TNFA/ TNFR2* | TNF-1031 and -308 | Colombia | | 154 | 159 | | | 39 |
| *TNF* | TNF-308 and -238 | Brazil | 132 | 53 | 66 | | | 40 |
| *TNF* | TNF-308 and -238 | Mexico | 169 | 27 | 27 | | | 41 |
| *TNF* | TNFa microsatellite and -308 | Brazil | | | 42 | | | 42 |
| *TNF* | TNFa microsatellite and -308 | Brazil | | 80 | 166 | | | 43 |
| *TNF.* | TNF microsatellites x5 | Brazil | 221 | 33 | 71 (17/54) | 25 | 33 | 44 |
| *TNF/LTA* | TNF-308 and -238/ LTA+252 | Peru | 87 | 52 | 33 | | | 45 |
| *LTA* | LTA+80 and +252 | Brazil | | 76 | 169 | | | 46 |
| *LTA* | LTA+252 | Brazil | 161 | 53 | 70 | | | 47 |
| *CYP21A2* | 1 SNP | Bolivia | | 133 | 60 | 81 | | 48 |
| *BAT1* | 2 SNPs | Brazil | | 76 | 154 | | 17 | 49 |
| *IKBL* | 2 SNPs | Brazil | | 76 | 169 | | | 50 |

The less polymorphic *HLA-G*, *MICA*, and *MICB* have also been studied,[24,28,29] as have the Killer cell Immunoglobulin-like Receptor (KIR) loci on chromosome 19, together with the genes coding for their HLA ligands on chromosome 6.[27] A Spanish study examined HLA associations with cutaneous reactions to benznidazole, used to treat CD.[1,11,37]

Although there is no consistent pattern of associations for either class I or class II loci, it seems likely that further investigations will prove useful. Of course bona fide associations with the MHC would carry clear biological implications, e.g., suggest the importance of a key pathogenic epitope triggering autoimmunity, restricted by a single HLA specificity.

## Focusing on the MHC class III region

Two of the most widely investigated loci in the context of susceptibility to infectious disease are *TNF* and *LTA* within the MHC class III region. Indeed there is well known LD between these two loci. Studies of class III loci and susceptibility to CD, mostly on ethnically mixed populations from Brazil, are summarized in Table 27.2. All studies, bar one, address at a minimum susceptibility to CCC. The variation examined is SNPs except for *TNF* where three Brazilian studies utilize microsatellite markers.[42–44] Whereas the *TNF-308* polymorphism is widely used, and has a literature debating its functional relevance, it has the major problem of being uninformative, with a MAF of <0.1 in many populations. This together with the small sample sizes of some studies means that a failure to detect association may merely reflect lack of information. The highly polymorphic microsatellites provide much greater information than SNPs, although integrating SNP-based and microsatellite-based findings is not always straightforward.

For *TNF*, associations were reported at positions -1031 in Colombia,[39] -308 in Colombia and Mexico,[39,41] -238 in Brazil,[40] and for microsatellite markers in Brazil.[44] However others reported no association at positions -308 in Brazil,[38,40,43] -238 in Mexico,[41] and for microsatellite markers in Brazil.[43] Only a minority of studies considered LD and haplotypes.[39,44] There is insufficient data, even for *TNF-308*, for conclusive meta-analysis. *LTA+252\*G* and the *LTA+80\*C+252\*G* haplotype were associated with CCC in Brazilian populations,[46,47] although *LTA+252* was not associated in a small Peruvian study.[45] Some of these studies have attempted to correlate expression/production of TNF-$\alpha$ with polymorphisms,[40,46,47] and one study with survival.[42] *TNF-238\*A* carriers had high levels of TNF-$\alpha$,[40] whereas *LTA+80\*A* homozygotes produced low levels.[46]

## Chemokines and their receptors

Interest in variation in genes coding for chemokines and their receptors has doubtless been stimulated by the extensive work with respect to susceptibility to HIV-1, the *CCR5Δ32* deletion and copy number variation in *CCL3L1*. CCL3L1 and CCL5, otherwise known as Rantes, are ligands of CCR5. However such loci are also biologically relevant, for example in controlling uptake of trypanosomes by macrophages. *CCR5Δ32* and the *59029A/G* promoter polymorphism have been used in several studies of susceptibility to CCC, whereas others have employed SNPs across *CCR5* (Table 27.3). Whilst the *CCR5Δ32* is undoubtedly of interest, its low information content in some populations means that there is little information provided by small studies. In contrast the 59029-promoter polymorphism is more informative, and there are some suggestive associations with this and other SNPs in *CCR5*.[51−57]

*CCR2* and the gene coding for its ligand *CCL2* both show possible associations (*CCR2*,[54,55] *CCL2*[56,58]). *CCL5* together with *CXCL8* (*IL8*), *CXCL9*, *CXCL10*, and *MIF* also have a little data reported (Table 27.3). However, the limited numbers of individuals and polymorphisms used to date mean that confirmation of any preliminary findings would be required in independent studies.

# Cytokines and their receptors

There are a number of reports that have addressed the role of genetic variation in cytokine genes in relation to susceptibility to CD per se and to CCC (Table 27.4). Some utilize polymorphisms reported to be functionally relevant. Few of these CD studies provide complementary functional information. Perhaps surprising is the lack of studies on cytokine receptor genes. Rare variation in genes, inherited in a Mendelian fashion, including *IFNGR1*, *IFNGRII*, *IL12B*, and *IL12RB1*, are well known for predisposing to severe mycobacterial infection,[72] and there has been a widespread view that common variation in such loci may predispose to more common disease. These genes all are involved in IFN-γ related immunity. Single SNPs in *IL12B* and *IFNG* have shown some association in Colombian populations, but more remains to be done.[66,70]

The *IL1A/IL1B/IL1RN* gene cluster on chromosome 2, similar to *TNF* and *LTA* in the MHC class III region on chromosome 6, has received attention for many diseases since the genes code for the major proinflammatory cytokines. In the first of two studies across *IL1A/IL1B/IL1RN*, the *IL1B+5810*G* allele was overrepresented in CCC, and *IL1B* haplotypes showed association.[60] Notably the second study, across *IL1B/IL1RN*, used 50 cardiac patients of the 159 seronegative controls in an effort to provide appropriate controls for study of CCC.[61] One polymorphism in *IL1RN* was associated with infection and development of CCC.[61] Similarly *IL17A* has been associated with several pro-inflammatory conditions. A recent substantial Colombian study showed one of five SNPs tested, rs8193036 in the promoter region of *IL17A*, was associated with protection against infection ($P = 0.017$) and CCC ($P = 0.0065$).[67] IL-18 is an important cytokine in promotion of Th1 cytokine responses and hence provides a good candidate for investigation. Investigation of these Colombian samples for six SNPs in *IL18* showed four to be associated when

**Table 27.3 Chemokines and their receptors**

| Gene | Genotyping | Population | Seronegative | Asymptomatic | CCC (mild/severe) | Digestive | Mixed | Ref. |
|---|---|---|---|---|---|---|---|---|
| CCR5 | Δ32 and 59029 A/G | Brazil | 172 | | 131 | 109 | | 51 |
| CCR5 | Δ32 and 59029 A/G | Peru | 87 | 53 | 32 | | | 52 |
| CCR5 | Δ32 and 59029 A/G | Venezuela | | 34 | 73(38/35) | | | 53 |
| CCR2/CCR5 | 2/7 SNPs | Colombia | | 206 | 270(96/174) | | | 54 |
| CCR2/CCR5/ CCL5/CXCL8 | 1 SNP/7 SNPs + Δ32/2 SNPs/1 SNP | | | 239 | 368(111/257) | | | 55 |
| CCR5/CCL2 | 3/6 SNPs | Brazil | | 118 | 315 | | | 56 |
| CXCL9/CXCL10/CCR5 | 1 SNP per gene | Brazil | | 146 | 174(79/95) | | | 57 |
| CCL2 (=MCP-1) | 1 SNP | Brazil | | 76 | 169 | | | 58 |
| MIF | 1 SNP | Colombia and Peru | 199 + 85 | 115 + 48 | 125 + 26 | | | 59 |

Table 27.4 Cytokines and their receptors

| Gene | Genotyping | Population | Seronegative | Asymptomatic | CCC (mild/ severe) | Digestive | Mixed | Ref. |
|---|---|---|---|---|---|---|---|---|
| IL1A/IL1B/ IL1RN | 2/4/3 SNPs | Colombia | | 130 | 130 | | | 60 |
| IL1B/IL1RN | 5 polymorphisms | Mexico | 159 | 28 | 58 | | | 61 |
| IL4 | Whole gene sequencing | Bolivia | 36 | 76 | | | | 62 |
| IL4/IL4RA/ IL10 | 1/4/3 SNPs | Colombia | | 130 | 130 | | | 63 |
| IL6 | 1 SNP | Colombia and Peru | 399 | 113 + 50 | 117 + 28 | | | 64 |
| IL10 | 1 SNP | Brazil | 43 | 58 | 97(44/53) | | | 65 |
| IL2B | 1 SNP | Colombia | 200 | 130 | 130 | | | 66 |
| IL17A | 5 SNPs | Colombia | 595 | 175 | 401 | | | 67 |
| IL8 | 1 SNP | Brazil | | 202 | 849(366/333) | | | 68 |
| IL8 | 6 SNPs | Colombia | 595 | 175 | 401 | | | 69 |
| IFNG | 1 SNP | Colombia | 282 | 116 | 120 | | | 70 |
| TGFB1 | 5 SNPs | Colombia and Peru | 279 | 175 | 172 | | | 71 |

comparing seronegative to seropositive individuals, but not in development of CCC, and further analysis suggested rs360719 was key.[69] In contrast, a previous Brazilian study tested only *IL18* rs2043055 and had suggested some relevance to progression of CCC.[68]

*IL4* has been examined in two studies, although one of these studies used a single SNP.[63] The more detailed Bolivian study, addressing susceptibility to CD per se, illustrates some of the benefits and problems of sequence-based approaches.[62] Achieving statistical significance with small sample sizes and large numbers of variants is difficult. Forty-five polymorphic sites were found, 3 of which were in the coding sequence and present in affected only, 16 singleton variants appeared in affected only, and *IL4 590\*T* was a marker of haplotypes conferring protection against infection.[62]

*IL10* and *TGFB1* code for "downregulators" of inflammation. Several SNPs in each of these genes have been tested, and analyses of haplotypes carried out, over a number of years for a wide range of other disorders. A small Brazilian study focusing on the potentially functional *IL10-1082* polymorphism, where the "A" allele determined low IL-10 production, found weak association.[65] However, a Colombian study, using 3 SNPs and haplotypic analyses, failed to show genetic association, but for 10 patients where IL-10 production was correlated with LVEF.[63] Susceptibility to CD and/or CCC for other cytokine loci are examined in single studies, in some instances using single SNPs, and further investigation is required (Table 27.4).

# Other genes

Other genes that have been studied for susceptibility to CD per se and chronic disease are summarized in Table 27.5. These genes were selected as candidates for a variety of reasons, and some have been thoroughly investigated in the context of other infectious diseases. They include genes coding for Toll-like receptors, and related molecules such as TIRAP, responsible for pathogen recognition by the innate immune system. Others are involved in the complement cascade such as *MASP2* and *MBL2*, also targeting *T. cruzi*. Some have alleles widely recognized to determine different levels of protein production, also supported by experimental data.[73,74]

More than half the studies in Table 27.5 suggest an association, although some are of borderline significance. Importantly, there are no good replicate studies, and many of the loci have been investigated using only a single SNP. The only genes with more than one publication suggesting association are *MBL2*[74,75] and *TIRAP*.[56,77]

Of note is preliminary information by Juiz et al., since this refers to a study of susceptibility to congenital CD.[89] Candidate loci are the gene coding for placental alkaline phosphatase (*PLAP*) and two metalloproteinase genes (*MMP2* and *MMP9*). Although a very small study, it will hopefully be the first of many, since knowledge of susceptibility to congenital CD is one area that may lend itself to translation into clinical practice.

## Table 27.5 Other genes

| Gene | Genotyping | Population | Seronegative | Asymptomatic | CCC (mild/severe) | Digestive | Mixed | Ref. |
|---|---|---|---|---|---|---|---|---|
| MASP2 | 6 SNPs | Brazil | 300 | 81 | 76 | 19 | 28 | 73 |
| MBL2 | Promoter and exon 1 sequencing | Brazil | 404 | 144 | 148 | 40 | 54 | 74 |
| MBL2/TLR4/TLR1/TLR2/TLR6/TIRAP | 4/2/1/1/1/1 SNPs | Chile | 45 | 61 | 64 | | | 75 |
| TLR4/TLR2 | 2/1 SNPs | Colombia | 200 | 132 | 143 | | | 76 |
| TLR1/TLR2/TLR4/TLR5/TLR9/TIRAP | 1/1/1/1/2/1 SNPs | Brazil | | 76 | 169 | | | 77 |
| TIRAP | 6 SNPs | Brazil | | 118 | 315 | | | 56 |
| HP | ASP | Brazil | 142 | 36 | 71(48/23) | | | 78 |
| HP | ASP | Venezuela | 120 | 30 | 66(30/36) | | | 79 |
| FUT2/ABO | 1 SNP and hemagglutination | Brazil | | | 120 | 120 | | 80 |
| ACTC1 replicate | 18 SNPs | Brazil | | 118 | 315 | | | 81 |
| | | | | 36 | 102 | | | |
| SOD-Mn | 1 SNP | Argentina | 326 | 81 | 90 | 67 | 39 | 82 |
| CTLA4/PDCD1 | 3/1 SNPs | Brazil | 305 | 88 | 96 | 23 | 33 | 83 |
| FCN2 | 4 SNPs | Brazil | 93 | 8 | 8 | | | 84 |
| MTHFR/eNOS | 1/1 SNPs | Argentina | 85 | 8 | 32 | | | 85 |
| NRAMP1 | 4 polymorphisms | Peru | 85 | 51 | | | | 86 |
| PTPN22 | 1 SNP | Colombia and Peru | 435 + 85 | 113 + 44 | 126 + 28 | | | 87 |
| CTLA4 | 1 SNP | Venezuela | 98 | 34 | 73(28/35) | | | 88 |
| PLAP/MMP2/MMP9 | 2/2/1 SNPs + 1CA repeat | Argentina | 103 | 88[a] | | | | 89 |

[a]Congenital infection.

# Genome-wide association studies

Across all multifactorial disorders, the last decade has seen a rapid rise in the number of publications of genome-wide association studies (GWASs) with a large number of associated loci. This reflects changing technologies and use of SNP chips, with association relying on LD between genotyped SNPs and causal variants (which may be imputed) and a strategy known as haplotype tagging. Studies are mainly case control design. As for candidate gene studies, replication is key and a good proportion of GWASs incorporate a second dataset to test for reproducibility.

Areas endemic for CD are often ethnically mixed, including populations with sub-Saharan African ancestry, and hence it is important to note that African populations show reduced LD across the genome since they are genetically more diverse. This means that SNP coverage needs to be denser for these populations to achieve the appropriate level of resolution. It has been estimated that only a third to a half of additive genetic variation is tagged by GWAS SNPs.[90] However the density of SNP chips is increasing and next generation sequencing technologies may eventually take the place of SNP chips.

Approaches required to interrogate different regions of the genome may vary. For example the MHC is a region of the genome containing many potentially relevant genes and variants, and coverage of this region may need to be thorough. Genetic models for analysis also may depend on the region of study. For classical HLA molecules there is great diversity at the population level and heterozygosity at the level of the individual may be optimal. For cytokine loci, alleles determining high or low levels of cytokine production, and therefore homozygosity, might be important for CD outcome.

There are a number of sites cataloguing GWAS results to enable scientists to see genes highlighted in multiple studies (GWAS Central at www.gwascentral.org and https://www.ebi.ac.uk/gwas/). As described earlier, diseases with an immune component often "share" genes with other conditions, and such sites raise awareness of commonalities. Results from GWASs may stimulate more targeted candidate gene approaches. Many of the issues relating to GWASs mirror those seen for candidate gene studies. The GWAS approach is described further by Bush et al.[91] and the first 5 years reflected on by Visscher et al.[90]

There is only a single reported GWAS for CD, specifically for cardiomyopathy in *T. cruzi* seropositive subjects.[92] It included 499 Brazilian *T. cruzi* seropositive blood donors and 101 patients with CD cardiomyopathy. Of the 600 samples, 221 were classified as having CCC, 311 had no cardiomyopathy, and 68 inconclusive. These 600 samples were genotyped on an Affymetrix array with more than 800,000 SNPs. Finally 675,718 genotyped SNPs were analyzed, and a further 5 million SNPs imputed for 580 samples. Seven phenotypes were analyzed including anti-*T. cruzi* antibody levels, cardiomyopathy, and parameters from ECG. For cardiomyopathy the final analysis was on 207 CCC and 306 non-CCC samples. This population was highly admixed and ancestry was quantified for each individual. On publication, two SNPs were highlighted in *SLCO1B1* with respect to cardiomyopathy. This gene codes for a solute carrier that plays a role in drug metabolism and has been implicated previously in myopathy. A total of 46 SNPs were described as associated with the seven traits, spread over novel genes not previously investigated by a candidate gene approach. However, none of the SNPs reached accepted genome-wide significance levels and this is almost certainly due to the low power of this dataset. More typical numbers for a GWAS would be 2000 cases and 2000 controls, with additional numbers for a replicate dataset. So this is a study waiting to be tackled. It will certainly rely on a collaborative approach.

For those diseases where large-scale GWASs have been executed, questions that are being asked concern whether all the heritability been accounted for, i.e., have all the genes making up the genetic contribution been identified? Has all variation been tagged in the study design? Do the common associated variants identified have biological relevance? GWASs are expensive for individual laboratories, the sample sizes needed to give adequate power are large, and population differences need to be accounted for. Arguably expenditure is still small for the potential yield of information, although the large sample numbers required and cost mean that it is impractical for all but consortium groups.

# The future

Despite nearly 30 years of interest in the genetics of susceptibility to CD per se and chronic disease such as CCC, we are still in the early stages of investigation, and the literature is relatively small compared to a number of other tropical diseases. Although estimates of heritability are encouraging that the search for genes contributing to disease susceptibility will be possible and prove useful, the numbers of studies indicating a genetic component to phenotypic variance are few.

Candidate gene studies may be providing some clues as to potentially contributory loci. Nevertheless, ethnic diversity in regions where CD is endemic, and the problems of collecting suitable numbers of samples, when chronic disease may be slow to develop, are evident. All studies published to date have too few samples and polymorphisms tested to exclude as contributory loci currently showing no association. Changing technologies should enable investigators to replicate and expand the number of candidate genes considered and improve coverage of these loci. The development of next generation sequencing technologies will ensure that laboratory and analytical methods change and with this, new questions will be asked.

Undoubtedly larger GWASs would be worthwhile. Since GWASs often detect new loci, but have been known to miss proven susceptibility loci, candidate gene and GWAS approaches can be regarded as complementary. It appears unlikely that a single gene will account for a large proportion of the heritability and the risk conferred by each contributing locus will be small.

To date, the genetics of susceptibility to CD in mammalian reservoir hosts has not been considered. The rise in availability of genome data for other species now makes GWASs possible. Notably canine genetics determining susceptibility to visceral leishmaniasis has been studied in domestic dogs.[93,94]

Implicit in the approaches used is that common variants cause common disease, with the corollary that rare variants cause rare disease. The possibility has been raised that rare variants might cause common disease, with a different selection of rare variants in each individual. An estimate that an individual genome carries around 400 damaging variants and maybe two bona fide mutations for diseases will not simplify the interpretation of data, particularly when variants contributing to multifactorial conditions are likely to be less damaging than those resulting in Mendelian disorders.[95] Tennessen et al. studying >1000 Europeans and >1000 African exomes showed that of >500,000 single nucleotide variants, 86% had a MAF <0.5%, i.e., were not polymorphic, 82% were novel, 82% were population specific, and >95% of functionally important variants were rare.[96] If the role of rare variants is thought to be important, then sample numbers will need to increase greatly and analytical methods change further. Perhaps we should focus on exomes to minimize problems from filtering away key variants in whole genome data? GWASs to date have often identified noncoding changes. However, many of the robust well replicated changes associated with infectious disease susceptibility are changes in coding sequence.

Hopefully, through genetics, we will gain a better understanding of disease mechanisms, and genetics will have a place in development of new therapeutic targets and approaches. Gradual identification of genes predisposing to severe and maybe rare manifestations of disease could be useful. As described above, better understanding of congenital transmission of *T. cruzi* is needed. The two existing drugs, nifurtimox and benznidazole, have side effects and although satisfactory for treatment of acute CD, their usefulness for the chronic phase of disease is less conclusive.[1,11] One CD study has already identified a role of the HLA region in determining drug reactions.[37] Pharmacogenetics should identify individuals with varying abilities to metabolize drugs. As an example, efavirenz is an RT inhibitor used to treat HIV infection. This drug is metabolized by CYP2B6 and a polymorphism of this gene is associated with CNS side effects.[97] Combined studies of host pharmacogenetics and pathogen genetic diversity may prove to be particularly relevant.[98] As vaccines are developed, variation in the MHC may determine efficacy in different populations. With all these considerations in mind, we can aspire to bringing aspects of personalized medicine to the control of CD.

# References

1. Ribeiro AL, Nunes MP, Teixeira MM, Rocha MOC. Diagnosis and management of Chagas disease and cardiomyopathy. *Nat Rev Cardiol* 2012;**9**:576−89.
2. Carlier Y, Truyens C, Deloron P, Peyron F. Congenital parasitic infections: a review. *Acta Trop* 2012;**121**:55−70.
3. Carlier Y, Sosa-Estani S, Luquetti AO, Buekens P. Congenital Chagas disease: an update. *Mem Inst Oswaldo Cruz* 2015;**110**:363−86.
4. Williams-Blangero S, VandeBerg JL, Blangero J, Correa-Oliveira R. Genetic epidemiology of Chagas disease. *Adv Parasitol* 2011;**75**:147−67.

5. Fernandez-Villegas AC, Thomas MC, Carrilero B, Tellez C, Maranon C, et al. The innate immune response status correlates with a divergent clinical course in congenital Chagas disease of twins born in a non-endemic country. *Acta Trop* 2014; **140**:84−90.

6. Barbosa CAA, Morton NE, Rao DC, Krieger H. Biological and cultural determinants of immunoglobulin levels in a Brazilian population with Chagas-disease. *Human Genet* 1981;**59**:161−3.

7. Zicker F, Smith PG, Netto JCA, Oliveira RM, Zicker EMS. Physical-activity opportunity for reinfection, and sibling history of heart-disease as risk-factors for Chagas cardiopathy. *Am J Trop Med Hyg* 1990;**43**:498−505.

8. Williams-Blangero S, Vandeberg JL, Blangero J, Teixeira ARL. Genetic epidemiology of seropositivity for *Trypanosoma cruzi* infection in rural Goias, Brazil. *Am J Trop Med Hyg* 1997;**57**:538−43.

9. Silva-Grecco RL, Balarin MAS, Correia D, Prata A, Rodrigues Jr. V. Familial analysis of seropositivity to *Trypanosoma cruzi* and of clinical forms of Chagas disease. *Am J Trop Med Hyg* 2010;**82**:45−8.

10. Junqueira C, Caetano B, Bartholomeu DC, Melo MB, Ropert C, Rodrigues MM, et al. The endless race between *Trypanosoma cruzi* and host immunity: lessons for and beyond Chagas disease. *Exp Rev Mol Med* 2010;**12**:e29.

11. Bern C. Chagas' Disease. *N Engl J Med* 2015;**373**:456−66.

12. Bonney KM, Engman DM. Autoimmune pathogenesis of Chagas heart disease looking back, looking ahead. *Am J Pathol* 2015;**185**:1537−47.

13. Chatelain E, Konar N. Translational challenges of animal models in Chagas disease drug development: a review. *Drug Design Dev Therapy* 2015;**9**:4807−23.

14. Rothfuchs AG, Roffe E, Gibson A, Cheever AW, Ezekowitz RAB, Takahashi K, et al. Mannose-binding lectin regulates host resistance and pathology during experimental infection with *Trypanosoma cruzi*. *PLoS ONE* 2012;**7**:e47835.

15. Vorraro F, Cabrera WHK, Ribeiro OG, Jensen JR, de Franco M, Ibanez OM, et al. *Trypanosoma cruzi* infection in genetically selected mouse lines: genetic linkage with quantitative trait locus controlling antibody response. *Med Inflamm* 2014;952857.

16. Pennisi E. Genomics. New database links regulatory DNA to its target genes. *Science* 2015;**348**:618−19.

17. Rockett KA, Clarke GM, Fitzpatrick K, Hubbart C, Jeffreys AE, Rowlands K, et al. Reappraisal of known malaria resistance loci in a large multicenter study. *Nat Genet* 2014;**46**:1197−204.

18. Cunha-Neto E, Chevillard C. Chagas disease cardiomyopathy: immunopathology and genetics. *Med Inflamm* 2014;683230.

19. Ayo CM, Dalalio MMO, Visentainer JEL, Reis PG, Sippert EA, Jarduli LR, et al. Genetic susceptibility to Chagas disease: an overview about the infection and about the association between disease and the immune response genes. *BioMed Res Int* 2013;284729.

20. Vasconcelos RHT, Montenegro SML, Azevedo EAN, Gomes YM, Morais CNL. Genetic susceptibility to chronic Chagas disease: an overview of single nucleotide polymorphisms of cytokine genes. *Cytokine* 2012;**59**:203−8.

21. Henao-Martinez AF, Schwartz DA, Yang IV. Chagasic cardiomyopathy, from acute to chronic: is this mediated by host susceptibility factors? *Trans R Soc Trop Med Hyg* 2012;**106**:521−7.

22. Layrisse Z, Fernandez MT, Montagnani S, Matos M, Balbas O, Herrera F, et al. HLA-C*03 is a risk factor for cardiomyopathy in Chagas disease. *Human Immunol* 2000;**61**:925−9.

23. Fernandez-Mestre MT, Layrisse Z, Montagnani S, Acquatella H, Catalioti F, Matos M, et al. Influence of the HLA class II polymorphism in chronic Chagas' disease. *Parasit Immunol* 1998;**20**:197−203.

24. Dias FC, Mendes-Junior CT, Silva MC, Tristao FSM, Dellalibera-Joviliano R, Moreau P, et al. Human Leucocyte Antigen-G (HLA-G) and its murine functional homolog Qa2 in the *Trypanosoma cruzi* infection. *Med Inflamm* 2015;595829.

25. Llop E, Rothhammer F, Acuna M, Apt W, Arribada A. HLA antigens in Chagasic heart-disease—new evidence based on a case control study. *Rev Med Chile* 1991; **119**:633−6.

26. Lllop E, Rothhammer F, Acuna M, Apt W. HLA antigens in cardiomyopathic Chilean Chagasics. *Am J Human Genet* 1988;**43**:770−3.

27. Ayo CM, Reis PG, de Oliveira Dalalio MM, Visentainer JEL, de Freitas Oliveira C, de Araujo SM, et al. Killer cell immunoglobulin-like receptors and their HLA ligands are related with the immunopathology of Chagas disease. *PLoS NTD* 2015;**9**:e0003753.

28. Reis PG, Sell AM, Ayo CM, Oliveira CF, Dalalio MMO, Visentainer JV, et al. MHC class I polypeptide-related sequence A genes and linkage disequilibrium with HLA-B in Chagas disease. *Tissue Antigens* 2014;**84**:163.

29. del Puerto F, Nishizawa JE, Kikuchi M, Roca Y, Avilas C, Gianella A, et al. Protective Human Leucocyte Antigen haplotype, HLA-DRB1*01-B*14, against chronic Chagas disease in Bolivia. *PLoS NTD* 2012;**6**:e1587.

30. Cruz-Robles D, Reyes PA, Monteon-Padilla VM, Ortiz-Muniz AR, Vargas-Alarcon G. MHC class I and class II genes in Mexican patients with Chagas disease. *Human Immunol* 2004;**65**:60−5.

31. Deghaide NHS, Dantas RO, Donadi EA. HLA class I and II profiles of patients presenting with Chagas' disease. *Digest Dis Sci* 1998;**43**:246−52.

32. Fae KC, Drigo SA, Cunha-Neto E, Ianni B, Mady C, Kalil J, et al. HLA and beta-myosin heavy chain do not influence susceptibility to Chagas' disease cardiomyopathy. *Microbes Infect* 2000;**2**:745−51.

33. Garcia Borras S, Racca L, Cotorruelo C, Biondi C, Beloscar J, Racca A. Distribution of HLA-DRB1 alleles in Argentinean patients with Chagas' disease cardiomyopathy. *Immunol Invest* 2009;**38**:268−75.

34. Borras SG, Diez C, Cotorruelo C, Pellizon O, Biondi C, Beloscar J, et al. HLA class II DRB1 polymorphism in Argentinians undergoing chronic *Trypanosoma cruzi* infection. *Ann Clin Biochem* 2006;**43**:214−16.

35. Colorado IA, Acquatella H, Catalioti F, Fernandez MT, Layrisse Z. HLA class II DRB1, DQB1, DPB1 polymorphism and cardiomyopathy due to *Trypanosoma cruzi* chronic infection. *Human Immunol* 2000;**61**:320−5.

36. Nieto A, Beraun Y, Collado MD, Caballero A, Alonso A, Gonzalez A, et al. HLA haplotypes are associated with differential susceptibility to *Trypanosoma cruzi* infection. *Tissue Antigens* 2000;**55**:195−8.

37. Salvador F, Sanchez-Montalva A, Martnez-Gallo M, Sala-Cunill A, Vinas L, Garcia-Prat M, et al. Evaluation of cytokine profile and HLA association in Benznidazole related cutaneous reactions in patients with Chagas disease. *Clin Infect Dis* 2015;**61**:1688−94.

38. Alves SM, Lannes Vieira J, Arnez LEA, Moraes MO, Oliveira WA, Sarteschi C, et al. Chagas cardiomyopathy: prognostic value of genetic polymorphisms of TNF-alpha. *Eur J Heart Failure* 2014;**16**:250.

39. Criado L, Florez O, Martin J, Gonzalez CI. Genetic polymorphisms in *TNFA/TNFR2* genes and Chagas disease in a Colombian endemic population. *Cytokine* 2012;**57**: 398–401.

40. Pissetti CW, Correia D, de Oliveira RF, Llaguno MM, Balarin MAS, Silva-Grecco RL, et al. Genetic and functional role of TNF-alpha in the development *Trypanosoma cruzi* infection. *PLoS NTD* 2011;**5**:e976.

41. Rodriguez-Perez JM, Cruz-Robles D, Hernandez-Pacheco G, Perez-Hernandez N, Murguia LE, Granados J, et al. Tumor necrosis factor-alpha promoter polymorphism in Mexican patients with Chagas' disease. *Immunol Lett* 2005;**98**:97–102.

42. Drigo SA, Cunha-Neto E, Ianni B, Cardoso MRA, Braga PE, Fae KC, et al. TNF gene polymorphisms are associated with reduced survival in severe Chagas' disease cardiomyopathy patients. *Microbes Infect* 2006;**8**:598–603.

43. Drigo SA, Cunha-Neto E, Ianni B, Mady C, Fae KC, Buck P, et al. Lack of association of tumor necrosis factor-alpha polymorphisms with Chagas disease in Brazilian patients. *Immunol Lett* 2007;**108**:109–11.

44. Campelo V, Dantas RO, Simoes RT, Mendes-Junior CT, Sousa SMB, Simoes AL, et al. TNF microsatellite alleles in Brazilian Chagasic patients. *Digest Dis Sci* 2007;**52**:3334–9.

45. Beraun Y, Nieto A, Collado MD, Gonzalez A, Martin J. Polymorphisms at tumor necrosis factor (TNF) loci are not associated with Chagas' disease. *Tissue Antigens* 1998;**52**:81–3.

46. Ramasawmy R, Fae KC, Cunha-Neto E, Muller NG, Cavalcanti VL, Ferreira RC, et al. Polymorphisms in the gene for lymphotoxin-alpha predispose to chronic Chagas cardiomyopathy. *J Infect Dis* 2007;**196**:1836–43.

47. Pissetti CW, de Oliveira RF, Correia D, Nascentes GAN, Llaguno MM, Rodrigues Jr V. Association between the lymphotoxin-alpha gene polymorphism and Chagasic cardiopathy. *J Int Cytokine Res* 2013;**33**:130–5.

48. del Puerto F, Kikuchi M, Nishizawa JE, Roca Y, Avila C, Gianella A, et al. 21-Hydroxylase gene mutant allele CYP21A2*15 strongly linked to the resistant HLA haplotype B*14:02-DRB1*01:02 in chronic Chagas disease. *Human Immunol* 2013; **74**:783–6.

49. Ramasawmy R, Cunha-Neto E, Fae KC, Muller NG, Cavalcanti VL, Drigo SA, et al. *BAT1*, a putative anti-inflammatory gene, is associated with chronic Chagas cardiomyopathy. *J Infect Dis* 2006;**193**:1394–9.

50. Ramasawmy R, Fae KC, Cunha-Neto E, Borba SCP, Ianni B, Mady C, et al. Variants in the promoter region of *IKBL/NFKBIL1* gene may mark susceptibility to the development of chronic Chagas' cardiomyopathy among *Trypanosoma cruzi*-infected individuals. *Mol Immunol* 2008;**45**:283–8.

51. de Oliveira AP, Bernardo CR, Camargo AV, Ronchi LS, Borim AA, Brandao de Mattos CC, et al. Genetic susceptibility to cardiac and digestive clinical forms of chronic Chagas disease: involvement of the CCR5 59029A/G polymorphism. *PLoS ONE* 2015;**10**:e0141847.

52. Calzada JE, Nieto A, Beraun Y, Martin J. Chemokine receptor CCR5 polymorphisms and Chagas' disease cardiomyopathy. *Tissue Antigens* 2001;**58**:154–8.

53. Fernandez-Mestre MT, Montagnani S, Layrisse Z. Is the CCR5-59029-G/G genotype a protective factor for cardiomyopathy in Chagas disease? *Human Immunol* 2004;**65**: 725−8.

54. Machuca MA, Suarez EU, Echeverria LE, Martin J, Gonzalez CI. SNP/haplotype associations of *CCR2* and *CCR5* genes with severity of chagasic cardiomyopathy. *Human Immunol* 2014;**75**:1210−15.

55. Florez O, Martin J, Gonzalez CI. Genetic variants in the chemokines and chemokine receptors in Chagas disease. *Human Immunol* 2012;**73**:852−8.

56. Frade AF, Pissetti CW, Ianni BM, Saba B, Wang HTL, Nogueira LG, et al. Genetic susceptibility to Chagas disease cardiomyopathy: involvement of several genes of the innate immunity and chemokine-dependent migration pathways. *BMC Infect Dis* 2013;**13**:587.

57. Nogueira LG, Barros Santos RH, Ianni BM, Fiorelli AI, Mairena EC, Benvenuti LA, et al. Myocardial chemokine expression and intensity of myocarditis in Chagas cardio-myopathy are controlled by polymorphisms in *CXCL9* and *CXCL10*. *PLoS NTD* 2012;**6**: e1867.

58. Ramasawmy R, Cunha-Neto E, Fae KC, Martello FG, Muller NG, Cavalcanto VL, et al. The monocyte chemoattractant protein-1 gene polymorphism is associated with cardio-myopathy in human Chagas disease. *Clin Infect Dis* 2006;**43**:305−11.

59. Torres OA, Calzada JE, Beraun Y, Morillo CA, Gonzalez CI, Gonzalez A, et al. Association of the macrophage migration inhibitory factor-173G/C polymorphism with Chagas disease. *Human Immunol* 2009;**70**:543−6.

60. Florez O, Zafra G, Morillo C, Martin J, Gonzalez CI. Interleukin-1 gene cluster poly-morphism in Chagas disease in a Colombian case−control study. *Human Immunol* 2006;**67**:741−8.

61. Cruz-Robles D, Pablo Chavez-Gonzalez J, Magdalena Cavazos-Quero M, Perez-Mendez O, Reyes PA, Vargas-Alarcon G. Association between IL-1B and IL-1RN gene poly-morphisms and Chagas' disease development susceptibility. *Immunol Invest* 2009;**38**:231−9.

62. Arnez LEA, Venegas EN, Ober C, Thompson EE. Sequence variation in the *IL4* gene and resistance to *Trypanosoma cruzi* infection in Bolivians. *J Allergy Clin Immunol* 2011;**127**:279−82.

63. Florez O, Martin J, Gonzalez CI. Interleukin 4, interleukin 4 receptor-alpha and interleu-kin 10 gene polymorphisms in Chagas disease. *Parasit Immunol* 2011;**33**:506−11.

64. Torres OA, Calzada JE, Beraun Y, Morillo CA, Gonzalez A, Gonzalez CI, et al. Lack of association between *IL-6*-174G/C gene polymorphism and Chagas disease. *Tissue Antigens* 2010;**76**:131−4.

65. Costa GC, da Costa Rocha MO, Moreira PR, Menezes CAS, Silva MR, Gollob KJ, et al. Functional IL-10 gene polymorphism is associated with Chagas disease cardiomyopathy. *J Infect Dis* 2009;**199**:451−4.

66. Zafra G, Morillo C, Martin J, Gonzalez A, Gonzalez CI. Polymorphism in the 3' UTR of the *IL12B* gene is associated with Chagas' disease cardiomyopathy. *Microbes Infect* 2007;**9**:1049−52.

67. Leon Rodriguez DA, Echeverria LE, Gonzalez CI, Martin J. Investigation of the role of *IL17A* gene variants in Chagas disease. *Genes Immunity* 2015;**16**:536−40.

68. Nogueira LG, Frade AF, Ianni BM, Laugier L, Pissetti CW, Cabantous S, et al. Functional IL18 polymorphism and susceptibility to chronic Chagas disease. *Cytokine* 2015;**73**:79−83.

69. Rodriguez DAL, Carmona FD, Echeverria LE, Gonzalez CI, Martin J. *IL18* gene variants influence the susceptibility to Chagas disease. *PLoS NTD* 2016;**10**:e0004583.

70. Torres OA, Calzada JE, Beraun Y, Morillo CA, Gonzalez A, Gonzalez CI, et al. Role of the IFNG + 874T/A polymorphism in Chagas disease in a Colombian population. *Infect Genet Evolut* 2010;**10**:682−5.

71. Calzada JE, Beraun Y, Gonzalez CI, Martin J. Transforming growth factor beta 1 (TGF beta 1) gene polymorphisms and Chagas disease susceptibility in Peruvian and Colombian patients. *Cytokine* 2009;**45**:149−53.

72. Bustamante J, Boisson-Dupuis S, Abel L, Casanova JL. Mendelian susceptibility to mycobacterial disease: genetic, immunological, and clinical features of inborn errors of IFN-gamma immunity. *Semin Immunol* 2014;**26**:454−470.

73. Boldt ABW, Luz PR, Messias-Reason IJT. MASP2 haplotypes are associated with high risk of cardiomyopathy in chronic Chagas disease. *Clin Immunol* 2011;**140**:63−70.

74. Luz PR, Miyazaki MI, Neto NC, Padeski MC, Barros ACM, Boldt ABW, et al. Genetically determined MBL deficiency is associated with protection against chronic cardiomyopathy in Chagas disease. *PLoS NTD* 2016;**10**:e0004257.

75. Weitzel T, Zulantay I, Danquah I, Hamann L, Schumann RR, Apt W, et al. Short report: mannose-binding lectin and Toll-like receptor polymorphisms and Chagas disease in Chile. *Am J Trop Med Hyg* 2012;**86**:229−32.

76. Zafra G, Florez O, Morillo CA, Echeverria LE, Martin J, Gonzalez CI. Polymorphisms of toll-like receptor 2 and 4 genes in Chagas disease. *Mem Inst Oswaldo Cruz* 2008;**103**:27−30.

77. Ramasawmy R, Cunha-Neto E, Fae KC, Borba SCP, Teixeira PC, Ferreira SCP, et al. Heterozygosity for the S180L variant of *MAL/TIRAP*, a gene expressing an adaptor protein in the Toll-like receptor pathway, is associated with lower risk of developing chronic Chagas cardiomyopathy. *J Infect Dis* 2009;**199**:1838−45.

78. Jorge SEDC, Abreu CF, Guariento ME, Sonati MdeF. Haptoglobin genotypes in Chagas' disease. *Clin Biochem* 2010;**43**:314−16.

79. Fernandez NM, Fernandez-Mestre M. The role of haptoglobin genotypes in Chagas disease. *Dis Markers* 2014;793646.

80. de Mattos L, Bernardo CR, Oliveira AP, Camargo AVS, Brandao de Mattos CC, Cavasini CE, et al. The expression of B blood group carbohydrate under control of FUT2 gene (19q13.3) increases the risk for digestive Chagas disease. *Immunology* 2012;**137**:SI562.

81. Frade AF, Teixeira PC, Ianni BM, Pissetti CW, Saba B, Wang LHT, et al. Polymorphism in the alpha cardiac muscle actin 1 gene is associated to susceptibility to chronic inflammatory cardiomyopathy. *PLoS ONE* 2013;**8**:e83446.

82. D'Arrigo M, Gerrard G, Lioi S, Diviani R, Ceruti MJ, Beloscar J. Gene polymorphisms of oxidative stress enzymes in Chagasic patients. *Vox Sanguinis* 2013;**105**:SI192.

83. Dias FC, Medina TdaS, Mendes-Junior CT, Dantas RO, Pissetti CW, Rodrigues Jr V, et al. Polymorphic sites at the immunoregulatory CTLA-4 gene are associated with chronic Chagas disease and its clinical manifestations. *PLoS ONE* 2013;**8**:e78367.

84. Luz PR, Boldt ABW, Grisbach C, Kun JFJ, Velavan TP, Messias-Reason IJT. Association of L-ficolin levels and FCN2 genotypes with chronic Chagas disease. *PLoS ONE* 2013;**8**:e60237.

85. D'Arrigo M, Lioi S, Gerrard G, Ensinck A, Zumoffen C, Corbera M, et al. Association among antioxidant enzymes levels, ENOS (G894T), MTHFR (C677T) polymorphisms and Chagas heart disease. *Vox Sanguinis* 2010;**99**:312.

86. Calzada JE, Nieto A, Lopez-Nevot MA, Martin J. Lack of association between NRAMP1 gene polymorphisms and *Trypanosoma cruzi* infection. *Tissue Antigens* 2001;**57**:353−7.

87. Robledo G, Gonzalez CI, Morillo C, Martin J, Gonzalez A. Association study of PTPN22 C1858T polymorphism in *Trypanosoma cruzi* infection. *Tissue Antigens* 2007;**69**:261−4.

88. Fernandez-Mestre M, Sanchez K, Balbas O, Gendzekhzadze K, Ogando V, Cabrera M, et al. Influence of CTLA-4 gene polymorphism in autoimmune and infectious diseases. *Human Immunol* 2009;**70**:532−5.

89. Juiz NA, Cayo NM, Bua J, Longhi SA, Schijman AG. Searching for human genetic polymorphisms associated with congenital transmission of Chagas disease. *Placenta* 2015;**36**:483−4.

90. Visscher PM, Brown MA, McCarthy MI, Yang J. Five years of GWAS discovery. *Am J Human Genet* 2012;**90**:7−24.

91. Bush WS, Moore JH. Chapter 11: Genome-wide association studies. *PLoS Comput Biol* 2012;**8**:e1002822.

92. Deng X, Sabino EC, Cunha-Neto E, Ribeiro AL, Ianni B, Mady C, et al. Genome wide association study (GWAS) of Chagas cardiomyopathy in *Trypanosoma cruzi* seropositive subjects. *PLoS ONE* 2013;**8**:e79629.

93. Utsunomiya YT, Ribeiro ES, Quintal APN, Sangalli JR, Gazola VR, Paula HB, et al. Genome-wide scan for visceral leishmaniasis in mixed-breed dogs identifies candidate genes involved in T helper cells and macrophage signaling. *PLoS ONE* 2015;**10**:e0136749.

94. Quilez J, Martinez V, Woolliams JA, Sanchez A, Pong-Wong R, Kennedy LJ, et al. Genetic control of canine leishmaniasis: genome-wide association study and genomic selection analysis. *PLoS ONE* 2012;**7**:e35349.

95. Xue Y, Chen Y, Ayub Q, Huang N, Ball EV, Mort M, et al. Deleterious- and disease-allele prevalence in healthy individuals: insights from current predictions, mutation databases, and population-scale resequencing. *Am J Human Genet* 2012;**91**:1022−32.

96. Tennessen JA, Bigham AW, O'Connor TD, Fu W, Kenny EE, Gravel S, et al. Evolution and functional impact of rare coding variation from deep sequencing of human exomes. *Science* 2012;**337**:64−9.

97. Mukonzo JK, Owen JS, Ogwal-Okeng J, Kuteesa RB, Nanzigu S, Sewankambo N, et al. Pharmacogenetic-based efavirenz dose modification: suggestions for an African population and the different CYP2B6 genotypes. *PLoS ONE* 2014;**9**:e86919.

98. Paganotti GM, Gallo BC, Verra F, Sirima BS, Nebie I, Diarra A, et al. Human genetic variation is associated with *Plasmodium falciparum* drug resistance. *J Infect Dis* 2011;**204**:1772−8.

# Clinical phases and forms of Chagas disease

*A. Rassi[1], J.M. de Rezende[1,†], A.O. Luquetti[1] and A. Rassi Jr[2]*
[1]Federal University of Goias, Goias, Brazil, [2]Anis Rassi Hospital, Goias, Brazil

## Chapter Outline

## Introduction

Chagas disease is characterized by an acute and a chronic phase of infection. In the acute phase most patients have the unapparent (asymptomatic) form, while the remaining infected individuals usually show a nonspecific febrile disease. In the chronic phase two well-defined forms of disease are distinguished: indeterminate (latent, preclinical) and determinate (clinical), which is subdivided into cardiac, digestive (usually expressed as megaesophagus and/or megacolon), and cardiodigestive forms. Cardiac disease is further classified into stages, and esophageal Chagas disease into groups (Fig. 28.1).

Any febrile illness in an endemic area should lead to suspicion of acute Chagas disease, which is confirmed by the demonstration of parasites in the peripheral blood. The chronic phase is suspected from clinical findings, mainly in the cardiac and digestive systems, supported by epidemiological evidence and confirmed serologically.

Chagas disease is clinically silent in most patients (mainly in the acute phase, but also during the chronic phase), and the diagnosis should be confirmed by the results of laboratory tests. Very often the diagnosis is made fortuitously; e.g., when individuals donate blood, during health screening examination, during self-referral testing, and in patients with a strong positive family history or epidemiological antecedents.

---

† Deceased

American Trypanosomiasis Chagas Disease. DOI: http://dx.doi.org/10.1016/B978-0-12-801029-7.00029-0

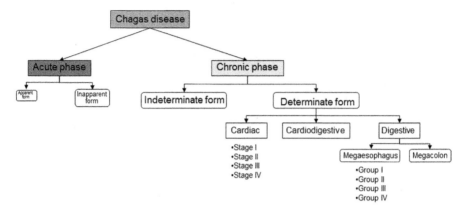

**Figure 28.1** Chagas disease: clinical phases, forms, stages and groups. Evolutionary and temporal relationships are not represented.

It has been estimated that more than 95% of all acute cases of Chagas disease are not diagnosed.[1] This observation is based on the patient's past medical history: when chronic chagasic individuals are asked about their signs and symptoms of acute infection, almost all cannot reply. In the chronic phase, it is well known that at least half of the infected individuals do not have either manifestations of disease or visceral lesions that can be identified by routine tests, such as the electrocardiogram (ECG), chest radiography, and barium studies of esophagus and colon (indetermined form).

The acute and chronic phases of Chagas disease are associated with distinct clinical findings that do not overlap. The initial phase of infection with *T. cruzi* lasts for 4–8 weeks, and the chronic phase persists for the host's life span. Symptomatic manifestations of the acute phase usually disappear within 60 days, even if the infection is not treated with a trypanocidal agent. However, manifestations of the chronic phase, if present, persist, and in some patients become more severe with time. There is no well-defined laboratorial marker, patient characteristic, or clinical measure that reliably predicts Chagas disease progression.

There are few or no geographic differences in the clinical findings of the acute phase, but in the chronic phase the differences are remarkable. The benefit of specific treatment is more accentuated and easily demonstrable when given during the acute phase. Once at the chronic phase, the response will depend on the time elapsed since the acute infection.[2,3] Evolution to death is rare in the acute phase but common during the chronic phase in patients with severe cardiac lesions.

As a large proportion of individuals are asymptomatic during the chronic phase, they are not referred to as patients, but as infected persons. Most individuals with the chronic form of the disease are actively working, and do not know that they are infected. For those who find out about their infection, most may continue working at the same job. Some individuals (e.g., 13% in the 21- to 30-year-old age group) may have cardiac symptoms that need further investigation, and may incapacitate them for work. Very few (approximately 2%) in the same age group need to retire because of severe cardiomyopathy (Table 28.1).

**Table 28.1** **Chronic phase: theoretical model of the clinical form of 100 people infected with *T. cruzi* according to age (*T. cruzi* II, Central Brazil)**

| Age group (years) | Indeterminate form | Cardiac form | | Digestive form | Cardiodigestive form | Total |
|---|---|---|---|---|---|---|
| | | Mild/moderate | Severe[a] | | | |
| 01−10 | 96 | 2 | 1 | 1 | 0 | 100 |
| 11−20 | 90 | 2 | 1 | 5 | 2 | 100 |
| 21−30 | 75 | 7 | 2 | 10 | 6 | 100 |
| 31−40 | 60 | 15 | 3 | 12 | 10 | 100 |
| 41−50 | 55 | 19 | 3 | 13 | 10 | 100 |
| >51 | 50 | 23 | 3 | 13 | 11 | 100 |

[a]Severe cardiac form includes complex ventricular arrhythmias, complete atrioventricular block, atrial fibrillation, echocardiogram with an ejection fraction <35%, cardiomegaly, and congestive heart failure.

In relation to the subclassification of individuals in the chronic phase, Carlos Chagas proposed dividing them into two large groups: those without clinical manifestations and without abnormalities in routine tests, and those with symptoms and/or other abnormalities in one or more tests. This classification was convenient for its simplicity, feasibility, and applicability to most endemic regions since no sophisticated or expensive tests were needed. It was also noted early that a certain number of patients with Chagas disease would progress from one group to the other each year. The importance of this classification was supported by the results of autopsy studies,[4] which showed that in patients with sudden cardiac death a previous abnormal ECG was seen in all. Moreover, in patients with a normal ECG, the probability of severe cardiopathy in the short and medium term is almost zero. Since the disease may progress, annual follow-up should be carried out to search for new ECG abnormalities that, if present, indicate the need for further investigation with other tests for proper risk stratification and work capacity evaluation.[5,6]

This multistep evaluation is affordable, cost-effective, and has been applied in several specialized outpatient clinics in Latin America. Obviously, each case needs to be assessed with regard to the patient's occupation, daily work performed, and other potential risks. For example, a worker who lifts heavy weights every day, if classified with the indeterminate form, needs to be further investigated by an exercise testing or perhaps a 24-h Holter monitoring. These tests are usually not indicated for individuals who work solely at home or as executives.

# Acute phase

The acute phase of vector-borne Chagas disease is observed mainly in the first or second decades of life. Clinical manifestations appear around 8−10 days after the penetration of the parasite.[7] In transfusion-transmitted Chagas disease this period

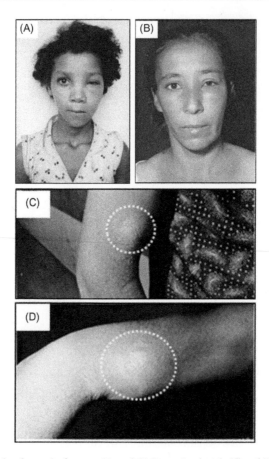

**Figure 28.2** Signals of portal of entry. (A and B) Romaña signal. (C and D) Chagoma in the arm (circle).

may be longer (20−40 days). The acute phase is not clinically recognized in most cases. The experience of those who work in endemic areas is that there is one diagnosed acute case for every 100 chronic patients. When the concentration of the inoculum is small, an atypical clinical picture, not recognized by the patient or the physician, may ensue. Alternatively, the disease may appear as a chronic infection since the beginning.

Romaña's sign is the most typical sign of portal of entry of the parasite. It is characterized by a painless swelling of one or both eyelids of one eye (Fig. 28.2A and B).

The eyelids turn a bluish color, and conjunctival congestion and hypertrophy of satellite lymph nodes (usually preauricular) frequently occur. The edema may spread to half of the face; sometimes dacryoadenitis and diminished conjunctival secretion are observed. Inoculation chagoma is another sign of portal of entry (through the skin), characterized by a maculonodular erythematous lesion, consistent, painless, surrounded by swelling and increased volume of satellite lymph nodes, more often found on open areas and sometimes ulcerated (Fig. 28.2C and D).

Fever is a constant sign, frequently accompanied by malaise, asthenia, anorexia, and headache. Fever is usually higher in children, may be continuous or intermittent, and the temperature may be more elevated during the afternoon.

Lymph node enlargement, hepatomegaly, splenomegaly, and subcutaneous edema are the principal systemic signs, together with cardiac and neurologic alterations. Lymph node enlargement is frequent, of slight or moderate intensity, isolated or contiguous, with a smooth surface, painless, hard and nonadherent, and not fistulous. Hepatomegaly and splenomegaly are also frequent, with characteristics similar to that of lymph nodes.

The edema, whose exact mechanism is unknown, may be generalized or restricted to the face and lower limbs. It is seen most frequently in children. Meningoencephalitis and myocarditis (sometimes with associated pericarditis) are the most severe neurological and cardiological manifestations.[7]

ECG and radiological alterations are not frequently observed during the acute phase if compared with the histopathological findings, but they may become more evident when these tests are repeated (Fig. 28.3).

A disproportional increase in heart rate may be seen in the recovery phase, when fever is no longer present, a finding well described by Carlos Chagas, who also noticed the rarity of cardiac rhythm disturbances in the acute phase, in contrast with their high prevalence during the chronic phase. Other investigators subsequently confirmed these observations. The most common ECG alterations during the acute phase are: sinus tachycardia, low QRS voltage, primary ST-T changes (Fig. 28.4), prolonged electrical systole, and first-degree atrioventricular block.

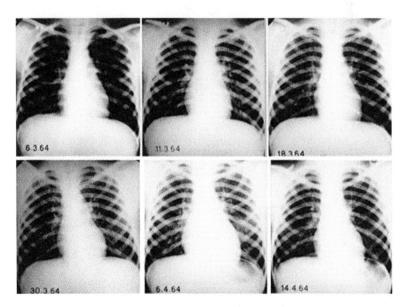

**Figure 28.3** Acute phase of Chagas disease. Importance of serial radiography in the detection of cardiac involvement which is observed only in chest radiography of April 06, 1964.

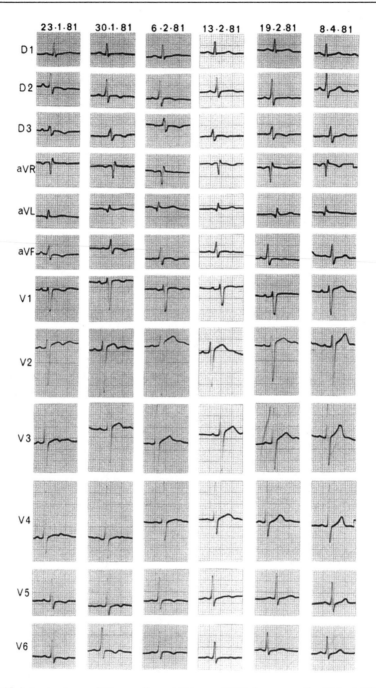

**Figure 28.4** Acute phase of Chagas disease. Primary ST-T changes on the 12-lead ECG that start to normalize on the ECG registered on February 13, 1981.

The chest radiograph may reveal variable degrees of global cardiomegaly.[7] Echocardiography was recently introduced, which explains the lack of information about its performance during the acute phase (since most cases were reported before this method was available). Nevertheless, a recent publication[8] described the echocardiographic findings in 108 of 158 patients during the acute phase of the disease. The main abnormalities were variable degrees of pericardial effusion, mitral or tricuspid valve regurgitation, and concentric hypertrophy of the left ventricle, often with more than one abnormality seen in the same patient.

Other less frequent manifestations observed mainly in Argentina are squizotripanides (a morbilliform, urticariform, and macular exanthema),[9] orchiepididymitis (*T. cruzi* in the fluid produced by the vaginal tunics), and hematogenic chagomas, described by Mazza and Freire.[10] Hematogenic chagomas are flat formations or nodules on the skin and subcutaneous tissues, without color alteration, nonadherent, painless, and of variable size (the size of a coin or larger) that are more palpable than visible.[11]

The mortality in the acute phase used to be around 5% of all symptomatic cases, often as a consequence of meningoencephalitis or myocarditis. However, nowadays this percentage has decreased as the result of use of specific drugs. Spontaneous cure, although exceptional, may occur as has been described by Zeledon et al.[12] and Francolino et al.[13]

Mild to moderate leukocytosis may occur during the acute phase of the disease, with lymphocytosis (atypical lymphocytes), plasmocytosis, and relative neutropenia. Eosinophilia may be observed during the evolution of the disease. The hemosedimentation rate is slightly increased and C-reactive protein is also elevated. Plasma protein electrophoresis usually shows hypoalbuminemia and increased levels of alpha-2 and gamma-globulins. When meningoencephalitis is present, the spinal fluid shows hypercellularity with lymphocytosis (>100 cells/mL), low glucose level, and a slight increase in protein level. It is possible to find trypomastigote forms of *T. cruzi* after centrifugation and specific staining.[7]

The natural evolution of the acute phase in about 90−95% of infected individuals is to pseudocure, when all clinical symptoms and signs disappear spontaneously in approximately 2 months. A direct progression from the acute phase to a clinical form of Chagas disease has been recorded in a few patients (5−10%).

Diagnosis in the acute phase is based on the demonstration of the parasite in peripheral blood, via a wet smear, or after staining (thick smear) or via concentration methods (Strout, microhematocrit).

Identification by these methods is generally possible only during the initial weeks of the disease. Other methods used for diagnosis are skin biopsy of a suspected chagoma, lymph node, and skeletal muscle. Xenodiagnosis with an early examination of the parasites (5−10 days after the blood meal), the search for specific IgM class antibodies by indirect immunofluorescence and the polymerase chain reaction (PCR) are alternative methods. PCR assays may also be used to monitor for acute *T. cruzi* infection in the recipient of an infected organ or after accidental exposure.

# Chronic phase

The chronic phase begins 2 months after the initial infection when the clinical manifestations (if any) of the acute phase disappear, and parasitemia falls to undetectable levels. In most cases, the chronic phase presents as an indeterminate form, which may evolve to the cardiac, digestive, or cardiodigestive forms after years or decades. The diagnosis is made by serological tests, such as indirect hemagglutination, indirect immunofluorescence, and ELISA, all of which have high sensitivity (around 98%) and acceptable specificity. The historical complement fixation reaction (Guerreiro−Machado) is no longer used because of its complexity and because it is no more sensitive or specific than the other tests. According to WHO recommendation,[14] diagnosis should be based on the positivity of at least two of the tests mentioned above.

Demonstration of the parasite in blood may be performed by xenodiagnosis, with the classic (4 boxes with 10 triatomines in each) or the artificial method; the latter has several advantages (is more comfortable for the patients, avoids skin reactions to the triatomine bites, and has equal or superior sensitivity than the classical xenodiagnosis). Another method for parasitological diagnosis is hemoculture, which shows positivity in about 50% of cases. Positivity of these techniques increases when the examination is performed two or more times.

The PCR method is useful for diagnosis of the chronic phase, mainly in those cases with dubious results on serology.

## Indeterminate form

The concept of the indeterminate form was not based on histological findings, but on the fact that visceral lesions could not be detected through clinical examination and complementary routine exams in a significant proportion of patients in the chronic phase of Chagas disease. According to a consensus of experts published in 1985, during the first meeting of applied research in Chagas disease (Araxá, Brazil), in order to be classified in the indeterminate form, the patients should meet all the following criteria: positive serological and/or parasitological tests; absence of signs and symptoms of disease; normal 12-lead ECG; and normal radiological examination of chest, esophagus, and colon. This strict definition provides a good opportunity to categorize patients in epidemiological surveys. In cross-sectional studies conducted in endemic areas, about half of the patients with chronic Chagas disease have the indeterminate form. Recognition of the indeterminate form delimits a group of patients with a favorable prognosis, low morbidity, capable of performing any type of activity, and having the same mortality as that of the general population.

A serious conceptual error frequently observed in the medical literature is to assume that Chagas disease has three phases (acute, indeterminate, and chronic), instead of considering "indeterminate" as one of the forms of the chronic phase. By definition, "chronic" is the time period that follows any acute condition, and where patients with the indeterminate form are situated. Otherwise, we should not consider as being at the chronic phase of the disease an asymptomatic individual who has been infected with *T. cruzi* for a long time.

Although a variable proportion of patients with the indeterminate form present some structural and/or functional abnormalities when they are fully evaluated by more sensitive methods (usually for research purpose), such as ergometry, 24-h Holter monitoring, vectorcardiography, echocardiography, radioisotopic techniques, cardiac magnetic resonance imaging, hemodynamic study, electrophysiologic study, endomyocardial biopsies, autonomic tests, and esophageal and colonic manometric studies, these abnormalities are often subtle and frequently isolated. Moreover, they can occasionally be found also in healthy individuals, and are not related to a decrease in life expectancy. Of note, most studies that have assessed tests of higher sensitivity in patients with chronic Chagas disease did not include the use of contrast media in the examination of the esophagus and colon because of the difficulty of carrying out such tests in asymptomatic individuals. So, it is quite possible that some of these patients had the digestive and not the indeterminate form of the disease.

Some of us studied 103 patients with the indeterminate form, who performed an exercise testing, an echocardiogram, and a 24-h Holter monitoring and had their results compared with that of 20 healthy controls.[15] All chagasic patients fulfilled the rigid definition of the indeterminate form and had a normal barium swallow and enema done. The 2D echocardiogram—only left ventricular systolic function was analyzed—was normal in all patients of both groups. The ambulatory Holter monitoring showed frequent or complex ventricular arrhythmias in 20% of chagasics versus 25% of controls. In the exercise testing, the prevalence of ventricular arrhythmias or an abnormal inotropic or chronotropic response was 16% in the chagasics versus 10% in normal individuals. This controlled study suggests that chagasic patients with the indeterminate form have similar performance when compared with normal population. Discrepancies in the results of studies investigating the role of highly sensitive tests in patients with the indeterminate form may reflect variations in sample size, lack of a normal control group, differences in the definition of abnormal responses, lack of radiological study of esophagus and/or colon, and use of plain abdominal X-ray in substitution of a barium enema.

Although patients with the indeterminate form (inclusive of those with any abnormality on more sensitive tests) have good prognosis, epidemiological studies in endemic areas have shown that 1−3% of them evolve each year from the indeterminate to a clinical (determinate) form of the disease.[16,17] Whether these abnormalities are a reliable early marker of disease progression or an innocent bystander remains to be determined. The subsequent follow-up of patients with the indeterminate form should rely on annual history, physical examination, and 12-lead ECG tracing.

An individual chronically infected with *T. cruzi* remains in the indeterminate form, generally for a period of 10−30 years. Nevertheless, the finding of older people (far from endemic regions for decades) with antibodies against *T. cruzi* and no evidence of visceral involvement indicates that a proportion of the infected people (50−60%) remain in this form for longer periods of time, or even for life.

There have been few pathological studies focusing on individuals with the indeterminate form. Necropsy studies of patients who died from accidental causes revealed mild myocarditis with scattered small foci of interstitial infiltration by lymphocytes, macrophages, and plasma cells, together with a limited reduction in the number of cardiac neurons and myenteric plexuses that are insufficient to produce clinical manifestations.[4] Intact parasites are rarely seen, but *T. cruzi* DNA can be demonstrated in the samples of myocardium, by PCR[18] or other techniques, even in the absence of local inflammation. Whether these lesions represent sequelae of the acute phase, a parasite—host state of equilibrium, or are cumulative, progressing to diffuse myocardial damage remain elusive.

## Cardiac form

The cardiac form is the most serious and frequent manifestation of chronic Chagas disease. It develops in 20—30% of individuals and manifests as three major syndromes that may coexist in the same patient: arrhythmic, heart failure, and thromboembolism (systemic and pulmonary).[19] Clinical presentation varies widely according to the extent of myocardial damage.

Arrhythmias are very common and of different types, frequently in association (Fig. 28.5), and cause palpitations, presyncope, syncope, and Stokes—Adams syndrome; sometimes arrhythmias are asymptomatic.

Frequent, complex, ventricular premature beats, including couplets and runs of nonsustained ventricular tachycardia, are a common finding on 24-h Holter monitoring or stress testing (Fig. 28.6).

They correlate with the severity of ventricular dysfunction, but can also occur in patients with relatively well-preserved ventricular function. Episodes of nonsustained ventricular tachycardia are seen in approximately 40% of patients with mild wall motion abnormalities and in virtually all patients with heart failure, an incidence that is higher than that observed in other cardiomyopathies.[20] Sustained ventricular tachycardia is another hallmark of the disease. This life-threatening arrhythmia can be reproduced during programmed ventricular stimulation in approximately 85% of patients and seems to result from an intramyocardial or subepicardial re-entry circuit usually located at the inferior—posterior—lateral wall of the left ventricle.[21,22]

Heart failure is often a late manifestation of Chagas heart disease. It is usually biventricular with a predominance of right-sided failure (peripheral edema, hepatomegaly, and ascites more prominent than pulmonary congestion) at advanced stages. Nocturnal paroxysmal dyspnea, cardiac asthma, and acute pulmonary edema are all rare. Gallop rhythm is infrequent. Once cardiomegaly appears, a systolic murmur of functional mitral or tricuspid regurgitation may be heard. Isolated left heart failure can be seen in the early stages of cardiac decompensation.[23,24] Heart failure of chagasic etiology is associated with higher mortality than is heart failure from other causes.[25] Systemic and pulmonary embolisms arising from mural thrombi in the cardiac chambers are quite frequent.[26] Clinically, the brain is by far the most frequently recognized site of embolisms (followed by

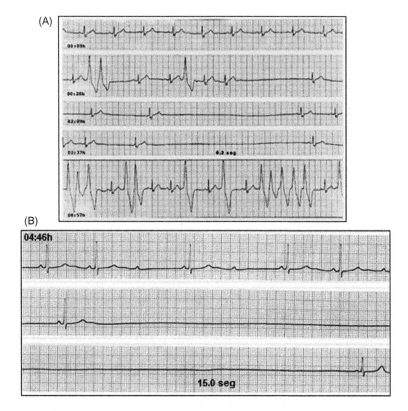

**Figure 28.5** Associated arrhythmias in patients with Chagas heart disease (24-h Holter monitoring). (A) Sinus pauses and nonsustained ventricular tachycardia; (B) second degree atrioventricular block (Mobitz 2) and sinus pause of 15.0 s of duration (during sleep).

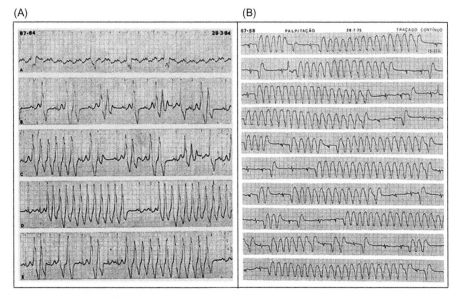

**Figure 28.6** Frequent episodes of nonsustained ventricular tachycardia on stress testing (A) and on 24-h Holter monitoring (B) in patients with Chagas heart disease.

limbs and lungs), but at necropsy, embolisms are found more frequently in the lungs, kidneys, and spleen. Chagas disease is an independent risk factor for stroke in endemic areas.[27]

Sudden death is the main cause of death in patients with Chagas heart disease, accounting for nearly two-thirds of all deaths, followed by refractory heart failure (25–30%) and thromboembolism (10–15%).[28] Sudden cardiac death can occur even in patients who were previously asymptomatic. It is usually associated with ventricular tachycardia and fibrillation or, more rarely, with complete atrioventricular block or sinus node dysfunction. Leading causes of death vary depending on the stage of disease, with a clear predominance of sudden death at early stages, and a slight predominance of death from pump failure at advanced stages.

Electrocardiographic alterations are varied, but the most frequent and important are ventricular premature beats (monomorphic or polymorphic, isolated or in pairs), complete right bundle branch block (CRBBB), left anterior fascicular block, primary ST-T changes, Q waves, different degrees of atrioventricular block, manifestations of sinus node dysfunction (sinus bradycardia, sinoatrial block, and sinus arrest), atrial fibrillation, and nonsustained or sustained ventricular tachycardia. All these alterations may be isolated or associated. A frequent association is CRBBB and left anterior fascicular block, and when this occurs in an endemic area, it strongly suggests chronic Chagas heart disease (Fig. 28.7).

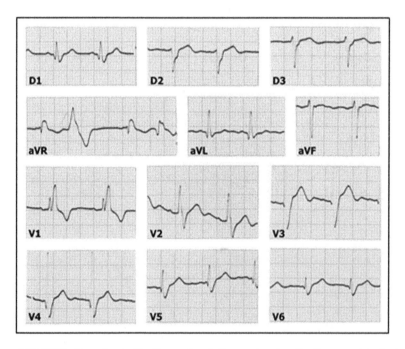

**Figure 28.7** ECG of a patient with Chagas heart disease showing the three most typical alterations: right bundle branch block, left anterior fascicular block, and ventricular extrasystole.

On radiological examinations, the cardiac size is generally normal in the initial phase of the cardiopathy and even when important electrocardiographic changes are present. The cardiac size may be slightly, moderately, or severely increased, in all chambers (Fig. 28.8). In nearly half of the cases with heart failure, the manifestations of pulmonary congestion are poor or even absent.

The echodopplercardiogram may be abnormal even in patients with a normal ECG and normal chest radiograph. Echo shows wall motion abnormalities in two main areas of the left ventricle: the apex and the posterior—inferior wall. The most characteristic findings are apical aneurysms (with or without thrombi) (Fig. 28.9) and akinesia or hypokinesia of the posterior wall of the left ventricle (with preservation of the atrioventricular septum).

Ambulatory ECG monitoring (Holter system) is an excellent method for investigating patients with Chagas heart disease.[29-31] It may be used to identify complex ventricular arrhythmias, evaluate antiarrhythmic therapy, diagnose transitory arrhythmias, identify the association of tachyarrhythmias with bradyarrhythmias, evaluate people for job activities, and establish whether an artificial pacemaker is working properly. It is performed routinely for a 24-h period. In some cases a special device (event recorder) is used that registers ECG activity for several days.

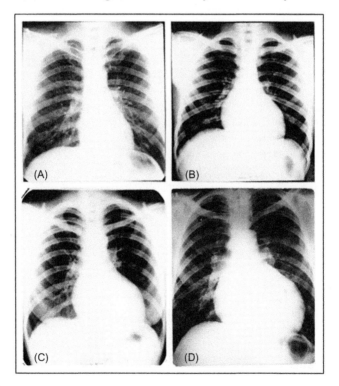

**Figure 28.8** Chest radiography of four patients with Chagas heart disease. (A) Normal; (B) mild cardiomegaly; (C) moderate cardiomegaly; and (D) severe cardiomegaly without pulmonary congestion.

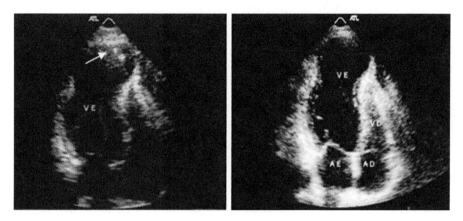

**Figure 28.9** Two-dimensional echocardiogram showing left ventricular apical aneurysm with (arrow) and without thrombus.

The exercise testing evaluates the functional capacity of the patient, qualifies and quantifies ventricular premature beats, and may verify the efficacy of antiarrhythmic drugs.

Intracardiac electrophysiological studies evaluate the sinus node function, identify the location of atrioventricular and intraventricular blocks precisely, and investigate the inducibility of ventricular tachyarrhythmias, as well as their place of origin. It is of great value in the evaluation of presyncope and syncope of unknown origin, in indicating the need for an artificial pacemaker, as well as evaluating alternative methods of treatment of sustained ventricular tachycardia (e.g., catheter ablation). Because of its invasive nature, it should be performed only in selected patients or after all other noninvasive methods have been tried, such as Holter monitoring and exercise testing.

More recently, cardiac magnetic resonance has become an important tool in the assessment of cardiac function and myocardial structure. Not only segmental contractility, ventricular aneurysms, intracavitary thrombus, and left and right ventricular ejection fraction and volumes can be well defined, but also myocardial perfusion at rest and under stress are precisely determined. In addition, the myocardial areas of necrosis and/or fibrosis can be analyzed noninvasively and related to clinical aspects of Chagas cardiomyopathy, such as severe ventricular arrhythmias, symptoms of heart failure, sudden death, and other major events.[32]

Chagas heart disease can be divided schematically into four stages[33] (Table 28.2).

In stage I, patients are usually symptom free and show mild and nonspecific ECG alterations. Left ventricular systolic function is preserved, but diastolic abnormalities may be found. Complex ventricular arrhythmias on 24-h Holter monitoring are rare. In stage II, manifestations include more specific conduction abnormalities, most frequently right bundle branch block, left anterior fascicular block (or both), complex ventricular arrhythmias, and segmental left ventricular wall motion abnormalities. Manifestations of later stages (III and IV)

**Table 28.2 Stages of chronic Chagas heart disease**

| | Cardiac symptoms[a] | NYHA class | ECG changes | Chest X-ray (cardiomegaly) | 24-h Holter (complex VA[b]) | 2D Echocardiogram | | Thrombo-embolism | Sustained VT | Sudden death |
|---|---|---|---|---|---|---|---|---|---|---|
| | | | | | | LV wall motion abnormalities | LV apical aneurysms | | | |
| Stage I | Absent or minimal | – | Not specific | Absent | Rare | Rare | Very rare | Very rare | Rare | Rare |
| Stage II | Fairly common | I/II | RBBB ± LAFB, mono VPBs, diffuse ST-T Changes, 1°, 2° AV block | Absent or mild | Common | Absent or segmental | Common | Fairly common | Common | Common |
| Stage III | Common | I/II/III | + q waves, poli VPBs, advanced AV block, severe bradycardia, low QRS voltage | Mild to moderate | Very common | Segmental or diffuse (mild to moderate) | Common | Fairly common | Common | Common |
| Stage IV | Common | II/III/IV | + atrial flutter/fibrillation | Moderate to severe | Very common | Diffuse (severe) | Fairly common | Common | Fairly common | Fairly common |

2D, two-dimensional; AV, atrioventricular; ECG, electrocardiogram; LAFB, left anterior fascicular block; LV, left ventricular; mono, monomorphic; NYHA, New York Heart Association; poli, polymorphic; RBBB, right bundle branch block; VA, ventricular arrhythmias; VPBs, ventricular premature beats; VT, ventricular tachycardia.

*Schematic classification based on the authors' own experience and review of the literature with aim of helping physicians better understand the heterogeneous clinical course of chronic Chagas disease; minor interchanges in some characteristics among the different stages of cardiac disease are possible.

§ Megaesophagus and/or megacolon without apparent heart disease; mixed (cardiodigestive) form of chronic Chagas disease, which is defined as the association of megaesophagus and/or megacolon with any one of the stages of cardiac disease, is not included in the table because of the multiplicity of possible combinations. Incomplete RBBB, incomplete LAFB, mild bradycardia, minor increase in PR interval, minor $T$-$T$ changes.

[a]Palpitations, presyncope, syncope, atypical chest pain, fatigue, and edema.
[b]Couplets and/or episodes of nonsustained VT.

are: (1) sinus node dysfunction, usually leading to severe bradycardia; (2) high-degree heart block; (3) pathologic Q waves, low QRS voltage, and atrial fibrillation, compatible with extensive areas of myocardial fibrosis; (4) pulmonary and systemic thromboembolic phenomena due to thrombus formation in the dilated cardiac chambers or aneurysm; (5) cardiomegaly; and (6) progressive dilated cardiomyopathy with marked impairment of systolic function and congestive heart failure.

Improved understanding of prognostic factors in Chagas heart disease has helped clinicians to identify patients' risk, choose appropriate treatment, and direct patient counseling. Some of us used a rigorous multivariate analysis to develop a risk score for mortality prediction in 424 outpatients from a regional Brazilian cohort and the score has been validated[34,35] successfully in two external cohorts. Several demographic, clinical, and noninvasive variables were tested, and six were identified as independent predictors of mortality and were assigned points according to the strength of their statistical association with the outcome. From addition of the points to provide the risk score, patients can be classified into groups of low, intermediate, and high risk (Fig. 28.10).

Subsequently, two systematic reviews[5,36] integrated the results of all previous studies in which multivariable regression models of prognosis were used and a clearly defined outcome (all-cause mortality, sudden cardiac death, or cardiovascular death) was analyzed. According to these reviews, the strongest and most consistent predictors of mortality are New York Heart Association (NYHA)

| A          Risk Factor | Points |
|---|---|
| NYHA class III or IV | 5 |
| Cardiomegaly (chest X-ray) | 5 |
| Segmental or global WMA (2D echo) | 3 |
| Nonsustained ventricular tachycardia (24-h Holter) | 3 |
| Low QRS voltage (ECG) | 2 |
| Male sex | 2 |

| Total Points | Total Mortality (%) | | Risk |
|---|---|---|---|
|  | 5 Years | 10 Years |  |
| 0–6 | 2 | 10 | Low |
| 7–11 | 18 | 44 | Intermediate |
| 12–20 | 63 | 84 | High |

**Figure 28.10** Prognostic factors in Chagas heart disease. Rassi score for prediction of total mortality. Echo, echocardiogram; NYHA, New York Heart Association; WMA, wall motion abnormality.

functional class III or IV, cardiomegaly on chest radiography, impaired left ventricular systolic function on echocardiogram or cineventriculography, and nonsustained ventricular tachycardia on 24-h Holter monitoring. On the basis of these findings, a risk stratification model for mortality, which can assist treatment in patients with Chagas heart disease, is proposed in Table 28.3.

With the exception of some peculiarities, the general principles that guide the symptomatic treatment of chronic Chagas heart disease are the same as those established for heart disease of other causes. Bradyarrhythmias are treated with pacemaker implantation. As a general rule, a pacemaker is indicated for all patients with symptomatic bradyarrhythmias or for those at high risk of complete atrioventricular block. The electrode should be placed in the subtricuspid zone[37] avoiding the apex of the right ventricle, which may be thin, fibrotic, and contain thrombus.

**Table 28.3 Stratification of risk of death associated with Chagas heart disease and recommended therapy**

| Risk of death | Risk factor | | | Recommended treatment |
|---|---|---|---|---|
| | NYHA class III/IV | LV systolic dysfunctions (echo) and/or cardiomegaly (chest X-ray) | Nonsustained VT (24-h Holter) | |
| Very high | Present[a] | Present | Present | ACE inhibitor, espironolactone, amiodarone, diuretics, digitalis, betablocker,[b] cardiac transplant,[c] ICD? |
| High | Absent | Present | Present | ACE inhibitor, amiodarone diuretic,[c] betablocker,[b] ICD? |
| Intermediate | Absent | Present | Absent | ACE inhibitor, betablocker, diuretic[c] Antiparasitic drug? |
| | Absent | Absent | Present | Amiodarone Antiparasitic drug? |
| Low | Absent | Absent | Absent | Antiparasitic drug[c] |

ACE, angiotensin-converting enzyme; echo, echocardiogram; ICD, implantable cardioverter-defibrillator; LV, left ventricular; NYHA, New York Heart Association; VT, ventricular tachycardia.
[a]Nearly 100% of patients with Chagas heart disease in NYHA class III or IV also have LV systolic dysfunction on echo and nonsustained VT on 24-h Holter monitoring.
[b]If clinically tolerated.
[c]For selected patients.

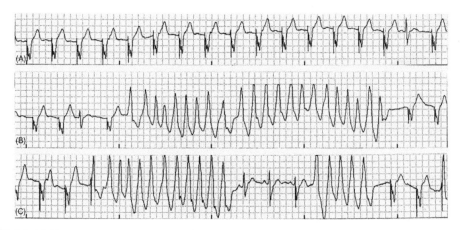

**Figure 28.11** (A) 24-h Holter monitoring in a patient with Chagas heart disease after pacemaker implantation showing (B and C) episodes of nonsustained ventricular tachycardia.

However, the management of rhythm disorders does not end with the implant of a pacemaker. Ventricular arrhythmias should also be promptly searched in patients with a pacemaker using the 24-h Holter monitoring and/or an exercise testing (Fig. 28.11), and treated accordingly.[20]

Ventricular arrhythmias are treated mainly with amiodarone; sotalol and beta blockers are second choice drugs. Propafenone and mexiletine have been used in some symptomatic patients with normal ventricular function based exclusively on their antiectopic activity. Quinidine, procainamide, and disopiramide do not have adequate antiarrhythmic activity; nevertheless, the use of procainamide when given intravenously for the treatment of paroxysmal ventricular tachycardia is highly effective. Monomorphic sustained ventricular tachycardia may also be amenable to percutaneous endocardial or pericardial ablation using catheter-delivered radiofrequency or cumulative high-energy fulguration in selected patients with mappable arrhythmia. The use of implantable cardioverter-defibrillators in patients with Chagas heart disease is hampered by the lack of controlled data to establish precise indications and efficacy[38] as well as by socioeconomic limitations. A Brazilian randomized trial (CHAGASICS) is currently recruiting patients for a comparison of amiodarone versus the implantable cardioverter-defibrillator for primary prevention of death in patients with nonsustained ventricular tachycardia and a Rassi score of 10 or more points.[39] For secondary prevention of sudden cardiac arrest or sustained ventricular arrhythmias, the implantable cardioverter-defibrillator is usually recommended, especially for patients with an ejection fraction less than 35%. When cardiac failure is present, it may be necessary to use higher doses of diuretics; angiotensin-converting enzyme inhibitors, espironolactone, and digoxin are also commonly used, and in special situations, betablockers are used.[33] In some individuals, such as those with intractable cardiac failure following optimized treatment, a cardiac transplant is necessary; in this situation, the patient should usually receive specific treatment before or shortly after the surgical procedure. Palliative procedures, such as dynamic cardiomyoplasty and partial left ventriculectomy, are contraindicated because of unsatisfactory results. Cardiac resynchronization is another form of treatment for heart failure, and is mostly for patients with left bundle branch block. Remarkably few data support its use in patients with right bundle branch block, which is much more common in patients with Chagas heart disease. The potential benefit of transplantation of bone marrow cells for treatment of Chagas heart failure was assessed in a multicenter randomized controlled trial sponsored by the Brazilian Health Ministry (MiHeart study), but it failed to show additional benefits over standard therapy in patients with severe heart failure.[40]

Because of the high occurrence of thromboembolic phenomena in Chagas heart disease, oral anticoagulants are recommended for patients with atrial fibrillation, previous embolic episodes, and apical aneurysm with thrombus. If poor social and economic factors limit the implementation of anticoagulant therapy, because of the increased risk of bleeding, the use of acetylsalicylic acid is considered a reasonable alternative.

## Digestive form

The digestive form of Chagas disease is characterized by alterations in the motor, secretory, and absorptive functions of the gastrointestinal tract. Lesions of the enteric nervous system are pivotal in the pathogenesis of Chagas digestive megasyndromes. The myoenteric plexus of Auerbach, which is located between the longitudinal and circular muscular layers of the digestive tract, is the main one affected.[41] Although most of the damage to the neurons of this plexus and the nervous fibers occurs during acute infection, further neuronal loss occurs slowly over an extended period of the chronic phase. There is a marked reduction in the number of nervous cells of the Auerbach's plexus as demonstrated by Koberle[42] in quantitative studies performed on several segments of the digestive tract, in humans, and in experimental animals infected with *T. cruzi*. Denervation occurs to variable degrees, is irregular and noncontinuous, and probably depends on both parasite and host factors.

Variations in *T. cruzi* strains related to the pathogenicity for the enteric nervous system probably explain the regional differences associated with Chagas disease (i.e., why the digestive form is seen only in some geographical areas), its unpredictable evolution, and its multiplicity of clinical manifestations.

The medical literature indicates a higher prevalence of the digestive form in the central region of Brazil. It has also been described in other countries of South America, but is not seen in countries above the equatorial line, where only a few cases with esophageal motor alterations have been described.[43]

Prevalence studies of the chagasic digestive form in Brazil (the country with the highest rates) have been performed based on radiological findings of the esophagus as an indicator of the involvement of the digestive tract. In seven radiological surveys performed in endemic areas and blood banks by abreugraphy (roentgenphotography, a radiograph of 35 or 70 mm, used as screening for tuberculosis), the prevalence rates of esophagopathy ranged from 7.1% to 18.3% (mean 8.8%) among 3073 infected individuals.[44]

Although intrinsic denervation can be found along the entire digestive tract, with variable intensity and distribution, the esophagus and the distal colon, because of their physiology, are the most frequently involved segments. As a consequence of denervation, motor uncoordination and achalasia of the sphincters occur, making it difficult for these segments to empty semisolid material, and leading to dilatation with time; this is the pathophysiological mechanism underlying chagasic megaesophagus and megacolon.

It has been observed that the frequency of megaesophagus is higher than that of megacolon in outpatient clinics or institutions caring for chagasic patients.

A survey conducted at the Hospital das Clinicas of the Federal University of Goias, between 1976 and 1997, showed that 1761 patients had megaesophagus at the first consultation (56.8% males and 43.2% of females; ages ranging from 2 to 102 years, of whom 75% were 20–70 years old). The association with megacolon was investigated by barium enema in 765 patients, and 365 of them (45.5%) also had megacolon.[45]

Serological tests for Chagas disease were performed on 1271 sera from patients with megaesophagus, including 362 with associated megacolon. Positive results were found in 91.3% of patients with megaesophagus and in 99.4% of patients with associated megacolon.[44]

Association of the cardiac and digestive form may vary according to peculiarities in each region and these data have limited value. In a region of central Brazil, this association was evaluated in 1313 patients. A normal ECG was found in 48.2% ($n = 633$), nonspecific ECG alterations were found in 21.1% ($n = 277$), and characteristic alterations (i.e., CRBBB) in 30.7% ($n = 403$). Only 14 out of 403 patients had severe alterations. The more frequent ECG abnormalities were CRBBB with or without left anterior fascicular block and ventricular premature beats.[44]

The clinically more interesting entities in the digestive form are esophagopathy and colopathy. In those cases with higher denervation, evolution is to ectatic forms of megaesophagus and megacolon.

## Megaesophagus

The main complaints presented by patients at consultation are dysphagia, regurgitation, and esophageal pain. Other less frequent symptoms are hiccups, pyrosis, and hypersalivation accompanied by parotid hypertrophy. Malnutrition is observed with the progression of the disease.

Dysphagia is often the first and the most frequent symptom in the natural history of idiopathic achalasia or chagasic megaesophagus. It may be mild, moderate, or severe, and the intensity varies with type of food ingested, its temperature, and the emotional status of the patient.

Regurgitation may be active, occurring during or immediately after meals with the conscious participation of the patient, or passive, when the patient is lying in bed sleeping, generally at night. The regurgitated material is expelled through the mouth and narines and may enter the respiratory tract, causing coughing and suffocation. Regurgitation is a common cause of pulmonary complications, mainly aspirative bronchopneumonia.

Esophageal pain may be spontaneous or associated with food ingestion, when it is called odynophagia. Spontaneous pain is localized at the level of the xiphoid appendix or below the sternum and propagates in an ascending direction up to the base of the neck, and radiates to the interscapulovertebral region and upper limbs. The pain is of the burning type, constrictive, tearing, or colicky, and is alleviated or abolished with the ingestion of water or other liquids.

Radiological examination is essential to confirm the diagnosis and to stage the disease (based on the morphofunctional characteristics of the esophagus), which is very important for the selection of the most appropriate therapy. Although there are several radiological classifications, we recommend the one by Rezende et al.,[46] which identifies four groups (Fig. 28.12).

> Group I: Normal diameter of esophagus; minimal contrast retention; presence of a residual air column above the contrast
> Group II: Moderate dilatation, with some contrast retention; increase in uncoordinated motor activity; relative hypertony of the inferior third of the esophagus
> Group III: Large increase in diameter and great contrast retention; hypotonic esophagus with weak or absent motor activity
> Group IV: Large increase in volume, atonic, elongated esophagus, lying on the right diaphragmatic dome.

Radiological examination should be combined with fluoroscopy to assess esophageal motility and emptying. The examination is performed with the patient in the upright position, preferentially at right anterior oblique view. In this position, the cardiac shadow projects to the front and the column to the back, allowing for better discrimination of the contrasted esophageal image.

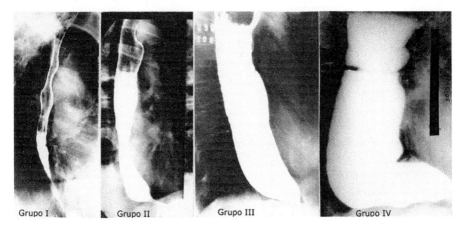

Grupo I   Grupo II   Grupo III   Grupo IV

**Figure 28.12** Radiological classification of chagasic megaesophagus in four groups according to the stage of disease.[46]

The amount of contrast medium should be sufficient to generate an ideal height and pressure column that promotes the passage of contrast to the stomach, when the shape, diameter, wall contour, and mainly the contractile activity of the esophagus can be clearly seen. It is also important to search for eventual tertiary waves, which are uncoordinated and nonpropulsive contractions. The distal esophagus should be carefully observed. The last X-ray should be done after all the contrast medium has passed through the cardia.

For the detection of cases in group I, in which the diameter of the esophagus is normal, a special technique, known as retention test (analysis of two consecutive radiographs, the first immediately after ingestion of barium, and the second 1 min later), is recommended. The test is positive when incomplete emptying is observed on the second radiograph producing a level of residual contrast, and the esophagus remains open by the presence of an air column. A differential diagnosis should be established with other diseases that may display the same image, such as presbyesophagus, hiatus hernia, esophagitis, systemic sclerosis, neoplasia, and the use of anticholinergic drugs before the barium swallow.

There is significant correlation between symptoms and the evolution of megaesophagus. In group I, dysphagia is generally the only complaint. In group II, besides more severe dysphagia, there is active regurgitation and esophageal pain. In groups III and IV, passive regurgitation and malnutrition are frequent.

The evolution of chagasic esophagopathy to worsening of symptoms and progression of radiological and manometric parameters is not uniform in all cases; and if it occurs, it evolves slowly over time.

In a longitudinal study performed in an endemic area (Mambai, Goias State, Brazil) the prevalence of megaesophagus was assessed in 1006 individuals with positive serology. A chest abreugraphy (roentgenphotography, 70 mm) was taken after a barium meal of 75 mL contrasted the esophagus; a second abreugraphy was done 1 min later. Megaesophagus was detected in 71 (7%) of these patients: 43 were classified as group I, 18 as group II, 5 as group III, and 5 as group IV. Twenty-one patients with megaesophagus were reexamined 25 years later with the same technique. Progression was observed in 10 cases.[47]

Esophagealgastroduodenal endoscopy should be routinely performed after the radiological examination of the esophagus for evaluation of the mucosa and detection of associated lesions, mainly esophageal cancer, and cancer of the esophagealcardiotuberosity region.

For the differential diagnosis of chagasic megaesophagus with other esophagopathies, if there are any doubts, esophageal manometry is indicated using at least three pressure channels. The abnormalities seen in patients with chagasic megaesophagus vary depending on the stage of the disease. There is a loss of peristaltic activity at the body of the esophagus (aperistalsis), with synchronic waves and failure or incomplete aperture of the lower esophageal sphincter with ingestion (achalasia). In groups III and IV contractions are of low amplitude.

Manometry is particularly useful in the differential diagnosis of the hyperkinetic forms of megaesophagus and diffuse esophageal spasm, and for evaluation of the basal pressure of the lower sphincter of the esophagus before and after dilatation or surgery.

Idiopathic achalasia and chagasic megaesophagus are both risk factors for the development of esophageal cancer, because of chronic irritation of the mucosa caused by residual food. The prevalence of this association varies widely from 0.4% to 9.3%.[45] The duration of the disease may be more important than the age of the patient. Higher prevalence of megaesophagus has been described by surgical services, probably because patients who need surgery are those with more advanced disease.

Treatment of chagasic megaesophagus and idiopathic achalasia may be clinical, instrumental, or surgical. Clinical treatment is indicated only for group I, or when other types of treatment are contraindicated for groups II, III, or IV. Clinical treatment is based on hygiene and dietary measures, and, eventually, the use of drugs such as isosorbitol dinitrate or nifedipine given before meals to relax the lower esophageal sphincter.

Instrumental treatment may be performed by dilatation of the cardioesophageal junction with a mercury-filled dilator (bougies of Hurst or Maloney) to temporarily alleviate the dysphagia, or by a pneumatic or hydrostatic balloon that reduces the pressure of the lower esophageal sphincter and usually shows satisfactory results. For older patients, the injection of botulinum toxin into the muscular layer of the esophagus−gastric transition may be performed as an alternative procedure and has an effect that lasts, on average, for 1 year.

The preferential treatment for groups II and III is surgery, using the Heller extra-mucosal cardiomyotomy technique via videolaparoscopy. For group IV, different types of surgery, including resection of the esophagus with cervical esophagogastric anastomosis, are indicated.

## Megacolon

The prevalence of megacolon is hard to estimate, because of difficulties related to its diagnosis, which involves the realization of a barium enema. Megacolon is seldom the only manifestation of the digestive tract; in most cases it is associated with megaesophagus.

The most common symptoms are constipation, meteorism, dyskesia, and less often, abdominal colicky pain. Constipation may even be absent in 25−30% of individuals who have radiological dilatation of the colon.[44,48]

On physical examination, an increase in the abdominal volume is observed. Since the distal colon is the most affected segment, the distended sigmoid occupies a large part of the abdominal cavity and may be localized by palpation and percussion outside its normal topography.

Prolonged retention of feces in the distal colon leads to formation of fecaloma, which may be diagnosed by simple abdominal palpation, as an elastic tumor that can be molded by pressure. Rectal examination will detect a fecaloma at the rectal ampulla. Radiological examination is necessary to confirm the diagnosis, and should begin with a noncontrasted plain abdominal radiograph, which may show increased intestinal air and, if fecaloma is present, a bread-like image. After the noncontrasted X-ray, a barium enema is performed, which usually involves the use of intestinal cleansing or purgatives, as well as the introduction of air into the colon to achieve double contrast. These maneuvers, however, modify the original morphology of the colon and may induce false results. The colon is an elastic organ with capacity for distension or contraction, depending on the fecal contents as well as the endogenous or exogenous stimuli. Purgatives are irritants and increase the tonus and enterocolic contractility. The introduction of air into the colon causes distension of its wall that is proportional to the injected pressure, increasing the diameter of the distal colon, mainly the sigmoid colon. As a result, a false picture of the anatomical dimensions of the distal colon is obtained.

To avoid these pitfalls, a simplified technique is recommended, which has been shown to be satisfactory for the diagnosis of chagasic megacolon in endemic regions.[49] Barium enema is performed without previous preparation and double contrast, using 300 mL of barium sulfate diluted up to 1200 mL with water. This preparation is delivered at a height of 1 m with the patient in ventral decubitus position, without any pressure effect. Then the patient moves to the right lateral decubitus position for 5 min. The first radiograph is taken in the dorsal decubitus position, and the second in the ventral decubitus position, using a $30 \times 40$ mm X-ray film. Another film, $24 \times 30$ mm, is taken with the patient in the right lateral decubitus position to image the rectum. The distance between the source of X-rays and the film (focus-film distance) should be 1 m. The presence of fecaloma is not an obstacle to this simplified technique. If there is suspicion that another disease of the colon is present, enema should be repeated with the conventional technique.

When the colon is largely dilated, the diagnosis is easy. When it is not, doubts may arise, because there is no clear-cut division among normal and abnormal patterns. The diameter and the dimension of sigmoid and rectal ampoule as well as the total length of the colon varies widely in normal subjects and in infected people. For this reason, the limits of normality need to be established for a given population. In an endemic region of Central Brazil, the application of the technique mentioned above in 72 nonchagasic individuals allowed to establish the following values as the upper limits of normal for radiological films: 7 cm for the diameter of sigmoides in an anteroposterior view; 11 cm for rectum diameter; and 70 cm for the length of distal colon, including rectum and sigmoides. By employing these parameters, the prevalence of megacolon in 225 infected individuals in this area was 6.2%.[50]

Dilation is usually located at the distal colon, including sigmoid and rectum (Fig. 28.13A). Rarely a dilatation is found in other segments or in the entire colon (Fig. 28.13B). Very often dilatation is associated with an increase in colon length, the dolicomegacolon.

Obviously, diagnosis of the nondilated colopathy cannot be performed by radiological examination and requires other methods, such as manometry and pharmacological tests of denervation.

Differential diagnosis should be made with other colonic dilatations of obstructive or functional origin, such as neoplasias, stenosis, extrinsic compressions, and rectosigmoid endometriosis. Among dilatations of functional origin, the psychogenic megacolon of the infancy, the andine megacolon (without lesions of the myoenteric plexus), the toxic megacolon that occurs as a complication of inflammatory bowel

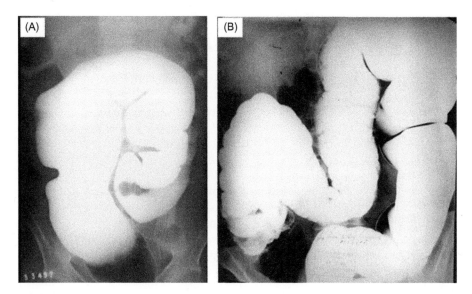

**Figure 28.13** Chagasic megacolon. (A) Dilatation is mainly at the rectum and sigmoid. (B) Total megacolon (rare).

diseases, and the atonic colon due to the action of drugs leaving to a secondary dilatation should always be remembered.

Differential diagnosis with Hirschsprung disease, also called congenital megacolon, is usually easy because chagasic megacolon is exceptional in low-age children.

Two other complications, apart from fecaloma formation, may occur: the fecal impactation and sigmoid volvulus, both with a clinical syndrome of intestinal occlusion. Fecal impactation may be solved with fecaloma emptying. Volvulus, depending on the degree of torsion and the aspect of the mucosa, may be treated by endoscopy distortion. If signals of suffering of mucosa are present at the local of torsion, surgical treatment is indicated.

Differently from megaesophagus, cancer of colon is rarely seen in patients with megacolon.

Treatment of megacolon may be clinical or surgical. In oligosymptomatic patients, when constipation is mild to moderate, a treatment based on osmotic laxatives (saline, lactulose, macrogol 3350) or emollients (mineral oil) is indicated, together with appropriate hygienic and dietary measures. An additional aid may be the inclusion of glycerol in enemas or in suppositories. The same conservative procedure is indicated for patients waiting for surgery and for those with a high surgical risk.

Surgical treatment is indicated in symptomatic patients with persistent constipation and clear evidence of dilatation of the distal colon in the radiological examination, as well as in those with previous complications. There are several surgical techniques, but the most frequently used (because of the results) is the resection of the dilated segment and lowering of the retrorectal portion of colon, leaving the rectum without function (technique of Duhamel—Haddad).

## Other organs of the digestive tract

Other segments and organs of the digestive system may be compromised in Chagas disease, causing functional alterations that may be detected by different investigation methods, but with a lower impact than the lesions involving esophagus and colon.[45]

Chagasic gastropathy was initially suspected based on clinical evidence only.[51] Gastric involvement is found in nearly 20% of patients with megaesophagus. On radiological examination the gastric volume is extremely variable, and the absence of air in the stomach of patients with advanced megaesophagus is very typical (Fig. 28.14).

In patients with the digestive form, hypersensitivity of the muscle layer of the gastric wall in response to cholinergic pharmacological stimuli, as well as alterations in both motility and secretion, may be detected by several methods. In these cases there is rapid gastric emptying for liquids and delayed for solids. A lower adaptative relaxation of the stomach in response to distension is also usually found. An alteration of the gastric electric rhythm has recently been demonstrated by electrogastrography.[52]

Another alteration seen in patients with Chagas disease is a lower basal and stimulated (under different stimuli such as histamin, histalog, pentagastrin, and calcium ion infusion) gastric acid secretion. However, when a stimulus with a cholinergic substance is added, an increase of hydrochloric acid or pepsin secretion

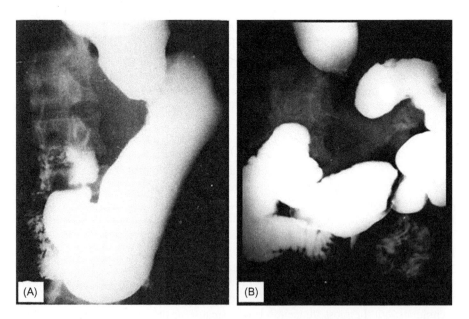

**Figure 28.14** (A) megaesophagus group IV associated with megastomach; (B) Megaesophagus of group III associated with dilatation of stomach, bulb, and duodenal archade.

is obtained. This demonstrates that hyposecretion is mainly due to intrinsic denerva-tion of the stomach and not due to reduction in the number of secretory cells. Fast and postprandial hypergastrinemia is another finding.

Besides these secretory and motor alterations, chronic gastritis of variable intensity is frequently found. Multiple etiopathogenic factors may be involved, such as biliary duodenogastric reflux and infection by *Helicobacter pylori.*

Hypertrophy of pyloric muscle is usually seen in cases with severe difficulty in gastric emptying, formerly known as pylorus achalasia. In these cases pyloroplastia is indicated as a complement to cardiomyotomy for the surgical treatment of megaesophagus.

Duodenum is, after the esophagus and colon, the segment that most often shows dilatation (Fig. 28.15).

Megaduodenum is nearly always associated with other visceromegaly. The dilatation may be localized only at the bulb (megabulb), at the second and third segments, or involve the entire duodenal arcade. Even when no dilatation is present, dyskinesia and hyperreactivity to cholinergic stimuli are common, due to enteric denervation. Symptoms caused by megaduodenum may be confused with dyspepsia of gastric origin, of the dysmotility type.

Histopathological studies have shown less degree of denervation at the small intestine than at esophagus and colon. Dilatation of jejunum or ileum characterizing megajejunum or megaileum is rare, with few published cases (Fig. 28.16).

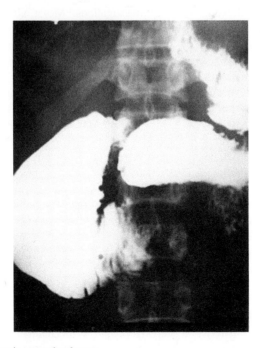

**Figure 28.15** Chagasic megaduodenum.

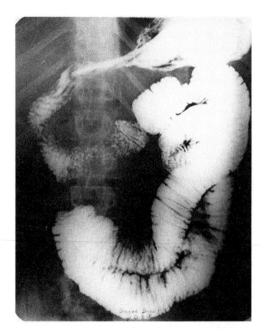

**Figure 28.16** Megajejunum in a patient with megaesophagus of group II.

The evidence of chagasic enteropathy is not readily apparent by clinical means, but may be detected using specific investigations. Motor alterations have been described in radiological and manometric studies. Patients with other manifestations of the digestive form usually show abnormalities in the interdigestive motor migratory complex. As a consequence, it is possible to have an increase in bacterium flora growth, which in some cases is similar to that seen in the syndrome of stagnant loop.

Studies in patients with the digestive form have also demonstrated an abnormal increase in the absorption of glucose and other sugars. As a consequence, the tolerance to glucose oral test may show abnormal glycemic curves, with transitory hyperglycemia in the first hour. In association with hyperabsorption of glucose a modest hypoabsorption of fats may be seen, although not sufficient to reduce the fecal fat excretion rate. Both alterations are partially due to abnormalities in gastric emptying.

An intrinsic denervation of the gallbladder may also be observed, leading to motor alterations in gallbladder filling and emptying. Manometric alterations were also described at the Oddi sphincter. Nevertheless, colecistomegaly and choledocho dilatation are not frequent (Fig. 28.17).

A higher prevalence of colelithiasis in chagasic patients with megaesophagus and/or megacolon has been described.

Salivary glands, mainly parotids, are hypertrophic in patients with megaesophagus, a common finding in any obstructive esophageal disease as a consequence of the esophageal−salivary reflex that produces hypersalivation. Chagasic patients also have a higher sensitivity of salivary glands to mechanical stimuli of mastication and to the pharmacological stimuli by pilocarpin. Interestingly, the

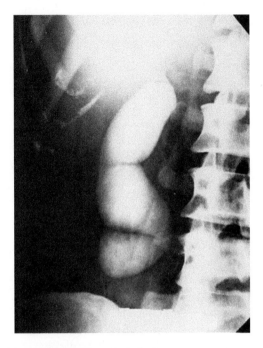

**Figure 28.17** Colecistomegaly in a chagasic patient.

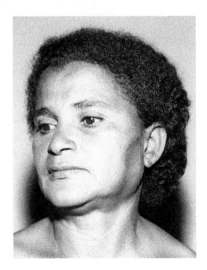

**Figure 28.18** Hypertrophic parotids in a patient with chagasic megaesophagus.

hypersalivation and parotid hypertrophy persist in esophagectomized patients, showing that these alterations are not exclusively due to the esophagus–salivary complex, but that there may also be some inervation involvement of salivary glands in Chagas disease (Fig. 28.18).

Regarding the exocrine pancreas, its functional capacity is preserved in relation to direct stimuli of the organ. However, in consequence of alterations in the delivery of duodenojejunal hormones, a secretory deficiency by indirect stimuli may be found.

## Cardiodigestive form

The association of heart disease with megaesophagus or megacolon, or both defines the cardiodigestive form of Chagas disease. In most countries the development of megaoesophagus usually precedes heart and colon disease, but the exact prevalence of the cardiodigestive form is not known because of the scarcity of appropriate studies.

# Concluding remarks

Individuals with Chagas disease may be seen in two distinct phases: acute, seldom diagnosed as such, and chronic. The diagnosis of the chronic phase is based mainly on the presence of IgG antibodies against *T. cruzi* in patients with high suspicion of the disease or in those with a compatible clinical syndrome. Chronic Chagas infection is silent for life in more than half of the individuals. In order to define the clinical form of disease, a complete search for cardiovascular and gastrointestinal symptoms and a resting 12-lead ECG are essential. Although barium swallow and enema are needed for final diagnosis of the digestive form, these tests are usually not recommended as standard practice for patients without gastrointestinal symptoms. Asymptomatic patients with a normal ECG and no gastrointestinal tract or cardiovascular symptoms have a favorable prognosis and should be followed up every 12–24 months, since about 2% of these patients progress to a clinical form of the disease each year. There are no known markers of disease progression. Patients with ECG changes consistent with Chagas heart disease should undergo a routine cardiac assessment to establish the stage of disease. Ambulatory 24-h Holter monitoring is used to detect arrhythmias; combined chest radiography and 2D echocardiography refine the assessment of cardiac size and function, and provide additional prognosis. If complaints of dysphagia or constipation are present, the routine contrasted X-rays are indicated. Most patients can be followed by a general practitioner. Labor restrictions are limited according to the degree of heart involvement. Of note, even if a reasonable proportion of patients with Chagas heart disease die early, a similar number may have irrelevant disease until elderly ages.

# Glossary

**24-h Holter monitoring (ambulatory Holter monitoring)** A portable device used for 24 h that continuously records the patient's ECG during usual daily activity.
**Abnormal chronotropic response** Inadequate increase in heart rate during exercise testing.

**Abnormal inotropic response** Inadequate increase in systolic blood pressure during exercise testing.

**Achalasia** An esophageal motility disorder in which the smooth muscle layer of the esophagus loses normal peristalsis (muscular ability to move food down the esophagus), and the lower esophageal sphincter fails to relax properly in response to swallowing.

**Atrial fibrillation** An abnormality in the heart rhythm that involves irregular and often rapid beating of the heart and is related to thromboembolic phenomena.

**Cardiac resynchronization (biventricular pacing)** A treatment for heart failure that uses a three-lead biventricular pacemaker implanted in the chest. The pacemaker sends tiny electrical impulses to the heart muscle to coordinate (resynchronize) the pumping of the chambers of the heart, improving the heart's pumping efficiency. Both ventricles are paced to contract at the same time. This can reduce the symptoms of heart failure.

**Complete atrioventricular block** Also known as third-degree heart block, it is a rhythm disorder in which the impulse generated in the sinus node in the atrium does not propagate to the ventricles.

**Couplets** Two ectopic beats occurring one after the other.

**Dyskesia (dyschezia)** Pain with defecation.

**Fecaloma** A tumor made of feces.

**First-degree atrioventricular block** A disease of the electrical conduction system of the heart in which the PR interval is lengthened beyond 0.20 s.

**Gallop rhythm** A usually abnormal rhythm of the heart on auscultation. It includes three or four sounds, thus resembling the sounds of a gallop.

**Intracardiac electrophysiological study** Placement of multiple catheter electrodes into the heart for the diagnosis and management of selected cardiac conditions. This procedure has been used mainly for identifying the mechanisms, site, and severity of brady-or tachyarrhythmias.

**Low QRS voltage** Voltage of entire QRS complex in all limb leads of the ECG <5mm.

**New York Heart Association functional class** A functional classification of heart failure into four stages according to the type of activity causing shortness of breath I (intense physical activity); II (moderate physical activity); III (mild physical activity); and IV (rest).

**Nonsustained ventricular tachycardia** A period of three or more ventricular ectopic beats lasting less than 30 s.

**Primary ST-T changes** ST-T wave changes that are independent of changes in ventricular activation and that may be the result of global or segmental pathologic processes that affect ventricular repolarization.

**Programmed ventricular stimulation** A minimally invasive procedure which tests the electrical conduction system of the heart to assess its electrical activity and conduction pathways.

**Sinus node dysfunction** A group of abnormal heart rhythms presumably caused by a malfunction of the sinus node (the heart's primary pacemaker).

**Stokes−Adams syndrome** Sudden collapse into unconsciousness due to a disorder of heart rhythm in which there is a slow or absent pulse resulting in syncope (fainting) with or without convulsions.

**Transcatheter ablation** An invasive procedure used to remove a faulty electrical pathway responsible for some cardiac arrhythmias. Catheters are advanced toward the heart and high-frequency electrical impulses are used to induce the arrhythmia, and then ablate (destroy) the abnormal tissue that is causing it.

**Volvulus** A bowel obstruction in which a loop of bowel has abnormally twisted on itself.

**Xenodiagnosis** Procedure allowing the feeding of laboratory-reared triatomine bugs (known to be infection-free) the blood of patients suspected of having Chagas disease; after several weeks, the bug feces are checked for the presence of *Trypanosoma cruzi*.

# References

1. Teixeira MGLC. *Doenca de Chagas, Estudo da forma aguda inaparente*. Rio de Janeiro: Faculdade de Medicina, UFRJ; 1977.
2. Cancado JR. Long term evaluation of etiological treatment of Chagas disease with benznidazole. *Rev Inst Med Trop Sao Paulo* 2002;**44**(1):29−37.
3. Coura JR, de Castro SL. A critical review on Chagas disease chemotherapy. *Mem Inst Oswaldo Cruz* 2002;**97**(1):3−24.
4. Lopes ER, Chapadeiro E, Andrade ZA, Almeida HO, Rocha A. Pathological anatomy of hearts from asymptomatic Chagas disease patients dying in a violent manner. *Mem Inst Oswaldo Cruz* 1981;**76**(2):189−97.
5. Rassi Jr A, Rassi A, Marin-Neto JA. Chagas heart disease: pathophysiologic mechanisms, prognostic factors and risk stratification. *Mem Inst Oswaldo Cruz* 2009;**104**(Suppl 1):152−8.
6. Rassi Jr. A, Dias JC, Marin-Neto JA, Rassi A. Challenges and opportunities for primary, secondary, and tertiary prevention of Chagas' disease. *Heart* 2009;**95**(7):524−34.
7. Rassi A, Rassi Jr A, Rassi GG. Fase Aguda. In: Brener Z, Andrade ZA, Barral Netto M, editors. *Trypanosoma cruzi e Doença de Chagas*. 2nd ed. Rio de Janeiro; 2000.
8. Pinto AY, Valente SA, Valente Vda C, Ferreira Junior AG, Coura JR. [Acute phase of Chagas disease in the Brazilian Amazon region: study of 233 cases from Para, Amapa and Maranhao observed between 1988 and 2005]. *Rev Soc Bras Med Trop* 2008;**41** (6):602−14 [in Portuguese].
9. Mazza S, Basso G, Basso R, Freire R, Miyara S. Esquizotripanides. *M.E.P.R.A* 1941; **52**:31.
10. Mazza S, Freire RS. Manifestaciones cutaneas de inoculacion, metastaticas y hematogenas en Enfermedad de Chagas. Chagomas de inoculacion, chagomas metastaticos y chagomas hematogenos. *M.E. P.R.A* 1940;**46**:3−38.
11. Lugones HS. *Enfermedad de Chagas. Diagnostico de su faz aguda*. Santiago del Estero, Argentina: Univ. Catolica Santiago del Estero; 2001.
12. Zeledon R, Dias JC, Brilla-Salazar A, de Rezende JM, Vargas LG, Urbina A. Does a spontaneous cure for Chagas' disease exist? *Rev Soc Bras Med Trop* 1988;**21**(1): 15−20.
13. Francolino SS, Antunes AF, Talice R, Rosa R, Selanikio J, de Rezende JM, et al. New evidence of spontaneous cure in human Chagas' disease. *Rev Soc Bras Med Trop* 2003;**36**(1):103−7.
14. Committee WHO. Control of Chagas disease. *World Health Organ Tech Rep Ser* 2002;**905**(i-vi):1−109, back cover.

15. Rassi A, Rassi Jr A, Rassi AG, Rassi Jr L, Rassi SG. Avaliacao da forma indeterminada da doenca de Chagas. *Arq Bras Cardiol* 1991;**57**(Suppl):140.

16. Dias JC. The indeterminate form of human chronic Chagas' disease: a clinical epidemiological review. *Rev Soc Bras Med Trop* 1989;**22**(3):147−56.

17. Storino R. Evolucion natural y estudios longitudinales. In: Storino R, Milei J, editors. *Enfermedad de Chagas*. Bueno Aires: Doyma Argentina Editorial; 1994. p. 593−604.

18. Jones EM, Colley DG, Tostes S, Lopes ER, Vnencak-Jones CL, McCurley TL. Amplification of a *Trypanosoma cruzi* DNA sequence from inflammatory lesions in human chagasic cardiomyopathy. *Am J Trop Med Hyg* 1993;**48**(3):348−57.

19. Rassi A, Luquetti AO, Rassi Jr A, Rassi SG, Rassi AG. Chagas' disease: clinical features. In: Wendel S, Brener Z, Camargo ME, Rassi A, editors. *Chagas' disease (American Trypanosomiasis): Its impact on transfusion and clinical medicine*. Sao Paulo: Editora ISBT; 1992. p. 81−101.

20. Rassi Junior A, Gabriel Rassi A, Gabriel Rassi S, Rassi Junior L, Rassi A. [Ventricular arrhythmia in Chagas disease. Diagnostic, prognostic, and therapeutic features]. *Arq Bras Cardiol* 1995;**65**(4):377−87 [in Portuguese].

21. Sosa E, Scanavacca M, D'Avila A, Piccioni J, Sanchez O, Velarde JL, et al. Endocardial and epicardial ablation guided by nonsurgical transthoracic epicardial mapping to treat recurrent ventricular tachycardia. *J Cardiovasc Electrophysiol* 1998;**9**(3):229−39.

22. d'Avila A, Splinter R, Svenson RH, Scanavacca M, Pruitt E, Kasell J, et al. New perspectives on catheter-based ablation of ventricular tachycardia complicating Chagas' disease: experimental evidence of the efficacy of near infrared lasers for catheter ablation of Chagas' VT. *J Interv Card Electrophysiol* 2002;**7**(1):23−38.

23. Rassi Jr. A, Rassi A, Little WC. Chagas' heart disease. *Clin Cardiol* 2000;**23**(12):883−9.

24. Marin Neto JA, Rassi Jr A, Maciel BC, Simoes VL, Schmidt A. Chagas heart disease. In: Yusuf S, Cairns JA, Camm AJ, Fallen EL, Gersh BJ, editors. *Evidence-based cardiology*. 3rd ed. London: BMJ Books; 2010. p. 823−41.

25. Freitas HF, Chizzola PR, Paes AT, Lima AC, Mansur AJ. Risk stratification in a Brazilian hospital-based cohort of 1220 outpatients with heart failure: role of Chagas' heart disease. *Int J Cardiol* 2005;**102**(2):239−47.

26. Samuel J, Oliveira M, Correa De Araujo RR, Navarro MA, Muccillo G. Cardiac thrombosis and thromboembolism in chronic Chagas' heart disease. *Am J Cardiol* 1983;**52**(1):147−51.

27. Carod-Artal FJ, Vargas AP, Horan TA, Nunes LG. Chagasic cardiomyopathy is independently associated with ischemic stroke in Chagas disease. *Stroke* 2005;**36**(5):965−70.

28. Rassi Jr. A, Rassi SG, Rassi A. Sudden death in Chagas' disease. *Arq Bras Cardiol* 2001;**76**(1):75−96.

29. Rassi A, Perini GE. Valor da eletrocardiografia dinamica (sistema Holter) no estudo da Cardiopatia Chagasica Cronica. *Ars Cvrandi Cardiol* 1979;**2**:31−54.

30. Rassi A, Lorga AM, Rassi S. Abordagem diagnostica e terapeutica das arritmias na cardiopatia chagasica cronica. In: Germiniani H, editor. *Diagnostico e Terapeutica das Arritmias Cardiacas*. 3rd ed. Rio de Janeiro: Guanabara Koogan; 1990. p. 225−44.

31. Rassi A, Lorga AM, Rassi SG. Diagnostico e tratamento das arritmias na cardiopatia cronica. In: Cancado JR, Chuster M, editors. *Cardiopatia Chagasica*. Belo Horizonte: Imprensa Oficial do Estado de Minas Gerais; 1985. p. 274−88.

32. Belisario Falchetto E, Costa SC, Rochitte CE. Diagnostic challenges of Chagas cardiomyopathy and CMR imaging. *Glob Heart* 2015;**10**(3):181−7.

33. Rassi Jr. A, Rassi A, Marin-Neto JA. Chagas disease. *Lancet* 2010;**375**(9723):1388−402.

34. Rassi Jr. A, Rassi A, Little WC, Xavier SS, Rassi SG, Rassi AG, et al. Development and validation of a risk score for predicting death in Chagas' heart disease. *N Engl J Med* 2006;**355**(8):799−808.

35. Rocha MO, Ribeiro AL. A risk score for predicting death in Chagas' heart disease. *N Engl J Med* 2006;**355**(23):2488−9, author reply 90-1.

36. Rassi Jr. A, Rassi A, Rassi SG. Predictors of mortality in chronic Chagas disease: a systematic review of observational studies. *Circulation* 2007;**115**(9):1101−8.

37. Korman DS, Jatene AD. Triangulo eletrodo-vertebro-diafragmatico no posicionamento de eletrodo endocavitario para marca-passos cardiacos. *Arq Bras Cardiol* 1977;**30**(Suppl. 2).

38. Rassi Jr. A. Implantable cardioverter-defibrillators in patients with Chagas heart disease: misperceptions, many questions and the urgent need for a randomized clinical trial. *J Cardiovasc Electrophysiol* 2007;**18**(12):1241−3.

39. Martinelli M, Rassi Jr. A, Marin-Neto JA, de Paola AA, Berwanger O, Scanavacca MI, et al. Chronic use of Amiodarone aGAinSt Implantable cardioverter-defibrillator therapy for primary prevention of death in patients with Chagas cardiomyopathy Study: rationale and design of a randomized clinical trial. *Am Heart J* 2013;**166**(6):976−82.

40. Ribeiro Dos Santos R, Rassi S, Feitosa G, Grecco OT, Rassi Jr. A, da Cunha AB, et al. Cell therapy in Chagas cardiomyopathy (Chagas arm of the multicenter randomized trial of cell therapy in cardiopathies study): a multicenter randomized trial. *Circulation* 2012;**125**(20):2454−61.

41. Koberle F. Patogenia da molestia de Chagas. Estudo dos orgaos musculares ocos. *Rev. Goiana Med.* 1957;**3**:155−80.

42. Koberle F. Pathology and pathological anatomy of Chagas' disease. *Bol Oficina Sanit Panam* 1961;**51**:404−28.

43. Rezende JM. Chagasic mega syndromes and regional differences. *PAHO Scientific Publication* 1975;**318**:195−205.

44. Rezende JM, Luquetti AO. *Chagasic megavisceras. Nervous system in Chagas disease*. Washington: PAHO/OMS; 1994. p. 149−71.

45. Rezende JM, Moreira H. Forma digestiva da doenca de Chagas. In: Castro LP, Coelho LCV, editors. *Gastroenterologia*. Rio de Janeiro: Editora Medica e Cientifica Ltda; 2004. p. 325−92.

46. Rezende JM, Lauar KM, de OA. Clinical and radiological aspects of aperistalsis of the esophagus. *Rev Bras Gastroenterol* 1960;**12**:247−62.

47. Penaranda-Carrillo R, Castro C, Rezende J, Prata A, Macedo V. Radiographic study of the oesophagus of chagasic patients in 25 years of the Mambai Project. *Rev Soc Bras Med Trop* 2006;**39**(2):152−5.

48. Vaz MGMR JM, Ximenes CA, Luquetti AO. Correlacao entre a sintomatologia e a evolucao do megaesofago. *Rev. Goiana Med* 1996;**41**:1−15.

49. Ximenes CA, Rezende JM, Moreira H, Vaz MGM. Tecnica simplificada para o diagnostico radiologico do megacolo chagasico. *Rev. Soc. Bras. Med. Trop* 1984;**17**:23.

50. Castro C, Hernandez EB, Rezende J, Prata A. Radiological study on megacolon cases in an endemic area for Chagas disease. *Rev Soc Bras Med Trop* 2010;**43**(5):562−6.

51. Porto C. Gastropatia chagasica cronica. *Rev. Goiana Med* 1955;**1**(1):43−54.

52. Rezende Filho J, De Rezende JM, Melo JR. Electrogastrography in patients with Chagas' disease. *Dig Dis Sci* 2005;**50**(10):1882−8.

# Diagnosis of *Trypanosoma cruzi* infection

A.O. Luquetti[1] and G.A. Schmuñis[2]

[1]Federal University of Goias, Goias, Brazil, [2]Regional Office of the World Health Organization for the Americas

## Chapter Outline

## Introduction

This review describes the different methodologies and techniques that made possible the laboratorial diagnosis of Chagas disease since the first test was described in 1913. It has been a long journey and still there are questions without answer.

American Trypanosomiasis Chagas Disease. DOI: http://dx.doi.org/10.1016/B978-0-12-801029-7.00030-7

With the globalization of the infection by the protozoan *Trypanosoma cruzi* with thousands of infected individuals all over the world,[1] the role of the laboratory is even more important than before. We will describe here how the possible few cases of recent *T. cruzi* infection that may appear today in special circumstances would be diagnosed using parasitological techniques. Taking into account that the vast majority of infected individuals are at the chronic asymptomatic phase, their only marker would be the presence of *T. cruzi* antibodies, mainly of the IgG class. Therefore, their accurate serological diagnosis is a must, either for exclusion or for confirmation of the infection. This is the only way medical personnel can handle the patients correctly. Special attention is given to the advantages and limitations of the different diagnostic methods as well as different examples on how these diagnostic tools may be applied by physicians in real-life situations.

## History of diagnosis in Chagas disease

Four years after the discovery of the parasite *T. cruzi* by Carlos Chagas, as well as the disease it produces in humans and the epidemiology of the infection, the complement fixation (CF) or Bordet—Gengou test was adapted by Guerreiro and Machado[2] to the serological diagnosis of what is now known as Chagas disease.

The CF test was the only one routinely used for diagnosis for more than 50 years, using as a source of antigen, organs of infected animals.[3] Later on, extracts of in vitro cultured epimastigotes were employed. These extracts were treated with benzene, ether, or acetone[4−9] in order to remove the lipids that could cross-react with serum samples positive for syphilis. The final reagent was suspended in water or methanol and kept with glycerol at −20°C or lyophilized at 4°C. Throughout this time, the whole crude extract of epimastigotes was replaced by proteins or polysaccharides derived from it.[6,10−13]

The CF test was cumbersome to perform. The amount of complement available, the temperature, and the time of incubation were all crucial for this test, and these variables were not always followed by the laboratories that performed the test. The diversity of antigens available also made the test difficult to standardize. In any case, it was the only test available and continuous efforts to improve standardization made the CF test reliable when in the hands of those laboratories that complied with the strict norms necessary to obtain the maximum reactivity.[14−16] In these conditions, the CF had from 90% to 100% sensitivity,[17,18] and cross-reactivity was mainly with visceral and tegumentary leishmaniasis. Another problem was the variable number of samples in which the serum was anticomplementary, which made the results inconclusive. Doing the CF and the indirect hemagglutination test (IH) on thousands of serum samples, agreement among the two tests was 96.5−98.5%. There were also 1.5−3.5% of samples that were doubtful because there was no agreement among the tests or because anticomplementary results were obtained with the CF test.[19]

**Table 29.1 Tests for diagnosis of Chagas disease 1940s−1970s[a]**

| Year | Test for diagnosis |
|------|--------------------|
| 1913 | Complement fixation |
| 1914 | Xenodiagnosis |
| 1944 | Agglutination |
| 1944 | Precipitation |
| 1949 | Conditioned hemolysis |
| 1952 | Immobilization test |
| 1955 | Indirect Coombs |
| 1958 | Immunofluorescence with epimastigotes |
| 1959 | Dye test |
| 1962 | Indirect hemagglutination test |
| 1964 | Immunofluorescence with amastigotes |
| 1967 | Trypanolysis |
| 1970 | Latex test |
| 1971 | Direct agglutination test |

[a]Modified from Cerisola, 1972

The xenodiagnosis is another old diagnostic method described by Brumpt.[20] The principle is to reproduce the natural cycle in the vector host by feeding bugs in infected individuals. Several variables have been adjusted with time, which were standardized by Cerisola et al.[21] It was used in the past mainly in Brazil, Argentina, and Chile and is now available in only a handful of laboratories in the world.

From the early 1940s until the end of the 1970s, other diagnostic tests appeared based on the detection of antibodies (Table 29.1). With exception of the indirect immunofluorescence antibody test (IFA) and the IH, none of the others survive as tests for routine use. The IFA was used as a test for many infectious diseases, but the first reports applied to Chagas disease using epimastigotes as antigen by Fife and Muschel[22]; it started to be widely used some years later after the standardization by Camargo.[13] The first publication on the IH was from Cerisola et al. in Argentina[23] and Knierim and Saavedra[24] from Chile. Because of its simplicity, it was quickly adopted as one of the methods of choice for diagnosis.

# Diagnosis of *T. cruzi* infection

Diagnosis of infection by *T. cruzi* should include, as in any infectious disease, clinical data, supported by the epidemiology and confirmed or not by laboratory tests.

This general statement has some pitfalls in Chagas disease, mainly because more than half of the infected individuals may have no complaints and clinical

Table 29.2 **Relation among positive serology for Chagas disease and some characteristic symptoms in infected patients**

| Alteration | Positive serology | % | Negative serology | % | Total |
|---|---|---|---|---|---|
| Complete Right Bundle Branch Block[a] | 847 | 98.0 | 18 | 2.0 | 865 |
| Megaesophagus | 1575 | 93.3 | 114 | 6.7 | 1689 |
| Megacolon | 916 | 94.6 | 52 | 5.4 | 968 |

[a]As a single or combined EKG alteration. Patients were all less than 61 years old. No children included.
*Source*: Laboratorio de doença de Chagas, Hospital das Clinicas, UFG; Rezende JM, Luquetti AO. Chagasic megavisceras. *Nervous system in Chagas disease*. Washington: PAHO/OMS; 1994. p. 149–71.

examination, as well as some exams, such as electrocardiogram (ECG), chest X-ray, barium swallow, and barium enema, may be normal.[25] In these cases, the suspicion may arouse from the epidemiological background of the patient. Past residence in endemic areas, infected mother or siblings, or work with this pathogen may be recorded and evaluated, and laboratory examinations used for exclusion or confirmation. The third aspect of diagnosis, laboratory tests, may be the only proof of disease and thus should be properly done.

On the other hand, some clinical alterations are so frequent in those patients with symptoms of Chagas disease that a negative laboratory result should be taken with caution and a request to repeat the exam, may be advisable. We refer to complete right bundle branch block (CRBBB), an ECG alteration which is typical (but not pathognomonic) of Chagas disease (Table 29.2). Less than 20% of infected individuals have digestive tract manifestations, as megaesophagus and/or megacolon. These alterations are also not frequent in the general population. If present, they strongly suggest Chagas disease. In fact more than 90% of the patients with any one of these disturbances, in an endemic area, have positive serological tests for *T. cruzi*[26] (Table 29.2).

Laboratory diagnosis includes parasitological and serological tests. Infected individuals/patients may look for medical care during the acute phase or, more often, during the chronic phase. Laboratory tests to be ordered depend on the suspected phase of the disease. For those unusual cases during the acute phase, which lasts only for 2 months, parasitological tests are mandatory. On the other hand, in the chronic phase which lasts for life, serological tests are the diagnostic method of choice. These principles are explained by the natural history of Chagas disease, with easily detected parasites during the acute phase, which is defined because of the presence of them. Weeks after symptoms start, the immune response will destroy the majority (but not all) the parasites and they will be no longer easily detectable. By this time (4 weeks) IgG antibodies should be present, with higher affinity as time goes on, and they will hold for the rest of life, unless the patient would receive anti-*T. cruzi* treatment.[27]

In summary, to confirm or exclude an acute infection by *T. cruzi*, parasitological tests should be performed as the first choice. When the suspicion is of a chronic infection, serological tests must be performed.

# Parasitological tests

## Overview

The natural course of Chagas infection starts with an acute phase, whose manifestations, if present, will arise some days after the entrance of the parasites. Parasites multiply exponentially until the antibody response starts, which becomes evident 10−20 days later. As a consequence, the number of parasites begins to decline, and, at the end of the first month, they are scarce. This phase lasts for 2 months, and is defined by the easy detection of the parasite, which becomes more difficult to find after the first weeks. For diagnosis of this phase, parasitological tests should be employed.[27]

At this stage, it is useful to include as acute cases all the following conditions, independent of the mechanism of transmission: acute phase by vector transmission, congenital infection, transfusion or by organ transplantation, oral route, accidental infection, and reactivation by immunosuppression. Even if the finding of parasites is the hallmark, clinical manifestations may be different. In those infected by vector contamination, most of them will not be recognized. Those infected through transfusion may also not have been diagnosed, and the manifestations may appear with a longer incubation period, the reasons for which have not been understood yet.[28] Congenital transmission may also remain undiagnosed, because most of the cases are born with normal weight and without any other features, apart from the infected mother. Oral route may have digestive manifestations, probably because of the large inoculum and the multiplication of parasites at the digestive tract. For these reasons, many acute cases are not diagnosed at this phase, but many years later by chance (i.e., during a blood donation).[29]

After the acute phase, which is estimated to be asymptomatic in more than 95% of the infected individuals, even without diagnosis or treatment, the infected person enters the chronic phase, usually in the indetermined form (no symptoms or signs, no ECG, or X-ray abnormalities) which lasts for the entire life. Spontaneous cure has been reported but is certainly highly unusual.[30] Circulating parasites are scarce, never found by direct observation (see section: Chronic phase) and may be absent for circulation for some periods. It has been said[27] that parasitemia at the chronic phase is variable, not constant, and present at a given moment only in a few mL of the 5 L of blood that a human being has. This fact explains several observations made in the natural history of the infection: transmission by transfusion is successful only in 20% of the cases, up to 50% in hyperendemic areas.[31−34]

When performing several parasitological methods (see section: Chronic phase) at the same time, it is normal to find parasites only with one of them; by using xenodiagnosis (40 bugs), positive bugs are only $1-3$ of them, the others remain negative because they did not ingest a single parasite.[21] Cerisola et al. observed that each bug is as a "single microhemoculture processed at the digestive tract of each bug," hence the chances to find positive bugs increase as more bugs are included.[21]

## Indications

For all the earlier reasons, parasitological methods should not be used for diagnosis of chronic phase of Chagas disease because most of the results will be negative. A negative parasitological result has no value in terms of diagnosis. On the other hand, a positive test has tremendous value, even when antibodies are present in low titers. For diagnosis of the chronic phase, parasitological examination should not be used.

Parasites are easily detected only in the acute phase or during the reactivation of the chronic phase because of immune suppression. Actually, this is the definition of acute phase. What does "easily detected" mean? This is when finding of parasites by direct observation or by concentration techniques (see later) is possible. These tests are easy to perform and cheap, but only available in specialized laboratories in the field. There is no need to buy them, because they use simple tools that any laboratory has (glass slides, tubes, centrifuges, microscopes). However, there is a need to have personnel with expertise to search and diagnose *T. cruzi* and at the same time, avoid being infected by live parasites (see section: Prophylaxis to avoid accidental contamination).

There are methods for the detection of *T. cruzi* when it is present in low numbers (i.e., the chronic phase). These methods are based on another principle: the multiplication of parasites that are not easily found in the sample (usually peripheral blood). For this multiplication, the conditions offered to the parasite should be optimal.

Methods most used are classic xenodiagnosis and hemoculture, and the relatively recent[35−37] polymerase chain reaction (PCR), a molecular test, based on the amplification of DNA or RNA present in *T. cruzi* through probes. Xenodiagnosis and hemoculture have common features; they are not commercially available, demand some time to get multiplication of the parasites (weeks, months), are time-consuming, and need expertise from technicians. In addition, the former demands a colony for growing bugs, which is available in less than a handful of laboratories in the world; and the latter needs to be processed in absolute sterility and at $4°C$, conditions difficult to find in the field. As both have been in use for decades, they are properly standardized.[21,38]

PCR may be performed in a few hours, but is more expensive, requires special skills, and attempts for standardization and validation have only recently been made. This technique has been applied for *T. cruzi* since the early 1990s, with high interest after the first publications indicating 100% positivity.[39] Further studies revealed much lower figures, depending on the population group studied. When analyzing the first results, they were performed with patients who previously had positive xenodiagnosis, so a bias was introduced (Borges-Pereira, personal communication). The technique revealed variable sensitivity depending not only on the characteristics of the population analyzed but also from the test itself, the volume and conservation of samples, DNA extraction method, parasite sequences used, primers, reagents, and thermo-cycling conditions.[40]

The need for a standardization was recently stressed (2011) in a multicenter evaluation sponsored by TDR/WHO and performed in two steps. In the first, 29 research groups were invited to participate and received three sets of samples blind. The first set comprised five 10-serial dilutions of *T. cruzi* DNA from 3 reference stocks. The second were blood samples spiked with 10-fold dilution of culture parasites and the third was a panel of 40 clinical samples (10 from noninfected persons) from several countries. Each laboratory performed its own method with the same samples. From the 49 different strategies used by the 29 laboratories, only 4 methods were selected, on the basis of their performance with a specificity of 100% and a sensitivity of 56−63%. In the second step, 18 participants, selected by their better performance, participated in a workshop, performing the analysis of the clinical samples with the same reagents and methods. Silica gel column extraction followed by satellite-based PCR was more specific and sensitive than other methods, and a standard operating procedure was defined for the test.[41]

There are two main questions regarding PCR. The first is because of the natural history of the parasitemia at the chronic phase. As written above, some infected individuals may be free of circulating parasites for long periods of time, so PCR could not find DNA of nonexisting parasites, and this fact may explain why several recent reports[42] cannot reach the 100% sensitivity predicted years ago. The other main question relates to the reliability of PCR diagnosis, with a high frequency of false positives due to contamination observed in some studies, as well as false negatives due to inhibitory substances in the lysate.[40]

## Conclusions

For all the reasons exposed, these multiplication methods have several limitations and a short range of applications like the follow-up of treated patients to check treatment failure and, in research, for isolation of parasites. These situations are seen in very specialized laboratories devoted to the study of the disease, but up to now not for routine diagnosis.

Nevertheless, in the best conditions, parasitemia can be found in a number of individuals at the chronic phase. Statistics are different according to geographical area (i.e., lower in Piaui, Brazil),[43] age of the patients (higher parasitemia before 11 and after 60 years old), pregnancy (increases),[44] and use of specific treatment (decreases). Because of the lower parasitemia, the chance to find parasites increases with the number of examinations. All the studies show that figures are higher in the same individual, if the same method is performed two or more times.[42,45] Also, if more than one method is applied, the chance of obtaining parasites increases.[43] Recent studies show that a single hemoculture or xenodiagnosis may be positive in 24−52% of the patients. The same sort of studies show that if more examinations are performed, the figures increase to a maximum of 65%.[46] It is clear from these studies that some patients are always negative, irrespective of the number of tests applied. On the other side, some positives always turn out that way (around 8−12% depending on the study). These are classified as having high parasitemia (each test applied is positive). Another way to measure the degree of parasitemia is to record the number of positive tubes of hemocultures[44,47] or the number of positive bugs, which allow you to classify the degree of parasites present. These studies are particularly useful when a new drug is tested.[48]

## Acute phase (direct and concentration methods)

Several easy methods are available to search for parasites when they are present in large numbers, as in the acute phase. They could be divided in direct tests and concentration methods.

## Direct tests

The simplest and cheapest direct test is the fresh blood smear. A drop of peripheral blood from the patient is collected from the ear, fingertip, foot, or from a vein through a syringe. 10 µL of blood are immediately deposited on a smear and a cover slip (22 × 22 mm) covers the drop. The amount of 10 µL is ideal for a nice preparation (i.e., a very thin smear that allows seeing red blood cells separated from each other). The preparation should be mounted in a microscope with an objective of 40 × and ocular of 10 × (i.e., 400×). If *T. cruzi* is present, it will be seen as a refringent body with very quick movements, disturbing the quiet red blood cells. It is advisable to have some previous training, which may be just an observation for some minutes of such a preparation. As an exercise, this could be prepared from infected mouse blood in those laboratories that work with *T. cruzi*. This parasite easily contaminates humans, so all measures to avoid a laboratory accident should be taken, like the use of gloves and facial mask (personal protection equipment).[49,50] More than 100 laboratory accidents have been documented and published and probably a similar number of cases have not been recorded.[49]

In cases of vector transmission, with less than 20 days from the start of symptoms, it is common to find one parasite every 10−50 fields. The smear should be looked at for 100−400 fields before being informed as negative. The test may be performed in several smears or on different days. If a single examination is negative, concentration methods may be applicable if the clinical suspicion persists. In some transfusional cases[27] or immunosuppression, several parasites may be seen in one field.

If a motile, refringent flagellate is found, the diagnosis is made. No further analysis is necessary. Check if clinical data are available (i.e., fever of unknown origin, recent transplantation or transfusion). The preparation may be dried and stained, but for better visualization, a proper smear as for differential count of leukocytes is preferable.

## Other direct tests

The dry smear as for differential count has a much lower sensitivity, and will be positive only when a large number of parasites are present, equivalent to more than one parasite per field with the fresh smear. It is not recommended because of that. The thick smear, as used for malaria diagnosis, also has lower sensitivity but is better than the dry smear. The morphology of the parasite is generally not well preserved, but is an excellent option when used in the field in malaria regions. If negative for hematozoan, the presence of a flagellate could be diagnostic. Many otherwise nondiagnosed cases were found by malaria control program personnel, after proper training, in Brazil and other countries.

## Concentration methods

Two are most used: the Strout technique and microhematocrit.

### Strout (1962)

The Strout[51] technique is very simple. Centrifuge tubes, a centrifuge, and a microscope will suffice. Blood (3−5 mL) is collected without anticoagulant and left to clot, at room temperature, or quicker, at 37°C. Once the clot is formed (15−60 min) the blood exudate is transferred with a pipette to a centrifugal tube and spun down at low speed (i.e., 50 g, 500 rpm according to the radius of the centrifuge) for 5 min. This will allow for the separation of most (but not all) red blood cells that remain at the bottom of the tube. Take all the supernatant (approximately 1 mL) and transfer to another centrifuge tube and spin hard (i.e., 500*g*, around 2000 rpm) for 10 min. This will clear the suspension, having a clear supernatant. Take nearly all the supernatant and store for serology. Now, with the last drop remaining at the bottom of the tube, resuspend it and apply 10 μL to a glass slide and cover slip, with the same methodology as the fresh blood smear explained above. Look on the microscope. Parasites are there. The rationale of this method is that all the parasites escape from the clot to the serum. By separating most of the red blood cells with the first spin, we get rid of them. By the second spinning, parasites are forced to remain at the bottom of the tube. *Hint*: Do not delay in preparing the smear after the centrifuge stops, otherwise the parasites will swim to the sera and will be lost.

### Microhematocrit

Microhematocrit is very useful for congenital infection, because of the need for only 100 μL of blood for each test. Ideally collect from the plantar region of the baby's foot, four glass capillaries (heparinized, to avoid clot).[52] Spin down as for hematocrit in a proper centrifuge. Look at the interface of the capillary. Hematocrit will have an upper layer of plasma, the interface where leukocytes and *T. cruzi* are, and a lower layer of packed red blood cells. It is not necessary to break the capillary tube, but if necessary it could be done. In this case, take strict care to avoid accidental contamination, as described before.

## Other methods for concentration

Several other methods have been described, as the separation by Ficoll-Hypaque,[53] on the same layer as mononuclear cells, but in practical terms the two already described are the top choices.

## Chronic phase

### Xenodiagnosis

The main variables are species of bug to be used; number of bugs to be applied; stage of bug; time for application on patient; number of examinations to be performed; days of fast before application; method of examination of bugs; temperature and humidity to preserve alive bugs; ideal time for examination after feeding; method of examination; individual or pool examination; number of readings; and expression of results. After many publications on the subject, a standardization was published by Cerisola et al.[21] which has been followed until now. Some variables are still a matter of discussion, such as if it is better to use an autochthonous species of bug. After Cerisola et al., xenodiagnosis is performed as follows: for *Triatoma infestans*, 40 bugs, third instar, 15 days fast, divided in 4 boxes (10 bugs in each), each box in arms and/or legs, applied for 30 min, bugs stored in chambers at 25–30°C, humidity 70%, examined at 30 and 60 days. Results may be expressed as number of positive boxes (i.e., 1/4). The number of examinations will depend on the investigator. Several improvements were developed later, mainly the use of artificial xenodiagnosis, because allergic reactions were observed in some patients, and the risk of contamination from the bugs, in immunocompromised host, mainly after the era of AIDS.[54] Artificial xenodiagnosis consists in feeding bugs through a membrane (condom) with warm heparinized blood from the patient. This last variation allowed use of a large number of bugs, up to 360 with 10–30 mL of venous blood, increasing the chances of positivity.[54,55]

There are several limitations of this technique. There is a need for a large insectary, with more than 100 female and male adult bugs, in order to provide enough eggs to perform the examination. Bugs (adults and nymphs) need to be fed on hens or other birds, every 15 days. Colonies of bugs may be contaminated with *Blastochritidiae triatoma*, morphologically similar to *T. cruzi*, and if this happens all the bugs should be eliminated and the research started from scratch.[56] The examination of bugs is time-consuming and requires a proper infrastructure. Results will be ready after 60 days or more. The advantages of this technique are that it may be performed in the field (it is only necessary to transport bugs with 15 days on fast), does not require sterile handling, and allows for inoculation in animals. Very few laboratories in the world have the capacity to maintain such an infrastructure and those who need to isolate parasites are moving to hemoculture, whenever possible. Nowadays, the preferred method is artificial xenodiagnosis.

## Hemoculture

Developed many years after xenodiagnosis, for a time hemoculture had a lower yield in terms of positivity.[57] Some improvements developed mainly by Chiari et al.[38] helped make it the current method of choice. Variables, as with xenodiagnosis, include the amount of blood to be collected, anticoagulant to be used, separation/inclusion of plasma, medium to be used, relation inoculum/medium, number of tubes to be used, temperature for maintenance, timing and number of readings, and method of examination. After the standardization, the conditions were: 30 mL of peripheral blood with heparin handled quickly (less than 2 h) at 4°C, spin down at 4°C to get rid of plasma, wash in medium liver infusion tryptose (LIT), made 6 replicates by 1 mL washed blood and 3 mL of LIT each, maintain at 26°C, examine every 30 days for 5 consecutive months. Results may be expressed as number of positive tubes (i.e., 2+/6).[44,47]

The main limitation is sterility, because blood needs to be processed in several steps. The medium (LIT) should be prepared (not commercially available) and has several variables which are out of the scope of this chapter.

## Animal inoculation

Rarely used nowadays, animal inoculation was once employed in the field. It is essential to use a susceptible animal, often mice (Balb C), which should be young (up to 30 days of age) and male, as they are more susceptible. Examination of the tail blood should be done daily or every 3 days, since parasites may be present for very short periods. It is time-consuming, and animal house facilities should be available. It may be used in combination with xenodiagnosis by inoculation of positive bug feces in order to isolate a stock for further characterization. After the first passage, mice could be treated with immunosuppressors (i.e., cyclophosphamide) to increase parasitemia.[58]

## Antigenuria

This method was once more popular[59] but has several disadvantages, such as the need for concentrating large volumes of urine.

## Polymerase chain reaction

As discussed earlier (see "Indications of Parasitological Tests"), PCR is the newest parasitological test in use. It has higher sensitivity than the other multiplication methods, but like the others it is not 100%.[60] The goal is now to assure that the specificity of this technique is 100%.[40] As it is an *in house* test, it is not commercially available.

# Serological tests

## Antigenic makeup

The kinetoplastid *T. cruzi* has many antigens distributed on its surface (cytoplasmic membrane and flagellum), and from the different organelles at the cytoplasm and nucleus. Some of these antigens are exposed when the parasite is circulating, as a trypomastigote, and others will be presented to the immune system after it is dead. A different set of antigens may be excreted. This parasite may also shed antigens and after some time internalize antigens that were previously exposed.

The antigenic makeup of *T. cruzi* from different geographical areas is rather similar, as demonstrated in several publications that used reagents made from *T. cruzi* circulating in the Southern Cone to diagnose serum from patients of Mexico.[61] As known, *T. cruzi* is heterogeneous, and two main *T. cruzi* are recognized: *T. cruzi* I and *T. cruzi* II. The former has been isolated from silvatic regions in the United States and also from humans infected above the Amazon River. The second, now split into five groups, is found to the south of the Amazon River. A recent classification[62] expanded to six groups defined as discrete typing units (DTU), from TcI to TcVI. Antigenic differences among those six *T. cruzi* genotypes are currently under study.

There is another trypanosome, *T. rangeli*, which is not pathogenic for humans but may be present in the same geographical regions as *T. cruzi* and may share some antigens. Several studies show that infected humans with this parasite, diagnosed by hemoculture, do not have anti-*T. cruzi* antibodies, at least with the high titer seen in those with Chagas infection. The reasons are probably due to the short contact with humans in their brief life spans.[63,64]

The other genus that has human pathogenic parasites is *Leishmania*, and again, some antigens may be shared. Several leishmanias are recognized to be present at the same geographical areas as *T. cruzi*, such as the agents of mucocutaneous leishmaniasis (*Leishmania mexicana* and *Leishmania braziliensis*) and *Leishmania donovani chagasi*, the American agent of visceral leishmaniasis (kalazar). Both diseases are quite different: in the former, amastigotes remain inside macrophages mainly on the skin and mucosal surfaces. The immune response is mainly by cell-mediated immunity and antibody responses are poor, making the serological diagnosis of mucocutaneous leishmaniasis difficult. On the contrary, visceral leishmaniasis is a severe disease, with a poor prognosis if not diagnosed and treated. As known, *L. donovani* parasites are widely distributed in bone marrow, liver, spleen, and in circulation. It is also well known that this parasite stimulates B lymphocytes in a polyclonal activation, with a huge increase in antibodies of several classes and subclasses, leading to a polyclonal hypergammaglobulinemia. As a consequence, in advanced stages, antibodies to an array of antigens are present. In relation with the diagnosis of Chagas disease, nearly any reagent used with sera from kalazar patients will be positive. It is our experience that, in laboratory terms, it is not possible to differentiate a kalazar patient, serologically, from a chagasic one. All the difference is on the clinical setup, which must be evaluated by the clinician. The kalazar patient who shows a positive serology for Chagas disease is severely ill, with fever, liver and spleen enlargement, edema, hemorrhagic lesions, and with a complete blood count that shows pronounced anemia, leukopenia, and plaquetopenia. Furthermore an electrophoresis of plasmatic proteins will show a large increase of gammaglobulin. Not one of these alterations is present in the chronic phase of Chagas disease. The laboratorial diagnosis of kalazar is confirmed by bone marrow aspiration, which should be conducted if this diagnosis is suspected. So, in this case, diagnosis should be clinical, epidemiological, and supported by the laboratory.

## Antibody response

As part of the life of *T. cruzi* is in the circulation, the immune system is continuously stimulated by an array of antigens, and the production of antibodies of high affinity is the rule. Because of this, most of the infected individuals mount a strong antibody response against it. Some antibodies may kill trypomastigotes by a complement dependent mechanism, as shown in vitro by the antibody-dependent complement-mediated lysis test.[65] This is probably one of the mechanisms that maintains the parasitemia at low levels in vivo, but not so efficiently, because some parasites evade it and may be found alive, as demonstrated in xenodiagnosis or hemocultures.

Other antibodies may be directed to shed antigens, such as shed acute phase antigen (SAPA), present mainly during the acute phase of the disease, and evanish both antigens and antibodies after few months.[66]

The antibody response at the acute phase is possible to detect after 1−2 weeks, mainly by the presence of specific IgM class antibodies. It should be emphasized again that the diagnosis at this phase is by parasitological methods. Only when parasites are not found and the clinical suspicion persists should the search for IgM anti-*T. cruzi* begin. These antibodies may be detected by a few techniques, most commonly indirect immunofluorescence (IIF), and direct agglutination with 2-ME has been employed as well. There is no commercial kit available for IIF-IgM or ELISA-IgM. An additional difficulty is obtaining positive controls. There are several pitfalls with in house IIF, mainly the presence of rheumatoid factor, which may yield a false-positive result.[67] Also, some chronic phase patients may have IgM anti-*T. cruzi*[68] (Table 29.3). It has not been recommended for diagnosis of congenital infection, since several infected children have shown negative results.[69] Serological conversion should also be considered when a negative result with IgG is obtained followed, days after, by a positive one. In such cases the conversion indicates an acute phase. Shortly after IgM responses arise, specific IgG will be detectable, with lower titers in the first month, increasing progressively after that. These IgG antibodies are first detected by IIF and HA and later by ELISA tests.[27] By the end of the second month after symptoms start, most infected individuals have a detectable IgG response, which will last for life, unless interventions (i.e., specific treatment) are performed.

In viral diseases transmitted through transfusion, there is a window period in which recently infected individuals are asymptomatic and serologically negative by

**Table 29.3 IgM detection in Chagas disease, by indirect immunofluorescence**

| Titers | Clinical phase and form | | | | |
|---|---|---|---|---|---|
| | Acute phase | Congenital | Chronic phase | | |
| | | | Adults nonpregnant | Pregnant | Older (>70 years old) |
| <1/5 | 8 | 8 | 336 | 372 | 238 |
| 1/5 | 1 | | 13 | 22 | 13 |
| 1/10 | 1 | | 11 | 14 | 20 |
| 1/20 | 2 | | 38 | 35 | 46 |
| 1/40 | 3 | 1 | 45 | 33 | 65 |
| 1/80 | 4 | | 29 | 17 | 74 |
| >1/80 | 49 | 1 | 28 | 7 | 44 |
| Total | 69 | 10 | 500 | 500 | 500 |

Each figure is the number of sera with a given titer. Some of these sera have rheumatoid factor.
*Source*: Laboratory for Chagas disease, Goiania, Brazil.

the assays usually used in Latin America for the screening, but they may transmit the infection. This window period is 20–25 days for HIV, up to 84 days for HBV, and 51 days for HCV. The possibility that this may happen in *T. cruzi* infection is remote. Most recent infections occur in childhood or adolescence and in rural areas. In addition, those recently infected will have fever, so they should not be accepted as donors.[70]

## Different serological tests

Serological tests may be divided into conventional and nonconventional methods. The first group comprises the classical methods used for diagnosis since the discovery of the disease. They use antigenic mixtures, most are commercialized and able to diagnose most infected individuals. Great experience in all endemic countries has been achieved with time and many groups of investigation published results comparing their performance. Nonconventional methods were introduced since 1980, but most are not available for universal use (not commercially available) and experiences with their results are restricted to a few groups.

## Conventional methods

### The complement fixation test (CF)

This was the first test employed for diagnosis, very soon after the discovery of the disease.[2] Most of reagents were prepared *in house* and the test was time-consuming when a large amount of samples were necessary to test, as in blood banks. By the time that standardization was ready, other simpler tests were progressively substituting for the CF (mainly HA and IIF). By 1985 most laboratories abandoned the CF, moving to simpler tests. Nowadays, no commercial kits are available anymore.

## The indirect hemagglutination test (IH)

This is one of the methods of choice for diagnosis. It has several advantages which hold up to now, such as few steps (dilution of sera and contact with sensitized red blood cells), low cost, no equipment, and quick results (1–2 h). The substitution of tubes for microplates was a further advantage, allowing researchers to process more samples in a shorter time. For all these reasons, different manufacturers started to produce and sell kits, containing microplates, sensitized red blood cells, and dilution media. Several brands were on the market by 1985, mainly produced in South America (Argentina, Brazil, and Chile). Specificity was high (98–99%) and often higher than ELISA or IIF at that time, but it was perceived that sensitivity of tests from different manufacturers varied widely.[71–73] This made the test unacceptable in situations where sensitivity was essential, as in blood banks. Nevertheless, it is still considered a good test for confirmation of the infection.

Even with the advantage of simplicity, there are a few details that should be kept in mind: some sera have a nonspecific reaction with some kits (natural antibodies), and it is recommended in these cases that serum should be treated with 2-mercaptho-ethanol (2-ME) (incubation of 30 min at 37°C with a dilution of 1/100) before. Depending on the source of red blood cells, some sera have antibodies against some species of animals, and the kits should include nonsensitized red blood cells in case of a discrepancy with the other tests (positive only in HA).

There is also a discussion in relation to the better bottom of the microplates to facilitate the reading, and manufacturers sell the kits with V or U bottom, but this last allows a better reading. The cutoff point depends on the kit, but positive results with dilutions higher than 1/40 are considered reactive. The common titers obtained in 95% of infected individuals are higher than $1/128-1/160$[27].

Finally, there are a few brands on the market, because the test is cheaper and the industry is not interested to invest in it, as the main customer, blood banks, do not use it. As a consequence, marked differences in specificity and sensitivity are seen among brands and the selection of a good one is necessary.

## The direct agglutination test

The direct agglutination test[74] is also a simple test which has been widely used in some countries, but now it is not commercially available. The principle is the agglutination of the parasite by antibodies, if present. It has advantages, like the HA, and the possibility to search for IgM anti-*T. cruzi* if samples are run in parallel with and without 2-ME. If differences of more than two titers occur, there is a strong possibility that they are due to IgM. This test has been applied with success during the acute phase.[75] The disadvantages are mainly related to the reading because of the clear color of epimastigotes. Titers obtained with this test are higher than 1/32 in most infected people. Typical results of serum from acute phase are 1/256 without and 1/16 with 2-ME.[76]

## The indirect immunofluorescence (IIF)

Indirect immunofluorescence is used mainly in research laboratories or diagnostic centers that handle a limited amount of samples per day. One of the advantages for laboratories is that the same conjugate (antihuman IgG) may be used for the diagnosis of several diseases and the ability to use the same equipment (fluorescence microscope). This test is conducted by reacting serum with smear fixed epimastigotes and, after washing, incubating with conjugate. The smears are read in the fluorescence microscope. The key advantage of this test is very high sensitivity. It is quite hard to find a serum from an infected individual which does not react. However, a disadvantage is that this same extreme sensitivity may lead to cross-reactions with several diseases. These cross-reactions are observed mainly in lower titers (1/40−1/80) and a higher one is quite characteristic of Chagas disease, unless visceral leishmaniasis is present.

This test has several steps and each may be critical, so it should be performed by a skilled technician. Among the variables, the growing phase of the epimastigotes, the pH of phosphate buffered saline, the pH of glycerol buffer, the concentration of conjugate, and the life of the microscopic light need to be checked for top performance. The reading is subjective, and after examination of more than 20 smears (200 wells), results may not be reliable because of exhaustion of the technician. Nevertheless, in good hands this is an excellent test. In a recent search, in an analysis of 1302 sera from infected individuals with typical clinical alterations, 92.7% had a titer of 1/320 or higher. More than two-thirds of this group had high titers of 1/1280 or more.[77] The cutoff region is between 1/20 and 1/40 and some individuals of the noninfected population may be reactive in these low titers (Table 29.4).

Table 29.4 **Titers obtained in 1302 sera from nontreated chronic phase patients, by indirect immunofluorescence**[1]

| Titer | Nr | % |
|-------|------|-------|
| 1/40 | 0 | 0.0 |
| 1/80 | 27 | 2.1 |
| 1/160 | 67 | 5.2 |
| 1/320 | 135 | 10.4 |
| 1/640 | 220 | 16.9 |
| 1/1280 | 331 | 25.4 |
| 1/2560 | 315 | 24.2 |
| 1/5120 | 84 | 6.5 |
| 1/10,240 | 52 | 4.0 |
| 1/20,480 | 71 | 5.5 |
| Total | 1,302 | 100.2 |

All patients have had cardiopathy (CRBBB), and/or megaesophagus and/or megacolon.[77]
*Source*: Laboratory for Chagas disease, Goiania, Brazil.

## The immunoenzymatic test of ELISA (Enzyme-Linked ImmunoSorbent Assay)

This test was first applied for Chagas infection in 1975 in a study on filter paper.[78] It is rather similar to IIF, because it has many steps, needs a well-trained technician, and has extreme sensitivity, which is one advantage, but carries the problem of a more limited specificity. On the other hand, the advantages over IIF are the objective readings (spectrophotometer) and the possibility of automatization for handling hundreds of samples at a time. The classic technique described by Voller et al.[78] had several steps and the time to run a plate was 6 h. Now kits have improved the incubation time and the same plate may be ready in 2 h. As with the IIF, it is difficult to have a sample of serum from an infected individual that yields a negative result. Cutoff should be calculated as per technical instructions, but a curve with negative, low-positive, and high-positive controls is useful for the range of responses. Once the cutoff has been calculated, it is accepted that positive samples should be considered as such when Optical Density (OD) is at least 10% higher than the cutoff. In order to compare results in the follow-up of treated patients, it is useful to express results as an index, obtained through the division of the OD of the sample and the OD of the cutoff of the plate. Results below 0.9 are negative, from 0.9 to 1.2 are borderline, and above 1.2 positive.

In a recent study performed by the Ministry of Health, Brazil, 12 different brands of commercially available ELISA kits, approved by the sanitary authorities, were tested with 150 positive and negative sera, including sera of low reactivity, by four independent laboratories. Results showed that the sensitivity for all of them was high (97−100%) but specificity was low (60−98%).[79] The interpretation was that kits were tailored to fulfill the needs of the main client (blood banks) and acceptable for them, but not good enough for the serological diagnosis of an individual patient (see Table 29.5).

To summarize, the ELISA test is excellent for the purpose of screening blood donors, but in order to confirm the infection, other tests of higher specificity should be employed in parallel. We will come back to these issues when the indications of serological tests are discussed.

## Nonconventional methods

### Radio-immunoprecipitation assay (RIPA)

This test was developed in the United States by Kirchhoff et al.[80] and is claimed to be the gold standard for serology.[81] It is not widely available as it is only performed in few research institutions, is expensive, time-consuming, and uses radioisotopes, which make its application as a standard procedure remote. One study compared their results with conventional tests[82] and, although sensitivity compared well with IFI, HA, and ELISA of several brands, the number of negative sera used in this study ($n = 19$) was not enough to evaluate specificity.

### Western blot (including TESA-blot)

These tests have been widely used in research institutions, and several publications are available.[83−85] They are time-consuming and costly (estimated at US$20.00 per

Table 29.5 **Sensitivity and specificity of different commercial ELISA tests for screening for *T. cruzi* infection in blood donors, 2006**

| Kits | Kappa | % Sensitivity | CI 95% | % Specificity | CI 95% |
|------|-------|---------------|--------|---------------|--------|
| Adaltis | 0.71 | 100 | 94.0−100.0 | 60 | 46.0−73.2 |
| Bio-manguinhos[a] | 0.95 | 100 | 94.0−100.0 | 93 | 82.2−97.7 |
| Bio-manguinhos[b] | 0.97 | 97 | 89.7−99.5 | 98 | 89.7−99.9 |
| Biomerieux | 0.97 | 100 | 94.0−100.0 | 95 | 85.4−98.7 |
| Biochile | 0.98 | 99 | 91.9−99.9 | 98 | 89.9−99.9 |
| Biozima Chagas | 0.98 | 100 | 93.9−100.0 | 97 | 87.3−99.4 |
| Ebram | 0.97 | 99 | 91.5−99.9 | 97 | 87.5−99.4 |
| Hemagen | 0.98 | 100 | 93.9−100.0 | 97 | 87.5−99.4 |
| Patozime-Chagas | 0.97 | 99 | 91.3−99.9 | 97 | 87.5−99.4 |
| REM Gold | 0.97 | 99 | 91.8−99.9 | 97 | 87.0−99.4 |
| Wama diagnostica | 0.98 | 99 | 91.5−99.9 | 98 | 89.9−99.9 |
| Wiener | 0.97 | 100 | 94.0−100.0 | 95 | 85.4−98.7 |

CI, Confidence interval.
[a]Recombinant.
[b]Conventional.
*Source*: Ministerio da Saude, Brazil, 2006.

sample). Several antigens have been employed, among them the TESA-blot, a trypomastigote excreted-secreted antigen.[86] This test has been employed with eluates of filter paper in a serological survey of children less than 5 years old in Brazil to learn if insecticide spraying to kill the vector was effective to halt the transmission.[87] Eighty thousand seven hundred eighty-eight samples were run in the laboratory that was the quality control of the study (105,000 samples were collected)[88] and results were excellent in terms of specificity and sensitivity. This test is now commercially available (TESAcruzi, Biomerieux[®])

## Lytic assays including flow cytometry

The complement-mediated lysis of trypomastigotes test, developed by Krettli and Brener in the 1980s,[65] was used as a diagnostic tool and evaluation of treated patients. The rationale of this test was to screen for lytic antibodies, present in infected individuals, but absent in those successfully treated. This antibody would disappear before those detected by conventional tests.[89] In practice it is a rather simple test that reacts alive trypomastigotes from irradiated mice with sera. If lytic antibodies are present, the parasites will be killed after the addition of complement when counted in a cytometer (Neubauer chamber). This apparently simple test has several drawbacks that made it unsuitable for routine use. Among them, the use of irradiated mice or cell lines to grow trypomastigotes poses a problem and the use of living parasites makes it potentially dangerous. The use of complement adds more problems, similar to those described with the CF test.

More recently, the adaptation of this test with flow cytometric techniques shows good results with the group of treated patients, but the test has been employed only in one research institution and is not available in the market.[90−92]

## Chemiluminescence

The combination of a purified antigen analyzed by chemiluminescence has been used by Almeida et al.[93] and applied as a diagnostic tool for evaluation of treatment success on treated patients. Antibodies against this specific antigen disappear before the crude antigens employed in conventional tests.[94] The problem is that the preparation of the antigen is difficult and the need of a microplate chemiluminescent apparatus makes this test difficult to be used as a routine test. It is not commercially available.

A combination with chemiluminiscence and an array of recombinant antigens has been developed for Blood Banks and is currently used in United States and several laboratories thorough the world (Chemiluminiscent Microparticle Immuno Assay, CMIA ARCHITECT Chagas® Abbott). It has been proved very sensitive and specific, but occasionally false positives are found, so to label an individual as infected, again, it is necessary to have a second test.

## *Rapid tests*

A new generation of rapid tests became available at the end of the 1990s. They had several applications (pregnancy, diabetes, HIV) and several advantages apart from speed. You do not need a skilled worker to perform them. They are very important in rural areas devoid of specialized laboratories when a diagnosis of *T. cruzi* infection may be crucial (i.e., in an emergency for a blood transfusion). Also, in serological surveys, and in some remote places that require such costly displacement that the possibility to give a result at once, solve problems of public health. Some laboratories have so few samples per day to test, that the possibility to use a rapid test may, in the end, reduce costs.

The industry quickly became aware of this niche and responded in kind. Devices were produced with recombinant antigens and, in a quick run (10−20 min) after a drop of serum and buffer are placed, results were obtained. A positive control band should be seen in negative and positive sera, indicating that the system did work. Otherwise, the result is not validated. In a few years, several rapid tests were available on the market and became extensively used in some areas, such as Central America and Bolivia. Several papers indicated good sensitivity and specificity, but they should not be used as a single test for a case confirmation.[95,96] Main brands available are Stat-Pack and Inbios.

More recently Sanchez-Camargo et al.[97] carried a comparative evaluation of 11 commercialized rapid diagnostic tests (RDT) for detecting *Trypanosoma cruzi* antibodies from areas of endemicity and nonendemicity. The evaluation was performed on 474 positive and negative samples tested before by at least three different techniques, at 10 national reference laboratories from nine countries. It was found that eight of the RDT were appropriate for field work, with lower performances than disclosed by manufacturers. Sensitivity of 97.2% and specificity of 94% were the best obtained.

## Antigens

*T. cruzi*, as with most pathogens, has an array of antigens of different origins. In antibody detection systems, as with serology, the selection of a proper antigen is essential in order to get a reliable result. The selection of antigens also depends on what investigators want to know. If the point is to diagnose the disease, any antigen or group of antigens present in the parasite will suffice. Antigens selected should be exclusively from *T. cruzi* and not present in other pathogens.[98] Historically the easiest antigens to use were extracts of the full parasite. Obviously some of them may cross-react with other pathogens. This led to purifying antigens from different structures, obtaining better results in terms of specificity. A further step to gain specificity was the use of recombinant antigens and immediately after that, the use of synthetic peptides. Excreted antigens were also found and used. It was soon clear that as the antigens selected were more restricted, some infected people have no responses against some of them. Then, the idea to sum up several recombinants or peptides was considered. So, the tendency now is to have a mixture of now-refined antigens.

## Crude preparations

Crude preparations were first employed in 1914 and remained popular until the 1980s. The extraction procedure varied in order to select antigens present mainly in this parasite (see historical section). The source of *T. cruzi* also should be considered. Cultures are rich in epimastigote forms (with 5% trypomastigotes; this percentage increases in old cultures), with a relatively easy growth, which facilitates large amounts of antigen, making it the preferred option. Preferred medium is LIT and best temperature at 26°C. Cross-reactions may occur with other pathogens. One of the issues is that this form is not present in human tissues or blood. Another option is to employ trypomastigotes, which are more difficult to grow, mainly because a lineage of cell culture should be used and maintained in a $CO_2$ incubator at 37°C to reproduce the cycle in humans. It has been shown that these preparations are more specific. Some authors tried to use amastigotes,[99] which are also difficult to prepare in large numbers, but again, results were better than with epimastigotes.

## Purified antigens

As a need to have better tools for diagnosis grew, in the 1980s several purified antigens were tested with panels of well-characterized sera. The first attempts used surface glycoproteins, theoretically more exposed to the immune system. Several publications using antigens of 25,[100] 90,[101] and 72 kDa[102] did show that results improved, with higher specificity and without loss of sensitivity. The problem was that preparation of these antigens required special technical conditions and manufacturers were not interested. These purified antigens have been tested mainly in ELISA systems.

## Recombinant proteins

By the end of 1980s, recombinant protein technology had grown and several laboratories published an array of candidate antigens for use in diagnostic tests, claiming good specificity and sensitivity. Even if most of them were different proteins, some proved to be homologous. The real value of these recombinant proteins was tested with the support of TDR/WHO in 10 laboratories that received 50 coded sera.[103] Results showed that a single recombinant have few chances to detect all the infected samples. Therefore the tendency was to mix several recombinants.[104] The better mixture (FRA and CRA) was used in kits which have been distributed to all government laboratories in Brazil.

Other recombinant proteins have been produced by several manufacturers and are widely available (i.e., Wiener ELISA Recombinante®, Immuno Comb II Chagas®, ARCHITECT Chagas®) with good results. Interestingly, some of these kits may have occasional false-positive results, probably due to reactions to remaining antigens in the process of fabrication. These recombinant antigens have also been used in combination to make rapid tests, several of which are available in the market.

## Synthetic peptides

These have been synthesized and used with panels of sera, and again, part of the infected population do not respond to a single antigen, so an array of them is necessary to get good sensitivity.[104,105] They have been applied in different supports and some were available as rapid tests (PaGia®).[106] This test has now been withdrawn from the market.

## Different supports

The first serological tests were devised to be used in glass tubes where the sera would be mixed, in several dilutions, with the antigens in ideal proportions. Glass smears were used for agglutination and demarked smears for immunofluorescence. With the era of plastics, polypropylene tubes were used, with the advantage of a single use and discard, avoiding the time-consuming and imperfect process of washing.

Very shortly after, plastic (polypropylene or other) microplates were applied in serology, with easy handling of hundreds of samples. Their use was routine by the time ELISA was described.[78] Antigens in ELISA were fixed in the wells by special buffers, and all the reactions were faster. Later, for those laboratories that process a few samples of sera a day, detached rows of the plate (strips) were available.

When purified antigens, recombinant proteins, and synthetic peptides were available, spots in filter papers (or different materials) were used, substituted in blots by nitrocellulose membranes.

## Filter paper

To collect some drops of blood from a finger prick directly on a filter paper, has certainly several operational advantages on the field. It is simple, straightforward, avoids mistakes of identification, and allows to follow this procedure in hundreds of individuals on the same day. It avoid steps such as refrigeration, centrifugation, and transfer of sera to further tubes. Filter papers may be stored for days at room temperature and processed later at a central laboratory. But eluates obtained are dirty preparations which often gave borderline results. Not all kits are prepared to handle these sorts of samples. The quality of the filter should be of high standards and any positive result should be confirmed by collecting venous blood. This type of support is ideal for large epidemiological work, at the field.[88]

### Membranes

Nitrocellulose membranes are commonly used for Western blot tests. Recently one became available for the market (TESAcruzi, Biomerieux®). Tests are expensive and time-consuming, requiring several steps to complete and with a few samples used in each run. The subjective reading of faint bands may be another difficulty.

### Gels

The use of gels in microtubes separated the mixture of antigens and reagents by centrifugation. If reaction occurs, the complex does not come down and in negative samples, the reagent (generally colored) passes through to the bottom.[106]

## Blood banks, serology, and quality control for Chagas disease

Transfusion of blood and blood products is an essential part of health care for patients deficient in one or more blood components. In order to avoid transfusion of tainted blood, every country should have an organized blood transfusion service based on a national blood policy, including relevant legislation, rules, and regulations, which in turn must be an integral part of any national health policy. For practical purposes, the status of the blood supply may depend on: (1) the existence of a pool of healthy donors, making the supply sufficient to cover the country's needs; (2) mandatory screening of blood donors for infectious diseases, following quality assurance procedures; and (3) appropriate use of blood. This is especially important for Chagas disease, as the second most common way of transmission of *T. cruzi* was considered to be, for many years, transfusion of blood or blood products. In fact, the minimum screening of blood donors in Latin America includes HIV, HVB, HVC, syphilis, and *T. cruzi*.[107−109]

In the 1980s and early 1990s transfusion infection was also considered a public health problem. At that time there were a high number of blood transfusions as well as a few countries mandating serology for *T. cruzi* for screening blood donors. Danger may come not only from whole blood, but also from packed red cells, platelets, white cells, fresh frozen plasma, and cryoprecipitate. On the other hand, the use of lyophilized products seemed to be safe.[110−112]

In the 1970s, with 4 million transfusions yearly, an annual incidence of 10,000−20,000 cases was thought to occur in Brazil.[113,114] At that time it was also assumed that 10,000 cases occurred in the Sao Paulo metropolitan area yearly.[115]

These numbers were revised downward in the early 1990s. The number of donors with positive serology for *T. cruzi* in that country was estimated at 55,000, of whom 11,000 were not screened. Taking into account that the probability of getting a *T. cruzi* infection after receiving an infected unit was considered to be 20%,[31] the number of infected cases by blood transfusion would be 1500−3000 individuals.[116] In fact, the real incidence of *T. cruzi* acquired through blood was unknown, because most cases are unapparent or *T. cruzi* is not recognized as the etiological agent.[117]

The risk of receiving *T. cruzi*-infected blood will increase in proportion to the prevalence of the infection in the donor population and the number of transfusions received. Therefore, polytransfused individuals like hemophiliac patients, those with other hematologic disorders, or patients undergoing dialysis are at greater risk. Fifty percent of hemophiliacs became infected after receiving 30 or more transfusions from a blood bank with a 2% prevalence of positive serology for *T. cruzi*.[32] Another study showed that 15% of individuals who had multiple transfusions had positive serology for *T. cruzi*, while the general population was 2% positive.[118] Polytransfused individuals from a blood bank with 2% positive serology for *T. cruzi* were 8.7 times more likely to be positive than individuals who did not receive transfusions.[34]

Thousands of immigrants from Latin American endemic countries living in Europe created a Chagas disease problem there. In France, blood donors born in *T. cruzi*-endemic areas or from a mother coming from an endemic area must be screened. Donors returning from endemic areas are deferred from blood donation for 4 months, and blood used in French Guyana comes directly from France.[119] In Spain, the country in Western Europe that received the most Latin American immigrants, a Royal Decree[120] deferred permanently as donors those individuals with positive serology for *T. cruzi*. If tests for screening of blood donors are not available, individuals born in endemic areas, newborns from mothers coming from endemic areas, and those who received transfusions in endemic areas need to be excluded from donating blood for labile components. These individuals may donate blood only when having a negative serological test for *T. cruzi*.

The regulatory system in the United States is based on private initiatives, either the Red Cross or community-based nonprofit organizations. They are responsible for obtaining and processing the blood and blood products, under strong government and professional society supervision.[121] In Canada, implementation of activities related to blood and blood products belonged to the Canadian Red Cross until the responsibility switched to the central Canadian Blood Services (CBS) and one provincial government (Hema-Quebec) after a scandal in the 1990s led to safety concerns.[122] In the United States, the three main organizations dealing with blood (American Red Cross, Council of Community Blood Centers, and America Blood Centers) for many years reported blood-related accidents and incidents. The Red Cross alone covers 50% of the hospitals in United States and collects information for hemovigilance in those hospitals. The Food and Drug Administration (FDA) also has a thorough collection of data related to the use of blood and blood products. In addition, information from other sources, like the Retrovirus Epidemiology Donor Survey, provides data used for establishing residual risk.[121]

The FDA introduced a concept of "zero risk blood supply" as the industry goal and regulatory agencies require blood donor screening laboratories, blood banks, and transfusion services to establish and follow a quality control and quality assurance program for their licensing, certification, and accreditation.[123] All errors and accidents must be reported to the FDA promptly.[124]

In order to prevent transfusion transmission of *T. cruzi* infection, it is recommended (but not mandatory) that the donor pool be screened for *T. cruzi*. Positive units must be removed from distribution and the donor not allowed to make donations.[125] The US Food and Drug Administration[126] recommended testing of blood donors with an approved ELISA assay. It is estimated that about 65% of the blood supply is being screened. The AABB (formerly known as the American Association of Blood Banks) recommends that blood donations that have repeatedly tested reactive by ELISA should be quarantined and removed from distribution, and the donor be kept from making donations.[125] Recipients of blood components from donors who tested positive should be identified and tested for *T. cruzi* infection. Those who tested positive for *T. cruzi*, their at-risk family members, children from infected mothers, and potentially infected recipients should receive a comprehensive clinical assessment.[125]

Laws, decrees, norms, and/or regulations related to blood transfusion began to appear in the 1960s (Argentina, Brazil, Chile, Costa Rica); 1970s (Bolivia, Colombia, Ecuador, Paraguay, Uruguay, Venezuela); 1980s (Honduras, Mexico, Nicaragua); and 1990s (Guatemala, Panama, Peru).[127,128] They began because of concerns about transmission of infectious diseases like syphilis and Chagas disease. They were followed by worries about hepatitis in the 1970s, and then HIV in the 1980s. They have evolved through time, from focusing at the beginning only on disease screening to later mandates on voluntary donations and quality assurance. Enforcement varied from stringent to weak, and most countries do not have a well-trained group of inspectors to make mandatory visits to independent laboratories or blood banks that do the serological screening. In addition, in some countries there are so many blood banks that process a small number of blood donors that visiting all of them annually or even every 2 years is a daunting (and expensive) task.

The first Expert Committee on Chagas disease from WHO (1991)[107] recommended that screening for *T. cruzi* in blood donors should be conducted in all countries where *T. cruzi* was endemic using at least two serological tests based on different principles (e.g., a HA and ELISA, or a IIF and a HA, or an ELISA and a IFI). There should be a ban on paid blood donors and a program of quality control for serology must be implemented.[107] At that time, only two countries, Argentina and Brazil, had mandatory tests for *T. cruzi* screening, and several of the other countries did not screen for *T. cruzi* in all donors, and a few did not screen blood donors at all. Even for the two countries in which two tests were mandatory, both tests were not always employed.

Before 1993 there was no nationwide official information system in any Latin American country on indicators of the status of blood supply, including the prevalence of infectious diseases markers. Data became available from nine countries in 1993, four more in 1994, one each in 1995 and 1997, and two more in 1999. This allows an analysis of the overall situation: how safe was the donor pool? The answer is based on the percentage of different categories of blood donors from the country; repeat voluntary donors are the safest, replacement donors should be avoided, and paid donors must be banned.[109] Information available on: (1) the total number of donors; (2) the total number of donors screened; and (3) the prevalence of *T. cruzi* infection made it possible to estimate the risk of blood receptors of receiving an infected unit or potentially acquire a *T. cruzi* infection.[70,129–131]

From 1993 to 2005, it was assumed that reagents used for routine screening for *T. cruzi* antibodies, either ELISA or HA, had a sensitivity of 90% and a specificity of 95%.[129] Later, commercial reagents improved, and some but not all of those used for the ELISA or HA test had sensitivity and specificity equal or higher than 90%.[132,133] This fact stressed the need that government agencies, or any technical group in which the government delegates this activity, test the different diagnostic reagents and vouch for their usefulness. Tables 29.5−29.7 show the sensitivity and specificity of different commercial reagents and the differences in sensitivity and specificity.

Tables 29.8 and 29.9 show the number of donors, the percentage of donors screened, and the prevalence of *T. cruzi* infection in donors from Latin American countries from 1993 to 2007.[70,129–131,134]

The second WHO Expert Committee[108] faced the reality that 9 years after the first Expert Committee, only in Argentina and Brazil were two tests for the screening of blood donors mandatory for *T. cruzi* antibodies. The fact that several ELISA in the market had high sensitivity and specificity and could be used in an automated

**Table 29.6 Sensitivity and specificity of hemagglutination and agglutination tests[a]**

| Indirect hemagglutination, 1997[a] | | |
|---|---|---|
| **KIT** | **% Sensitivity** | **% Specificity** |
| Imunoserum | 94.64 | 95.42 |
| Ebran | 88.69 | 59.92 |
| Wama | 100.00 | 95.80 |
| Hemagen | 93.45 | 87.79 |
| Biolab | 99.40 | 97.33 |
| **Particle agglutination, 2006[b]** | | |
| Serodia | 100 | 97.71 |
| ID PaGIA | 98.81 | 98.85 |

[a]Saez-Alquezar et al., 1997.
[b]Schmuñis, 2007.

**Table 29.7 Antibodies anti-*T. cruzi* in 1455 blood donors from the Province of Chaco, Argentina (2006−07)**

| Tests | % Reactive | % Agreement |
|---|---|---|
| Chagatek (EIABioM) | 25.2 | − |
| Chagas BiosChile (EIA BiosCh) | 23.5 | 98.1 |
| BioZima Chagas (EIA BioZ) | 24.4 | 98.4 |
| Chagatest rec. (EIA Wrec) | 24.7 | 97.0 |
| Chagas Serodia (PA) | 20.6 | 95.2 |
| Chagas HAI (IHA) | 18.9 | 92.1 |
| HAI LC (IHA LC) | 18.8 | 88.0 |

*Source*: Remezar MC, Gamba C, Colaianni IF, Puppo M, Sartor PA, Murphy EL et al. Estimation of sensitivity and specificity of several *Trypanosoma cruzi* antibody assays in blood donors of Argentina. *Transfusion* 2009. doi:1111/ j1537-2995.2009.02301.

system, as well as that the cost of two tests were not affordable for several countries, weighed in the decision that mandatory screening for Chagas disease in blood donors could be made using a single test and this should be an ELISA test of high sensitivity.[108]

The simplest way to follow up progress in this area is to establish the number of countries with 100% screening for *T. cruzi* in blood donors. Table 29.9 shows how these figures were improved from 1993 to 2005. In 1993, 2 out of 9 countries reported 100% screening coverage for *T. cruzi*, 7 out of 16 in 1999, and 9 out of 17 in 2005. Among the 17 Latin American countries from the Continental Western Hemisphere, in which *T. cruzi* was endemic, 13 countries in 2013 screened 100% of their blood donors for *T. cruzi* including: Argentina, Brazil, Colombia, Costa Rica, EL Salvador, Guatemala, Honduras, Panama, Paraguay, Peru, Nicaragua, Uruguay, and Venezuela. During 2013, Bolivia did not screen 8507 blood donors, Chile 5359, Ecuador 8638, and Mexico 111,169.[135] In any case, 100% screening in blood donors alone may not be enough. It is necessary also to have reagents of excellent quality; to follow manufacturer's guidelines; and that laboratories follow good laboratory practices[136] (see section: Quality Control in Serology).

An international performance evaluation program on serology for infectious diseases with participation, depending on the year, of 13 to 21 national reference centers from 11 to 16 Latin American countries was active from 1997 to 2008.[137,138] The program sent out panels with positive or negative samples for HIV, HBV, HCV, syphilis, and *T. cruzi*. Five panels with 24 unknown samples each, 2−3 of which were negative samples, were sent to participating institutions in 1997−2000; 81% of them sent the results of the five panels back; and 87−100% of the institutions responded on time (within 60 days of receiving the panel).[137] Results regarding *T. cruzi* serology showed false-negative results in 3.2% of 527 positive tests for *T. cruzi*, and 0.73% of 2329 samples positives for *T. cruzi* were false positive.[137,138] Since 2010, the Brazilian National Programme of quality control promotes the implementation of internal and external quality control and a monthly frequency for laboratory assessment of blood banks.[139]

## Table 29.8 Number of donors, screening coverage and prevalence (in thousands) of serology for *T. cruzi* in blood donors, 1993–99

| Year | 1993 | | | 1995 | | | 1997 | | | 1999 | | |
|---|---|---|---|---|---|---|---|---|---|---|---|---|
| Country | # Donors | Screen[a] % | Serologic prevalence T. cruzi | # Donors | Screen[a] % | Serologic prevalence T. cruzi | # Donors | Screen[a] % | Serologic prevalence T. cruzi | # Donors | Screen[a] | Serologic prevalence T. cruzi |
| ARG | | | | 811,850 | 96.0 | 49.0 | 742,330 | 100 | 44.0 | 810,259 | 100.00 | 55.0 |
| BOL | 37,948 | 29.40 | 147.9 | 22,146 | 66.0 | 137.0 | 40,056 | 44 | 172.0 | 20,628 | 23.18 | 454.6 |
| BRA | | | | | | | | | | 1,663,857 | 100.00 | 7.6 |
| CHI | 217,312 | 76.70 | 12.0 | 370,815 | 46.0 | 13.0 | 228,801 | 77 | 9.7 | 218,371 | 87.00 | 1.0 |
| COL | 352,316 | 1.40 | 12.0 | 45,311 | 13.0 | 8.0 | 425,359 | 99.2 | 11.0 | 353,991 | 99.89 | 10.0 |
| COR | 50,692 | 0.00 | 8.0 | 100,774 | 75.0 | 1.0 | 58,436 | 7 | 25.8 | | | |
| ECU | | | | | | | 110,619 | 72 | 1.3 | 103,448 | 90.30 | 1.3 |
| ELS | 48,048 | 42.50 | 14.7 | 52,365 | 99.0 | 23.0 | 55,069 | 100 | 22.0 | 67,224 | 100.00 | 25.0 |
| GUT | 45,426 | 75.00 | 14.0 | | | | 40,732 | 100 | 3.1 | 31,939 | 100.00 | 8.1 |
| HON | 27,885 | 100.00 | 12.4 | 31,937 | 90.0 | 17.0 | 32,670 | 99 | 11.9 | 40,933 | 99.36 | 20.5 |
| MEX | | | | | | | 936,662 | | | 1,092,741 | 13.18 | 3.8 |
| NIC | 46,001 | 58.40 | 2.4 | 48,030 | 51.0 | 1 | 46,539 | 62.1 | 39 | 45,000 | 100.00 | 3.5 |
| PAN | | | | 40,325 | 11.0 | 12 | 42,342 | 0.7 | 17.0 | 43,921 | 17.00 | 14.0 |
| PAR | | | | 34,216 | 83.0 | 58 | 40,721 | 97.99 | 37.7 | 45,597 | 99.80 | 47.0 |
| PER | | | | 82,656 | 4.0 | 0 | 205,826 | 60 | 2.0 | 311,550 | 99.80 | 1.4 |
| URU | | | | 111,518 | 100 | 6 | 115,490 | 100 | 6.5 | 116,626 | 100.00 | 4.5 |
| VEN | 204,316 | 100.00 | 13.2 | 202,515 | 100 | 8 | 262,295 | 100 | 7.8 | 302,100 | 100.0 | 6.0 |

Cell blank: No information or incomplete information.
[a]Screening coverage. Argentina (ARG); Bolivia (BOL); Brazil (BRA); Chile (CHI); Colombia (COL); Costa Rica (COR); Ecuador (ECU); El Salvador (ELS); Guatemala (GUT); Honduras (HON); Mexico (MEX); Nicaragua (NIC); Panamá (PAN); Paraguay (PAR); Perú (PER); Uruguay (URU); Venezuela (VEN).

## Table 29.9 Number of donors, screening coverage and prevalence (in thousands) of serology for *T. cruzi* in blood donors, 2001–07[a]

| Country | 2001 | | | 2003 | | | 2005 | | | 2007 | | |
|---|---|---|---|---|---|---|---|---|---|---|---|---|
| | # Donors | % Screen | Serologic prevalence | # Donors | % Screen | Serologic prevalence | # Donors | % Screen | Serologic prevalence | # Donors | % Screen | Serologic prevalence |
| ARG | 804,018 | 100 | 45.0 | 780,440 | 100 | 45.0 | | | | 54,951 | 99.84 | 25.3 |
| BOL | 24,747 | 86.09 | 99.1 | 38,621 | 79.58 | 76.5 | 46,764 | 99.26 | 86.10 | | | |
| BRA | 1,763,130 | 100 | 6.5 | 2,931,813 | 100 | 6 | 3,738,580 | 100 | 6.10 | 238,124 | 72.28 | 3.4 |
| CHI | 210,403 | 81.42 | 6.1 | 173,814 | 67 | 5.1 | 178,079 | 68.7 | 2.70 | | | |
| COL | 399,171 | 99.8 | 6.7 | 495,004 | 99.9 | 4.1 | 527,711 | 99.99 | 4.10 | | | |
| COR | 55,737 | 6.17 | 5.8 | 48,625 | 93 | 2.4 | 54,170 | 100 | 0.90 | | | |
| ECU | 65,496 | 94.05 | 0.8 | 79,204 | 100 | 3.6 | 124,724 | 100 | 0.10 | 144,600 | 100 | 4.3 |
| ELS | 72,545 | 100 | 37.0 | 76,142 | 100 | 33 | 80,142 | 100 | 24.00 | 81,246 | 100 | 2.9 |
| GUT | 43,622 | 92.27 | 14.8 | 68,626 | 99.82 | 12.3 | 77,290 | 100 | 14.00 | 76,485 | 100 | 6.9 |
| HON | 36,781 | 100 | 14.0 | 48,783 | | 13 | 52,317 | 100 | 14.70 | 52,497 | 99.31 | 4.3 |
| MEX | 1,135,397 | 13.3 | 0.5 | 1,136,047 | 32.67 | 4.4 | 1,351,204 | 36.34 | 5.00 | 1,493,674 | 53.31 | 6.6 |
| NIC | 49,346 | 94 | 5.6 | 46,558 | 94.2 | 6.3 | 54,117 | 100 | 9.00 | 59,755 | 94.5 | 6.2 |
| PAN | 42,867 | 33 | 9.0 | 46,176 | 95.5 | 1.3 | 42,771 | 97.64 | 1.20 | 46,947 | 99.5 | 9.0 |
| PAR | 48,406 | 99.15 | 44.6 | 29,718 | 96.1 | 41.4 | 47,060 | 99.83 | 33.00 | 54,538 | 100 | 7.2 |
| PER | 347,250 | 100 | 2.9 | 145,665 | 96.36 | 8.4 | 179,721 | 76.46 | 5.70 | | | |
| URU | | | | 99,675 | 100 | 3.6 | 95,686 | 100 | 2.60 | | | |
| VEN | 345,953 | 100 | 6.7 | 342,526 | 100 | 6.5 | 465,653 | 100 | 6.10 | | | |

Cell blank. No information or incomplete information.

[a]Organización Panamericana de la Salud, 2009. Screening coverage: Argentina (ARG); Bolivia (BOL); Brazil (BRA); Chile (CHI); Colombia (COL); Costa Rica (COR); Ecuador (ECU); El Salvador (ELS); Guatemala (GUT); Honduras (HON); Mexico (MEX); Nicaragua (NIC); Panamá (PAN); Paraguay (PAR); Perú (PER); Uruguay (URU); Venezuela (VEN).

Up to 2001, 11 Latin American countries had programs of performance evaluation for the serology of infectious diseases in blood banks: Argentina, Bolivia, Brazil, Colombia, El Salvador, Guatemala, Honduras, Mexico, Nicaragua, Paraguay, and Venezuela.[137,138] Another was later implemented in Ecuador. In Chile, all blood banks participate in a proficiency testing program for clinical laboratories.[137] It is unfortunate, however, that not all blood banks in most of the countries participate—less than 50% do in Argentina, Colombia, and Venezuela, up to 90% or more in El Salvador and Paraguay.[137]

These results show the usefulness of a program for performance evaluation as well as that the performance of some laboratories should improve. Another aspect that should improve is the management of the program. In order to properly evaluate performance, the samples should be tested in the same time period used in the routine of the participating laboratories. Usually, it takes less than 18 h for the routine serology to provide results that allow the blood unit to be liberated. So, to give the participating laboratories in the performance evaluation 30 days or more to reply is too much. Even if they respond without errors, there is no relation to what happens in the daily routine, so it gives a false sense of security.

# Application of diagnostic tests in different contexts

As explained in the beginning of this chapter, Chagas disease has two main phases, acute and chronic, and diagnostic tests should be applied according to the suspected phase. During acute phase, parasitological tests are preferred and serological tests are used only if the former were negative and suspicion persists. For the chronic phase, serological tests are the option, and parasitological only used in special circumstances. Even if major groups of tests are parasitological and serological, other tests which are not routinely used have been employed. Search for antigen during the acute and chronic phase has been the subject of a few investigations. Skin tests have been tried without success[140,141] and, as an invasive procedure, may have ethical consequences, mainly when there are other tests that are easier to perform.

Furthermore, there is the context of the clinical situation to consider. For example, there is the confirmation of a suspected case against exclusion of a donor. A responsible diagnostic laboratory should concentrate all efforts to demonstrate or exclude the presence of the infection. The hematologists need to be sure that the blood is not infected. If there is any suspicion, even if not confirmed after, blood should be discarded. There are other situations in which a special array of tests or timing is necessary, such as epidemiological surveys and congenital transmission. Each one of these situations needs to be analyzed. For a better handling some examples are given below, including in each the clinical context, epidemiology, laboratory tests to be requested, and action to be done.

## Parasitological and serological tests in the acute phase and reactivation

### Vectorial transmission

1. Clinical situation: Person with fever, of some days/weeks of evolution. Common causes of fever discarded. Not severely ill. Few nonspecific findings on examination. Sometimes a portal of entry (one eye, both eyelids) or skin.
2. Epidemiology: Living or has been recently in endemic area for Chagas disease.
3. Laboratory: Ask for fresh blood smear, looking for motile flagellates. Ask for Strout or microhematocrit technique.
4. Action: If positive, the diagnosis is acute phase of Chagas disease, probably by vector contamination. Start treatment at once.

If negative and the clinical suspicion persists, try to collect further blood mainly during febrile peaks. If negative persist, ask for IgM antibodies, by IIF. If positive, decide with the clinician if the clinical picture, evolution and this result may justify etiological treatment.

*Hints*: Romaña sign and other eventual portal of entry, will remain for several weeks. Conjunctivitis will disappear in few days. Differential diagnosis with visceral leishmaniasis should be made if negative parasitological results are obtained, mainly if the evolution of the patient is to a progressive worsening.

### Transmission by transfusion or transplantation

1. Clinical picture: Generally at hospital, with severe disease (or not), started with fever of unknown origin. Frequent causes have not been found.
2. Epidemiological fact: Received transfusion recently (last 2 months) or transplantation (bone marrow, other organs) and has fever after, unknown causes.
3. Laboratory: Perhaps some laboratory technician saw strange pathogens in the smear, during a routine differential count. Try to identify the parasite. Ask for a fresh blood smear. If negative, ask for Strout or microhematocrit technique. Transfusional transmitted cases have easily detected parasitemias.
4. Action: If positive, the diagnosis is acute phase of Chagas disease, by transfusion or transplantation in a patient with other disease, which motivates the transfusion/transplantation. Start specific treatment.

### Oral transmission

1. Clinical picture: Several people living at the same house or neighbors who participate recently in some festivity, and used the same food, became febrile after some days. A disease transmitted by foods is suspected. Some have digestive manifestations, even with hematemesis (blood vomiting). Some patients may look severely ill. Liver tests may show alterations (bilirubins, transaminases).
2. Epidemiological fact: Endemic region or not endemic, that uses fresh foods from endemic regions.
3. Laboratory: Ask for a fresh blood smear. If negative, ask for Strout or microhematocrit technique.

**4.** Action: If positive, the diagnosis is acute phase of Chagas disease, by oral route. Start treatment and diagnose the other similarly affected. Direct diagnosis should be made in all the persons that eat or drink the identified food (if any identified).

## Laboratory acquired infection

**1.** Clinical picture: Normal person working in a health service, laboratory, or research institution start with fever of unknown origin. Usual causes have been discarded.

**2.** Epidemiological fact: Works with reduviid bugs, or with *T. cruzi*, in cultures, mice, or other animals. May be working in a nonendemic region. Surgeon or technician of necropsy personnel.

**3.** Laboratory: Ask for a fresh blood smear. If negative, ask for Strout or microhematocrit technique.

**4.** Action: If positive, the diagnosis is acute phase of Chagas disease, by laboratory accident. Start treatment and collect a sample of blood at once. Perhaps in endemic regions, the worker is already infected.

## Reactivation of chronically infected

**1.** Clinical picture: Patient with known HIV infection or with diagnosed cancer or other disease (autoimmune) which requires, as part of the treatment, large doses of corticoid or other immunosuppressors. During the course of the disease or the treatment, not expected skin lesions and/or nervous system involvement, which was not present, mainly with loss of consciousness. Any other not predicted clinical manifestation.

**2.** Epidemiological fact: Has had Chagas disease diagnosed years ago, or was born/lived in endemic areas for Chagas disease.

**3.** Laboratory: Ask for a fresh blood smear. If negative, ask for Strout or microhematocrit technique.

**4.** Action: If parasitological tests are positive, the diagnosis is reactivation of chronic phase of Chagas disease, by immune suppression, which is in fact an acute phase, because the criteria of having easily detectable parasites is fulfilled. Start treatment and collect a sample of blood at once for serology. This serology should be positive, because the patient was in the chronic phase.[142]

The congenital route is a special situation that behaves as an acute phase and is described in other chapter.

## Tests in the chronic phase

Application of tests in the situations that follow are always serological for routine purposes. Parasitological tests are performed only for research.

### Confirmation of a clinical case

The most common situation is the confirmation or exclusion in a particular case. This case may arrive at the clinician by several channels: (1) an outpatient consultation as a routine checkup; (2) from a blood bank because of exclusion as a donor; (3) during a selection for a job in a country in which screening for *T. cruzi* is mandatory and an infection was found; (4) patient has relatives with Chagas and wants to exclude/confirm the infection; and (5) a gynecologist may send the pregnant patient for evaluation of risk to have the infection and then to investigate for congenital transmission.

In any case, the physician should look for symptoms and signs common in Chagas disease, ask for epidemiological background (an infected mother is important), and ask for laboratory tests for confirmation or exclusion. These serological tests should be very specific and performed in parallel, with at least two tests of different principles (i.e., ELISA and HA; IFI and HA, recombinant ELISA and HA). The results should be expressed in titers for IFI, HA, and OD of the sample and of the cutoff of the plate for ELISA, together with a table with the normal values for the population of the region. If results demonstrate anti-*T. cruzi* antibodies in high titers in both tests, the chances of error are minimized.

The serological confirmation of *T. cruzi* infection ought to be done with two tests of different principles. A common mistake made by the clinicians is to accept the result of a single rapid test or a single recombinant ELISA result or a single chemiluminiscence result (i.e., CMIA Architect). Rapid tests lack the specificity and sensitivity necessary to make or exclude the serological diagnosis.[97] The single recombinant ELISA and the single chemiluminiscence tests have a very high sensitivity, but not the required specificity to assure diagnosis; false positives may be found. A second assay will confirm or exclude the infection. If results are discordant (one positive, the other negative) a detailed search of the true situation is necessary.

An error at this stage may have legal consequences. A false-negative result may lead the physician to look for other diseases or believe the patient is noninfected. Perhaps a false positive may be even worse, because he/she will have the stigma of a severe disease that may be fatal. This person may even have had relatives dead from Chagas disease.

## Epidemiological surveys

Serology is used in epidemiological surveys for prevalence purposes and as a tool to measure efficacy of control. In order to know the prevalence of Chagas disease in different endemic areas, governments and research groups in some countries launched serological surveys. Results obtained would help to focus prophylaxis on the affected areas, which is basically application of insecticides to kill domiciliated bugs.

These surveys involve a large number of samples, on the order of thousands, after a proper statistical selection of the regions to be studied. It is not possible to obtain venous blood from thousands of individuals in a short period of time in rural areas. The need for centrifugation on the same day, as well as the possibility of misrotulations, the need for a cold chain, and problems of space made this common way to obtain clinical samples nonpractical for these purposes. The alternative in this situation is blood collection by finger prick, collecting the blood on filter paper, which is easier and quicker. It allows collection of hundreds of samples per day that can be stored at room temperature in small containers, to be tested in central laboratories weeks or months later. It could even be transported by postal services, avoiding the expensive costs of transportation.

Once at the laboratory, filter papers should be cut to a proper size and eluted with saline buffer overnight. The eluate obtained may be then tested with the reagents, mainly conventional tests. Even if results are not so clear cut as those obtained with sera, positive samples are detected and the confirmation may be done later by a proper venous blood collection. The number of tests applied may vary according to the question to be solved, but there is consensus to employ tests of high sensitivity.

The most well-known example was a survey conducted in Brazil in 1975−80. A single IIF was used, collecting more than 1,200,000 samples covering all the states of Brazil but Sao Paulo, which was previously studied. To the best of our knowledge, this has been the largest survey in the world for Chagas disease. A map was built with the prevalence of the infection all over the country to delineate endemic areas.[143]

In other surveys, it was possible to estimate the prevalence in urban workers[144] and compare filter paper and venous blood results. In another example, now in rural communities, in order to establish the efficacy of specific treatment in children, the population was visited in their schools, and it was possible to select and treat those infected, confirming results with venous blood.[94]

Other uses of epidemiological surveys in Chagas disease are to check if prophylactic measures (insecticide spraying of houses) were really effective. In this approach, the goal will be to detect infected people born after the colonization of bugs in homes was controlled. To this end, another national survey was launched, also in Brazil, from 2001 until 2008, in all states but Rio de Janeiro, from children born after the insecticide spraying (i.e., less than 5 years old). More than 105,000 samples were collected and processed with two tests of recognized high sensitivity, IIF and ELISA. Quality control was performed in another laboratory with 10% of the samples. This survey detected 110 positive samples, from which 45 were confirmed as passive transmission from the infected mother, 20 were considered cases of vertical transmission, and 11 originated from vectors other than *T. infestans* which was the target of the elimination campaign.[88]

## Follow up of specifically treated patients

Tests that follow up of specifically treated patients (serology for cure and parasitological tests for failure) have revealed that specific treatment is effective in nearly all infected by congenital route, in 60−80% of acute phase patients, children, and early chronic phase, and in 25−30% of those treated during the chronic phase.[145,146] Treatment is mandatory for first two groups and optional for the last. The follow-up of treated patients to know if they were cured is performed through serological and parasitological tests, though the latter is not essential. Cure is attained when antibodies, formerly present, disappear. Parasitological tests are useful only when positive and indicate treatment failure.[48]

In Chagas disease, antibodies demand different amounts of time to disappear, related to the phase of the disease and to the type of *T. cruzi*. In congenital infection, nearly all treated are cured, and 1 year follow-up is enough. Acute and chronically infected individuals with less than 10 years of evolution (mainly children) are cured at a lower rate (60−80%) and the antibodies may take 2−10 years to disappear.[146] It has been recently demonstrated that the type of parasite present is of utmost importance.[147] In those countries where *T. cruzi* I predominates (Mexico, Central America, Colombia, and Venezuela), the antibody responses vanish by 16 months in children. Where *T. cruzi* II predominates, as in Brazil, the same group of patients takes more than 5 and often 10 years to be free of antibodies.[147]

Those treated during the chronic phase usually take longer: no studies with large series of adults are available from *T. cruzi* I region, but below the equator line (*T. cruzi* II) it usually takes 15−30 years to obtain a negative serology and the number cured is no higher than 30%. This long time is probably due to the time the immune memory would forget a parasite which was in circulation for decades.[148]

Antibody response should be measured by conventional tests as described. The use of recombinant antigens may yield equivocal results. In some already cured, the responses to recombinant antigens is still high when there are no more anti-*T. cruzi* antibodies found by ELISA, IIF, and HA. A number of nonconventional tests show that antibodies measured by these systems could indeed have a quicker shift and decrease after shorter periods of time.[149,150]

# Quality control in serology

Although serological diagnosis is relatively simple to perform considering the complex tasks that involve the activities of the modern diagnostic laboratory, some principles should be followed in order to guarantee either a correct screening or a final diagnosis: use of diagnostic reagents of proven quality. Validation of the reagents available in the market should be performed by a competent authority or an institution in which this validation is delegated. For *T. cruzi* screening a sensitivity of at least 99.8% and a specificity of 99.5% are appropriate, but there is still room for improvement; internal quality assurance of the equipment, procedures, and diagnostic reagents; complete records of all activities verified through periodic audit (at least every 2 years); continuous training of staff; and mandatory participation in performance evaluation schemes for which unknown samples are tested together with the routine work and results informed with the same celerity.

The inclusion of an international standard serum is also desirable. In the past, this was not possible for *T. cruzi* infection, because it was not available. In 2007, the *WHO Program on Blood Products and Related Biologicals/Quality and Safety: Medicines Team*, convened the First WHO Consultation on International Biological Reference Preparations for Chagas Diagnostic Tests.[151] During this meeting it was agreed on two preparations, one representing countries where Tc1 was prevalent and the other from regions where Tc2 was prevalent. After a WHO collaborative study involving 24 laboratories from 16 countries, the 2 preparations (09/186 and 09/188) were approved and are available from WHO.[152]

# Prophylaxis to avoid accidental contamination

As this chapter is intended to be useful to personnel from diagnostic laboratories, some guidelines for prophylaxis of accidental contamination are included. Accidental contamination with *T. cruzi* has been reported in more than 100 cases.[49,50] Contamination may be of laboratory staff who works with infected bugs, with inoculated animals, cultures for antigen production, cryopreserved samples, and blood from acute phase patients. Also surgeons and staff in surgical procedures or necropsies may be contaminated if handling infected patients. However, there are guidelines to help avoid this danger. It is advisable that all personnel working with this parasite have a sample of blood collected and serum stored each year. This is useful to know if someone was infected before arrival at the laboratory, and to compare antibody levels in the case of an accident or recognize an otherwise unnoticed contamination. The main measures to avoid an accident are, in order of importance: (1) eye and mouth protection, by using a mask, (2) gloves and covered shoes (no sandals allowed), (3) do not work alone; and (4) concentration on the task. Some of these are obvious and a part of good laboratory practices, which should be followed nowadays in any laboratory together with personal protection equipment (PPE).

# Future perspectives

The serological diagnosis has had profound advances in the last decade. Most infected individuals are correctly diagnosed. The main problems are due to poor control in two main variables: quality kits and laboratory practices. In any case a few sera (up to 2%) have doubtful results. Diagnosis ought to be handled by a clinician who decides based on clinical findings and serology results.

Although recent research showed that with the tests we have, most treated children will have negative serology in less than 15 months in areas of TcI, proving that conventional tests are good enough, and that the long time required for negativation is more dependent on the type of *T. cruzi* than the tests, new tests capable of measuring antibodies that assess cure or other approaches nonantibody dependent (proteomics) are needed.

Progress also could be made in diagnosis in rural areas, and rapid tests should help with this goal. Some efforts were performed to have several recombinants at the same device, but this will increase costs. Another advance would be development of a PCR kit that could be commercially available and used at the field, with enhanced sensitivity and specificity.

# References

1. Schmunis GA. Epidemiology of Chagas disease in non-endemic countries: the role of international migration. *Mem Inst Oswaldo Cruz* 2007;**102**(Suppl. 1):75−85.
2. Guerreiro C, Machado A. Da reacao de Bordet e Gengou na molestia de Carlos Chagas como elemento diagnostico. *Bras. Med.* 1913;**27**:225−6.
3. Camargo ME, Takeda GK. Diagnostico de laboratorio. In: Brener Z, Andrade ZA, editors. *Trypanososma cruzi e doenca de Chagas*. Rio de Janeiro: Guanabara Koogan; 1979. p. 175−98.
4. Freitas JLP, Almeida JO. Nova tecnica de fixacao do complemento para molestia de Chagas. Reacao quantitativa com antigeno gelificado de culturas de *Trypanosoma cruzi*. *Hospital (Rio J)* 1949;**35**:787−800.
5. Batista SM, Santos UM. Methyl antigen from a "Schizotrypanum cruzi" culture. *Hospital (Rio J)* 1959;**56**:1045−51.
6. Fife Jr. EH, Kent JF. Protein and carbohydrate complement fixing antigens of *Trypanosoma cruzi*. *Am J Trop Med Hyg* 1960;**9**:512−17.
7. Maekelt GA. The complement fixation reaction in Chagas' disease. *Z Tropenmed Parasitol* 1960;**11**:152−86.
8. Baracchini O, Costa A, Carloni J. Use of heat and methanol in the preparation of antigen from "*Trypanosoma cruzi*." *Hospital (Rio J)* 1965;**67**(6):1313−19.
9. Maekelt GA. Diagnostico de laboratorio de la Trypanosomiasis Americana. *Rev Venez Sanid* 1964;**29**:1−18.
10. Goncalves JM, Yamaha T. Immunochemical polysaccharide from *Trypanosoma cruzi*. *J Trop Med Hyg* 1969;**72**(2):39−44.
11. Bergendi L, Knierim F, Apt W. *Trypanosoma cruzi*: immunological properties of a soluble extract of culture forms. *Exp Parasitol* 1970;**28**(2):258−62.
12. Gonzalez Cappa SM, Kagan IG. Antigenicity of fractions of a somatic antigen of *Trypanosoma cruzi*. *J Parasitol* 1973;**59**(6):1080−4.
13. Camargo ME. Fluorescent antibody test for the serodiagnosis of American trypanosomiasis. Technical modification employing preserved culture forms of *Trypanosoma cruzi* in a slide test. *Rev Inst Med Trop Sao Paulo* 1966;**8**(5):227−35.
14. De Almeida Oliveira J. Isofixation curves as a method of standardizing quantitative complement-fixation tests. *J Immunol* 1956;**76**(4):259−63.
15. Siqueira AF. Comparacao de antigenos de *Trypanosoma cruzi* para reacoes quantitativas de fixacao do complemento. II. Analise sequencial de probabilidade direta aplicada ao sistema molestia de Chagas. *Rev Inst Med Trop Sao Paulo* 1964;**6**:268−76.
16. Almeida JO, Fife Jr. EH. *Metodos de fijacion del complemento estandarizado cuantitativamente para la evaluacion critica de antigenos preparados con* Trypanosoma cruzi. Washington, DC: Org. Panam. Salud Publ; 1976.
17. Freitas JLP. Reacao de fixacao do complemento para o diagnostico da molestia de Chagas pela tecnica quantitativa. *Arch Hig (Sao Paulo)* 1951;**16**:55−94.
18. Salgado Ade A, Mayrink W, Dias JC. Comparative study between the complement fixation test with methyl and benzene-chloroformium antigens and xenodiagnosis. *Rev Inst Med Trop Sao Paulo* 1970;**12**(1):36−40.
19. Cerisola JA. *Valor del inmunodiagnostico en la infeccion Chagasica. Proc. Simposio Internacional sobre Enfermedad de Chagas*. Buenos Aires; 1972.
20. Brumpt E. Le xenodiagnostic. Application au diagnostic de quelques infections parasitaires et en particulier a la Trypanosomose de Chagas. *Bull. Soc. Pat. Exot.* 1914;**7**:706−10.

21. Cerisola J.A., Rohwedder R., Segura E.L., Del Prado C.E., Alvarez M., Martini G.J.W. *El xenodiagnostico*. Buenos Aires: Imp. Inst. Nac. Invest. Cardiovasc; 1974.

22. Fife Jr. EH, Muschel LH. Fluorescent-antibody technic for serodiagnosis of *Trypanosoma cruzi* infection. *Proc Soc Exp Biol Med* 1959;**101**(3):540−3.

23. Cerisola JA, Fatala Chaben M, Lazzari JO. Hemagglutination test for the diagnosis of Chagas' disease. *Prensa Med Argent* 1962;**49**:1761−7.

24. Knierim F, Saavedra P. Hemagglutination test applied to the serological diagnosis of parasitic diseases. *Bol Chil Parasitol* 1966;**21**(2):39−44.

25. Rassi A, Luquetti AO, Rassi Jr A, Rassi SG, Rassi AG. Chagas' disease: clinical features. In: Wendel S, Brener Z, Camargo ME, Rassi A, editors. *Chagas' Disease (American Trypanosomiasis): its impact on transfusion and clinical medicine*. Sao Paulo: Editora ISBT; 1992. p. 81−101.

26. Rezende JM, Luquetti AO. *Chagasic megavisceras. Nervous system in Chagas disease*. Washington: PAHO/OMS; 1994. p. 149−71.

27. Luquetti AO, Rassi A. Diagnostico Laboratorial da Infeccao pelo *Trypanosoma cruzi*. In: Brener Z, Andrade AZ, Barral-Neto M, editors. *Trypanosoma cruzi e Doenca de Chagas*. 2nd ed. Rio de Janeiro: Guanabara Koogan; 2000. p. 344−78.

28. Amato-Neto V. Comentarios sobre caso de transmisso da doenca de Chagas por transfusao de sangue e longo periodo de incubacao. *Rev. Soc. Bras. Med. Trop*. 1969;**3**:273−5.

29. Luquetti AO, Ferreira AW, Oliveira RA, Tavares SB, Rassi A, Dias JC, et al. Congenital transmission of *Trypanosoma cruzi* in Brazil: estimation of prevalence based on preliminary data of national serological surveys in children under 5 years old and other sources. *Rev Soc Bras Med Trop* 2005;**38**(Suppl. 2):24−6.

30. Zeledon R, Dias JC, Brilla-Salazar A, de Rezende JM, Vargas LG, Urbina A. Does a spontaneous cure for Chagas' disease exist? *Rev Soc Bras Med Trop* 1988;**21**(1):15−20.

31. Rohwedder RW. Chagas' infection in blood donors and the possibility of its transmission by blood transfusion. *Bol Chil Parasitol* 1969;**24**(1):88−93.

32. Cerisola JA, Rabinovich A, Alvarez M, Di Corleto CA, Pruneda J. Enfermedad de Chagas y la transfusion de sangre. *Bol Of Sanit Panam* 1972;**73**:203−21.

33. Zuna H. *Estudio de la importancia de la transmision de la enfermedad de Chagas por via transfusional. Experiencia de Santa Cruz, 1982−1983*. Proc. Coloquio Internacional Enfermedad de Chagas. Bolivia: Santa Cruz de la Sierra; 1983.

34. Atias A, Lorca M, Canales M, Mercado R, Reyes V, Child R. Enfermedad de Chagas: transmision por transfusion sanguinea en Chile. *Bol. Hosp. San Juan Dios. (Santiago)* 1984;**31**:301−6.

35. Gonzalez A, Prediger E, Huecas ME, Nogueira N, Lizardi PM. Minichromosomal repetitive DNA in *Trypanosoma cruzi*: its use in a high-sensitivity parasite detection assay. *Proc Natl Acad Sci USA* 1984;**81**(11):3356−60.

36. Ashall F, Yip-Chuck DA, Luquetti AA, Miles MA. Radiolabeled total parasite DNA probe specifically detects *Trypanosoma cruzi* in mammalian blood. *J Clin Microbiol* 1988;**26**(3):576−8.

37. Sturm NR, Degrave W, Morel C, Simpson L. Sensitive detection and schizodeme classification of *Trypanosoma cruzi* cells by amplification of kinetoplast minicircle DNA sequences: use in diagnosis of Chagas' disease. *Mol Biochem Parasitol* 1989;**33** (3):205−14.

38. Chiari E, Dias JC, Lana M, Chiari CA. Hemocultures for the parasitological diagnosis of human chronic Chagas' disease. *Rev Soc Bras Med Trop* 1989;**22**(1):19−23.

39. Avila HA, Pereira JB, Thiemann O, De Paiva E, DeGrave W, Morel CM, et al. Detection of *Trypanosoma cruzi* in blood specimens of chronic chagasic patients by

polymerase chain reaction amplification of kinetoplast minicircle DNA: comparison with serology and xenodiagnosis. *J Clin Microbiol* 1993;**31**(9):2421−6.

40. Schijman A. RT-PCR in the diagnosis of Chagas disease: an overview of the workshop sponsored by PAHO/WHO. *Rev. Patol. Trop* 2009;**38**:1411−12.

41. Schijman AG, Bisio M, Orellana L, Sued M, Duffy T, Mejia Jaramillo AM, et al. International study to evaluate PCR methods for detection of *Trypanosoma cruzi* DNA in blood samples from Chagas disease patients. *PLoS NTD* 2011;**5**(1):e931.

42. Castro AM, Luquetti AO, Rassi A, Rassi GG, Chiari E, Galvao LM. Blood culture and polymerase chain reaction for the diagnosis of the chronic phase of human infection with *Trypanosoma cruzi*. *Parasitol Res* 2002;**88**(10):894−900.

43. Junqueira AC, Chiari E, Wincker P. Comparison of the polymerase chain reaction with two classical parasitological methods for the diagnosis of Chagas disease in an endemic region of north-eastern Brazil. *Trans R Soc Trop Med Hyg* 1996;**90**(2):129−32.

44. Siriano LR, Luquetti AO, Avelar JB, Marra NL, de Castro AM. Chagas disease: increased parasitemia during pregnancy detected by hemoculture. *Am J Trop Med Hyg* 2011;**84**(4):569−74.

45. Rassi A, Lustosa ES, Carvalho MESD, Nascimento MD, Ferrioli Filho F, Luquetti AO. Sensibilidade do xenodiagnostico em pacientes na fase cronica da doenca de Chagas. Resultados preliminares. *Rev. Soc. Bras. Med. Trop.* 1991;**24**:36−7.

46. Luz ZM, Coutinho MG, Cancado JR, Krettli AU. Hemoculture: sensitive technique in the detection of *Trypanosoma cruzi* in chagasic patients in the chronic phase of Chagas disease. *Rev Soc Bras Med Trop* 1994;**27**(3):143−8.

47. de Castro AM, Luquetti AO, Rassi A, Chiari E, Galvao LM. Detection of parasitemia profiles by blood culture after treatment of human chronic *Trypanosoma cruzi* infection. *Parasitol Res* 2006;**99**(4):379−83.

48. Rassi A, Luquetti AO, Rassi Jr. A, Rassi GG, Rassi SG, IG, et al. Specific treatment for *Trypanosoma cruzi*: lack of efficacy of allopurinol in the human chronic phase of Chagas disease. *Am J Trop Med Hyg* 2007;**76**(1):58−61.

49. Brener Z. *Laboratory-acquired Chagas' disease: an endemic disease among parasitologists? Genes and antigens of parasites: a laboratory manual.* Rio de Janeiro: Fundacao Oswaldo Cruz; 1984. p. 3−9.

50. Ministerio da Saude FNdS, Gerencia Tecnica de Doenca de Chagas. Normas de seguranca para infeccoes acidentais com o *Trypanosoma cruzi*, agente causador da doenca de Chagas. *Rev Patol Trop* 1997;**26**:129−130.

51. Strout RG. A method for concentrating hemoflagellates. *J Parasitol* 1962;**48**:100.

52. Freilij H, Muller L, Gonzalez Cappa SM. Direct micromethod for diagnosis of acute and congenital Chagas' disease. *J Clin Microbiol* 1983;**18**(2):327−30.

53. Budzko DB, Kierszenbaum F. Isolation of *Trypanosoma cruzi* from blood. *J Parasitol* 1974;**60**(6):1037−8.

54. dos Santos AH, da Silva IG, Rassi A. A comparative study between natural and artificial xenodiagnosis in chronic Chagas' disease patients. *Rev Soc Bras Med Trop* 1995;**28**(4):367−73.

55. Franco YB, Silva IG, Rassi A, Rocha AC, Silva HH, Rassi GG. Correlation among the positivity of the artificial xenodiagnosis and the amount of blood and triatomines used in the exam, in chronic chagasic patients. *Rev Soc Bras Med Trop* 2002;**35**(1):29−33.

56. Cerisola JA, Rohwedder R, Bozzini JP, Del Prado CE. *Blastocrithidia triatomae* n. sp. found in *Triatoma infestans* from Argentina. *J Protozool* 1971;**18**(3):503−6.

57. Chiari E, Brener Z. Contribution to the parasitological diagnosis of human Chagas' disease in its chronic phase. *Rev Inst Med Trop Sao Paulo* 1966;**8**(3):134−8.

58. Oliveira EC, Stefani MM, Luquetti AO, Vencio EF, Moreira MA, Souza C, et al. *Trypanosoma cruzi* and experimental Chagas' disease: characterization of a stock isolated from a patient with associated digestive and cardiac form. *Rev Soc Bras Med Trop* 1993;**26**(1):25−33.

59. Corral RS, Altcheh J, Alexandre SR, Grinstein S, Freilij H, Katzin AM. Detection and characterization of antigens in urine of patients with acute, congenital, and chronic Chagas' disease. *J Clin Microbiol* 1996;**34**(8):1957−62.

60. De Winne K, Buscher P, Luquetti AO, Tavares SB, Oliveira RA, Solari A, et al. The *Trypanosoma cruzi* satellite DNA OligoC-TesT and *Trypanosoma cruzi* kinetoplast DNA OligoC-TesT for diagnosis of Chagas disease: a multi-cohort comparative evaluation study. *PLoS NTD* 2014;**8**(1):e2633.

61. Luquetti AO, Espinoza B, Martinez I, Hernandez-Becerril N, Ponce C, Ponce E, et al. Performance levels of four Latin American laboratories for the serodiagnosis of Chagas disease in Mexican sera samples. *Mem Inst Oswaldo Cruz* 2009;**104**(5):797−800.

62. Zingales B, Andrade SG, Briones MR, Campbell DA, Chiari E, Fernandes O, et al. A new consensus for *Trypanosoma cruzi* intraspecific nomenclature: second revision meeting recommends TcI to TcVI. *Mem Inst Oswaldo Cruz* 2009;**104**(7):1051−4.

63. D'Alessandro-Bacigalupo A, Saravia NG. *Trypanosoma rangeli*. In: Kreier JP, editor. *Parasitic protozoa*. New York: Academic Press; 1992. p. 1−54.

64. Vasquez JE, Krusnell J, Orn A, Sousa OE, Harris RA. Serological diagnosis of *Trypanosoma rangeli* infected patients. A comparison of different methods and its implications for the diagnosis of Chagas' disease. *Scand J Immunol* 1997;**45**(3):322−30.

65. Krettli AU, Brener Z. Resistance against *Trypanosoma cruzi* associated to anti-living trypomastigote antibodies. *J Immunol* 1982;**128**(5):2009−12.

66. Affranchino JL, Ibanez CF, Luquetti AO, Rassi A, Reyes MB, Macina RA, et al. Identification of a *Trypanosoma cruzi* antigen that is shed during the acute phase of Chagas' disease. *Mol Biochem Parasitol* 1989;**34**(3):221−8.

67. Cabral HR. Rheumatoid factors and Chagas' disease. *Science* 1983;**219**(4589):1238.

68. Luquetti AO, Tavares SBN, Oliveira RA, Oliveira EC, Vaz MGM, Rassi A. Presenca de anticorpos especificos da classe IgM nas diferentes formas clinicas da fase cronica da doenca de Chagas. *Rev. Soc. Bras. Med. Trop.* 1996;**29**:134−5.

69. Carlier Y, Torrico F. Congenital infection with *Trypanosoma cruzi*: from mechanisms of transmission to strategies for diagnosis and control. *Rev Soc Bras Med Trop* 2003;**36**(6):767−71.

70. Schmunis GA, Cruz JR. Safety of the blood supply in Latin America. *Clin Microbiol Rev* 2005;**18**(1):12−29.

71. Lorca M, Child R, Garcia A, Silva M, Osorio J, Atias A. Evaluation of commercially available reagents for diagnosis of Chagas disease in Chilean blood banks. I. Selection of reagents. *Rev Med Chil* 1992;**120**(4):420−6.

72. Lorca M, Child R, Garcia A, Silva M, Martinez L, Jerez G, et al. Evaluation of commercial kits used for Chagas disease diagnosis in blood banks in Chile. II. Routine application. *Rev Med Chil* 1994;**122**(8):925−31.

73. Saez-Alquezar A, Luquetti AO, Borges-Pereira J, Furtado EM, Gadelha MFS, Garcia-Zapata MT. Estudo multicentrico: avaliacao dodesempenho de conjuntos diagnosticos de hemaglutinacao indireta, disponiveis no Brasil, para o dianostico sorologico da infeccao pelo *Trypanosoma cruzi. Rev. Patol. Trop.* 1997;**26**:343−74.

74. Vattuone NH, Yanovsky JF. *Trypanosoma cruzi*: agglutination activity of enzyme-treated epimastigotes. *Exp Parasitol* 1971;**30**(3):349−55.

75. Schmunis GA. A resposta imune-humoral na infeccao humana recente pelo *Trypanosoma cruzi. Rev. Patol. Trop.* 1991;**20**:51−146.

76. Peralta JM, Magalhaes TC, Abreu L, Manigot DA, Luquetti A, Dias JC. The direct agglutination test for chronic Chagas's disease. The effect of pre-treatment of test samples with 2-mercaptoethanol. *Trans R Soc Trop Med Hyg* 1981;**75**(5):695–8.
77. Luquetti AO, Tavares SBN, Oliveira RA, Siriano LR, Costa DG, Oliveira EC. Sorologia como criterio de cura em pacientes tratados com benznidazol. Titulos obtidos em chagasicos nao tratados por imunofluorecencia indireta. *Rev. Soc. Bras. Med. Trop.* 2008;**41**:242–3.
78. Voller A, Draper C, Bidwell DE, Bartlett A. Microplate enzyme-linked immunosorbent assay for Chagas' disease. *Lancet* 1975;**1**(7904):426–8.
79. *Resultado da avaliacao dos kits para diagnostico da doenca de Chagas.* Brasilia: Ministerio da Saude; 2006.
80. Kirchhoff LV, Gam AA, Gusmao RA, Goldsmith RS, Rezende JM, Rassi A. Increased specificity of serodiagnosis of Chagas' disease by detection of antibody to the 72- and 90-kilodalton glycoproteins of *Trypanosoma cruzi*. *J Infect Dis* 1987;**155**(3):561–4.
81. *Anti-Trypanosoma cruzi assays: operational characteristics.* Geneva: World Health Organisation; 2010.
82. Leiby DA, Wendel S, Takaoka DT, Fachini RM, Oliveira LC, Tibbals MA. Serologic testing for *Trypanosoma cruzi*: comparison of radioimmunoprecipitation assay with commercially available indirect immunofluorescence assay, indirect hemagglutination assay, and enzyme-linked immunosorbent assay kits. *J Clin Microbiol* 2000;**38**(2):639–42.
83. Stolf AM, Umezawa ES, Zingales B. Simultaneous identification of *Trypanosoma cruzi* surface and internal antigens reactive to different immunoglobulin classes (radio-immunoblotting). *Rev Inst Med Trop Sao Paulo* 1990;**32**(5):379–83.
84. Teixeira MG, Borges-Pereira J, Netizert E, Souza ML, Peralta JM. Development and evaluation of an enzyme linked immunotransfer blot technique for serodiagnosis of Chagas' disease. *Trop Med Parasitol* 1994;**45**(4):308–12.
85. Mendes RP, Hoshino-Shimizu S, Moura da Silva AM, Mota I, Heredia RA, Luquetti AO, et al. Serological diagnosis of Chagas' disease: a potential confirmatory assay using preserved protein antigens of *Trypanosoma cruzi*. *J Clin Microbiol* 1997;**35** (7):1829–34.
86. Umezawa ES, Nascimento MS, Kesper Jr. N, Coura JR, Borges-Pereira J, Junqueira AC, et al. Immunoblot assay using excreted-secreted antigens of *Trypanosoma cruzi* in serodiagnosis of congenital, acute, and chronic Chagas' disease. *J Clin Microbiol* 1996;**34**(9):2143–7.
87. Frade AF, Luquetti AO, Prata A, Ferreira AW. Western blotting method (TESAcruzi) as a supplemental test for confirming the presence of anti-*Trypanosoma cruzi* antibodies in finger prick blood samples from children aged 0–5 years in Brazil. *Acta Trop* 2011;**117**(1):10–13.
88. Ostermayer AL, Passos AD, Silveira AC, Ferreira AW, Macedo V, Prata AR. The national survey of seroprevalence for evaluation of the control of Chagas disease in Brazil (2001–2008). *Rev Soc Bras Med Trop* 2011;**44**(Suppl. 2):108–21.
89. Galvao LM, Nunes RM, Cancado JR, Brener Z, Krettli AU. Lytic antibody titre as a means of assessing cure after treatment of Chagas disease: a 10 years follow-up study. *Trans R Soc Trop Med Hyg* 1993;**87**(2):220–3.
90. Martins-Filho OA, Pereira ME, Carvalho JF, Cancado JR, Brener Z. Flow cytometry, a new approach to detect anti-live trypomastigote antibodies and monitor the efficacy of specific treatment in human Chagas' disease. *Clin Diagn Lab Immunol* 1995;**2**(5):569–73.
91. Vitelli-Avelar DM, Sathler-Avelar R, Wendling AP, Rocha RD, Teixeira-Carvalho A, Martins NE, et al. Non-conventional flow cytometry approaches to detect anti-*Trypanosoma cruzi* immunoglobulin G in the clinical laboratory. *J Immunol Methods* 2007;**318**(1-2):102–12.

92. Matos CS, Coelho-Dos-Reis JG, Rassi A, Luquetti AO, Dias JC, Eloi-Santos SM, et al. Applicability of an optimized non-conventional flow cytometry method to detect anti-*Trypanosoma cruzi* immunoglobulin G for the serological diagnosis and cure assessment following chemotherapeutic treatment of Chagas disease. *J Immunol Methods* 2011;**369**(1-2):22–32.

93. Almeida IC, Rodrigues EG, Travassos LR. Chemiluminescent immunoassays: discrimination between the reactivities of natural and human patient antibodies with antigens from eukaryotic pathogens, *Trypanosoma cruzi* and *Paracoccidioides brasiliensis*. *J Clin Lab Anal* 1994;**8**(6):424–31.

94. de Andrade AL, Zicker F, de Oliveira RM, Almeida Silva S, Luquetti A, Travassos LR, et al. Randomised trial of efficacy of benznidazole in treatment of early *Trypanosoma cruzi* infection. *Lancet* 1996;**348**(9039):1407–13.

95. Luquetti AO, Ponce C, Ponce E, Esfandiari J, Schijman A, Revollo S, et al. Chagas' disease diagnosis: a multicentric evaluation of Chagas Stat-Pak, a rapid immunochromatographic assay with recombinant proteins of *Trypanosoma cruzi*. *Diagn Microbiol Infect Dis* 2003;**46**(4):265–71.

96. Ponce C, Ponce E, Vinelli E, Montoya A, de Aguilar V, Gonzalez A, et al. Validation of a rapid and reliable test for diagnosis of Chagas' disease by detection of *Trypanosoma cruzi*-specific antibodies in blood of donors and patients in Central America. *J Clin Microbiol* 2005;**43**(10):5065–8.

97. Sanchez-Camargo CL, Albajar-Vinas P, Wilkins PP, Nieto J, Leiby DA, Paris L, et al. Comparative evaluation of 11 commercialized rapid diagnostic tests for detecting *Trypanosoma cruzi* antibodies in serum banks in areas of endemicity and nonendemicity. *J Clin Microbiol* 2014;**52**(7):2506–12.

98. Stolf AMS. Serological diagnosis—*Trypanosoma cruzi* antigens in serodiagnosis. In: Wendel S, Brener Z, Camargo ME, Rassi A, editors. *Chagas disease (American Trypanosomiasis), its impact on tranfusion and clinical medicine*. Sao Paulo: Sociedade Brasileira de HematologiaeHemoterapia; 1992. p. 195–205.

99. Primavera KS, Umezawa ES, Peres BA, Camargo ME, Hoshino-Shimizu S. Chagas'disease: IgA, IgM and IgG antibodies to *T. cruzi* amastigote, trypomastigote and epimastigote antigens in acute and in different chronic forms of the disease. *Rev Inst Med Trop Sao Paulo* 1990;**32**(3):172–80.

100. Scharfstein J, Luquetti A, Murta AC, Senna M, Rezende JM, Rassi A, et al. Chagas' disease: serodiagnosis with purified Gp25 antigen. *Am J Trop Med Hyg* 1985;**34**(6):1153–60.

101. Schechter M, Luquetti AO, Rezende JM, Rassi A, Miles MA. Further evaluation of lectin affinity purified glycoprotein (GP90) in the enzyme linked immunosorbent assay (ELISA) for diagnosis of *Trypanosoma cruzi* infection. *Trans R Soc Trop Med Hyg* 1985;**79**(5):637–40.

102. Schechter M, Stevens AF, Luquetti AO, Snary D, Allen AK, Miles MA. Prevalence of antibodies to 72-kilodalton glycoprotein (GP72) in patients with Chagas' disease and further evidence of zymodeme-associated expression of GP72 carbohydrate epitopes. *Infect Immun* 1986;**53**(3):547–52.

103. Moncayo A, Luquetti AO. Multicentre double blind study for evaluation of *Trypanosoma cruzi* defined antigens as diagnostic reagents. *Mem Inst Oswaldo Cruz* 1990;**85**(4):489–95.

104. da Silveira JF, Umezawa ES, Luquetti AO. Chagas disease: recombinant *Trypanosoma cruzi* antigens for serological diagnosis. *Trends Parasitol* 2001;**17**(6):286–91.

105. Peralta JM, Teixeira MG, Shreffler WG, Pereira JB, Burns Jr. JM, Sleath PR, et al. Serodiagnosis of Chagas' disease by enzyme-linked immunosorbent assay using two synthetic peptides as antigens. *J Clin Microbiol* 1994;**32**(4):971−4.

106. Rabello A, Luquetti AO, Moreira EF, Gadelha Mde F, dos Santos JA, de Melo L, et al. Serodiagnosis of *Trypanosoma cruzi* infection using the new particle gel immunoassay−ID-PaGIA Chagas. *Mem Inst Oswaldo Cruz* 1999;**94**(1):77−82.

107. *Control of Chagas' disease report of a WHO Expert Committee*. Geneva: World Health Organization; 1991.

108. *Control of Chagas' disease report of a WHO Expert Committee*. Geneva: World Health Organization; 2002.

109. *Elegilibilidad Para la Donacion de* sangre. Washington, DC.: Organizacion Panamericana de la Salud; 2009.

110. Schlemper Jr BR. Estudos experimentais de quimioprofilaxia da transmissao da doenca de Chagas por transfussao sanguinea. *Rev. Patol. Trop* 1978;**7**:55−111.

111. Schmunis GA. *Trypanosoma cruzi*, the etiologic agent of Chagas' disease: status in the blood supply in endemic and nonendemic countries. *Transfusion* 1991;**31**(6):547−57.

112. Contreras MC, Schenone H, Borgono JM, Salinas P, Sandoval L, Rojas A, et al. Chagasic infection in blood donors from hospitals in endemic regions of Chile (1982−1987). Epidemiological impact of the problem. *Bol Chil Parasitol* 1992;**47** (1-2):10−15.

113. Dias JCP, Brener S. Chagas' disease and blood transfusion. *Mem. Inst. Oswaldo Cruz* 1984;**79**(Suppl.):139−47.

114. Wendel S., Pinto Dias J.C. Transfusion transmitted Chagas' disease. *Chagas' disease (American Trypanosomiasis): its impact on transfusion and clinical medicine*, Sao Paulo; 1992. 103−33.

115. Dias JCP. Mecanismos de transmissao. In: Brener Z, Andrade ZA, editors. *Trypanosoma cruzi e doenca de Chagas*. Rio de Janeiro: Guanabara Koogan; 1979.

116. Amato Neto V. Conduta frente ao doador Chagasico. *Rev. Soc. Bras. Med. Trop. 26* 1993;**26**:86−7.

117. Bergoglio RM. Enfermedad de Chagas postransfusional. Experiencia clínica de 48 casos. *Prensa Med. Argent* 1984;**71**:49−52.

118. Lorca M, Lorca J, Child R, Atias A, Canales M, Lorca E, et al. Prevalence of infection by *Trypanosoma cruzi* in patients with multiple blood transfusions. *Rev Med Chil* 1988;**116**(2):112−16.

119. Assal A, Aznar C. Chagas disease screening in the French blood donor population. Screening assays and donor selection. *Enf. Emerg* 2007;**9**(Suppl. 1):38−40.

120. Decreto Real 1088/2005. In: Espania MdSyCd, ed. *Boletin Oficial del Estado del 20 de Septiembre 2005*. Vol. 225. Spain; 2005:31288−304.

121. Goodman C, Chan S, Collins P, Haught R, Chen YJ. Ensuring blood safety and availability in the US: technological advances, costs, and challenges to payment--final report. *Transfusion* 2003;**43**(8 Suppl.):3S−46S.

122. *Government action on Krever Commission recommendations*. Available at: http://www. hcsc.gc.ca/english/media/relerases/1998/9889bke1.htm; 1998.

123. Du K. The quest for quality blood banking program in the new millennium the American way. *Int. J. Hematol.* 2002;**76**(Suppl. 2):258−62.

124. Engelfriet CP, Reesink HW, Brand B, Levy G, Williamson LM, Menitove JE, et al. Haemovigilance systems. *Vox Sang* 1999;**77**(2):110−20.

125. Centers for Disease C, Prevention. Blood donor screening for Chagas disease−United States, 2006−2007. *MMWR Morb Mortal Wkly Rep* 2007;**56**(7):141−3.

126. *FDA approves first test to screen blood donors for Chagas disease.* 2006; Available at: http://www.fda.gov/bbs/topics/NEWs/2006/NEW01524.html [accessed 10.03.07], 2007.

127. Rios C.R. Regimen Legal de Bancos de Sangre en America Latina: Malaria, Chagas y Hepatitis B. *Organizacion Panamericana de la Salud, Serie Informes Tecnicos No. 18*; 1992.

128. Bolis M. *Comparativo de Legislaciones Sobre Sangre Segura.* 2009; Available at: http://new.paho.org/hq/index.php?option=com_content&task=view&ld=1466&Itemid=1270&lang=en.THS/EV-2005/009 [accessed 3.12.09], 2009.

129. Schmunis GA, Zicker F, Pinheiro F, Brandling-Bennett D. Risk for transfusion-transmitted infectious diseases in Central and South America. *Emerg Infect Dis* 1998;**4**(1):5−11.

130. Schmunis GA, Zicker F, Segura EL, del Pozo AE. Transfusion-transmitted infectious diseases in Argentina, 1995 through 1997. *Transfusion* 2000;**40**(9):1048−53.

131. Schmunis GA, Zicker F, Cruz JR, Cuchi P. Safety of blood supply for infectious diseases in Latin American countries, 1994−1997. *Am J Trop Med Hyg* 2001;**65**(6):924−30.

132. Oelemann WM, Teixeira MD, Verissimo Da Costa GC, Borges-Pereira J, De Castro JA, Coura JR, et al. Evaluation of three commercial enzyme-linked immunosorbent assays for diagnosis of Chagas' disease. *J Clin Microbiol* 1998;**36**(9):2423−7.

133. Saez-Alquezar A, Otani MM, Sabino EC, Ribeiro-dos-Santos G, Salles N, Chamone DF. Evaluation of the performance of Brazilian blood banks in testing for Chagas' disease. *Vox Sang* 1998;**74**(4):228−31.

134. Salud OPdl. Suministro de Sangre Para Transfusiones en los Paises del Caribe y Latinoamerica en 2005. *Organizacion Panamericana de la Salud*; 2007.

135. Salud OPdl. Suministro de sangre para transfusiones en los paises de Latinoamerica y del Caribe 2012 y 2013. *Organizacion Panamericana de la Salud*; 2015.

136. Organizacion Panamericana de la Salud DdDdSdS. *Estandares de Trabajo Para Bancos de Sangre.* Washington, DC; 1999.

137. Otani MM. *Programa de avaliacao externa para os testes de triagem sorologica de doadores de banco de sangue dos centros de referencia da America Latina: utilizacao de multipainel especifico.* Sao Paulo: University of Sao Paulo; 2003.

138. Saez-Alquezar A, Otani MM, Sabino EC, Salles NA, Chamone DF. External serology quality control programs developed in Latin America with the support of PAHO from 1997 through 2000. *Rev Panam Salud Publica* 2003;**13**(2−3):91−102.

139. Saez-Alquezar A, Albajar Vinas P, Valpassos Guimaraes A, Correa Abol J. Quality control in screening for infectious diseases at blood banks. Rationale and methodology. *J. Int. Fed. Clin Chem. Lab Med.* 2015;**26**:278−85.

140. Zeledon R, Ponce C. Letter: a skin test for the diagnosis of Chagas's disease. *Trans R Soc Trop Med Hyg* 1974;**68**(5):414−15.

141. Teixeira AR, Figueiredo F, Rezende Filho J. Delayed hypersensitivity to *Trypanosoma cruzi* antigen. II−Use of the skin test with T12E antigen for the diagnosis of Chagas disease. *Rev Soc Bras Med Trop* 1995;**28**(3):259−65.

142. Luquetti AO, Ferreira MS. Diagnostico da doença de Chagas na coinfecção *T. cruzi*/HIV. In: Almeida EA, editor. *Epidemiologia e clínica da coinfecção Trypanosoma cruzi/HIV.* Campinas, Brazil: Editora Universidade Estadual de Campinas; 2015. p. 205−14.

143. Camargo ME, da Silva GR, de Castilho EA, Silveira AC. Serological survey of the prevalence of Chagas' infection in Brazil, 1975/1980. *Rev Inst Med Trop Sao Paulo* 1984;**26**(4):192−204.

144. Zicker F, Smith PG, Luquetti AO, Oliveira OS. Mass screening for *Trypanosoma cruzi* infections using the immunofluorescence, ELISA and haemagglutination tests on serum samples and on blood eluates from filter-paper. *Bull World Health Organ* 1990;**68** (4):465−71.

145. Rassi A, Luquetti AO. Therapy of Chagas disease. In: Wendel S, Brener Z, Camargo ME, Rassi A, editors. *Chagas disease (American Trypanosomiasis), its impact on tranfusion and clinical medicine.* Sao Paulo: Sociedade Brasileira de Hematologia e Hemoterapia; 1992. p. 237−47.

146. Rassi A, Luquetti AO. Specific treatment for *Trypanosoma cruzi* infection (Chagas disease). In: Tyler KM, Miles MA, editors. *American Trypanosomiasis.* Boston: Kluwer Academic Publishers; 2003. p. 117−25.

147. Yun O, Lima MA, Ellman T, Chambi W, Castillo S, Flevaud L, et al. Feasibility, drug safety, and effectiveness of etiological treatment programs for Chagas disease in Honduras, Guatemala, and Bolivia: 10-year experience of Medecins Sans Frontieres. *PLoS NTD* 2009;**3**(7):e488.

148. Luquetti AO, Rassi A. Tratamiento específico de la enfermedad de Chagas en la fase cronica: Criterios de cura convencionales: xenodiagnostico, hemocultivo y serologia. *Rev. Patol. Trop.* 1998;**27**(Suppl):37−51.

149. Almeida IC, Covas DT, Soussumi LM, Travassos LR. A highly sensitive and specific chemiluminescent enzyme-linked immunosorbent assay for diagnosis of active *Trypanosoma cruzi* infection. *Transfusion* 1997;**37**(8):850−7.

150. Sosa Estani S, Segura EL, Ruiz AM, Velazquez E, Porcel BM, Yampotis C. Efficacy of chemotherapy with benznidazole in children in the indeterminate phase of Chagas' disease. *Am J Trop Med Hyg* 1998;**59**(4):526−9.

151. *WHO Consultation on International Biological Reference Preparations for Chagas Diagnostic Tests WHO.* 2007; Available at: http://www.who.int/bloodproducts/ref_materials/WHO_Report_1st_Chagas_BRP_consultation_7-2007_final.pdf; 2011.

152. Otani M., Hockley J., Guzmán-Bracho C., Rijpkema S., Luquetti A.O., Duncan R., et al. Evaluation of two International Reference Standardrs for antibodies to *Trypanosoma cruzi* in a WHO collaborative study. WHO/BS/2011.2181, Geneva. p. 2011.

# AIDS and Chagas' disease

*M. Corti and M.F. Villafañe*
Infectious Diseases Hospital "F. J. Muñiz," Buenos Aires, Argentina

## Chapter Outline

## Introduction

Chagas' disease or American Trypanosomiasis is a zoonotic disease caused by the flagellated protozoan *Trypanosoma cruzi*, which was first identified by Carlos Chagas in 1909 in Minas Gerais, Brazil. Generally, this zoonotic disease is transmitted to humans and animals by *Triatoma infestans* (vectors) known as "vinchucas" in Argentina and "barbeiros" in Brazil. Less frequently, *T. cruzi* can be transmitted by transfusion of infected blood, via the transplacental route and organ transplantation from an infected donor. Sharing intravenous needles with an infected person with parasitemia is another possible source of infection.[1] Rarely, the oral route including breast milk and laboratory accidents can be an alternative source of infection.[2]

Several authors have observed the occurrence of severe forms of Chagas' disease, such as meningoencephalitis and myocarditis in patients with severe immunodepression. The majority of cases have been described in Brazil and in the other countries in which this parasitosis is endemic. Generally, the clinical manifestations of the reactivation of *T. cruzi* infection in immunosupressed patients result in the

American Trypanosomiasis Chagas Disease. DOI: http://dx.doi.org/10.1016/B978-0-12-801029-7.00031-9

reactivation of chronic and previously asymptomatic or oligosymptomatic disease.[3] Chagasic patients infected with the human immunodeficiency virus (HIV) present episodes of reactivation of the *T. cruzi* infection. Acute exacerbation of chronic Chagas' disease is more frequent in AIDS than in other immunocompromised patients. Reactivation of Chagas' disease in AIDS is possible in those patients with a CD4 T cell count less than 200 cell/μL and the highest risk occurs with a CD4 T cell count less than 50 cell/μL.

## Epidemiology of Chagas' disease in Latin America and Argentina

Chagas' disease is an important health problem in these areas of the world. In America, Chagas' disease is observed from the south of the United States to the south of Argentina. According to the World Health Organization (WHO) there are 100 million people at the risk of infection with 10−12 million people infected and 50,000 deaths per year, the majority due to dilated myocarditis.[4] Urban migration transformed Chagas' disease into a health problem in nonendemic countries. In the United States (US) approximately 50,000 to 100,000 Latin American residents have evidence of chronic *T. cruzi* infection[5] and in the last years many multifactorial associated cases were diagnosed in the United States, Canada, and Europe.[6] According to estimates, the prevalence of *T. cruzi* in Latin American immigrants is 16/1000 in Australia, 9/1000 in Canada, 25/1000 in Spain, and 8−50/1000 in the United States.[7] The rural and urban migration, the contamination of donated blood products, intravenous drug abuse, laboratory accidents, and congenital transmission increase the diagnosis of this parasitosis in great cities. Since 2007, blood transfusions have been screened for Chagas' disease in the United States.[8]

In Argentina, there are 7 million people exposed to the risk of *T. cruzi* infection with approximately 2.5−3 million infected and 400,000 patients with different grades of cardiomyopathy.[4] Cardiac involvement become evident 20−30 years after the first infection but 5−10% of the patients can develop symptomatic myocarditis in the acute phase of the disease.[9]

According to the Centers for Diseases Control and Prevention (CDC) of the United States, only 3 of the 12 diseases defining AIDS opportunistic infections are parasitoses: toxoplasmosis, cryptosporidiosis, and isosporidiosis. In endemic areas, reactivation of *T. cruzi* infection should be included among the potential opportunistic pathogens indicative of AIDS.[4]

## Natural history of Chagas' disease

*T. cruzi* populations include multiclonal strains with different biological properties such as replication rates, drug susceptibility, virulence, and tissue tropism, which may be implicated in the clinical forms of the disease.[10,11] *T. cruzi* is an obligate intracellular parasite. Among immunocompetent individuals the clinical course of Chagas' disease is usually divided into three stages: acute, indeterminate, and chronic. The indeterminate phase usually extends 10−20 years, but in the majority of the patients it lasts a lifetime.[12,13] As well as in immunocompromised patients, in some subjects, during the acute phase of the disease, it is probable to show signs and symptoms associated with parasitemia (Fig. 30.1). These patients can present clinical manifestations of acute myocarditis or meningoencephalitis.[14−16] When *T. cruzi* invade the myocardial cells it induces a diffuse and severe neutrophilic and monocytic inflammatory infiltrate and myofibrillar lesions with or without fibrosis that can be seen in endomyocardial biopsies. Also, during the acute phase of the disease, cardiac parasympathetic neurons are damaged by the parasite.[17] Meningoencephalitis occurs mainly in acute Chagas' disease in children under 2 years. After the acute phase, the majority of cases progress to a subclinical and latent period named as the indeterminate phase.[18,19] Finally, 10−30% of seropositive individuals developed three different syndromes in the context of symptomatic chronic Chagas' disease. These are the chronic cardiomyopathy with frequent and marked cardiac arrhythmias, especially sinus bradycardia with right bundle branch block and other electrocardiographic abnormalities. In other patients, the destruction of visceral autonomic neurons of the digestive tract leads to progressive enlargement of visceral organs (especially megaesophagus and megacolon) named as megasyndromes or chronic gastrointestinal Chagas' disease. Megaesophagus and

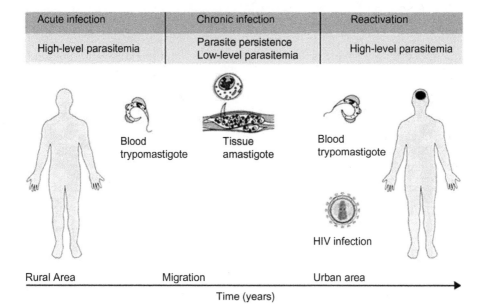

| Acute infection | Chronic infection | Reactivation |
|---|---|---|
| High-level parasitemia | Parasite persistence Low-level parasitemia | High-level parasitemia |

Blood trypomastigote     Tissue amastigote     Blood trypomastigote

HIV infection

Rural Area          Migration          Urban area

Time (years)

**Figure 30.1** Natural history of HIV and Chagas' disease coinfection.
*Source*: Taken from DíazGranados CA, Saavedra-Trujillo CH, Mantilla M, Valderrame S, Alquichire C, Franco-Paredes C. Chagasic encephalitis in HIV patients: common presentation of an evolving epidemiological and clinical association. *Lancet Infect Dis* 2009;**9**:324−30.[14]

megacolon may or may not be associated with the cardiac involvement and occur in 10 to 20% of cases according to the area considered.[20,21] A small number of patients develop different grades of neuropsychiatric compromise.

## Pathogenic mechanisms of Chagas' disease reactivation in AIDS patients

The diversity of clinical manifestations of Chagas' disease in humans has been attributed to the host's immune response and to the genetic heterogeneity of the parasite which may be formed by a multiclonal population with various biological profiles.[10,22] The preferential location of T. cruzi in the central nervous system (CNS) may be associated with the presence of subpopulations with neurotropic characteristics that may be reactivated during the immunosupresion of the host. Patients with HIV infection, does not lead to new T. cruzi genotypes, because T. cruzi stocks isolated from these patients were closely related to clonal genotypes previously identified (genotypes 30 or 32) in 89% and 94% of the stocks isolated from HIV-positive and HIV-negative patients, respectively.[23] Reactivation of Chagas' disease does not occur spontaneously and is strongly associated with immunosupresion in patients who have onchohematologic neoplasms,[24] those chronically treated with high doses of corticosteroids, and those with advance HIV-AIDS disease.[25] In these groups of immunocompromised patients chronically infected by T. cruzi, it is possible that the parasite load can increase and the detection of parasitemia is more frequent.[26,27]

In this context, and especially in AIDS patients, the high level of parasitemia is related to the development of acute CNS or heart disease. However, the relation between T. cruzi parasitemia and organ damage is not absolute; sometimes we can see that severe disease is associated without detectable parasitemia. In these patients it is necessary to obtain biopsy smears to achieve a definitive diagnosis.[14,25,28]

T. cruzi displays a relevant genetic variability demonstrated by at least six discrete typing units (DTUs) from TcI to TcVI. Evidence of the impact of this genetic variability on HIV coinfection is scarce. However, some studies have suggested a differential tissue tropism of the infecting DTUs; these studies have reported mixed infections in coinfected patients, observing TcI and TcII, or TcI, TcV, and TcVI in blood, and only monoclonal TcI in cerebrospinal fluid (CSF) or brain tissue.[29]

## AIDS and Chagas' disease

Reactivation of chronic stage of Chagas' disease is uncommon; acute exacerbations of a latent or chronic infection due to T. cruzi can occur in individuals with involvement of cellular immunity, especially in those with advanced HIV/AIDS disease, prolonged corticosteroid use, or other immunosuppressive therapies and transplant-associated immunosupresion.[30,31]

In a prospective study that included patients in the pre and post highly active antiretroviral therapy (HAART) era the frequency of reactivation of *T. cruzi* infection was approximately 20%.[32]

In patients coinfected with HIV, the reactivation of Chagas' disease may be related to the selected cellular immune depletion or to the characteristics of the parasite. This situation has been demonstrated by the presence of *Trypomastigotes* in blood by microhematocrit of quantitative buffy-coat (QBC) and by the invasion of the CNS or the heart.[33–35]

# Clinical aspects

The majority of the patients present with CNS or myocardial involvement; less frequent clinical manifestations include the digestive tract, especially the esophagus and the colon.[33] Skin lesions,[34] peritoneum involvement,[35] and cervix uteri compromise[36] are described infrequently.

Generally, the majority of AIDS patients with reactivated of Chagas' disease have CD4 T cell counts below 200 cell/μL and, especially, less than 50 cells/μL.

In contrast with heart transplant recipients with reactivated of chronic Chagas' disease in whom myocarditis is the predominant clinical form of presentation, in AIDS patients, CNS manifestations occur frequently and can include meningoencephalitis or brain masses (named as chagomas). The CNS involvement represents 80–90% of total episodes of reactivation of chronic Chagas' disease in AIDS patients.[37] In patients with cerebral masses, neurological symptoms and signs include headaches, fever, cognitive changes, seizures, or neurological focal signs depending on the number, size, and location of these lesions. On the other hand, patients who develop diffuse meningoencephalitis present with fever, headaches, meningism, and altered mental status.

The CNS tumor-like lesions are, in our experience, the most common clinical manifestation and these are indistinguishable from other opportunistic infections, such as toxoplasmosis or neoplastic process, as primary central nervous system lymphoma (PCNSL) that can involve the CNS in AIDS patients.[24]

Cerebral chagomas are contrast-enhancing single or multiple focal brain lesions with hypodense areas of perilesional edema and mass effect on the middle line structures (Fig. 30.2). Generally, lesions due to *T. cruzi* are located in the white matter and occasionally involve the cerebral cortex. In a study by Cordova et al.[38] which included 15 patients with reactivation of Chagas' disease with CNS involvement, the most frequent findings were a single supratentorial hypodense lesion compatible with abscess and involving predominately the white matter of brain lobes (Fig. 30.3). On the contrary, the lesions caused by *Toxoplasma gondii* frequently compromise the brain cortex, thalamus, and the basal ganglia. In both cases, histopathological examination reveals necrotic encephalitis; however, the multifocal identification of parasites is more frequent in the reactivation of Chagas' disease than in *Toxoplasma* encephalitis.

The second most frequent expression of the reactivation of *T. cruzi* infection in the CNS is the diffuse meningoencephalitis. In these patients the diagnosis is

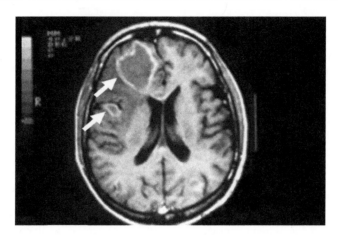

**Figure 30.2** Axial T1-weighted MRI image shows two large lesions in the right parietal and frontal lobes (*arrows*), with contrast enhancement, perilesional edema, and mass effect on the middle line structures.

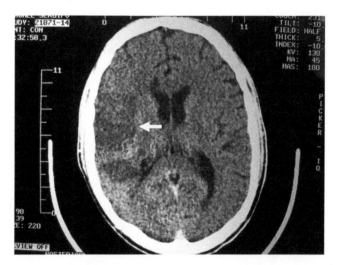

**Figure 30.3** CT of the brain showing a single hypodense lesion in the right temporoparietal lobe, with minimum contrast enhancement, no displacement of normal structures, and edema (*arrow*).

easily confirmed by the lumbar puncture and the centrifugation of cerebrospinal fluid (CSF) with the detection of *Trypomastigotes* with a Giemsa smear. Lumbar puncture has a high sensitivity for the diagnosis of chagasic meningoencephalitis and should always be performed in the absence of contraindication for it. Cordova et al.[38] showed that the sensitivity of this technique was 85%. CSF examination showed typical parasitic meningitis with leptomeningeal involvement and lymphomononuclear pleocytosis.[39]

Pagano et al.[40] studied 10 patients with AIDS and Chagas' disease. All patients presented cerebral tumor-like lesions and six of them developed intracranial hypertension syndrome. In addition, Cordova et al.[38] in 15 patients showed only 2 patients with meningoencephalitis as a unique clinical expression of the disease.

In Argentina, the myocardium is, after the CNS, the second target organ in patients with reactivation of chronic Chagas' disease and AIDS. Acute myocarditis with arrhythmias and refractory congestive heart failure, with rapid and generally fatal evolution, represents the most frequent clinical presentation.[27,41,42] Diagnosis of this complication should be suspected in HIV patients with dilated cardiomyopathy, epidemiological antecedents, and positive serologic tests for *T. cruzi* antibodies. Symptoms and signs are identical to other dilated cardiomyopathies.[6,43]

Less frequent, medical literature describes the existence of patients with chronic diarrhea and amastigotes of *T. cruzi* in duodenal biopsy smears prolonged fever and parasitemia.

A high rate of the disease reactivation in the coinfected population may be observed with the central nervous system as the main site of reactivation, representing more than 70% of cases. Some of the predictors of the occurrence of Chagas' disease reactivation are the detection of parasitemia, low CD4 T lymphocyte values ($<200$ cells/mm$^3$), and high viral load of HIV, although these are not essential to its occurrence.[44]

## Laboratory diagnosis

Laboratory diagnosis of Chagas' disease in immunocompromised patients is based on the same methods used in the immunocompetent population. Diagnostic methods include serological tests and the direct detection of the parasite (Fig. 30.4). However, the knowledge of the natural history of Chagas' disease is important to determine the stage and to interpret the laboratory findings (Fig. 30.1). The reactivation of Chagas' disease in an AIDS patient with chronic infection due to *T. cruzi* includes the following laboratory findings: (1) serological tests to detect specific antibodies to *T. cruzi*; (2) detection of the parasite in fresh blood by QBC, Strout method, or microhematocrit[45]; (3) in patients with meningoencephalitis the detection of the parasite by microscopic examination of CSF with Giemsa smear; and (4) the detection of *T. cruzi* amastigotes with an acute and necrotic inflammatory infiltration in tissue by biopsies obtained in patients with chagomas or myocarditis.[46]

Reactivation of Chagas' disease in AIDS patients are usually associated with the detection of *T. cruzi* trypomastigote forms by direct microscopic examination of

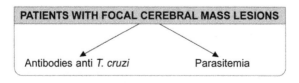

**Figure 30.4** Diagnosis algorithm of focal brain lesions in AIDS patients.

blood. High levels of *T. cruzi* parasitemia can precede the clinical manifestations or may be found later, during the reactivation. The dynamics of *T. cruzi* parasitemia in HIV-coinfected patients may play an important role in the reactivation of the disease. *T. cruzi* parasitemia was detected more frequently in HIV-seropositive patients with chronic Chagas' disease than in HIV-negative individuals. HIV-coinfected patients also had higher levels of parasitemia.[47] According to the number of triatomines fed, Sartori et al.[47] classified the parasitemia level in three categories: (1) very high parasitemia; (2) high parasitemia; and (3) low parasitemia when trypomastigotes of *T. cruzi* were detected by direct examination of blood or CSF.

More recently, different studies have reported a higher sensitivity of polymerase chain reaction (PCR) to detect the DNA of *T. cruzi* in laboratory samples. PCR appears to be a specific and highly sensitive laboratory method to inform the number of DNA copies present in the sample examination.[20,48] In order to investigate the reactivation of *T. cruzi* infection in immunosupressed patients, in 2005, the *Brazil Consensus of Chagas' disease* proposed that PCR should be performed directly from the patient's fresh blood.[49]

In patients with AIDS, the differential diagnosis between acute encephalitis due to *T. gondii* and *T. cruzi* may be difficult; in this context, PCR in peripheral blood and brain tissue obtained by stereotactic biopsy, provided a rapid differential and sensitive diagnosis method of *T. cruzi* reactivation, allowing the prompt administration of specific therapy which can modify the poor prognosis of this kind of patients.[50]

Qualitative parasitological techniques, such as xenodiagnosis and hemoculture (the gold standard of laboratory Chagas' disease diagnosis), have a low value in AIDS patients with suspected Chagas' disease reactivation (Fig. 30.5).[51]

---

**Suspicion of Chagas´ disease reactivation in immunosuppressed patients Techniques proposed for the laboratory diagnosis**

**1 -** direct microscopic examination, buffy coat examination (alternatively Strout), and PCR of fresh blood

**2 -** depending on the laboratory availability:

A - xenodiagnosis coupled to microscopic examination and to PCR of triatomines feces, performed on days one to five (two or three tests), 10 and/or 15 (one or two tests), 30 and 60 days after blood meal.

and/or

B - hemoculture coupled to microscopic examination and to PCR of hemoculture aliquots, performed on days one to five (two or three tests), 10 and/or 15 (one or two tests), 30 and 60 after seeded.

Model for the investigation of Chagas disease reactivation in immunosuppressed patients.

**Figure 30.5** Laboratory diagnosis of suspected Chagas' disease reactivation in AIDS patients.
*Source*: Taken from Almeida Braz, LM, Amato Neto V, Okay TS. Reactivation of *Trypanosoma cruzi* infection in immunosupressed patients: contributions for the laboratorial diagnosis standardization. *Rev Inst Med trop S Paulo* 2008;**50**:65−6.[52]

# Diagnosis of chagasic meningoencephalitis

CNS compromise is the most frequent manifestation of the acute reactivation of chronic infection due to *T. cruzi* in AIDS patients and can include meningoencephalitis or brain mass. The CSF may be normal or can be associated with mild to moderate pleocytosis with prevalence of mononuclear cells and low to mild protein levels. For these reason, in our opinion, all CSF samples from AIDS patients should be routinely sent to the parasitology laboratory for the detection of trypomastigotes. Diagnosis of meningoencephalitis is confirmed by the direct observation of trypomastigotes in CSF by Giemsa smear. Centrifugation of the CSF enhances the sensibility of this test.[37]

Current tests for diagnosis of CNS invasion in Chagas' disease have a low sensitivity and, in some situations, they do not allow to establish the etiology. In these cases, when there exists a strong diagnosis suspect, a rapid and specific technique, such as PCR, which can detect minimal quantities of the parasite DNA, may be useful for early diagnosis and for monitoring treatment.[25,53,54] Recently, several studies have reported a higher sensitivity of PCR to the laboratory diagnosis of Chagas' disease.[52]

Despite its low sensibility, the first approach in the laboratory diagnosis of Chagas' disease in HIV + patients depends on the microscopic demonstrations of *T. cruzi* trypomastigotes in samples of blood and CSF. Alternatively, when the physicians have access to the more modern technological resources, serological and molecular techniques for the detection of *T. cruzi* antigens or genes, respectively, are very useful. PCR methods using formalin-fixed- (FF-) and paraffin-embedded- (PE-) tissues can achieve specific amplification of trypanosome and *T. cruzi* DNA sequences and can show the presence of an amplicon band of 330 bp corresponding to the amplification of minicircle kinetoplast DNA of trypanosomes. However, an accurate molecular identification of amastigotes from CNS lesions can be also achieved with a PCR technique for the amplification of repeated sequences of satellite DNA.[55] In conclusion, PCR appears as a complementary method for the rapid, differential, and sensitive diagnosis of Chagas' disease reactivation in HIV/AIDS patients.[56]

Anatomopathological findings associated with Chagas' disease meningoencephalitis in AIDS patients include the presence of lymphomonocytic meningitis with the presence of *T. cruzi* amastigotes in the meninges and generalized cerebral edema with hemorrhagic necrosis.[26]

# Diagnosis of chagasic tumor-like lesions

In patients with cerebral mass lesions, neuroimages typically show one or more ring-enhancing lesions involving both gray and white matter, the cerebellum and the brain steam.[56–58] Magnetic resonance imaging (MRI) and cranial computed tomography (CT) reveal single or multiple tumor-like lesions with hypodense or

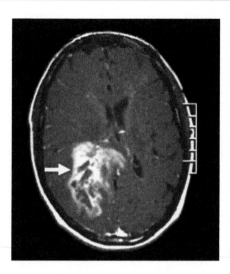

**Figure 30.6** Axial T1-weighted MRI showing a heterogeneous right parieto-occipital lesion with irregular gadolinium enhancement, mass effect on the middle line structures, and perilesional edema (*arrow*).

hypointense centers, with or without contrast enhancement, with or without areas of perilesional edema, and with or without effect on the middle line structures (Fig. 30.6). This imaging pattern of brain chagoma is similar and indistinguishable to that cerebral toxoplasmosis.[39,40,54] MRI spectroscopy showed a significant increase in choline/creatine ratios (Cho/cr) associated with an increased membrane synthesis and the pathological evidence of lipid or lactate signals related to the presence of anaerobiosis or necrosis in the central area of the abscess (Fig. 30.7). In endemic areas for *T. cruzi* infection, all HIV patients presenting with cerebral brain lesions should be evaluated for specific anti-*T. cruzi* antibodies and for parasitemia (Fig. 30.4).[59]

When *T. cruzi* trypomastigotes cannot be demonstrated in the CSF, a cerebral biopsy of focal brain lesions may be necessary. Histopathological findings include a granulomatous abscess with necrosis, cerebral edema with focal necrotizing and hemorrhagic encephalitis with uni- or multifocal lesions of undefined limits containing amastigotes of *T. cruzi* in Giemsa smears (Fig. 30.8).[60] The most striking finding is the presence of many small organisms within the macrophages (amastigotes). Electron microscopic features of the organism include parallel microtubules under the cell membrane, a kinetoplast, and a flagellar pocket containing a rudimentary flagellae.[61] These lesions are generally localized at the brain periphery, affecting the gray and, especially, the white matter. Lesions can also occur in the brainstem and in the cerebellum.[62]

The absence of anti-*Toxoplasma* antibodies in patients with HIV infection who have one or more expansive lesions should raise clinical suspicion of alternative diseases, including Chagas disease. The presence of anti-*T. cruzi* antibodies is

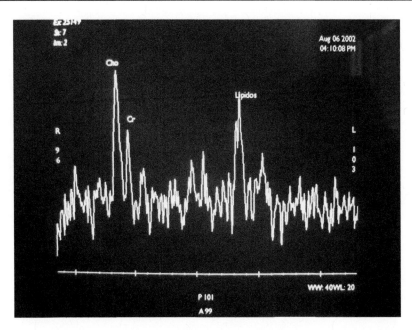

**Figure 30.7** MRI spectroscopy in axial T1-weighted with a single voxel localized at the lesion and corresponding to the patient of Fig. 30.6. Significant increase in choline/creatine ratios (Cho/cr) associated with an increased membrane synthesis and the pathological evidence of lipid signal related to the presence of anaerobiosis or necrosis.

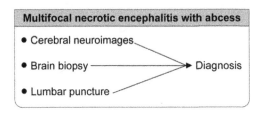

**Figure 30.8** Diagnosis algorithm of cerebral abscesses in AIDS patients.

important in the initial approach. The mortality rate is approximately 85%, even in patients receiving treatment, mainly due to delayed diagnosis and severe immunosuppression.[63]

# Diagnosis of heart compromise

The diagnosis of Chagas' cardiomyopathy in AIDS patients should be suspected in those with epidemiologic and positive serologic tests and signs and symptoms of myocardial involvement. The frequency of cardiomyopathy is almost 30–40%. In

AIDS patients the most common clinical presentation is the acute dilated myocarditis characterized by symptoms and signs of heart failure or severe arrhythmias. In some cases, the only clinical expression is the electrocardiographic alterations or the histopathological findings of myocarditis. The most frequent electrocardiographic pattern is the right bundle branch block with or without left anterior fascicular block, sinus bradycardia, or malignant arrhythmias. Bidimensional echocardiogram shows a dilated cardiomyopathy, segmental contractile abnormalities, apical aneurysms, which are frequently associated with mural thrombus, and pericardial effusion. MRI can detect myocardial fibrosis, wall motion abnormalities, and compromise of the left ventricular function.[64] Diagnosis is confirmed by the histopathological examination which reveals cardiomegaly with a dilated myocarditis associated with the ruptures of myofibrils and inflammatory infiltration with plasma cells, lymphocytes, and macrophages in myocardial tissue obtained by endomyocardial biopsies or autopsy studies. Also, it is possible to observe an intense parasitism of cardiac fiber cells with numerous amastigotes of *T. cruzi*. Epicarditis and endocarditis can also be observed in these patients.[65] Using light and electron microscopy, abundant amastigotes of *T. cruzi* with a nucleus, a kinetoplast. and a rudimentary flagellae were seen in the cytoplasm of the macrophages in muscle fibers.[65,66]

## Differential diagnosis

Diffuse chagasic meningoencephalitis should be included in the differential diagnosis of other opportunistic infections that can cause CNS encephalitis in AIDS patients. This syndrome may be caused by various opportunistic pathogens including *Cryptococcus neoformans, Mycobacterium tuberculosis*, neuroherpesvirus, and *Treponema pallidum.*

The focal neurological disease or chagomas should be included in the differential diagnosis of toxoplasmosis, CNS primary lymphoma, tuberculomas, piogenic abscesses due to *Nocardia* species and *Mycobacterium tuberculosis*, and finally the progressive multifocal leukoencephalopathy.

Differential diagnosis of myocarditis includes HIV, *Toxoplasma gondii*, cytomegalovirus, and other herpesvirus.

## Treatment

At this moment, there are only two effective drugs for the treatment of Chagas' disease: nifurtimox and benznidazole. These two drugs are particularly useful in the acute and early phase of the infection and in the reactivation observed in immunocompromised patients.[16,67] Nifurtimox and benznidazole have a greatly limited use related to their frequent and occasionally severe side effects and the necessary long-term treatment.

Other drugs such as allopurinol, ketoconazole, fluconazole, and itraconazole have been used for the reactivation treatment by some authors with apparent success but they are not recommended as first-line therapy.[68,69]

In consequence, drugs usually used for the therapy of Chagas' disease in AIDS patients are identical to those that we use in immunocompetent patients. Nifurtimox and benznidazole are the only two drugs effective in killing this parasite in blood and tissues. In the majority of South American countries these drugs are not commercially available for patients in pharmacies. Nifurtimox is unavailable in Argentina and the distribution of Benznidazole depends on the Health Ministry.

The majority of the patients with CNS reactivation of Chagas' disease associated with AIDS have a poor prognosis and a high mortality related with a delay in the diagnosis and specific therapy. However, the mortality rate diminishes to approximate 20% in patients with at least 30 days of specific treatment.[70] Both drugs induce significant side effects and some strains of *T. cruzi* are resistant to treatment.[70]

Nifurtimox is a nitrofuran derivate that is used at the dose of 8−10 mg/kg per day divided into 2 or 3 doses daily, orally, for 60−90 days. The mechanism of action of nifurtimox involves the production of nitro-anion radicals which, in the presence of oxygen, leave *T. cruzi* incapable of detoxifying free radicals.[71]

In countries where nifurtimox is commercialized, the drug has a similar efficacy as benznidazole.

The most frequent adverse side effects observed include anorexia, weight loss, psychological and psychiatric changes (excitability, muscle tremors, somnolence, and hallucinations), and digestive manifestations, such as nausea, vomiting, abdominal pain, and diarrhea. The side effects can be controlled by administrating diazepam, metoclopramide, antihistamines, and other symptomatic medications.

Benznidazole is a nitroimidazole derivate that is administrated orally at the dose of 5 mg/kg per day in two doses for a period of 60 days. The action of benznidazole is related to the introduction of components of the DNA and kDNA of *T. cruzi* and the lipids and proteins of the parasite.[72] Side effects of benznidazole generally occur in the first days of therapy and include cutaneous eruption (including dermatitis, generalized angioedema, and Stevens Johnson syndrome), peripheral neuropathy, and bone marrow depletion (granulocytopenia, thrombocytopenia with purpura). The side effects can be controlled with antihistamines, corticosteroids, and, in severe cases, with the necessary suspension of the treatment (Fig. 30.9).[3]

After remission of the clinical manifestations, a second prophylaxis is recommended, because further reactivations can occur later. In this aspect, an expert committee recommended the use of benznidazole at the dose of 5 mg/kg per day three times a week up to immune reconstitution associated to antiretroviral therapy (Fig. 30.10).

Highly active antiretroviral therapy should be systematically indicated to these patients in order to achieve the immune reconstitution.[66]

Primary prophylaxis in chagasic patients infected with HIV is not recommended.

PCR is more sensitive than parasitological tests and could provide earlier evidence of therapeutic failure. Therapeutic efficacy was checked with periodic PCR, hemoculture, and conventional serology.[73]

```
┌─────────────────────────────────────────────────────────┐
│                      TREATMENT                          │
├─────────────────────────────────────────────────────────┤
│  ● Nifurtimox: 8 to 10 mg/kg per day, 3 times daily,    │
│                during 60–90 days.                       │
│    Seizures, polineuropathy, psychiatric disorders,     │
│    anorexia.                                            │
│                                                         │
│  ● Benznidazol: 5 mg/kg per day twice daily, during     │
│    60 days. Skin reactions, peripheral neuropathies.    │
│                                     ┌  Itraconazol      │
│                                     │  Fluconazol       │
│  ● Therapeutic Alternatives  ──────<                    │
│                                     │  Gamma Interferon  │
│                                     └  Allopurinol       │
└─────────────────────────────────────────────────────────┘
```

**Figure 30.9** Therapeutic alternatives for reactivation of Chagas' disease.

```
┌─────────────────────────────────────────────────────────┐
│  ● Considered primary prophylaxis in patients with      │
│    chronic Tripanosoma cruzi infection and CD4 counts   │
│    < 200 cells/μL.                                      │
│                                                         │
│  ● Secondary prophylaxis with benznidazol or nifurtimox │
│    during a long time after the acute episode of        │
│    meningoencephalitis.                                 │
└─────────────────────────────────────────────────────────┘
```

**Figure 30.10** Primary and secondary prophylaxis in patients with AIDS and *T. cruzi* infection.

# Conclusion

We come to the conclusion that the identification of latent *T. cruzi* infection in HIV/AIDS patients is highly important. In our opinion, this recommendation should be considered both in endemic and nonendemic areas of Chagas' disease. The effective control of viremia by HAART associated with a period of maintenance treatment of 6–12 months associated with increased CD4$^+$ T lymphocytre count and negative PCR in the blood may represent sufficient parameters for discontinuation of antiparasitic therapy. Early diagnosis of reactivation of chronic Chagas' disease with CNS involvement followed by specific antiparasitic therapy may modify the poor prognosis of this kind of patient.

# Glossary of specialized terms of this chapter

| | |
|---|---|
| **AIDS** | acquired immune deficiency syndrome |
| **CDC** | Centers for Diseases Control and Prevention, USA |
| **CNS** | central nervous system |
| **CSF** | cerebrospinal fluid |

CT computed tomography
**HAART** highly active antiretroviral therapy
**HIV** human immunodeficiency virus
**MRI** magnetic resonance imaging
**PCNSL** primary central nervous system lymphoma
**PCR** polymerase chain reaction
**QBC** quantitative buffy coat
*T. cruzi* *Trypanosoma cruzi*
**WHO** World Health Organization

# References

1. Almeida EA, Ramos Junior AN, Correia D, Shikanai-Yasuda MA. Coinfection *Trypanosoma cruzi*/HIV: systematic review (1980–2010). *Rev Soc Bras Med Trop* 2011;**44**:762–70.
2. Coura JR. Transmissão da infecção chagásica por via oral na história natural da doença de Chagas. *Rev Soc Bras Med Trop* 2006;**39**(Suppl. IV):113–17.
3. Ferreira MS, Borges AS. Some aspects of protozoan infections in immunocompromised patients. A review. *Mem Inst Oswaldo Cruz* 2002;**97**:443–57.
4. Corti M. AIDS and Chagas' disease. *AIDS Patient Care and STDs* 2000;**14**:581–8.
5. Maguire JH. Chagas' disease—can we stop the deaths? *N Engl J Med* 2006;**335**:760–1.
6. Dobarro D, Gomez-Rubin C, Sanchez-Recalde A, Olias F, Bret-Zurita M, Cuesta-Lopez E, et al. Chagas' heart disease in Europe: an emergent disease? *J Cardiovasc Med (Hagerstown)* 2008;**9**:1263–7.
7. Centers for Disease Control and Prevention. Blood donor screening for Chagas' disease – United States, 2006–2007. *MMWR Morb Mortal Wkly Rep* 2007;**56**:141–3.
8. Leiby DA, Read EJ, Lenes BA, Yund AJ, Stumpf RJ, Kirchhoff LV, et al. Seroepidemiology of *Trypanosoma cruzi*, etiologic agent of Chagas' disease in US blood donors. *J Infect Dis* 1997;**176**:1047–52.
9. Punukollu G, Gowda RM, Khan IA, Navarro VS, Vasavada BC. Clinical aspects of the Chagas' heart disease. *Int J Cardiol* 2007;**115**:279–83.
10. Macedo AM, Machado CR, Olivera R, Pena SDJ. *Trypanosoma cruzi*: genetic structure of populations and relevance of genetic variability to the pathogenesis of Chagas' disease. *Mem Inst Oswaldo Cruz* 2004;**99**:1–12.
11. Macedo AM, Pena SDJ. Genetic variability of *Trypanosoma cruzi*: implications from the pathogenesis of Chagas' disease. *Parasitol Today* 1998;**14**:119–23.
12. Marin-Nieto J.A., Cunha-Neto E., Maciel B.C., Simões M.V. Pathogenesis of chronic Chagas' heart disease. *Circulation* 1997;**115**:1109–23.
13. Texeira AR, Nascimento RJ, Strurm NR. Evolution and pathology in Chagas' disease—a review. *Mem Inst Oswaldo Cruz* 2006;**101**:147–56.
14. DiazGranados CA, Saavedra-Trujillo CH, Mantilla M, Valderrame S, Alquichire C, Franco-Paredes C. Chagasic encephalitis in HIV patients: common presentation of an evolving epidemiological and clinical association. *Lancet Infect Dis* 2009;**9**:324–30.
15. Bern C, Montgomery SP, Herwaldt B. Evaluation and treatment of Chagas' disease in the United States: a systematic review. *JAMA* 2007;**298**:2171–81.
16. Shinakai-Yasuda MA, Lopes MH, Tolezano JE. Acute Chagas' disease: transmission routes, clinical aspects and response to specific therapy in diagnosed cases in an urban centre. *Rev Inst Med Trop Sao Paulo* 1990;**32**:16–27.

17. Rassi Jr A, Rassi A, Little WC, Xavier SS, Rassi SG, Rassi AG, et al. Development and validation of a risk score for predicting death in Chagas' heart disease. *N Engl J Med* 2006;**355**:799–808.

18. Pinto Dias JC. The treatment of Chagas' disease (South American Trypanosomiasis). *Ann Intern Med* 2006;**144**:772–4.

19. Rossi MA, Bestetti RB. The challenge of chagasic cardiomyopathy. The pathologic roles of autonomic abnormalities, autoimmune mechanisms and microvascular changes, and therapeutic implications. *Cardiology* 1995;**86**:1–7.

20. Barret MP, Burchmore RJ, Stich A, Lazzari JO, Frasch AC, Cazzulo JJ, et al. The trypanosomiases. *Lancet* 2003;**362**:1469–80.

21. Prata A. Clinical and epidemiological aspects of Chagas' disease. *Lancet Infect Dis* 2001;**1**:92–100.

22. Macedo AM, Martins MS, Chiari E, Pena SDJ. DNA fingerprinting of *Trypanosoma cruzi*: a new tool for characterization of strains and clones. *Mol Biochem Parasitol* 1992;**55**:147–54.

23. Rocha A, de Meneses AC, Silva AM. Pathology of patients with Chagas' disease and acquired immunodeficiency syndrome. *Am J Trop Med Hyg* 1994;**50**:261–8.

24. Gluckstein D, Ciferri F, Ruskin J. Chagas' disease: another cause of cerebral mass in the acquired immunodeficiency syndrome. *Am J Med* 1992;**92**:429–32.

25. Lazo JE, Meneses AC, Rocha A. Chagasic meningoencephalitis in the immunodeficient. *Arq Neuropsiquiatric* 1998;**56**:93–7.

26. Karp CL, Neva FA. Tropical infectious diseases in human immunodeficiency virus-infected patients. *Clin Infect Dis* 1999;**28**:947–65.

27. Rocha A, Ferreira MS, Nishioka SA, Silva AM, Burgarelli MK, Silva M, et al. *Trypanosoma cruzi* meningoencephalitis and myocarditis in a patient with acquired immunodeficiency syndrome. *Rev Inst Med Trop Sao Paulo* 1993;**35**:205–8.

28. Skiest DJ. Focal neurological disease in patients with acquired immunodeficiency syndrome. *Clin Infect Dis* 2002;**34**:103–15.

29. Burgos JM, Begher S, Silva HM, Bisio M, Duffy T, Levin MJ, et al. Molecular identification of *Trypanosoma cruzi* tropism for central nervous system in Chagas reactivation due to AIDS. *Am J Trop Med Hyg* 2008;**78**:294–7.

30. Ferreira MS, Nishioka SA, Silvestre MT, Vorges AS, Nunes Araujo FR, Rocha A, et al. Reactivation of Chagas' disease in patients with AIDS: report of three new cases and review of the literature. *Clin Infect Dis* 1997;**25**:1397–400.

31. Ferreira MS. Chagas disease and immunosupression. *Mem Inst Oswaldo Cruz* 1999;**94**:325–7.

32. Ministerio Da Saude. Secretaria de Vigilancia em Saude. Recomendações para diagnóstico, tratamento e acompanhamento da co-infecção *Trypanosoma cruzi*-vírus da imunodeficiência humana. *Rev Soc Bras Med Trop* 2006;**39**:392–406.

33. Fontes Rezende RE, Lescano MA, Zambelli Ramalho LN, de Castro Figueiredo JF, Oliveira Dantas R, Garzella Meneghelli U, et al. Reactivation of Chagas' disease in a patient with non-Hodgkin's lymphoma: gastric, oesophageal and laryngeal involvement. *Trans R Soc Trop Med Hyg* 2006;**100**:74–8.

34. Sartori AM, Sotto MN, Braz LM, Oliveira Júnior Oda C, Patzina RA, Barone AA, et al. Reactivation of Chagas' disease manifested by skin lesions in a patient with AIDS. *Trans R Soc Trop Med Hyg* 1999;**93**:631–2.

35. Sartori AM, Neto JE, Visone Nunes E, Braz LM, Caiaffa-Filho HH, Oliveira Oda Jr C, et al. *Trypanosoma cruzi* parasitemia in chronic Chagas' disease: comparison between human immunodeficiency virus (HIV)-positive and HIV-negative patients. *J Infect Dis* 2002;**186**:872–5.

36. Concetti H, Retegui M, Perez G, Perez H. Chagas' disease of the cervix uteri in a patient with acquired immunodeficiency syndrome. *Hum Pathol* 2000;**31**:120−2.
37. Ferreira MS, Nishioka AS, Rocha A, Silva AM, Ferreira RG, Olivier W, et al. Acute fatal *Trypanosoma cruzi* meningoencephalitis in a hemophilic patient. *Am J Trop Med Hyg* 1991;**45**:723−7.
38. Cordova E, Boschi A, Ambrosioni J, Cudos C, Corti M. Reactivation of Chagas' disease with central nervous system involvement in HIV-infected patients in Argentina, 1992−2007. *Int J Infect Dis* 2008;**12**:587−92.
39. Livramento JA, Machado LR, Spina-Franca A. Cerebrospinal fluid abnormalities in 170 cases of AIDS. *Arq Neuropsiquiatr* 1989;**47**:326−31.
40. Pagano MA, Segura MJ, Di Lorenzo GA, Garau ML, Molina HA, Cahn P. Cerebral tumor-like American trypanosomiasis in acquired immunodeficiency syndrome. *Ann Neurol* 1999;**45**:403−6.
41. Lages-Silva E, Crema E, Macedo AM, Pena SD, Chiari E. Relationship between *Trypanosoma cruzi* and human chagasic megaesophagus: blood and tissue. *Am J Trop Med Hyg* 2001;**65**:435−41.
42. Sartori AM, Ibrahim KY, Nunes Westphalen EV, Braz LM, Oliveira Jr OC, Gakiya E, et al. Manifestations of Chagas' disease in patients with HIV/AIDS. *Ann Trop Med Parasit* 2007;**101**:31−50.
43. Sartori AMC, Shikanai Yasuda MA, Amato Neto V, Lopes MH. Follow up of 18 patients with human immunodeficient virus infection and chronic Chagas' disease, with reactivation of Chagas' disease causing cardiac disease in three patients. *Clin Infect Dis* 1998;**26**:177−9.
44. Schmunis GA. Epidemiology of Chagas' disease in non endemic countries: the role of international migration. *Mem Inst Oswaldo Cruz* 2007;**102**(Suppl. 1):75−85.
45. Luquetti AO, Rassi A. Diagnóstico laboratorial da infecção pelo *Trypanosoma cruzi*. In: Brener Z, Andrade ZA, Barral-Netto M, editors. Trypanosoma cruzi e doença *de Chagas*. Rio de Janeiro: Guanabara Koogan; 2000. p. 344−79.
46. Sartori AM, Lopes MH, Benvenuti LA, Caramelli B, di Pietro A, Nunes EV, et al. Reactivation of Chagas' disease in a human immunodeficiency virus-infected patient leading to severe heart disease with a late positive direct microscopic examination of the blood. *Am J Trop Med Hyg* 1998;**59**:784−6.
47. Sartori AM, Lopes MH, Caramelli B, Duarte MI, Pinto PL, Neto V, et al. Simultaneous occurrence of acute myocarditis and reactivated Chagas' disease in a patient with AIDS. *Clin Infect Dis* 1995;**21**:1297−9.
48. Gomes ML, Macedo AM, Vago AR, Pena SD, Galvão LM, Chiari E. *Trypanosoma cruzi*: optimization of polymerase chain reaction for detection in human blood. *Exp Parasitol* 1998;**88**:28−33.
49. BRASIL. MINISTÉRIO DA SAÚDE. SECRETARIA DE VIGILÂNCIA EM SAÚDE-Consenso Brasileiro em Doença de Chagas. Rev Soc Bras Med Trop 2005;**38** (Suppl. III):1−29.
50. Burgos JM, Begher SB, Freitas JM, Bisio M, Duffy T, Altcheh J, et al. Molecular diagnosis and typing of *Trypanosoma cruzi* populations and lineages in cerebral Chagas' disease in a patient with AIDS. *Am J Trop Med Hyg* 2005;**73**:1016−18.
51. Shikanai Yasuda MA, Teixeira de Fretas VL, Ibrahim KY, Furuchó C. Diagnostico laboratorial da doença de Chagas em imunodeprimidos. *Rev Soc Bras Med Trop* 2006;**39**:110−11.
52. Braz LM, Amato Neto V, Okay TS. Reactivation of *Trypanosoma cruzi* infection in immunosupressed patients: contributions for the laboratorial diagnosis standardization. *Rev Inst Med Trop Sao Paulo* 2008;**50**:65−6.

53. Avila H, Sigman DS, Cohen LM, Millikan RC, Simpson L. Polymerase chain reaction amplification of *Trypanosoma cruzi* kinetoplast minicircle DNA isolated from whole blood lysates: diagnosis of chronic Chagas' disease. *Mol Biochem Parasitol* 1991;**48**:211−22.

54. Hoff R, Texeira RS, Carvalho JS, Mott KE. *Trypanosoma cruzi* in the cerebrospinal fluid during the acute stage of Chagas' disease. *N Engl J Med* 1978;**298**:604−6.

55. Rossi Spadafora MS, Céspedes G, Romero S, Fuentes I, Boada-Sucre AA, Cañavate C, et al. *Trypanosoma cruzi* necrotizing meningoencephalitis in a Venezuelan HIV + - AIDS patient: pathological diagnosis confirmed by PCR using formalin-fixed- and paraffin-embedded-tissues. *Analyt Cell Pathol* 2014.

56. Corti M, Yampolsky C. Prolonged survival and immune reconstitution after chagasic meningoencephalitis in a patient with acquired immunodeficiency syndrome. *Rev Soc Bras Med Trop* 2006;**39**:85−8.

57. Di Lorenzo GA, Pagano MA, Taratuto AL, Garau ML, Meli FJ, Pomsztein MD. Chagasic granulomatous encephalitis in immunosupressed patients: computed tomography and magnetic resonance imaging findings. *J Neuroimaging* 1996;**6**:94−7.

58. Walker M, Zunt JR. Parasitic central nervous system infections in immunocompromised hosts. *Clin Infect Dis* 2005;**40**:1005−15.

59. Brito AM, Castilho EA, Szwarcwald CL. AIDS e infecçao pelo HIV no Brasil: uma epidemia multifacetada. *Rev Soc Bras Med Trop* 2001;**34**:207−17.

60. Labarca J, Acuña G, Saavedra H, Oddó D, Sepúlveda C, Ballesteros J, et al. Enfermedad de Chagas en el síndrome de inmunodeficiencia adquirida: casos clínicos. *Rev Med Chil* 1992;**120**:174−9.

61. Perez-Ramírez L, Barnabe C, Sartori AM, Ferreira MS, Tolezano JE, Nunes EV, et al. Clinical analysis and parasite genetic diversity in human immunodeficiency virus/ Chagas' disease coinfections in Brazil. *Am J Trop Med Hyg* 1999;**61**:198−206.

62. Nijjar SS, Del Bigio MR. Cerebral trypanosomiasis in a incarcerated man. *CMJA* 2007;**176**:448.

63. Cordova E, Maiolo E, Corti M, Orduna T. Neurological manifestations of Chagas' disease. *Neurol Res* 2010;**32** 238−4.

64. Rochitte CE, Oliveira PF, Andrade JM, Ianni BM, Parga JR, Avila LF, et al. Myocardial delayed enhancement by magnetic resonance imaging in patients with Chagas' disease: a marker of disease severity. *J Am Coll Cardiol* 2005;**46**:1553−8.

65. Oddo' D, Casanova M, Acuña G, Ballesteros J, Morales B. Acute Chagas' disease (trypanosomiasis americana) in acquired immunodeficiency syndrome: report of two cases. *Hum Pathol* 1992;**23**:42−4.

66. Karp CL, Auwaerter PG. Coinfection with HIV and tropical infectious diseases: protozoal pathogens. *Clin Infect Dis* 2007;**45**:1208−13.

67. Jannin J, Villa L. An overview of Chagas' disease treatment. *Mem Inst Oswaldo Cruz* 2007;**102**:95−7.

68. Montero A, Cohen JE, Martinez DP, Giovannoni AG. Tratamiento empírico antitoxoplasma en sida y chagas cerebral: relato de dos casos, revisión de la bibliografía y propuesta de un algoritmo. *Medicina (Buenos Aires)* 1998;**58**:504−6.

69. Nishioka SA, Ferreira MS, Rocha A, Borges AS. Reactivation of Chagas' disease successfully treated with benznidazole in a patient with acquired immunodeficiency. *Mem Inst Oswaldo Cruz* 1993;**88**:851−3.

70. Coura JR. Present situation and new strategies for Chagas' disease chemotherapy—a proposal. *Mem Inst Oswaldo Cruz* 2009;**104**:549−54.

71. Do Campo R, Moreno SNJ. Free radical metabolism of antiparasitic agents. *Fed Proceed* 1986;**45**:2471−6.
72. Polak A, Richie R. Mode of action of 2-nitroimidazole derivative benznidazole. *Ann Trop Parasitol* 1978;**72**:228−32.
73. Lacunza CD, Olga Sánchez Negrette O, Mora MC, García Bustos MF, Basombrío MA. Use of the polymerase chain reaction (PCR) for the therapeutic control of chronic *Trypanosoma cruzi* infection. *Rev Patol Trop* 2015;**44**:21−32.

# Treatment of Chagas disease

**31**

*W. Apt*
University of Chile, Santiago, Chile

## Chapter Outline

## Introduction

Chagas disease has existed for at least 9000 years. Of the desiccated human mummies from coastal valley sites in northern Chile and Peru, 41% were found to be positive by polymerase chain reaction (PCR) and hybridization probes for kDNA of *Trypanosoma cruzi*. These tissue extracts correspond to the cultural groups that lived from 7000 BC to 1500 AD. These findings confirm that the sylvatic animal cycle of Chagas disease was well established by that time.[1]

American Trypanosomiasis Chagas Disease. DOI: http://dx.doi.org/10.1016/B978-0-12-801029-7.00032-0

**Table 31.1 Drugs administered from 1940 to 1975 to laboratory animals and Chagas disease patients which produced a reduction of the parasitemia but not a parasitological cure**

| |
|---|
| 8 Aminoquinolines (Primaquine) |
| Bisquinaldines (Bayer 7602) |
| Arsenebenzenes (Spirotrypan) |
| Fenantridines (Cardibium) |
| Emetine and derivatives |
| Nitrofurans and derivates |
| Nitroimidazole and derivatives |
| Piperazine and derivatives |
| Triphenylmethane |
| Triaminoquinazolines |
| 2-Acetamide-5-nitrodiazole |

*Source*: Adapted from Brener Z. Terapéutica experimental na doença de Chagas. En: Brener Z, Andrade Z, Barral-Neto M, editors. Trypanosoma cruzi e Doença de Chagas. Río de Janeiro, Brazil: Guanabara Koogan; 2000. p. 379−88.

Although Chagas disease is an old zoonosis, its treatment is recent. The present human treatment with nifurtimox (NF) and benznidazole (BZN) dates from the 1970s and is based on an empirical therapy.[2−4]

There are several drugs which act in vitro on *Trypanosma cruzi*, in cultures of epimastigotes and trypomastigotes, tissue cultures of amastigote forms, and in vivo in different species of infected animals with diverse strains (subpopulations) of the parasite. It is important to point out that the drugs used in Chagas disease therapy must have an effect on the intracellular amastigote forms, which are the reproductive forms in the vertebrate host. The epimastigote and trypomastigote forms of these hosts derive from the amastigotes, and for this reason their response to different drugs has less importance.[5,6] In Table 31.1 several drugs are described that were empirically applied to *T. cruzi* in experiments on animals and humans between 1940 and 1975. With the majority of these drugs a decrease of the parasitemia and lethality may be obtained, but not a parasitological cure.[7]

# Drugs which inhibit protein or purine synthesis

A rational therapy of *T. cruzi* should be based on drugs that inhibit protein or purine synthesis. One of these drugs is allopurinol. *T. cruzi* is not able to synthesize purines de novo as human do. Allopurinol (4-hydroxypirazol (3,4-d) pyrimidine) HPP (Fig. 31.1) is an analog of hypoxanthine, which decreases uric acid and the conversion of hypoxanthine to xanthine.

For this reason it is used to treat gout, which is characterized by the deposit of uric acid in the joints. HPP inhibits the epimastigote forms in culture. In mice infected with *T. cruzi* and treated with allopurinol, an important reduction of the

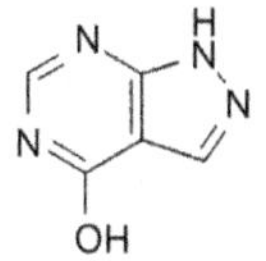

**Figure 31.1** Chemical structure of allopurinol (4-hydroxypirazol (3,4-d) pyrimidine).

parasitemia is obtained, although some parasite strains are resistant to the drug.[8] *T. cruzi* changes HPP to APP (4-aminopyrazol (3,4-d) pyrimidine), which is 15 times more powerful against epimastigotes than HPP. If APP is administered to infected *T. cruzi* mice a suppression of the parasitemia is obtained with a dose 400 times lower than allopurinol.[9] In patients with acute Chagas disease treated with allopurinol at high doses (20–30 mg/day) for 60 days, no reduction of the parasite burden was obtained. In a multinational study performed in Argentina, Brazil, and Bolivia in patients with chronic Chagas disease treated with 900 mg/day for 60 days, no parasitological cure was obtained. This drug was well tolerated in a number of studies performed in patients with chronic Chagas disease, and in some of these an improvement of the electrocardiographical alterations in Chagas cardiopathy (CCC) was demonstrated.[10] It has been used in heart transplantation in Chagas patients with good results.[11] In a combined treatment in chronic chagasic patients with 600 mg of allopurinol daily for 3 months followed by 30 days of benznidazole good results have been obtained.[12] In exceptional cases it has been necessary to suspend the treatment due to the secondary effects of allopurinol.[13]

Megazole (CL 641855), 2-amino-5-(methyl-5-nitro-2-inidazole)-1,3,4-thiazole, is a nitroimidazole-thiadiazol derivative that inhibits the protein synthesis of *T. cruzi*. With this drug a cure of mice inoculated with Y[20] strains and Colombian *T. cruzi* was obtained. The parasitological cure was demonstrated by hemocultures, reinoculations, and an indirect immunofluorescence (IF) test. The drug has not been used in human clinical studies, since the experimental survey in animals demonstrated that it was mutagenic.[14,15]

MK-436 is a compound, 3-(methyl-5-nitroimidazole-2-yl)-3α,4,5,6,7,7α-hexahydro-1,2-benzisoxazole, that is a substitute for 5-nitroinidazole and its derivative dihydro (L-634, 549). It affects amastigotes in culture tissue, and in acute and chronic infections in mice. With this drug a parasitological cure of the treated animals is obtained. To date it has not been used in human patients with Chagas disease.

# Inhibitors of ergoesterol

Diverse azolic products have been used with success in human and veterinary medicine. These drugs interface in sterol synthesis, and together with other heterocyclic nitrogenated compounds belong to the group of drugs that inhibit ergosterol synthesis. *T. cruzi* has ergosterol; the antimycotic prevents its synthesis without affecting the human host, who has cholesterol. Cholesterol differs from ergosterol by the presence of a 24-methyl group and double bonds in 7A and 22A. The three enzymes that produce the methylation and the double bonds of ergosterol do not have counterparts in mammalian cholesterol synthesis. Several of these azolic products have been studied for Chagas disease treatment: miconazole, econazole, ketoconazole, itraconazole, fluconazole, ravuconazole, and posaconazole (Fig. 31.2). With these drugs a parasitological cure has been obtained in mice with acute and chronic Chagas disease.[16]

Ketoconazole, itraconazole, and DO 870 inhibit cytochrome P450-dependent lenosterol C14 demethylase, thus reducing ergoesterol synthesis. Although mammals have this enzyme; it is much less sensitive to the drugs than those of fungi or of *T. cruzi*. Itraconazole has been applied in the treatment of chronic indeterminate Chagas disease and CCC. The drug prevents cardiopathy, compared to controls without therapy, and improves 50% of the electrocardiographic alterations of patients with CCC. Twenty percent of these cases are "cured" of parasites, determined by xenodiagnosis, PCR in blood, hybridization probes in blood, PCR in dejections, and hybridization probes in dejections of triatomines

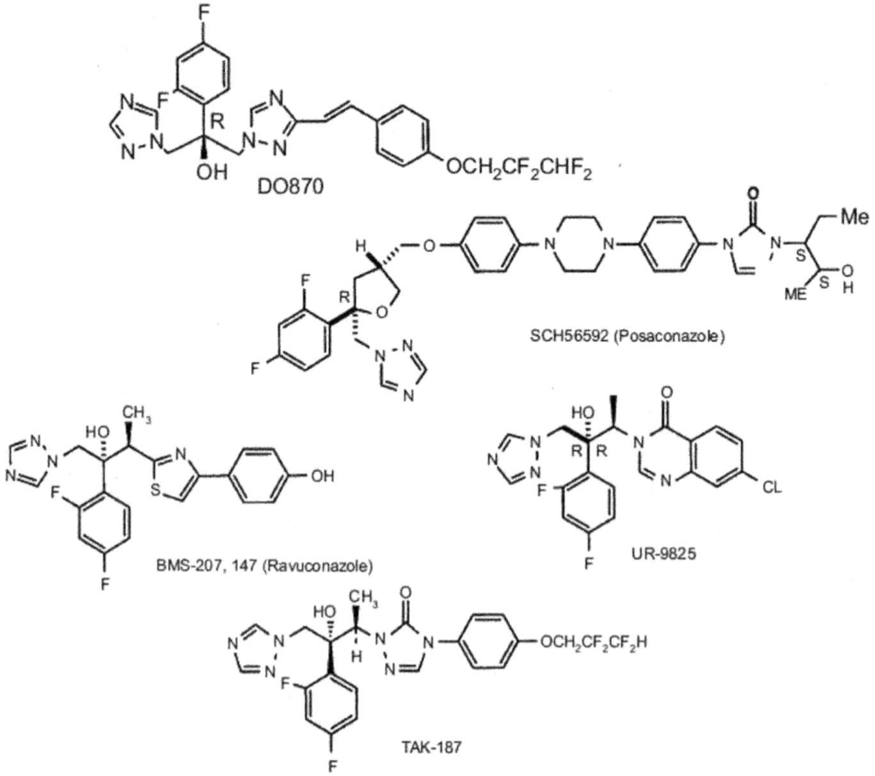

**Figure 31.2** Chemical structure of triazole derivatives, inhibitors of *Trypanosoma cruzi* sterol C14α sterol demethylase.

applied to these patients. However, none of the "cured" cases presented a negative conventional serology (indirect hemagglutination [HAI], indirect IF, or ELISA) for *T. cruzi*.[10,17,18] When the drug DO 870 was administered to mice with acute infection ($10^5$ *T. cruzi* Y strain), the treated animals lived longer than the controls without treatment or treated with NF or ketoconazole, 105 days survival versus 21. A 60% cure was obtained by control of parasitemia, hemocultures, and PCR. When this therapy was applied to mice with chronic infection ($10^4$ *T. cruzi* Bertoldo strain), after 40−50 days 50% of the controls survived and 30% of these had negative PCR, while the parasitological cure was 80−90% in the treated group.[16] Today DO 870 has been discontinued, but posaconazole (SCH 56592), MS-207, 147 (Ravuconazole), VR-9825, and TAK-187 have demonstrated activity against *T. cruzi* in vitro and in vivo. Of these compounds, posaconazole has proved to be efficient, and have very good tolerance in studies performed in patients with oropharyngeal candidiasis.[19] It has been observed that the majority of these compounds (Posaconazole, Ravuconazole, VR-9825, and TAK-187) have activity against *T. cruzi* strains partially resistant to NF, benznidazole (BNZ), and in which ketaconazole does not function.[20] Posaconazole with amiodarona, an antiarrhythmic drug, has a synergistic activity against *T. cruzi* in vitro and in vivo.[21]

A multinational study started in 2011 with 145 chronic chagasic patients with an indeterminate period treated with posaconazole (POS) for 60 days. The patients were divided into four groups: (1) Received POS 400 mg twice a day; (2) Received POS 400 mg twice a day plus 200 mg BNZ twice a day; (3) Received placebo 400 mg twice a day; and (4) Received BNZ 200 mg twice a day plus placebo 400 mg twice a day. The results of the efficiency of the drugs will be ready in 2016 (Stop Chagas Phase II 2011).[22,23]

In 2011 a study in Spain started with 79 patients with chronic indeterminate Chagas disease treated with BNZ or POS for 60 days (Chagasazol). The patients were divided into three groups: (1) received BNZ 150 mg twice a day; (2) received POS 400 mg twice a days (high dose); and (3) POS 100 mg twice day (low dose). The treatment failure at 12 months of follow up was 38.4% for BNZ, 80.7% and 92.3% for POS high and low dose, respectively.

In 2011 in Cochabamba and Tarija, Bolivia, a survey was performed with ravuconazole (RAV, compound E1224) phase II for 60 days in chronic chagasic patients with an indeterminate period. 230 patients were divided into five groups of 46 patients each. Group I, II, and III received RAV in high, middle, and low doses, respectively. The group IV received placebo and the group V received BNZ. The adherence of the drug was good, the secondary effects were scarce, but the compliance of the drug (RAV) in acute cases was 30% lower than the 70−75% obtained with NF and BNZ, respectively[24] (Table 31.2).

# Ofloxacine

Ofloxacine is an inhibitor of topoisomerase II, an essential enzyme for bacteria. This drug blocks the differentiation of amastigotes in tissue cultures.

Table 31.2 **Comparative efficacy of posaconazole, ravuconazole, and benznidazole for the treatment of chronic indeterminate Chagas disease**

| Trial | Chagasazol | Stop Chagas | E1224 (Ravuconazole) |
|---|---|---|---|
| No. patients | 79 | 160[a] | 231 |
| BNZ | 150 mg b.i.d[b] 60 days | 200 mg b.i.d 60 days | 200 mg b.i.d. 60 days |
| Azole (High dose) | POS: 400 mg b.i.d 60 days | POS: 400 mg b.i.d. 60 days | E 1224[c] 60 days |
| Azole (Low dose) | POS 100 mg b.i.d. 60 days | – | E1224[c] 60 days |
| Other | – | POS 400 mg b.i.d + BNZ 200 mg b.i.d. 60 days | E1224[c] 30 days |
| Treatment failure (*) (at 12 months follow up) BNZ | 38.4% | (d) | 19% |
| Azole ⎰ High dose | POS 80.7% | (d) | E1224 71.1% |
| Azole ⎱ Low dose | POS 92.3% | (d) | E1224 91.7% |
| Other | – | (d) | E1224 89.1% |

*Positive *T. cruzi* PCR. [a] Estimated; [b] Twice daily; [c] Amount not specified; [d] Study ongoing.
*Source*: Modified from Keenan M, Chaplin J. A new era for Chagas disease drug discovery? In: Lawton G, Witty D, editors. *Progress in medicinal chemistry*, vol. 54; 2015. p. 185–230.

Ultramicroscopy shows morphological alterations of the kinetoplast of *T. cruzi*, suggesting that ofloxacine destroys the parasites. In vivo experiments did not confirm the utility of this enzymatic inhibitor.

# Inhibitors of trypanothione metabolism

Trypanothione ($N^1$, $N^8$-*bis*-(glutatyonil)-spermidine) (Fig. 31.3) and trypanothione reductase are unique systems in the kinetoplastid protozoa which replace intracellular glutathion and glutathion reductase, the principal mechanism of the thyol-redux system.

Although trypanothione reductase is an essential enzyme in *Leishmania donovani* and *L. mayor*, the overexpression of the enzyme in *L. donovani* and *L. mayor* does not alter its sensitivity in vitro to agents that induce oxidative stress such as NF, nitrofurazone, and gentian violet. Inhibitors of trypanothione metabolism, such as buthionine sulfoximine (BS0), are ideal potential candidates as drugs against *T. cruzi* alone, or jointly with free radical-producing drugs such as NF and BNZ[25] (Fig. 31.4).

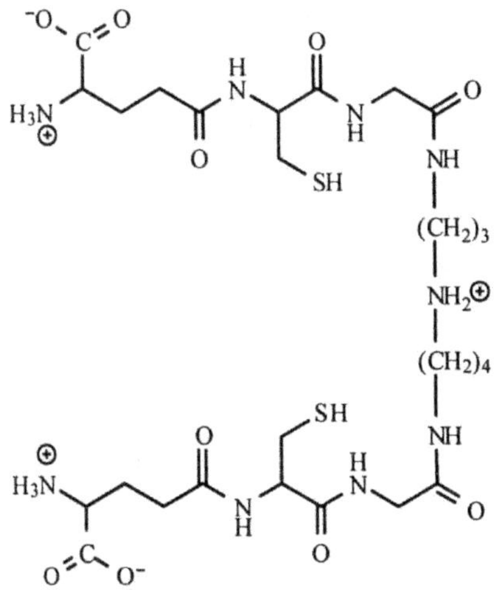

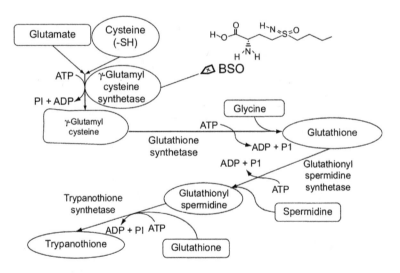

**Figure 31.3** Chemical structure of trypanothione ($N^1$, $N^8$-bis (glutationyl) spermidine).

**Figure 31.4** Biosynthesis of glutathione and trypanothione in *Trypanosoma cruzi*: glutathione is synthesized by the consecutive action of γ-glutamylcysteine synthetase and glutathione synthetase in an ATP-dependent reaction. In *T. cruzi*, two molecules of glutathione are conjugated with spermidine to synthesize trypanothione ($N^1$, $N^8$-bisglutathionyl spermidine, $T(SH)_2$). The host is unable to synthesize $T(SH)_2$. γ-Glutamylcysteine synthetase is the step-limiting enzyme in this process and can be inhibited by buthionine sulfoximine (BSO).

*Source*: Adapted from Maya J, Cassels B, Iturriaga-Vasquez P, Ferreira J, Faundez M, Galanti N, et al. Mode of action of natural and synthetic drugs against *Trypanosoma cruzi* and their interaction with the mammalian host. Comp *Biochem Physiol* 2006;146:601−20.

## Inhibitors of cysteine protease (CPI)

Cruzipain (cruzain, gp 51/57) is a simile of catepsine L-cysteine protease responsible for the proteolytic activity in all the life stages of *T. cruzi*. The genes which code for this protein have been cloned and expressed. A recombinant enzyme has been elaborated and different drugs have been studied that specifically inhibit the CPI protease in vitro, blocking the proliferation of epimastigotes and amastigotes and arresting metacyclogenesis. It has been demonstrated that these drugs such as vinyl-sulphone, vinyl-sulphone-phenyl derivatives block the development of cruzipain and its transport by lysosomes. These facts indicate that cruzipain is an ideal target; but to date, although CPI has been applied in murine models with acute and chronic infection, obtaining parasitological cure with minimal toxicity, the short half-life of the drug, which requires high and increasing doses, inhibits its use in clinical practice.[26,27]

Recently reversible and selective cruzipain inhibitors containing an amino nitride "war-pead" demonstrated good results in vitro and in a murine model, being considered promising anti-*T. cruzi* chemotherapeutic agents.[28,29]

## Inhibitors of phospholipids

Alkyl-lysophospholipids (ALP) are synthetic analogs of lysophospholipids that have been shown to be effective in vitro and in vivo on *T. cruzi* and trypanosomatides. Miltefosine, one of its representatives, has been used orally in visceral leishmaniasis with good results. ALP blocks selectively the biosynthesis of phosphatydil-coline (PC) of *T. cruzi* through the transmethylation of the Greenberg pathway, in contrast to the vertebrate host where the Kennedy pathway of CDP choline is predominant.[20]

## Inhibitors of pyrophosphate metabolism

The inorganic pyrophosphates ($P_2 O_7^{4-}$; PPi) and other short-chain tri- and tetra-polyphosphates are those that have the greatest energy of phosphate compounds in trypanosomatides (*T. cruzi*, *T. brucei*, and *L. mexicana*) and apicomplexa parasites (*Toxoplasma gondii*). They have 10−15 times more energy than ATP. PPi is distributed throughout the cell, but is concentrated in the acidocalcisomes, specialized acid vacuoles with large quantities of $Ca^{2+}$. PPi enzymes of *T. cruzi*, such as a proton-translocating pyrophosphose in acidocalcisomes and pyruvate phosphate dikinase in glycosomes, suggest that PPi has an important role in parasite survival. This has been confirmed by the observation that pamidronate, alendronate, and risedronate, contain biphosphonates, nonmetabolizable pyrophosphate analogs currently used in human medicine in alterations of bone reabsorption, which selectively inhibit the proliferation of intracellular amastigotes and tachyzoites of *T. gondii*. It has been demonstrated that residronate (Ris) acts in vitro on epimastigotes and cell cultures of amastigotes of *T. cruzi*, also reducing the infection in mice with acute infection, eliminating almost completely the parasitemias and intracellular amastigote forms. This drug inhibits farnesyl pyrophosphate synthase of the parasite, blocking the biosynthesis of polyisoprenoids.[30] It has not yet been used in humans. One inhibitor of farnesyltransferase, Tipifarnib (R115777), which inhibits cytochrome P450 sterol demethylase (CYP$_{51}$), is a potential target against *T. cruzi*, but in spite of its success in experimental animals it has not been applied to humans.[31]

The sterol 14-demethylase of *T. cruzi* has been studied (TCCYP51). It is related catalytically to the CYP51 of animal fungi.[32,33] Inhibition by obtusifoliol and its analogs enormously reduces enzyme activity. TCCYP51 constitutes a potential target against *T. cruzi*; however, to date no experimental surveys have performed to establish its efficacy in animals.

# Natural drugs

A great spectrum of natural products has been used against *T. cruzi*, but very few are useful at a concentration of 10 μg/mL, considering that the IC$_{50}$ for NF and BNZ is less than 3 μg/mL. Some products block the respiratory chain of the parasite, such as boldo (*Peumos boldus*) alkaloids, and naphthoquinone, extracted from *Calceolara sessilis*.[34] Other alkaloids extracted from Brazilian plants that have isoquinoline have an effect on *T. cruzi*.[35] Some natural drugs inhibit the response of *T. cruzi* to oxidative stress by producing superoxide radicals.[25] The triterpenes of *Arrabidae triplinervia* and their derivatives, such as diterpenes, komaroviquinone, and terpenoids isolated from *Pinus oocarpa*, have action on epimastigotes and trypomastigotes of *T. cruzi*.[36–38] In the majority of the natural drugs the exact mechanism of action is not known. The great majority of them have effects on epimastigote forms and some on culture amastigotes. Very few have been used in experimental studies in murines, and none have been used in clinical surveys. To date no natural product that acts on *T. cruzi* transialidase has been studied, although this enzyme is an optimal target. Only one natural drug has been used on cysteine protease (CPI), inhibiting cruzipain synthesis, this product is a 164 residue amino acid protein extracted from the seeds of *Bahuinia bauhinioides*. No experimental investigations have been performed with this product.[39] Oleic palmitic and stearic acids obtained from seeds of *Carica papaya* have demonstrated good compliance against trypomastigotes and amastigotes forms of *T. cruzi*. None of these acids have been used in clinical studies.[40] Metabolites of hydroethanolic extracts from *Aristeguietia glutinosa* inhibited the mitochondrial dehydrogenases and the biosynthesis of sterol membranes of *T. cruzi*.[41]

# Other drugs

Recently it has been demonstrated that MCPs, methylcarboxypeptidases that belong to the M32 peptidase family, are present in the cytosol of *T. cruzi*. Previously it was thought that these enzymes only existed in bacteria and prokaryotes. *T. cruzi* has two MCPs: TcMCP-1 and TcMCP-2. The former is found in all stages of the parasite, while TcMCP-2 only exists in epimastigotes and trypomastigotes. Because this enzyme does not exist in humans, its inhibition could represent an effective therapy against *T. cruzi*.[42,43] In the last 3 years there have been many studies of drugs against *T. cruzi*, among those who have had good compliance both in vitro and or in animal experiments we can mentionate: fexinidazole,[44] vinylsulfone,[27] glycosyl disulfider,[45] fenarimol and analogs,[46] novel quinoxaline,[47] novel 3-nitro-1-(1-1,2,4,treazole),[48] pentamidine,[49] squaramides,[50] hydroxamic acid and derivatives,[51] and lanthanide complexes.[52] None of these drugs has been used in human infections yet.

# Treatment of human infection

Treatment with NF and BNZ began in the 1970s and is based on an empirical treatment.[53–55] NF is 4-([5-nitrofurfuryledene] amino) 3 methylthiomorpholine-1, 1-dioxide (Fig. 31.5).

It acts by the production of free radicals, superoxide anions, hydrogen peroxide, and electrophilic metabolites. It has been demonstrated that in addition to the metabolic action of the drug on *T. cruzi*, its incorporation and transport by the parasite is of great importance. There are strains with some resistance to NF that differ due to a lower intake and transportation of the drug, rather than by the amount of free radical production. *T. cruzi* in the presence of NF increases oxygen consumption, $H_2O_2$, and superoxide radical production (Fig. 31.6).

The drug BNZ (*N*-benzyl-2 nitroimidazole-1-acetamide) was introduced in human clinical use in 1978. The drug inhibits protein synthesis, originating a degradation of macromolecule biosynthesis. Reduced metabolites of BNZ in covalent unions with macromolecules interact with the DNA of the parasite.[25] The drug inhibits the respiratory chain. The free radical production is lower than with NF.

## Current drug therapy

Chagas disease must always be treated in the acute period, as well as in the initial, middle determinate, and indeterminate chronic periods. The only exceptions from the etiological treatment are those patients with chronic infections with *Core bovis* and terminal cardiac insufficiency. The indication to apply specific therapy in chronic cases is the demonstration of parasites by PCR when they are not detected by optical microscopy. In these cases, therapy is effective. Today it is accepted that a precocious treatment is able to modify the natural evolution of the disease. This is

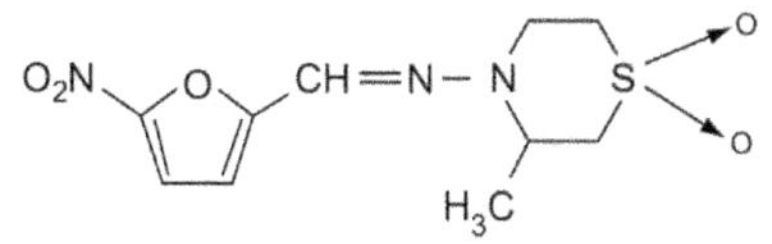

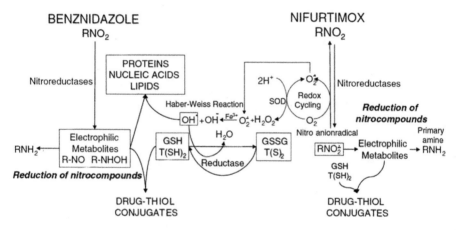

**Figure 31.5** Chemical structure of nifurtimox and benznidazole.

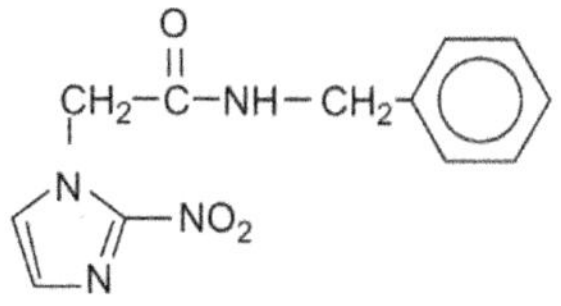

**Figure 31.6** Role of glutathione and trypanothione in the action and metabolism of the antichagasic drugs nifurtimox and benznidazole. The nitro group of both antichagasic drugs is reduced to free radicals or electrophilic metabolites by *T. cruzi* cytochrome P450-related nitroreductases. The nifurtimox-derived free radicals may undergo redox cycling with oxygen and $H_2O_2$ is produced by the further action of superoxide dismutase (SOD). The produced oxygen-derived free radicals and electrophilic metabolites bind to intracellular macromolecules and damage them. In the parasite, trypanothione $(T(SH)_2)$ and glutathione (GSH) neutralize the nifurtimox and benznidazole-derived metabolites by conjugation producing drug−thiol conjugates that will be further metabolized to mercapturates in the mammal host. Free radicals are neutralized by oxidation of reduced GSH or $T(SH)_2$. Trypanothione reductase reduces oxidized trypanothione $(T(S)_2)$.

*Source*: Adapted from Maya J, Cassels B, Iturriaga-Vasquez P, Ferreira J, Faundez M, Galanti N, et al. Mode of action of natural and synthetic drugs against *Trypanosoma cruzi* and their interaction with the mammalian host. *Comp Biochem Physiol* 2006;**146**:601−20.

why, due to the number of patients in countries where infection is prevalent, its treatment is a public health problem.[18,56−59]

## Acute cases

Patients with clinical manifestations must receive treatment. This includes those with an infection of less than 4 months, as well as the acute cases with easy detection of parasites in fresh samples and smears, and those with positive conventional serology: IHA, CF, IF, ELISA, and immunoblotting (IB) with positive IgM. The idea is to treat these cases with NF 8 mg/kg/day for 30−60 days in adults and 10 mg/kg/day for the same period in children. This daily quantity must be divided into three doses taken after meals (every 8 h). In Brazil, where NF is not available, BNZ is used: 5 mg/kg/day with a maximum daily dose of 300 mg, for 60 days in adults, and 5−10 mg/kg/day (7.5 mg/kg/day) for 60 days in children, divided into two or three doses (every 8 or 12 h) after meals. In an investigation performed in Santiago del Estero (Argentina) in 470 cases, the majority (84.4%) of children aged 1−9 years with acute Chagas disease presented with an ophthalmic lymph node complex, 367 were treated with 25 mg/kg of NF for 15 days and continued with 15 mg/kg for another 77 days; 40 received placebo; and another 20 other antichagasic drugs. Drug tolerance was greater in small children and the 15-mg dose was better tolerated than the 25-mg. After 60 days of treatment the direct parasitological tests were negative in both groups who received therapy; however, in the placebo group there were 28.6% positive cases. After 18 months there was 69% seroconversion of the treated patients; in other words, they passed from positive to negative. However, the placebo group maintained positive serology (IHA, CF, and IF).[60] With BNZ in acute acquired cases, a 76% cure is obtained (Table 31.3).[61]

## Congenital infection

Treatment must begin as soon as the diagnosis is performed, when the clinical suspicion is confirmed by observation of the parasite in fresh samples of blood smears, microstrout, etc. Sometimes the diagnosis is confirmed when the child is in the chronic period (8 or more months) by persistent positive serology after this period. Better therapeutic results are obtained when the diagnosis is more precocious. It is important to perform a clinical, serological, and parasitological follow-up of the treated newborn. Recently the utility of PCR in the precocious diagnosis of congenital Chagas disease in neonates has been confirmed. Its effectiveness is greater than that of xenodiagnosis.[62,63] This technique has great utility as has been demonstrated by Paraguayan investigators and others in the follow-up of treated cases. In an investigation performed in the maternity ward of the Clinical Hospital of Asunción and in the Regional Hospital of San Pedro, Paraguay, the newborn of chagasic mothers were studied. Three percent were positive by microscopy, which increased to 10 percent when they added the cases with persistent positive serology at 6 months. Of 58 newborn, in two cases T. cruzi was observed at birth and four presented positive PCR with negative microscopic investigation. All the positive cases

**Table 31.3 Adverse reactions to nifurtimox and benznidazole**

***Digestive alterations***
Gastric upset
Nausea
Vomiting

***Hematologic alterations (by hypersensitivity)***
Leukopenia
Thrombocytopenia
Agranulocytosis

***Dermatological alterations***
Erythematus, light-sensitive rash
Atopic dermatitis (mild or severe)
Occasionally Stevens-Johnson syndrome, which requires the suspension of therapy

***Neurological alterations***
Polyneuropathy, dose dependent
In general it appears in schedules of high dosages
In the usual dose of 5 mg/kg/day of benznidazole, 10—30% of the patients present
  neuropathies, especially at the end of treatment

were treated with BNZ and followed for 4 years by conventional serology and PCR.

In another study performed in an endemic area of Paraguay, of 1865 neonates with chagasic mothers, there were 104 cases where congenital infection was demonstrated by direct microscopic observation, PCR, and serology: ELISA, ELISA AIDS, and IF. PCR was the most sensitive test.[64]

All congenital cases must be treated, since up to 98% of such treatments may produce negative serology and parasitemia; the earlier the treatment is begun, the better the response obtained. NF must be administered in doses of 8—10 mg/kg/day for 60 days, taken every 8 or 12 h, or BNZ 5—10 mg/kg/day for 60 days. In a survey performed in Cochabamba, Bolivia, in 2013, success was obtained in congenital cases treated with 7.5 mg/kg/day during 30 days. If this result is confirmed by other investigations, we could have a shorter treatment with low cost.[65] To avoid secondary effects (convulsions) it is recommended to associate phenobarbital in therapeutic doses during the first 15 days of treatment. In case of secondary dermatological reactions, it is suggested to add antihistamines. Adverse reactions in neonates are fewer than in adults.

It is important to perform a precocious diagnosis of congenital cases to treat them as quickly as possible.[66] In pregnant women, conduct a serological test jointly with other tests such as VDRL during the first trimester of pregnancy and conduct follow-up of the positive cases until the diagnosis of congenital infection is confirmed or discarded. This activity must be performed in all women of fertile age, in pregnant women from endemic areas, and in women with a history of having lived in these zones.

In a newborn, run a serological study for *T. cruzi* infection, together with VDRL and other tests. In the positive cases a follow-up must be realized until confirmation or refutation of the diagnosis.

## Accidental Chagas disease

All accidental cases must be treated with the same drugs as the acute infections acquired from the vector, for 15 days. In this group the transfusion by error from a chagasic donor must be considered. In persons who work in laboratories and have a puncture accident with contaminated samples of infective *T. cruzi* forms, the confirmation of the contamination of the object with the parasite and the posterior infection of the patient (serology and PCR) must be performed. If there are positive results, immediate treatment must be undertaken with BNZ 5 mg/kg/day (adults) or 7−10 mg/kg/day (children) for 15 days, depending on the immunological state of the person. A serological study must be done at 15−30 and 60 days.

## Organ transplants

A transplant where the donor or recipient has Chagas disease must always be treated, when it is possible before the transplant with NF 8 mg/kg/day in adults and 10 mg/kg/day in children for 60 days, or BNZ 5 mg/kg/day in adults and 5−10 mg/kg/day in children ($\Sigma$7.5 mg/kg/day) for 60 days. In cases with a transplant from a chagasic patient without knowing, e.g., a kidney from a corpse, they will receive treatment only if there is a reactivation (20−30% of the cases).[67] In bone marrow transplants with *T. cruzi* infections (which relapse in 40% of the cases) the treatment must be maintained for 2 years and in solid organ recipients treatment must be given for the period in which sufficient CD4 lymphocytes for an adequate immune response are present (more than 200 lymphocytes per mL). In these patients the most commonly prescribed drugs are the traditional NF and BNZ. In the model of patients exposed by organ transplant a number of situations may be produced, such as primoinfections and reactivations; thus it is important to perform a good screening of donor and recipient before the transplant. The clinical manifestations of reactivation usually differ from that of the acute phase (primoinfection), for this reason the monitoring of patients after the transplant is relevant. In both situations, the recipient who receives an organ from a chagasic donor or a chagasic reactivated recipient, therapy must be initiated with NF or BNZ.

## Reactivations of chronic Chagas disease and treatment of Chagas disease in immunosuppressed patients

Patients with chronic Chagas disease who acquire AIDS or in whom immunosuppressor therapy is administered must receive treatment at the same dose as the group mentioned above for 5 or more months. In these cases the most suitable strategy is prevention, performing serology for Chagas disease in all AIDS patients. In the primoinfection by *T. cruzi* in AIDS patients, the same treatment schedule must be prescribed as in reactivations. The same classic antiparasitic drugs are used in the standard doses until the immune response of the host is reconstituted (in some cases 60 or more days). Once the alteration of the immune system is normalized, including the ratio of CD4/CD8, the antiparasitic schedule is changed to every 3 days, balancing the parasiticide effects with the adverse effects. The patients with AIDS without retroviral treatment are the most severely affected. In these patient, once the CD4 levels are normalized with specific antiviral treatment, maintenance schedules may be used.

## Evaluation and follow-up of specific therapy

The principal objection to the treatment of Chagas disease is its long duration. The treatment must be maintained at least for 60 days and the cure criteria depend on several factors.[56] Some authors consider serological conversion as necessary, but this sometimes happens 10−20 years or more after the end of treatment of chronic Chagas disease,[68] and there are cases in which former patients die without seroconversion. Recently it has been published that in treated cured mice experimentally infected with *T. cruzi* in which no parasites and no *T. cruzi* antigens could be demonstrated, CD8 central memory cells maintain a positive serology for more than a year.[69] We do not know if this process occurs in humans, but if it does, we can explain why cures in chronic cases could be reached without seroconversion.

Others consider the following parameters as cure criteria of the chronic period: the conversion of the xenodiagnosis from positive to negative; conversion of qualitative PCR from positive to negative; the incapacity to demonstrate parasites by quantitative PCR; and in cardiopaths the elimination of the electrocardiographic alterations. These changes must always be permanent and must persist for 12 or more years independent of the conventional serological results. There must be at least two parasitological and one or more clinical parameters to confirm the cure.[10] In the acute indeterminate and determinate chronic periods a follow-up must be performed with hemocultures, quantitative PCR for *T. cruzi*,[70,71] hemogram, biochemical profile, and/or xenodiagnosis. It must be kept in mind that serological tests in severe immunosuppressed patients usually have negative results and for this reason do not serve to follow up the treatment. A prolonged persistent negativity of PCR with these characteristics for *T. cruzi* is considered as a cure criterion. Some authors give value to the disappearance of lytic antibodies as a complement to improve the criterion.

# Resistance of *T. cruzi* to drugs

In vitro and in vivo it has been demonstrated that certain *T. cruzi* strains are resistant to NF and BNZ. This is valid especially for *T. cruzi* clones isolated from sylvatic animals or vectors. It is important to emphasize that we do not know if what we observe in murine models happens in humans. Furthermore, in many publications the strains of *T. cruzi* have not been well characterized by isozymes (zymodemes), nuclear restriction enzymes (schizodemes), genetic composition, etc.[72] No consensus exists on the relation between the sensitive or resistant strains and virulence. Andrade et al.[73] claimed that there is a relationship and the resistant strains are more virulent, while Filardi and Brener[74] did not find this association. In relation to the genetic composition of *T. cruzi* and resistance to drugs, it has been demonstrated in vitro that a relation exists between genetic distances and biological differences, among the latter is the resistance to NF and BNZ. This is true for epimastigotes and amastigotes. Trypomastigotes are the exception, since in them a relation between genetic distances and sensitivity to drugs does not exist. It is necessary to make better genotypic studies of *T. cruzi* in relation to resistance to drugs. It has been demonstrated that patients with chronic Chagas disease treated with itraconazole or allopurinol who did not respond to the specific therapy (there is no parasitological cure) were infected with the TcI lineage of *T. cruzi*, while those that responded to the therapy with itraconazole had the lineage TcIIb (now TcV)[75] suggesting that TcI is resistant to these drugs and TcIIb (TcV) is sensitive.[76]

## Critical comments

At present there is no effective therapy for the majority of the patients who have chronic Chagas disease in the indeterminate (60−70%) and determinate (10−30%) periods. In the acquired acute period 70−75% of the cases are cured and in newborn and suckling children with congenital Chagas disease a 98−100% cure is obtained.

The compliance of beznidazole in chronic chagasic cardiopathy as well as its efficiency in these cases was determinate in September 2015 by the BENEFIT project.[77,78] In this randomized double blind, placebo-controlled trial, 1423 patients were treated with BNZ, 300 mg/day, and 1423 with placebo during 60 days. After a mean of 5.4 years of follow-up (5−7 years) the PCR *T. cruzi* conversion rate was 62.2% in the BNZ group and 33.5% in the placebo group. However, despite the significant difference in parasitemia of both groups no differences were observed in the clinical outcome. The people with Chagas disease have low economic resources. Chagas disease is one of the "neglected diseases" and for this reason is not of interest to the pharmaceutical companies.[79] What will happen when the current supply of NF is exhausted? Bayer is not interested in continuing its production. Since ROCHE did not want to continue production of BNZ, it assigned the process to Brazilian and Argentinean laboratories. Recently a pediatric formula of nifurtimox and benznidazole has been produced, and in the last few years new drugs have been developed against *T. cruzi* that can be applied to humans. So there is a hope that in the near future chronic chagasic patients could be treated with new drugs or a combination of drugs.[80]

# Glossary

**Chinchorro culture** Earliest humans in Latin America. They lived from 9000 to 450 years B.P. They were infected by *T. cruzi*.

**MCPs** Methylcarboxypeptidases. *T. cruzi* has two MCPs: TcMCP-1 and TcMCP-2. The last one exists only in epimastigote and trypomastigote and the former in all stages of the parasite.

# References

1. Aufderheide AC, Salo W, Madden M, Streitz J, Buikstra J, Guhl F, et al. 9000-year record of Chagas' disease. *Proc Natl Acad Sci USA*. 2004;**101**:2034–9.
2. Pinto Dias J. Tratamiento etiológico de la enfermedad de Chagas. En XII Reunión de la Comisión Intergubernamental del Cono Sur para la eliminación de *Triatoma infestans* y la interrupción de la transmisión transfusional de la Tripanosomiasis Americana (INCOST/Chagas). Washington DC. *Pan American Health Organization* 2004;**2004**:129–34.
3. Coura R. Chagas disease: clinical and therapeutic features. *Enf Emerg* 2005;**8**:18–24.
4. Steverding D, Tyler K. Novel antitrypanosomal agents. *Expert Opin Investig Drugs* 2005;**14**:939–55.
5. Andrade Z, Andrade S. Patología Da Doença de Chagas. In: Brener Z, Andrade Z, Barral-Neto M, editors. Trypanosoma cruzi e *doença de Chagas*. Río de Janeiro, Brazil: Guanabara Koogan; 2000. p. 201–30.
6. Teixeira A, Nascimento R, Sturn N. Evolution and pathology in Chagas disease: a review. *Mem Inst Oswaldo Cruz* 2006;**101**:463–91.
7. Brener Z. Terapéutica experimental na doença de Chagas. In: Brener Z, Andrade Z, Barral-Neto M, editors. Trypanosoma cruzi e *Doença de Chagas*. Río de Janeiro, Brazil: Guanabara Koogan; 2000. p. 379–88.
8. Avila J, Avila A. *Trypanosoma cruzi* allopurinol in the treatment of mice with experimental acute Chagas disease. *Exp Parasitol* 1981;**51**:204–8.
9. Avila J, Avila A, Muñoz E, Monzon H. *Trypanosoma cruzi:* 4-aminopyrazolopyrimidine in the treatment of experimental Chagas disease. *Exp Parasitol* 1983;**56**:236–40.
10. Apt W, Arribada A, Zulantay I, Solari A, Sánchez G, Mundaca K, et al. Itraconazole an Allopurinol in the treatment of chronic American tripanosomiasis: the results of clinical and parasitological examinations 11 years post treatment. *Ann Trop Med Parasitol* 2005;**99**:733–41.
11. Tomimori-Yamashita J, Deps P, Almeida D, Enokihara M, De Seixas M, Freymuller E. Cutaneous manifestation of Chagas disease after heart transplantation: successful treatment with allopurinol. *Br J Dermatol* 1997;**137**:626–30.
12. Perez-Mazliah D, Alvarez M, Cooley G, Lococo B, Bertocchi G, Petti M, et al. Sequential combined treatment with allopurinol and benznidazole in the chronic phase of *Trypanosoma cruzi* infection: a pilot study. *J Antimicrob Chemother* 2013;**68**:424–37.
13. Apt W, Aguilera X, Arribada A, Pérez C, Miranda C, Sánchez G, et al. Treatment of chronic Chagas disease with itraconazole and allopurinol. *Am J Trop Med and Hyg* 1988;**59**:133–8.

14. Enanga B, Ariyanayagam M, Stewart M, Barret M. Activity of megazol, a trypanocidal nitroimidazole is associated with DNA damage. *Antimicrob Agents Chemother* 2003;**47**:3368−70.
15. Nesslany F, Brugier S, Mouries M, Le Curieux F, Marzin D. In vitro and in vivo chromosomal aberrations induced by megazol. *Mutat Res* 2004;**560**:147−58.
16. Urbina J. Chemotherapy of Chagas disease. *Curr Pharm Des* 2002;**8**:287−95.
17. Zulantay I, Apt W, Gil LC, Rocha C, Mundaca C, Solari A, et al. The PCR-based detection of *Trypanosoma cruzi* in the faeces of *Triatoma infestans* fed on patients with chronic American trypanosomiasis gives higher sensitivity and a quicker result than routine xenodiagnosis. *Ann Trop Med Parasitol* 2007;**101**:673−9.
18. Apt W, Arribada A, Zulantay I, Rodríguez J, Saavedra M, Muñoz A. Treatment of Chagas' disease with itraconazole: electrocardiographic and parasitological conditions after 20 years of follow-up. *J Antimicrob Chemother* 2013;**68**:2164−9.
19. Skies D, Vazquez J, Anstead G, Greybill J, Reynes J, Ward D, et al. Posaconazole for the treatment of azole-refractory oropharyngeal and esophaged candidiasis in subjects with HIV infection. *Clin Infect Dis* 2007;**44**:607−14.
20. Urbina J. New chemotherapeutic approaches for the treatment of Chagas disease (American Trypanosomiasis). *Expert Opin Ther Patents* 2003;**13**:661−9.
21. Benaim G, Sanders J, Garcia-Marchán Y, Colina C, Lira R, Caldera A, et al. Amiodarone has intrinsic anti-*Trypanosoma cruzi* activity and acts synergistically with posaconazole. *J Med Chem* 2006;**49**:892−9.
22. Morillo C. *Actualización Estudio Clínico Stop-Chagas Study of oral posaconazole in the treatment of asymptomatic chronic Chagas disease. VIII Taller sobre la enfermedad de Chagas importada. Avances en el tratamiento antiparasitario.* ISI Global Barcelona; 2012. p. 17−20.
23. Keenan M, Chaplin J. A new era for Chagas disease drug discovery? In: Lawton G, Witty D, editors. *Progress in medicinal chemistry*, vol. 54; 2015. p. 185−230.
24. Torrico F, Ribeiro I, Alonso-Vega C, Alves F, Pinazo M, Ortiz L, et al. Justificación y diseño de un estudio de fase II de prueba de concepto del E1224, nuevo fármaco candidato para el tratamiento de pacientes adultos con enfermedad de Chagas crónica. VIII Taller sobre la enfermedad de Chagas importada. Avances en el tratamiento antiparasitario IS Global Barcelona; 2012. p. 22−4.
25. Maya J, Cassels B, Iturriaga-Vasquez P, Ferreira J, Faundez M, Galanti N, et al. Mode of action of natural and synthetic drugs against *Trypanosoma cruzi* and their interaction with the mammalian host. *Comp Biochem Physiol* 2006;**146**:601−20.
26. Cazzulo J. Proteinases of *Trypanosoma cruzi:* potential targets for the chemotherapy of Chagas desease. *Curr Top Med Chem* 2002;**2**:1261−71.
27. Choy J, Bryant C, Calvet C, Doyle P, Gunatilleke S, Leung S, et al. Chemical−biological characterization of a cruzain inhibitor reveals a second target and a mammalian off-target. *Beilstein J Org Chem* 2013;**9**:15−25.
28. Ndao M, Beaulieu C, Black W, Isabel E, Vasquez-Camargo F, Nath-Chowdhury M, et al. Reversible cysteine protease inhibitors show promise for a Chagas disease cure. *Antimicrob Agents Chemother* 2014;**58**:1167−78.
29. Ferreira R, Dessoy M, Pauli I, Souza M, Krogh R, Sales A, et al. Synthesis, biological evaluation, and structure-activity relalationships of potent noncovalent and nonpeptidic cruzain inhibitors as anti-*Trypanosoma cruzi* agents. *J Med Chem* 2014;**57**:2380−92.
30. Garzoni L, Waghabi M, Baptista M, de Castro S, Meirelles M, Britto C, et al. Antiparasitic activity of risedronate in a murine model of acute Chagas disease. *Int J Antimicrob Agents* 2004;**23**:286−90.

31. Hucke O, Gelb M, Verlinde C, Buckner F. The protein farnesyltransferase inhibitor Tipifarnib as a new lead for the development of drugs against Chagas disease. *J Med. Chem* 2005;**48**:5415−18.

32. Lepesheva G, Zaitseva N, Nes W, Shou W, Arase M, Liu J, et al. CYP51 from *Trypanosoma cruzi*: a phyla-specific residue in the B′ helix defines substrate preferences of sterol 14 alpha-demethylase. *J Biol Chem* 2006;**281**:3577−85.

33. Lepesheva G, Waterman M. Structural basis for conservation in the CYP51 family. *Biochim Biophys Act* 2011;**1814**:88−93.

34. Morello A, Lipchenca I, Cassels B, Speisky H, Aldunate J, Repetto Y. Trypanocidad effect of boldine and related alkaloids up on several strains of *Trypanosoma cruzi*. *Comp Biochem Physiol* 1994;**90**:1−12.

35. Tempone A, Borborema S, de Andrade Jr. H, de Amorim N, Yogi A, Carvalho C, et al. Antiprotozoal activity of Brazilian plant extracts from isoquinoline alkaloid-producing families. *Phytomedicine* 2005;**12**:382−90.

36. Rubio J, Calderon J, Flores A, Castro C, Céspedes C. Trypanocidad activity of oleoresin and terpenoids isolated from *Pinus oocarpa*. *Naturforsch* 2005;**60**:711−16.

37. Uchiyama N, Kabututu Z, Kubata B, Kiuchi F, Ito M, Nakajima-Shimada J, et al. Antichagasic activity of komaroviquinone is due to generation of reactive oxygen species catalyzed by *Trypanosoma cruzi* old yellow enzyme. *Antimicrob Agents Chemother* 2005;**49**:5123−6.

38. Leite J, Oliveira A, Lombardi J, Filho J, Chiari E. Trypanocidad activity of triter-penes from *Arrabidaea triplinervia* and derivatives. *Biol Pharm Bull* 2006;**29**:2307−9.

39. de Oliveira C, Santana L, Carmona A, Cezari M, Sampaio M, Sampaio C, et al. Structure of cruzipain/cruzain inhibitors isolated from *Bauhinia bauhinioides* seeds. *Biol Chem* 2001;**382**:847−52.

40. Jiménez-Coello M, Guzman-Marín E, Ortega-Pacheco A, Perez-Gutierrez S, Acosta-Viana K. Assessment of the anti-protozoal activity of crude *Carica* papaya seed extract against *Trypanosoma cruzi*. *Molecules* 2013;**18**:12621−32.

41. Varela J, Serna E, Torres S, Yaluff G, de Bilbao N, Miño P, et al. In vivo anti-*Trypanosoma cruzi* activity of hydro-ethanolic extract and isolated active principles from *Aristeguietia glutinosa* and mechanism of action studies. *Molecules* 2014;**19**:8488−502.

42. Niemirowicz G, Parussini F, Aguero F, Cazzulo J. Two metallocarboxypeptidases from the protozoan *Trypanosoma cruzi* belong to the M32 family, found so far only in prokar-yotes. *Biochem J* 2007;**401**:399−410.

43. Rawlings N. Unusual phyletic distribution of peptidases as a tool for identifying poten-tial drug targets. *Biochem J* 2007;**401**:5−7.

44. Bahia M, de Andrade I, Martins T, do Nascimento A, Diniz L, Caldas I, et al. Fexinidazole: a potential new drug candidate for Chagas disease. *PLoS NTD* 2012;**6**:e1870.

45. Gutiérrez B, Muñoz C, Osorio L, Fehér K, Illyés T, Papp Z, et al. Aromatic glycosyl disulfide derivatives: evaluation of their inhibitory activities against *Trypanosoma cruzi*. *Bioorg Med Chem Lett* 2013;**23**:3576−9.

46. Keenan M, Chaplin J, Alexander P, Abbott M, Best W, Khong A, et al. Two analogues of fenarimol show curative activity in an experimental model of Chagas disease. *J Med Chem* 2013;**56**:10158−70.

47. Torres E, Moreno-Viguri E, Galiano S, Devarapally G, Crawford P, Azqueta A, et al. Novel quinoxaline 1,4-di-N-oxide derivatives as new potential anti-chagasic agents. *Eur J Med Chem* 2013;**66**:324−34.

48. Papadopoulou M, Blooner W, Rosenzweig H, Ashworth R, Wilkinson S, Kaiser M, et al. Novel 3-nitro-1H-1,2,4-triazole-based compounds as potential anti-chagasic drugs: in vivo studies. *Future Med Chem* 2013;**5**:1763−76.

49. Díaz M, Miranda M, Campos-Estada C, Reigada C, Maya J, Pereira C, et al. Pentamidine exerts *"in vitro"* and *"in vivo"* anti *Trypanosoma cruzi* activity and inhibits the polyamine transport in *Trypanosoma cruzi*. *Acta Trop* 2014;**134**:1−9.

50. Olmo F, Rotger C, Ramírez-Macías I, Martínez L, Marin C, Carreras L, et al. Synthesis and biological evaluation of N,N'-squaramides with high in vivo efficacy and low toxicity: toward a low-cost drug against Chagas disease. *J Med Chem* 2014;**57**:987−99.

51. Rodriguez G, Feijó D, Bozza M, Pan P, Vullo D, Parkkila S, et al. Design, synthesis, and evaluation of hydroxamic acid derivarives as promising agents for the management of Chagas disease. *J Med Chem* 2014;**57**:298−308.

52. Caballero A, Rodríguez-Diéguez A, Salas J, Sánchez-Moreno M, Marín C, Ramírez Macías I, et al. Lanthanide complexes containing 5-methyl-1,2,4-triazolo[1,5-a] pyrimidin-7(4H)-one and their therapeutic potential to fight leishmaniasis and Chagas disease. *J Inorg Biochem* 2014;**138**:39−46.

53. Prata A. Abordagem general do paciente chagasico. In: Coura Pinto Dias J, editor. *Clinica e terapeutica do doença de Chagas. Um manual practico para o clínico general.* Río de Janeiro: Fio Cruz; 1997. p. 115−26.

54. Rassi A, Rassi Jr A, Rassi S. Cardiopatía crónica: arritmias. In: Coura Pinto Dias J, editor. *Doença de Chagas. Um manual para o clínico general.* Río de Janeiro: Fio Cruz; 1997. p. 201−22.

55. Pinto Dias J. The treatment of Chagas disease (South American tripanosomiasis). *Ann Int Med* 2006;**144**:772−4.

56. Viotti R, Vigliano C, Lococo B, Bertocci G, Petti M, Alvarez M, et al. Long-term cardiac outcome of treating chronic Chagas disease with benznidazole versus no treatment: a nonrandomized trial. *Ann Intern Med* 2006;**144**:724−34.

57. Apt W, Heitman I, Jercic MI, Jofre L, del Muñoz PC V, Noemí I, et al. Guidelines for the Chagas disease: Part VI. Antiparasitic treatment for Chagas disease. *Rev Chilena Infectol* 2008;**25**:384−9.

58. Viotti R, Alarcón de Noya B, Araujo-Jorge T, Grijalva M, Guhl F, López M, et al. Towards a paradigm shift in the treatment of chronic Chagas disease. *Antimicrob Agents Chemother* 2014;**58**:635−9.

59. Urbina J. Recent clinical trials for the etiological treatment of chronic Chagas disease: advances, challenges and perspectives. *J Eukaryot Microbiol* 2015;**62**:149−56.

60. Cerisola J. Evolución serológica de pacientes con enfermedad de Chagas aguda tratados con Bay 2502. *Bol Chile Parasitol* 1969;**24**:54−9.

61. Cançado R. Tratamiento etiológico do doença de Chagas pelo benznidazol. In: Brener Z, Andrade Z, y Barral-Neto M, editors. Trypanosoma cruzi e doença de Chagas. Río de Janeiro, Brazil: Guanabara Koogan; 2000. p. 389−405.

62. Virreira M, Torrico F, Truyens C, Alonso-Vega C, Solano M, Carlier Y, et al. Comparison of polymerase chain reaction methods for reliable and easy detection of congenital *Trypanosoma cruzi* infection. *Am J Trop Med Hyg* 2003;**68**:574−82.

63. Sánchez O, Mora M, Basombrio M. High prevalence of congenital *Trypanosoma cruzi* infection and clustering in Salta, Argentina. *Pediatrics* 2005;**115**:668−72.

64. Russomando G, Almiron M, Candra N, Franco L, Sanchez Z, Guileen Y. Implementation and evaluation of a locally sustainable system of prenatal screening that allows the detection of cases of congenital transmission of Chagas disease in endemic zone of Paraguay. *Rev Soc Bras Med Trop* 2005;**38**:49−54.

65. Chippaux J, Salas-Clavijo A, Postigo J, Schneider D, Santalla J, Brutus L. Evaluation of compliance to congenital Chagas disease treatment results of a randomised trial in Bolivia. *Trans R Soc Trop Med Hyg* 2013;**107**:1−7.

66. Carlier Y, Truyens C, Deloron P, Peyron F. Congenital parasitic infections: a review. *Acta Trop* 2012;**121**:55−70.

67. Huprikar S, Bosseman E, Patel G, Moore A, Pinney S, Anyanwu A, et al. Donor-derived *Trypanosoma cruzi* infection in solid organ recipients in the United States, 2001−2011. *Am J Transplant* 2013;**13**:2418−25.

68. Lacunza C, Negrete O, Mora M, Bustos M, Basombrio M. Uso de la reacción en cadena de la polimerasa para el control terapéutico de la infección crónica por *Trypanosoma cruzi*. *Rev Patol Trop* 2015;**44**:21−32.

69. Bustamante J, Bixby L, Tarleton R. Drug induced cure drives conversion to a stable and protective CD8$^+$ T central memory response in chronic Chagas disease. *Nat Med* 2008;**14**:542−50.

70. Duffy T, Bisio M, Altcheh J, Burgos I, Diaz M, Levin M, et al. Accurate real-time PCR strategy for monitoring bloodstream parasites loads in Chagas disease patients. *PLoS NTD* 2009;**3**:419−29.

71. Britto C. Usefulness of PCR-based assays to assess drug efficacy in Chagas disease chemotherapy: value and limitations. *Mem Inst Oswaldo Cruz* 2009;**104**:122−35.

72. Solari A, Muñoz S, Venegas J, Wallace A, Aguilera X, Apt W, et al. Characterization of Chilean, Bolivian and Argentinian *Trypanosoma cruzi* populations by restrictive endonuclease and isoenzime analysis. *Exp Parasit* 1992;**75**:187−95.

73. Andrade S, Magalhaes J, Pontes A. Evaluation of chemotherapy with benznidazole and nifurtimox in mice infected with *Trypanosoma cruzi* strains of different types. *Bull World Health Organ* 1985;**63**:721−6.

74. Filardi L, Brener Z. Susceptibility and natural resistance of *Trypanosoma cruzi* strains to drugs used clinically in Chagas disease. *Trans Roy Soc Trop Med Hyg* 1987;**81**:755−9.

75. Zingales B, Andrade S, Briones M, Campbell D, Chiari E, Fernandes O, et al. A new consensus for *Trypanosoma cruzi* intraspecific nomenclature: second revision meeting recommends TcI to TcVI. *Mem Inst Oswaldo Cruz* 2009;**104**:1051−4.

76. Coronado X, Zulantay I, Rozas M, Apt W, Sánchez G, Rodríguez J, et al. Dissimilar distribution of *Trypanosoma cruzi* clones in humans alter chemotherapy with allopurinol and itraconazole. *J Antimicrob Chemother* 2006;**58**:216−19.

77. Marin-Neto J, Rassi Jr A, Morillo C, Avezum A, Connolly S, Sosa-Estani S, et al. BENEFIT Investigators. Rationale and design of a randomized placebo-controlled trial assessing the effects of etiologic treatment in Chagas' cardiomyopathy: the Benznidazole Evaluation For Interrupting Trypanosomiasis (BENEFIT). *Am Heart J* 2008;**156**:37−43.

78. Morillo C, Marin-Neto J, Avezum A, Sosa-Estani S, Rassi Jr A, Rosas F, et al. BENEFIT Investigators. Randomized trial of benznidazole for chronic Chagas' cardiomyopathy. *N Engl J Med* 2015;**373**(14):1295−306.

79. Rassi Jr A, Dias JC, Marin-Neto J, Rassi A. Challenges and opportunities for primary, secondary, and tertiary prevention of Chagas' disease. *Heart* 2009;**95**:524−34.

80. Fagi M, Kaiser M, Tanner M, Schneiter R, Mäser P, Guan X. Match-making for posaconazole through systems thinking. *Trends Parasitol* 2015;**31**:46−51.

# Vaccine development for Chagas disease

A.M. Padilla[1,] *, C.P. Brandan[2,] * and M.A. Basombrío[2]
[1]University of Georgia, Athens, GA, United States, [2]Universidad Nacional de Salta, Salta, Argentina

## Chapter Outline

## Introduction

Vaccines have had an indisputable impact on the control of many important human and veterinary diseases and unquestionably have shaped the health landscape of the last generations. Nevertheless the crucial benefits obtained with vaccines for diseases like smallpox and poliomyelitis, many tropical diseases, commonly referred to as neglected diseases, suffer the lack of an effective vaccine. Chagas disease is one of these neglected diseases and it is a major health problem in Latin America countries, especially the poorest ones. The advantages of having a vaccine that prevents Chagas disease have been estimated to be significant not just in terms of public health but also in terms of economic and social development.[1] Although some important advances on the comprehension of human immune response to *Trypanosoma cruzi* infection have been done, the vast majority of our knowledge about immune mechanisms and protective response comes from experimental animal models.

---

* Both authors contributed equally to this chapter.

American Trypanosomiasis Chagas Disease. DOI: http://dx.doi.org/10.1016/B978-0-12-801029-7.00033-2

# Immune mechanisms associated with protection against *Trypanosoma cruzi* infection

In recent years increasing knowledge about the immune response associated with Chagas disease has been invaluable for the design and testing of vaccination approaches, although still fundamental questions remain obscure. We need to define the immune response against *T. cruzi* to better understand the protective mechanisms involved, in order to improve them as well as to identify the weaknesses in the response that allows parasite persistence in the chronic infection.

*Trypanosoma cruzi* infection is naturally initiated by the invasion of the parasite through mucosa or skin lesions that get in contact with the parasite-containing feces deposited by the insect vector. Once the parasite crosses the skin barrier it encounters the host tissue cells at the site of entry and the normal immune cells that populate that tissue or are recruited there by the lesion. In *T. cruzi* infection it is possible that the first immune cells to be recruited at the site of entry are also neutrophils as in *Leishmania* infection[2] but probably the majority of the parasites directly infect tissue cells at the site rather than recruited immune cells. This notion is supported by the little parasite migration to surrounding tissues or draining lymph nodes and the evidence of parasite proliferation at the site of infection.[3] Therefore, infecting trypomastigotes probably invade host tissue cells at the site of infection (e.g., fibroblasts), transform to cytoplasmic amastigotes forms, and proliferate, with very few parasites spread to some other adjacent tissues or draining lymph nodes.[4] It is not well established if the few parasites that get access to the draining lymph nodes right after infection make their way by themselves or are passively transported by immune cells like dendritic cells that migrate to the lymph nodes after acquiring antigen in the periphery. Ultimately, after several rounds of replication inside tissue cells, parasites would be released to gain access to other distant organs through the bloodstream. Thereupon, parasites that arrive to the draining lymph node right after the initial infection do not seem to be effectively presented to trigger an adaptive immune response, which is developed only after the first week postinfection, coincident with the release of parasites that replicate at the site of infection.[3,5]

Several factors seem to be involved in this delay in the onset of the adaptive immune response during the first days postinfection, including the parasite number and the activation signals provided to the antigen presenting cells that will initiate the adaptive response. This early period seems to be a rather immunologically "silent" one with very few immune mechanisms that reveal the infectious process going on. A vaccination approach that shortens this response time could have a favorable impact controlling the first parasite proliferation at the site of infection. However if during this "silent" period, parasites are not "visible" to the immune system due to an insufficient activation of the antigen presenting cells that display the relevant antigens, the presence already of memory cells from a previous vaccine may not drastically modify this initial response time. On this sense, some evidence suggests that reinfecting parasites may be rapidly controlled by a fully activated immune response maintained by an ongoing infection (premunition), but this parasite control at the site of infection may be delayed when the previous infection has been resolved leaving resting memory cells that need to be reactivated by antigen presentation. It could be suggested that the delay in the generation of the adaptive response would allow the parasites to reach other tissues like muscle or adipose tissue where immunological or metabolic factors could allow them to chronically persist.[6,7] Based on the hypothesis that an insufficient activation of the antigen presenting cells during *T. cruzi* infection could influence the speed of the origination of the immune response, vaccines based on live-attenuated parasites should incorporate additional immune activating molecules to those originally provided by the parasites. So far some *T. cruzi* molecules have been shown to activate Toll-like receptors TLR2 and TLR9,[8] although these TLR ligands, GPI anchors, and DNA may not be freely available in live parasites initiating the infection which would reduce their activating effect on antigen presenting cells.[9] In agreement with this hypothesis, parasites genetically modified to express TLR ligands from other pathogens induce an earlier immune response.[10]

Once generated, the adaptive immune response is highly efficient in controlling the parasite level, even though this strong response does not reach the total clearance of the parasites. This adaptive immune response is mainly characterized by the presence of specific antibodies, some of which have the capacity to lyse trypomastigote forms and are generically called lytic antibodies.[11] The cellular branch of this adaptive immune response is characterized by CD4$^+$ and CD8$^+$ T cells, both of them crucial for parasite control.[12,13] Our knowledge about the specific CD8$^+$ T cells response notably increased due to the identification of specific parasite epitopes recognized by these immune cells and the application of new immunological techniques.[14,15] Among these specific epitopes, the TSKB20 peptide (ANYKFTLV) present in some proteins of the transialidase superfamily has been successfully used to follow the kinetics of the CD8$^+$ T cell response by staining with MHC class I complexes containing this peptide. The CD8$^+$ T cell response against TSKB20 is one of the highest responses described so far involving approximately 20−30% of the total CD8$^+$ T cell population at its peak.[14] After the contraction, these CD8$^+$ T cells persist in low levels with characteristics predominantly of an effector memory population[16] and a smaller subset of cells displaying central memory markers.[17] Despite the strong humoral and cellular response mounted against *T. cruzi* in the acute phase, parasites manage to avoid clearance and persist chronically. The reasons for the incapability of the immune system to completely eliminate parasites are not fully understood and represent an important aspect to be covered for the rationale of developing an effective vaccine. Recently a lower "fitness" of the CD8$^+$ T cells generated during *T. cruzi* infection compared to those generated by a *T. cruzi* gene-expressing adenovirus vaccine has been suggested as a possible explanation for parasite persistence, however the precise mechanisms required to drive the CD8$^+$ T cell response toward a more effective one are not clear.[18]

Even though a strong CD8$^+$ T cell response is elicited against *T. cruzi* and the relevance of this lymphocyte population for host survival, the precise mechanisms by which these cells control the infection are not completely understood. Depletion or lack of CD8$^+$ T cells leads to high susceptibility and mortality of infected mice[19] and it has been shown that cytotoxic CD8$^+$ T cells from infected animals are able to identify and destroy cells loaded with parasite peptides or parasite infected ones.[20] However, it has not been clearly demonstrated yet the importance of these cells to recognize and destroy parasite infected cells in vivo, specially cells known to be chronically infected like muscle fibers or adipocytes, nor that this cytotoxic lysis of infected cells is an effective mechanism to control parasite load in vivo. Furthermore, experiments with perforin-deficient mice yielded contradictory results in terms of susceptibility to the infection.[15,21] Therefore, the development of a vaccine that stimulates a strong CD8$^+$ T cells response against intracellular parasites is desirable, even when the mechanistic bases of the protection conferred by those cells is still not fully defined.

Other important effector function exerted by CD8$^+$ T cells is IFN-gamma production. This cytokine is also produced by CD4$^+$ T cells and NK among others cells. IFN-$\gamma$ has been shown crucial in directing the development of naïve CD4$^+$ T cells toward a Th-1 phenotype as well as activating macrophages. IFN-$\gamma$ is considered a key cytokine involved in the control of T. cruzi because mice deficient in this cytokine are highly susceptible to the infection and succumb in the acute phase. Therefore, it is a generally accepted notion that a vaccine against T. cruzi should induce a response with a Th-1 cytokine profile.[22] Regardless of its demonstrated involvement in the resistance to infection and its activation effect on macrophages, there is no clear mechanism linking IFN-$\gamma$ production and parasite control in vivo.

Although there is some contradiction about the importance of the CD4$^+$ T cells in the development of the CD8$^+$ T cell response during T. cruzi infection,[5,23] their role in the control of the parasite is clearly demonstrated by the high susceptibility of mice defective in CD4$^+$ T cells which do not survive the acute phase of the infection.[24] The helper functions of the CD4$^+$ lymphocyte subset in the maturation of the antibody producing B lymphocytes as well as orchestrating the cytokine profile make them a fundamental branch of the immune response. However, relatively little is known about their priming characteristics during T. cruzi infection or other antiparasitic features that would be advantageous to develop during a vaccination protocol. Recently, a new subset of noncirculating memory cells called T resident memory cells has shown promising features as a first line of defense in skin and mucosa, which are common infection routes for many pathogens including T. cruzi. The capacity of these cells induced by vaccination to confer protection has been demonstrated in experimental infections with the closely related parasite Leishmania major.[25]

As mentioned before, despite the strong immune response against T. cruzi mounted in the acute phase, parasites survive and settle down to a chronic infection. How do parasites avoid the complete clearance by the immune system? How can we boost or modify this response by prophylactic vaccination to block the progression of the infection and prevent the persistence of the parasites?

One of the mechanisms suggested to participate in the chronic persistence of parasites is the apparent dysfunction of the CD8$^+$ T cells infiltrating the infected muscle tissue. As demonstrated by Leavey and Tarleton,[6] these cells have a lower capacity to produce IFN-γ after restimulation in vitro than their counterparts isolated from spleen. However, this dysfunction does not seem to be induced by T regulatory cells or TGF-β.[26,27] Although chronic infecting parasites cannot be efficiently removed by the immune system, they can successfully be eliminated by the administration of the trypanomicidal drug Benznidazole.[28] After clearance of the parasites, the CD8[+] T cells populations specific against parasite epitopes change their phenotype from effector to central memory cells. This change in the phenotype agrees with the current opinion that the pathogen persistence continuously stimulates the cells, turning them antigen addictive and avoiding the development of a central memory population. Therefore, the expression of central memory markers (e.g., CD62L and CD127) in the specific CD8[+] T cell population has been proposed as an indirect evidence of the efficacy of the drug treatment in this mouse model of *T. cruzi* infection. Unfortunately, the cure by drug treatment does not provide sterile immunity and cured mice displaying specific central memory CD8[+] T cells are able to better control a subsequent infection but unable to completely eliminate the totality of the reinfecting parasites.[29] This poses a considerable challenge for the development of a vaccine against *T. cruzi* infection that provides sterile immunity, since such a vaccine should stimulate and maintained protective mechanisms that are not obtained after the cure of a natural infection. Regarding this matter, the immune response elicited and maintained by a current infection is usually strong enough to provide protection against a second infection. So an ideal vaccine should elicit and keep a response as strong as the one produced by a virulent infection but lacking the pathogenic effects produced by persistent parasites. So far some experimental vaccines with attenuated live parasites have been shown to provide a strong protection against a subsequent reinfection with more virulent parasites, although the parasites from the secondary infection are rarely completely cleared. Also it is highly probably that the maintenance of the protective effect is associated with the persistence of the vaccinating parasites. Moreover, commonly the strength of the immune response originated by the attenuated live parasites used as a vaccine is lower than a response induced by fully virulent parasites.

Here is another paradox of the immune response in *T. cruzi* infection: How is the immune response maintained in the chronic phase so strong as to provide protection against a reinfection but at the same time so inefficient to clear the chronic parasites from the previous infection? How can we boost or redirect the chronic immune response to recognize and eliminate the persistent parasites? Can we design a therapeutic vaccine to modify the already established immune response?

These specific responses persist during the chronic phase and the CD8[+] T cells specific against TSKB20 do not seem to suffer exhaustion, a common phenomenon seen in other chronic infections which results in the loss of the effector functions of the cells and their final deletion.[30] This characteristic of the chronic CD8[+] T cell response in *T. cruzi* opens the possibility for a therapeutic vaccine that could boost the immune response to achieve the complete clearance of the chronic parasites. However, choosing the right antigens against which to restimulate the response and turn the chronic parasites "targetable," as well as modifying the already established immunodominance hierarchy, could be a complicated task. Currently a consortium of academic and industrial partners is working on the development of a therapeutic vaccine based on two recombinant *T. cruzi* antigens,[31] although the capacity of this approach to prevent or delay the onset of Chagasic pathology in human patients is under debate.

# DNA vaccination in experimental models of *Trypanosoma cruzi* infection

In the past two decades, the development of recombinant techniques allowed the production of different immunogens ranging from recombinant proteins to DNA and adenovirus vaccines for experimental *T. cruzi* infection.[32−34] Recombinant proteins allowed testing of several well-defined antigens, but the main immune feature induced by these antigens is the production of specific antibodies. Unfortunately, antibodies are not as effective in controlling *T. cruzi* infection as they are in other infections. Parasites can persist as amastigotes inside host cells avoiding direct contact with antibodies and even after release from infected cells, parasites can survive and be readily detected in the bloodstream of chronically infected animals and patients despite the high level of specific antibodies circulating. In this context a cellular response able to detect and eliminate infected cells seems more suitable for *T. cruzi* control. However, vaccination with native or recombinant proteins generally elicits a considerable antibody response but a limited cellular immunity. This is mainly due to the limited efficacy of exogenous antigens to be directed to the MHC class I pathway which activates cytotoxic T lymphocytes. Therefore, during last years, vaccines that induce a cellular response as DNA vaccines have become more important in Chagas research.

During DNA vaccination an eukaryotic expression plasmid containing the gene of interest is delivered either by intramuscular injection or subcutaneously using a gene-gun. This plasmid is incorporated by antigen presenting cells that produce the protein codified in the gene and direct it to the MHC class I pathway for antigen presentation. Besides developing a strong cellular response, DNA vaccines have the potential for easy manufacturing and broad administration as well as non cold-chain requirements, key features for vaccines intended for the poor countries where tropical diseases are endemic. Also the cytokine profile of the immune response generated by DNA vaccination can be directed toward a strong cellular Th-1 response which is considered to be protective against *T. cruzi* infection, by adding in the vaccine formulation genes codifying for costimulatory proteins like cytokine IL-12.[35,36]

Albeit sterile immunity after the challenge has not been reported in DNA vaccine experiments, vaccination protocols were successful at decreasing parasitemia, tissue damage, and mortality in mouse models immunized with different *T. cruzi* genes.[37] Primarily CD8[+] and CD4[+] T cells have been described as the effector mechanisms responsible for protective immunity in mice vaccinated with *T. cruzi* genes, since the depletion of these cells subpopulations resulted in the abrogation of the protection.[35,38] The genes tested in DNA vaccines belong mainly to the large trans-sialidase superfamily of surface proteins expressed in amastigotes or trypomastigotes with a few example of other unrelated genes. Immunization experiments carried out by different laboratories demonstrated the efficacy of DNA vaccines containing genes encoding Amastigote Surface Proteins and Trans-Sialidase proteins to confer protection against *T. cruzi* infection.[38–40] However, broad vaccination approaches based on antigens belonging to superfamilies with several different genes and high variability among parasite strains could be difficult due to the elevated chances of mutation on the antigen structure that could render the immune response against them ineffective.[41]

Several *T. cruzi* genes have been tested and provided protection against the infection opening the possibility of a multivalent vaccine composed of different parasite genes and costimulatory molecules.[42] Heterologous priming and boosting protocols combining DNA vaccines with recombinant proteins or viral vectors have been successfully explored. Usually the immunogenic and protective characteristics of the combined protocols were improved over the single individual methodologies. In this sense, the recombinant proteins reinforced the CD4$^+$ and B cell activation of DNA vaccines while the boost with viral vectors strengthened the CD8$^+$ response in a more efficient way than a homologous DNA vaccine boost.[43] This last combined immunization approach is highly interesting due to the induction of a CD4$^+$ and CD8$^+$ T cell mediated protection which was demonstrated to be dependent on IFN-$\gamma$ and perforin.

Even more, DNA vaccines have been used not just as preventive vaccines before the challenge infection but also as therapeutic vaccines administered to chronically infected animals. These experiments demonstrate the capacity of DNA vaccines not only to protect against a posterior virulent challenge but to reduce the immunopathology associated with an existing infection.[44] Zapata Estrella et al.[45] were able to dramatically reduce the parasitemia and the cardiac tissue damage as well as rapidly increase the number of CD4$^+$ and CD8$^+$ T cells of mice injected in the acute phase with a DNA vaccine encoding two different *T. cruzi* antigens. Even though DNA vaccines with therapeutic properties are promising, not all the antigens used are equally efficient.[46] Recently, the therapeutic effect of DNA vaccines has been evaluated in experimentally infected dogs.[47] This study suggests that therapeutic DNA vaccines may be a promising novel therapy for Chagas disease in dogs which are the principal domestic reservoirs for *T. cruzi* in endemic areas.

Many of the genes tested in DNA vaccines have been chosen for being present in the infective amastigote or trypomastigote forms.[48] The currently accepted opinion is that the immune response should be directed against these parasite stages present in the mammalian host, rather than the epimastigote extracts used in earlier times containing proteins expressed in the insect vector that could not be relevant for protection. Nowadays, the availability of the *T. cruzi* genome, transcriptome, and proteome[49–51] allows the screening for genes in the entire genome and to choose specific genes which codify for proteins with peptides that are predicted to bind specific MHC molecules as well as genes of proteins that have been identified as specific for a parasite stage. This detailed information about possible vaccine candidates and new technologies open an unprecedented opportunity for the rational development of new vaccination strategies.[52]

One important advantage over other vaccination approaches used in experimental *T. cruzi* infection is the safety of DNA vaccines. They do not integrate into the genome as viral vector vaccines do and have been proved to be safe in clinical trials for other diseases.[53] Also unlike the attenuated or genetically modified live parasites, they are not autoreplicative organisms that could revert to a virulent phenotype or trigger the pathology associated with Chagas disease. Considering these aspects, DNA vaccines may be the most promising approach for a vaccine against *T. cruzi* infection applicable to humans. However, the protection level obtained with these vaccines is still very limited and more research has to be performed in order to improve their efficacy.

A broader and stronger immune response than that obtained with DNA vaccines can be achieved by immunization with live-attenuated or genetically modified parasites. Nevertheless the inoculation of live parasites in humans entails obvious ethical and practical problems, making its human application very unlikely. Still vaccination with genetically modified parasites could be eventually implemented for domestic animals involved in the transmission cycle of *T. cruzi*. The rationale for this intervention is to target domestic animals which are reservoirs of the parasite for the infection of the insect vectors. Dogs have been pointed out as the best candidates for this sort of vaccine intended to block the transmission to humans, mainly for the preponderant role of dogs as sources of parasites in the domestic environment.[54] The dog population is also the target of several vaccine formulations against visceral leishmaniasis due to its role as main domestic reservoir, some of these approaches have shown to confer protection and been registered as commercial canine vaccines.[55]

# Vaccination with attenuated parasites (premunition)

## Basic laboratory studies on premunition against Typanosoma cruzi

In 1952, Pizzi[56] published that mice that had been inoculated with a *T. cruzi* epimastigote culture presenting low virulence became resistant to reinoculations of virulent parasites. From 1965 to 1990, Menezes published a series of papers based on the vaccination of mice against virulent *T. cruzi* infection by means of preinoculations with an avirulent strain (PF), derived from the virulent Y strain.[57–59] Animals inoculated with cultures where epimastigote forms predominated, became resistant and survived lethal *T. cruzi* inoculations.[60] The experiments were replicated in dogs where the levels of parasitemia and mortality rates were significantly reduced. Moreover, electrocardiographic determinations and histopathological studies of the myocardium showed a clear prevention of functional and anatomic lesions of the heart.[61] Dr. Menezes' preclinical and Phase I clinical studies were completed with inoculations into *Callitrix* monkeys and humans, including himself.[62] Most inoculations used by Menezes for experimental vaccination contained mostly epimastigotes, with a low proportion of trypomastigotes. The term "avirulent" was challenged by Chiari,[63] who demonstrated infections by means of hemoculture in mice inoculated with doses as low as 5000 metacyclic trypomastigotes from PF cultures, although direct blood examination was negative. Since Menezes himself had acknowledged exceptional cases of demonstrated infection in PF strain-inoculated animals, the term "attenuated" seemed more adequate to describe *T. cruzi* strains of very low infectivity.

Some other attenuated *T. cruzi* strains with protective activity have been described. Cultures of the "Corpus Christi" strain were unable to establish apparent infections when $10^7$ live culture forms were inoculated into C3H(He) mice. Mice preinoculated with this strain developed resistance against a further infection with the virulent Brazil strain. Moreover, this resistance could be also obtained in naïve mice by transfer of spleen cells from immunized mice to nonimmunized receptor ones. Depletion of the B cell population but not of the T cell components abrogated the adoptive transfer of resistance.[64]

The group of Gattas made a series of presentations to the Brazilian Meetings of Basic Research in Chagas Disease reporting the apparent lack of infectivity of a *T. cruzi* clone derived from the CL strain of *T. cruzi* and named the clone CL-14. Inoculations of $2 \times 10^6$ metacyclic forms into highly susceptible, newborn BALB mice produced no detectable parasitemias and protected against virulent challenge in a time- and dose-dependent manner, as shown by blood parasite counts and detailed histological observations.[65] Further studies with more sensitive methods such as hemoculture and xenodiagnosis also failed to reveal infection with metacyclic forms of this clone, whether they were derived from vectors or from axenic cultures.[66] The specific antibody levels were much lower in mice inoculated with clone CL-14 than in those inoculated with the parental strain CL. Furthermore CL-14 infected mice did not produce the polyclonal response which is characteristic of *T. cruzi* infection.[67]

Some partial insights into the mechanisms of attenuation of the CL-14 clone were obtained by the group of Yoshida et al.[68] They carried out a series of comparisons between the attenuated CL-14 and the "wild-type" CL strain dominant surface glycoproteins. The ability of this attenuated clone to infect HeLa cells in vitro was reduced four-fold and no intracellular replication was observed. The expression of GP82, a dominant surface glycoprotein known to play an important role in infectivity, was shown to be close to 10-fold lower, as measured by fluorescent antibody-labeled parasites analyzed by flow cytometry. The genomic organization of the GP82 gene family, as shown by the hybridization patterns of GP82-labeled probes that did not show remarkable differences in the attenuated clone when compared to the original CL parental strain. However, chromosomal mapping of the gene family, which displayed a wide distribution across several pulse-field electrophoretically separated chromosomes, revealed some distinct patterns in CL-14 as compared with CL.

Other metacyclic trypomastigote surface molecules known to interact with host cells, such as cruzipain (GP 57-51), trans-sialidase (TS), and the mucin-like GP

35-50, were examined in the CL-14 clone. The expression of cruzipain was higher, a finding consistent with determinations by Paiva et al.[69] for clone CL-14. However, in three other attenuated strains (TCC, Tul 0, and Y-null), a clear reduction of cruzipain gelatinolytic activity as compared with three virulent strains was detected.[70] Regarding TS, its activity in CL-14 was 1.6-fold higher than in the CL wild-type strain,[68] confirming previous studies by Gattas et al.[71] Similarly, a remarkable increase in TS activity was detected in the TCC-attenuated strain. The relative increase, in strains of low infectivity, of proteins known to play a role in infection may seem, in principle, paradoxical. However, the existence of multiple isoforms of these proteins, many of which may be inactive or irrelevant for infection, may explain their overexpression or rebound production in parasites of low infectivity.

A long-term culture, named TCC (*Trypanosoma cruzi* de Cultivo) was shown to be unable to persistently infect mice or rabbits.[72] It was cloned twice, in 1980 and 1990, and characterized after 2000 as belonging to *T. cruzi* I lineage. The attenuated phenotype was stable, since no virulent sublines could be derived by either mouse culture or insect vector passage, tested repeatedly until lines were extinguished. Since strains of very low virulence but unexpectedly displaying high pathogenicity have been described,[73] this possibility was examined for the TCC strain. Mice inoculated with cultures were subjected to long-term histopathological studies. This strain was unable to trigger immunopathological responses or to induce histopathological alterations in immunocompetent mice.[72] Experiments involving laboratory conditions to enforce infection (high trypomastigote inocula into newborn or immunosuppressed animals) allowed the demonstration of infections with extremely low density; however, attempts to propagate these infections indefinitely from mouse to mouse, always failed.

Leguizamón et al.[74] examined the process of attenuation by prolonged passage in culture in an originally virulent *T. cruzi* strain, named RA. They demonstrated a correlation between the attenuation of infectivity and the time the parasites were propagated in axenic culture (up to 2 years). Even though the original line was highly virulent, after 2 years in culture, inocula of $10^7$ epimastigotes were unable to produce detectable parasitemia in immunocompetent, susceptible BALB mice. However, reactivation of virulence was shown by serial passage in athymic mice. Conversely, similar serial passages were attempted with the attenuated TCC strain but inocula of $10^5$ TCC trypomastigotes into *nu/nu* athymic mice rarely caused detectable blood parasitemia, although parasite tissue nests were found more often in urinary bladder and heart atria. Homogenates of these tissues, where the presence of parasites was verified, were thus used routinely for serial passage and weakly infective TCC sublines could be recovered, but not serially propagated in immunodeficient mice.

Serological studies in mice[75,76] and dogs[77] indicated antibody titer regression to negative values in most animals, although some mice remained seropositive after 1 year. Inoculation of live TCC epimastigotes afforded protection, not only against acute infection, but also against late development of chronic pathology induced by either the Tulahuen laboratory strain or also by 17 wild isolates obtained in a broad endemic area of Argentina.[78] Electrocardiographic studies in mice showed that

TCC preinoculations before virulent infection significantly reduced functional alterations of the heart, such as sinus bradycardia, supraventricular tachycardia, and atrioventricular blocks.[79]

## Field studies on premunition in guinea pigs and dogs

In contrast with the short-term resistance induced by nonreplicating immunogens, the TCC culture induced long-lasting resistance over a year after inoculation.[80] TCC-induced protection was not restricted to laboratory mice and was also demonstrated in an ecologic field model of *T. cruzi* transmission consisting of standard corrals of loose bricks surrounded by mosquito net tents, where guinea pigs and *Triatoma infestans* shared an entomologically isolated, seminatural environment. Experiments involving large numbers of guinea pigs showed that TCC parasites did not propagate in a natural vector–host cycle. Moreover, TCC inoculations protected these domestic reservoir animals against naturally transmitted infection and the trafficking of parasites from hosts to vectors was significantly reduced, acting as a transmission-blocking vaccine.[80,81]

Measurement of the efficiency of insect vectors to transmit *T. cruzi* infection to mammalian hosts is cumbersome since variables such as parasite load and frequency of bites, and also behavioral and physiologic factors are involved. Nevertheless, the systematic measurement of several transmission variables in guinea pig yards, such as number of hosts, number of vectors, days of exposure, proportion of fed vectors and proportion of infected vectors, allowed to estimate the "number of bites necessary for infection" (NBNI).[82] This estimation showed that vaccination with TCC parasites produced an average 4.28-fold increase in NBNI in several independent experiments.

Experiments with naturally infected dogs[77] also indicated a transmission-blocking effect of the TCC live-attenuated vaccine. TCC-immunized dogs displayed a lower proportion of infected animals after 1 year of exposure to natural infection in an endemic area, as shown by serologic-xenodiagnostic parameters. A different parameter, the average percentage of bugs that became infected after feeding on vaccinated or control dogs exposed for 2 years to natural infection, also showed lower values in vaccinated dogs, indicating that vaccination apparently exerted a transmission-blocking effect: lower parasite load and reduced capacity to disseminate the parasite through vectors. A similar effect of vaccination has been confirmed by Basso et al.[83] in dogs immunized with killed *T. rangeli* and challenged with *T. cruzi*.

## Generation of attenuated parasites by genetic manipulation and their use as potential vaccines against Chagas disease

Despite the good short-term immunization results achieved with nonreplicating experimental immunogens against *T. cruzi*[40,84−89] and based on the quality and length of the protection achieved, the inoculation and infection by live-attenuated parasites seem to confer so far the best vaccine effect. These attenuated strains have been shown to yield substantial protection in murine models against a virulent challenge. However, the genetic background and the potential of reversion to a virulent phenotype cannot be foretold, turning them unsuitable for use in human vaccination trials. Nevertheless, the generation of gene transfer experiments as well as the development of new molecular techniques for endogenous gene manipulation has offered the possibility of a better understanding of trypanosomatid genetics and biology. We are now able to identify specific genes in silico, and then, by gene target deletion through homologous recombination, remove them from the parasite genome. This alternative is tempting and promising, since genes related to virulence or persistence could be specifically and permanently deleted or altered. In malaria, the use of genetically modified parasites as experimental vaccines has been well studied.[90−92] In different *Plasmodium*—mouse models, it has been shown that infections with genetically manipulated malaria parasites conferred sterile protection against lethal challenge.[93−96] Vaccination approaches based on genetically altered live parasites are also currently under study for Leishmaniasis.[97−99] However, in comparison to what has been published for other parasitic organisms, there are relatively few genes which have been genetically manipulated in *T. cruzi*. The first report of stable transfection of a plasmid vector by homologous recombination in *T. cruzi* was done in 1993.[100] Since then and to our knowledge, there are not many proteins that have been studied in *T. cruzi* through gene-targeted deletion,[101−113] due initially to the lack of more straightforward methods for gene manipulation needed for reverse genetic studies in this organism. However, and until recently, homologous recombination was the only method available for gene suppression or downregulation, since RNA interference has, to date, failed in *T. cruzi*.[114] Recently, advanced and more efficient gene-editing methods have been applied. The CRISPR-Cas9 system was adapted to *T. cruzi*, demonstrating rapid and efficient downregulation of multiple endogenous genes, including essential genes. This progress holds the promise of developing a variety of genetically defined, mutant *T. cruzi* strains for immunization.[115,116]

Most mutants were studied in in vitro systems in order to elucidate metabolic pathways, resistance or susceptibility to different anti-*T. cruzi* compounds, differentiation of life cycle stages, etc. Only a few *T. cruzi* mutants have been evaluated in in vivo models and even fewer are the ones evaluated as potential vaccines.[117,118]

One of the *T. cruzi* proteins which has been well characterized by reverse genetic studies is the surface glycoprotein GP72. This protein is proposed to be involved in the differentiation of life cycle stages of the parasite[119]; although its precise role in this process is not completely understood. Parasites carrying a targeted deletion of the gene coding for the GP72 protein were generated (Y-null) and an unexpected altered morphology on the general shape of the parasite was observed as a result of this gene deletion.[106] Contrary to that observed for Y wild-type parasites, Y-null parasites could not easily be detected when injected in highly susceptible mouse models.[120] PCR reactions carried out in order to determine *T. cruzi* presence, as well as serological reactions for specific antibodies indicated that Y-null infections were no longer detectable after 90 days postinfection, suggesting that the GP72 protein is essential for sustaining latent infections in immunocompetent animals. Inoculation of Y-null mutant parasites strongly protected adult Swiss mice against a challenge with virulent blood trypomastigotes, as shown by a decrease in parasite load in mice preinoculated with the mutant parasites. Even though the protective effect was detectable and significant up to 14 months, the longest interval tested after priming, a weakening of the protection was observed.[121] In this sense, and as mentioned before, the duration of the protective effect could be directly related to the antigenic offer at which the immune system is constantly exposed.

In another approach, a monoallelic mutant clone for the calmodulin-ubiquitin (*cub*) gene (TulCub8) was obtained from the highly virulent Tulahuen strain of *T. cruzi*. Genetic manipulation of the cub gene resulted in a remarkable reduction in parasite virulence as shown in a murine model; since the mutant clone could only be propagated in mice by means of highly sensitive, hemoculture recovery. Swiss mice were inoculated subcutaneously with doses of TulCub8 epimastigotes and later challenged with virulent wild-type Tulahuen blood trypomastigotes. In this case, a strong protection, based on a reduction in parasite burden in mice preinoculated with TulCub8 epimastigotes, was observed.[122]

The third *T. cruzi* mutant tested in protection assays was the *T. cruzi* clone L16, a *Lyt1*[−/−] null mutant carrying a biallelic deletion of the gene. The infective and protective behavior of the biallelic knockout clone L16 in a murine model was analyzed by Zago et al.[123] A significant reduction in the infective capacity of clone L16 was observed in adult Swiss mice, determined by fresh blood mounts, spleen index, and tissue parasite load. Furthermore, a considerable reduction in the muscle inflammatory response elicited by the L16 clone as compared to wild-type parasites was detected. However, a latent and persistent infection with this mutant clone was shown by positive *T. cruzi* DNA detection in blood samples until 12 months postinfection. Long-term protection was also observed in Swiss mice inoculated with L16 epimastigotes. Fourteen months later, these animals were still strongly protected against a challenge with Tulahuen wild-type blood trypomastigotes as shown by a reduction in the parasite load in blood.[123]

Another set of genes involved in amastigote energy metabolism is the one encoding the putative enoyl-coenzyme A hydratase/isomerase proteins (ECH1 and ECH2). Mutants carrying only one copy of the *ech1* gene and none of the *ech2* genes failed to establish persistent infections in mice. However, oral gavage of *ech* mutants in mice induced a systemic muscle tissue infection and a potent *T. cruzi* specific CD8[+] T cell response.[124] Protection conferred by these mutant parasites was obtained after three doses of $10^5$ trypomastigotes administered 2 weeks apart by oral route. Challenge was performed in the footpad using fluorescent trypomastigotes[125] 45 days after the last immunization dose. A high number of activated CD8[+] T cells in peripheral blood of *ech* mutant vaccinated group was detected and it was in concordance with a strong protective response, indicating thus T cell proliferation could be a good indicator of the effectiveness of the vaccine.

Since the molecular basis of attenuation in the wild-type TCC strain of *T. cruzi* is still unknown, attempts to introduce targeted gene deletions into this clone, as a safety mechanism against eventual reversion to the virulent phenotype were carried out. A TCC monoallelic mutant clone for the dihydrofolate reductase—thymidylate synthase gene (*dhfr-ts*) was generated.[112] In trypanosomatids, dihydrofolate reductase—thymidylate synthase (*dhfr-ts*) is a single-copy gene encoding an important enzyme involved in the thymidine biosynthesis pathway and, therefore, in the DNA synthesis. Besides showing some delay in growth rate in axenic cultures, TCC *dhfr-ts*[+/−] parasites also showed a striking attenuation in in vivo models. A remarkably low percentage of *T. cruzi* specific CD8[+] T cell was detected in mice inoculated with TCC *dhfr-ts*[+/−] parasites. This is not ideal, since the generation of genetically attenuated parasites capable of inducing a strong CD8[+] T cell response is desirable. However, these mutant parasites retained their protective effect against a virulent *T. cruzi* challenge in different mouse strains. Even more, these mutant parasites retained their protective effect against a virulent challenge with virulent fluorescent trypomastigote parasites even after a year postinoculation. In all experiments performed, the protection induced by mutant parasites did not differ from that obtained with wild-type parasites, suggesting that the deletion of one *dhfr-ts* allele did not alter the protective capacity of the original wild-type live immunogen.[112]

The TCC strain was also genetically manipulated at the *crt* locus[113] since mutant parasites with a monoallelic deletion of the TcCRT gene were generated. *T. cruzi* Calreticulin is a calcium-binding chaperone involved in the quality control of endoplasmic reticulum nascent proteins. After being translocated to the flagellum pocket, TcCRT inhibits the activation of the classical and lectin complement pathways evading the lytic action of the complement in the host blood system. TcCRT mutant epimastigotes parasites have a high susceptibility to the lytic action of the complement system, compared with the wild-type strain and displayed a stable loss of virulence.[113] Mice receiving a prime and boost immunization regimen of $10^5$ mutant or wild-type TCC metacyclic tripomastigotes were protected against a virulent challenge with a *T. cruzi* field isolate[126] after 120 days of the last immunization dose. Mice immunized with TcCRT mutant and TCC wild-type parasites displayed, after challenge, a significantly lowered parasite density in peripheral blood. Necropsies at day 60 postinfection revealed that mice immunized with mutant parasites showed reduced inflammatory response in heart and muscle tissues, compared to controls. Also, the spleen index was significantly reduced in mutant and wild-type TCC-immunized mice.[127]

To our knowledge, the studies mentioned above are the only ones involving knockout *T. cruzi* clones in protection assays. These studies included control groups where mice preinoculated with the "wild-type," nonengineered *T. cruzi* strain were challenged with virulent parasites. Inhibition of acute phase parasitemia was as strong as with the mutants, but this "protection" (or premunition) was obtained at the expense of a previous infection with heavy parasite load and development of disease. These control groups thus showed that the mutated parasites retained the immunogenic effects of a mild infection, sparing the untoward effects of a previous acute and chronic phase disease. However, the immune bases of the protection elicited by these genetically modified parasites, as well as the presence of inflammatory infiltrates or amastigote nests in target organs after challenge was not always fully evaluated. However, these results reinforce the possibility of generating transgenic experimental vaccines that combine the immunogenicity of live vaccines and a genetically supported built-in safety modification, currently absent in naturally attenuated parasites.

Also attractive is the generation of mutant parasites expressing foreign genes such as specific immune factors. CD40 is a cell surface receptor belonging to the TNF family and its ligand, CD40L, is a costimulatory protein belonging to the same family. The CD40/CD40L complex not only presents immunomodulatory properties but is also involved in the humoral and cellular response.[128] It has been previously shown that *T. cruzi* parasitemia and mortality rate could significantly be reduced in infected mice by the inoculation of CD40L-transfected fibroblasts together with *T. cruzi* parasites.[129] Mice infected with transgenic *T. cruzi* parasites carrying a plasmid encoding the gene CD40L were able to better control infection than those infected with wild-type *T. cruzi* ones. IFN-$\gamma$ production and lymphocyte proliferation was observed by immunization with CD40L-parasites. Even more important is the protective capacity conferred by these parasites. A very low or even null level of parasites was detected in the group of mice first infected with the transgenic parasites, suggesting that the infection by these parasites is able to induce protection against a subsequent virulent infection.[130]

In summary, *T. cruzi* is an organism where gene-targeted deletion and gene silencing have so far not been as successfully applied as in bacteria or even as in other trypanosomatids, such as *Trypanosoma brucei* and *Leishmania*. Studies where *T. cruzi* mutants were compared with wild-type parasites using infectivity measurements, almost invariably revealed a change toward attenuation. Sometimes this change has been profound and sometimes partial. Therefore, targeted deletion of specific genes can be conceived as a potential procedure to generate clones able to develop in culture, but less efficient to invade and persist in vivo, providing a potential for mass production coupled with a built-in safety device against reversion to the virulent phenotype. The use of *T. cruzi* attenuated parasites is very appealing since the infection obtained thereof is much alike to a natural infection and may consequently lead to the establishment of a protective immune response. However, genome manipulation could lead to a loss of the protective immunity, either because such genetically modified parasites no longer express antigen epitopes essentials for triggering a good immune response or because they are not able to persist long enough to fully activate the immune system. In this sense, a wide spectrum of specific individual genes or a combination of them, as well as different *T. cruzi* strains should be evaluated.

Considering the recent improvements in genetic manipulation, a live-genetically attenuated parasite vaccine applicable to dogs and other mammals, which act as natural reservoirs, and with capacity to reduce the intensity and spread of the disease seems to be a possible and realistic achievement. An important factor to be considered is the presence of antibiotic-resistant genes in the genome of these "vaccine" parasites and the possible implications that this could bring. Drug resistance genes are the common mechanism to select genetically modified parasites; nonetheless the release of drug-resistant parasites to the environment implies an undesirable and potential risk. Hence, one of the main objectives for these mutant parasites is to make them incapable of persistence in the host and completely unable to be spread or transmitted to the insect vectors. Another approach to tackle the drug resistance problem is a new strategy exploited in the generation of *Leishmania* mutant parasites, in which after the target deletion, the drug-resistant gene is removed from the parasite genome.[131] Furthermore, the generation of *T. cruzi* parasites genetically modified in order to "commit suicide" as a response to external stimulus is also an appealing alternative.[132] In this approach, genetically modified parasites could be inoculated and allowed to infect the mice until a fully immune response is developed before being induced to die. This technology has been well documented in other parasitic organisms such as *Leishmania*.[133,134] Based on this, genetically modified *T. cruzi* parasites could be achieved and safely used as live vaccines.

The recent elucidation of the trypanosomatids genomes and the identification of new targets for genetic manipulation open the possibility of generating a wide variety of mutant parasites that could be evaluated as potential vaccines against Chagas disease. The generation of parasites carrying more than one gene deletion or a combination of gene deletions and/or expression of foreign genes could also be feasible. The strategy of superimposing attenuating mutations into already naturally attenuated and protective strains might provide additional mechanisms against reversion to virulent phenotypes.

# Final considerations

In the last decades repeated insecticide spraying in several endemic regions in South America resulted in a considerable control of the insect vectors for Chagas disease as well as in a reduction in the natural transmission of the parasite to humans. It has also become more evident that Chagas disease, as well as other neglected diseases, is a "poverty-disease" and that basic improvements in the housing conditions and economical development of the endemic areas would have a huge impact on its control. Considering this, we might wonder: do we really need a vaccine against Chagas disease? The answer to this question seems to be yes, even more now than before. Unfortunately, the economic and social conditions of the rural areas in South America where the disease is endemic are unlikely to remarkably improve at least in the next 10 years. Additionally, the current occurrence of insecticide-resistant populations of vectors jeopardizes the achievements of the massive spraying and active control successfully implemented in some regions. Clearly, a human vaccine or a veterinary one intended to block the transmission of *T. cruzi* is not going to solve the problem of Chagas disease by itself. But unquestionably, the availability of a vaccine combined with effective insecticide spraying and improvement in the dwellings will have a remarkable impact on the health and social development of the people living in endemic areas.

# Acknowledgments

We thank Dr. Mirella Ciaccio for first introducing to our laboratory the Molecular Biology techniques necessary for gene-targeted deletion, for characterizing some of the mutants here described and for teaching these methods to new generations of researchers in our group. We thank also all the past and present technicians and researchers of the Instituto de Patología Experimental for their continuous efforts to investigate the biology and genetics of *T. cruzi* and the immune response elicited during its infection.

# References

1. Hotez PJ, Ferris MT. The antipoverty vaccines. *Vaccine* 2006;**24**(31−32):5787−99.
2. Ritter U, Frischknecht F, van Zandbergen G. Are neutrophils important host cells for Leishmania parasites? *Trends Parasitol* 2009;**25**(11):505−10.
3. Padilla AM, Simpson LJ, Tarleton RL. Insufficient TLR activation contributes to the slow development of CD8[+] T cell responses in *Trypanosoma cruzi* infection. *J Immunol* 2009;**183**(2):1245−52.
4. Giddings OK, Eickhoff CS, Smith TJ, Bryant LA, Hoft DF. Anatomical route of invasion and protective mucosal immunity in *Trypanosoma cruzi* conjunctival infection. *Infect Immun* 2006;**74**(10):5549−60.
5. Tzelepis F, Persechini P, Rodrigues M. Modulation of CD4 T cell-dependent specific cytotoxic CD8 T cells differentiation and proliferation by the timing of increase in the pathogen load. *PLoS ONE* 2007;**2**(4):e393.
6. Leavey JK, Tarleton RL. Cutting edge: dysfunctional CD8+ T cells reside in nonlymphoid tissues during chronic *Trypanosoma cruzi* infection. *J Immunol* 2003;**170**(5):2264−8.
7. Combs TP, Nagajyothi, Mukherjee S, de Almeida CJ, Jelicks LA, Schubert W, et al. The adipocyte as an important target cell for *Trypanosoma cruzi* infection. *J Biol Chem* 2005;**280**(25):24085−94.
8. Bafica A, Santiago HC, Goldszmid R, Ropert C, Gazzinelli RT, Sher A. Cutting edge: TLR9 and TLR2 signaling together account for MyD88-dependent control of parasitemia in *Trypanosoma cruzi* infection. *J Immunol* 2006;**177**(6):3515−19.
9. Tarleton R. Immune system recognition of *Trypanosoma cruzi*. *Curr Op Immun* 2007;**19**:430−4.
10. Kurup SP, Tarleton RL. Perpetual expression of PAMPs necessary for optimal immune control and clearance of a persistent pathogen. *Nat Commun* 2013;**4**:2616.
11. Krautz G, Kissinger J, Krettli A. The targets of the lytic antibody response against *Trypanosoma cruzi*. *Parasitol Today* 2000;**16**(1):31−4.
12. Kumar S, Tarleton RL. Antigen-specific Th1 but not Th2 cells provide protection from lethal *Trypanosoma cruzi* infection in mice. *J Immunol* 2001;**166**(7):4596−603.
13. Padilla A, Bustamante J, Tarleton R. CD8+ T cells in Chagas disease. *Curr Opin Immun* 2009;**21**:1−6.
14. Martin D, Weatherly D, Laucella S, Cabinian M, Crim M, Sullivan S, et al. CD8[+] T-Cell responses to *Trypanosoma cruzi* are highly focused on strain variant transialidase epitopes. *PLoS Pathogens* 2006;**2**(8):e77.
15. Tzelepis F, de Alencar BC, Penido ML, Gazzinelli RT, Persechini PM, Rodrigues MM. Distinct kinetics of effector CD8[+] cytotoxic T cells after infection with *Trypanosoma cruzi* in naive or vaccinated mice. *Infect Immun* 2006;**74**(4):2477−81.

16. Martin D, Tarleton R. Antigen-specific T cells maintain an effector memory phenotype during persistent *Trypanosoma cruzi* infection. *J Immun* 2005;**174**:1594−601.

17. Bixby L, Tarleton R. Stable CD8$^+$ T cell memory during persistent *Trypanosoma cruzi* infection. *J Immunol* 2008;**181**:2644−50.

18. Dos Santos Virgilio F, Pontes C, Dominguez MR, Ersching J, Rodrigues MM, Vasconcelos JR. CD8(+) T cell-mediated immunity during *Trypanosoma cruzi* infection: a path for vaccine development? *Mediators Inflamm* 2014;**2014**:243786.

19. Tarleton RL, Koller BH, Latour A, Postan M. Susceptibility of beta 2-microglobulin-deficient mice to *Trypanosoma cruzi* infection. *Nature* 1992;**356**(6367):338−40.

20. Low HP, Santos MA, Wizel B, Tarleton RL. Amastigote surface proteins of *Trypanosoma cruzi* are targets for CD8$^+$ CTL. *J Immunol* 1998;**160**(4):1817−23.

21. Kumar S, Tarleton R. The relative contribution of antibody production and CD8$^+$ T cell function to immune control of *Trypanosoma cruzi*. *Parasite Immunol* 1998;**20** (5):207−16.

22. Hoft DF, Eickhoff CS. Type 1 immunity provides both optimal mucosal and systemic protection against a mucosally invasive, intracellular pathogen. *Infect Immun* 2005;**73** (8):4934−40.

23. Padilla A, Xu D, Martin D, Tarleton R. Limited role for CD4$^+$ T-cell help in the initial priming of *Trypanosoma cruzi*-specific CD8$^+$ T Cells. *Infect Immun* 2007;**75**(1):231−5.

24. Tarleton RL, Grusby MJ, Postan M, Glimcher LH. *Trypanosoma cruzi* infection in MHC-deficient mice: further evidence for the role of both class I- and class II-restricted T cells in immune resistance and disease. *Int Immunol* 1996;**8**(1):13−22.

25. Glennie ND, Yeramilli VA, Beiting DP, Volk SW, Weaver CT, Scott P. Skin-resident memory CD4 + T cells enhance protection against *Leishmania major* infection. *J Exp Med* 2015;**212**(9):1405−14.

26. Kotner J, Tarleton R. Endogenous CD4(+) CD25(+) regulatory T cells have a limited role in the control of *Trypanosoma cruzi* infection in mice. *Infect Immun* 2007;**75** (2):861−9.

27. Martin DL, Postan M, Lucas P, Gress R, Tarleton RL. TGF-beta regulates pathology but not tissue CD8$^+$ T cell dysfunction during experimental *Trypanosoma cruzi* infection. *Eur J Immunol* 2007;**37**(10):2764−71.

28. Bustamante J, Bixby L, Tarleton R. Drug-induced cure drives conversion to a stable and protective CD8$^+$ T central memory response in chronic Chagas disease. *Nat Med* 2008;**14**(5):542−50.

29. Bustamante J, Tarleton R. Reaching for the Holy Grail: insights from infection/cure models on the prospects for vaccines for *Trypanosoma cruzi* infection. *Mem Inst Oswaldo Cruz* 2015;**110**(3):445−51.

30. Shin H, Wherry EJ. CD8 T cell dysfunction during chronic viral infection. *Curr Opin Immunol* 2007;**19**(4):408−15.

31. Dumonteil E, Bottazzi ME, Zhan B, Heffernan MJ, Jones K, Valenzuela JG, et al. Accelerating the development of a therapeutic vaccine for human Chagas disease: rationale and prospects. *Expert Rev Vaccines* 2012;**11**(9):1043−55.

32. Garg N, Bhatia V. Current status and future prospects for a vaccine against American trypanosomiasis. *Expert Rev Vaccines* 2005;**4**(6):867−80.

33. Cazorla S, Frank F, Malchiodi E. Vaccination approaches against *Trypanosoma cruzi* infection. *Expert Rev Vaccines* 2009;**8**(7):921−35.

34. Arce-Fonseca M, Rios-Castro M, Carrillo-Sanchez Sdel C, Martinez-Cruz M, Rodriguez-Morales O. Prophylactic and therapeutic DNA vaccines against Chagas disease. *Parasit Vectors* 2015;**8**:121.

35. Katae M, Miyahira Y, Takeda K, Matsuda H, Yagita H, Okumura K, et al. Coadministration of an interleukin-12 gene and a *Trypanosoma cruzi* gene improves vaccine efficacy. *Infect Immun* 2002;**70**(9):4833−40.

36. Miyahira Y, Akiba H, Katae M, Kubota K, Kobayashi S, Takeuchi T, et al. Cutting edge: a potent adjuvant effect of ligand to receptor activator of NF-kappa B gene for inducing antigen-specific CD8$^+$ T cell response by DNA and viral vector vaccination. *J Immunol* 2003;**171**(12):6344−8.

37. Rodrigues MM, de Alencar BC, Claser C, Tzelepis F, Silveira EL, Haolla FA, et al. Swimming against the current: genetic vaccination against *Trypanosoma cruzi* infection in mice. *Mem Inst Oswaldo Cruz* 2009;**104**(Suppl. 1):281−7.

38. Vasconcelos JR, Hiyane MI, Marinho CR, Claser C, Machado AM, Gazzinelli RT, et al. Protective immunity against *Trypanosoma cruzi* infection in a highly susceptible mouse strain after vaccination with genes encoding the amastigote surface protein-2 and trans-sialidase. *Hum Gene Ther* 2004;**15**(9):878−86.

39. Garg N, Tarleton RL. Genetic immunization elicits antigen-specific protective immune responses and decreases disease severity in *Trypanosoma cruzi* infection. *Infect Immun* 2002;**70**(10):5547−55.

40. Fralish BH, Tarleton RL. Genetic immunization with LYT1 or a pool of trans-sialidase genes protects mice from lethal *Trypanosoma cruzi* infection. *Vaccine* 2003;**20** (21−22):3070−80.

41. Haolla FA, Claser C, de Alencar BC, Tzelepis F, de Vasconcelos JR, de Oliveira G, et al. Strain-specific protective immunity following vaccination against experimental *Trypanosoma cruzi* infection. *Vaccine* 2009;**27**(41):5644−53.

42. Bryan MA, Norris KA. Genetic immunization converts the *Trypanosoma cruzi* B-cell mitogen proline racemase to an effective immunogen. *Infect Immun* 2010;**78**(2): 810−22.

43. de Alencar BC, Persechini PM, Haolla FA, de Oliveira G, Silverio JC, Lannes-Vieira J, et al. Perforin and gamma interferon expression are required for CD4$^+$ and CD8$^+$ T-cell-dependent protective immunity against a human parasite, *Trypanosoma cruzi*, elicited by heterologous plasmid DNA prime-recombinant adenovirus 5 boost vaccination. *Infect Immun* 2009;**77**(10):4383−95.

44. Dumonteil E, Escobedo-Ortegon J, Reyes-Rodriguez N, Arjona-Torres A, Ramirez-Sierra MJ. Immunotherapy of *Trypanosoma cruzi* infection with DNA vaccines in mice. *Infec Immun* 2004;**72**(1):46−53.

45. Zapata Estrella H, Hummel Newell C, Sanchez Burgos G, Escobedo Ortegon J, Ramirez Sierra MJ, Arjona Torres A, et al. Control of *Trypanosoma cruzi* infection and changes in T-cell populations induced by a therapeutic DNA vaccine in mice. *Immun Lett* 2006;**103**(2):186−91.

46. Sanchez-Burgos G, Mezquita-Vega RG, Escobedo-Ortegon J, Ramirez-Sierra MJ, Arjona-Torres A, Ouaissi A, et al. Comparative evaluation of therapeutic DNA vaccines against *Trypanosoma cruzi* in mice. *FEMS Immunol Med Microbiol* 2007;**50**(3):333−41.

47. Quijano-Hernandez IA, Bolio-Gonzalez ME, Rodriguez-Buenfil JC, Ramirez-Sierra MJ, Dumonteila E. Therapeutic DNA vaccine against *Trypanosoma cruzi* infection in dogs. A pilot clinical trial. *An Biodiv Emer Dis* 2008;**1149**:343−6.

48. Silveira EL, Claser C, Haolla FA, Zanella LG, Rodrigues MM. Novel protective antigens expressed by *Trypanosoma cruzi* amastigotes provide immunity to mice highly susceptible to Chagas' disease. *Clin Vaccine Immunol* 2008;**15**(8):1292−300.

49. Atwood III JA, Weatherly DB, Minning TA, Bundy B, Cavola C, Opperdoes FR, et al. The *Trypanosoma cruzi* proteome. *Science* 2005;**309**(5733):473−6.

50. El-Sayed N, Myler P, Bartholomeu D, Nilsson D, Aggarwal G, Tran A, et al. The genome sequence of *Trypanosoma cruzi*, etiologic agent of Chagas disease. *Science* 2005;**309**(5733):409−15.

51. Minning TA, Weatherly DB, Atwood 3rd J, Orlando R, Tarleton RL. The steady-state transcriptome of the four major life-cycle stages of *Trypanosoma cruzi*. *BMC Genomics* 2009;**10**:370.

52. Dumonteil E. Vaccine development against *Trypanosoma cruzi* and *Leishmania* species in the post-genomic era. *Infect Genet Evol* 2009;**9**(6):1075−82.

53. Ledgerwood JE, Graham BS. DNA vaccines: a safe and efficient platform technology for responding to emerging infectious diseases. *Hum Vaccin* 2009;**5**(9):623−6.

54. Basombrio MA, Segura MA, Mora MC, Gomez L. Field trial of vaccination against American trypanosomiasis (Chagas' disease) in dogs. *Am J Trop Med Hyg* 1993;**49**(1):143−51.

55. Gradoni L. Canine Leishmania vaccines: still a long way to go. *Vet Parasitol* 2015;**208**(1-2):94−100.

56. Pizzi T, Prager R. Immunity to infection induced by culture of *Trypanosoma cruzi* of atenuated virulence; preliminary communication. *Bol Inf Parasit Chil* 1952;**7**(2):20−1.

57. Menezes H. Histological lesions in vaccinated mice with nonvirulent strain of *Trypanosoma cruzi*. *Rev Bras Med* 1968;**25**(3):160−5.

58. Menezes H. Protective effect of an avirulent (cultivated) strain of *Trypanosoma cruzi* against experimental infection in mice. *Rev Inst Med Trop Sao Paulo* 1968;**10**(1):1−4.

59. Menezes H. Active immunization of mice with the avirulent Y strain of *Trypanosoma cruzi* against heterologous virulent strains of the same parasite. *Rev Inst Med Trop Sao Paulo* 1969;**11**(5):335−42.

60. Menezes H. Immunizacao ativa contra a tripanosomose sul-americana. Sintese da nossa experiencia. *Rev Bras Med* 1972;**29**:1−6.

61. Menezes H. Active immunization of dogs with a non virulent strain of *Trypanosoma cruzi*. *Rev Inst Med Trop Sao Paulo* 1969;**11**(4):258−63.

62. Menezes H. A vacinacao de seres humanos com vacina viva avirulenta de *Trypanosoma cruzi*. Seguimento do dois primeiros casos durtante 21 anos. *Rev Pat Trop (Brazil)* 1990;**19**:159−61.

63. Chiari E. Infectivity of *Trypanosoma cruzi* metacyclic trypomastigotes from cultures kept in laboratory for different periods of time. *Rev Inst Med Trop Sao Paulo* 1974;**16**(2):61−7.

64. Rowland EC, Ritter DM. Corpus Christi strain-induced protection to *Trypanosoma cruzi* infection in C3H(He) mice: transfer of resistance to Brazil strain challenge with lymphocytes. *J Parasitol* 1984;**70**(5):760−6.

65. Lima MT, Rondinelli R, Sarno EN, Barcinski MA, Gattas CR. Preliminary studies on the infection of BALB/c mice with a clone of *Trypanosoma cruzi*. *Mem Inst Oswaldo Cruz* 1986;**81**:124.

66. Lima M, Lenzi H, Rondinelli E, Gattas C. *Trypanosoma cruzi*: immunogenicity of a non-infective clone. *Mem Inst Oswaldo Cruz* 1992;**81**:159.

67. Pyrrho AS, Goncalves R, Pecanha LMT, Gattas CR. Immunoglobulin isotypes in *Trypanosoma cruzi* vaccinated mice. *Mem Inst Oswaldo Cruz* 1994;**89**:151.

68. Atayde VD, Neira I, Cortez M, Ferreira D, Freymuller E, Yoshida N. Molecular basis of non-virulence of *Trypanosoma cruzi* clone CL-14. *Int J Parasitol* 2004;**34**(7):851−60.

69. Paiva CN, Souto-Padron T, Costa DA, Gattass CR. High expression of a functional cruzipain by a non-infective and non-pathogenic *Trypanosoma cruzi* clone. *Parasitology* 1998;**117**(Pt 5):483−90.

70. Duschak VG, Ciaccio M, Nassert JR, Basombrio MA. Enzymatic activity, protein expression, and gene sequence of cruzipain in virulent and attenuated *Trypanosoma cruzi* strains. *J Parasitol* 2001;**87**(5):1016–22.

71. Gattas CR, Costa DA, Andrade AB, Souto Padron T. Transsialidase expression by a non-infective clone of *Trypanosoma cruzi*. *Mem Inst Oswaldo Cruz* 1994;**89**:57.

72. Basombrio MA, Besuschio S, Cossio PM. Side effects of immunization with liver attenuated *Trypanosoma cruzi* in mice and rabbits. *Infect Immun* 1982;**36**(1):342–50.

73. Romaña C, Borel JF. Experimental chronic myocarditis without previous acute phase caused by a non-virulent strain of *Trypanosoma cruzi*. *Rev Fed Argentina Cardiol* 1989;**18**:71–4.

74. Leguizamon MS, Campetella OE, Orn A, Cappa SM. Reversion of culture-induced virulence-attenuation in *Trypanosoma cruzi*. *Mem Inst Oswaldo Cruz* 1993;**88**(1):161–2.

75. Basombrio MA, Segura MA, Nasser JR. Relationship between long-term resistance to *Trypanosoma cruzi* and latent infection, examined by antibody production and polymerase chain reaction in mice. *J Parasitol* 2002;**88**(6):1107–12.

76. Basombrio MA, Arredes H. Long-term immunological response induced by attenuated *Trypanosoma cruzi* in mice. *J Parasitol* 1987;**73**(1):236–8.

77. Basombrio MA, Segura MA, Mora MC, Gomez L. Field trial of vaccination against American trypanosomiasis (Chagas' disease) in dogs. *Am J Trop Med Hyg* 1993;**49**(1):143–51.

78. Basombrío MA, Arredes HR, Rossi R, Molina de Raspi E. Histopathological and parasitological evidence of immunization of mice against challenge with 17 wild isolates of *Trypanosoma cruzi*. *Int J Parasitol* 1986;**16**(4):375–80.

79. Cuneo CA, Molina de Raspi E, Basombrio MA. Prevention of electrocardiographic and histopathologic alterations in the murine model of Chagas' disease by preinoculation of an attenuated *Trypanosoma cruzi* strain. *Rev Inst Med Trop Sao Paulo* 1989;**31**(4):248–55.

80. Basombrio MA, Arredes H, Uncos DA, Rossi R, Alvarez E. Field trial of vaccination against American trypanosomiasis (Chagas' disease) in domestic guinea pigs. *Am J Trop Med Hyg* 1987;**37**(1):57–62.

81. Basombrío MA, Nasser JR, Segura MA, Gomez LE. *Trypanosoma cruzi:* effect of immunization on the risk of vector-delivered infection in guinea pigs. *J Parasitol* 1997;**83**(6):1059–62.

82. Basombrío MA, Gorla D, Catalá S, Segura MA, Mora MC, Gómez L, et al. Number of vector bites determinig the infection of guinea pigs with *Trypanosoma cruzi*. *Mem Inst Osw Cruz* 1996;**91**(4):421–4.

83. Basso B, Castro I, Introini V, Gil P, Truyens C, Moretti E. Vaccination with *Trypanosoma rangeli* reduces the infectiousness of dogs experimentally infected with *Trypanosoma cruzi*. *Vaccine* 2007;**25**(19):3855–8.

84. Fontanella GH, De Vusserb K, Laroyb W, Daurelioa L, Nocitoc AL, Revelli S, et al. Immunization with an engineered mutant trans-sialidase highly protects mice from experimental *Trypanosoma cruzi* infection: a vaccine candidate. *Vaccine* 2008;**26**(19):2322–34.

85. Cazorla SI, Frank FM, Becker PD, Corral RS, Guzmán CA, Malchiodi EL. Prime-boost immunization with cruzipain co-administered with MALP-2 triggers a protective immune response able to decrease parasite burden and tissue injury in an experimental *Trypanosoma cruzi* infection model. *Vaccine* 2008;**26**(16):1999–2009.

86. Cazorla SI, Becker PD, Frank FM, Ebensen T, Sartori MJ, Corral RS, et al. Oral vaccination with Salmonella enterica as a cruzipain-DNA delivery system confers protective immunity against *Trypanosoma cruzi*. *Infect Immun* 2008;**76**(1):324–33.

87. Martinez-Campos V, Martinez-Vega P, Ramirez-Sierra MJ, Rosado-Vallado M, Seid CA, Hudspeth EM, et al. Expression, purification, immunogenicity, and protective efficacy of a recombinant Tc24 antigen as a vaccine against *Trypanosoma cruzi* infection in mice. *Vaccine* 2015;**33**(36):4505−12.

88. Bontempi IA, Vicco MH, Cabrera G, Villar SR, Gonzalez FB, Roggero EA, et al. Efficacy of a trans-sialidase-ISCOMATRIX subunit vaccine candidate to protect against experimental Chagas disease. *Vaccine* 2015;**33**(10):1274−83.

89. Serna C, Lara JA, Rodrigues SP, Marques AF, Almeida IC, Maldonado RA. A synthetic peptide from *Trypanosoma cruzi* mucin-like associated surface protein as candidate for a vaccine against Chagas disease. *Vaccine* 2014;**32**(28):3525−32.

90. Vaughan AM, Wang R, Kappe SH. Genetically engineered, attenuated whole-cell vaccine approaches for malaria. *Hum Vaccin* 2010;**6**(1):107−13.

91. VanBuskirk KM, O'Neill MT, De La Vega P, Maier AG, Krzych U, Williams J, et al. Preerythrocytic, live-attenuated *Plasmodium falciparum* vaccine candidates by design. *Proc Natl Acad Sci USA* 2009;**106**(31):13004−9.

92. Keitany GJ, Vignali M, Wang R. Live attenuated pre-erythrocytic malaria vaccines. *Hum Vaccin Immunother* 2014;**10**(10):2903−9.

93. Aly AS, Downie MJ, Mamoun CB, Kappe SH. Subpatent infection with nucleoside transporter 1-deficient Plasmodium blood stage parasites confers sterile protection against lethal malaria in mice. *Cell Microbiol* 2010;**12**(7):930−8.

94. Mueller AK, Deckert M, Heiss K, Goetz K, Matuschewski K, Schluter D. Genetically attenuated *Plasmodium berghei* liver stages persist and elicit sterile protection primarily via CD8 T cells. *Am J Pathol* 2007;**171**(1):107−15.

95. Keitany GJ, Sack B, Smithers H, Chen L, Jang IK, Sebastian L, et al. Immunization of mice with live-attenuated late liver stage-arresting *Plasmodium yoelii* parasites generates protective antibody responses to preerythrocytic stages of malaria. *Infect Immun* 2014;**82**(12):5143−53.

96. van Schaijk BC, Ploemen IH, Annoura T, Vos MW, Foquet L, van Gemert GJ, et al. A genetically attenuated malaria vaccine candidate based on *P. falciparum* b9/slarp gene-deficient sporozoites. *Elife* 2014;**3**. Available from: http://dx.doi.org/10.7554/eLife.03582.

97. Selvapandiyan A, Dey R, Nylen S, Duncan R, Sacks D, Nakhasi HL. Intracellular replication-deficient *Leishmania donovani* induces long lasting protective immunity against visceral leishmaniasis. *J Immunol* 2009;**183**(3):1813−20.

98. Silvestre R, Cordeiro-da-Silva A, Ouaissi A. Live attenuated Leishmania vaccines: a potential strategic alternative. *Arch Immunol Ther Exp (Warsz)* 2008;**56**(2):123−6.

99. Fiuza JA, Dey R, Davenport D, Abdeladhim M, Meneses C, Oliveira F, et al. Intradermal immunization of *Leishmania donovani* Centrin knock-out parasites in combination with salivary protein LJM19 from sand fly vector induces a durable protective immune response in hamsters. *PLoS NTD* 2016;**10**(1):e0004322.

100. Hariharan S, Ajioka J, Swindle J. Stable transformation of *Trypanosoma cruzi*: inactivation of the PUB12.5 polyubiquitin gene by targeted gene disruption. *Mol Biochem Parasitol* 1993;**57**:15−30.

101. Ajioka J, Swindle J. The calmodulin-ubiquitin (CUB) genes of *Trypanosoma cruzi* are essential for parasite viability. *Mol Biochem Parasitol* 1996;**78**(1-2):217−25.

102. Allaoui A, Francois C, Zemzoumi K, Guilvard E, Ouaissi A. Intracellular growth and metacyclogenesis defects in *Trypanosoma cruzi* carrying a targeted deletion of a Tc52 protein-encoding allele. *Mol Microbiol* 1999;**32**(6):1273−86.

103. Annoura T, Nara T, Makiuchi T, Hashimoto T, Aoki T. The origin of dihydroorotate dehydrogenase genes of kinetoplastids, with special reference to their biological

significance and adaptation to anaerobic, parasitic conditions. *J Mol Evol* 2005;**60** (1):113−27.

104. Caler E, Vaena de Avalos S, Haynes P, Andrews N, Burleigh B. Oligopeptidase B-dependent signaling mediates host cell invasion by *Trypanosoma cruzi*. *EMBO J* 1998;**17**(17):4975−86.

105. Conte I, Labriola C, Cazzulo J, Docampo R, Parodi A. The interplay between folding-facilitating mechanisms in *Trypanosoma cruzi* endoplasmic reticulum. *Mol Biol Cell* 2003;**14**:3529−40.

106. Cooper R, de Jesus AR, Cross GA. Deletion of an immunodominant *Trypanosoma cruzi* surface glycoprotein disrupts flagellum-cell adhesion. *J Cell Biol* 1993;**122** (1):149−56.

107. Gluenz E, Taylor MC, Kelly JM. The *Trypanosoma cruzi* metacyclic-specific protein Met-III associates with the nucleolus and contains independent amino and carboxyl terminal targeting elements. *Int J Parasitol* 2007;**37**:617−25.

108. MacRae JI, Obado SO, Turnock DC, Roper JR, Kierans M, Kelly JM, et al. The suppression of galactose metabolism in *Trypanosoma cruzi* epimastigotes causes changes in cell surface molecular architecture and cell morphology. *Mol Biochem Parasitol* 2006;**147**:126−36.

109. Manning-Cela R, Cortes A, Gonzalez-Rey E, Van Voorhis WC, Swindle J, Gonzalez A. LYT1 protein is required for efficient in vitro infection by *Trypanosoma cruzi*. *Infect Immun* 2001;**69**(6):3916−23.

110. Wilkinson SR, Taylor MC, Horn D, Kelly JM, Cheeseman I. A mechanism for cross-resistance to nifurtimox and benznidazole in trypanosomes. *Proc Nat Acad Sci USA* 2007;**105**(13):5022−7.

111. Xu D, Perez Brandan CM, Basombrio MA, Tarleton RL. Evaluation of high efficiency gene knockout strategies for *Trypanosoma cruzi*. *BMC Microbiol* 2009;**9**:90.

112. Perez Brandan C, Padilla AM, Xu D, Tarleton RL, Basombrio MA. Knockout of the dhfr-ts gene in *Trypanosoma cruzi* generates attenuated parasites able to confer protection against a virulent challenge. *PLoS NTD* 2011;**5**(12):e1418.

113. Sanchez Valdez FJ, Perez Brandan C, Zago MP, Labriola C, Ferreira A, Basombrio MA. *Trypanosoma cruzi* carrying a monoallelic deletion of the calreticulin (TcCRT) gene are susceptible to complement mediated killing and defective in their metacyclo-genesis. *Mol Immunol* 2013;**53**(3):198−205.

114. DaRocha WD, Otsu K, Teixeira SMR, Donelson JE. Tests of cytoplasmic RNA interference (RNAi) and construction of a tetracycline-inducible T7 promoter system in *Trypanosoma cruzi*. *Mol Biochem Parasitol* 2004;**133**:175−86.

115. Lander N, Li ZH, Niyogi S, Docampo R. CRISPR/Cas9-induced disruption of paraflagellar rod protein 1 and 2 genes in *Trypanosoma cruzi* reveals their role in flagellar attachment. *MBio* 2015;**6**(4):e01012.

116. Peng D, Kurup SP, Yao PY, Minning TA, Tarleton RL. CRISPR-Cas9-mediated single-gene and gene family disruption in *Trypanosoma cruzi*. *MBio* 2015;**6**(1): e02097−14.

117. Perez Brandan C, Basombrio MA. Genetically attenuated *Trypanosoma cruzi* parasites as a potential vaccination tool. *Bioengineered* 2012;**3**(4):242−6.

118. Sanchez-Valdez FJ, Perez Brandan C, Ferreira A, Basombrio MA. Gene-deleted live-attenuated *Trypanosoma cruzi* parasites as vaccines to protect against Chagas disease. *Expert Rev Vaccines* 2015;**14**(5):681−97.

119. Sher A, Snary D. Specific inhibition of the morphogenesis of *Trypanosoma cruzi* by a monoclonal antibody. *Nature* 1982;**300**(5893):639−40.

120. Basombrio MA, Gomez L, Padilla AM, Ciaccio M, Nozaki T, Cross GA. Targeted deletion of the gp72 gene decreases the infectivity of *Trypanosoma cruzi* for mice and insect vectors. *J Parasitol* 2002;**88**(3):489—93.

121. Basombrío MA, Segura MA, Ciaccio M, editor. Duration of the protection maintained in mice by a gp72 null mutant of *Trypanosoma cruzi*, unable to sustain persistent infection. XXIX annual meeting on basic research in Chagas' disease. *XVIII Meeting of the Brazilian Society of Protozoology* 2002, Caxambu, Brasil.

122. Barrio AB, Van Voorhis WC, Basombrio MA. *Trypanosoma cruzi*: attenuation of virulence and protective immunogenicity after monoallelic disruption of the cub gene. *Exp Parasitol* 2007;**117**(4):382—9.

123. Zago MP, Barrio AB, Cardozo RM, Duffy T, Schijman AG, Basombrio MA. Impairment of infectivity and immunoprotective effect of a LYT1 null mutant of *Trypanosoma cruzi*. *Infect Immun* 2008;**76**(1):443—51.

124. Collins MH, Craft JM, Bustamante JM, Tarleton RL. Oral exposure to *Trypanosoma cruzi* elicits a systemic CD8(+) T cell response and protection against heterotopic challenge. *Infect Immun* 2011;**79**(8):3397—406.

125. Canavaci AM, Bustamante JM, Padilla AM, Perez Brandan CM, Simpson LJ, Xu D, et al. In vitro and in vivo high-throughput assays for the testing of anti-*Trypanosoma cruzi* compounds. *PLoS NTD* 2010;**4**(7):e740.

126. Ragone PG, Perez Brandan C, Padilla AM, Monje Rumi M, Lauthier JJ, Alberti D'Amato AM, et al. Biological behavior of different *Trypanosoma cruzi* isolates circulating in an endemic area for Chagas disease in the Gran Chaco region of Argentina. *Acta Trop* 2012;**123**(3):196—201.

127. Sanchez-Valdez FJ, Perez Brandan C, Ramirez G, Uncos AD, Zago MP, Cimino RO, et al. A monoallelic deletion of the TcCRT gene increases the attenuation of a cultured *Trypanosoma cruzi* strain, protecting against an in vivo virulent challenge. *PLoS NTD* 2014;**8**(2):e2696.

128. van Kooten C, Banchereau J. CD40—CD40 ligand. *J Leukoc Biol* 2000;**67**(1):2—17.

129. Chaussabel D, Jacobs F, de Jonge J, de Veerman M, Carlier Y, Thielemans K, et al. CD40 ligation prevents *Trypanosoma cruzi* infection through interleukin-12 upregulation. *Infect Immun* 1999;**67**(4):1929—34.

130. Chamekh M, Vercruysse V, Habib M, Lorent M, Goldman M, Allaoui A, et al. Transfection of *Trypanosoma cruzi* with host CD40 ligand results in improved control of parasite infection. *Infect Immun* 2005;**73**(10):6552—61.

131. Denise H, Coombs GH, Mottram JC. Generation of *Leishmania* mutants lacking antibiotic resistance genes using a versatile hit-and-run targeting strategy. *FEMS Microbiol Lett* 2004;**235**(1):89—94.

132. Ma Y, Weiss LM, Huang H. Inducible suicide vector systems for *Trypanosoma cruzi*. *Microbes Infect* 2015;**17**(6):440—50.

133. Ghedin E, Charest H, Zhang WW, Debrabant A, Dwyer D, Matlashewski G. Inducible expression of suicide genes in *Leishmania donovani* amastigotes. *J Biol Chem* 1998;**273**(36):22997—3003.

134. Muyombwe A, Olivier M, Harvie P, Bergeron MG, Ouellette M, Papadopoulou B. Protection against *Leishmania major* challenge infection in mice vaccinated with live recombinant parasites expressing a cytotoxic gene. *J Infect Dis* 1998;**177**(1):188—95.

# Index